W9-ATL-028

Community/ Public Health Nursing Practice

HEALTH FOR FAMILIES AND POPULATIONS

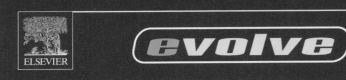

∴ *To access your Resources, visit:*

http://evolve.elsevier.com/maurer/community/

Evolve Resources for Maurer/Smith: ***Community/Public Health Nursing Practice:
Health for Families and Populations,*** **fourth edition,** offer the following features:

- **Quizzes**
  NCLEX-style questions for each chapter, with answers and rationales provided.
- **Web Scenarios**
  Clinically-based exercises that take you to the Internet to find information and answers.
- **Critical Thinking Questions and Answers for Case Studies**
  Questions based on the Case Studies in the chapters, with answers provided.
- **Website Resources**
  Materials such as assessment tools, detailed tables, and additional information that
  supplement the chapter content.
- **Care Plans**
  Plans, based on *The Nursing Process in Practice* features in the text, that provide additional
  nursing diagnoses, goals, interventions, and outcomes for each case.
- **WebLinks**
  Links to hundreds of websites carefully chosen to supplement the content of the textbook.
- **Healthy People Updates**
  The latest updates on *Healthy People 2010,* with current information on recent developments
  as it becomes available.
- **Glossary**
  Key Terms and their definitions.

http://evolve.elsevier.com/maurer/community/

Fourth Edition

Community/ Public Health Nursing Practice

HEALTH FOR FAMILIES AND POPULATIONS

FRANCES A. MAURER, MS, RN, C
Community Health Nursing Educator and Consultant
Baltimore, Maryland

CLAUDIA M. SMITH, RN-BC, MPH, PhD
Assistant Professor
School of Nursing
University of Maryland
Baltimore, Maryland

SAUNDERS

ELSEVIER

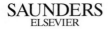

11830 Westline Industrial Drive
St. Louis, Missouri 63146

COMMUNITY/PUBLIC HEALTH NURSING PRACTICE: HEALTH FOR FAMILIES AND POPULATIONS

ISBN: 978-1-4160-5004-9

Copyright © 2009, 2005, 2000, 1995 by Saunders, an imprint of Elsevier Inc.

Unit opener photograph credits:
Unit 1: *Historical—Nurse surrounded by children*: Instructive Visiting Nurse Association, Richmond, Virginia; *Group of children from Sri Lanka*: Gene Dailey, American Red Cross
Unit 2: *Factory with smokestacks*: Elsevier Inc. *Japanese family on bridge*: Photos.com.
Unit 3: *Family in front yard*: CLG Photographics Inc.; *Mother and two daughters*: Elsevier Inc.
Unit 4: *Cityscape*: Elsevier Inc.; bottom: *Rural landscape*: Photos.com
Unit 5: *Nurse taking man's blood pressure*: Elsevier Inc.; *Classroom presentation about tobacco*: Elsevier Inc.
Unit 6: *Homeless mother and child*: CLG Photographics Inc.; *Disaster scene with American Red Cross worker*: Gene Dailey, American Red Cross
Unit 7: *Children on playground bars*: Photos.com; *Wheelchair track event*: Department of Veterans Affairs
Unit 8: *Nurse giving medications to elderly woman*: CLG Photographics Inc.; *Migrant workers*: Photos.com.

All rights reserved. No part of this publication may be reproduced or transmitted in any form or by any means, electronic or mechanical, including photocopying, recording, or any information storage and retrieval system, without permission in writing from the publisher. Permissions may be sought directly from Elsevier's Rights Department: phone: (+1) 215 239 3804 (US) or (+44) 1865 843830 (UK); fax: (+44) 1865 853333; e-mail: healthpermissions@elsevier.com. You may also complete your request on-line via the Elsevier website at http://www.elsevier.com/permissions.

Notice

Neither the Publisher nor the Authors assume any responsibility for any loss or injury and/or damage to persons or property arising out of or related to any use of the material contained in this book. It is the responsibility of the treating practitioner, relying on independent expertise and knowledge of the patient, to determine the best treatment and method of application for the patient.

The Publisher

Previous editions copyrighted 2005, 2000, and 1995.

Library of Congress Cataloging-in-Publication Data
Community/public health nursing practice : health for families and
populations / [edited by] Frances A. Maurer, Claudia M. Smith.—4th ed.
    p. ; cm.
    Includes bibliographical references and index.
    ISBN 978-1-4160-5004-9 (pbk. : alk. paper)
  1. Community health nursing. 2. Public health nursing. I. Maurer,
Frances A. II. Smith, Claudia M.
    [DNLM: 1. Community Health Nursing—United States. 2. Public Health
Nursing—United States. WY 106 C73593 2009]
    RT98.C65623 2009
    610.73'43—dc22   2008035238

ISBN: 978-1-4160-5004-9

Managing Editor: Linda Thomas
Developmental Editor: Carlie Bliss Irwin
Publishing Services Manager: Jeff Patterson
Project Manager: Clay S. Broeker

Working together to grow
libraries in developing countries

www.elsevier.com | www.bookaid.org | www.sabre.org

ELSEVIER   BOOK AID International   Sabre Foundation

Printed in Canada

Last digit is the print number: 9 8 7 6 5 4 3 2

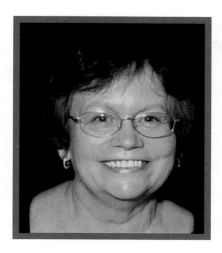

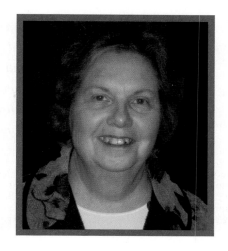

FRANCES A. MAURER MS, RN, C

CLAUDIA M. SMITH, RN-BC, MPH, PhD

Frances A. Maurer is a community health consultant. She is retired from the University of Maryland School of Nursing, where her primary focus was baccalaureate community health nursing. Ms. Maurer received her diploma in nursing from St. Joseph's Hospital School of Nursing and her BSN from California State University at Long Beach. Her MS is from the University of Maryland in Baltimore, Maryland, and her post-master's education has been at the University of Maryland in the field of Health Policy.

For more than 35 years, Ms. Maurer's career in nursing has focused on community health services, both as an educator and clinician. She has supervised students in a variety of clinical situations and service populations, including general health services, prenatal care, child health, and communicable disease. She has had extensive experience in curriculum development and has participated in major curriculum revisions and curriculum evaluations.

She is the educator for a statewide program, funded by the Maryland Department of Health and Mental Hygiene, to facilitate accurate tuberculosis control. She is also involved in several national studies, directed by the Centers for Disease Control and Prevention, to help determine how best to facilitate immigrant access to tuberculosis diagnosis and treatment and to improve identification and treatment for multi-drug resistant tuberculosis. Her primary interests are in developing equitable access and health services for vulnerable populations and those with communicable diseases. She has written on health policy and finance issues and developed curriculum for and served as a consultant to both local and state health departments.

Dr. Claudia M. Smith is currently Assistant Professor at the University of Maryland School of Nursing and Co-Director of the Community/Public Health Nursing Masters specialty. She has been a community/public health nurse for over four decades and an educator for over 35 years. For 8 years she served in a multi-county health resources planning agency. She teaches in both undergraduate and graduate courses. She earned her BS in Nursing from the University of Maryland and her MPH with a major in Public Health Nursing from the University of North Carolina at Chapel Hill. Her PhD in Education is from the University of Maryland, College Park, with a major in Education Policy and Leadership. She is a curriculum consultant regarding undergraduate public/community health education.

Dr. Smith is committed to working with low-income and underserved populations, especially families with young children. She co-developed the Family Needs Model for family health nursing in community/public health. She has supervised numerous community assessments and over 65 community-focused interventions, including those targeting school children, the elderly in home health, Spanish-speaking immigrants, maternal/child health populations, and teenagers. She was Director of a Healthy Homes Project funded by the federal Department of Housing and Urban Development (HUD); this project demonstrated that lead dust and selected allergens can be reduced safely in occupied homes without displacing families.

Her research interests include improving access to health promotion activities and promoting safer environments, especially in low-income communities. Through qualitative research, she has explored the experiences of joy for low-income women with preschool children; despite difficult life experiences, their "hearts blossom with vulnerability and strength," especially in their relationships with their children.

DEDICATION

This book is dedicated to
former community/public health nurses
and to contemporary and future
community/public health nurses, students, educators, and researchers,
who, in partnership with community members, contribute energy, insight, and compassion
directed towards a vision of
healthful families, populations, and communities.

ACKNOWLEDGMENTS

Many people have contributed to our exploration of community/public health nursing practice, including colleagues, faculty, and community members. We are especially indebted to the community/public health nursing students with whom we have worked over the years. We are grateful for our relationships with community/public health graduates, practicing community/public health nurses, and community/public health nursing researchers who have taught us much. They have provided the inspiration for exploring community/public health nursing from empirical, experiential, ethical, and critical perspectives.

Without the contributors and their expertise, this book could never have been written. They have shared their knowledge, beliefs, experiences, and visions. Our conscientious reviewers affirmed our strengths; challenged us when we were unclear, inaccurate, parochial, or too narrow in our focus; and made constructive suggestions.

Dr. Theresa Nagy and Ms. Mary Rees provided technologic computer support for the fourth edition.

Our families have continued to extend their support to this fourth endeavor. Fran Maurer's husband, Dick, served as research assistant locating and distributing relevant materials to the editors and contributors. Her daughter, Jennifer Maurer Kliphouse, provided the fresh perspective of a recently graduated registered nurse. Claudia Smith's husband, Tony Langbehn, and mother, Gerry Smith, continue to encourage us and take pride in our accomplishment. All of these family members have contributed encouragement and support of our pursuit of an excellent fourth edition.

We thank Elsevier for transforming our manuscripts into a coherent publication, especially Linda Thomas, Carlie Irwin, and Clay Broeker.
Thank you.

Margaret M. Andrews, PhD, RN, CTN, FAAN
Director and Professor of Nursing
University of Michigan—Flint, School of Health Professions and
    Studies
Flint, Michigan
Chapter 10: Relevance of Culture and Values in Community/
    Public Health Nursing

Mary L. Beachley, MS, RN, CNAA
Chief, Division of Health Facilities and Special Programs
Maryland Institute for Emergency Medical Services Systems
Baltimore, Maryland
Chapter 22: Disaster Management: Caring for Communities in
    an Emergency

Angeline Bushy, PhD, RN, FAAN
Professor and Bert Fish Chair
University of Central Florida College of Nursing
Daytona Beach, Florida
Chapter 32: Rural Health

Verna Benner Carson, PhD, PMHCNS-BC
President
C&V Senior Care Specialists, Inc.
Fallston, Maryland
Chapter 33: Community Mental Health

Marcia L. Cooley, APMH, RN, MS, PhD
Associate Professor
York College of Pennsylvania
York, Pennsylvania
Chapter 12: A Family Perspective in Community/Public Health
    Nursing
Chapter 14: Multiproblem Families

Roslyn Pollack Corasaniti, RN, PhD, CRRN
Professional Development Coordinator
Kernan Orthopaedic and Rehabilitation Hospital
Baltimore, Maryland
Chapter 26: Rehabilitation Clients in the Community

Sara Groves, DrPH, APRN
Assistant Professor
Johns Hopkins University School of Nursing
Baltimore, Maryland
Chapter 30: School Health

Mary R. Haack, PhD, FAAN
Professor
Department of Family and Community Health
University of Maryland School of Nursing
Baltimore, Maryland
Chapter 25: Substance Use Disorders

Sarah Hargrave, RN, BSN, MS
Quality Assurance/Quality Improvement Nurse Consultant II
State of Alaska, Department of Health and Social Services,
    Division of Public Health, Section of Public Health Nursing
Juneau, Alaska
Chapter 29: State and Local Health Departments

Gail Ann DeLuca Havens, PhD, RN
Owner and Principal
INSIGHT: Consultative Services in Healthcare Ethics
Bluffton, South Carolina
Ethics in Practice boxes

Gail L. Heiss, RN, BC, MSN
MRSA Prevention Coordinator
VA Maryland Health Care System
Baltimore, Maryland
Chapter 18: Health Promotion and Risk Reduction in the
    Community
Chapter 19: Screening and Referral
Chapter 20: Health Teaching

Gayle Hofland, MSN, RN
Assistant Professor of Nursing
Dickinson State University
Dickinson, North Dakota
Table 8-3: Communicable Diseases, Community Health
    Concerns, and Treatment

Jennifer Maurer Kliphouse, RN, BA, BSN
Staff Nurse
Morristown Memorial Hospital
Morristown, New Jersey
The Nursing Process in Practice boxes

Helen R. Kohler, RN, PhD
Visiting Professor
University of Eastern Africa
Baraton, Kenya
Chapter 5: International Health

Joan E. Kub, PhD, MA, APRN
Associate Professor
Johns Hopkins University School of Nursing
Baltimore, Maryland
Chapter 30: School Health

David R. Langford, RN, DNSc
Associate Professor
University of North Carolina at Charlotte
    School of Nursing
Charlotte, North Carolina
Chapter 23: Violence: A Social and Family Problem

Corrine Olson, RN, BSN, MS
Deputy Chief
State of Alaska, Department of Health and Social Services
Division of Public Health, Section of Public Health
    Nursing
Juneau, Alaska
Chapter 29: State and Local Health Departments

Donna S. Raimondi, RN, MS
Director, Quality and Professional Development
Kernan Hospital
Baltimore, Maryland
Chapter 26: Rehabilitation Clients in the Community

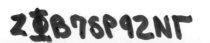

Anne Rath Rentfro, MSN, RN
Associate Professor
University of Texas at Brownsville Nursing Department
Brownsville, Texas
Chapter 27: Children in the Community

Robyn Rice, PhD, RN
Nurse Educator
Lutheran School of Nursing
St. Louis, Missouri
Staff Nurse, Hospice
Gateway Regional Medical Center
Granite City, Illinois
Chapter 31: Home Health Care

Gina Castelnovo Rowe, MSN, MPH, CRNP
Clinical Instructor
University of Maryland School of Nursing
Baltimore, Maryland
Chapter 7: Epidemiology: Unraveling the Mysteries of Disease and Health

Barbara Sattler, RN, DrPH, FAAN
Professor and Director
Environmental Health Education Center
University of Maryland School of Nursing
Baltimore, Maryland
Chapter 9: Environmental Health Risks: At Home, at Work, and in the Community

Meredith Wallace, PhD, APRN
Associate Professor
Yale University School of Nursing
New Haven, Connecticut
Chapter 28: Older Adults in the Community

Susan Wozenski, JD, MPH
Vice Chair and Assistant Professor
Family and Community Health
University of Maryland School of Nursing
Baltimore, Maryland
Chapter 6: Legal Context for Community/Public Health Nursing Practice

John W. Young, MBA, RN
Director of Hospital Programs
Maryland Institute for Emergency Medical Services Systems
Baltimore, Maryland
Chapter 22: Disaster Management: Caring for Communities in an Emergency

ANCILLARY CONTRIBUTORS

Jennifer Maurer Kliphouse, RN, BA, BSN
Staff Nurse
Morristown Memorial Hospital
Morristown, New Jersey
Care Plans for the Nursing Process in Practice boxes

Virginia Nehring, PhD, RN
Professor Emeritus
Wright State University College of Nursing and Health
Dayton, Ohio
Test Bank

Stephanie Powelson, RN, MPH, EdD
Chair, Nursing Department
Truman State University
Kirksville, Missouri
PowerPoint Slides

Anna K. Wehling Weepie, MSN, RN
Assistant Professor of Nursing
Allen College
Waterloo, Iowa
Quiz

REVIEWERS

Pamela Ark, PhD, RN
Assistant Professor
University of Central Florida School of Nursing
Orlando, Florida

Susan L. Fogarty, RN, MSN
Associate Professor
Ferris State University School of Nursing
Big Rapids, Michigan

Stephanie Powelson, RN, MPH, EdD
Chair, Nursing Department
Truman State University
Kirksville, Missouri

Julie Bertelson St. Clair, RN, MSN
Instructor, Nursing Program
University of Southern Indiana
College of Nursing and Health Professions
Evansville, Indiana

When the first edition of this text was published, we had just celebrated the 100th anniversary of modern community/public health nursing in the United States. The second edition anticipated the arrival of the twenty-first century, which brought both practical and symbolic implications for the future of community/ public health nursing. As the fourth edition is published, the nation confronts global health issues including global warming, food shortages and maldistribution, refugee health, exposure to environmental chemicals, and disabilities and deaths from conflicts, and warfare. Our county continues to confront a crisis in health care delivery that calls for creative ways to improve the health and well-being of our citizens and communities.

Anniversaries and transitions offer time to reflect on the past and present, as well as to clarify directions and strategies for the future. Among our historic roots are ethical values, commitments, principles, theories and concepts, experiences, models for nursing and health care delivery, and research findings that inform our nursing practice. The health care system is undergoing dramatic changes that will affect both consumers and providers of health care services in dramatic ways. This fourth edition explores our history and present practice, and contemplates our future. The title: *Community/ Public Health Nursing Practice: Health for Families and Populations* reflects the practice arena of community/public health, emphasizing the *application of content to nursing practice,* and shows the broad scope of community-based and community-focused practice.

Throughout this text, emphasis is placed on the core of "what a community/public health nurse needs to know" to practice effectively in the context of a world, nation, society, and health care system that are ever changing. This text is intended for baccalaureate nursing students taking courses related to community/public health nursing, including registered nurses returning for their baccalaureate degrees. Beginning practitioners in community/public health nursing will also find much useful information. The term *community/public health nursing* is used in this text to remind the reader that community-orientated nursing practice is broad based and aimed at improving the health of families, groups, and populations. To save space in the text, the term *community health nurse* may sometimes be used in place of *community/public health nurse.* The term *client* is used to reflect individual, group, and population recipients of nursing care, while the term *patient* is used selectively to denote individuals under care in intense clinical and hospital-based practice.

Changes in the delivery and financing of health care services affect professional practice as well as individuals, families, populations, and communities. Therefore in this edition we explore past and present efforts at health service and funding reform, critique progress toward stated reform goals, and identify current and future areas of concern for health care providers and communities.

Unlike 100 years ago, the major causes of death in the United States today are not communicable diseases. Rather, the major causes today are chronic diseases, such as heart disease, cancer, stroke, pulmonary diseases, and diabetes, and, at all ages, unintentional injury. Much of the premature death and disability is preventable through control of environmental and personal risk factors, such as smoking and obesity. Health promotion and prevention have been historic aims of community/ public health nursing. Today, the *National Health Objectives for the year 2010* identify measurable targets for reduction in death and disability. Because community/public health nurses are in the forefront of helping families and communities identify and reduce their risk factors, the *Healthy People 2010* objectives and progress toward goal attainment are included in all appropriate chapters.

Reducing health disparities is a foremost national goal. Health, illness, and health care are unevenly distributed among people. The relevance of population-focused nursing emerges when the unmet health needs of populations are recognized. For example, numbers of homeless, chronically mentally ill, injured veterans, and poor children are increasing. The poor have higher rates of illness, disability, and premature death. The cost of health care and absent or inadequate health insurance coverage combine to also increase the numbers of medically indigent, such as survivors of accidental head and spinal trauma. This text explores the commitments and activities of community/public health nursing in improving the health of such vulnerable families, groups, and populations. Research studies discussed throughout the text illustrate the success of nursing interventions with vulnerable populations in communities and provide a basis for evidence-based practice.

To identify the health-related strengths and problems of a community, it is necessary to assess the demographic and health statistics of the community's population and to explore the existing community structures, functions, and resources. In this text, we stress the importance of developing partnerships with community members, present a community assessment tool with several case studies showing its application, and discuss varied perspectives for planning and evaluating nursing care within communities. The tool is applied to both geopolitical and phenomenological communities.

Community/public health nurses recognize that much of a person's attitude and behavior toward health is learned initially in his or her own family. Family-focused health promotion and prevention is an important community/public health nursing strategy. As was true in previous centuries, some families today experience multiple problems with unhealthy environments, disabled or chronically ill members, developmental issues, breakdowns in family communication, and weak support systems.

The text reflects the increasing demand for community/public health nursing in home health care for the ill. Hospital cost-containment measures that began in the 1980s have resulted in a decrease in the average length of stay of patients in hospitals. As was true 100 years ago, families today are caring for ill members at home and are requiring assistance from community health nurses. In response to client needs, newer structures of nursing care delivery also have emerged, including hospice and medical daycare centers. A family focus and care for clients in their daily settings—homes, schools, and worksites— are traditional aspects of community/public health nursing. Community/public health nursing acknowledges the importance of caring for the family caregivers as well as for ill family members and of strengthening community support services.

The community/public health nurse's involvement with contemporary public health problems—substance abuse and addictions, violence, and newly emerging or persistent communicable diseases (including HIV/AIDS, MRSA, SARS, multi-drug resistant tuberculosis, and West Nile Virus)—is thoroughly covered. As a response to recent events, the disaster chapter provides greater emphasis on disaster prevention and management. Adolescent sexuality and the health risks associated with sexual activity for both adolescents and their infants are explored. Chapters on vulnerable populations and community mental health examine two areas of increasing concern for community/public health nursing. Toxic substances in home, work, and community environments are identified as special health risks.

Changes in the age composition of our country's residents poses concerns related to the ratio of dependent persons. More elderly persons and, in selected subpopulations, more children make up the population. Special emphasis is given in the text to a discussion of the support networks with which community/public health nurses work as they provide nursing care with elderly people, children, and persons with disabilities.

LEVEL OF LEARNER

This book is intended as a basic text for baccalaureate students in community/public health nursing. It is appropriate for basic baccalaureate students, registered nurses returning for baccalaureate degrees, and baccalaureate graduates who are new to community/public health employment. It assists the learner in the practical application of community/public health nursing content.

Additionally, the text can benefit registered nurses without baccalaureate degrees who are changing their practice settings because of health care system changes. For example, in some places, registered nurses with strong technological medical-surgical or pediatric skills are being employed in home care. These nurses, their supervisors, and/or in-service education directors can use this text to provide background information, especially in relation to the context of practice, family-focused care, home visiting, and scope of community resources.

The text has a descriptive focus, including both historical changes in practice and the relative magnitude of community/public health nursing problems and solutions today. The text also is structured to promote further inquiry related to each subject and to connect information with examples of practice. Thus, the text includes abstractions and concepts, as well as questions and examples, to promote critical thinking and application of the information.

We are pleased with student comments about the strengths of previous editions and have maintained these positive characteristics in the fourth edition:

• The text is very readable.
• The writing style maintains interest.
• Tables are clear and useful.
• Explanations discuss the relevance of ideas to practice.
• Examples show practical application.
• Evidence-based practice examples are integrated throughout.
• Each chapter is self-contained, without the need to refer to the appendixes.

This text builds on prerequisite knowledge and skills related to application of the nursing process, interpersonal relationships, and nurse/client communication skills. Other prerequisites are knowledge of human development, basic concepts of stress and adaptation, and nursing care with individuals. While a basic general systems language is used with family and community theory, terms are defined for those who have not had formal instruction in these concepts.

ORGANIZATION OF TEXT

The text is organized into eight units. *Unit One, Role and Context of Community/Public Health Nursing Practice*, describes the ethical commitments underlying community/public health nursing practice as well as the scope and context of community/ public health nursing practice. We explore how the structure and function of our complex health care system and legal and economic factors influence communities and community/public health nursing practice. A chapter on international health provides a broader perspective of the concepts of health and illness and their relationship to the globalization of health.

Unit Two, Core Concepts for the Practice of Community/Public Health Nursing, presents basic concepts necessary for effective community/public health practice. An understanding of the process of epidemiology, including the impact and control of communicable diseases, is essential to community/public health nursing practice. A chapter on environmental issues at home, at worksites, and in geopolitical communities identifies specific health risks. Culturally competent nursing care depends on understanding the impact of culture and values on health and health behaviors and understanding the impact that diversity in culture and values among clients and health providers may have on the nurse-client relationships.

Unit Three, Family as Client, presents a broad theory base related to family development, structure, functioning, and health. A family assessment tool is provided, and sources for additional tools are identified. Specific case studies demonstrate the application of the nursing process with families. Special emphasis is given to working with families in crisis and "multiproblem" families.

Nurses with baccalaureate degrees belong to one of a few professions whose members learn to care for people at home as a part of their educational experiences. Many nurses without baccalaureate degrees who desire to transfer from hospital to home care settings must learn on the job. Consequently a chapter is devoted to home visiting, a continuing facet of community/public health nursing.

Unit Four, Community as Client, presents the community and population approach that is unique to community/public health nursing. Communities may be characterized as geopolitical or phenomenological (communities of belonging). Assessment tools are presented for each type of community and case examples provided to illustrate the application of the nursing process with communities. Numerous measures for evaluating the outcomes of community/public health nursing programs are discussed. Additionally, process and management evaluations are examined.

Unit Five, Tools for Practice, develops three strategies for population-focused intervention used frequently by community/ public health nurses:

- Health promotion and risk reduction
- Screening and referral
- Health teaching

Specific tools are included that can be used to help individuals identify risk factors for illness and identify more healthful personal behavior. Detailed instructions are provided for conducting health screening. Also included are the current recommended schedules for health screening for males and females of various age groups. These specific practice skills may be applied with individuals, families, and populations.

Unit Six, Contemporary Problems in Community/Public Health Nursing, focuses on contemporary problems encountered in community/public health nursing practice. Demographic and epidemiologic data help identify populations most at risk for specified health problems. A chapter is devoted to each of the following:

- Vulnerable populations, including people in poverty, the homeless, and migrant populations
- Disaster management
- Family and community violence
- Adolescent sexual activity and teenage pregnancy
- Substance use disorders

The impact of poverty on health is explored in depth. The health risks of vulnerable groups are explored. Societal and personal factors contributing to health problems are identified, including psychologic and family stress related to homelessness, poverty, and a migrant lifestyle.

The disaster chapter emphasizes the importance of preplanning and outlines the roles of both public and private organizations in disaster relief. Common disaster scenarios for both natural and manmade disasters are presented. Changes in disaster preparation and management to improve community response to terrorism are outlined, and potential terrorist threats are identified.

Unit Seven, Support for Special Populations, discusses three vulnerable populations: persons with disabilities, children, and elderly persons. Prevalence of health problems, common nursing interventions, and importance of community support services are discussed.

Unit Eight, Settings for Community/Public Health Nursing Practice, describes state and local health departments, school, home health agencies, rural communities, and community mental health as settings for community health nursing practice. Each chapter includes a day or a week in the life of a community/public health nurse or a case study to help students experience the reality of working in that setting.

CHANGES TO THE FOURTH EDITION

The fourth edition expands and updates content from the third edition, which was widely acclaimed. New content is also included and listed below. The chapter on Environmental Health Risks has been moved to Unit Two as a core concept for community/public health nursing practice.

Expanded Content in this Edition:
- Clinical examples that are related to the chapter content and are common in the practice of community/public health nurses
- The most current version of the *Healthy People 2010* objectives, including the *MidCourse Review,* with *Healthy*

People 2010 boxes related to appropriate clinical practice areas for each chapter in which they are presented
- Internet resources for both faculty and students on the book's Evolve website, including additional links to Community Resource for Practice organizations (the website icon indicates each place where book content has corresponding website material)
- Social justice
- Managed care, health care reforms, and universal health care initiatives
- Core public health functions
- The role of state health departments
- Local health departments and emphasis on public-private partnerships
- Third-party reimbursement for nurse practitioners and clinical nurse specialists
- Cultural competency
- Health disparities and health care disparities
- Family case management in community/public health
- A model of family nursing in community/public health
- Clinical examples in the family and community units to promote application of learning
- Nursing interventions and communication with families
- Examples of epidemiologic studies and their application in public health practice
- Emerging problems with communicable diseases
- Guidelines for screening
- Migrant health problems
- Disaster management practices in the context of terrorist threats
- Interventions directed at improving responsible teen sexual behaviors
- Contemporary tools for addictions screening
- Health problems of older children and adolescents
- Environmental aspects of school health

Throughout the Text We Have Updated the Following:
- Demographic statistics
- Epidemiologic statistics
- Standards for practice
- Initiatives to improve access to health care
- Effects of managed care on groups and aggregates
- Current evidenced-based findings
- References and recommended readings
- Community resources

New Content in this Edition:
- The Minnesota Wheel of Public Health Nursing Interventions
- Trends in employer-provided health insurance
- Cost-sharing impacts on access to health care
- Medicare Part D—Prescription Drug Plan and Medicare Advantage
- Informed consent requirements
- Role of expert witnesses in legal suits
- Informatics: health information systems
- Comparison of pharmacology and toxicology
- Asthma risks posed by chemicals in health care environments
- Nanotechnology

- Global warming and health
- Chemical policies
- Evidence-based home visiting programs
- Mobilizing Action Through Partnerships and Planning (MAPP)
- Geographic information systems (GIS)
- Evidence-based practice examples of community planning and intervention
- Evidence-based practice examples of community health program evaluations
- New health risk appraisal tools
- Nursing interventions related to the Transtheoretical Model—Stages of Change
- SMOG formula to determine readability of print materials
- Sample health education lesson plan
- Prison populations: Characteristics and health issues
- Disparities between minimum wage income and income needed for housing
- Role of Department of Homeland Security in preparation for and management of disasters
- Fatalities associated with weather-related disasters
- Changes in sexual practices among adolescents
- Effectiveness of sexual education programs for adolescents by type of program
- Fetal alcohol spectrum disorders (FASDs)
- Disability prevalence by age
- Impact of No Child Left Behind on schools and students
- Major challenges for public health in the twenty-first century
- National goals for the community mental health system

CHAPTER ORGANIZATION TO PROMOTE LEARNING

Each chapter has the following features:

Focus Questions
Outline
Key Terms (boldfaced in the text)
Chapter narrative
Key Ideas
Learning by Experience and Reflection
References
Suggested Readings

The majority of chapters also present one or more of the following special features to aid learning:

Case Study
The Nursing Process in Practice
Community Resources for Practice
Ethics in Practice

Focus Questions at the beginning of each chapter and Key Ideas at the end help the reader focus on the material presented. The questions encourage the reader to approach learning from the perspective of inquiry. Key Ideas summarize the important ideas. Where appropriate, epidemiologic data are presented to describe the magnitude of the health problems and the populations in which they occur more frequently.

Case Studies and The Nursing Process in Practice encourage application of the chapter material. Most chapters provide an example of the nursing process applied with a family or community or a case study in which the chapter concepts may be applied.

Learning by Experience and Reflection at the end of each chapter is designed to foster student learning through inquiry and a variety of ways of knowing—empirical knowledge and logic, interpersonal learning experiences, ethics, and greater awareness of personal preferences (aesthetics). Guidelines may promote reflection and self-awareness, observation, analysis, and synthesis. Each chapter includes guidelines for learning appropriate to most students as well as suggestions for those who are interested in further evaluation and creativity.

Community Resources for Practice boxes appear in many chapters throughout the book. The WebLinks on the book's website provides a link to all listed resources where additional contact information may be found.

Suggested Readings have been selected with the level of student in mind. Some readings expand on concepts and tools of practice mentioned in the chapter. Other readings provide descriptions of community/public health nursing programs or descriptions of nurses' experiences related to their professional practice.

Ethics in Practice is a special feature appearing predominantly in chapters in Units Five and Six. A situation involving a community/public health nurse is used to identify ethical questions, related ethical principles, and the actions of the specific nurse. These situations provide the opportunity for student/faculty dialogue to explore one's own ethical decision-making. Several of the situations demonstrate the tension between the rights of individuals and the rights of the public at large; other situations depict competing values.

ANCILLARY PACKAGE

A complete teaching and learning package is available on the book's dedicated Evolve website at http://evolve.elsevier.com/Maurer/community/. This website offers materials for both students and instructors.

STUDY AIDS FOR STUDENTS

Quiz: 10 NCLEX-format questions per chapter, with answers.

Web Scenario: Exercises that involve using the Internet to explore or find information about a situation or question related to each chapter.

Critical Thinking Questions and Answers for Case Studies: These correspond to the Case Studies in the textbook.

Care Plans: Additional care plans that supplement The Nursing Process in Practice feature in the textbook. These care plans present relevant nursing diagnoses for the particular case described, and the corresponding goals, interventions, and outcomes.

WebLinks: Organized by chapter, these are hyperlinks to numerous websites related to the chapter content, including those of the organizations listed in Community Resources for Practice.

Healthy People Updates: Highlights of new information and findings that occur in community/public health after publication of the book, to stay current with trends and new developments.

Website Resources: These are tools, forms, and other resources referenced in particular chapters.

Glossary: Comprehensive list of all Key Terms and their definitions.

FOR INSTRUCTORS

PowerPoint Slides: Slides of bulleted information that highlight key chapter concepts to assist with classroom presentation and lecture.

Teaching Strategies for Learning by Experience and Reflection: Detailed plans and suggested activities for implementing the Learning by Experience and Reflection exercises in the book.

Test Bank: Over 800 NCLEX-style questions, with cognitive level, topic, rationale, and text page reference provided. One question in each chapter is presented in the newer innovative item format.

Discussion of Focus Questions: Short answers to the questions that introduce each chapter.

Image Collection: Contains illustrations selected from the textbook.

Frances A. Maurer
Claudia M. Smith

CONTENTS IN BRIEF

CONTENTS

UNIT SIX

Contemporary Problems in Community/Public Health Nursing, 531

UNIT SEVEN

Support for Special Populations, 665

Role and Context of Community/ Public Health Nursing Practice

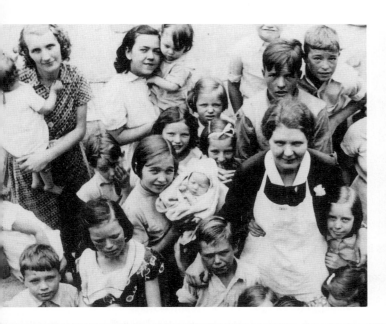

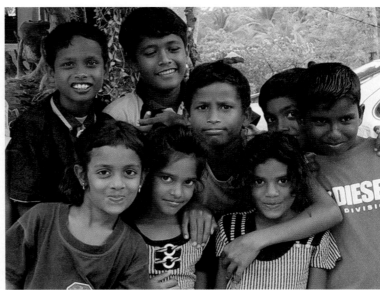

1 Responsibilities for Care in Community/ Public Health Nursing

Claudia M. Smith

FOCUS QUESTIONS

What is the nature of community/public health nursing practice?

What values underlie community/public health nursing?

How is empowerment important in community/public health nursing?

What health-related goals are of concern to community/public health nurses?

Who are the clients of community/public health nurses?

What are the basic concepts and assumptions of general systems theory?

What is meant by the terms *population-focused care* and *aggregate-focused care?*

What are the responsibilities of community/public health nurses?

What competencies are expected of beginning community/public health nurses?

How are community/public health nurse generalists and specialists similar and different?

CHAPTER OUTLINE

KEY TERMS

Aggregate
Commitments
Community-based nursing
Community health nursing
Community/public health nurse
Distributive justice

General systems theory
Group
Population
Population-focused
Professional certification
Public health nurse

Public health nursing
Risk
Social justice
Visions

Imagine that you are knocking on the door of a residential trailer, seeking the mother of an infant who has been hospitalized because of low birth weight. You are interested in helping the mother prepare her home before the hospital discharge of the infant. Or, imagine that you are conducting a nursing clinic in a high-rise residence for the elderly. People have come to obtain blood pressure screening, to inquire whether tiredness is a side effect of their antihypertensive medications, or to validate whether their recent food choices have reduced their sodium intake. Or, picture yourself sitting at an office desk. You are telephoning a physical therapist to discuss the progress of a school-aged child who has mobility problems secondary to cerebral palsy.

Now, imagine yourself at a school parent-teacher association (PTA) meeting as a member of a panel discussion on the prevention of human immunodeficiency virus (HIV) transmission. Think about developing a blood pressure screening and dietary education program for a group of predominantly African American, male employees of a publishing company. Picture yourself reviewing the statistics for patterns of death in your community and contemplating with others the value of a hospice program.

Who would you be to participate in all these activities, with people of all ages and all levels of health, in such a variety of settings—homes, clinics, schools, workplaces, and community meetings? It is likely you would be a community health nurse, and you would have specific knowledge and skills in public health nursing.

Notice that we have used the terms *community health nursing* and *public health nursing*. In the literature, and in practice, there is often a lack of clarity in the use of these terms. Also, the use of these terms changes with time (see Chapter 2). Both the American Nurses Association (ANA, 1980) and the Public Health Nurses Section of the American Public Health Association (APHA, 1980, 1996) agree that the type of involvement previously described is a synthesis of nursing practice and public health practice. What the ANA called *community health nursing*, the APHA called *public health nursing* (Box 1-1).

In 1984, the Division of Nursing, Bureau of Health Professions of the Health Resources and Services Administration of the U.S. Department of Health and Human Services (USDHHS), sponsored a national consensus conference. Participants were invited from the APHA, the ANA, the Association of State and Territorial Directors of Nursing, and the National League for Nursing. The purpose was to clarify the educational preparation needed for public health nursing and to discuss the future of public health nursing. It was agreed that "the term 'community health nurse' is … an umbrella term used for all nurses who work in a community, *including* those who have formal preparation in public health nursing (Box 1-2 and Figure 1-1). In essence, **public health nursing** requires specific educational preparation, and **community health nursing** denotes a setting for the practice of nursing" (USDHHS, 1985, p. 4) (emphasis added). The consensus conference further agreed that educational preparation for beginning practitioners in public health nursing should include the following: (1) epidemiology, statistics, and research; (2) orientation to health care systems; (3) identification of high-risk populations; (4) application of public health concepts to the care of groups of culturally diverse persons; (5) interventions

---

BOX 1-1   Recent Definitions of Community/Public Health Nursing

American Nurses Association

Community health nursing is a synthesis of nursing practice and public health practice applied to promoting and preserving the health of populations. The practice is general and comprehensive. It is not limited to a particular age group or diagnosis, and it is continuing, not episodic. The dominant responsibility is to the population as a whole; nursing directed to individuals, families, or groups contributes to the health of the total population. … The focus of community health nursing is on the prevention of illness and the promotion and maintenance of health.

American Public Health Association

Public health nursing is the practice of promoting and protecting the health of populations using knowledge from nursing, social, and public health sciences. … Public health nursing practice includes assessment and identification of subpopulations who are at high risk for injury, disease, threat of disease, or poor recovery and focusing resources so that services are available and accessible. … [Public health nurses work] with and through relevant community leaders, interest groups, employers, families, and individuals, and through involvement in relevant social and political actions.

Quad Council of Public Health Nursing Organizations

Public health nursing is population-focused, community-oriented nursing practice. The goal of public health nursing is the prevention of disease and disability for all people through the creation of conditions in which people can be healthy.

Data from American Nurses Association. (1980). *A conceptual model of community health nursing* (pp. 2, 11). Washington, DC: Author; American Public Health Association, Public Health Nursing Section. (1996). *The definition and role of public health nursing: A statement of APHA Public Health Nursing Section* (pp. 1, 4). Washington, DC: Author; and Quad Council of Public Health Nursing Organizations. (1999). *Scope and standards of public health nursing practice.* Washington, DC: American Nurses Association.

---

with high-risk populations; and (6) orientation to regulations affecting public health nursing practice (USDHHS, 1985). This educational preparation is assumed to be complementary to a basic education in nursing.

Following the logic of the consensus statements, a registered nurse who works in a noninstitutional setting and has either received a diploma or completed an associate-degree nursing education program can be called a *community health nurse* and practices **community-based nursing** because he or she works outside of hospitals and nursing homes. However, this nurse would *not* have had any formal education in public health nursing. Such a nurse may provide care directed at individuals or families, rather than populations (ANA, 2007b).

Public health nurses provide **population-focused** care. Assessment, planning, and evaluation occur at the population level. However, implementation of health programs and services may occur at the level of individuals, families, groups, communities, and systems (ANA, 2007b; Minnesota Department of Health, 2001; Quad Council of Public Health Nursing Organizations, 2004). The ultimate question is: *Has the health and well-being of the population(s) improved?*

Large numbers of registered nurses are employed in home health agencies to provide home care for clients who are ill. This text can assist those without formal preparation in public

---

Box 1-2   Where Are Community Health Nurses Employed?

1. More than 360,000 registered nurses are employed in community health in the United States (see Figure 1-1), who constitute 15% of all employed registered nurses.
2. Between 1980 and 2000, the numbers of nurses employed in community health nursing settings increased by 155% compared with an increase of 55% in nurses working in hospitals.
3. The largest percentage (38%) of community health nurses work in home health and hospice agencies to provide nursing care to ill, injured, or disabled individuals and their families.
4. Almost one in five community health nurses is employed by a local or state health department or community health or rural health center. These nurses provide primary care services, promote health, and prevent illnesses, injury, and premature death.
5. Other community health nurses work with populations associated with a specific age group or type of organization: youth in public and parochial schools, students in colleges and universities, and adults at work sites.
6. It is not the place of employment that determines whether a nurse is a community/public health nurse, however. Instead, community/public health nurses are distinguished by their education and by the community/population focus of their practice.

Data from U.S. Department of Health and Human Services. (2006). *The registered nurse population: Findings from the March 2004 National Sample Survey of Registered Nurses.* Washington, DC: Health Resources and Services Administration, Bureau of Health Professions, Division of Nursing.

health nursing to expand their thinking and practice to incorporate knowledge and skills from public health nursing.

For those currently enrolled in a baccalaureate nursing education program, this text can assist in integrating public health practice with nursing practice as part of the formal educational preparation for community/public health nursing.

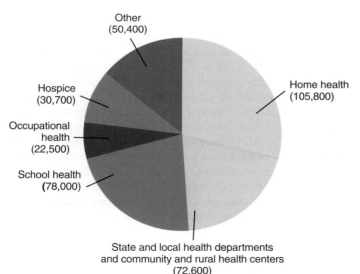

FIGURE 1-1 Community health nurses by work sites—2004 (total community health nurses = 360,000). (Data from U.S. Department of Health and Human Services. [2006]. *The registered nurse population: Findings from the March 2004 National Sample Survey of Registered Nurses.* Washington, DC: Health Resources and Services Administration, Bureau of Health Professions, Division of Nursing.)

The terms **community/public health nurse** and **public health nurse** are used in this text to denote a nurse who has received formal public health nursing preparation. Community/public health nursing is population-focused, community-oriented nursing. *Population focused* means that care is aimed at improving the health of one or more populations. To save space in the narrative of this text, the term *community health nurse* is sometimes used instead of community/public health nurse.

VISIONS AND COMMITMENTS

When describing an object, we often discuss what it looks like, what its component parts are, how it works, and how it relates to other things. Although knowledge of structure and function is important, in interpersonal activities the exact form is not as important as the purpose of the exchange. And the quality of our specific, purposeful relationships derives from our visions of what might be as well as our commitments to work toward these visions.

Visions are broad statements describing what we desire something to be like. They derive from the ability of human beings to imagine what does not currently exist. **Commitments** are agreements we make with ourselves that pledge our energies for or toward our visions.

As a synthesis of nursing and public health practice, community/public health nursing accepts the historical commitments of both. By definition and practice, our caring for clients who are ill is part of the essence of nursing. Likewise, we bring from nursing our commitment to help the client take responsibility for his or her well-being and wholeness through our genuine interest and caring. We add, from public health practice, our role as health teacher to provide individuals and groups the opportunity to see their own responsibility in moving toward health and wholeness.

Community/public health nurses are concerned with the development of human beings, families, groups, and communities. Nursing provides us our commitment to assist individuals developmentally, especially at the time of birth and death. Public health expands our commitment beyond individuals to consider the development and healthy functioning of families, groups, and communities.

Public health practice makes its unique contribution to community/public health nursing by adding to our commitments. These commitments include the following:
1. Ensuring an equitable distribution of health care
2. Ensuring a basic standard of living that supports the health and well-being of all persons
3. Ensuring a healthful physical environment

These commitments require our involvement with the public and private political and economic environments.

Boxes 1-3 and 1-4 list the commitments of nursing and public health, respectively, that are grounded in their historical developments. These commitments are the foundations on which specific professional practices, projects, goals, and activities can be created.

Because our culture is biased toward "doing" (being active, being busy, and producing), we often are not conscious of our visions of what might be. We study, exercise, go out with friends, cook, clean, play with children, invest money, and shop. We can get bogged down in "doing" the activities and projects appropriate to our commitments. For example, if you

Box 1-3	**Commitments of Nursing**

1. Patterning an environment of safety and asepsis that promotes health and protects clients.
2. Promoting health for individuals by caring for them when they are not able to do so themselves because of age, illness, disability, or dysfunction.
3. Promoting health for individuals and support for families related to developmental stages (pregnancy, labor and delivery, and care of newborns; care of dependent family members; care of dependent elderly; care of the dying).
4. Promoting wellness and integration during illness, disability, and dying.
5. Treating clients equitably without bias related to age, race, gender, socioeconomic class, religion, or cultural preferences.
6. Calling forth the client's commitment to his or her own well-being and wholeness.

are committed to having relationships with friends, recall a time when a meeting with friends felt like a duty and obligation. You were going through the motions of being together, but you were not genuinely relating to your friends. At that moment, you were not creating the relationship from your commitment; you probably felt burdened rather than enlivened.

Likewise, it is possible to get bogged down professionally by doing the "right" things that public health nurses are supposed to do but not feeling satisfied. We are disappointed that results do not show up quickly or that suffering persists. We create too many professional projects and feel spread too thin. We burn out.

Working on activities directed toward the commitments underlying community/public health nursing does not guarantee that we will achieve our visions. But not working toward our visions and giving up on our commitments guarantees that we are part of the problem rather than part of the solution in our communities. Not working toward our visions also results in dissatisfaction and disconnectedness.

Remaining in touch with the reasons we are doing something empowers us. Our vision of healthy, whole, vital individuals, families, and communities, and our related commitments, can provide a renewing source of energy. And it is hope and energy on which we draw to empower our professional practice and bring vitality to our relationships with individuals, families, and groups.

Box 1-4	**Commitments of Public Health**

1. Patterning of an environment that promotes health.
2. Promotion of health for families and populations.
3. Assurance of equitable, just distribution of health care to all.
4. Creation of a just economic environment to support health and vitality of individuals, families, and groups.
5. Prevention of physical and mental illnesses as a support to the wholeness and vitality of individuals, families, and groups.
6. Provision of the greatest good for the greatest number—thinking collectively on behalf of human beings.
7. Education of others to be aware of their own responsibility to move toward health, wholeness, and vitality.

Expressing our visions and commitments to others provides them an opportunity to become partners in working *for* what might be. By having partners we gain support not only for our visions but also for specific projects.

Janel, the mother in a young family consisting of a mother, a father, and a 2-year-old son with cerebral palsy, called the health department during her second pregnancy. She requested that nurse assist her in having a healthy second child. No one could guarantee that vision, but Janel's willingness to seek a partner in the commitment provided an opportunity for a nurse-client relationship that would increase the likelihood of a healthy newborn. The nurse, Shari, and Janel developed specific projects related to, among other things, financial access to prenatal care, nutrition, prenatal monitoring, and anxiety management.

Community/public health nurses often have visions about health that others do not know are possible. Nurses can educate and speak about visions of health and specific commitments that can increase the likelihood of particular health possibilities.

Amos and Joice, a married couple in their sixties, were committed to remaining self-sufficient. Both had diabetes, and Joice had had a stroke that resulted in right hemiparesis and expressive aphasia. When Joice had to retire from her job, their income declined dramatically. Amos worked two jobs and was rarely home to be a companion to his wife. The couple fought about money, and, because her verbal communication was very slow and unclear, for the first time in their marriage they resorted to expressing frustration and anger by hitting each other. Initially, the family did not ask Cassandra, the community/public health nursing student, for assistance. On one visit, Cassandra recognized that the wife was angry and began to explore the family stressors. The student's vision that "families can solve problems through communication" made it possible to discuss the problem with the spouses and solicit their commitment to explore alternatives with her. The family eventually agreed to turn to their extended family, social service agencies, and a bank for additional sources of revenue. In this situation it was the nurse who initiated the discussion of her vision and enlisted the family members' commitment to exploring possibilities.

We have discussed two examples of expressing a vision as a basis for creating commitments in nurse-client relationships and in relationships between the nurse and other service providers. It is helpful for each nurse to express his or her visions and commitments to peers and supervisors. As nurses, we need colleagues to encourage us, work with us, and coach us. Work groups whose members can identify some visions common to their individual practices and can agree on some common commitments have a vital source of energy. When we know what we are *for*, we can assertively invite others to participate with us. When others are working with us, more possibilities are created for synergistic effects.

DISTINGUISHING FEATURES OF COMMUNITY/PUBLIC HEALTH NURSING

Community/public health nurses are expected to use the nursing process in their relationships with individuals, families, groups, populations, and communities (ANA,

2007b). Community/public health nursing is the care provided by educated nurses in a particular place and time and directed toward promoting, restoring, and preserving the health of the total population or community. Families are recognized as an important social group in which values and knowledge are learned and health-related behaviors are practiced.

HEALTHFUL COMMUNITIES

What aspects of this definition are different from definitions of nursing in general? The explicit naming of families, groups, and populations as clients is a major focus. Community-based health nurses care for individuals and families. Community/public health nurses also may care for individuals and families; however, they are cared for in the context of a vision of a healthful community. Beliefs underlying community/public health nursing summarized from Chapter 2 are presented in Box 1-5. Community/public health nursing is nursing for social betterment.

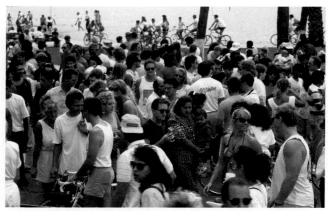

Community health nursing focuses on the health of a group, community, or population.

Box 1-5 Beliefs Underlying Community/Public Health Nursing

- Human beings have rights and responsibilities.
- Promoting and maintaining family independence is healthful.
- Environments have an impact on human health.
- Nurses can make a difference and promote change toward health for individuals, families, and communities.
- Vulnerable and at-risk populations/groups/families need special attention, especially the aged, infants, and disabled, ill, and poor persons.
- Poverty and oppression are social barriers to achievement of health and human potential.
- Interpersonal relationships are essential to caring for others.
- Hygiene, self-care, and prevention are as important as care of the sick.
- Community/public health nurses can be leaders and innovators in developing programs of nursing care and programs for adequate standards of living.
- Community/public health nursing care should be available to all, not just the poor.

Community/public health nurses seek to empower individuals, families, groups, community organizations, and other health and human service professionals to participate in creating healthful communities. The prevailing theory about how healthful communities develop has been that individuals and social groups clarify their identities first and then protect their own rights while also considering the rights of others. More recent studies on the moral development of women in the United States suggest that women first participate in a network of relationships of caring for others and then consider their own rights (Gilligan, 1982).

The ideal for a healthful community is a balance of individuality and unity. Community/public health nurses seek to promote healthful communities in which there is individual freedom *and* responsible caring for others. It is impossible for an individual to consider only his or her desires without infringing on the freedom of others. For collective well-being to exist, we must also be concerned about caring accountability. We must "ask about justice, about ... each person having space in which to grow and dream and learn and work" (Brueggemann, 1982, p. 50). We must ask about the conditions that promote health.

EMPOWERMENT FOR HEALTH PROMOTION

Because community/public health nurses often work with persons who are *not* ill, emphasis is placed on promoting and preserving health in addition to assisting people to respond to illnesses. Although not all illnesses can be prevented and death cannot be eliminated, community health nurses seek to empower human beings to live in ways that strengthen resilience; decrease preventable diseases, disability, and premature death; and relieve experiences of illness, vulnerability, and suffering.

Empowerment is the process of assisting others to uncover their own inherent abilities, strengths, vigor, wholeness, and spirit. Empowerment depends on the presence of hope. Power is not actually provided by the community/public health nurse. Empowerment is a process by which possibilities and opportunities for the expression of an individual's being and abilities are revealed. Nurses can assist in this process by fostering hope and by removing barriers to expression.

Community/public health nurses use the information and skills from their education and experiences in medical-surgical, parent-child, and psychiatric–mental health nursing to assist individuals, families, and groups in creating *opportunities* to make choices that promote health and wholeness. In community/public health nursing, nurses rarely make the choices for others. Instead, as a means of expanding opportunities for others, community/public health nurses provide information about interpersonal relationships and alternative ways of doing things. This is especially true when community/public health nurses instruct others in how to care for those with illnesses or how generally to support the growth and development of other members of families or groups. For example, a husband might be shown how to safely transfer his wife from the bed to a chair, or a young father might be taught how to praise his son and set limits without resorting to threats and frequent punishment.

Being related to people can invite a person to risk being connected and to trust in the face of his or her fears. This is particularly true for those who have experienced intense or patterned isolation, abuse, despair, or oppression. A nurse is said to be "present" with a client when the nurse is both physically near and psychologically "being with" the person (Gilje, 1993). Various ways a community/public health nurse can be "present" are revealed in the case study at the end of this chapter.

Culturally competent care is essential in both public health and nursing practice (ANA, 2007b; Campinha-Bacote et al., 1996; USDHHS, 1997). Community/public health nurses must recognize the diverse backgrounds and preferences of the individuals, families, populations, and communities with whom they work. Cultural influences on health problems, health promotion and disease prevention activities, and other health resources should be assessed. In addition, cultural differences must be considered when developing and adapting nursing interventions.

THEORY AND COMMUNITY/PUBLIC HEALTH NURSING

Nursing practice is based on the concepts of human beings, health and illness, problem-solving and creative processes, and the human-environment relationship (Hanchett, 1988; Marriner-Tomey & Alligood, 2006). Our environment includes physical, social, cultural, spiritual, economic, and political facets.

Our knowledge of these concepts evolves from several routes, including personal experience, logic, a sense of right and wrong (ethics), empiric science, aesthetic preferences, and an understanding of what it means to be human (Marriner-Tomey & Alligood, 2006). *Concepts* are labels or names that we give to our perceptions of living beings, objects, or events. *Theories* are a set of concepts, definitions, and hypotheses that help us describe, explain, or predict the interrelationships among concepts (Marriner-Tomey & Alligood, 2006).

Although Florence Nightingale began the formal development of nursing theory, most theory development in nursing has occurred since the 1960s (Choi, 1989). Marriner-Tomey and Alligood (2006) describe the work of numerous nursing theorists. (Obviously, we cannot discuss all of them here.) In community/public health nursing, general systems theory provides a way to link many of the concepts related to nursing. The nursing theories of Johnson (1989), King (1981), Neuman and Fawcett (2002), and Roy (1984) rely in part on general systems theory. Perspectives on client-environment relationships from these theories are discussed later in this chapter.

GENERAL SYSTEMS THEORY

An *open system* is a set of interacting elements that must exchange energy, matter, or information with the external environment to exist (Katz & Kahn, 1966; von Bertalanffy, 1968). Open systems include individuals as well as social systems such as families, groups, organizations, and communities with whom the community/public health nurse must work (Figure 1-2). Systems theory is especially useful in exploring the numerous and complex client-environment interchanges. For example, a community/public health nurse might provide postpartum home visits to a woman and her newborn, simultaneously focusing on the adjustment of the entire family to the birth. The same nurse might also teach teen parenting classes in a high school and monitor the birth rates in the community, identifying those populations at statistical risk of having low-birth-weight infants.

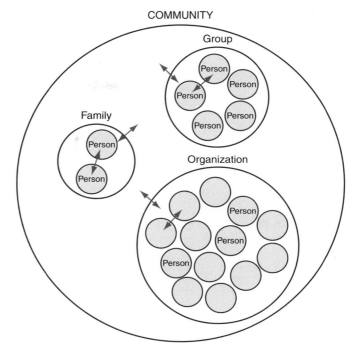

FIGURE 1-2 Social systems.

Compared with inpatient settings, the environments in community/public health nursing practice are more variable and less controllable (Kenyon et al., 1990). **General systems theory** provides an umbrella for assessing and analyzing the various clients and their relationships with dynamic environments. In this text, family and community assessments are approached from a general systems framework.

Each open system has the same basic structures (Smith & Rankin, 1972) (Figure 1-3, *A*). Figure 1-3, *B* is an example of application of the open system model to a specific organization. The *boundary* separates the system from its environment and regulates the flow of energy, matter, and information between the system and its environment. The *environment* is everything outside the boundary of the system. The skin acts as a physical boundary for human beings. A person's preference for relatedness is a more abstract boundary that helps determine the pattern of interpersonal relationships. Family boundaries might be determined by law and culture, such as a rule that a family consists of blood relatives. A family can have more open boundaries and define itself by including persons not related by blood. Groups, organizations, and some communities have membership criteria that assist in defining their boundaries. Other community boundaries might be geographic and political, such as city limits.

Outcomes are the created products, energy, and information that emerge from the system into the environment. Health behaviors and health status are examples of outcomes. *External influences* are the matter, energy, and information that come from the environment into the system. External influences can be resources for or stressors to the system. Each system uses the external influences together with internal resources to achieve its purposes and goals. *Feedback* is information channeled back into the system from its environment that describes the condition of the system. When a nurse tells a mother that her child's blood pressure is higher than the desired range,

ZDB75P92NT

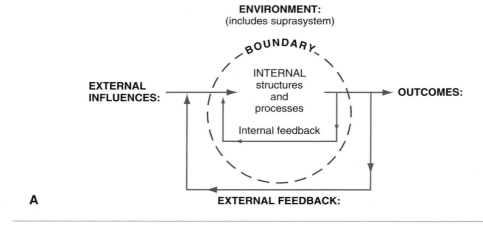

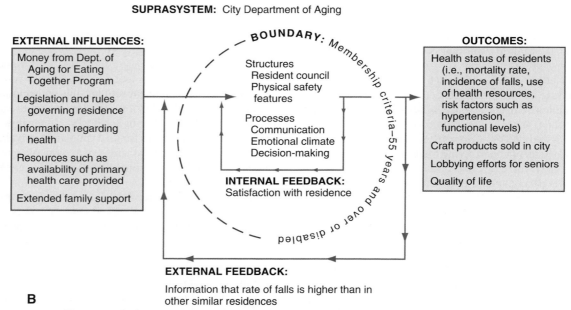

FIGURE 1-3 A, Model of an open system. **B,** Residence for the elderly viewed as an open system.

the nurse is providing health information as feedback to the mother. Feedback provides an opportunity to modify system functioning. The mother can then decide when and where to seek medical evaluation.

Each system is composed of parts called *subsystems*. Subsystems have their own goals and functions and exist in relationship with the other subsystems. In a human being, the gastrointestinal system is an example of a subsystem. In social systems, the subsystems might be structural or functional. Structural subsystems relate to organization. Examples of structural subsystems are a mother-child dyad in a family or the nursing department in a local health department. Functional subsystems are more abstract and relate to specific purposes. For example, the subsystems of organizations have been conceptualized as production, maintenance, integration, and adaptation (Katz & Kahn, 1966). Subsystems of

a community are often named by their function, such as the health care subsystem, the educational subsystem, and the economic subsystem.

Systems might relate as separate entities that interact, or they might create a variety of partnerships and confederations. Systems might be hierarchical. The *suprasystem* is the next larger system in a hierarchy. For example, the suprasystem of a county is the state; the suprasystem of a parochial school might be the church or the diocese that sponsors the school.

The assumptions that relate to all open systems (von Bertalanffy, 1968) are similar to those underlying holism in nursing (Allen, 1991) and the ecologic model of health in public health (Institute of Medicine, 2003):

1. A system is greater than the sum of its parts. One cannot understand a system by studying its parts in isolation. For example, we cannot make inferences about the health status

of a family unless we inquire about the health status of each member. However, knowing the health history and present status of individual members does not tell us how the family addresses its health concerns. Knowing the parts is necessary, but not sufficient, to describe the health of the family system.

2. The primary focus of systems theory is the relationship of the parts, not the parts per se. Life is dynamic. When nurses assess a family or community at a specific time, the assessment is more like a photograph than a movie. Exploring how the system has changed, how the individual members affect each other, and how the system interacts with the environment helps the assessment to become more like a movie.

3. A change in one part of a system affects the whole system. Change is a part of life. It might be accompanied by suffering because of either the type of change (an accident) or the quantity of the change (too many changes exceed the resources). At other times, change brings relief and strengthened resources.

4. Elements of one system can also be parts of another system. For example, a college student also belongs to a family, social groups, and perhaps a religious organization.

5. Exchanges between a system and its environments tend to be circular or cyclical. Interaction exists between the system and its environment. For example, in a community with a high percentage of hazardous occupations, a high accident rate might increase the rates of disability and unemployment within families. Because the unemployed pay less income tax, the money available to develop services for the disabled within a community with a high disability rate is reduced. Such a community has fewer resources, and, therefore, new businesses might find it a less attractive location. Although a single cause and effect relationship cannot usually be established, health problems are interconnected with social concerns. In the community just described, accident rates might be related to unemployment and economics.

6. Human beings and social systems seek to survive and to avoid disorganization and randomness (or *entropy*). As social systems develop, they tend to become more complex, with specialized structures and functions. Organizations often change their goals rather than disband when they have achieved their original goals. A multitude of health care professions, services, programs, and equipment have developed within the U.S. health care system. Community/public health nurses must recognize this complexity when helping others access health care and when proposing changes.

7. Systems operate with *equifinality,* meaning that the same end point can be reached from a variety of starting points and through various paths. There is not one right way. Culture influences child-rearing practices among families, for example, and local communities organize their health services differently.

NURSING THEORY

Nursing theories are based on a range of perspectives about the nature of human beings, health, nursing, and the environment. Most nursing theories have been developed with individual clients in mind (Hanchett, 1988). However, many concepts from the different nursing theories are applicable to nursing that addresses families and communities. The concepts of self-care and environment are introduced here.

Self-Care

Self-care is "the production of actions directed to self or to the environment in order to regulate one's functioning in the interests of one's life, integrated functioning, and well-being" (Orem, 1985, p. 31). Self-care depends on knowledge, resources, and action (Erickson et al., 1983). The concept of self-care is consistent with the community/public nursing focus on empowerment of persons and groups to promote health and to care for themselves.

Although each person is responsible for his or her own health habits, the family and community have responsibilities to support self-care (USDHHS, 1995). The family is the immediate source of support and health information. The community has responsibilities to provide safe food, water, air, and waste disposal; enforce safety standards; and create and support opportunities for individual self-care (USDHHS, 1995). When the focus is on self-care, the family and community are viewed primarily as suprasystems to individuals.

Client-Environment Relationships

Nursing theories acknowledge that humans live within an environment (Marriner-Tomey & Alligood, 2006). Nurses are caring professionals within the clients' environments who influence the clients through direct physical care, provision of information, interpersonal presence, and environmental management. Nursing theories that build on general systems theory tend to place more emphasis on the environment than do other nursing theories (Hanchett, 1988). The continuously changing environment requires that the client expend energy to survive, perform activities of daily living, grow, develop, and maintain harmony or balance. Clients must adapt within a dynamic environment (Table 1-1). (Also see Chapter 9 on environment.)

PUBLIC HEALTH THEORY

Public health theory is concerned with the health of populations of human beings. Public health is a practice discipline that applies knowledge from the physical, biologic, and social sciences to promote health and to prevent disease, injury, disability, and premature death. Epidemiology is the study of health in human populations and is explored in more detail in Chapter 7. Population, prevention, risk, and social justice are among the concepts from public health theory that are important to community health nursing. The first three concepts are discussed here, and justice is discussed later in this chapter.

Populations and Risk

Population has two meanings: people residing in an area, and a group or set of persons under statistical study. The word **group** is used here to mean a set or collection of persons, not a system of individuals who engage in face-to-face interactions, which is the definition of *group* used in discussion of systems theory. The fact that there are many definitions for *population* and *group* leads to lack of clarity and fosters debate and dialogue.

Both definitions of population are used in public health and community health nursing. The initial goal of public health was to prevent or control communicable diseases that were the major causes of death within human populations (i.e., the people living in specific geographic or political areas). Today, for example, a director of nursing in a city health department is concerned with the health of the population within the city limits. When used in this way, *population* means all the people

TABLE 1-1 Perspectives on Client-Environment Relationships in Selected Nursing Theories

Theorist	Relationship of Client and Environment
Dorothy Johnson	Clients attempt to adjust to environmental factors. Strong inputs from the environment might cause imbalance and require excess energy to the point of threatening the existence of the client. Stable environments help clients conserve energy and function successfully.
Sister Callista Roy	Clients attempt to adjust to immediate environmental excesses or absences within a background of other stimuli. Successful adaptation allows survival, growth, and improved ability to respond to the environment.
Imogene King	Clients interact purposefully with other people and the environment. Health is the continuous process of using resources to function in daily life and to grow and develop.
Betty Neuman	Clients continuously interact with people and other environmental forces and seek to defend themselves against threats. Health is balance and harmony within the whole person.

Data from Marriner-Tomey, A. & Alligood, M. (2006): *Nursing theorists and their work*, (6th ed.). St. Louis: Mosby

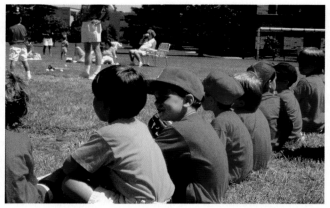

Children in a sports league are one example of a group, because they have one or more characteristics in common as well as a face-to-face relationship.

in the area or community. The noun *public* is often used as a synonym for this definition of population.

Because not everyone has the same health status, the second definition of population—a set of persons under statistical study—is especially important in public health practice. Using this definition, a *population* is a set of persons having a common personal or environmental characteristic. The common characteristic might be anything thought to relate to health, such as age, race, sex, social class, medical diagnosis, level of disability, exposure to a toxin, or participation in a health-seeking behavior, such as smoking cessation. It is the researcher or health practitioner who identifies the characteristic and set of persons that make up this population. In epidemiology, numerous sets of persons are studied clinically and statistically to identify the causes, methods of treatment, and means of prevention of diseases, accidents, disabilities, and premature deaths. In community/public health nursing, epidemiologic information is used to identify populations at higher risk for specific preventable health conditions. **Risk** is a statistical concept based on probability. Community/public health nursing is concerned with human risk of disease, disability, and premature death. Therefore, community/public health nurses work with persons within the population to reduce their risk for developing a health condition.

Aggregate is a synonym for the second definition of population. Aggregates are people who do not have the relatedness necessary to constitute an interpersonal group (system) but who have one or more characteristics in common, such as pregnant teenagers (Schultz, 1987). Williams (1977) focused attention on the aggregate as an additional type of client with whom community/public health nurses apply the problem-solving process. For example, aggregates can be identified by virtue of setting (those enrolled in a well-baby clinic), demographic characteristic (women), or health status (smokers or those with hypertension) (APHA, 1980, 1996). It is the community/public health nurse who identifies the aggregate by naming one or more common characteristics.

The terminology regarding statistical groups and aggregates is confusing. Although there are subtle differences, the terms *at-risk population, specified population,* and *population group* are used to mean *aggregate.* The APHA (1980, 1996) uses the term *at-risk population* in place of the term *aggregate.* In its description of community health nursing, the ANA (1980) uses the term *specified population.* Others use *population group* to mean a population that shares similar characteristics but has limited face-to-face interaction (Porter, 1987). It is important to remember that regardless of which of these terms is used, such a population is not a system. The individuals within these populations are not classified because of interaction or common goals. It is the community/public health nurse who conceptually classifies, collects, or aggregates the individuals into such a population. The individuals within such a population often might not even know one another. The nurse has identified the population to focus intervention efforts toward health promotion and prevention.

Prevention

Prevention is a complex concept that also evolved from an attempt to control diseases among the public. Epidemiology is a science that helps to describe the natural history of specific diseases, their causes, and their treatments. The natural history of a disease includes a presymptomatic period, a symptomatic period, and a resolution (death, disability, complications, or recovery) (Friedman, 1994). The broad concept of prevention has three levels: primary, secondary, and tertiary. The goal of *primary prevention* is the promotion of health and prevention of the occurrence of the disease. Activities of primary prevention include environmental protection (such as maintaining asepsis and providing clean water) and personal protection (such as providing immunizations and avoiding smoking). The goal of *secondary prevention* is the detection (screening) and treatment of the disease as early as possible during the natural history of the disease. For example, Papanicolaou (Pap) smear testing allows cervical cancer to be detected earlier in the disease process so that cure is more likely. *Tertiary prevention* is geared toward preventing disability, complications, and death from the disease. Tertiary prevention includes rehabilitation.

All levels of prevention can be accomplished through work with individuals, families, and groups. Prevention can also be accomplished by targeting changes in the behaviors of specified populations, changes in social functioning of communities (law, social mores), and changes in the physical environment (waste disposal). The well-being and health of the entire population within the community is the ultimate goal of public health.

GOALS FOR COMMUNITY/PUBLIC HEALTH NURSING

Care is always in the here and now, responsive to the needs of specific persons, in a specific place, at a specific time. It is always personal and intimate. Even when community/public health nurses work with other professionals and community groups, the care is expressed through recognition of the uniqueness of each of the others.

There are several major goals for community health nursing (Box 1-6). Table 1-2 identifies examples of health outcomes for each of the goals for each category of client. All nurses address these goals, but most do so with individuals, hospitalized individuals and their families or friends, and small groups. In addition to formulating these goals with individuals, community/public health nurses do the same with families, groups, aggregates, populations, and organizations/systems within the community.

Box 1-6   Major Goals for Community/Public Health Nursing

- Care of the ill, disabled, and suffering in nonhospital settings.
- Support of development and well-being throughout the life cycle.
- Promotion of human relatedness and mutual caring.
- Promotion of self-responsibility regarding health and well-being.
- Promotion of relative safety in the environment while conserving resources.
- Reduction of health disparities among populations.

From Smith, C. M. (1985). Unpublished data. Baltimore: University of Maryland School of Nursing.

NURSING ETHICS AND SOCIAL JUSTICE

The goals of community health nursing reflect the values and beliefs of both nursing and public health. Each profession has an ideology, or set of values, concepts, ideas, and beliefs, that defines its responsibilities and actions (Hamilton & Keyser, 1992). Ideologies are linked closely with ethics—study of and thinking about what one ought to do (i.e., right conduct).

Public health and nursing are based on the same ethical principles: respecting autonomy, doing good, avoiding harm, and treating people fairly (Fry, 1983; Last, 1998) (Table 1-3). These principles are sometimes in conflict. Issues related to application of these principles are discussed in case examples in *Ethics in Practice* boxes (see Chapters 8, 9, 21, 23, 24, 26, 27, and 28).

TABLE 1-2   Examples of Health Outcomes Related to Goals to Community/Public Health Nursing

	Care of the Ill	Support of Development	Support of Relatedness	Promotion of Self-Responsibility	Promotion of Healthful Environment
Individual	Individual learns self-management of diabetes mellitus	Teenage mother adjusts to newborn care	Adult joins group for socialization	Adult-child of alcoholic seeks counseling	Homeless person seeks shelter
Family	Family cares for member with terminal cancer	Extended family decides how best to care for aging grandparents	Family with disabled child seeks out other such families	Family identifies preferences of members	Elderly couple improves safety in the home
Group	Children with physical disabilities are cared for in school	Junior high school students explore responsibility regarding sexual activity	Several women in a residence start a sharing group	Women at a mother and children's center take on responsibilities in the center	Mothers Against Drunk Driving advocates laws against driving while intoxicated
Aggregate	Barriers are identified in a number of clients regarding failure to return for tests of cure after antibiotics	Worksite program regarding preretirement planning is established	*	Worksite program for counseling for health risk reduction is initiated	Curriculum is developed for schools regarding burn prevention
Community	Hospice program is initiated in a city	Regulations for safe daycare are passed as country ordinance	A network of case management is established for discharged psychiatric clients	Crisis hotline is established	Waste recycling program is established

*By definition, aggregates are individuals or families with common characteristics who are identified as such by the community health nurse or other professional. If such clients become known to one another and develop a sense of belonging or support, the aggregate would become a group or community.

TABLE 1-3	Basic Ethical Principles in Health	
Principle	**Definition**	**Example**
Altruism	Concern for the welfare of others	Being present
Beneficence	Doing good	Providing immunizations
Nonmaleficence	Avoiding harm	Not abandoning client
Respect for autonomy	Honoring self-determination (i.e., right to make one's own decisions; respecting privacy)	Allowing client to refuse treatment, informed consent; maintaining confidentiality
Veracity	Truth-telling	Communicating authentically and not lying
Fidelity	Keeping promises	Arriving on time for home visit
Justice	Treating people fairly	Providing nursing services to all, regardless of ability to pay

Data from American Association of Colleges of Nursing. (1986). *Essentials of college and university education for professional nursing,* Washington, DC: The Association; and Beauchamp, T., & Childress, J. (2001). *Principles of biomedical ethics* (5th ed.). New York: Oxford University Press.

ETHICAL PRIORITIES

Historically, the *ANA Code for Nurses* (ANA, 1985, p. 2) stated that the most important ethical principle of nursing practice is "respect for the inherent dignity and worth ... of human existence and the individuality of all persons" (Box 1-7). However, because public health is concerned with the well-being of the entire population, the foremost ethical principle of public health practice is doing good for the greatest number of persons with the least amount of harm. Consequently, in community health nursing, there is a tension between an individual-focused ethic

BOX 1-7   Code of Ethics for Nurses

1. The nurse, in all professional relationships, practices with compassion and respect for the inherent dignity, worth, and uniqueness of every individual, unrestricted by considerations of social or economic status, personal attributes, or the nature of health problems.
2. The nurse's primary commitment is to the client, whether an individual, family, group, or community.
3. The nurse promotes, advocates for, and strives to protect the health, safety, and rights of the client.
4. The nurse is responsible and accountable for individual nursing practice and determines the appropriate delegation of tasks consistent with the nurse's obligation to provide optimum client care.
5. The nurse owes the same duties to self as to others, including the responsibility to preserve integrity and safety, to maintain competence, and to continue personal and professional growth.
6. The nurse participates in establishing, maintaining, and improving health care environments and conditions of employment conducive to the provision of quality health care and consistent with the values of the profession through individual and collective actions.
7. The nurse participates in the advancement of the profession through contributions to practice, education, administration, and knowledge development.
8. The nurse collaborates with other health professionals and the public in promoting community, national, and international efforts to meet health needs.
9. The profession of nursing, as represented by associations and their members, is responsible for articulating nursing values, for maintaining the integrity of the profession and its practice, and for shaping social policy.

From American Nurses Association. (2001). *Code of ethics for nurses with interpretive statements.* Washington, DC: Author.

and a society-focused ethic (Fry, 1983; Hamilton & Keyser, 1992). Community/public health nurses consider both ethical perspectives.

How does a nurse respect the autonomy of individuals while securing health for many? There is no single "right" answer. The question needs to be asked often and answered anew as circumstances change. At times, the community/public health nurse's decision will be to protect the autonomy of an individual while working for environmental changes that seek to protect many. For example, a community/public health nurse honors a teenager's autonomy and does not force him or her to avoid cigarette use. However, the nurse can lobby for higher cigarette taxes that decrease consumption, for enforcement of laws prohibiting cigarette sales to minors, and for substance-free recreation centers. Both nursing and public health ideologies value education and environmental modifications over coercion.

The ANA (2001, p. 9) acknowledges that there are "situations in which the right to individual self-determination may be outweighed or limited by the rights, health and welfare of others, particularly in relation to public health considerations." For example, in an airplane disaster, one individual already close to death might be allowed to die to save several others. Individual autonomy might also be curtailed by involuntary confinement if a person is threatening to commit suicide or to abuse or kill another, or if the person has a drug-resistant form of tuberculosis. Community quarantine may be necessary to prevent the spread of an outbreak of avian flu.

DISTRIBUTIVE JUSTICE

A more difficult issue emerges when we consider the number of individuals with competing interests and needs. Does everyone have a right to health care? If so, what kind and how much? Nursing is working to "ensure the availability and accessibility of high-quality health services to all persons whose health needs are unmet" (ANA, 1985, p. 16).

How are health care, nursing, and other social services to be distributed within the population? How are healthful environments to be created and hazards reduced? *Justice* is an ethical concept concerned with treating human beings fairly. Nurses are to provide competent, personalized care, regardless of an individual client's financial, social, or personal characteristics (ANA, 2007b). **Distributive justice** is the ethical concept concerned with the fair provision of opportunities, goods, and services to populations of people. Because the nursing code of ethics focuses primarily on care of individuals, community health nurses also need other perspectives of justice in helping to provide ethical care to populations (Fry, 1985).

There are two perspectives for determining justice when working with populations: egalitarian (equal) and utilitarian (Fry, 1985). In an *egalitarian* system of justice, each person has equal access to equal health services. Providing every person in a country with access to basic health services is an example of egalitarian justice. In a *utilitarian* system of justice, resources are distributed so as to provide the greatest good for the greatest number with the least amount of harm. When resources are limited, the utilitarian perspective is helpful. At times, individuals might be harmed under the utilitarian perspective. The airplane disaster mentioned earlier is an example of utilitarian decision making. With utilitarian justice, it is important to try to determine the benefits and risks of an action (Last, 1998). A health care system does not meet the criterion for justice if health care services are provided only to those who can pay. Instead, health care is provided unequally (only to those who can afford it), and the good of the entire population is not considered.

SOCIAL JUSTICE

Our public health ethic goes further. Not only is health care considered a right, but "a basic standard of living necessary for health" is also a right (Winslow, 1984). Furthermore, a healthful environment and protection from environmental hazards are prerequisites for health (Kotchian, 1995). Because environmental risks are greater for some individuals, groups, families, and populations, environmental issues have been framed as social justice issues (Lum, 1995). If hazardous waste is dumped primarily in low-income communities, justice is not achieved.

Social justice is explicitly defined in the most recent edition of *Public Health Nursing: Scope and Standards of Practice*:

> [*Social justice* is] the principle that all persons are entitled to have their basic human needs met, regardless of differences in economic status, class, gender, race, ethnicity, citizenship, religion, age, sexual orientation, disability or health. This includes the eradication of poverty and illiteracy, the establishment of sound environmental policy, and equality of opportunity for healthy personal and social development. (ANA, 2007b, p. 43)

As discussed in the history of public health nursing in Chapter 2, public health nursing is rooted in social justice. However, social justice has not been consistently described in recent national nursing documents (Bekemeier & Butterfield, 2005). Fahrenwald and colleagues (2007, p. 190) advocate for public health nursing faculty to assist "students to understand and participate in social justice actions that aim to amend … the social conditions that influence health and the delivery of health care." Other public health nursing scholars recommend that social justice "from a population vantage point" be recognized as the central concept in public health nursing (Schim et al., 2007).

Creating a just society and a just health care system in a context of limited resources is a major challenge in the twenty-first century. Questions that are being asked to determine health care priorities for populations are, for example, the following: Who decides what is good? What are the benefits and risks? How do we weigh the short-term and long-term benefits and risks? How do we determine who has a reasonable chance of benefiting? In our democratic society, there are competing interests, and the process is ongoing. Potentially, all community members, government leaders, nurses, and other health care professionals contribute to priority setting. Community/public health nursing practice and research contribute information to help answer these questions. An ethic that includes social justice also helps to focus priorities.

There is a constant tension between facilitating the freedom of individuals and nurturing a community in which people feel connected enough to care for one another. One of our challenges as community/public health nurses is to foster communities in which people experience their interconnection and treat one another justly. In the remainder of this chapter, the specific responsibilities and competencies that assist community/public health nurses in working for social betterment are explored.

THE NURSING PROCESS IN COMMUNITY/ PUBLIC HEALTH

Public Health Nursing: Scope and Standards of Practice (ANA, 2007b) was developed in concert with the steps of the nursing process and indicates that community/public health nurses are to apply the entire nursing process to promote the "health of the public" (p. 88). To improve the health of one or more populations, baccalaureate-prepared community/public health nurses often implement programs with individuals, families, and groups to promote health and wellness (Box 1-8). Masters-prepared community/public health nurses "develop and evaluate programs and policy designed to prevent disease and promote health for populations at risk" (ANA, 2007b, pp. 88-89). These standards describe both a competent level of nursing care provided to clients (see Box 1-8) and a competent level of behavior within the profession (discussed later in the chapter under Quality Assurance). Therefore, standards of clinical community/public health nursing practice help define the scope and quality of community/public health nursing care; they also help to distinguish community/public health nursing from other nursing specialties. One of the particular features of the specialty is that community/public health nurses are concerned with the health of communities.

How do community/public health nurses work with communities? Community/public health nurses use demographic and epidemiologic data to identify health problems of families, groups, and populations; community/public health nurses incorporate knowledge of community structure, organization, and resources in developing solutions to meet the needs of families, groups, and populations (Quad Council, 1999). From this point of view, the community might be seen as part of the environment or suprasystem of the families, groups, and populations.

The ANA (1980) makes a distinction between direct and indirect care in community health nursing. *Direct* community/public health nursing care is the application of the nursing process to individuals, families, and groups and involves face-to-face relationships. Direct care includes management and coordination of care. For example, a community/public health nurse who performs a developmental assessment of an infant, teaches the mother about age-appropriate play, and administers

Box 1-8 **Standards of Care of Public Health Nursing Practice**

Standard 1: Assessment
The public health nurse collects comprehensive data pertinent to the health status of populations.

Standard 2: Population Diagnosis and Priorities
The public health nurse analyzes the assessment data to determine the population diagnoses and priorities.

Standard 3: Outcomes Identification
The public health nurse identifies expected outcomes for a plan that is based on population diagnoses and priorities.

Standard 4: Planning
The public health nurse develops a plan that reflects best practices by identifying strategies, action plans, and alternatives to attain expected outcomes.

Standard 5: Implementation
The public health nurse implements the identified plan by partnering with others.

Standard 5A. Coordination
The public health nurse coordinates programs, services, and other activities to implement the identified plan.

Standard 5B. Health Education and Health Promotion
The public health nurse employs multiple strategies to promote health, prevent disease, and ensure a safe environment for populations.

Standard 5C. Consultation
The public health nurse provides consultation to various community groups and officials to facilitate the implementation of programs and services.

Standard 5D. Regulatory Activities
The public health nurse identifies, interprets, and implements public health laws, regulations, and policies.

Standard 6: Evaluation
The public health nurse evaluates the health status of the population.

From American Nurses Association. (2007). *Public health nursing: Scope and standards of practice.* Silver Spring, MD: Author.

immunizations is engaged in direct care. *Indirect* community/public health nursing does not involve interpersonal relationships with all persons who benefit from care. Priorities are determined after assessing the health status of the entire population and aggregates, the existing resources, the environment, and the social mechanisms for solving problems (American Association of Colleges of Nursing [AACN], 1986). Goals include promotion of self-help and appropriate use of health resources by community members, development of new services, and provision of effective, adequate direct nursing care services (ANA, 1980). Indirect care also includes the use of political, social, and economic means to ensure a basic standard of living for community members. A nurse who writes a grant proposal for providing primary health care to a rural population is engaged in indirect community/public health nursing care.

All professional nurses are expected to collaborate with their peers to improve nursing care and to collaborate with others to develop new health resources and "ensure safe, legal, and ethical healthcare practices" (AACN, 1986, p. 18). Therefore, we might ask: How is community/public health nursing distinct from other specialties? One distinction is that community/public health nursing has a broader perspective and is concerned with the health of the entire community and all of the aggregates within it. A second difference is that the direct care in community health is *targeted* toward individuals, families, groups, and aggregates based on those at risk (Quad Council, 1999). Care is not just provided to those who seek it. It is the responsibility of community/public health nurses to identify those who might benefit from health promotion and health prevention, as well as those with illnesses and disabilities, who are not receiving care.

RESPONSIBILITIES OF COMMUNITY/PUBLIC HEALTH NURSES

Community/public health nurses have a basic set of responsibilities regardless of where they work. The traditional historical responsibilities of community/public health nurses (see Chapter 2) are summarized in Box 1-9. At present, the Minnesota model for public health nursing practice, known as the *interventions wheel* or the *Minnesota wheel,* describes 17 public health interventions that may be focused on (or targeted to) several levels of practice: individuals/families, communities, and systems that impact population health (Minnesota Department of Health, 2001). Although these interventions are also used by other public health disciplines, the constellation of interventions and the levels of practice "represent public health nursing as a specialty practice of nursing" (Minnesota Department of Health, 2001, p. 1). The Public Health Nursing Section of the Minnesota Department of Health developed this practice-based model and with a grant from the federal Division of Nursing identified supporting evidence from literature, research, and expert opinion (Keller et al., 2004a, 2004b). The interventions wheel is presented in Figure 1-4. Table 1-4 includes definitions of each of the interventions. This model is

Box 1-9 **Responsibilities of Community/Public Health Nurses**

1. Providing care to the ill and disabled in their homes, including teaching of caregivers.
2. Maintaining healthful environments.
3. Teaching about health promotion and prevention of disease and injury.
4. Identifying those with inadequate standards of living and untreated illnesses and disabilities and referring them for services.
5. Preventing and reporting neglect and abuse.
6. Advocating for adequate standards of living and health care services.
7. Collaborating to develop appropriate, adequate, acceptable health care services.
8. Caring for oneself and participating in professional development activities.
9. Ensuring quality nursing care and engaging in nursing research.

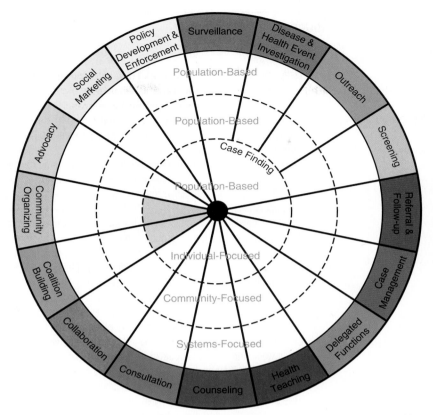

FIGURE 1-4 Minnesota Public Health Interventions Wheel (March, 2001). (From Minnesota Department of Health, Division of Community Health Services, Public Health Nursing Section. [2001]. *Public health interventions: Applications for public health nursing practice.* St. Paul: Author.)

being used to strengthen public health nursing practice, education, and management (Keller et al., 2004a, 2004b). (See the WebLinks feature on the book's Evolve website for the link to the Minnesota Department of Health's website to obtain more information about this model.)

Several responsibilities stand out as being of great importance for baccalaureate-prepared community/public health nurses: (1) identification of unmet needs; (2) advocacy and referral to ensure access to health and social services; (3) teaching, especially for health promotion and prevention; (4) screening and case finding; (5) environmental management; (6) collaboration and coordination; and (7) political action to advocate for adequate standards of living and health care services and resources. In the following discussion of nursing responsibilities in community/public health, direct care of the clients who are ill is discussed first because it is the responsibility with which nurses are most familiar. (See Chapter 19 for in-depth discussion of screening and case finding and Chapter 13 for family care management.)

DIRECT CARE OF ILL, INFIRM, SUFFERING, AND DISABLED CLIENTS

"Doing for" those who cannot do for themselves because of illness, infirmity, suffering, or disability is the historical basis of nursing. Hospitals and nursing homes have been the places where most nursing care has been provided in the United States during the twentieth century. However, home care of ill persons by nurses preceded hospital care. Since the mid-1960s, care for ill clients in the home has reemerged as a significant mode of care. Reasons for this include the aging of the population,

the relatively high prevalence of chronic diseases, reimbursement for skilled nursing care in the home (see Chapter 31), and the decreased length of hospital stays resulting from efforts to reduce hospital costs.

Care of individuals in the home today builds on care that nurses have learned to provide in institutional settings. Whatever theoretic framework is used for viewing the needs and health problems of individuals, with creativity it can be transferred to the home setting. Generally speaking, a family's access to 24-hour home nursing care for sick family members depends on the family's ability to pay for such services. Most insurance policies limit payment for nursing care for the ill in their homes to the intermittent performance of specific treatment procedures and to the nurse's instructing a family member or other caregiver in 24-hour care.

As is discussed in Unit Three, a distinguishing feature of community/public health nursing is that care is provided from a family-focused model, which is broader than and qualitatively different from an individual-focused model. The community health nurse is concerned not only with the health of the identified client but also with the health of other family members, especially the caregiver, and the family as a unit.

Populations also can experience illness and suffering as a result of natural or human-caused disasters, such as Hurricane Katrina in New Orleans. Chapter 22 discusses emergency preparedness and nursing in disasters.

REFERRAL AND ADVOCACY

Community/public health nurses often encounter individuals who have significant concerns, untreated diseases, or unmet

TABLE 1-4   Public Health Interventions with Definitions

Public Health Intervention	Definition
Surveillance	Describes and monitors health events through ongoing and systematic collection, analysis, and interpretation of health data for the purpose of planning, implementing, and evaluating public health interventions. (Adapted from MMWR, 1988.)
Disease and other health event investigation	Systematically gathers and analyzes data regarding threats to the health of populations, ascertains the source of the threat, identifies cases and others at risk, and determines control measures.
Outreach	Locates populations-of-interest or populations-at-risk and provides information about the nature of the concern, what can be done about it, and how services can be obtained.
Screening	Identifies individuals with unrecognized health risk factors or asymptomatic disease conditions in populations.
Case-finding	Locates individuals and families with identified risk factors and connects them with resources.
Referral and follow-up	Assists individuals, families, groups, organizations, and/or communities to identify and access necessary resources to prevent or resolve problems or concerns.
Case management	Optimizes self-care capabilities of individuals and families and the capacity of systems and communities to coordinate and provide services.
Delegated functions	Direct care tasks a registered professional nurse carries out under the authority of a health care practitioner as allowed by law. Delegated functions also include any direct care tasks a registered professional nurse entrusts to other appropriate personnel to perform.
Health teaching	Communicates facts, ideas and skills that change knowledge, attitudes, values, beliefs, behaviors, and practices of individuals, families, systems, and/or communities.
Counseling	Establishes an interpersonal relationship with a community, a system, family or individual intended to increase or enhance their capacity for self-care and coping. Counseling engages the community, a system, family or individual at an emotional level.
Consultation	Seeks information and generates optional solutions to perceived problems or issues through interactive problem solving with a community, system, family or individual. The community, system, family, or individual selects and acts on the option best meeting the circumstances.
Collaboration	Commits two or more persons or organizations to achieve a common goal through enhancing the capacity of one or more of the members to promote and protect health. (Adapted from Henneman, Lee, Cohen [1995]. Collaboration: A concept analysis, *J. Advanced Nursing, 21,* 103-109.)
Coalition building	Promotes and develops alliances among organization or constituencies for a common purpose. It builds linkages, solves problems, and/or enhances local leadership to address health concerns.
Community organizing	Helps community groups to identify common problems or goals, mobilize resources, and develolp and implement strategies for reaching the goals they collectively have set. (Adapted from Minkler, M [ed]. *Community organizing and community buildings for health.* New Brunswick, NJ: Rutgers University Press, 1997, 30.)
Advocacy	Pleads someone's cause or act on someone's behalf, with a focus on developing the community, system, individual or family's capacity to plead their own cause or act on their own behalf.
Social marketing	Utilizes commercial marketing principles and technologies for programs designed to influence the knowledge, attitudes, values, beliefs, behaviors, and practices of the population-of-interest.
Policy development	Places health issues on decision-maker's agendas, acquires a plan of resolution, and determines needed resources. Policy development results in laws, rules and regulations, ordinances, and policies.
Policy enforcement	Compels others to comply with the laws, rules, regulations, ordinances, and policies created in conjunction with policy development.

From Minnesota Department of Health, Section of Public Health Nursing, March 2001.

needs related to a basic standard of living (food, clothing, shelter, transportation) or who have experienced oppression, such as neglect or abuse. The community/public health nurse is not expected to independently solve all existing problems. When problems cannot be managed solely by the nurse and client, the community/public health nurse assists the client in seeking appropriate resources.

Referral is the process of directing someone to another source of assistance. The community health nurse is expected to make assessments with clients, discuss the possible significance of such findings, explore the meaning of the experience with the client, and refer the client to appropriate resources. This process is discussed in more depth in Chapter 19.

To facilitate a match between the client's need and the available resources, the community health nurse must be aware of the channels for accessing that help. Assessing the presence and quality of other health and social resources is a skill that community/public health nurses learn. There are some resources, such as welfare departments, faith communities, and schools, that exist in all geopolitical areas. There are other resources, such as drug detoxification units, that may not be found within easy traveling distance or have waiting lists. A community/public health nurse should not be surprised if it takes up to 6 months to feel knowledgeable about the resources in a specific community. Keeping abreast of the changes in the resources, their services, and contact persons is an ongoing activity.

Unless a service requires that a referral be initiated by a health professional, clients are usually encouraged to initiate the contact. At times, clients will be reluctant to pursue a referral because they are afraid or do not know how to make requests for themselves. Others might be unable to pursue the referral because of limits in functioning or inadequacy of means (such as lack of fluency in English or absence of a telephone). In such instances, community/public health nurses attempt to empower the client to overcome barriers and initiate referral contacts.

Community/public health nurses have the option of advocating for the client. *Advocacy* is the action of speaking or writing on behalf of someone else and using persuasion in support of another. This requires the skill of assertive communication and the knowledge of communication channels within and among organizations. Especially in large, bureaucratically administered programs, special channels for complaints and appeals exist if services have been denied. Clients have general legal rights as health consumers that can be inquired about through a state attorney general's office. In addition, administrators of health programs can provide information about client rights related to specific programs (such as Medicare insurance for the elderly).

In some circumstances, families, groups, or populations do not have access to a health or social service. Community/public health nurses can advocate for a population by networking with others for the development of such services. For example, a community/public health nurse might work with other professionals, religious leaders, welfare-rights advocates, and homeless persons to develop a primary health care site for the homeless. Advocacy is linked with being a leader in collaborating with others.

TEACHING

Teaching is the process of imparting cognitive knowledge, skills, and values. Nurses have information and skills that make them specialists in caring for the ill; preventing disease, illness, disability, suffering, and premature death; and promoting wellbeing. "Self-determination, independence, and choice in decision-making in health matters" is of "highest regard" to nurses (ANA, 1980, p. 18). Because community/public health nurses work with people in various stages of wellness, community health nurses have special opportunities to foster human development and capabilities through client education. The teaching process is discussed in more depth in Chapter 20. *Anticipatory guidance* is education that occurs before the client is expected to need to act on the information.

Following Nursing and Medical Plans

Community/public health nurses have always imparted information and demonstrated to family members how to care for the ill at home, especially in relation to nutrition, comfort, and maintaining a healthful, clean home. For practical reasons, it is mandatory that family members or other caregivers both provide nursing care and follow the medical treatment plan for the sick person. Community health nurses have provided this teaching and continue to do so today, especially in home health care. For example, individuals newly diagnosed with hypertension and their families or significant others are taught about taking multiple medications, modifying dietary intake, and employing relaxation techniques.

Preventing Illness and Injury

All life involves risk of disease, injury, and premature death. However, individuals have choices that affect their risks. Nurses' knowledge of these risks depends on the prevailing evidence about the natural history of diseases, epidemiology, modalities for early detection and treatment, methods of protection and prevention, and determinants of human behavior. Community/public health nurses apply this information in education for prevention of disease, injury, and premature death.

For example, we know that smoking is a risky behavior related to cancer, heart disease, and lung disease and that alcohol consumption harms the fetus. Treatment of childhood asthma reduces the number of days missed from school. Use of bicycle helmets and automobile seat belts reduce head injuries. Safer sex practices and sexual abstinence reduce the likelihood of transmission of HIV. A basic truth about the teaching-learning process is that information alone is *not* sufficient to change human behavior. Telling someone what to do or how to do it will not result in modified behavior unless the person can relate the behavior to his or her values and goals and believes that the behavior change will contribute to the achievement of aspirations. Consequently, the clarification of values is a primary strategy in identifying and changing people's health-related attitudes (see Chapter 10).

Promoting Wellness and Transcendence of Suffering

A primary responsibility of community/public health nurses is teaching to promote health (see Chapter 18). Each of us has a perception of what is necessary to promote health, which depends in part on our definition of health (Benner & Wrubel, 1989). If health is viewed as the ability to fulfill our social roles, we will be interested in learning about what will support us in performing activities of daily living, communicating, thinking, problem solving, and relating to others. If we define health as a commodity, we will be interested in learning what will repair or replace our deficiencies, and what will cure or "fix" us. If we define health as the ability to adapt, we will be interested in learning about stress-reduction techniques, the resources available for support, and methods of environmental control. If we view health as well-being, we will be interested in learning to create meaning and a sense of belonging in our lives and to accept that total control and autonomy are not possible. For example, a family with a child who has severe developmental delays might focus on providing loving care for each family member, even though they cannot predict exactly what the child might be able to learn to do as he or she develops.

Nurses working in acute care settings with the critically ill and dying have opportunities to promote well-being by helping clients and family members to find meaning and interpersonal connectedness. Community/public health nurses also have opportunities to address well-being with those dying at home or in hospices. Steeves and Kahn (1987, p. 116) discuss ways to reduce suffering by establishing conditions for "experiences of meaning." Meaning cannot be imparted through providing information or skills; rather, through discussions, meaning might be discovered as a possibility by the client. When the nurse attends carefully to the verbal and nonverbal messages of the client and family members, the nurse might help to discover what will provide meaning within the experience of suffering and death (Callanan & Kelley, 1993). See Chapter 31 for more about hospice care.

In community/public health nursing, there are circumstances besides illness and a client's impending death that evoke the need for meaning. The death of a loved one, divorce, abuse by a family member, unemployment, neglect, loss of one's home by fire, and acts of prejudice are examples.

SURVEILLANCE, MONITORING, AND EVALUATION

Community health nurses monitor the health of individuals, families, populations, and communities. *Monitoring* is the verification of the state or condition of health, and *evaluation* is the determination of the significance or value of this information. *Assessment* also denotes determination of the state of health and involves the collection and analysis of data; *reassessment* might occur at a later time. A distinction between monitoring and reassessment is that monitoring implies either a continuous process or short intervals between episodes of data collection and evaluation.

Monitoring the health of individuals in their homes and in clinics differs from monitoring patients in hospitals. In inpatient settings, many individual patients are monitored continuously because of the acuteness and instability of their diseases and illnesses. When sick people are cared for at home, the family is taught what to monitor and what is significant to report to the nurse or other health professional. The nurse, in collaboration with the physician and other health professionals, determines the frequency of monitoring by the health professionals.

In clinics, protocols are often used to schedule the next appointment. For example, individuals receiving antibiotics are often scheduled to return after 10 days for evaluation of treatment effectiveness; women are rescheduled annually for Pap testing.

When providing family-centered care, the community/public health nurse determines the frequency of monitoring based on the health status of the family, the preferences of the family, and agency policy. When determining the frequency of contact with families, the nurse must always consider any life-threatening situation and the family's perception of priorities.

Monitoring the health of groups, aggregates, and communities involves collecting and evaluating information about populations. Monitoring the health of populations and communities is called *surveillance* (Minnesota Department of Health, 2001). Demographic and epidemiologic data are used to determine age distributions, mortality, morbidity, and risky behavior of populations (see Chapter 7). Surveillance is an ongoing process to detect trends in health status. *Disease and other health event*

investigation involves identification of cases and determination of control measures. Unit Two discusses data important for determining the availability, accessibility, and acceptability of health and other community resources. Community/public health nurses often analyze data collected by others and can participate in data collection, especially as it relates to the need for and client responses to nursing care. Monitoring the health of communities is an interdisciplinary process.

Both objective and subjective information are collected during monitoring. Because nursing is concerned with "human experiences and responses" (ANA, 2003, p. 4), it is insufficient for community health nurses to monitor objective information such as physiologic outcomes, patterns of death and illness, health-related behavior, and the presence and quality of community resources. Subjective meaning and life experiences also must be explored. What do clients think about their health status? What health concerns are foremost? Interviews, conversations, and surveys are some of the ways community health nurses learn how clients view their own health needs.

POLICY ENFORCEMENT

Because our culture values individual autonomy highly, and because nursing and public health both value human growth and self-actualization, most health-related interventions do not involve coercion. However, there are instances in which the rights of the majority take precedence over the rights of individuals. To protect the health of the family or community, individual autonomy might be limited. Most states have laws that protect nurses from liability for reporting neglect, abuse, and threats of bodily harm by clients to themselves or others. Many states also provide forced treatment or curtailed behavior for individuals who have a specified communicable disease, such as tuberculosis, and who refuse to protect others from exposure. In these circumstances, community health nurses develop skill in balancing persuasion with enforcement, empowerment with coercion (Zerwekh, 1992b).

Community/public health nurses employed by local or state health departments have special responsibilities as agents of the government to enforce selected public health laws (see Chapter 6). For example, if a source of food poisoning has been attributed to an infected food handler, it will likely be the community health nurse who explains to the restaurant employee why stool cultures (with negative results for specific microorganisms) are required before his or her return to work.

ENVIRONMENTAL MANAGEMENT

Environmental management means (1) the control of those things in the immediate surroundings to protect human beings from disease and injury, or (2) the promotion of a place conducive to healing and well-being. Environmental management also includes the conservation of resources and limitation of pollution in the environment (see Chapter 9). Providing asepsis and safety are basic ethical and legal responsibilities of all nurses in managing the physical aspects of environment. The ANA *Code of Ethics* (2001) also calls for nurses to relate to clients in ways that promote their dignity and respect their religious, cultural, and political preferences. Nurses are to foster interpersonal and social environments that recognize cultural differences and promote the dignity of all persons.

Institutional Environments

Some community/public health nurses are employed by local or state governments to inspect daycare centers (for children and adults), nursing homes, and residential care settings as part of quality control of the environment (see Chapter 29). School nurses, employed by health departments or school boards, also seek to promote healthful environments, especially to prevent communicable diseases, injuries, substance abuse, and violence (see Chapter 30).

Home Environments

Community/public health nurses who make home visits and those who work in clinics have special responsibility for assisting families to provide safe home environments. The kinds of injuries that can occur depend in part on the ages of the family members, characteristics of housing structures, limitations in activities of daily living, knowledge of prevention by family members, and presence of specific hazards. Falls, burns, poisoning, and gunshot wounds are prevalent injuries in U.S. homes.

Clean, orderly physical environments and safe, adequate food, water, and waste disposal are to be provided in hospitals and other institutions. In homes, families have that immediate responsibility. Some families might need information on what constitutes safe preparation and storage of food. For example, parents might not realize that their infants can become ill from microorganisms growing in improperly stored formula. Community/public health nurses can provide information about proper formula preparation and storage. At other times, families might not have sufficient food because of chronic poverty or an emergency. Community/public health nurses assist the family in obtaining the necessary resources in such circumstances.

To promote development and well-being, community/public health nurses instruct family members in such tasks as providing stimulation for infants, communicating with bed-bound family members, and exploring the meaning of health and well-being with those who experience pain or isolation.

Occupational Environments

Chapter 9 describes occupational health nursing as a subspecialty of community health nursing. As part of their practice, occupational health nurses seek to limit hazards in the workplace and to promote safer working habits.

Community Environments

The environmental responsibilities of community/public health nurses do not stop at the physical boundaries of homes or institutions. Through observations in communities and discussions with clients and others, community/public health nurses are in special positions to observe hazards and the environmental concerns of community members (Afzal, 2007; Lum, 1995). Community/public health nurses can collaborate with others, such as sanitarians, environmental scientists, and environmental advocacy groups (see Chapter 9).

The view of the environment primarily as a suprasystem to be controlled and used for human consumption is evolving to a view that the survival of humans as a global community is inextricably linked with the environment. There is more focus on living not in, but in relationship with, the environment (Kotchian, 1995). Rather than focusing solely on the use of environmental resources for humans, the need to focus on conservation and regeneration of natural resources where possible has been recognized.

Health professionals are recognizing that the social environment is especially important when considering such concerns as teenage pregnancy, poverty, homicide, suicide, and substance abuse. Community/public health nurses are exploring ways to strengthen human connectedness, promote a basic standard of living, and reduce dependence on violence as a means of conflict resolution.

CASE MANAGEMENT, COORDINATION OF CARE, AND DELEGATION

Coordination is bringing together the parts or agents of a plan or process into a common whole. Community/public health nurses work within complex community networks of resources to coordinate care for clients in a variety of ways. Community/public health nurses coordinate or manage care through case management, caseload management, site management, and coordination of teams.

Case management refers to the development and coordination of a plan of care for a selected client, usually an individual or family. In community/public health nursing, it includes both coordination of care and service provision (Minnesota Department of Health, 2001). This is similar to the concept of primary nursing in the hospital. Case management depends on the nurse's ability to accurately assess client needs and community resources. The community/public health nurse works with the client and the other disciplines and resources involved to create and manage a coherent plan of care that neither overwhelms the client nor results in the overlooking of some needs; in addition, the plan of care is cost effective and efficient (see Chapter 13). Goals of case management include promoting client self-care, facilitating access to resources, and creating new services (Bower, 1992). Within managed care organizations, cost containment is also a goal of case management (see Chapter 4).

Caseload management refers to the coordination of care for a number of clients for whom the community/public health nurse is accountable. Caseload management involves the community/public health nurse's self-management, time management, and resource management for numerous clients during a specified period. Community/public health nurses often schedule their own workdays and determine who will receive home visits, who will be scheduled for clinic appointments, when phone calls and meetings will be held, and how much time will be devoted to each activity. Travel time must also be considered. Community/public health nurses need to make certain that they have sufficient supplies, such as forms for documentation, health teaching materials, and biologics for immunization.

Site management refers to the coordination of nursing effort at a specific geographic place, such as a clinic, school, or office for community/public health nurses, where nursing care is planned and provided. Although community/public health nursing supervisors usually manage nursing administrative offices, community/public health nurses might be responsible for the equipment, cleanliness, and efficiency of clinic sites and nursing areas in schools.

Community/public health nurses are often the *coordinators of direct care teams*. Management of nursing teams is the coordination of care provided by nurses, nursing assistants, licensed practical nurses (LPNs) (called *licensed vocational nurses* in some states), nurse practitioners, homemakers, and parent aides. This is identical to the concept of team nursing in inpatient settings except that the community/public health nurse is not always immediately available to the nursing team member. Management often occurs via telephone calls, meetings, and intermittent on-site supervisory visits. Community/public health nurses might *delegate* to nonbaccalaureate registered nurses, LPNs, nursing assistants, and others such as homemakers, parent aides, and community workers.

Coordination of personnel in multiple disciplines can occur within a single organization. For example, within a health department immunization clinic, there might be nurses, secretaries or receptionists, social workers, and dietitians. The community/public health nurse might be the designated coordinator of services. At other times, the community/public health nurse might emerge as coordinator because he or she is the one who initiates the interdisciplinary communications across two or more organizations. The latter often occurs because the community/public health nurse has frequent contact with the client and has developed a meaningful relationship with the client. Coordination occurs through phone calls, meetings, and sharing of written client records. As coordinator, the nurse needs to ensure that written records of discussions and decisions are kept and shared with team members, consistent with confidentiality laws and policies.

PARTNERSHIP/COLLABORATION

Collaboration means working together and denotes that the participants have relatively equal influence. Collaboration can occur informally or formally. It takes place among nursing peers, community members, and interdisciplinary professional teams.

Peer sharing occurs when nurses share their experiences, both successful and disappointing, in providing care. It is an educational process and a means for giving and receiving support.

Networking means the establishment and maintenance of relationships with other professionals and community leaders for the purpose of solving common problems, creating new projects or programs, identifying experts for future consultation, maintaining mutual support, or enlisting others to work toward common goals.

Community/public health nurses can be *team members* of multidisciplinary teams that plan and provide direct care. The care is organized, but not through one coordinator. Rather, each team member is seen as having something to contribute that is of equivalent value, and the team is accountable for results. In practice, influence varies among the members, but influence is not dependent on a designated leader or coordinator.

Membership in community planning groups is essential for collaborating with interagency and community-wide planning groups. Such groups exist to assess the health status and needs of the entire community or populations, to target recipients of direct care, to develop additional health care services, and to evaluate the quality of existing care. Individuals who are seen as influential in their respective fields are usually included as members. They are expected to contribute their perspective to collaborative planning. Community/public health nurses have relevant contributions because they know about nursing, and they can advocate for client needs as well.

Community health nurses also help create *professional-community partnerships* to assist communities in planning to improve their health (Bushy, 1995; Flynn et al., 1992). The goal is to strengthen a community's competence to interact, develop solutions to community problems, and promote health.

CONSULTATION

Consultation means the seeking of advice, especially from an expert or professional. Community/public health nurses are experts in community health nursing by virtue of education and experience. Community health nurses also are experts on the health status and needs of families, population groups, aggregates, and the community with which they work. This is especially true in regard to the needs for nursing care services. Community/public health nurses have special knowledge of the meaning of health for the people they serve.

Legally, community/public health nurses can be called as *expert witnesses* to testify in courts about the quality of care rendered by other community health nurses. Some state nurses' associations establish criteria for expert witnesses and maintain lists of qualified nurses (Kelly & Joel, 1999) (see Chapter 6).

Community/public health nurses seek expert opinions from nurses, other professionals, agency representatives, key leaders or informants, and clients themselves. For example, if a parent is giving his or her child a chemical home remedy, the nurse might consult with a registered pharmacist about the clinical compounds and their actions, and perhaps with a community elder regarding the cultural meaning of the remedy.

SOCIAL, POLITICAL, AND ECONOMIC ACTIVITIES

The ANA (2003, p. 2) asserts that all of nursing derives from a social contract that permits autonomy within the profession as long as nurses act "responsibly, always mindful of the public trust." Community/public health nurses were the first nurses to focus on identifying the health needs of populations, promoting adequate standards of living, and facilitating and encouraging people to care for themselves.

Public health practice seeks to collectively "assure conditions in which people can be healthy" (Institute of Medicine, 1988, p. 7). The three *core public health functions* of government in fulfilling that mission are (1) assessment of the community, (2) assurance that services are provided, and (3) health policy development. Community health nurses are in key positions to contribute to these functions (APHA, 1996). See Chapter 29 for more detail.

Community/public health nurses, by virtue of their special commitment to the health of communities, are called on to be involved with the social power structures in the health care system and the larger community. What would be a more healthful balance of individual choices and social responsibility in our culture? How can nurses model and advocate for a more humane society? Community/public health nurses might work for change within existing systems and work to change the systems themselves. *Social action* is the influencing of decisions in a community.

Change within Existing Power Structures

Change is a continuous process. There is room for change within the existing organizations and governmental structures. Assessment of unmet health needs and creation of nursing services through social planning are one example (see Unit Four). Identification of population groups at special risk and development of outreach, screening, and educational programs for them is another example. Nurses exert influence to promote change.

Coalition building involves community/public health nurses' development of linkages or alliances among organizations or those persons with similar interests. Change is targeted primarily at health and other systems (Minnesota Department of Health, 2001).

Such changes can be encouraged through political and economic strategies. *Political action* depends on the use of power to influence decisions. Governments make many public health decisions. Community/public health nurses can support the election of those sympathetic to community needs.

Nurses can influence *policy development*, that is, the development of legislation and administrative rules and regulations. Policy development places health issues, plans of action, and provision of resources on decision makers' agendas (Minnesota Department of Health, 2001). This can be done by testifying at hearings, participating on task forces, supplying written testimony, and personally visiting legislators. Lawsuits can be initiated as an attempt to influence judicial decisions. For example, the APHA and the ANA worked together to challenge the first President Bush's executive order that temporarily prohibited health professionals from discussing abortion in clinics that received federal funding.

Political action also includes attempts to influence decisions made by nongovernmental groups. For example, a community/public health nurse employed by the health department might assist the local mental health association in obtaining grant money from a private foundation to establish a substance abuse hotline.

Economic action depends on the use of money to influence social decisions. Money is contributed to political action committees (PACs) to support those candidates for political office who espouse specific values and health programs. For example, the ANA PAC contributes money to the campaigns of those supportive of the nursing profession. Financial decisions also can affect business policy. For instance, some professionals boycotted imaging equipment made by a major company because it also made nuclear bombs; the boycott was ended when the company sold its defense business.

Becoming Part of Power Structures

Obtaining membership in decision-making groups is another way to increase influence. Having nurses in political office and as members of planning bodies increases the influence of the nursing profession. Community/public health nurses can recognize imbalances of power and injustices that oppress individuals and groups. Nurses can empower disenfranchised people, such as the poor, cultural minorities, and disabled, to become members of influential groups or to form their own organizations.

During the past 20 years, nurses have become better educated in business and economic areas so that they can participate as full partners in the business of health care. Equality in a flawed health care system has its value but also has its limits (Reverby, 1987). Although business participation increases nurses' power within existing structures, it is important that nursing also seeks to make the health care system more equitable and caring for clients.

Changing Power Structures

According to a former chief of nursing of the World Health Organization, the values underlying health for a community should include equity, empowerment, and cooperation (Maglacas, 1988). Although these values are inherent in care and responsibility, they are not dominant values in our culture. Dominant values within U.S. culture include preferences for quick fixes, action, production and technology, material goods, control of natural resources, individual autonomy, and hierarchical power structures. What would it take to transform our current structures of power to allow currently subordinate values to emerge? How can speaking about our values, and what we are for, transform the current structure into a more balanced and caring community? The specific answers to these questions are still being created.

Many nurses are speaking for more human connectedness and caring in our communities (Aroskar, 1987; Benner & Wrubel, 1989; Leininger, 1984; Maglacas, 1988; Moccia, 1988; Watson, 1988). National and state interest in health care reform provides an opportunity for nurses to advocate for equitable health care for all and to apprise policy makers of the contributions of community/public health nurses.

The process of "enabling people to increase control over and to improve their health" represents a mediating strategy between people and the environments in which they live, synthesizing personal choice and social responsibility to create a healthier future. (Maglacas, 1988, p. 68)

Nursing's role was always to extract from the bureaucracy its hidden humanity and use it to "civilize the system," to bring caring into interpersonal relations. (Jessie Scott, quoted in Moccia, 1988, p. 31)

A contextual question for each community health nurse might be: How does my practice further a more caring community?

In summary, all nursing is concerned with public and nongovernmental decisions that shape the health care services and delivery system and affect access to care. Community/public health nurses have special concerns related to adequate standards of living, appropriate and adequate health care and social services for the underserved and at-risk populations, environmental management and preservation, and empowerment of community members.

EMPOWERMENT FOR CREATIVITY

Empowerment depends on the presence of hope or an expectation that "what is not" could actually be. Empowerment is blocked by magical thinking, in which a desire or wish itself is held as the solution to a problem. Rather, empowerment involves the creation of a vision of what is desired and the development of a plan to work toward that vision. The planner should consider the reality of the circumstances.

Empowerment consists of more than solving problems or fixing what does not work. For example, a paraplegic man living in the community has hope that he can be more mobile and envisions himself as a participant in sports. A plan is created, depending on what sports he is interested in, and involves creation of equipment adapted to his physical capabilities and limitations. There is no ready-made means to achieve his vision, and he might not be able to achieve exactly what he envisioned. Yet, were it not for the original vision, even the current degree of exercising and participating in sports would not have come about.

At the community level, *community organizing* helps community groups identify common problems or goals and use strengths to mobilize resources to plan and implement strategies for goal achievement (Minnesota Department of Health, 2001). Communities take control of their lives and resources through collective action.

Empowerment allows creation of new ways of being and doing and provides for transformation—that is, going beyond the next obvious step to radical shifts. Fritz (1989) discusses how individuals can move from reaction and response to the circumstances of life to creativity. Chinn (2008) describes a process by which caring communities can be created in groups. Duncan (1996) includes political action and community development as strategies for empowering communities (see Unit Four). The possibility of a culture more balanced between autonomy and relatedness exists for the future.

Changing the structures of power and the dominant culture of our society depends on empowerment of ourselves and others to envision an equitable, cooperative society in which individuals have an opportunity to develop their uniqueness, regardless of age, race, gender, culture, sexual orientation, or economics and "to be" in a caring community. Does this sound like a magical wish? It might be—or it can be a vision of community toward which to strive.

SELF-CARE AND DEVELOPMENT

Professional development is a lifelong process. To continue to give accurate information to others, we must stay informed. To continue to stay in touch with our own concerns and commitments, we need caring professional partners and persons who will listen to and coach us when we have forgotten our calling. To continue to competently perform therapeutic treatments, we must have opportunities to learn from other nurses and practice new skills. To assist others in finding meaning in life's circumstances, we must continue to face our own imperfections, vulnerabilities, and mortality and to re-create meaning for our lives.

As humans, we are social beings. To care for others, we must be cared for (Wallinder, 1997). To be cared for, we must be in relationships with others who are able and willing to give to us, and we must be willing to receive (Karl, 1992). Nurses often are so committed to caring for others that a conscious effort must be made to include sufficient "being cared for." In our own lives, we must address the issues that also confront families and communities. Given the specific circumstances, what is a workable balance between your own individuality and "being in community"? You can ask yourself what balance you want to establish between professional and personal aspects of your life. There is no right way to work toward knowing ourselves and developing our empiric, experiential, and moral knowledge.

Carper (1978) proposed four patterns of knowing: empiric or factual knowledge; knowledge that emerges from experiential acquaintance with others; self-knowledge; and ethical knowledge, involving moral judgments. There are other schemes for thinking about knowing.

Table 1-5 describes some ways in which nurses can develop different patterns of knowing to promote professional development. Table 1-6 provides specific examples of knowledge that emerge from different ways of knowing.

Nursing, therefore, depends on the scientific knowledge of human behavior in health and in illness, the aesthetic perception of significant human experiences, a personal understanding of the unique individuality of the self, and the capacity to make choices within concrete situations involving particular moral judgments. (Carper, 1978, p. 22)

EXPECTED COMPETENCIES OF BACCALAUREATE-PREPARED COMMUNITY/PUBLIC HEALTH NURSES

Generalists in community/public health nursing are those prepared at the baccalaureate level (ANA, 2007b; APHA, 1996; Quad Council, 2004). Such community/public health nurses are expected to be able to apply the entire nursing process with individuals, families, and groups to promote health and

TABLE 1-5   Ways of Developing Patterns of Knowing

Factual	Experiential	Ethical	Self-Knowledge
Reading	Joining peer sharing groups, interest groups regarding professional experiences	Studying human rights	Participating in counseling
Studying logic and analysis		Studying codes of ethics	Clarifying values
Continuing education		Exploring values underlying goals and actions	Participating in spiritual study and worship
Extending formal education	Studying art, music, dance	Studying philosophy	Clarifying commitments
Participating in quantitative research	Perceiving own experiences	Studying ethical frameworks	Accepting uncertainty
Participating in study groups	Participating in qualitative research	Participating on ethics panels	
Observing and describing	Exploring meaning with clients	Continuing education/formal education regarding ethics	
	Seeking cross-cultural experiences, traveling	Exploring own ethical decisions	
	Becoming aware of own creativity		
	Envisioning personal desires		
	Continuing education regarding creativity		

Categories of knowing adapted from Carper, B.A. (1978). Fundamental patterns of knowing in nursing. *Advances in Nursing Science, 1*(1), 13–23.

| TABLE 1-6 | **Ways of Knowing Related to the Example of Infant Feeding** |

Knowledge Route*	Example
Experiential	
Personal and interpersonal experience	You have cared for a newborn and experienced your own alertness and anxiety when the infant cried. You have felt satisfaction when the infant quieted during feeding.
Factual	
Logic	You use knowledge of nutrition and physiology to assist infant in rooting and sucking formula or breast milk.
Empiric science	You ask whether there are different types of cries. You systematically observe infant crying patterns and read research reports.
Ethical	
Ethics	You wonder whether crying is good/helpful or bad/unhealthy for the infant.
Self	
Aesthetic preferences	You prefer a quiet environment, without infant crying.
Understanding of what it means to be human	You recognize that every culture has a way of caring for human infants, but the specific details might differ.

*Knowledge routes adapted from Carper, B.A. (1978). Fundamental patterns of knowing in nursing. *Advances in Nursing Science, 1*(1), 13-23: and Marriner-Tomey, A. & Alligood, M. (2006). *Nursing theorists and their work* (6th ed.) St.Louis: Mosby.

wellness. The individuals, families, and groups targeted for direct community/public health nursing care are to be selected on the basis of the results of population-focused and community-wide analysis. Baccalaureate-prepared nurses are expected to assist advanced practice community/public health nurses with master's degrees, interdisciplinary teams, and community members in conducting community-wide data collection, analyses, and priority setting. It is the generalist community/public health nurses who often implement the interventions that emerge from such community planning. Through direct delivery of care, coordination, health education and promotion, consultation, and regulatory activities (ANA, 2007b), the nurses ensure that health care is available and accessible (Quad Council, 1999). Generalist community health nurses also participate in collecting data used for evaluation of nursing care.

DIRECT CARE WITH INDIVIDUALS

In the direct care of individuals in nonhospital settings, new baccalaureate graduates are expected to apply the nursing process with limited supervision—that is, they have already learned to provide such care and need to validate their judgments and interventions with a nursing supervisor (AACN, 1986). Most employers of newly graduated community/public health nurses will provide a more experienced nurse who is available to validate adaptations to nonhospital settings. This is especially important when resources and environments are severely compromised, as occurs in some household settings. New baccalaureate-prepared community/public health nurses are expected to independently and proficiently use numerous

skills and to adapt them to client needs. Such skills include those related to medication use, treatment, management of the environment, asepsis, recording, and provision of assistance with activities of daily living (AACN, 1986).

The AACN expects recent baccalaureate graduates to seek supervision (validation of performance) when exercising the following skills (AACN, 1986, pp. 20-23):
1. Administering developmental, functional, and psychosocial screening tools
2. Using consultation skills
3. Monitoring psychologic crises and using crisis intervention skills
4. Analyzing results of evaluation tools, such as surveys of client satisfaction with nursing care
5. Resolving conflict
6. Using change strategies as coordinators of care and as members of the profession

DIRECT CARE WITH FAMILIES

Novice community health nurses with baccalaureate degrees are expected to apply the nursing process with limited supervision while adapting care to the "preferences and needs" of families (AACN, 1986). Goals of family care include providing support during a family member's dying, fostering "family growth during developmental transitions," and promoting "family integrity and autonomy" (AACN, 1986, pp. 11-12).

By conducting interviews and taking family histories, community health nurses should collect and analyze the following information about the family system (AACN, 1986, p. 9):
• Family development
• Structure and function
• Communication patterns
• Decision making
• Family dynamics and behavior
• Family dysfunction

Family assessment is the competency that community health nursing educators in baccalaureate programs have ranked "most important" (Blank & McElmurry, 1986).

The predominant intervention strategies used with families are primary care, health teaching (including anticipatory guidance), referral, and collaboration in and coordination of care (AACN, 1986). In their survey of all baccalaureate programs accredited by the National League for Nursing, Blank and McElmurry (1986) determined that educators emphasized these competencies regardless of geographic location and size or type of curriculum. Ability to perform these intervention strategies is consistent with the responsibilities of community/public health nurses in family case management and caseload management. Family care is explored further in Unit Three.

DIRECT CARE WITH GROUPS

Application of the nursing process with groups is also expected of baccalaureate-prepared community health nurses; limited supervision is to be available (AACN, 1986). Here, *group* means a system of individuals who engage in face-to-face interaction. Required nursing skills include the abilities to assess group dynamics and group dysfunction, to facilitate group process, to teach groups, and to solve coordination problems (AACN, 1986). Some emphasis on group leadership is provided in most baccalaureate community/public health nursing curricula, although it is not emphasized to the degree that it is stressed by professional organizations' definitions of community/public health nursing (Blank & McElmurry, 1986).

DIRECT CARE WITH AGGREGATES/ POPULATIONS

Since the early 1970s, as more community/public health nurses have become employed in agencies that serve a specific population rather than in agencies with a broad public health mandate, direct care of aggregates has become a more prevalent form of delivering community health nursing care. It is the responsibility of nurses in such settings to assess the entire caseload or clinic enrollment for common health needs, to target those who have not received services but who are eligible, and to plan interventions accordingly (ANA, 2007b; APHA, 1996).

Eileen, a nurse employed in a home health agency, recognized that many of the elderly she visited had limited socialization and recreation. She joined with a social worker and neighborhood groups to develop a more systematic survey of the elderly. Eventually, a senior center was established in the urban neighborhood, and the baccalaureate-prepared nurse was appointed to the board of directors, where she continued to assess the health-related needs of the center members. Besides assessing the unmet affiliation needs of the elderly and determining that inadequate resources existed, she collaborated to develop services, such as health screening. Eileen did not stop at serving the elderly enrolled in the home health agency or senior center. She knew that many elderly are at risk of social isolation and participated with others in publicizing the senior center and finding elderly who could benefit from attendance at the center.

Eileen was reaching out to those who were eligible for the program but were not using it. Such *outreach* is another distinguishing feature of community/public health (ANA, 2007b). In business language, this practice might be called *capturing market share;* however, the primary motivation of outreach is not revenue but provision of health care to the previously underserved.

Population-focused care and aggregate-focused care are ranked among the top 10 concepts that constitute the basis of baccalaureate-prepared community/public health nursing education (Blank & McElmurry, 1986). Community assessment is one of the basic competencies expected of baccalaureate-prepared community health nurses (AACN, 1986; ANA, 2007b; Blank & McElmurry, 1986). Community/public health nurses are to collect and analyze information, such as the following (AACN, 1986, p. 10):

- Epidemiologic data
- Risk factors
- Resources
- Environmental factors
- Social organization

Such nurses are expected to apply the nursing process with aggregates with limited supervision. Baccalaureate-prepared community/public health nurses are expected to be able to *collaborate with others* to assess the entire population and multiple aggregates in a geopolitical community. Unit Four provides more in-depth discussion of working with communities and aggregates.

LEADERSHIP IN COMMUNITY/PUBLIC HEALTH NURSING

Leaders in community health nursing have demonstrated a common set of concerns, skills, and actions (Box 1-10). Leaders are sensitive to the needs of others, are able to respond, and are willing to work toward their visions of what might be. All community/public health nurses have opportunities to be leaders for healthful communities. Specialists in community/public health nursing provide orientation, staff development, consultation, and professional leadership to nurse generalists. The ANA and APHA reserve the term *nurse specialist* for those who have graduate degrees in specific areas of nursing. Nurse specialists have both specialized and expanded knowledge and skills (ANA, 2003). *Generalists* are licensed professional nurses with a baccalaureate degree in nursing.

Community/public health nursing specialists usually have a master's degree in community health nursing/public health nursing from a school of nursing or a master's degree in public health (MPH) from a school of public health. Community/public health nurse specialists are capable of performing and might perform the functions of a community/public health nursing generalist and are competent to provide care to families and groups. However, community/public health nursing specialists usually focus their practices on communities, the entire population, or multiple aggregates. Such specialists are proficient in assessing the health of an entire community or population and in planning, implementing, and evaluating population-focused health programs (ANA, 2007b). Community/public health nursing specialists structure systems of data collection and evaluation. They target intervention strategies toward the health care delivery system, institutions, and organizations (Helvie, 1998; Kalb et al., 2006), including development of health and social policy, development and evaluation of health programs, and research and theory development (ANA, 1986).

All community/public health nurses can contribute to improving the quality of community/public health nursing practice by meeting qualifications for professional certification, participating in quality-assurance programs, and generating and disseminating new knowledge through nursing research (ANA, 2007b).

BOX 1-10   Leadership Characteristics in Community/Public Health Nursing

1. Ability to recognize and be present to human suffering.
2. Ability to create a vision of improvement in the health and well-being of people.
3. Commitment to action.
4. Ability to identify specific health problems and sources of suffering within a specific time and place.
5. Openness to possibilities to alleviate and prevent suffering and ability to develop a plan.
6. Ability to communicate with other people to enlist support and enroll partners.
7. Ability to create opportunities for people to help themselves
8. Commitment to advocacy to affect social policy.
9. Patience and persistence.

PROFESSIONAL CERTIFICATION

The ANA has a program of certification for community/public health nurses managed through the American Nurses Credentialing Center (ANCC). **Professional certification** is a process that validates an individual registered nurse's qualifications, nursing practice, and knowledge in a defined area of nursing (ANA, 2007a) and acknowledges that the nurse's education, experiences, and knowledge meet standards determined by the profession. Certification is voluntary.

Prior to 2005, nurse generalists (those with a bachelor of science in nursing) could become certified as *community/public health nurses* and use the credentials RN, BC (registered nurse, board certified). However, as of 2005, the ANCC no longer accepts new applications for this certification. Nurse generalists who were previously certified by the ANCC as a community/public health nurse, school nurse, college health nurse, or home health nurse can continue to be recertified. Nurses with a master's degree or a more advanced degree in nursing with a specialization in community/public health nursing and baccalaureate-prepared nurses who also have a master's degree in Public Health with a specialization in nursing are eligible to take an advanced examination. These nurse specialists can become certified as an *advanced public health nurse board certified* and use the credential APHN-BC.

Certification expires in 5 years and can be renewed. The nurse needs at least 1000 hours of practice during the previous 5 years and documentation of professional development or reexamination to become recertified (ANA, 2007a).

QUALITY ASSURANCE

Community/public health nurses have a responsibility to maintain and improve the quality and effectiveness of community health nursing practice. Community health nurses are expected to fulfill requirements for relicensure and participate in self-evaluation, continuing education, and peer review. In peer review, nurses "appraise the quality of nursing care in a given situation in accordance with established standards of practice" (ANA, 1980, p. 18).

Standards of professional performance for community/public health nurses call for nurses to engage in the following activities (ANA, 2007b):

- Systematic evaluation of nursing practice for populations to enhance quality and effectiveness
- Maintenance of up-to-date knowledge and competency in nursing and public health practice
- Evaluation of own nursing practice
- Establishment and maintenance of partnerships with community members, health professionals, and others
- Contribution to the professional development of students and colleagues
- Application of ethical standards for health care delivery and for advocacy for health and social policy
- Integration of research findings for evidence-based practice
- Use of resources safely, effectively, and efficiently to ensure "maximum possible health benefit to the population"
- Provision of leadership in nursing and public health
- Advocacy to protect the health, safety, and rights of the population

These standards help guide community/public health nursing practice and "describe competency in the professional role"

(ANA, 2007b, p. 13). For instance, public health nurses in the Los Angeles County Department of Health Services used the public health nursing standards to develop their *Public Health Nursing Practice Manual* (Sakamoto & Avila, 2004). This manual serves as a tool to standardize practice and monitor performance of baccalaureate-prepared public health nurses.

COMMUNITY/PUBLIC HEALTH NURSING RESEARCH AND EVIDENCE-BASED PRACTICE

Community/public health nurse generalists actively participate in research activities appropriate to their education and position. These activities may include, but are not limited to, identifying questions for investigation; participating in data collection; "participating in agency-based, organization-based or population-focused research" under the supervision of nurse or other researchers; implementing research protocols; and applying research findings to practice (ANA, 2007b, p. 36). *Participatory research* actively involves communities, populations, organizations, and others in the process.

Evidence-based practice is an approach to practice in which the "public health nurse is aware of the evidence in support of one's clinical practice, and the strength of that evidence" (ANA, 2007b, p. 42). Generalists are to use the "best available evidence, including research findings, to guide practice, policy and service delivery decisions" (ANA, 2007b, p. 36). Using this evidence in practice strengthens both nursing practice and the community's health. This text documents multiple sources describing evidence-based community/public health nursing practice. Integrated throughout this text are contemporary citations of best practices and nursing or public health research.

Community/public health nurse specialists collaborate or consult with researchers with doctoral degrees to engage in all phases of the research process (ANA, 1986). Community/public health nursing specialists ensure that research findings are disseminated and assist nurse generalists in interpreting and applying the research findings in their nursing practices.

Nurses at the National Institute of Nursing Research (NINR) collaborate with other nurses to identify a national agenda for nursing research. The agenda focuses on both nursing care delivery and specific nursing interventions. Many of the priorities in the national agenda are relevant to community/public health nurses. During the 1990s, nurse researchers studied ways to improve the health of the underserved as well as of those with HIV infection and acquired immunodeficiency syndrome, cognitive impairment, and chronic illness. In 2003, the NINR emphasized areas of research in which nursing had a base of previous funding and showed promise for additional contributions. These research emphasis areas were reaffirmed in 2006 (NINR, 2006):

- Promoting health and preventing disease, including changing lifestyle behaviors for better health
- Managing the effects of chronic illness to improve health and quality of life
- Identifying effective strategies to reduce health disparities
- Harnessing advanced technologies to serve human needs
- Enhancing end-of-life experience for clients and families

Specific topics related to community/public health nursing include research in family caregiving, culturally sensitive interventions to modify health disparities, prevention of cardiac and other chronic conditions, creative ways to use the Internet and telehealth for client education, and evaluation of cost-effective nursing interventions. Federal funding for nursing research is not limited to these topics.

Nursing research also helps to describe the scope of practice and to strengthen nursing theory. Often, nurses take much of their practice for granted and do not describe explicitly what they are doing and how they are relating to clients. Studies of the practice of community/public health nurses can uncover the details of nursing practice (Zerwekh, 1991, 1992a, 1992b). Community/public health nursing practice can be improved only when nurses are clear about their practice and how interventions explicitly relate to human health and client satisfaction (Deal, 1994; Kalb et al., 2006; Reutter et al., 1998).

Much research is needed to explore what encourages health-promoting and risk-reducing behavior. Even when interventions are based on existing scientific knowledge, attempts at assisting others, such as intravenous drug users, in modifying their behavior have not been very successful. Community/public health nurses need to study what works with specific aggregates and to learn more about targeting care to different populations (Reutter et al., 1998). Evaluation of environmentally oriented interventions is also vital. Involvement of community members in research methods, such as *participatory action research,* can contribute to community empowerment (ANA, 2007b; Reutter et al., 1998).

Because cost containment in health care continues to be a national goal, it is important for community/public health nurses to continue to document the cost of nursing care and the savings that nursing care can provide (Deal, 1994). Home care expanded because nurses demonstrated that quality care can be provided for some clients in the home at a lower cost than in the hospital (Brooten et al., 1986).

One example of cost savings involves maternal and infant health promotion. A prenatal and infancy home visitation program not only led to healthier infants, fewer injuries, less abuse, and improved maternal social outcomes, but also resulted in a net savings in government expenditures, such as cash assistance and food stamps (Olds et al., 1993).

A second example of cost savings relates to tuberculosis control. When community health nurses visit tuberculosis clients to directly administer antibiotics at homes, work sites, or shelters, it is less expensive than hospitalization. This practice has been named *directly observed therapy* (DOT). Furthermore, under this program the percentage of clients who complete a course of antibiotic therapy is increased, emergence of drug-resistant strains of tuberculosis is thereby prevented, and mortality is reduced (Lewis & Chaisson, 1993). Health outcomes are better when nurses are involved than when clients self-administer medications obtained from clinics or private physicians.

In summary, nurses are concerned with people's experiences and responses as they seek to restore or promote health (ANA, 2003). Community/public health nursing research needs to consider the degree to which clients become healthier (epidemiologic measures of outcomes) as well as how much nursing care costs. In addition, community/public health nursing research needs to describe the specific interventions that best facilitate modification of behavior and promote health. What helps to prevent illness and injury and to promote well-being? What helps people work collaboratively to improve their physical and social environments? Community/public health nurses will continue to be challenged by this inquiry during the twenty-first century.

KEY IDEAS

1. Community/public health nurses synthesize their knowledge of nursing and public health to promote the health of populations in communities. Nursing knowledge helps in the understanding of problem solving and creative empowerment, of human experiences and responses related to health and illness, and of relationships between people and their environment. Public health knowledge helps make clear the magnitude of disease, disability, and premature death in human populations and suggests methods of prevention.

2. Community/public health nurses seek to empower persons in families, groups, organizations, and communities to achieve their individual potentials *and* to care for one another. Empowerment is accomplished by using interpersonal relationships to create opportunities for people to promote their own health.

3. Health promotion involves decreasing preventable diseases, disability, and premature death; reducing experiences of illness, vulnerability, and suffering; and fostering experiences of human caring, connectedness, and fulfillment.

4. Baccalaureate-prepared community/public health nurses (generalists) apply the nursing process with individuals, families, groups, and populations as guided by *Public Health Nursing: Scope and Standards of Practice* (ANA, 2007b).

5. Generalists work with community/public health nurse specialists, other professionals, and community members to identify the populations or aggregates at greatest risk for compromised health.

6. General systems theory is useful in studying clients at multiple hierarchical levels. Individuals, families, groups, organizations, and communities are open systems that exchange energy with their environment to survive and develop. Population aggregates are not systems because the members are not related interpersonally. Instead, they have one or more health-related characteristics in common.

7. Physical, social, cultural, spiritual, economic, and political facets of our environment all have an impact on community health. Community/public health nurses need to be broadly educated to recognize human-environment interactions. Community/public health nurses seek healthful environments while preserving natural resources.

8. Prevention is a complex public health concept linked with the natural history of diseases. Primary prevention activities preclude the occurrence of a disease or injury. Secondary prevention activities focus on early identification and treatment of diseases. Tertiary prevention seeks to reduce negative consequences of illness and restore health as much as possible.

9. Community/public health nurses use a variety of nursing interventions. Identifying persons with unmet health and social needs, ensuring access to health and social services, teaching for health promotion, screening and case finding, promoting healthful environments, providing and coordinating direct care, and participating with others to influence community decisions and policy are especially important to community/public health nurse generalists.

10. Social justice is important in the promotion of community/public health. Concern for the "greatest good for the greatest number" sometimes allows community/public health nurses to force clients to do something (take antituberculosis medications), or not to do something (abuse a spouse), to protect others. However, education and empowerment are preferred to enforcement and coercion.

11. Mechanisms to ensure quality of nursing care include licensure, continued professional development, certification, quality assurance, research and evidence-based practice.

CASE STUDY Being Present

The community health nurse greeted a 30-year-old mother at the door of her apartment. They had met several times. The mother has a history of "crack" use, although she denies current use. She has had difficulty feeding her 2-year-old son because of his almost constant seizures.

The relationship between the mother and the community health nurse developed slowly. The nurse was aware that the child's pediatrician would not prescribe strong antiseizure medication because he did not trust the mother to give it appropriately and feared resultant liver damage in the child. The mother had refused to return to the pediatrician. The nurse knew that the only health service provider the mother had visited with regularity was the health department's well-child clinic where the nurse worked, which provided screening, education, and immunizations. The child's immunizations were also delayed because of the seizures.

The nurse spoke the mother's name, seated herself quietly, and took in what was happening in the room. The mother was ironing and had age-appropriate toys next to her developmentally delayed son. The nurse said hello to the boy, commenting that he seemed to be interested in the toy the mother had placed next to him. She followed the mother's lead as they discussed how the mother was providing stimulation for her son's development. The nurse commented that it must be difficult to feed a child with frequent seizures; the mother replied that she could not take all day to feed him because she had two other children to care for and she was afraid he would choke. The nurse realized that she would have similar feelings if the child were hers.

She acknowledged the mother's request to obtain seizure medication and indicated that she might find another pediatrician for the child.

Because of her resourcefulness and persistence, the nurse was able to find a second pediatric neurologist in another city, 40 miles away. With transportation arranged through volunteers, the mother and son were seen by this physician. The child was hospitalized for regulation of the seizure medication regimen, and the mother agreed to implantation in the child of a gastrostomy tube for feedings. Three months after the home visit described earlier, the mother had been taught to feed the child, and his seizures were sufficiently controlled for him to be accepted into a special education program in the public school system. The mother was beginning to talk about seeking job training.

The nurse could have judged the mother for having used cocaine, which might have caused her child's health problems. The nurse could have labeled the mother as noncompliant when she refused to return to the first pediatrician. Instead, the community health nurse was present to the mother; she was physically present in the home several times and psychologically present to acknowledge the mother's strengths and perspective of the circumstances. In addition, the community health nurse was spiritually there and could honestly say that she liked the mother, despite all of her troubles. She felt genuine positive regard for the mother as a human being, while not forgetting that her primary professional goal as a "child health nurse" was to promote the well-being of the child. Her presence demonstrated her genuine caring and led to new possibilities for this family.

WEB   See **Critical Thinking Questions** for this Case Study on the book's website.

LEARNING BY EXPERIENCE AND REFLECTION

1. Look through several copies of a major newspaper to find articles related directly or indirectly to human health. Describe any inequalities in access to health care, access to a basic standard of living, or exposure to environmental hazards. Identify implications for community/public health nursing practice.

2. Express your vision of a healthy family and of a healthy community. List some of your commitments related to your choice of nursing as a profession. As your experience in community/public health nursing broadens, consider modifying your list of commitments.

3. Express your vision of an empowering work environment. If you are a student, consider what an empowering clinical practice environment would be like for you. Identify what commitments you are willing to make for this vision. Share your visions and commitments with your work group or learning group in an attempt to identify some common visions and commitments as a basis for partnership.

4. Select a public health problem of interest to you, such as falls among the elderly, and describe primary, secondary, and tertiary prevention strategies.

5. Using the same health problem you identified in item 4, discuss how interventions might be directed toward individuals, families, groups, and the public. To whom would you target interventions and why? Explore evidence of best nursing practices related to this health problem and proposed interventions.

6. Interview or accompany a community/public health nurse to identify his or her professional responsibilities. To what degree does the nurse provide care to individuals, families, or groups? How does the nurse use data about the public or aggregates to target care? How does the nurse participate in continuing professional development and improvement of nursing care? What current research findings does the nurse use to strengthen evidence-based practice?

COMMUNITY RESOURCES FOR PRACTICE

Information about each of the following organizations is found on its website, which can be accessed through the **WebLinks** section of this book's website at http://evolve.elsevier.com/Maurer/community/.

WEB

American Association of Colleges of Nursing (AACN)
American Nurses Association (ANA)
American Nurses Credentialing Center (ANCC)

American Public Health Association (APHA)
Association of State and Territorial Directors of Nursing (ASTDN)
Institute of Medicine (IOM)
Minnesota Department of Health, Division of Community Health Services, Public Health Nursing Section (Information about the Minnesota model for public health nursing practice, known as the "interventions wheel," is found on the department's website.)
National Institute of Nursing Research (NINR)
U.S. Department of Health and Human Services (USDHHS)

STUDY AIDS   http://evolve.elsevier.com/Maurer/community/

Visit the Evolve website for this book to find the following study and assessment materials:

- Quiz
- Web Scenario
- Critical Thinking Questions and Answers for Case Studies

- Care Plans
- *Healthy People* Updates
- Glossary

REFERENCES

Afzal, B. (2007, May 31). Global warming: A public health concern. *OJIN: The Online Journal of Issues in Nursing, 12*(2), manuscript x. Retrieved January 4, 2008 from *http://www.nursingworld.org/MainMenuCategories/ANAMarketplace/ANAPeriodicals/OJIN/TableofContents/Volume122007/May31/GlobalWarming.aspx*.

Allen, C. (1991). Holistic concepts and the professionalization of public health nursing. *Public Health Nursing, 8*(2), 74-80.

American Association of Colleges of Nursing. (1986). *Essentials of college and university education for professional nursing: Final report*. Washington, DC: Author.

American Nurses Association. (1980). *A conceptual model of community health nursing*. Washington, DC: Author.

American Nurses Association. (1985). *Code for nurses with interpretive statements*. Washington, DC: Author.

American Nurses Association. (1986). *Standards of community health nursing practice*. Washington, DC: Author.

American Nurses Association. (1998). *American Nurses Credentialing Center certification catalog*. Washington, DC: Author.

American Nurses Association. (2001). *Code of ethics for nurses with interpretive statements*. Washington, DC: Author.

American Nurses Association. (2003). *Nursing's social policy statement*. Washington, DC: Author.

American Nurses Association. (2007a). *American Nurses Credentialing Center certification catalog*. Washington, DC: Author.

American Nurses Association. (2007b). *Public health nursing: Scope and standards of practice*. Silver Spring, MD: Author.

American Public Health Association, Public Health Nursing Section. (1980). *The definition and role of public health nursing in the delivery of health care*. Washington, DC: Author.

American Public Health Association. (1996). *The definition and role of public health nursing*. Washington, DC: Author.

Aroskar, M. A. (1987). The interface of ethics and politics in nursing. *Nursing Outlook, 35*(6), 268-272.

Bekemeier, B., & Butterfield, P. (2005). Unreconciled inconsistencies: A critical review of the concept of social justice in three national nursing documents. *Advances in Nursing Science, 28*(2), 152-162.

Benner, P., & Wrubel, J. (1989). *The primacy of caring*. Menlo Park, CA: Addison-Wesley.

Beauchamp, T., & Childress, J. (2001). *Principles of biomedical ethics* (5th ed.). New York: Oxford University Press.

Blank, J., & McElmurry, B. (1986). An evaluation of consistency in baccalaureate public health nursing education. *Public Health Nursing, 3*(3), 171-182.

Bower, K. (1992). *Case management by nurses*. Washington, DC: American Nurses Publishing.

Brooten, D., Kumar, S., Brown, L., et al. (1986). A randomized clinical trial of early hospital discharge and home follow-up of very low-birth-weight infants. *New England Journal of Medicine, 315*(15), 934-938.

Brueggemann, W. (1982). *Living toward a vision*. New York: United Church Press.

Bushy, A. (1995). Harnessing the chaos in health care reform with provider-community partnerships. *Journal of Nursing Care Quality, 9*(3), 10-19.

Callanan, M., & Kelley, P. (1993). *Final gifts*. New York: Bantam Books.

Campinha-Bacote, J., Yahle, S., & Langenkamp, M. (1996). The challenge of cultural diversity for nurse educators. *Journal of Continuing Education in Nursing, 27*(2), 59-64.

Carper, B.A. (1978). Fundamental patterns of knowing in nursing. *Advances in Nursing Science, 1*(1), 13-23.

Chinn, P. (2008). *Peace and power: Creative leadership for building community* (7th ed.). Sudbury, MA: Jones & Bartlett.

Choi, E. (1989). Evolution of nursing theory development. In A. Marriner-Tomey (Ed.), Nursing theorists and their work (pp. 51-61). St. Louis: Mosby.

Deal, L. (1994). The effectiveness of community health nursing interventions: A literature review. *Public Health Nursing, 11*(5), 315-323.

Duncan, S. (1996). Empowerment strategies in nursing education: A foundation for population-focused clinical studies. *Public Health Nursing, 13*(5), 311-317.

Erickson, H., Tomlin, E., & Swain, M. (1983). *Modeling and role-modeling: A theory and paradigm for nursing*. Englewood Cliffs, NJ: Prentice Hall.

Fahrenwald, N., Taylor, J., Kneipp, S., (2007). Academic freedom and academic duty to teach social justice: A perspective and pedagogy for public health nursing faculty. *Public Health Nursing, 24*(2), 190-197.

Flynn, B., Rider, M., & Bailey, W. (1992). Developing community leadership in healthy cities: The Indiana model. *Nursing Outlook, 40*(3), 121-126.

Friedman, G. (1994). *Primer of epidemiology* (4th ed.). New York: McGraw-Hill.

Fritz, R. (1989). *The path of least resistance: Learning to become the creative force in your own life*. New York: Fawcett Columbine.

Fry, S. (1983). Dilemma in community health ethics. *Nursing Outlook*, *31*(3), 176-179.

Fry, S. (1985). Individual vs. aggregate good: Ethical tension in nursing practice. *International Journal of Nursing Studies*, *22*(4), 303-310.

Gilje, F. (1993). Being there: An analysis of the concept of presence. In D. Gaut (Ed.), *The presence of caring in nursing* (pp. 53-67). New York: National League for Nursing.

Gilligan, C. (1982). *In a different voice*. Cambridge, MA: Harvard University Press.

Hamilton, P., & Keyser, P. (1992). The relationship of ideology to developing community health nursing theory. *Public Health Nursing*, *9*(3), 142-148.

Hanchett, E. (1988). *Nursing frameworks and community as client: Bridging the gap*. Norwalk, CT: Appleton & Lange.

Helvie, C. (1998). *Advanced practice nursing in the community*. Thousand Oaks, CA: Sage Publications.

Institute of Medicine. (1988). *The future of public health*. Washington, DC: National Academy Press.

Institute of Medicine. (2003). *The future of the public's health in the twenty-first century*. Washington, DC: National Academy Press.

Johnson, D. (1989). The behavioral system model for nursing. In J. Riehl & C. Roy (Eds.), *Conceptual models for nursing practice* (2nd ed.). New York: Appleton-Century-Crofts.

Kalb, K., Cherry, N., Kauzloric, J., et al. (2006). Competency-based approach to public health nursing performance appraisal. *Public Health Nursing*, *23*(2), 115-138.

Karl, J. (1992). Being there: Who do you bring to practice? In D. Gaut (Ed.), *The presence of caring in nursing* (pp. 1-13). New York: National League for Nursing Press.

Katz, D., & Kahn, R. (1966). *The social psychology of organizations*. New York: John Wiley & Sons.

Keller, L., Strohschein, S., Lia Hoagberg, B., et al. (2004a). Population-based public health interventions: Practice-based and evidence-supported. Part I. *Public Health Nursing 21*(5), 453-468.

Keller, L., Strohschein, S., Schaffer, M., et al. (2004b). Population-based public health interventions: Innovations in practice, teaching, and management. Part II. *Public Health Nursing 21*(5), 469-487.

Kelly, L., & Joel, L. (1999). *Dimensions of professional nursing* (8th ed.). New York: McGraw-Hill.

Kenyon, V., Smith, E., Vig Hefty, L., et al. (1990). Clinical competencies for community health nursing. *Public Health Nursing*, *7*(1), 33-39.

King, I. (1981). *Toward a theory for nursing: Systems, concepts, process*. New York: John Wiley & Sons.

Kotchian, S. (1995). Environmental health services are prerequisites to health care. *Family and Community Health*, *18*(3), 45-53.

Last, J. (1998). Ethics and public health policy. In R, Wallace (Ed.), *Maxcy-Rosenau-Last public health and preventive medicine* (14th ed.; pp. 35-43). Stamford, CT: Appleton & Lange.

Leininger, M. (1984). Care: A central focus of nursing and health care services. In M. Leininger (Ed.), *Care: The essence of nursing and health* (pp. 45-59). Thorofare, NJ: Slack.

Lewis, J., & Chiasson, R. (1993, September). *Tuberculosis: The reemergence of an old foe*. Paper presented at the Baltimore City Health Department 200th Anniversary Celebration Conference, Baltimore, MD.

Lum, M. (1995). Environmental public health: Future direction, future skills. *Family and Community Health*, *18*(1), 24-35.

Maglacas, A. (1988). Health for all: Nursing's role. *Nursing Outlook*, *36*(2), 66-71.

Marriner-Tomey, A., & Alligood, M. (2006). *Nursing theorists and their work* (6th ed.). St. Louis: Mosby/Elsevier.

Minnesota Department of Health, Division of Community Health Services, Public Health Nursing Section. (2001). *Public health interventions: Applications for public health nursing practice*. St. Paul: Author.

Moccia, P. (1988). At the faultline: Social activism and caring. *Nursing Outlook*, *36*(1), 30-33.

National Institute for Nursing Research. (2006). *The NINR strategic plan 2006-2011*. Bethesda, MD: The Institute. Retrieved November 28, 2007 from *http://www.ninr.nih.gov/AboutNINR/NINRMissionandStrategicPlan*.

Neuman, B., & Fawcett, J. (Eds.). (2002). *The Neuman systems model*. Upper Saddle River, NJ: Prentice Hall.

Olds, D., Henderson, C., Phelps, C., et al. (1993). Effect of prenatal and infancy nurse home visitation on government spending. *Medical Care*, *31*(2), 155-174.

Orem, D. (1985). *Nursing: Concepts of practice*. New York: McGraw-Hill.

Porter, E. (1987). Administrative diagnosis—Implications for the public's health. *Public Health Nursing*, *4*, 247-256.

Quad Council of Public Health Nursing Organizations. (1999). *Scope and standards of public health nursing practice*. Washington, DC: American Nurses Association.

Quad Council of Public Health Nursing Organizations. (2004). Public health nursing competencies. *Public Health Nursing*, *21*(5), 443-452.

Reutter, L., Neufeld, A., & Harrison, M. (1998). Nursing research on the health of low-income women. *Public Health Nursing*, *15*(2), 109-122.

Reverby, S. (1987). *Ordered to care: The dilemma of American nursing 1850-1945*. Cambridge, England: Cambridge University Press.

Roy, C. (1984). *Introduction to nursing: An adaptation model* (2nd ed.). Englewood Cliffs, NJ: Prentice-Hall.

Sakamoto, S., & Avila, M. (2004). The public health nursing practice manual: A tool for public health nurses. *Public Health Nursing*, *21*(2), 179-182.

Schim, S., Benkert, R., Bell, S., et al. (2007). Social justice: Added metaparadigm concept for urban health nursing. *Public Health Nursing*, *24*(1), 73-80.

Schultz, P. (1987). When client means more than one: Extending the foundational concept of person. *Advances in Nursing Science*, *10*, 71-86.

Smith, C., & Rankin, E. (1972). *General systems theory and systems analysis [Audiotape and study guide]*. Baltimore, MD: University of Maryland School of Nursing.

Smith, C. M. (1985). Unpublished data. Baltimore: University of Maryland School of Nursing.

Steeves, R. H., & Kahn, D. L. (1987). Experience of meaning in suffering. *Image: Journal of Nursing Scholarship*, *19*(3), 114-116.

U.S. Department of Health and Human Services. (1985). *Consensus Conference on the Essentials of Public Health Nursing Practice and Education: Report of the conference*. Rockville, MD: Author.

U.S. Department of Health and Human Services. (1995). *Healthy People 2000: Midcourse review and 1995 revisions*. Washington, DC: U.S. Government Printing Office.

U.S. Department of Health and Human Services. (1997). *The public health workforce: An agenda for the twenty-first century*. Washington, DC: Public Health Service, Public Health Functions Project.

U.S. Department of Health and Human Services. (2006). *The registered nurse population: Findings from the March 2004 National Sample Survey of Registered Nurses*. Washington DC: Health Resources and Services Administration, Bureau of Health Professions, Division of Nursing.

von Bertalanffy, L. (1968). *General systems theory*. New York: George Brazziller.

Wallinder, J. (1997). Supporting one another: The definition of PHN, awards, and the impromptu. *Public Health Nursing*, *14*(2), 77-80.

Watson, J. (1988). *Nursing: Human science and human care*. New York: National League for Nursing.

Williams, C. (1977). Community health nursing—What is it? *Nursing Outlook*, *25*(64), 250-254.

Winslow, C. -E. A. (1984). *The evolution and significance of the modern public health campaign. South Burlington, VT: Journal of Public Health Policy. (Original work published in 1923. New Haven, CT: Yale University Press.)*

Zerwekh, J. (1991). A family caregiving model for public health nursing. *Nursing Outlook, 39*(5), 213-217.

Zerwekh, J. (1992a). Laying the ground work for family self-help: Locating families, building trust, and building strength. *Public Health Nursing, 9*(1), 15-21.

Zerwekh, J. (1992b). The practice of empowerment and coercion by expert public health nurses. *Image: Journal of Nursing Scholarship, 24*(2), 101-105.

SUGGESTED READINGS

American Nurses Association. (2001). *Code of ethics for nurses with interpretive statements.* Washington, DC: Author.

American Nurses Association. (2003). *Nursing's social policy statement.* Washington, DC: Author.

American Nurses Association. (2007). *Public health nursing: Scope and standards of practice.* Silver Spring, MD: Author.

Beauchamp, D. (1985, December). Community: The neglected tradition of public health. *Hastings Center Report, 15*(6), 28-36.

Chinn, P. (2008). *Peace and power: Creative leadership for building community* (7th ed.). Sudbury, MA: Jones & Bartlett.

Deal, L. (1994). The effectiveness of community health nursing interventions: A literature review. *Public Health Nursing, 11*(5), 315-323.

Institute of Medicine. (1995). *Nursing, health, and the environment: Strengthening the relationship to improve the public's health.* Washington, DC: National Academy Press.

Kalb, K., Cherry, N., Kauzloric, J., et al. (2006). Competency-based approach to public health nursing performance appraisal. *Public Health Nursing, 23*(2), 115-138.

Keller, L., Strohschein, S., Lia-Hoagberg, B., et al. (2004). Population-based public health interventions: Practice-based and evidence-supported. Part I. *Public Health Nursing 21*(5), 453-468.

Keller, L., Strohschein, S., Schaffer, M., et al. (2004). Population-based public health interventions: Innovations in practice, teaching, and management. *Part II. Public Health Nursing 21*(5), 469-487.

Kuss, T., Proulx-Girouard, L., Lovitt, S., et al. (1997). A public health nursing model. *Public Health Nursing, 14*(2), 81-91.

McMurray, A. (1992). Expertise in community health nursing. *Journal of Community Health Nursing, 9*(2), 65-75.

Minnesota Department of Health, Division of Community Health Services, Public Health Nursing Section. (2001). *Public health interventions: Applications for public health nursing practice.* St. Paul: Author.

Quad Council of Public Health Nursing Organizations. (2004). Public health nursing competencies. *Public Health Nursing, 21*(5), 443-452.

Reverby, S. (1993). From Lillian Wald to Hillary Rodham Clinton: What will happen to public health nursing? *American Journal of Public Health, 83*(12), 1662-1663.

Salmon, M. (1993). Public health nursing—The opportunity of a century (editorial). *American Journal of Public Health, 83*(12), 1674-1675.

Salmon, M. (1995). Public health policy: Creating a healthy future for the American public. *Family and Community Health, 18*(1), 1-11.

Schorr, L. (1989). *Within our reach: Breaking the cycle of disadvantage.* New York: Doubleday.

Williams, C. (1995). Beyond the Institute of Medicine report: A critical analysis and public health forecast. *Family and Community Health, 18*(1), 12-23.

Zerwekh, J. (1993). Going to the people— Public health nursing today and tomorrow [Commentary]. *American Journal of Public Health, 83*(12), 1676-1678.

Zlotnick, C. (1992). A public health quality assurance system. *Public Health Nursing, 9*(2), 133-137.

2 Origins and Future of Community/ Public Health Nursing

Claudia M. Smith

FOCUS QUESTIONS

What are distinctions among visiting nursing, district nursing, public health nursing, home health care nursing, and community/public health nursing?

What are some historical roots of such nursing?

How did nursing leaders, such as Florence Nightingale and Lillian Wald, merge public health practice with nursing to create public health nursing?

What led to the renaming of *public health nursing* as *community health nursing,* as well as to the return to *public health nursing?*

How have subspecialties in community/public health nursing emerged from population-focused care?

What stimulated the expansion of community/public health nursing into rural areas of the United States?

How did the government sponsorship of community/public health nursing contribute to the field's dichotomy?

What are distinctions between *community-based care* and *population-* or *community-focused care?*

How does health care reform offer the opportunity for community/public health nursing to regain its holistic perspective for human health?

How can *Healthy People* goals and objectives for health promotion and disease prevention help guide community/public health nursing practice?

What issues persist in defining community/public health nursing practice?

CHAPTER OUTLINE

Roots of Community/Public Health Nursing
Visiting Nursing in Europe before 1850
Birth of District Nursing in England: 1859
District Visitors and Visiting Nurses in the United States
Trained Visiting Nurses in the United States
Associations for Visiting Nursing and District Nursing
Public Health Nursing: Nursing for Social Betterment
Definition of Public Health Nursing and Sanitary Reform
Urban Health
Military Health

Policy Reforms and Health Education Campaigns
Population-Focused Care and Subspecialties
School Nursing
Industrial Nursing
Child Health Nursing
Tuberculosis Nursing
Expansion into Rural America
Red Cross Rural Nursing Service
Metropolitan Life Insurance Company Visiting Nurse Service
Frontier Nursing Service
Government Employment of Public Health Nurses

Dichotomy in Public Health Nursing
Educational Preparation for Public Health Nurses
Community/Public Health Nursing: 1965 to 2000
Community/Public Health Nursing: Present and Future
Health Care Reform
National Health Objectives
Populations and Community/Public Health Nursing
Emerging and Reemerging Infections and Threats of Terrorism
Continuing Issues

KEY TERMS

Community health nursing
Community/public health nursing
District nursing

National Health Objectives
Primary health care
Public health

Public health nursing
Visiting nursing

Public health nursing: *Nursing for social betterment; nursing care for the health needs of the entire population or public; community-based, population-focused nursing*

Community health nursing: *Term developed in the 1960s to expand the term* public health nursing *because the term* public health *had become linked only with nurses employed by governments; a synonym for public health nursing*

Because **community health nursing** is a synthesis of nursing and public health, an exploration of the evolution of each of these will strengthen our understanding of the roots of practice. The care of the sick has always been influenced by the meaning given to illnesses, injuries, and human suffering by members of a given culture. Types and prevalences of injuries and illnesses have also influenced care. Other roots of community health nursing include health promotion and disease prevention and population-focused care from public health. Both nursing and public health have been concerned with the interrelationships among people and their physical and social environments.

Public health nursing evolved from visiting nursing and district nursing. Public health nursing included home health nursing. From the 1960s through the end of the twentieth century, the term *community health nursing* was often used in place of *public health nursing.* The beginning of the twenty-first century presents yet another transition. The terms *community health nursing* and *public health nursing are linked together in community/public health nursing,* and there is a movement to return to the classic name of *public health nursing* (American Nurses Association [ANA], 2007c; Quad Council of Public Health Nursing Organizations, 1999).

Community/public health nursing in the United States has generally evolved from several programs developed in Western Europe, particularly Great Britain. Many people have influenced the development of community/public health nursing. A synopsis of their commitments, ideas, and activities provides an understanding of the foundation of contemporary community health nursing. When possible, the names of specific nurses are included to demonstrate that the history of nursing is the result of the collective efforts of individual nurses. Other community leaders are identified to demonstrate that early community/public health nurses worked in partnerships to create services and obtain financial support. Inclusion of their names allows interested readers to engage in further research.

ROOTS OF COMMUNITY/PUBLIC HEALTH NURSING

Visiting nursing originated when concerned laypersons provided care to the sick in their homes. In Europe, the Catholic Sisters of Charity and Protestant deaconesses evolved from groups of such lay nurses. In the United States, organized visiting nursing tended to be provided by nonreligious organizations, such as benevolent and ethical societies.

District nursing was started in England in 1859 by William Rathbone, who proposed to Florence Nightingale that visiting nurses who had graduated from nursing school be assigned within a parish or district. In the United States, district nurses often labored in conjunction with physicians who worked in the local dispensary. This was the forerunner of neighborhood or city block nursing.

In the 1880s, nonprofit visiting nursing associations were formed in several U.S. cities to provide care to ill persons and to teach health promotion and disease prevention. Some associations assigned nurses by geographic districts, and others did not.

Lillian Wald included visiting nursing and district nursing within her broader concept of public health nursing. Public health nursing is nursing for social betterment and includes nursing in schools, in clinics, at work sites, and in community centers, as well as in homes. Whether it is called *public health nursing* or *community health nursing,* the practice combines caring and activism to promote the health of the public (Backer, 1993).

VISITING NURSING IN EUROPE BEFORE 1850

During the Middle Ages, warfare, famine, and plagues persisted in Europe and the Middle East. Hospitals existed for military personnel, and wealthy patients were cared for at home. People became concerned about providing care to the poor and less-well-off members of society. Table 2-1 highlights some of the efforts to address the issue.

The gradual movement toward societal concern for human welfare was hastened during the Industrial Revolution. As workers flocked to cities seeking employment, the cities experienced dramatic overcrowding. Overcrowded slums, lodgings, jails, and workhouses became centers for disease. It was in this environment that reformers sought to prevent deaths through improvement of living conditions.

Scientific knowledge (cause and effect) and the concern for the well-being of individuals provided the intellectual and philosophic basis for responding to the dehumanizing conditions of industrialized, urban Europe. For some, the motivation for reform was the attempt to reconcile Christian principles with the poverty, suffering, and premature deaths of poor persons. Businessmen were beginning to realize that a sick workforce affected production, and therefore economics provided another motivation.

BIRTH OF DISTRICT NURSING IN ENGLAND: 1859

Rathbone, a Quaker, merchant, and philanthropist, is considered the originator of *district nursing* (Brainard, 1985; Gardner, 1936; Monteiro, 1985). Rathbone was a visitor for the District Provident Society in Liverpool, England, and went to the homes of members of his district every week. He believed that personal contact with the poor could assist people out of poverty and that financial relief alone was insufficient. He persuaded the Liverpool Relief Society to adopt a system whereby the town was divided into districts and subdivided into sections; after a paid relief worker had assessed the situation initially, the "case" was turned over to the friendly visitor in the district for ongoing assistance.

During his wife's long illness, Rathbone employed a nurse, Mary Robinson, to comfort and care for her. After his wife's death in 1859, Rathbone realized that if nursing care could be such an asset to his wealthy family, it could be an even greater asset to families whose suffering was compounded by poverty and ignorance. His idea was to provide nursing care by district, as welfare relief was provided. He employed Robinson for a 3-month experiment in nursing sick poor persons in their own homes in a district of Liverpool

TABLE 2-1 **Nursing Efforts in Europe before 1850**

Year	Event
Visiting Nursing	
1617	Vincent de Paul founded the Society of Missionaries, a congregation of priests trained to work among the poor in France. In addition to the accepted concept of material relief, he added human sympathy and personal service. Concerned with the causes of poverty, he advocated employment as a method of helping the poor care for themselves (Brainard, 1985).
1617	Vincent de Paul founded the Dames de Charite, an order of women who provided visiting nurse services to the sick poor. These women were volunteers, not nuns, who provided care, medicines, and feeding to the ill, and comforted the dying and grief-stricken.
1822	Theodor Fliedner, a pastor in a small German village, visited richer Protestant parishes seeking financial aid for his poor parishioners. His wife, Frederika Fliedner started a women's society for visiting and nursing sick persons in their homes, based on the deaconess Mennonite groups based in Holland.
1839	Pastor Fliedner started a hospital and training school for deaconesses. The students needed to be 25 or older, of good character and health, and from the working class.
1850	Institutes for training deaconesses were established in Paris, Austria, and Switzerland. Mrs. Fry, a prison reformer in England, founded the Society of Protestant Sisters of Charity. These nurses provided home nursing care to *all classes*, including the poor.
Workhouse and Hospital Nursing in England 1825-1850	
1825	Hospitals. There were 154 hospitals maintained by private subscription (prepayment). Hospitals were used for teaching. The middle and upper classes were cared for at home by privately employed nurses and physicians. Hospitals were considered "death houses," and fatality rates were high (White, 1978). For example, 70% of patients with compound fractures died. Hospital nurses were supervised by sisters. The sisters provided the more technical care—for example, dressing changes and medication. Both sisters and nurses were supervised by matrons.
1825	Workhouses. Each parish had a poorhouse where poor sick were looked after by other poor persons in residence. English law allowed "the aged, infirm, handicapped, orphans, widows and poor sick" as valid candidates for poor relief (White, 1978, p. 7).
1834	Amendment to Poor Laws restricted poor relief to the most destitute poor (White, 1978).
1850	More than 50,000 sick and elderly lived in workhouses. Sickness was the basis for 70% of poverty, and tuberculosis was rampant (White, 1978). Lack of able-bodied poor to care for the ill led to "pauper nurses" who were allowed to live in workhouses to care for the sick. There were 500 pauper nurses by 1850. There were an additional 248 paid nurses in workhouses. The Poor Law Board redefined the duties of paid nurses to be comparable to ward sisters in hospitals (White, 1978).

Data from Brainard, M. (1985). *The evolution of public health nursing* (pp. 120-121) New York: Garland. White, R. (1978). *Social change and the development of the nursing profession: A study of the poor law nursing service 1848-1948.* London: Henry Kimpton.

(Brainard, 1985). In addition, she was to instruct the families to care for their own sick members and to provide personal and home cleanliness. Brainard reports that at the end of a month, Robinson felt hopeless about the intense "squalor" and asked to be relieved. Rathbone encouraged her to persist, and at the end of 3 months, she was able to see relief from suffering and improved circumstances for some families. She continued in this new field of work and was the first "district nurse."

Rathbone sought to expand the district nursing model by employing additional nurses in other areas of Liverpool. Two barriers immediately emerged: public resignation to poverty and suffering and an insufficient number of trained nurses. In 1861 he wrote to Nightingale, who had started a school to train nurses at St. Thomas's Hospital in London in 1860, to request her assistance in training nurses for Liverpool. She was already engaged in a project for sanitary reform in India, which she directed from England, and so referred him to the Royal Liverpool Infirmary to request that they open a school to train nurses for both the infirmary and district nursing (Monteiro, 1985). With Rathbone's financial support, such a school was

established the next year. A third objective was to provide nurses to care for the sick in private families (Brainard, 1985). By 1865, there were trained nurses in 18 districts of Liverpool (Brainard, 1985; Monteiro, 1985).

The district boundaries were often the same as parishes so that nursing care could be coordinated with the work of the clergy. When a new district was established, partnerships were formed. Meetings were held among clergy, physicians, residents, and philanthropists to educate them about the proposal, to enlist cooperation, and to recommend individuals in need of care.

The district nurse visited numerous homes of the sick poor for 5 to 6 hours per day. Brainard (1985) summarizes the nurse's duties (Box 2-1). Generally, district nurses did not care directly for persons with communicable diseases, to avoid transmission from one household to another. Instead, nurses taught family members how to perform necessary care and provided equipment "at the door."

The nurse was to provide nursing to the sick rather than to give relief in the form of money, food, clothing, or other charity. Nurses were not to make families dependent on

---

Box 2-1 **Duties of District Nurses in Liverpool, England: 1865**

- Investigate new referrals as soon as possible
- Report to the superintendent situations in which additional food or relief would improve recovery
- Report neglect of patients by family or friends to the superintendent
- Assist physicians with surgery in the home
- Maintain a clean, uncluttered home environment and tend fires for heat
- Teach the patient and family about cleanliness, ventilation, the giving of food and medications, and obedience to the physician's orders
- Set an example for "neatness, order, sobriety, and obedience"
- Hold family matters in confidence
- Avoid interference with the religious opinions and beliefs of patients and others
- Report facts to and ask questions of physicians
- Refer the acutely ill to hospitals and the chronically ill, poor without family to infirmaries

From Brainard, M. (1985). *The evolution of public health nursing* (pp. 120-121). New York: Garland. (Original work published in 1922. Philadelphia: W. B. Saunders.)

---

them by providing the necessities that the head of the family would ordinarily provide (Brainard, 1985; Monteiro, 1985).

That nurses should be trained was an essential point advocated by Rathbone and Nightingale. Nightingale wrote, "a District Nurse must … have a fuller training than a hospital nurse, because she has no hospital appliances at hand at all" (and because she is the only one to make notes and report to the doctor), quotes Monteiro (1985, p. 184). The nurses' relative autonomy was recognized.

The integration of the public health sanitary movement and nursing can also be seen in Nightingale's comments that a district nurse must "nurse the room" and report sanitary defects to the officer of health. Hygiene was seen as an empiric help for recovery from illness and prevention of disease. Environmental health nursing was born.

In 1874, Rathbone persuaded Nightingale to expand district nursing throughout London. The Metropolitan Nursing Association was established in 1875 with Florence Lees, a Nightingale graduate, as president. Its purpose was to provide "nursing to the sick poor at home" (Monteiro, 1985, p. 183). An evaluation of existing district nursing was undertaken. Surveys inquiring about nursing in their districts were sent to clergy and medical officers. Lees personally observed the nurses engaged in district nursing. Finding wide variability in nursing practice, the association sought to standardize the training for district nurses. Nurses were recruited from the class of "gentlewomen," and after a year of hospital training, they received 6 months of supervised district training (Brainard, 1985).

In 1893 at the International Congress of Nursing in Chicago, Florence Craven (née Lees) spoke about district nursing as requiring nurses of intelligence, initiative, and responsibility, with the ability to teach and the commitment to reduce the suffering of poor persons. District nursing had crossed the Atlantic from London. Table 2-2 presents milestones of U.S. community health nursing, many of which are discussed in greater detail throughout the chapter.

DISTRICT VISITORS AND VISITING NURSES IN THE UNITED STATES

The first organized lay visitors to sick poor persons in America were members of the Ladies' Benevolent Society of Charleston, South Carolina, founded in 1813 (Brainard, 1985). The society's formation was a response to the poverty and suffering brought about by a yellow fever epidemic and the trade embargoes during the War of 1812. The society adopted principles that did not appear in England until 40 years later. Membership transcended church and color lines, and the patient's religion was not interfered with. Although substantial amounts of food, clothing, fuel, bedding, and soap were distributed, money was not given out. The circumstances of sick poor persons were investigated, and attempts were made to furnish work for unemployed persons. Charleston was divided into districts that corresponded to election wards. Ladies visited for 3 months. The society existed until the Civil War. In 1881 it resumed work, and a trained nurse was employed in 1903.

In 1839, the Nurse Society in Philadelphia assigned lady visitors by districts. Responsible women were assigned to *act* as nurses under the direction of physicians and lady visitors (Brainard, 1985). Although these nurses are considered the "first to systematically care for the poor in their homes" in the United States, they were not trained. Neither did they visit multiple homes; rather, they stayed with one patient until discharged by the physician.

TRAINED VISITING NURSES IN THE UNITED STATES

Visiting nursing by *trained* nurses in the United States began in the industrialized cities of the Northeast almost 20 years after its inception in Liverpool (Waters, 1912). In 1877, the Women's Branch of the New York City Mission sent trained nurses into the homes of poor persons; 2 years later, the Society for Ethical Culture placed one nurse in a city dispensary for the purpose of home visiting. Both assigned nurses by districts (Brainard, 1985).

It is not known whether the New York City Mission spontaneously generated the idea of visiting nurses or whether members of their board had visited London (Brainard, 1985). Frances Root, a graduate of the first class of nurses educated at Bellevue Hospital, was the first *trained* visiting nurse in the United States. During the next year, the number of nurses expanded to five, and the salary of each was provided by a charitable lady. The philosophy of the New York City Mission focused on fulfilling a religious call, providing material relief, and caring for sick persons. There was little focus on instruction in hygiene, sanitation, or prevention.

Felix Adler, founder of the Society for Ethical Culture, was influenced by the New York City Mission but wanted nurses to provide care in a nonsectarian way. The nurses employed by the Society for Ethical Culture received their patient assignments from physicians in dispensaries; each nurse visited in the district served by a dispensary. Teaching of cleanliness and proper feeding of infants and children were included as aspects of preventive care.

In 1893, Lillian Wald (age 26 years) and Mary Brewster organized the Nurses' Settlement in New York City, also known as the Henry Street Settlement (Figure 2-1). An 1891 graduate of the New York Hospital Training School for Nurses,

TABLE 2-2   Dates in U.S. Community/Public Health Nursing History

Year	Event
Visiting Nursing	
1813	Ladies Benevolent Society first organizes visitation by women to sick poor persons, Charleston, SC
1819	Hebrew Female Benvolent Society of Philadelphia organizes volunteer nurses to the sick
1839	Nurse Society in Philadelphia assigns women visitors to care for ill poor persons at home
1861	Teachers Dorothea Dix and Clara Barton and other women organize a system of supplies and visiting nurses during the Civil War
1877	Womens' Branch of the New York City Mission assigns first educated nurses to homes of sick poor persons
1885-1886	Visiting nurse associations established in Boston, Buffalo, and Philadelphia
Public Health Nursing	
1893	Nurses Lillian Wald and Mary Brewster organize Henry Street Settlement in New York
1895	First occupational health nurse, Ada Stewart, employed by Vermont Marble Works
1902	School nursing established in New York City
1903	First home care program for tuberculosis patients established by Visiting Nurse Association of Baltimore
1906	First infants' clinic established by Visiting Nurse Association of Cleveland
1908	First child health visiting program in a local health department, New York City
1909	National survey of visition nursing associations conducted by Yssabella Waters: Visits no longer limited to the poor; nurse work with patients of more than one physician
Rural Expansion	
1909	Metropolitan Life Insurance Company employs visiting nurses for policyholders
1910	Collegiate education in public health nursing established at Columbia University, New York
1912	National Organization for public Health Nursing (NOPHN) formed
1912	Quarterly publication of the Cleveland Visiting Nurse Association and forerunner of the jornal *Public Health Nursing* given to the NOPHN
1912	Red Cross Town and Country Nursing Service established
1916	First public health nursing text written by Mary Gardner
1918	National League for Nursing Education recommends that aspects of public health nursing be included in nursing education
1919	Red Cross manages more than 2900 rural public health nursing services providing both sick care and prevention through their Town and Country Nursing Service
1919	More than 1200 occupational health nurses employed by industries
1925	Frontier Nursing Service established by Mary Breckinridge in Kentucky
Federal Public Health Nursing	
1934	First nurse (Pearl McIver) employed by U.S. Public Health Service
1952	NOPHN incorporation into the National League for Nursing (NLN)
Expanded Practice in Community Health Nursing	
1965	Public health pediatric nurse practitioner graduate program established by Loretta Ford at University of Colorado
1973	Federal Health Maintenance Organization Act recommends extended roles for nurses in primary care
1974	Formation of Nurses' Coalition for Action in Politics (N-CAP), political action committee of American Nurses' Association (ANA)
1975	Certification of community health nurses established by ANA
1980	ANA and the American Public Health Assocation (APHA) publish statements about public health and community health nursing
1984	Consensus Conference on the Essentials of Public Health Nursing Practice and Education
1988	National Center for Nursing Research (NCNR) established at the National Institutes of Health
1991	ANA publishes *Nursing's Agenda for Health Care Reform*
1993	National Insitute of Nursing Research replaces NCNR
1995	ANA releases draft *Scope and standards of population-focused and community-based practice*
1995	Insitute of Medicine publishes *Nursing, health, and the environment*
1996	APHA publishes *The definition and role of public health nursing*
1997	Third-party reimbursement approved under Medicare and and Medicaid for all nurse practitioners and advanced clinical specialists
Reclaiming the Name Public Health Nursing	
1999	ANA generalist certifications restricted to those with Bachelor of Science in Nursing degree
1999	ANA publishes *Scope and Standards of Public Health Nursing* written by the Quad Council of Public Health Nursing Organizations
2003	ANA publishes *Nursing's social policy statement*
2004	*Public Health Nursing Competencies* written by the Quad Council
2007	ANA publishes *Public Health Nursing: Scope and Standards* written by the Quad Council
2007	Certification exam revised for Clinical Nurse Specialist in Public/Community Health Nursing

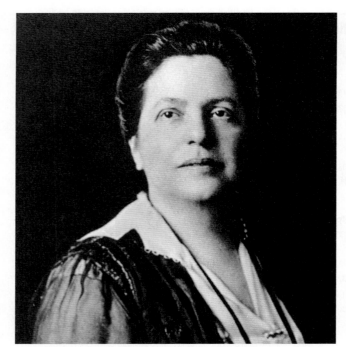

FIGURE 2-1 Lillian Wald (1867-1940), founder of the Henry Street Settlement and the Visiting Nurse Service of New York City, first coined the term *public health nurse.* (Courtesy Visiting Nurse Service of New York City.)

Wald cared for neglected children for a year at the New York Juvenile Asylum (Kraus, 1980). She entered the Women's Medical College and was asked to teach home nursing to a group of immigrant women. When she went to the home of a young girl who requested aid for her sick mother, Wald had an experience that changed the direction of her life. She left the medical college and enrolled Brewster, a nursing school classmate, in the idea of living on the East Side, a poverty-stricken neighborhood of Jewish immigrants. Mrs. Solomon Loeb, the wife of a wealthy banker, agreed to support the two nurses and provided $60 per month for each nurse and money for emergencies. During the summer of 1893, they lived in the College Settlement (started in 1889).

Settlements were part of a movement among university-educated young adults to reside in communities, to study the communities' problems through relationships with residents, and to reform the squalid conditions of urban workers (Kraus, 1980). Crowded tenements had insufficient ventilation and no toilets or baths. Fire escapes were also crowded with sleeping people. A police census in 1900 identified more than 2900 persons living in an area smaller than two football fields—approximately 1724 persons per acre (Kraus, 1980, p. 180). In this environment, Wald was committed to providing nursing services to sick poor persons. By 1900, there were 15 nurses; by 1909, there were 47 nurses on call; and by 1914, there were 82 affiliated nurses (Kraus, 1980). In 1913, the Henry Street Settlement reached 22,168 persons, or 1048 more than all persons admitted that year to Mt. Sinai Hospital, New York Hospital, and Presbyterian Hospital combined (Kraus, 1980, p. 176).

Alleviation of human suffering and illness was profound. The results in terms of creative nursing practice and the inception of new modes of health care delivery are with us today.

ASSOCIATIONS FOR VISITING NURSING AND DISTRICT NURSING

In 1886, inspired by district nursing in England, ladies in Boston and Philadelphia founded associations for the sole purpose of providing care by trained nurses to sick and poor persons in their homes (Brainard, 1985; Gardner, 1936). The Women's Education Association, encouraged by members Abbie Howes and Phoebe Adams, supported the *Instructive District Nursing Association of Boston,* so named to emphasize the importance of education in nursing work (Brainard, 1985).

The association adopted principles for working with the poor. For example, nurses were not to give money to patients or interfere with patients' religious beliefs and political opinions (Brainard, 1985). To prevent cross-infection, caring for patients with contagious diseases was limited. Instruction on hygiene, self-care, and prevention was as important as care of sick persons. Nurses reported to a single physician, who directed patient care. As the association expanded, professional nursing supervisors were employed, and nurses were expected to help community residents with fund-raising activities to support the association's work. By 1920, more than 36,000 patients were seen by association nurses each year; of these, 23% were maternity cases.

In Philadelphia, the *District Nurse Society,* later named the *Visiting Nurse Society of Philadelphia,* was established with the sponsorship of Mrs. Williams Jinks and other ladies. Like the Boston association, the Philadelphia society had a twofold mission: to care for the sick and to "teach cleanliness and proper care of the sick" (Brainard, 1985, p. 219).

The society employed nurses and attendants and added supervisory nurses in the first year. Fees of $0.50 to $1 were charged for each nurse visit, although services were provided free for those unable to pay. Initially only for poor persons, visiting nurse services expanded around 1918 to include others in need of nursing care. Nurses provided home visits or were available for care of longer duration at an hourly fee ($1.24 to $1.75 per hour) (Brainard, 1985, p. 224).

In the United States, such care was generally known by the term *visiting nursing* rather than by the English term *district nursing* (Brainard, 1985). The term *visiting nursing* was probably adopted because not all nurses were assigned to districts. Many types of organizations employed visiting nurses, including nursing associations, churches, hospitals, industries, and charity organizations. During the 1890s, the number of visiting nursing associations dramatically increased, especially in northeastern and midwestern cities.

In 1909, Ysabella Waters, a nurse with the Henry Street Settlement, undertook a national survey of organizations that employed trained nurses as visiting nurses. Waters reported a dramatic increase in visiting nursing associations since 1890. She noted that nurses served both the poor and those of greater economic means. A visiting nurse no longer worked primarily with one physician but could accept requests for services from all physicians.

Website Resource 2A depicts rules for nurses that were included in Waters's book; they incorporate the principles that first appeared in district nursing.

WE

PUBLIC HEALTH NURSING: NURSING FOR SOCIAL BETTERMENT

The demand for even more visiting nursing services led nursing leaders to consider the issue of standards for practice. There was concern that untrained nurses would be hired to meet the expanding demand and that nursing might revert to pre-Nightingale practices. In 1911, Ella Crandall, professor in the Department of Public Health and Nursing at Teachers College in New York, initiated correspondence with other nursing leaders to solicit their opinions about an "organization to protect the standards of visiting nursing" (Brainard, 1985, p. 326).

A joint committee appointed by the American Nurses Association (ANA) and the Society of Superintendents of Training Schools and chaired by Lillian Wald met to consider the issue. They sent letters to more than 1000 organizations in the United States that employed visiting nurses, inviting each to send a representative to a special meeting at the next ANA meeting in June 1912. Eighty replies were received, and 69 organizations agreed to send a delegate (Brainard, 1985; Fitzpatrick, 1975).

The report of the joint committee was accepted. A National Visiting Nurse Association was formed as a member of the ANA and recommended standards for organizations that employed visiting nurses were accepted (Brainard, 1985; Fitzpatrick, 1975).

The name of the association was debated at length because there had not been agreement within the joint committee. A majority had favored the *National Visiting Nurse Association,* but Crandall led a vocal minority advocating incorporation of Wald's term *public health nursing* (Brainard, 1985; Fitzpatrick, 1975). Reasons for selecting *visiting nursing* included the fact that it was the term commonly recognized by the public. *Public health nursing* was a broader term, which encompassed all nurses "doing work for social betterment" and was not limited to those who primarily did home visiting to provide bedside care (Brainard, 1985, p. 332). Public health nursing was general enough to include nurses in schools, tuberculosis programs, hospital dispensaries, factories, settlements, and child welfare organizations in addition to those providing bedside care through home visiting. Crandall argued that the public health movement would expand and that adoption of the term *public health nursing* provided a generic label under which new forms of practice could evolve. The organization was finally named the *National Organization for Public Health Nursing* (NOPHN). The word *for* was consciously selected to allow the participation of nonnurses in promoting the work of public health nursing (Brainard, 1985; Fitzpatrick, 1975). In 1952, the NOPHN merged with the National League for Nursing (NLN), which continues today.

DEFINITION OF PUBLIC HEALTH

C.-E. A. Winslow (1877-1957), the leading theoretician of the American public health movement, provided a definition of **public health** in 1920 (Box 2-2). He asserted that public health is a social activity that builds "a comprehensive program of community service" on the basic sciences of chemistry, bacteriology, engineering and statistics, physiology, pathology, epidemiology, and sociology (Winslow, 1984, p. 1).

Although his original definition of public health focused on the goal of physical health, by 1923 Winslow acknowledged

---

BOX 2-2   **Definition of Public Health**
Public health is the science and the art of preventing disease, prolonging life, and promoting physical health and efficiency through organized community efforts for the following purposes: 1. Sanitation of the environment 2. Control of community infections 3. Education of the individual in principles of personal hygiene 4. Organization of medical and nursing service for the early diagnosis and preventive treatment of disease 5. Development of the social machinery that will ensure a standard of living adequate for the maintenance of health for every individual in the community

Data from Winslow, C.-E. A. (1984). *The evolution and significance of the modern public health campaign* (p. 1). South Burlington, VT: Journal of Public Health Policy. (Original work published in 1923. New Haven, CT: Yale University Press.)

---

that prevention and treatment of mental illness was an expanding sector of the public health movement (Winslow, 1984). In 1945, Winslow predicted that "public health which was an engineering science and has now become a medical science must expand until it is in addition a social science" (Winslow, 1984, p. x). In 1953, the American Public Health Association (APHA) encouraged "collaboration between public health workers and social scientists to better promote the utilization of social science findings toward the solution of public health problems" (Suchman, 1963, p. 22). In 1963, Edward A. Suchman, professor of sociology at the University of Pittsburgh, described the application of sociology in the field of public health. He noted that both sociology and public health originated in the social reform movement, that both deal with populations of individuals, and that both employ statistical methods. The connection between social context and public health remains. It is especially important in the area of preventive mental health.

Winslow (1984) specifically named nursing services as an essential part of the organized community efforts that will prevent disease, prolong life, and promote health. He was an advocate for public health nursing, and in 1923 he agreed with William H. Welch (the founder of the Johns Hopkins School of Public Health) that public health nursing was one of two unique contributions that the United States had made to public health. Winslow (1984, p. 56) acknowledged public health nurses as "teachers of health par excellence" and recognized teaching as a responsibility additional to "care of the sick in their homes."

If the environment is healthful, if medical and nursing services are provided to assist ill persons, and if individuals are taught about health-related behavior and responsibilities, does a comprehensive community effort for health exist? "No," according to Winslow. There must also be "social machinery ... [to] ensure a standard of living adequate for the maintenance of health" (Winslow, 1984, p. 1). The science and art of public health is inherently concerned with standard of living.

Public health nursing, as a composite of nursing and public health, is committed to the existence of standards of living sufficient to maintain health. The fields of public health and public health nursing originated in social reform that occurred as a result of the collective commitment of individuals to the health and well-being of others.

Acknowledging this commitment can provide renewed energy and clarity of purpose. Community health nurses who are empowered by this commitment can continue to have an impact on the social and political power structures.

NURSING AND SANITARY REFORM

Before 1890, the primary public health measures to control communicable diseases in Europe and the United States were isolation of ill persons (quarantine) and enactment of laws governing food markets, water supplies, and sanitation (Duffy, 1990). As a result of the industrial revolution, many people moved to cities, where crowded conditions and poor sanitation helped to spread communicable diseases.

URBAN HEALTH

Descriptive epidemiologic studies laid the groundwork for sanitary reforms in England and the United States (Duffy, 1990). In 1842, Edwin Chadwick published a report on the unsanitary conditions among poor persons in cities in Great Britain. Lemuel Shattuck founded the American Statistical Society in 1839 and identified high death rates among workers in Boston. His *Report of the Sanitary Commission of Massachusetts* in 1850 called for the government to improve sanitary and social conditions to reduce disease and death. In 1854, the English physician John Snow demonstrated that the cases of cholera in an outbreak were linked to water from the same well. The germ theory of disease was only emerging. Table 2-3 lists other public health accomplishments in the United States.

MILITARY HEALTH

During this time, Nightingale in England and Dorothea Dix and Clara Barton, both teachers, in the United States, confronted the unsanitary conditions and high death rates from disease among military personnel (Hays, 1989; Pryor, 1987). In the 1850s, British troops entered the Crimean War in Turkey and occupied India. The Civil War (1861 to 1865) erupted in the United States.

Nightingale hypothesized that both environmental and behavioral factors increased the soldiers' risk of infectious disease (Hays, 1989). In Turkey, she organized and managed the nurses who cared for wounded soldiers, and she instituted reforms in sanitation, lifestyle, and data collection for monitoring disease. Sanitary reforms included improvements in drainage, laundries, hospital design, and kitchen cleanliness. She recommended a varied diet, reduced alcohol consumption, and activities to improve the soldiers' quality of life. As a result of her advocacy, libraries, athletic programs, and service projects were established for the troops in India.

Nightingale proposed new ways of reporting and analyzing *biostatistics* about the health of the British military. Although she never went to India, she established a uniform data collection system that she managed from England. She established population-based objectives and demonstrated that annual mortality rates dramatically declined from 70 per 1000 population to 19 per 1000 population after her reforms (Hays, 1989, p. 154).

Initially, there was no system for battlefield care during the American Civil War. Even with surgery, 90% of soldiers with abdominal wounds and 62% with other wounds died (Pryor, 1987, p. 94). More soldiers died of disease than of the effects of wounds. The Sanitary Commission was a relief agency started by northerners to supply the Union Army with equipment. Newspapers advertised for surgeons and male nurses.

Although Nightingale's work was known in America, public roles for women remained limited. Because of the magnitude of the need, however, numerous women's groups traveled to the battlefields to care for the wounded. Dix led a group of nurses in the Christian Commission, a branch of the Young Men's Christian Association (YMCA) (Pryor, 1987). She had gained national prominence for her work in reforming prisons and mental institutions, and she was appointed head of the Department of Female Nurses. Most of the nurses worked in hospitals in Washington, DC.

Barton also organized volunteers at the battlefields. Although not a trained nurse, she found her life's purpose in caring for the wounded (Pryor, 1987). She tended wounds, cooked, and collected relief supplies for the troops. She was an excellent organizer and enrolled others in providing enough supplies to fill several warehouses. For a while during the war, she continued to receive her salary as one of only a few women employees of the U.S. Patent Office. She was committed to providing relief in times of war and disaster and became an advocate for the International Red Cross, a relief organization started in Switzerland. In 1881, Barton was one of the founders of the American branch of the Red Cross.

POLICY REFORMS AND HEALTH EDUCATION CAMPAIGNS

By the last quarter of the nineteenth century, the discovery of microbes had carried the sanitary movement into the "golden age of public health" (1880 to 1910). General sanitary reforms were supplemented by specific actions aimed at preventing communicable diseases. These included pasteurization of milk, surgical asepsis, and immunization. The germ theory of disease also gave new impetus to campaigns for adequate housing, public water and sewage systems, pure food and drugs, and reporting systems for disease surveillance. Public health nurses continued to be leaders in educating the public about disease prevention. As the demand for public health nurses increased, specialization within community health nursing emerged.

POPULATION-FOCUSED CARE AND SUBSPECIALTIES

Public health nursing was for the entire public. Nurses in most rural communities and nurses assigned by districts in urban areas continued to practice as generalists. Generalists worked with families and incorporated health promotion and disease prevention into care of the sick.

At its first annual meeting in 1913, the NOPHN recognized seven specializations and interest areas within public health nursing: general visiting nursing, rural nursing, school nursing, tuberculosis nursing, infant welfare, mental hygiene, and industrial welfare (Fitzpatrick, 1975). No longer were urban poor persons and military personnel the only target population groups.

Two schemes of subspecialties emerged simultaneously in public health nursing, especially in urban areas. One scheme considered the aggregate of people served: school populations and industrial workers. The second scheme considered health problems: health supervision or preventive education,

TABLE 2-3 **Dates in U.S. Public Health History**

Year	Event
U.S. Beginnings	
1793	First local health department in Baltimore, MD
1798	New York City establishes street cleaning system
1813	Federal law to encourage smallpox vaccination
1842	Massachusetts Registration Act provides for collecting vital statistics
1850	*Report of the Sanitary Commission of Massachusetts* by statistician Lemuel Shattuck
1855	First state quarantine board in Louisiana
1869	First state board of health in Massachusetts
1872	American Public Health Association (APHA) established
1878	Federal Marine Service Hospital established for sick and disabled seamen
1881	American Red Cross founded by Clara Barton
1890	Federal Marine Hospitals authorized to inspect immigrants
Expansion of Local Health Departments	
1894	First medical inspection of schoolchildren in New York City
1900	38 states have health departments
1910	Tuberculosis programs included in local and state health departments
1912	U.S. Public Health Service (USPHS) established
1912	National Safety Council formed
1935	Federal Social Security Act institutes Social Security retirement, disability, and survivors' benefits
1945	Federal Hill-Burton Act funds building of community hospitals
Expansion of Access to Care	
1963	Federal Community Mental Health Centers Act
1965	Amendments to Social Security Act provide financial mechanisms to pay for health care for poor (Medicaid) and elderly (Medicare) persons
1965	Regional Medical Program established to disseminate research findings to public regarding prevention and treatment of heart disease, cancer, and stroke
Health Planning and Cost Controls	
1966	Comprehensive Health Planning Amendments to Public Health Service Act
1974	National Health Resources Planning and Development Act provided for system of community-based health planning for entire nation
1980	First national health objectives published
1980	Smallpox eradicated throughout the world via leadership of World Health Organization
1983	Health Resources Planning and Development Act not renewed: national health planning abolished
1983	Prospective payment system instituted under Medicare
Strengthening Public Health and Prevention	
1988	Institute of Medicine of the National Academy of Sciences publishes *The Future of Public Health*
1990	*National Health Objectives for the Year 2000* published
1993	National legislation introduced for health care reform
1995	Public health responsibilities and essential public health services described by Public Health Functions Steering Committee (Centers for Disease Control and Prevention)
2000	*Healthy People 2010* published
2003	Centers for Disease Control and Prevention provides funds for public health infrastructure to strengthen preparedness for bioterrorism and other emergencies
2004	Institute of Medicine recommends health insurance for all in the United States by 2010
2008	First exam for Certification in Public Health (CPH) for graduates from Council on Education for Public Health (CEPH)-accredited schools and programs

maternity, and illnesses (morbidity). Mental hygiene was not specifically mentioned in either scheme. By the early 1930s the NOPHN surveyed public health nurses according to these two classification systems (Gardner, 1936).

Health supervision overlapped with the population classification because some nurses worked with a specific age group to promote health and prevent illness. For example, some nurses worked exclusively with mothers and children, and others worked with school or employed populations. Maternity services encompassed prenatal care, labor and delivery (including home deliveries by physicians or midwives), and postpartum and neonatal care. As previously discussed, care of ill persons in their homes was the basis for visiting nursing care. Morbidity care expanded to include the care of those not confined to bed, especially those with tuberculosis, gonorrhea, and syphilis.

SCHOOL NURSING

School health nursing evolved as a specialty in visiting nursing in London in 1892 and in New York in 1902 (Brainard, 1985; Gardner, 1936). In London, the first school nurse visited a school weekly to oversee nutrition and remedy minor ailments. By 1898, the London School Nurses' Society was organized as a private charity. Five nurses served 500 elementary schools, with each visiting four schools per day and examining 100 children (Brainard, 1985, p. 264). Medical inspection of schoolchildren in the United States was instituted in Boston in 1894, long after such systems were initiated in France (1837), Germany, England, Russia, Chile, and Egypt (Gardner, 1936). Physicians excluded schoolchildren who had untreated communicable diseases from school.

Wald noticed that the children excluded from school often did not receive medical treatment and so remained out of school for long periods but transmitted microorganisms to other children while playing in the streets. Nurses from the Henry Street Settlement were determined to prove that children could remain in school, receive treatment, and not increase the transmission of disease. In 1902, more than 10,000 children were excluded from New York City schools; in 1903, after the school health nursing services had been introduced, slightly more than 1000 children were excluded (Gardner, 1936). Daily treatment of illnesses such as ringworm and impetigo by the school nurses not only reduced illnesses but also dramatically reduced absenteeism.

As a result of such successes, the New York Board of Health employed 12 nurses to continue the work. According to Brainard (1985, p. 270), these nurses are "called the first Public Health Nurses."

The goal of protecting school-aged children from communicable diseases expanded to include screening and examination for other treatable conditions, such as deficits in growth, vision, and hearing. School nurses focused on the correction of potentially handicapping conditions. Children were taught hygiene in the schools by the nurses as they provided first aid. During the first quarter of the twentieth century, school nurses worked with elementary teachers and parent associations to incorporate more group health education. Nursing with high school populations was to emerge later.

School nursing was introduced in other cities, often because the local visiting nurse association would "loan" a nurse to demonstrate the value of the service (Brainard, 1985). Frequently, either the local health department or the board of education became interested in continuing the service. Today, school nursing remains an important part of community health nursing practice in many communities (see Chapter 30).

INDUSTRIAL NURSING

Industrial nursing in the United States predated industrial nursing in England. The Vermont Marble Works is credited with having employed Ada Stewart, a trained visiting nurse, to care for sick employees and their families in 1895 (Brainard, 1985; Gardner, 1936). Industrial nursing grew slowly and was started independently in firms by employer or employee associations, or both (Gardner, 1936).

With the start of World War I in 1914, industrial nursing positions increased (Brainard, 1985). Federal government contracts for war-related goods stimulated manufacturing businesses and industrial nursing positions. Productivity was important. The National Safety Council had been formed in 1912. Industrial nursing was beneficial because factory efficiency was improved if workers were at work and healthy (Gardner, 1936). Gardner (1936) suggests that philanthropy, industrial justice, and fear of union movements were other motives for starting industrial nursing services. By 1919, there were more than 1200 industrial nurses in 871 industries in the United States (Brainard, 1985, p. 294).

Employee health was the initial concern and was addressed by providing advice and first aid to individual employees, teaching employees collectively about safety and sanitation, visiting at home to care for and instruct ill employees and their families, and initiating other public health services in the communities (Gardner, 1936). Ella Crandall in 1916 advocated that nurses also be involved directly in environmental safety and sanitation of plants as well as "social service for employees, including recreation, vacation homes, education, relief and general fitting of the man to the job" (Brainard, 1985, p. 295). *Occupational health nursing,* as it is called today, continues to grow slowly (see Chapter 9).

CHILD HEALTH NURSING

Among the humanitarian reforms during the nineteenth century was the beginning of concern for the health and welfare of infants and children. In 1817, the Englishman John Davis wrote a book in which he explored the causes of mortality in children and suggested that "benevolent ladies" visit homes to instruct mothers, inspect children, and report on their conditions (Brainard, 1985; Gardner, 1936). Little came of his idea. Concurrently, he founded a dispensary especially for children in London.

In Paris in 1844, the first day nursery for infants *(la crèche)* was started. A nurse cared for 12 infants in a poor community, and a physician visited daily (Brainard, 1985). In 1876, a society for nursing mothers established shelters in Paris to care for poor women during the last few weeks of their pregnancy. Breast-feeding was promoted, infants were observed monthly, and social work services were provided (Brainard, 1985; Gardner, 1936). A high rate of infant mortality persisted.

The pasteurization of milk allowed clean milk supplies for mothers who could not breast-feed. In 1892, milk stations were established in New York City and Hamburg, Germany, to provide sanitary milk supplies to sick infants (Brainard, 1985). Little accompanying instruction existed related to infant feeding.

In the same year in Paris, Boudin provided the foundation for the modern movement to combat infant mortality (Brainard, 1985). After infants were discharged from maternity hospitals, they were seen regularly on an outpatient basis for 2 years. Their growth was monitored, breast-feeding was encouraged, and hygienic bottle-feeding was taught to mothers who could not breast-feed. In 1894, Dufour prepared artificial feedings according to medical formulas and distributed them to the poor of Paris for use when breast-feeding could not be carried out (Brainard, 1985).

From the beginning of district nursing in England and visiting nursing in the United States, the nurses devoted much effort to the care of women, infants, and children. This was a part of their generalized practice.

Specialized infant nursing began in the United States in 1902, the same year as school nursing. In that year, special nurses were employed solely to visit sick children in a district of New York City, and other nurses visited infants born in the summer months of 1902 and 1903 (Brainard, 1985).

Following French and German models, the Infants' Clinic was established in 1906 by the Visiting Nurse Association of Cleveland and the Milk Fund Association (Brainard, 1985). Infants were examined until age 15 months by physicians in the dispensary; nurses provided home visits every 2 to 3 weeks to promote breast-feeding, supervise formula preparation and feeding when necessary, and support mothers to follow medical advice. These nurses specialized in teaching mothers to properly care for their infants. Visiting nurse associations around the country began to hire nurses solely for infant welfare work.

Local government became involved in 1908, with the formation of the Division of Child Hygiene in the New York City Department of Health. Nurses visited all newborns and sick infants in 89 districts (Brainard, 1985). After the annual meeting of the American Academy of Medicine in 1908, nurses met with physicians, social workers, and laypersons to form the American Association for the Study and Prevention of Infant Mortality (Brainard, 1985). Through the advocacy of Wald, visiting nurses were recognized as being qualified to work in infant dispensaries (the forerunners of well-child clinics) to instruct mothers in how to prevent illness (Brainard, 1985).

In 1912, the federal government created the Children's Bureau, which sought to reduce morbidity and mortality in the children of the United States. This body established policy to promote prenatal care and home visits to mothers and children, vaccination and immunization, provision of sanitary milk, and prompt medical care, especially for physical defects (Gardner, 1936). With World War I, death rates of adult males increased, and birth rates fell. Saving the lives of children became especially important for families (Gardner, 1936).

Currently, promoting maternal and child health remains an important goal of local and state health departments (see Chapter 29). Even in communities in which a high percentage of the population is enrolled in managed care, measures of maternal and child health, such as childhood immunization rates, are used as indicators of quality of care.

TUBERCULOSIS NURSING

Tuberculosis was a dreaded disease in the 1870s in the United States. It was known to be communicable and incurable. Tuberculosis was the primary cause of death among young and middle-aged adults (Gardner, 1936). Fresh air, rest, and healthy food had been recommended by physicians throughout the nineteenth century, but no one knew why the treatments worked. When Robert Koch discovered in 1882 that tuberculosis was caused by a microorganism transmitted by sputum that could be killed by exposure to sunlight and boiling, prevention was possible. To prevent the spread of disease, persons with tuberculosis were instructed to collect sputum for proper disposal, avoid sleeping with others in close quarters, and avoid sharing eating utensils.

Tuberculosis nursing originated in the United States in 1903 when William Osler, professor of medicine at the Johns Hopkins University School of Medicine, hired Reiba Thelin to provide home care and instruction to tuberculosis patients in Baltimore (Brainard, 1985). Thelin had never done visiting nursing before and resigned after a year to study at the Henry Street Settlement. Mrs. Osler was also an ardent supporter of the antituberculosis movement; she sent letters to all Baltimore residents, soliciting $1.00 to support tuberculosis nurses (Brainard, 1985). The money went to the visiting nurse association to pay for nurses especially assigned as tuberculosis nurses. Similarly, the visiting nurse associations in other urban areas provided tuberculosis care.

The National Tuberculosis Association was founded in 1904. Its members soon recognized that there was much overlapping and confusion in the provision of tuberculosis care; some programs were privately sponsored, and others were sponsored by municipalities. By 1910, coordination and standardization of tuberculosis programs were recommended, and the cities and states took over sponsorship of the antituberculosis programs (Brainard, 1985). By the 1930s, tuberculosis nursing had become a part of the generalized practice of nurses employed by health departments (Gardner, 1936), but more than 500,000 cases of tuberculosis still existed. Public health nurses cared for those with advanced disease, conducted tuberculin skin testing to identify infection in children, and taught good ventilation practices and sputum disposal as effective preventive actions.

Contemporary health departments are mandated to control communicable diseases within their jurisdictions. Drug-resistant tuberculosis, human immunodeficiency virus (HIV) infection, sexually transmitted diseases, and diseases caused by new infectious agents are of special concern today (see Chapter 8).

EXPANSION INTO RURAL AMERICA

Wald advocated that public health nursing services also be provided to rural Americans (Bigbee & Crowder, 1985; Hamilton, 1988; Haupt, 1953). Consequently, the Visiting Nurse Service of the Metropolitan Life Insurance Company (1909) and the Red Cross Rural Nursing Service (1912) were established. Economic support from business and private philanthropic sources now existed for nationwide systems of public health nursing (Figure 2-2).

RED CROSS RURAL NURSING SERVICE

Originally called the Town and Country Nursing Service, the Red Cross Rural Nursing Service (RNS) established more than 1000 local nursing services, one of which led to the establishment of public health nursing services on American Indian reservations (Bigbee & Crowder, 1985). The services were funded totally by local Red Cross chapters or by local chapters in partnership with other private and government agencies. Traveling nurses were sent by the national Red Cross to local communities for several months to stimulate interest.

The RNS supported high professional qualifications for its nurses, including graduation from a 2-year nursing school, registration (in states requiring it), previous public health experience or postgraduate education, and membership in a professional association (Bigbee & Crowder, 1985).

The national Red Cross provided scholarships and loans for nurses to obtain postgraduate education in public health nursing. The RNS designed a model curriculum for postgraduate

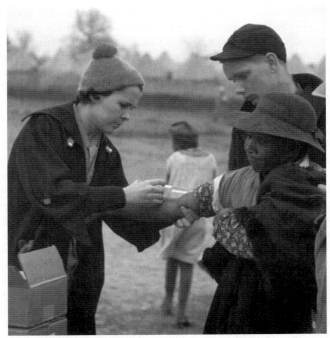

FIGURE 2-2 A public health nurse immunizes farm and migrant workers in the 1940s. (From Library of Congress, Washington, DC.)

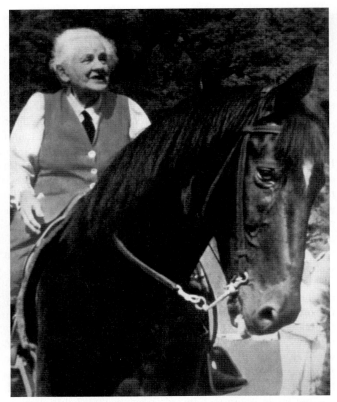

FIGURE 2-3 Mary Breckinridge, founder of the Frontier Nursing Service, on her horse Babette in the 1960s. (Courtesy Frontier Nursing Service, Wendover, Kentucky.)

courses in rural public health nursing (4 to 8 months' duration). The courses were first offered at Teachers College in New York City in 1913. Financial support for the RNS dwindled during the 1920s because of economic depression and the emergence of public health nursing programs in local and state health departments. However, hundreds of rural counties still did not have public health nursing services (Bigbee & Crowder, 1985).

METROPOLITAN LIFE INSURANCE COMPANY VISITING NURSE SERVICE

The Visiting Nurse Service of the Metropolitan Life Insurance Company (MLIC) was the prototype for business contracting for public health nursing services (Hamilton, 1988). The MLIC insured poor industrial workers who had high death rates. Lee Frankel of the company proposed that insurance agents provide health and safety teaching to their policyholders. When Wald persuaded him that public health nurses would be better health teachers, a 44-year partnership began between the company and public health nurses. Insurance agents provided publicity.

The MLIC contracted with existing visiting nurse associations to avoid duplication of services and to strengthen community-based agencies (Haupt, 1953). During its peak year, in 1931, more than 750,000 policyholders received more than 4 million home visits in more than 7000 cities in the United States and Canada (Hamilton, 1988; Haupt, 1953). Nurses also collected baseline health data in communities, started clinics, and gave immunizations (Hamilton, 1988). To stimulate the creation of nursing services where there were none, MLIC provided scholarships for nurses to attend college and university programs (Haupt, 1953). Statistics showed that public health nursing care resulted in decreased mortality and improved health among its policyholders.

The MLIC service ended in 1953 because the diminishing outcomes no longer justified the rising costs (Hamilton, 1988). By then, immunizations had reduced deaths from communicable diseases. The numbers of home visits had decreased because patients were now cared for in community hospitals, which were started as a result of the federal Hill-Burton Act (1945). Simultaneously the costs for home visits had risen, partly because of the increased education of nurses.

Funding from the Red Cross and the MLIC resulted in new instructive visiting nurse associations throughout the country. The nurses continued to combine preventive work with care for sick persons at home. Some visiting nurse associations entered into contracts with the MLIC. Other associations formed joint ventures and started demonstration projects (Buhler-Wilkerson, 1985). In joint ventures, another voluntary organization, such as the Red Cross, provided finances; in demonstrations, experimental programs were piloted on a small scale until their worth was proved, at which point someone else, such as a local health department, would take over the project. Until the 1920s, most public health nurses were employed by not-for-profit, nongovernmental agencies.

FRONTIER NURSING SERVICE

As a nurse-midwife, Mary Breckinridge made an extraordinary contribution to the health of women and children in the underserved rural area of eastern Kentucky through the establishment in 1925 of the Frontier Nursing Service, which continues to this day (Figure 2-3). (See the Case Study at the end of the chapter for more details about her life and nursing leadership.) Traveling by horseback through the mountainous areas, nurses provided general nursing care, bedside nursing, and midwifery to thousands of persons each year.

GOVERNMENT EMPLOYMENT OF PUBLIC HEALTH NURSES

By 1900, 38 states had established health departments (Hanlon & Pickett, 1984, p. 33). As the government took a more active role in public health, more nurses were employed by state and local governments, local health departments, and boards of education. As previously discussed, public hygiene measures implemented during the golden age of public health had successfully reduced sickness and death rates from infectious diseases in urban areas. Water was filtered, milk was pasteurized, garbage was removed, and housing codes were instituted. The rural sanitation movement of the 1920s stimulated the development of local health departments.

C.-E. A. Winslow (1984, p. 58) asserted that "the new public health movement" was to be based on "hygienic instruction, plus the organization of medical service for the detection and early treatment of incipient disease." Some physicians advocated that a new kind of public health worker who possessed knowledge of health, education, and social work be developed as a "health visitor" to perform the preventive activities normally carried out by public health nurses (Fitzpatrick, 1975). Winslow advocated for the public health nurse, who was already established in the homes. "Unlike the social worker, she knew the human body," its reactions, and "hygienic conduct of life"; unlike the physician, who focused on pathology, "she was trained to see the body as a whole" (Buhler-Wilkerson, 1985, pp. 1156-1157). The public health nurse was to be the educator for personal hygiene.

In 1916, the NOPHN supported "public health nursing under government auspices" as a means of extending health care services to more people (Fitzpatrick, 1975, p. 48). By the mid-1920s, more than 50% of public health nurses were government employees. By the late 1930s, all 48 states had public health nursing programs (Roberts & Heinrich, 1985). Many of the services provided by the RNS were taken over by local health departments. The federal government also stimulated the increase in public health nurses. Growth of state health departments was a result of the federal Sheppard-Towner Act of 1921, which sought improved maternal and child health.

Because of the Great Depression, many people were unemployed. The Federal Emergency Relief Act of 1933 identified bedside nursing care of poor persons as a relief service. Federal money was made available for contracting with nongovernmental visiting nurse associations to provide such services. The Civil Works Administration included relief projects for unemployed nurses themselves. By employing nurses in governmental agencies, the Civil Works Administration stimulated tax-supported public health nursing programs (Fitzpatrick, 1975).

During World War II, the U.S. Public Health Service temporarily employed 200 nurses and 35 supervisors to help prevent disease and provide health education to families of servicemen near military installations (Fitzpatrick, 1975, p. 65). Emphases were on childhood immunization, control of sexually transmitted diseases, and maternity care. As of 1984, 8.3% of all employed registered nurses in the United States were working in community health (101,430 registered nurses) or occupational health (22,890 registered nurses) (ANA, 1987, p. 101). About 36% were employed by local health departments, 30% by boards of education, and 21% by home health agencies. More than 66% of nurses in community health were government employees.

By 1996, the percentage of community health nurses who were government employees had dropped to 40% (U.S. Department of Health and Human Services [USDHHS], 1997). Although the total number of government-employed community health nurses increased between 1984 and 1996, the numbers of community health nurses employed in home health increased at a faster rate. Therefore, although there are more community health nurses in government employment today than in the 1980s, they comprise a smaller percentage of all community health nurses. (See Chapter 1 for the current distribution of community health nurses by work site.)

DICHOTOMY IN PUBLIC HEALTH NURSING

Early in the twentieth century, competition began to exist between health departments and nongovernmental organizations. Visiting nurse associations feared that health departments might take over. At the same time, there was conflict between the public health practitioners in health departments and the medical profession. Private physicians feared loss of income if health departments engaged in treating patients in addition to preventing illnesses. Thus, health officers made decisions that limited "publicly supported nurses to the prevention of disease, leaving the care of the sick to the visiting nurse associations" (Buhler-Wilkerson, 1985, p. 1159).

These decisions obviously acknowledged a place for nursing in both health departments and visiting nurse associations. However, the tragedy of these decisions was that they split nursing care of sick persons from preventive nursing activities. Public health nursing was no longer whole. Buhler-Wilkerson (1985) asserts that it was this division that has prevented public health nursing from achieving its potential as a delivery system for comprehensive health care. Many nursing leaders in the 1920s attempted to maintain a "framework that would allow the public health nurse to care for both the healthy and the sick" (Buhler-Wilkerson, 1985, p. 1159). In some communities, partnerships developed between the health department and the visiting nurse association to provide both types of nursing care through a "combined" administrative structure. Most of these structures did not survive.

In 1929, the NOPHN stressed that public health nursing was a nonprofit community service:

Public health nursing is an organized community nonprofit service, rendered by graduate nurses to the individual, family, and community. This service includes interpretation and application of medical, sanitary, and social procedures for the correction of defects, prevention of disease and the promotion of health; and may include skilled care of the sick in their homes. (Fitzpatrick, 1975, p. 102)

This definition included government-sponsored services as well as private, nonprofit services, such as visiting nurse associations. Preventive services were a necessary component of public health nursing, and skilled care of sick persons in their homes was permitted but not required.

In 1934, the NOPHN and APHA definitions of public health nursing were more general and included all nursing services that assisted with the "public health program."

Public health nursing includes all nursing services organized by a community or an agency to assist in carrying out any or all phases of the public health program. Services may be rendered on an individual, family, or community basis in the home, school, clinics, business establishment, or the office of the agency. (Fitzpatrick, 1975, p. 127)

By then, however, most public health programs were government sponsored.

The division in public health nursing in the United States occurred as a result of a basic schism within the health care system: the private sector versus the government-sponsored (public) sector. (See Chapter 3 for more about the health care system.) To manage competition and conflict between the two sectors, diagnosis and treatment of ill persons remained the domain of private physicians, and health promotion and disease prevention were the domain of state and local health departments. This division of responsibility was relatively clear and remained so until 1965, when, with the enactment of Medicare and Medicaid legislation, the government sector began paying for the health care of ill elderly and poor persons.

EDUCATIONAL PREPARATION FOR PUBLIC HEALTH NURSES

Before 1935, most public health nurses were trained nurses who learned about public health nursing from their on-the-job experience. By 1959, 20% of public health nurses had an academic degree.

In the early 1900s, some hospital schools placed students in private homes to provide nursing care and to increase revenues for the hospitals. However, most nurses in public health learned through apprenticeships with visiting nurse associations. In 1906, the Boston Instructive District Visiting Nurses Association developed a course for its nurses. For 4 months, nurses were closely supervised in their practice and received room and board but no salary (Brainard, 1985).

In 1910, Teachers College of Columbia University established the Department of Nursing and Health for postgraduate work for trained nurses. Western Reserve University in Cleveland and Simmons College in Boston soon followed their lead (Brainard, 1985). By 1922, there were 15 postgraduate schools of public health nursing (Goodnow, 1928, p. 240). Knowledge of hygiene and sanitation; prevention and control of health problems, such as tuberculosis and infant mortality; sociology; and social psychology were valuable to nurses promoting health (Brainard, 1985).

The NOPHN believed that effective nursing care for families was based on good general nursing. The National League for Nursing Education (NLNE) advocated that specialists in public nursing be prepared through university-sponsored courses for nurses who had graduated from training schools. The NLNE also advocated that training schools for nurses prepare generalists in public health by affiliating with visiting nurse associations and adding lectures in sociology, psychology, and public health nursing (Fitzpatrick, 1975). Electives in public health nursing were also encouraged in training schools.

By 1918, the NLNE had agreed on a standard curriculum that incorporated "social aspects of nursing" into the third year of basic diploma training schools (Fitzpatrick, 1975). Field practice was resisted by training schools, because the students were needed to staff hospitals. The NLNE and the NOPHN divided the duties of overseeing the incorporation of public health nursing content into curricula. The NLNE oversaw basic training schools, and the NOPHN was responsible for postgraduate and staff education (Fitzpatrick, 1975).

Despite the belief of the leadership that additional knowledge and experience were necessary for public health nurses, few nurses working in public health had the extra education. Correspondence courses were developed for those working in the field who were academically unprepared. The NOPHN endorsed the courses as appropriate staff education for those who had had 4 months of public health nursing experience (Fitzpatrick, 1975). Most public health nurses received additional information about their practice from publications supported by the NOPHN.

In 1924, after baccalaureate schools of nursing had become more prevalent, Alma Haupt, director of the MLIC Visiting Nurse Association and a member of the NOPHN Education Committee, proposed that public health nursing content be integrated into undergraduate education as a part of each specialized course, such as obstetric nursing. Each graduate would be able to "organize care, make nursing assessments, appreciate the home conditions of patients and learn about community resources [and] the concept of health as a community responsibility" (Fitzpatrick, 1975, p. 101). To avoid overburdening public health agencies with students, however, hospital schools were to place their students in clinics, with only observations in public health nursing agencies (Fitzpatrick, 1975).

Substantive increases occurred between 1935 and 1950 in the percentage of public health nurses having adequate academic preparation. Baccalaureate nursing programs were encouraged to include 8-week affiliations in public health agencies that met NOPHN standards; students were to "study health and sickness in one family over time" and understand the neighborhood factors that "influenced a family's health and socioeconomic situation" (Fitzpatrick, 1975, p. 129). The number of postgraduate courses approved by the NOPHN increased from 16 in 1935 to 26 in 1940 (Roberts & Heinrich, 1985, p. 1164). By 1950, 1 in 5 of the 25,000 public health nurses had one or more academic degrees; 56% of all supervisors and 70% of state-employed supervisors had degrees (Fitzpatrick, 1975, p. 193).

COMMUNITY/PUBLIC HEALTH NURSING: 1965 TO 2000

Several forces converged to promote the emergence of the term *community health nursing*. Hanlon and Pickett (1984) attribute the use of the term to the fact that numerous private, not-for-profit agencies evolved in the 1960s to address health needs that were not being met by local governments (the publicly sponsored agencies). As discussed previously, public health nursing had come to be associated with government-sponsored services; now that other agencies also were addressing health needs of neighborhoods and population groups, an expanded term was needed. The term *community health nursing* included nursing sponsored by both private, nonprofit organizations and governmental agencies (Hanlon & Pickett, 1984). For-profit agencies were not mentioned as being related to community health nursing. Simultaneously, the ANA began to develop the following divisions of nursing practice: community health, gerontologic, maternal and child health, medical-surgical, and psychiatric and mental health. Each division was to describe its scope and standards of practice.

Creation of the Division of Community Health Practice promoted the widespread use of the term *community health nursing* (USDHHS, 1985). The division included nurses working within a variety of community-based settings, including health departments; schools; work sites; private physicians' offices; private, nonprofit clinics; visiting nurse associations; and for-profit home health agencies. Therefore, the term included nurses employed by governmental, private nonprofit, and private for-profit agencies. For-profit (proprietary) home health agencies began to increase in number after 1965 when Medicare made skilled nursing care (home health care) financially accessible to homebound elderly persons (see Chapters 28 and 31). Today, agencies providing visiting nurses to care for ill persons in their homes are no longer sponsored primarily by the government and nonprofit private agencies.

The term *community health nursing,* in some respects, has reunited nursing both for the promotion of health and prevention of disease and for the care of ill persons at home. However, during the last half of the 1990s, an attempt emerged to distinguish community health nurses who have education and experience in nursing and public health practice from other nurses included within the ANA Division of Community Health Practice (ANA, 1995; Baldwin et al., 1998; Zotti et al., 1996). All nurses within the Division of Community Health Practice provide *community-based care,* meaning care outside an institution, such as a hospital or nursing home (Quad Council, 1999). As discussed in Chapter 1, many of these nurses provide individual-focused and/or family-focused care and do not have the educational preparation required for population- and community-focused care. Therefore, perhaps a better name for this ANA practice division would be *Division of Community-Based Practice* rather than *Division of Community Health Practice.*

The question remains: What name should be used for those community-based nurses who have education and experience in providing population- and community-focused care in addition to care of individuals and families? Some authors suggest that the term *community health nurse* be reserved for these practitioners (Zotti et al., 1996). Others use the term *community/public health nurse* to distinguish those community-based nurses who are population or community focused (Association of Community Health Nursing Educators, 1995; Baldwin et al., 1998).

Baldwin and colleagues (1998) recommend that the terms *community health nursing* and *public health nursing* be abandoned. They suggest that the term *population-focused nursing* or *population health nursing* be used to designate nurses whose practice is population focused. Although they retain the term *public health nursing,* nurses from the Minnesota Department of Health (1997, p. 7) assert that *population-based public health practice* is aimed at disease prevention and health promotion to "improve the health status of entire identified populations." Here, the word *based* does not refer to physical setting but means that on which the care is founded.

As discussed in Chapter 1, the APHA (1996, p. 4) also describes public health nursing as "nursing practice directed toward a population."

In 1999, the ANA replaced the 1986 ANA *Standards of Community Health Nursing Practice* with the *Scope and Standards of Public Health Nursing Practice.* These standards returned to the classic term *public health nursing.* This document continued to distinguish public health nursing as community- or population-focused care, as was discussed earlier in this chapter. The author of these standards was the Quad Council of Public Health Nursing Organizations, which comprises four associations: the ANA Council for Community, Primary, and Long-Term Care Nursing Practice; the Public Health Nursing Section of the APHA; the Association of Community Health Nursing Educators; and the Association of State and Territorial Directors of Nursing.

In 2007, the Quad Council authored the most recent standards, *Public Health Nursing: Scope and Standards of Practice* (ANA, 2007c). (See Chapter 1.) Dialogue about community/public health nursing practice continues. Whatever the terms used, the possibility exists for population-focused nursing in the twenty-first century to recapture the vitality and wholeness that existed in public health nursing in the late 1800s.

COMMUNITY/PUBLIC HEALTH NURSING: PRESENT AND FUTURE

The essence of public health is "organized community efforts" that ensure "conditions in which people can be healthy" (Institute of Medicine [IOM], 1988, pp. 7, 41). Safe environments, timely immunization, sound nutrition, attention to maternal and fetal health, responsible behaviors and self-care, and provision of health care services help create healthful conditions (Last, 1992). Social and health care needs cannot be met solely by making sure that everyone has financial access to medical care (IOM, 1988). Community health nurses as public health personnel are experts in "health problem identification, disease and disability prevention, and health promotion" (IOM, 1988, p. 153). Community/public health nurses are exemplars in "outreach and case finding, direct service delivery, and management of needs of multiproblem clients" (IOM, 1988, p. 153).

HEALTH CARE REFORM
Nursing's Agenda for Health Care Reform (ANA, 1991) called for a health care system that supports more nurses as primary care providers. **Primary health care** includes essential health care that is universally accessible to individuals and families within communities (ANA Council of Community Health Nurses, 1986b). Primary health care includes health promotion and disease prevention as well as a basic package of services for treatment of illnesses and injury. In 1997, third-party reimbursement under Medicare and Medicaid was expanded to all nurse practitioners and clinical nurse specialists (Keepnews, 1998).

In 2004, the Institute of Medicine recommended that health insurance be available to all persons in the United States by 2010. Even when almost everyone has financial access to a basic package of health care services, people still need to learn to gain access to that care, to cope with personal responses to their health status, and to understand how their own behavior can improve their well-being. These concerns are all within the domain of nursing practice. A variety of models for delivering nursing care in a changing health care system are under exploration (ANA Council, 1986a). Community/public health nurses, especially those employed by the government and charged with the health of entire populations, need to become more visible and vocal as leaders for health (Shalala, 1992; Ward, 1989).

We can look to nursing in other countries for nursing care delivery models that may fit our changing circumstances. For example, since the 1970s, some community health nurses in Canada and Britain have been employed by the government but "attached" to work with primary care physicians and their enrolled patients (Ciliska et al., 1992; McClure, 1984). As more Americans join health plans in which they designate a primary care provider, similar nursing care delivery models might be appropriate in the United States.

Not only universal access to primary health care services but also public-focused care services continue to be needed. Philip Lee (1993), Assistant Secretary of Health and Human Services, challenged public health leaders to (1) help develop data systems to monitor how well primary health care services support the health of populations, (2) engage in research about health care delivery and prevention, and (3) provide more primary health care workers (including community health nurses, nurse practitioners, and midwives) in underserved areas. He also called for more flexible outreach, support, and translation services to population groups that have previously been underserved. As new relationships are defined between public health departments and personal health care delivery organizations, including managed care organizations, community/public health nursing responsibilities will continue to evolve.

Community/public health nurses already are carrying out the core public health functions of assessment, policy development, and assurance (see Chapter 29). Community-wide services continue to be needed for the prevention and control of (1) communicable diseases and environmentally induced illnesses and injuries, such as HIV infection and violence; (2) premature deaths, especially among infants; and (3) chronic diseases and conditions, such as obesity. Community/public health nurses can stand on a century of nursing history to create nursing services for the future.

Knowledge of the structure and financing of U.S. health care is necessary if quality nursing is to exist in a climate of cost containment (Hamilton, 1988) (see Chapters 3 and 4). Making health insurance coverage available to more people is not the same as transforming the health care system into one that advocates health promotion and social betterment (Anderson, 1991).

NATIONAL HEALTH OBJECTIVES

National health objectives are developed and published in a series of documents called *Healthy People*. Each document is a decade-long action agenda to improve the health of all Americans. *Healthy People 2010* (USDHHS, 2000, 2006) establishes national health goals and objectives and provides a guide for community health nurses speaking with people about healthy communities (Figure 2-4). It is an effort to identify the most significant preventable threats to health and recommend

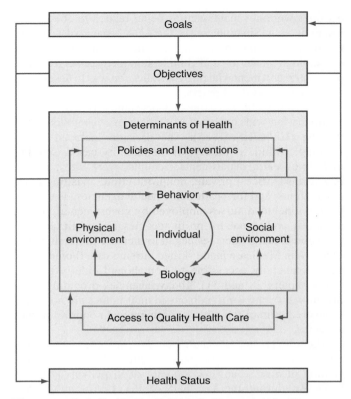

FIGURE 2-4 *Healthy People 2010:* Healthy people in healthy communities. (From U.S. Department of Health and Human Services. [2000]. *Healthy People 2010: Understanding and improving health.* Washington, DC: U.S. Government Printing Office.)

public and private-sector efforts to address these threats. There are two main goals:
- Increase quality and years of healthy life
- Eliminate health disparities

These broad goals are supported by four enabling goals: (1) promote healthy behaviors, (2) protect health, (3) provide access to quality health care, and (4) strengthen community prevention. *Healthy People 2010* is the U.S. contribution to the World Health Organization's plan "Health for All" (Maiese & Fox, 1998).

The national health objectives developed from these goals are distinguished from the plan for the previous decade, *Healthy People 2000,* by an effort to enhance the prevention science base, improve surveillance and data systems, and increase awareness of the need for public health services and quality health care for all. There is widespread recognition that changes in population demographics, science and technology, and disease spread will affect the public's health in the twenty-first century (USDHHS, 2000).

To achieve the goals, more than 450 objectives were developed to serve as the basis for action plans. Under the leadership of the U.S. Public Health Service, representatives from the health professions (including professional nursing organizations), state governments, consumers, and business leaders participated in the planning process. *Healthy People 2010* involves two types of objectives: measurable and developmental. *Measurable objectives* provide direction for action and use established data to set new targets. *Developmental objectives* set a vision for a desired outcome or health status but do not include specific targets because of a currently lack of adequate baseline data sources (USDHHS, 2000). An example of each type of objective follows:

Measurable objective: Reduce the infant mortality rate to no more than 4.5 per 1000 live births (baseline: 7.2 per 1000 live births in 1998)

Developmental objective: Increase the proportion of pregnant women who attend a series of prepared childbirth classes (no current baseline; target not yet set)

In 2005, tracking data were available for 281 of the objectives, baseline data were available for another 87 objectives, and some objectives were deleted because baseline data would not be available by 2010 (USDHHS, 2006).

Development and measurement of objectives is an ongoing process, starting with publication of a draft for public comment, continuing with publication of the final version, and proceeding with revisions and adjustments throughout the decade. The 2010 objectives were based on a projected profile of the U.S. population in the year 2010 and on knowledge of the existing health status of the public. This is presented in the *Healthy People 2010* box below. There are objectives for infants (younger than 1 year), children, adolescents and youth (15 to 24 years), adults, and older adults (65 years and older).

Objectives are organized into 28 focus areas as presented in the *Healthy People 2010* box on page 48. Within each of these focus areas, objectives address health status, risk reduction, and provision of services. Examples of the three kinds of objectives follow (USDHHS, 1998, 2000, 2006):

■ HEALTHY PEOPLE 2010 ■
Profile of the American People in the Year 2010

- The total population of the United States will have grown to nearly 290 million people from 254 million in 1990. The rate of growth between 2000 and 2010 is expected to be the slowest in the nation's history.
- Between 2000 and 2010, 8.2 million people will have migrated to the United States, primarily to the East and West Coasts.
- The population will be older, with the median age being more than 37.4 years (in 1990 it was 33 years). Persons 65 years and older will constitute 13.2% of the population; 5.6 million people will be older than 85 years.
- A smaller percentage of the population will be children younger than 5 years of age (20 million compared with 19.5 million in 1995, but 6.7% of the population compared with 7.5% in 1995).
- Average household size will be smaller at 2.55 people (compared with 2.62 in 1995).
- Racial and ethnic compositions will be different. The proportion of whites will decline from 73.6% in 1995 to 68% of the population. The proportion of blacks, Hispanics, and others (including American Indians, Native Alaskans, Asians, and Pacific Islanders) will increase to 32%. The Hispanic population will have grown at the fastest rate during the 2000s.

Data from U.S. Census Bureau. (1996a). *Population projections of the United States by age, sex, race, and Hispanic origin: 1995 to 2050* (CPR-P25–1130). Washington, DC: U.S. Government Printing Office; U.S. Census Bureau. (1996b). *Projections of the number of households and families in the United States: 1995 to 2010.* Washington, DC: U.S. Government Printing Office.

Health status: Reduce lung cancer deaths to a rate of no more than 44.3 per 100,000 people (age-adjusted baseline: 55.5 per 100,000 in 1999)

Risk reduction: Reduce cigarette smoking to no more than 12% among persons aged 18 years and older (baseline: 24.0% in 1998)

Services: Increase to at least 75% the proportion of primary care providers who routinely advise cessation and provide assistance, follow-up, and document charts for all their patients using tobacco (baseline example, nurse practitioners: 51% inquired about tobacco use; 20% discussed strategies to quit in 1992)

In many of the focus areas, population groups (aggregates) are identified and targeted because they have higher rates of risk. For example, children and teens are targeted for special attention in the smoking initiatives with education programs geared toward identifying the health risks of smoking and special efforts to discourage cigarette use during childhood and young adulthood. These particular groups are targeted because research indicates that most cigarette smokers started tobacco use as adolescents and young adults.

Unlike *Healthy People 2000,* the previous decade's national health objectives, *Healthy People 2010* does *not* establish specific target objectives for racial/ethnic population groups or aggregates, even when those groups might have greater risk factors for certain health problems (e.g., hypertension in African Americans). Instead, *Healthy People 2010* identifies a single target objective for the entire population, in an attempt to raise the health status of all groups to the target for the general population. Planners recognize that, in some instances, a certain racial/ethnic aggregate might already meet the national target objective whereas other groups might not meet the objective by 2010, although they make significant progress in improving health status or risk reduction. Health statistics will be collected and reported by racial/ethnic aggregates when possible to measure progress toward the targets.

Disparities in health status and access to quality health care were motivators in establishing a broad objective rather than separate objectives for subgroups of population at greater risk. Poorer health status is correlated with race/ethnicity and socioeconomic status (see Chapter 21). African Americans, Hispanics, American Indians and Alaska Natives, Pacific Islanders, and people with lower incomes are more likely to have serious health problems and die earlier than people who have white or Asian ancestry or people with middle or high incomes (USDHHS, 2000). The hope is that *Healthy People 2010*'s emphasis on improving access to quality health and health education, and improved public health infrastructure will reduce disparities among aggregates or subgroups in the population.

There is no single national plan for achieving the national health objectives. An agency of the federal government is assigned to provide leadership for each of the 28 focus areas (see the *Healthy People 2010* box on page 48). The national health objectives are used by federal, state, and local governments, as well as by nongovernmental groups interested in the health of communities. By 1998, 47 states, the District of Columbia, and Guam had developed their own Healthy People plans (USDHHS, 1998). Government funding can be targeted toward regional and national priorities for health promotion and disease prevention. For example, preventive mental health

■ HEALTHY PEOPLE 2010 ■
Objectives

Focus Area	Lead Agency
1. Access to quality health services programs	Agency for Healthcare Research and Quality
	Health Resources and Services Administration
	National Center for Chronic Disease Prevention and Health Promotion
2. Arthritis, osteoporosis, and chronic back conditions	Centers for Disease Control and Prevention
	National Institutes of Health
3. Cancer	Centers for Disease Control and Prevention
	National Institutes of Health
4. Chronic kidney disease	National Institutes of Health
5. Diabetes	Centers for Disease Control and Prevention
	National Institutes of Health
6. Disability and secondary conditions	Centers for Disease Control and Prevention
	National Institute on Disability and Rehabilitation Research, U.S. Department of Education
7. Education and community-based programs	Centers for Disease Control and Prevention
	Health Resources and Services Administration
8. Environmental health	Agency for Toxic Substances and Disease Registry
	Centers for Disease Control and Prevention
	National Institutes of Health
9. Family planning	Office of Population Affairs
10. Food safety	Food and Drug Administration
	Food Safety and Inspection Services, U.S. Department of Agriculture
11. Health communication	Office of Disease Prevention and Health Promotion
12. Heart disease and stroke	Centers for Disease Control and Prevention
	National Institutes of Health
13. Human immunodeficiency virus (HIV) infection	Centers for Disease Control and Prevention
	Health Resources and Services Administration
14. Immunization and infectious diseases	Centers for Disease Control and Prevention
15. Injury/violence prevention	Centers for Disease Control and Prevention
16. Maternal, infant, and child health	Centers for Disease Control and Prevention
	Health Resources and Services Administration
17. Medical product safety	Food and Drug Administration
18. Mental health and mental disorders	National Institutes of Health
	Substance Abuse and Mental Health Services Administration
19. Nutrition and overweight	Food and Drug Administration
	National Institutes of Health
20. Occupational safety and health	Centers for Disease Control and Prevention
21. Oral health	Centers for Disease Control and Prevention
	Health Resources and Services Administration
	Indian Health Service
	National Institutes of Health
22. Physical activity and fitness	Centers for Disease Control and Prevention
	President's Council on Physical Fitness and Sports
23. Public health infrastructure	Centers for Disease Control and Prevention
	Health Resources and Services Administration
24. Respiratory diseases	Centers for Disease Control and Prevention
	National Institutes of Health
25. Sexually transmitted diseases	Centers for Disease Control and Prevention
26. Substance abuse	National Institutes of Health
	Substance Abuse and Mental Health Services Administration
27. Tobacco use	Centers for Disease Control and Prevention
28. Vision and hearing	National Institutes of Health

From U.S. Department of Health and Human Services. (2000). *Healthy people 2010: Understanding and improving health* (2nd ed.). Washington, DC: U.S. Government Printing Office.

programs and other school-based services for children and adolescents can strengthen the overall health of adults in the future. *Healthy People 2010* objectives also can be used to measure progress of federally funded programs, such as the Indian Health Service and the Preventive Health and Health Services Block Grants. Not all the national objectives are relevant in every community.

Healthy People 2020 is scheduled to be released in two phases (USDHHS, 2007). The framework will be released by early 2009 and by January 2010, the specific goals, objectives, and action plans are scheduled to be released.

POPULATIONS AND COMMUNITY/PUBLIC HEALTH NURSING

To make progress toward our national vision of healthier people and communities, community/public health nurses must understand our historical roots. Earlier community health nurses recognized that people are whole human beings within complex social and physical environments. The betterment of human communities remains the goal of community health nursing. However, our specific objectives change with social and environmental conditions, types of illnesses present, and needs of specific populations.

Elderly, adolescent, low-income, and homeless persons are just some of the populations that can benefit from community/public health nursing care (Riportella-Muller et al., 1991). The elderly will make up an increasingly greater percentage of our national population. Elderly persons experience more illness than young persons and are in need of information on how to maintain their well-being and independence in the presence of chronic diseases and disabilities.

Attitudes and knowledge about health and health-promoting behaviors are learned within the family and community. Schools and peer groups are important social networks for children and adolescents. Although children tend to be physically healthier than their elders, issues of spiritual and emotional well-being are important. Obesity, teenage pregnancy, HIV infection, substance abuse, and violence are public health priorities for youth. Community/public health nurses working with families and in schools will continue to confront these challenges.

Poverty is stressful. Poor persons tend to have poorer health than their wealthier neighbors. The growing numbers of poor persons, especially women, children, and homeless persons, require coordinated assistance to meet their multiple needs. Sustained relationships are necessary for their empowerment (Schorr, 1989). Poverty rates tend to be higher in rural and inner-city communities, where fewer health care services are available. Although the largest number of poor in the United States are white, nonwhite populations suffer higher rates of poverty. Community/public health nurses have a long history of advocating for those who have not had equal access to health care and a basic standard of living, and they are challenged to continue to pursue justice (see Chapter 1).

Neonatal and infant illnesses and deaths are an important measure of a community's health. Infant mortality continues to decline in the United States. However, infant mortality is much higher among African Americans, Puerto Ricans, and some American Indian tribes than among whites. More than 100 years ago, community health nurses demonstrated their ability to reduce mortality among newborns and infants. Although communicable diseases are no longer the primary causes of death, community/public health nurses have shown their ability to work with parents to reduce rates of low birth weight in neonates and to prevent child abuse and accidents (Brooten et al., 1986; Olds et al., 1993). Special research opportunities exist for community/public health nurses to identify interventions that work best to reduce infant mortality among various socioeconomic, racial, and cultural populations.

Population-focused health promotion and primary prevention will be provided at community sites where individuals spend much of their time. Work sites will continue to be important places to assist people in changing their lifestyles and reducing their risk of such disorders as heart disease, cancer, diabetes, obstructive lung disease, and alcoholism. Community/public health nurses and other public health professionals will have opportunities to promote more healthful work environments, including improvement of indoor air quality. Occupational health nurses will be instrumental in preventing work site exposures to specific toxins and in teaching other nurses and the public about such hazards.

How do we organize and deliver public health nursing services in the public sector of health care? As local health departments reorganize to focus more on core public health functions, public health nursing is also reinvigorating itself. In some local health departments, public health nursing practice is moving away from primary health care clinic practice in order to strengthen its population-focused practice (Kosidlak, 1999). For instance, in Los Angeles County, California, 200 of 500 public health nurses were reassigned from categorical programs such as maternal child health or tuberculosis control to geographically defined service planning areas (Avila & Smith, 2003). As district public health nurses, they develop a community assessment database for their districts, expand practice beyond disease control, provide nursing consultation in the community, and participate in public health planning and community-level interventions.

Community/public health nurses have demonstrated that nursing care can be provided in the variety of other settings in which various populations spend much of their day (ANA Council, 1986a), such as medical daycare centers, child daycare centers, homeless shelters, prisons, and faith communities (Alexander-Rodriguez, 1983; ANA, 2005, 2007a). Community/public health nurses also provide communicable disease and safety consultation to in-home daycare providers (Lie, 1992). With the expected increases in the number of persons with acquired immunodeficiency syndrome (AIDS) and the number of elderly persons, hospice programs will become even more important (ANA, 2007b).

EMERGING AND REEMERGING INFECTIONS AND THREATS OF TERRORISM

A major activity of the governmental sector of health care is the control of communicable diseases in populations. The appearance of new infectious diseases, the reemergence of old infectious diseases, and the threat of bioterrorism are reasons that interest and support for communicable disease control has been increasing in recent years (Heymann, 2004). Examples of new diseases include Lyme tick disease, for which the infectious agent was identified only in 1982, and a global epidemic of severe acute respiratory syndrome (SARS) that occurred in 2003. International migration of diseases such as West Nile fever and malaria has expanded. Tuberculosis, thought to be controlled, reemerged as a secondary infection in persons with AIDS. The anthrax exposure of postal workers in the Washington, DC, area during 2001 underscores the need for effective public health measures to respond to terrorism (see Chapter 8). Community/public health nurses, especially those working for local and state health departments, are involved in developing plans for community-level preparedness and response to outbreaks of communicable diseases, whether caused by natural disaster or terrorism (see Chapter 22).

Specifically, new electronic surveillance systems have been developed to help health departments identify and monitor outbreaks of communicable diseases. Community/public health nurses are active in the effort to inform the public about risks and have helped develop the public health response to a bioterrorist attack. This strategy involves the stockpiling of effective antimicrobial agents and an efficient system for distributing these supplies to the affected areas. Because of the limited supply of personnel and funding, a tension exists between the use of these resources for homeland security and for other on-going, important public health problems.

Continuing Issues

The challenge continues for community/public health nurses to reunite aspects of practice, with focus on all levels of prevention. What is a practical balance between providing care for sick people in homes and providing health promotion and primary prevention within the community? Community/public health nurses continue to use their knowledge of epidemiology to identify vulnerable subpopulations within the entire population. However, much community/public health nursing care is provided to human beings as individuals and as members of families, groups, and organizations. The collective health of individual humans contributes to the health of the entire public. In addition, the network of social relationships contributes to the degree of connected caring. In community health nursing, there is always a tension of perspective. Unlike some planners and statisticians, community/public health nurses can attach human faces and personal stories to the numbers. Unlike many other nurses who choose to focus predominantly on the health of individuals, community/public health nurses think in terms of the health of populations.

Private businesses, rather than state and local governments, employ an increasing percentage of community health nurses. Health care reform is bringing changes in the organization and distribution of health care. Where will community/public health nurses fit in the scheme? Should community health nurses continue to be employed by others? Will more community/public health nurses consider starting private businesses and practices in which they contract with larger health care entities to provide community health nursing care?

How do we continue to provide quality community health nursing care? There are many nurses, especially in the subspecialty of home health care, who do not have formal community health nursing education. How can technologic competence be linked with competence in family-focused and population-focused care? These questions are similar to those that nurses in the 1920s asked themselves: How do we best provide on-the-job training, apprenticeships, formal education, and continuing education?

How can we work more effectively for social betterment in our communities? For vulnerable populations to become empowered, we must engage in sustained relationships that focus on the wholeness of persons and their communities (Erickson, 1996; Schorr, 1989). Community/public health nurses have known this for almost 150 years. Therefore, to truly improve the health of a community, community/public health nurses must provide holistic care, especially in underserved urban and rural communities. More nurses might need to return to district or neighborhood nursing (Avila & Smith, 2003). We also need to listen to the suffering of community members and respond to their needs. We need to commit to staying in nurse-client relationships for a while. We need to be more vocal and more visible in sharing our ideas about what works with other community leaders.

KEY IDEAS

1. Community/public health nursing has its roots in nursing and public health. The challenges of community/public health nursing evolve as changes occur in population characteristics, scientific knowledge and theory about health and illness, prevalent illnesses and causes of death, societal values, and economic and political systems.

2. Nursing's roots include visiting and district nursing to care for ill persons in their homes, health teaching and promotion with families, and "nursing the environment."

3. Public health's roots include the provision of a sanitary environment and the prevention of disease through immunization and personal responsibility for hygiene.

4. Population-focused nursing started with an interest in urban poor populations and British and American military personnel during the mid-1800s.

5. In 1912, visiting nurses in the United States named themselves *public health nurses* because they provided care to all members of the community—to the entire public—and were committed to social betterment.

6. As additional populations were identified as being at risk of illnesses and in need of nursing care, subspecialties of public health nursing emerged. These included maternal and child health, school health, and occupational health.

7. Under the leadership of Lillian Wald, public health nursing expanded into rural communities with the creation of the Visiting Nurse Service of the Metropolitan Life Insurance Company (1909) and the Red Cross Rural Nursing Service (1912). In 1925, Mary Breckinridge founded the Frontier Nursing Service in Kentucky, which survives today.

8. Public health nursing was originally sponsored by financial donations from the wealthy. As public health nursing demonstrated its effectiveness, it became institutionalized in health departments of local and state governments. The holism of public health nursing, with its focus on both sickness care and prevention, was broken when health departments sought not to threaten physicians' practices. Health departments took on the responsibility for health promotion and disease prevention, and visiting nurse agencies continued with care of sick persons in their homes (also called home health care).

9. The term *public health nursing* had become associated primarily with the work of those nurses employed by the government. Public health nurses working in new

community centers and for-profit home health agencies also needed to be included. Therefore, the term *community health nursing* emerged in the 1970s as the new name for public health nursing.

10. Because the term *community health nursing* can encompass all nurses working in community-based settings, some community health nurses have proposed clarifying that community health nurses are *population focused* or *community focused.*

11. With health care reform and the development of national health promotion goals, new opportunities exist to reunite care and prevention within community/public health nursing. New models are emerging to deliver community/public health nursing to the public. Issues of organizing and delivering community/public health nursing services are ongoing. The term *public health nursing* has reemerged to mean community-based, population-focused nursing care.

CASE STUDY   Mary Breckinridge: A Public Health Nursing Leader

Mary Breckinridge (1881-1965) initiated a study of the health needs of 29,000 people in three counties in eastern Kentucky in 1923. She rode more than 700 miles on horseback to interview 53 "granny women" or midwives, young mothers, schoolteachers, and those in charge of missions.

Her family had lived in Kentucky since 1790 and had been in public service since the time of Thomas Jefferson. Her father was minister to Russia under President Grover Cleveland. She spent 12 winters in Washington, DC, as a girl and 2 years in Russia with French and German governesses. A great-aunt established schools for mountain children in the southern United States. To prepare for service Mary "took the stiff training as a nurse at St. Luke's Hospital in New York."

Her husband died. Her second marriage was unhappy, and two children died. She went to France to care for children there during World War I. Her thoughts returned to Kentucky, where neonatal and maternal deaths and epidemics of hookworm, diphtheria, smallpox, typhoid, and tuberculosis ravaged the population. Her assessment emerged from her commitment to demonstrate "what intelligent nursing could do to safeguard the lives of mothers and children on our many forgotten frontiers" in the United States. To be able to address the health needs she had identified, she studied in London to become licensed as a nurse-midwife. She returned to Kentucky in 1925 to provide trained nurse-midwives "to deliver women in childbirth and safeguard the lives of little children, to care for the sick of all ages and take measures to prevent disease, and to work for economic conditions less inimical to health."

The Frontier Nursing Service was thus created. By 1931 "the staff included two assistant directors, three supervisors, relief nurses, three nurses and a physician in a small hospital ... and 21 nurses in the field." One nurse's report indicated that she had made rounds for 11 hours a day and during the week had visited 143 persons. In addi-

tion, patients were seen at the centers. All services were provided for only $10.92 per year per individual served. In the year ending May 1931, 7806 persons in 1675 families were cared for; this included bedside nursing provided in 459 cases of serious illness.

The nurses at the outlying stations lived in comfortable quarters with two nurses per station and a housekeeper-cook. One nurse was assigned general duty and one midwifery. Each nurse was assigned a district and could cover 80 square miles per day. Six weeks of vacation were earned each year, preferably taken in two 3-week periods. The work itself was demanding. The nurse had to be independent, capable of extensive horseback travel, unstopped by vagaries of weather, and available to respond to emergency illnesses. The nurses were committed to the people as well as their own professional practice.

Mary Breckinridge enlisted others to assist in addressing the multitude of problems. She organized a local committee of mountaineers so she could work with the people, rather than for them. She involved her relatives, physicians, experts in public health, and the Kentucky State Board of Health in planning the organization. The nurses avoided involvement in the mountaineer clan wars and served all who were wounded or in need. Breckinridge collaborated with federal and state authorities, the Rockefeller Foundation, and the Johns Hopkins and Vanderbilt universities. The American Child Health Association participated to cure hookworm. Graduates of the Forestry Department of Yale University were invited to survey logging practices and revitalize the forests to improve employment opportunities to reduce poverty.

Mary Breckinridge was a pioneer in community assessment, population-based planning, and partnership building. She created a system for rural nursing and used research to demonstrate its effectiveness. Her vision remains fulfilled in the Frontier Nursing Service, which continues today.

Data from Poole, E. (1932). *Nurses on horseback.* New York: Macmillan.

WEB   See **Critical Thinking Questions** for this Case Study on the book's website.

LEARNING BY EXPERIENCE AND REFLECTION

1. After reading the Case Study in this chapter regarding the work of Mary Breckinridge, describe how she displayed the leadership characteristics described in Chapter 1.
2. Read a biography of a community/public health nurse. Identify the health problems and the communities with which the community/public health nurse worked. Reflect on the degree to which both care of ill persons and health promotion and primary prevention were included in the nurse's practice.

Describe how the social and physical environment affected the clients and nursing practice. Identify the expressed and implied ethical commitments and values of the nurse.
3. Interview a retired community/public health nurse and compare her or his experiences with those of a contemporary community/public health nurse. Focus on similarities and differences.
4. Identify the *Healthy People* objectives applicable to a population or aggregate to which you belong, such as young adult Asian women; urban African American adult men;

rural, low-income white women. Notice your thoughts and feelings as you consider the objectives.

5. Discuss which populations/aggregates should receive the most nursing attention. Is your answer different depending on whether you consider the community in which you live, your state, or the entire nation?

6. Identify client needs that are not likely to be solved by financial access to medical care. Envision how community/public health nursing care might address these needs.

COMMUNITY RESOURCES FOR PRACTICE

Information about each of the following organizations is found on its website, which can be accessed through the **WebLinks** section of this book's website at http://evolve.elsevier.com/Maurer/community/.

American Nurses Association
American Public Health Association
Healthy Cities at Indiana University School of Nursing World Health Organization Collaborative Center in Healthy Cities
Healthy People 2010
Henry Street Settlement House (New York City)
Frontier Nursing Service (Kentucky)

STUDY AIDS   http://evolve.elsevier.com/Maurer/community/

Visit the Evolve website for this book to find the following study and assessment materials:

- Quiz
- Web Scenario
- Critical Thinking Questions and Answers for Case Studies

- Care Plans
- *Healthy People* Updates
- Glossary

WEBSITE RESOURCES

The following item supplements the chapter's topics and is also found on the Evolve site:

2A: Rules for Nurses from the Instructive Visiting Nurse Association of Baltimore, Maryland (1912)

REFERENCES

Alexander-Rodriguez, T. (1983). Prison health—A role for professional nursing. *Nursing Outlook, 31*(2), 115-118.

American Nurses Association. (1987). *Facts about nursing 86-87*. Washington, DC: Author.

American Nurses Association. (1991). *Nursing's agenda for health care reform*. Washington, DC: Author.

American Nurses Association. (1995). *Scope and standards of population-focused and community-based nursing practice (Draft)*. Washington, DC: Author.

American Nurses Association. (2005). *Faith community nursing: Scope and standards of practice*. Silver Spring, MD: Author.

American Nurses Association. (2007a). *Corrections nursing: Scope and standards of practice*. Silver Spring, MD: Author.

American Nurses Association. (2007b). *Hospice and palliative nursing: Scope and standards of practice*. Silver Spring, MD: Author.

American Nurses Association. (2007c). *Public health nursing: Scope and standards of practice*. Silver Spring, MD: Author.

American Nurses Association Council of Community Health Nurses. (1986a). *Community-based nursing services: Innovative models*. Washington, DC: Author.

American Nurses Association Council of Community Health Nurses. (1986b).

Standards of community health nursing practice. Washington, DC: Author.

American Public Health Association, Public Health Nursing Section. (1996). *The definition and role of public health nursing*. Washington, DC: Author.

Anderson, E. (1991). A call for transformation. *Public Health Nursing, 8*(1), 1-2.

Association of Community Health Nursing Educators. (1995). Community/public health advanced practice nurse position statement. *Newsletter, 13*(2), 13.

Avila, M., & Smith, K. (2003). The reinvigoration of public health nursing: Methods and innovations. *Journal of Public Health Management, 9*(1), 16-24.

Backer, B. (1993). Lillian Wald: Connecting caring with activism. *Nursing and Health Care, 14*(3), 122-129.

Baldwin, J., Conger, C., Abegglen, J., et al. (1998). Population-focused and community-based nursing—Moving toward clarification of concepts. *Public Health Nursing, 15*(1), 12-18.

Bigbee, J., & Crowder, E. (1985). The Red Cross Rural Nursing Service: An innovative model of public health nursing delivery. *Public Health Nursing, 2*(2), 109-121.

Brainard, A. M. (1985). *The evolution of public health nursing*. New York: Garland. (Original work published in 1922. Philadelphia: W. B. Saunders.)

Brooten, D., Kumar, S., Brown, L., (1986). A randomized clinical trial of early hospital discharge and home follow-up of very-low-birth-weight infants. *New England Journal of Medicine, 315*, 934-938.

Buhler-Wilkerson, K. (1985). Public health nursing: In sickness or in health? *American Journal of Public Health, 75*(10), 1155-1161.

Ciliska, D., Woodcox, V., & Isaacs, S. (1992). A descriptive study of the attachment of public health nurses to family physicians' offices. *Public Health Nursing, 9*(1), 53-57.

Duffy, J. (1990). *The saintarians: A history of American public health*. Urbana: University of Illinois Press.

Erickson, E. (1996). To pauperize or empower: Public health nursing at the turn of the twentieth and twenty-first centuries. *Public Health Nursing, 13*(3), 163-169.

Fitzpatrick, M. L. (1975). *The national organisation for public health nursing, 1912-1952: Development of a practice field*. New York: National League for Nursing.

Gardner, M. S. (1936). *Public health nursing* (3rd ed.). New York: Macmillan.

Goodnow, M. (1928). *Outlines of nursing history* (4th ed.). Philadelphia: W. B. Saunders.

Hamilton, D. (1988). Clinical excellence, but too high a cost: The Metropolitan Life Insurance Company Visiting Nurse Service (1909-1953). *Public Health Nursing, 5*(4), 235-240.

Hanlon, J. J., & Pickett, G. E (Eds.). (1984). *Public health: Administration and practice* (8th ed.). St. Louis: Mosby.

Haupt, A. (1953). Forty years of teamwork in public health nursing. *American Journal of Nursing, 53*(1), 81-84.

Hays, J. (1989). Florence Nightingale and the India sanitary reforms. *Public Health Nursing, 6*(3), 152-154.

Heymann, D (Ed.). (2004). *Control of communicable disease manual* (18th ed.). Washington, DC: American Public Health Association.

Institute of Medicine. (1988). *The future of public health*. Washington, DC: National Academy Press.

Keepnews, D. (1998). New opportunities and challenges for APRNs. *American Journal of Nursing, 98*(1), 62-64.

Kosidlak, J. (1999). The development and implementation of a population-based intervention model for public health nursing practice. *Public Health Nursing, 16*(5), 311-320.

Kraus, H. P. (1980). *The settlement house movement in New York City, 1886-1914*. New York: Arno Press.

Last, J. (1992). Scope and methods of prevention. In J. Last & R. Wallace (Eds.), *Public health and preventive medicine*. Norwalk, CT: Appleton & Lange.

Lee, P. (1993, September). *Key note: Health care reform and public health*. Paper presented at the Baltimore City Health Department 200th Anniversary Celebration Conference, Baltimore, MD.

Lie, L. (1992). Health consultation services to family day care homes in Minneapolis, Minnesota. *Journal of School Health, 62*(1), 29-31.

Maiese, D., & Fox, C. (1998). *Laying the foundation for "Healthy People 2010"—The first year of consultation*. Washington, DC: U.S. Department of Health and Human Services, Office of Disease Prevention and Health Promotion.

McClure, L. (1984). Teamwork, myth or reality: Community nurses' experience with general practice attachment. *Journal of Epidemiology and Community Health, 38*, 68-74.

Minnesota Department of Health, Division of Community Health Services, Section of Public Health Nursing. (1997). *Public health interventions: Examples from public health nursing*. St. Paul: Author.

Monteiro, L. A. (1985). Florence Nightingale on public health nursing. *American Journal of Public Health, 75*(2), 181-186.

Olds, D., Henderson, C., Phelps, C., et al. (1993). Effect of prenatal and infancy nurse home visitation on government spending. *Medical Care, 31*(2), 155-174.

Poole, E. (1932). *Nurses on horseback*. New York: Macmillan.

Pryor, E. (1987). *Clara Barton: Professional angel*. Philadelphia: University of Pennsylvania Press.

Quad Council of Public Health Nursing Organizations. (1999). *Scope and standards of public health nursing practice*. Washington, DC: American Nurses Association.

Riportella-Muller, R., Selby, M., Salmon, M., et al. (1991). Specialty roles in community health nursing: A national survey of educational needs. *Public Health Nursing, 8*(2), 81-89.

Roberts, D., & Heinrich, J. (1985). Public health nursing comes of age. *American Journal of Public Health, 75*(10), 1162-1172.

Schorr, L. (1989). *Within our reach: Breaking the cycle of disadvantage*. New York: Doubleday.

Shalala, D. (1992). Nursing and society—The unfinished agenda for the twenty-first century. In *National League for Nursing: Perspectives in nursing 1991-1993* (pp. 3-8). New York: National League for Nursing.

Suchman, E. A. (1963). *Sociology and the field of public health*. New York: Russell Sage Foundation.

U.S. Census Bureau. (1996a). *Population projections of the United States by age, sex, race, and Hispanic origin: 1995 to 2050 (CPR-P25–1130)*. Washington, DC: U.S. Government Printing Office.

U.S. Census Bureau. (1996b). *Projections of the number of households and families in the United States: 1995 to 2010*. Washington, DC: U.S. Government Printing Office.

U.S. Department of Health and Human Services. (1985). *Consensus Conference on the Essentials of Public Health Nursing Practice and Education: Report of the conference*. Rockville, MD: Author.

U.S. Department of Health and Human Services. (1997). *The Registered Nurse population 1996: Findings from the national Sample of Registered Nurses*. Washington, DC: Health Resources and Service Administration, Bureau of Health Professions, Division of Nursing.

U.S. Department of Health and Human Services. (1998). *Healthy People 2010: Draft for public comment*. Washington, DC: U.S. Government Printing Office.

U.S. Department of Health and Human Services. (2000). *Healthy People 2010: Understanding and improving health* (2nd ed.). Washington, DC: U.S. Government Printing Office.

U.S. Department of Health and Human Services. (2006). *Healthy People 2010: Midterm*. Washington, DC: U.S. Government Printing Office.

U.S. Department of Health and Human Services. (2007). *Healthy People 2020: The road ahead*. Retrieved November 10, 2007 from *http://www.healthypeople.gov/hp2020*.

Ward, D. (1989). Public health nursing and the future of public health. *Public Health Nursing, 6*(4), 163-168.

Waters, Y. (1912). *Visiting nursing in the United States*. New York: Russell Sage Foundation, Charities Publication Committee.

White, R. (1978). *Social change and the development of the nursing profession: A study of the poor law nursing service 1848-1948*. London: Henry Kimpton.

Winslow, C.-E. A. (1984). *The evolution and significance of the modern public health campaign*. South Burlington, VT: Journal of Public Health Policy. (Original work published in 1923. New Haven, CT: Yale University Press.)

Zotti, M., Brown, P., & Stotts, R. C. (1996). Community based nursing versus community health nursing: What does it all mean? *Nursing Outlook, 44*(5), 211-217.

Suggested Readings

Abrams, S. (2005). "The expectation gap": A look at the Sybil Palmer Bellos lecture by Ruth B. Freeman, 1970. *Public Health Nursing, 22*(1), 82-86.

American Nurses Association. (2000). *Public health nursing: A partnership for healthy populations*. Washington, DC: Author.

American Nurses Association. (2007). *Public health nursing: Scope and standards of practice*. Silver Spring, MD: Author.

Backer, B. (1993). Lillian Wald: Connecting caring with activism. *Nursing and Health Care, 14*(3), 122-129.

Barger, S., & Rosenfield, P. (1993). Models in community health care: Findings from a national study of community nursing centers. *Nursing and Health Care, 14*(8), 431-462.

Buhler-Wilkerson, K. (1993). Bringing care to the people: Lillian Wald's legacy to public health nursing. *American Journal of Public Health, 83*(12), 1778-1786.

Chinn, P. (2008). *Peace and power: Creative leadership for building community* (7th ed.). Sudbury, MA: Jones & Bartlett.

Erickson, E. (1996). To pauperize or empower: Public health nursing at the turn of the twentieth and twenty-first centuries. *Public Health Nursing, 13*(3), 163-169.

Fondiller, S. (1999). Virginia M. Ohlson: International icon in public health nursing. *Nursing Outlook, 47*(3), 108-113.

Keller, L., Strohschein, S., Lia-Hoagberg, B., et al. (1998). Population-based public health nursing interventions: A model from practice. *Public Health Nursing, 15*(3), 207-215.

King, M., & Erickson, G. (2006). Development of public health nursing competencies: An oral history. *Public Health Nursing, 23*(2), 196-201.

Knollmueller, R., & Abrams, S. (2005). Beverly C. Flynn, an oral history with a twentieth century activist. *Public Health Nursing, 22*(2), 180-185.

Milio, N. (1971). *9226 Kercheval: The store front that did not burn.* Ann Arbor: University of Michigan Press.

Minnesota Department of Health, Division of Community Health Services, Public Health Nursing Section. (2001). *Public health interventions: Applications for public health nursing practice.* St. Paul: Author.

Reverby, S (Ed.). (1984). *Lamps on the prairie: A history of nursing in Kansas.* New York: Garland. (Original work compiled by Works Projects Administration, Writer's Program, and published in 1942.)

Rosen, G. (1955). *A history of public health.* New York: MD Publications.

Salmon, M. (1993). Public health nursing—The opportunity of a century [Editorial]. *American Journal of Public Health, 83*(12), 1674-1675.

Salmon, M., & Peoples-Sheps, M. (1989). Infant mortality and public health nursing: A history of accomplishments, a future of challenges. *Nursing Outlook, 37,* 6-7, 51.

Wald, L. (1936). *Windows on Henry Street.* Boston: Little, Brown.

Zerwekh, J. (1993). Going to the people— Public health nursing today and tomorrow (commentary). *American Journal of Public Health, 83*(12), 1676-1678.

3

The United States Health Care System

Frances A. Maurer

FOCUS QUESTIONS

What are the basic features and components of the U.S. health care system?

What distinguishes the U.S. health care system from those of other developed countries?

Why do community/public health nurses need to understand the health care system?

What are the differences between direct and indirect services and public- and private-sector health care services?

What are the two competing foci of care? Is one focus of care more prevalent today?

Which agencies have the most important roles in health care issues at the federal, state, and local levels?

How is the private sector of health care delivery organized?

What type of private-sector organization is the major provider of health care services?

What are the major problems with the current health care delivery system?

How have problem-solving strategies impacted health care services, personnel, and cost?

What are the significant changes in health care delivery in the past decade?

What are some of the ongoing proposals for health care reform?

CHAPTER OUTLINE

Our Traditional Health Care System
 Key Features of the U.S. System
 Distinctions from Other Health Care Systems
Components of the U.S. Health Care System
 Organizational Structure
 Management and Oversight
 Financing Mechanisms
 Resources
 Health Services
 Consumer
Direct and Indirect Services and Providers
Public and Private Sectors
Public Sector: Government's Authority and Role in Health Care
 Federal Government
 State Governments

 Local Governments
Private-Sector Role in Health Care Delivery
 For-Profit Providers and Organizations
 Role of Insurance and Other Third-Party Payers
 Managed Care
 Voluntary Component of the Private Sector
Public and Private Health Care Sectors before 1965
 Providers of Health Care
 Focus of Care: Private Sector
 Focus of Care: Public Sector
Public and Private Sectors, 1965 to 1992
 Medicare and Medicaid
 Cost Concern and Containment Efforts
 Efforts at Health Planning
 Competing Focuses of Care: Prevention or Cure

 Emphasis on State Control and Administration of Health Programs
 Rising Number of Uninsured
Public and Private Sectors Today
 Continuing Shift in Federal and State Relationships
 Power Conflicts within the System
 Specialization and Fragmentation
 Quality-of-Care Concerns
 Strategies Employed to Address Problems
A National Health Care System?
 Single-Payer System
 All-Payer System
 States and Universal Coverage
 Integrated Delivery Systems: The Present Reality
 Vested Interests
Challenges for the Future

KEY TERMS

Decentralization
Direct care providers
Direct care services
Free market
Gross domestic product (GDP)
Health care system

Home care
Indirect care services
Out-of-pocket expenses
Primary prevention
Private sector
Public sector

Secondary prevention
Tertiary prevention
Third-party reimbursement
Universal coverage
Vested interests
Wellness centers

The United States is in the midst of dramatic changes in the organizational structure and delivery of health care. Mergers and acquisitions have consolidated medical service providers into fewer, but larger, corporate models (Harrington & Estes, 2008a). Managed care is becoming a more popular form of health care delivery service. Technology has expanded the boundaries of treatment for difficult medical conditions and increased the cost of treatment. State and federal budgets crises are forcing reductions in government support for health care services, at a time when the number of people without health insurance continues to climb. Quality-of-care issues are a rising public concern. The cost of care, the problems of access to care, and the increasing concerns over the quality of health care have renewed the debate over the question of whether this country should adopt some form of national health coverage for all citizens.

In 1994, President Clinton attempted national health care reform. Although there was popular support for change, there was also vigorous opposition. A significant public relations campaign led by health industry providers, such as health maintenance organizations (HMOs), hospitals, pharmaceutical companies, and other health-related businesses, were successful in defeating the initiative (Gold, 1999; Navarro, 1995). Ironically, there has been a substantial shift toward managed health care, one of the principle recommendations of President Clinton's Task Force (White House Domestic Policy Council, 1993). The main difference is in oversight responsibility. The Clinton Task Force envisioned oversight as a public-sector function; instead, it is a private-sector, corporate responsibility. Today, the U.S. health care delivery system remains a system in transition. Public concerns about access and quality of care have resulted in piecemeal legislative attempts to protect consumers' rights and improve health services.

A **health care system** is the organizational structure in which health care is delivered to a population. What kind of health care system does the United States have? What are its component parts? This chapter examines the current structure and principal areas of concern of the U.S. health care system. At the end of the chapter, potential directions for further change are explored.

Few people really stop to think about the health care system and the organizational structure that delivers care, unless they have an unsatisfactory personal encounter. Consumer and health professional dissatisfaction is building, leading to critical questions about the delivery system, identification of areas for change, and suggestions about how the system might change.

Until recently, most Americans, including most health professionals, have tended to view the health care system as inflexible and unchangeable. In fact, the system is responsive to outside influence (Figure 3-1). Changes and modifications occur, although change usually takes place slowly and *incrementally* because the system is so large. For example, the role of nurse practitioners was gradually expanded over a long period. Discontent periodically builds to such a peak that significant change occurs in a relatively short time. For example, dissatisfaction with the financial burdens and limited access to medical care for older Americans led to the enactment of the Medicare program in 1965. Concern over health care costs in the 1990s led to an increasing reliance on managed care organizations as health care providers. Currently, the country

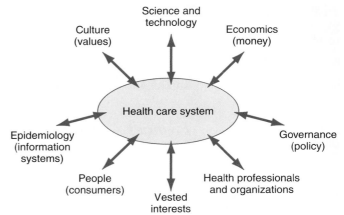

FIGURE 3-1 Influences on the health care system.

is again experiencing dissatisfaction with health care delivery (Mechanic, 2008; Patel & Rushefsky, 2006). President George W. Bush and the U.S. Congress have passed a prescription drug plan for Medicare recipients. **Primary prevention,** the promotion of healthy behaviors and reduction of health risks, is once again a popular concept. Former Congressman Newt Gingrich (2002), who helped defeat the Clinton health plan, is now espousing a more preventive, consumer-focused delivery system. Again, there exists a window of opportunity for health care change.

Health care professionals bear a responsibility to know and understand the system in which they function because it has considerable impact on both their behavior and the health behavior of the people they serve. Nurses should be cognizant of the issues that affect their nursing practice both in the workplace and in the broader context of the entire health care system. Beyond its influence on their personal nursing practice, community health nurses must understand the impact of the system on individual clients, groups, and communities.

Currently, health care is neither available nor accessible to everyone. Millions lack health insurance and are unable to pay for basic services. Every day, community health nurses see people who are denied basic services and others with serious illness who delay treatment because of cost. Because the professional practice of nursing is built around the promotion of health, the prevention of illness, and the restoration of health to all in need, it is hard for community health nurses to see people in need and know that, for some, they can offer no solution to the difficulties in accessing health care.

Ultimately, the real impact of any health care system must be measured in terms of the people it serves: How healthy is our population? How does our health status compare with that of other nations? Does our health care system prevent premature death and disability and provide good care to most of its citizens? Nurses need basic information about the health care system so that they can make informed judgments about the efficacy of the current system and the impact of suggested reforms.

OUR TRADITIONAL HEALTH CARE SYSTEM

When compared with health care systems in other developed countries, the delivery network in the United States seems disorganized and confusing (Sultz & Young, 2004). The U.S.

health care system has been defined as a system without a system, a fragmented system, and a nonsystem (Congressional Budget Office, 1992; Geyman, 2008; Harrington & Estes, 2008b; Shi & Singh, 2001). There is no central organization that plans and links the various elements into an integrated and purposeful whole. Some argue that as disjointed and decentralized as it might be, it is still a system—a system that continues to evolve in response to societal and market pressures (Patel & Rushefsky, 2006).

KEY FEATURES OF THE U.S. SYSTEM

Three prominent features of the U.S. system help explain, to some degree, the structure of the system and the manner in which it evolved. These features include highly decentralized governance, a strong emphasis on a laissez-faire philosophy, and an abundance of economic resources.

Decentralization

Consistent with other aspects of governance in the United States, legal governance and regulation of the health care delivery system are highly decentralized. The government was designed by individuals whose previous experiences led them to mistrust a highly centralized, autocratic system. Their solution was a decentralized federated system with checks and balances at each level. With **decentralization,** local communities, states, and the federal government share responsibilities for regulation and provision of services to the population; health care services are no exception. The United States has a delivery system in which funding, planning, regulation, and service delivery are influenced by city, county, state, and federal government policies, as well as by the policies of nongovernmental organizations, such as businesses.

Laissez-Faire Philosophy

The free market economy of the United States encourages a laissez-faire approach. There is no centralized planning structure. In a **free market,** private enterprise is allowed to develop goods and services as it chooses and to offer them to the clientele, or market, it selects. The health service market is no exception. Private individuals, groups, or corporations can plan, offer, and deliver health care to the target groups they wish to serve. Hospital owners or managers, physicians, and philanthropists, not the government, determine the organizational structure of U.S. health care. As with any business operation, payment is expected for service provided. In this country, a portion of the population cannot pay for service. For those unable to pay, the question of whether health care is a right or a privilege becomes critical. Debate on this question has raged since the nation's inception (Feldstein, 2005; Flint, 1997; Gebbie, 2007; Lindblom, 1953; Merrill, 1994; Reinhardt, 1986; Wilensky, 1975). Those who espouse a totally free market system support a laissez-faire attitude toward health care services. They consider health care a privilege, rather than a right, and would not support government intervention to ensure health care for those who cannot pay. Those who consider health care a right, rather than a privilege, would support action aimed at providing health care services to all.

In this country, health care is provided to the population by a combination of private and public means. Our bent toward a free market economy has encouraged development of a private, entrepreneurial delivery system and personal responsibility for

medical expenses (Sultz & Young, 2004). This private subsystem serves middle- and upper-income Americans who can afford to pay for their care.

Public concerns, however, do not allow a totally laissez-faire approach. Most Americans support the idea of basic health care services for all (Center on Policy Attitudes, 2000; Kover & Knickman, 2005). The public health community's commitment to the ethical position of providing the greatest good for the greatest number supports universal access to care rather than the laissez-faire approach. The government has gradually undertaken to provide some support to those persons who cannot afford to pay for health care. The public subsystem tends to care primarily for the poor and special populations.

Abundant Resources

Although the United States is a wealthy country, its economic resources for health care are limited. We spend more on health, in actual dollars, than most other countries. In 2005, health care expenditures were $1987.7 billion, or 16% of the gross domestic product (Centers for Medicare and Medicaid Services [CMS], 2007). The United States has devoted large sums of money to research and has led the way in development and use of complex and expensive medical procedures and equipment, such as organ transplantation, in vitro fertilization, and magnetic resonance imaging.

Decentralized governance, mass expenditures, and a free market philosophy have helped to shape the existing health care system. As various aspects of the system are examined in this chapter, it would be useful to attempt to identify how each of these elements has an impact on a particular area of practice or delivery of care to population subgroups.

DISTINCTIONS FROM OTHER HEALTH CARE SYSTEMS

Most developed countries have national health care programs administered by the government. The U.S. system is unique. It has neither a national health care plan nor a central administration to deliver health care to its people (Brown, 2001; Patel & Rushefsky, 2006). In Chapter 5, various health care models used by other developed countries are discussed.

Health Planning

Countries with national health care systems engage in more comprehensive health planning. Central planning is possible because the government has the means to influence services either by providing direct care or by reimbursing the cost of care for most of its citizens.

In contrast, the United States has engaged in little central health planning. The federal government is becoming more involved in national health planning and has established national health objectives. These objectives are only guidelines and do not have the force of law. Currently, those segments of the health care system not directly under federal control are free to ignore or address the objectives as they choose.

Health Insurance and Health Status

The most frequent criticism of our health care system is that delivery of "basic" (primary and preventive care) services is not readily available to the entire population (McKinsey and Company, 2007; Sultz & Young, 2004). Despite large health care expenditures, a significant segment of the population does not receive care. At least 50.4 million Americans have no health coverage (Roberts & Rhoades, 2007). The U.S. government provides fewer public monies for health care than does any other developed country (Rodwin, 2005; Torrens, 2002). Most commit more public funds and provide more services while spending less of their **gross domestic product (GDP)** on health care. GDP is a measure of all goods and services sold in the United States. Chapter 4 provides a more detailed discussion of health care spending and services in other countries.

If the U.S. system provided a better standard of health than the systems of other countries, the differences in expenditures of public funds would be more understandable. That is not the case, however. Comparison of infant mortality and life expectancy for eight selected countries indicates that the United States ranks lowest in life expectancy and highest in infant mortality (Figure 3-2). In fact, the United States ranks nineteenth of 19 industrialized nations in life expectancy and infant mortality (Hogberg, 2006; World Health Organization [WHO], 2007). In addition, the United States has a higher infant mortality rate than Andorra, the Czech Republic, Malta, Poland, and South Korea (WHO, 2007).

COMPONENTS OF THE U.S. HEALTH CARE SYSTEM

The U.S. health care system is complex, and it is difficult to reduce all of its elements, influences, and decision makers into a simple diagram. Figure 3-3 provides a basic model that identifies the essential components that form the basis of the U.S. system. The model illustrates some of the interrelationships. Each component is affected by and has impact on the others. Ultimately, the system links the consumer to health care services.

ORGANIZATIONAL STRUCTURE

In health care, structure significantly influences function. Structure determines how goods or resources are acquired and how services are dispersed or provided. The organizational structure of U.S. health care is a disjointed combination of public and private agencies, including government (federal, state, county, city, and local) and voluntary, charitable, entrepreneurial, and professional agencies and organizations. All of these agencies are involved in decisions that have an impact on the delivery of health care. Agencies sometimes operate with competing or overlapping objectives and functions. Because of the absence of a central organization, gaps exist in services and in population groups served. (It is helpful to keep this concept in mind as the discussion continues.)

MANAGEMENT AND OVERSIGHT

The three key features of our health care system were identified earlier. Two of these are important to the management aspect of health care. Both decentralized governance and a laissez-faire philosophy have created the environment within which oversight functions. A single overseer or manager is lacking, as is a central plan for organizing and delivering health care. Instead, multiple levels of government interrelate and interact with multiple levels of private-sector management in a bewildering arrangement. For example, in the State Children's Health Insurance Program (SCHIP), there is both federal and state funding and oversight. The health care services the children receive come from physicians, hospitals, managed care organizations, and other health providers. Those providers, in turn, must conform to Medicaid and SCHIP regulation and review.

Multiple Levels of Government

Within government itself, there are planning, legislative, and regulatory management efforts at the federal, state, and county levels. City government lends yet another level in some instances. Each layer directs services within its scope of operation. Because of the decentralized nature of American government, federal agencies usually manage specific programs by delegating day-to-day administration and oversight to local authorities. Federal agencies do so, however, only after devising guidelines or criteria that must be met by the specific program.

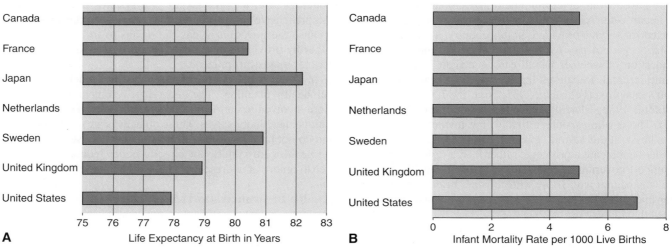

FIGURE 3-2 A, Life expectancy at birth, selected countries, 2005. **B,** Infant mortality rate per 1000 live births, selected countries, 2005. (Data from World Health Organization. [2007]. World health statistics: Core health indicators. Retrieved May 11, 2007 from *http://www.who.int/whosis/diatbase/core_select_process.cfm*.)

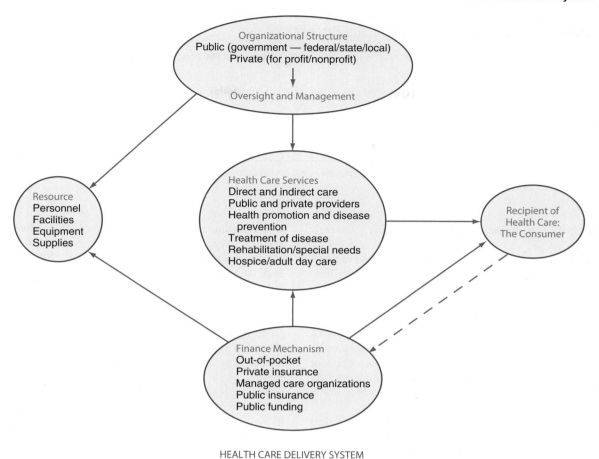

HEALTH CARE DELIVERY SYSTEM

FIGURE 3-3 Components of a health care delivery system.

For example, the Women, Infants, and Children (WIC) Program has multiple levels of managers and requirements. The WIC Program managers in the field, who actually provide service to the target groups, must comply with criteria that have been set at the federal and state levels. The WIC Program field director (county, city, or geographic district operation) reports to the state agency responsible for the program. The state manager, in turn, reports to an official in the U.S. Department of Agriculture. That individual, in turn, answers to both the President (executive branch) and the Congress (legislative branch) to ensure that management directives and budgeting requirements are followed.

Variety of Private Management Styles

Management, planning, and oversight methods of private organizations vary widely and are not easily categorized. They include centralized and decentralized, democratic and autocratic, and laissez-faire and extremely regulated management efforts. Most private facilities operate with a board of directors that influences the planning and administrative process.

Private facilities and organizations must comply with applicable federal, state, and local regulations, which place constraints on how they may operate, the types of services they may provide, and whether they may continue to offer services. State licensing is an example of regulatory activity. For instance, states conduct inspections and issue licenses for nursing homes and home care agencies. If the homes are not able to meet state standards, they are penalized by fines or forced to close. Failure to meet licens-

ing standards can also result in loss of revenue, because some reimbursement mechanisms are tied to continued licensure.

FINANCING MECHANISMS

The financing of health care services is discussed in detail in Chapter 4. In brief, financial support is derived from a variety of sources, both private and public (Figure 3-3). Private sources include personal expenditures of individuals and families, private insurance payments, corporate expenditures, and charitable contributions. Public sources are composed of federal, state, and local government revenues directed toward health care services.

RESOURCES

Health resources are considered essential for health care system functioning. These include (1) health professionals, who constitute the personnel who run the system; (2) facilities such as hospitals and other structural elements from which care is provided; and (3) health supplies and equipment. Because space is limited, only some of the relevant resources for health care delivery are highlighted in this chapter. Community health nurses need to know about health care resources, including the supply of other health care professionals, because resources influence the availability and accessibility of health care services to those in need.

Personnel

People are a crucial health care resource. Health professionals display considerable variety in education, skill, and practice setting. Table 3-1 presents some of the most common

TABLE 3-1   Comparisons of Selected Health Professions

Profession	Number	Supply per 100,000 Population	Average Salary ($)
Physician	567,000	204	166,420*
Dentist	150,000	54	129,920
Optometrist	34,000	12	88,410
Pharmacist	230,000	64	84,900
Physician assistant	62,000	22	69,410
Registered nurse	2,400,000	866	52,330

Data from U.S. Department of Labor, Bureau of Labor Statistics. (2006). *Occupational outlook handbook: 2006-2007 edition.* Washington, DC: Government Printing Office.
*Average salary for internal medicine.

health care professionals, their accessibility (supply), and their average salary levels.

Physicians. In the 1960s, both federal and state governments offered medical schools financial support and eased certification requirements for foreign-trained physicians to increase the number of practicing physicians. These actions increased the supply of physicians. Currently, there are 204 physicians per 100,000 population (U.S. Department of Labor, Bureau of Labor Statistics, 2006). Currently there are conflicting opinions on whether there will be long-term physician surplus or shortage. The projected supply is more than adequate to meet the needs of the population through 2030 (Blumenthal, 2004; Pew Commission, 1998).

Despite an adequate supply of doctors, accessibility to primary care service is problematic for many people. Two factors combine to restrict client access to primary care physicians: (1) geographic maldistribution and (2) specialization (Brewer, 2005). Physicians tend to concentrate in urban rather than rural areas. The Northeast and West have the highest ratios of physicians to population, and the South has the lowest. Most physicians (about 65%) specialize; only 35% are engaged in primary care practice (American Medical Association, 2004). In contrast, other developed countries restrict specialty practice, and 50% to 70% of physicians are engaged in primary care. Few American physicians specialize in community health medicine.

Registered Nurses. Registered nurses constitute the largest group of health professionals. There are 2.4 million licensed registered nurses in the United States (U.S. Department of Labor, Bureau of Labor Statistics, 2006). Most are salaried employees. Hospitals remain their largest single employer, although hospital-based nurse employment continues to decline (Figure 3-4). Government data are not current for all sources of nurse employment; Figure 3-4 represents employment areas found in a 2004 sample survey that lumps some areas into a single category—for example, extended-care facilities. Community-based employment opportunities for registered nurses continue to expand, although the proportion practicing in public health have declined (see Chapter 1).

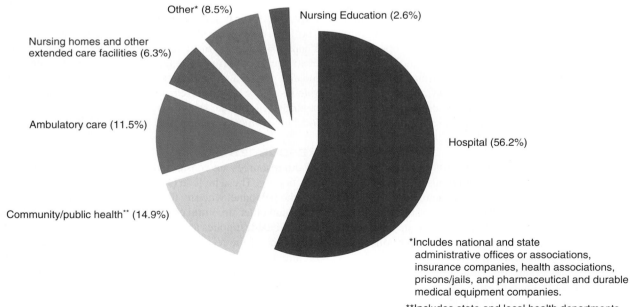

Other* (8.5%)
Nursing Education (2.6%)
Nursing homes and other extended care facilities (6.3%)
Ambulatory care (11.5%)
Hospital (56.2%)
Community/public health** (14.9%)

*Includes national and state administrative offices or associations, insurance companies, health associations, prisons/jails, and pharmaceutical and durable medical equipment companies.

**Includes state and local health departments, visiting nursing services and other health agencies, community health centers, student health services, and occupational services.

FIGURE 3-4 Registered nurse practice settings. (Data from U.S. Department of Health and Human Services, Health Resources and Services Administration, Bureau of Health Professionals, Division of Nursing. [2006]. *National sample survey of registered nurses, 2004.* Washington DC: U.S. Government Printing Office.)

Approximately 15% of registered nurses practice some form of community health nursing. Another 11.5% are involved with ambulatory care facilities that offer some community-related services.

Federal government estimates project a decline in the proportion of registered nurses practicing in hospital settings and an increased need for registered nurses prepared in community-type practice, including public health and ambulatory care. If health care reform initiatives continue to stress community- and home-based care, the need for community-based nursing services will create additional demand.

There have been cyclical shortages in the supply of registered nurses, but there is serious concern that the current shortfall may be more protracted and difficult to remedy (Unruh & Fottler, 2008). In the past, shortages have been alleviated by a combination of increase in salaries and increased enrollment of students in nursing programs (Brewer, 2005). Today enrollment in nursing programs is not expanding to meet the need. This is coupled with an aging registered nurse workforce. The average age of registered nurses in the workforce is 45.2 years (Health Resources and Services Administration [HRSA], 2006). These two factors may increase the length and severity of the current shortage period.

Nonphysician Practitioners/Extenders. Nonphysician practitioners/extenders are professionals who are trained to provide primary care in place of physicians and are either physician's assistants or advanced nurse practitioners. Physician's assistants are usually nonnurses with advanced education and certification.

Advanced nurse practitioners include nurse anesthetists, nurse clinical specialists, nurse practitioners, and nurse midwives. In most states, the Nurse Practice Act allows independent practice and direct reimbursement for nurse practitioners and nurse midwives, although some limitations persist (Brewer, 2005; Pulcini & Hart 2007a). Of the approximately 203,000 physician extenders, approximately 69% are nurse practitioners (HRSA, 2006; U.S. Bureau of the Census, 2007). Many nonphysician practitioners

serve populations that do not attract physicians, especially the poor and chronically ill (Brewer, 2005; Sultz & Young, 2004). Advanced nurse practitioners are especially good at working with the chronically ill because of their background in health teaching and their interest in health promotion and health maintenance. Nurse practitioners and nurse midwives are commonly employed in community health centers and other community agencies. Studies indicate that physician extenders compare favorably with physicians in quality of care delivered and patient satisfaction with service (see Chapter 4).

Other Professional Personnel. The supply of *dentists, pharmacists,* and *optometrists* is sufficient to meet demand into the future. Most do not work in public health. Dental care is expensive; as a result the poor and uninsured frequently do not receive dental care. If dental care were to become part of the Medicare/Medicaid programs, then the demand for dentists would outstrip the current supply. The demand for optometrists is expected to grow because of the lens correction needs of aging baby boomers.

Allied Health Professionals. During the past several decades, a variety of new health care workers have emerged to assist the more established professional groups in providing care to the population. A list of selected allied health workers and the approximate numbers in each category are given in Figure 3-5. Their specialized occupational activities are wide ranging. The allied health worker most often involved in substantial direct client care is the *licensed practical nurse (LPN)* or *licensed vocational nurse.* Historically, the practical nurse assisted registered nurses, but licensed vocational and practical nurses have assumed responsibilities once thought to be the sole province of professional nurses. In some states and clinical situations, LPNs administer medications, manage units, and take verbal orders from physicians. LPNs have limited experience in public health settings, although they are employed in ambulatory care and home health agencies.

Nursing aides provide personal care services in a variety of settings. They work under the direct supervision of registered

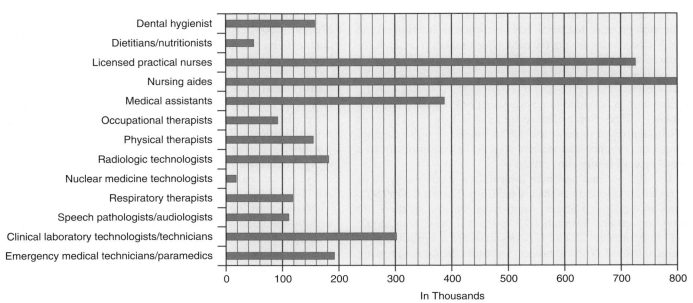

FIGURE 3-5 Supply of allied health professionals. (Data from *Occupational outlook handbook, 2006-2007.* [2006]. Washington DC: U.S. Department of Labor, Bureau of Labor Statistics.)

BOX 3-1   Types of Health Care Facilities

Inpatient
General hospitals
Special hospitals
Psychiatric residential treatment centers
Nursing homes:
    Skilled nursing facilities
    Intermediate care facilities
Resident care facilities
Other types of residential homes:
    Adult homes
    Halfway houses

Outpatient
Hospital-based clinics and emergency rooms
Local health departments and clinics
Specialty programs and services
Alcoholism programs and services
Birth centers
Drug programs and services
Mental health programs and services
Women's clinics
Family planning centers
Ambulatory care walk-in facilities
Physician practices:
    Solo
    Group
    Partnership
Professional corporations
Short-stay surgical centers
Renal dialysis centers
Rehabilitation centers
Hospice/respite care
Home health agencies
Wellness and health promotion centers
Workplace health services

---

nurses or LPNs. Some aides are certified through a formal education process, but many have informal instruction on the job. Nursing aides are poorly paid, which makes it difficult for agencies to retain competent, reliable employees.

Facilities

Health care is provided in a wide variety of inpatient and outpatient facilities. Some of these are listed in Box 3-1. The types of care delivered in facilities can be limited or wide ranging, simple or complex, and tailored to specific conditions or to a broad span of health concerns.

Box 3-2 outlines pertinent information about and services provided by selected health care facilities. There are 5759 hospitals in the United States. Approximately 90% of these are short-stay general hospitals (U.S. Bureau of the Census, 2007, p. 114). More than 85% of U.S. hospitals are nonprofit or government owned. Nursing homes constitute the fastest growing segment of this care market. Earlier hospital discharges and an ever-increasing population of elderly persons are the reasons for rapid growth of nursing homes. There are 16,081 nursing homes, three times the number of acute care hospitals (U.S. Bureau of the Census, 2007, p. 113).

Before 1960, *mental care/psychiatric hospitals* were separate facilities operated primarily by state and local governments. Starting in the 1960s, efforts to provide psychiatric patients with the least restrictive environment resulted in a large number of discharges from these institutions. Chapter 33 provides a more detailed discussion of the changes in mental health services. Deinstitutionalization did not result in the closing of many facilities, but most state and local hospitals significantly reduced bed capacity.

Primary care in clinics has always been provided to serve poor populations, but it is now becoming popular with other consumer groups. The greatest number of new *ambulatory care clinics* have been those set up to attract middle-class consumers rather than low-income or public assistance clients. Consumers who find the clinics particularly attractive are those with no regular physician who want quick treatment for a specific complaint. Hospitals, health corporations, or physicians in group partnership generally sponsor the new facilities.

Payment at time of service is a common feature of the newer clinics. Many do not process insurance forms as direct payment. Consumers are usually expected to file health insurance and Medicare claims to receive reimbursement for **out-of-pocket expenses** (those expenses paid for directly by the consumer), which may be covered by their insurance carrier.

Wellness centers promote healthy behavior and assist consumers in eliminating or reducing risky behaviors. Wellness centers (also known as *health promotion centers*) and *alternative medicine services* are geared to niche markets, primarily middle-class and wealthy individuals who can afford to pay. Health insurance and employers pay for limited numbers of these services. Some examples of services for which insurance pays are employer exercise programs, smoking cessation programs, and stress reduction programs. In the alternative medicine area, acupuncture is the most frequently covered service.

Home care, care of the client in his or her own home, has surged as the number of elderly grows. Home care is popular because it is cost efficient and often preferred to other types of care (see Chapter 4). Today there are more than 11,160 home care and hospice agencies in the United States, serving over 3.7 million clients (Hospice Association of America, 2007; MedPac, 2006). Approximately 60% of hospices are independent, and the remainder are operated by home health agencies, hospitals, or skilled nursing facilities.

Equipment and Supplies

Health equipment and supplies are another health resource. Materials used in the diagnosis and treatment of specific illnesses, prosthetic devices, eyeglasses, hearing aids, and drugs constitute just a partial list of the types of equipment in this category. The industry is enormous. For example, in 2005 the cost of eyeglasses and medical appliances was $24 billion (CMS, 2007).

Medications are the largest single category. Drugs are a multibillion-dollar industry. In 2005, $234.8 billion was spent on drugs and other nondurable medical supplies (CMS, 2007). Approximately 75% of the drugs sold are prescription medications. Prescription drugs are protected by patent for 17 years. Drug companies derive greater profits from the sale of brand name (patent) drugs, so there is clear incentive to protect and maintain patent rights as long as possible. Most companies, although they could, do not manufacture generic versions of

---

Box 3-2   Selected Health Care Facilities and Services

Hospitals
- Short stay (30 days or less) or long stay (more than 30 days).
- Provide generalized or specialized health care services.
- Control or ownership is nonprofit, for-profit, or governmental.
  - Nonprofit hospitals are controlled by local communities or voluntary organizations (e.g., a religious or charitable organization). They operate at no profit, and expenses must equal revenues each fiscal year. Most offer limited service to nonpaying clients.
- Proprietary hospitals are privately owned, for-profit enterprises. They do not generally accept nonpaying clients.
- Publicly owned hospitals are owned and operated by various levels of government such as the state, county, or city; a few are run by federal agencies. Most were set up to serve indigent clients, although they accept paying clients. Some publicly owned hospitals, especially in larger cities, are teaching hospitals or hospitals with ties to medical schools. Two of the more widely known are Cook County Hospital in Chicago and Bellevue Hospital in New York City.

Long-Term Care Facilities
- Provide care to chronically ill persons or to those needing rehabilitation after discharge from a general hospital. Types of facilities include long-term care hospitals, nursing homes, and rehabilitation centers. The bulk of nursing homes are proprietary, for-profit establishments.

Residential Care Facilities
- Have both a health and social welfare focus.
- Examples include homes for aged persons, custodial residential schools for blind and deaf persons, hospice care for terminally ill persons, halfway houses for mentally ill persons, and alcohol and drug abuse treatment residential units.

Psychiatric Hospitals
- Both publicly and privately managed, provide both short- and long-term care to mentally ill persons.
- Since 1960, there has been growth in privately owned and operated psychiatric facilities. Service is directed primarily to persons who can afford to pay.

- State and local government facilities provide the bulk of care for patients who cannot afford private care.

Ambulatory and Community Care Facilities
- Ambulatory care facilities provide a broad range of both services and health care professionals under one roof.
- There are several types: hospital sited, hospital sponsored offsite, and independent non–hospital affiliated.
- General hospitals provide primary care to patients who do not require hospital admission. Recently, to reduce costs and entice new customers, outpatient services have been promoted heavily as a substitute for inpatient care. Hospitals are now engaged in home health, rehabilitation, health promotion, and other enterprises such as sponsoring walking clubs and mediation classes.
- In addition to hospital outpatient clinics, there are public health, employer-sponsored, school health, charitable, private proprietor owned, and health maintenance organization–operated clinics providing ambulatory care.

Wellness or Health Promotion Centers
- Might be hospital based or free standing.
- Programs offer primary and secondary prevention health-promoting activities.
- Some are narrowly focused on a single issue, such as smoking cessation, breast cancer screening, or pregnancy.
- Others have a broader focus, identifying all health risks to individuals and designing programs tailored to promote or enhance individual health.

Alternative Medicine Service
- Services include acupuncture, aromatherapy, herbal medicine, meditation, and healing touch.

Home-Based Care
- Provides care at home for those with acute and chronic diseases.
- Includes occupational/rehabilitation therapy, custodial care, and skilled nursing care.

---

their own patent drugs until after the 17-year patent limit has expired.

HEALTH SERVICES

Perhaps more important than the system is the final product. What does the system provide for consumers (refer to Figure 3-3)? A complete and comprehensive health system should provide certain essential health care services (Torrens, 2002, p. 20):

- Health promotion/disease prevention
- Emergency medical care
- Ambulatory care
- Inpatient care
- Long-term care
- Services for social and psychologic conditions
- Rehabilitative services
- Dental services
- Pharmaceutical services
- Transportation to services as needed

The U.S. health care system contains most of these elements. However, not every community or individual has easy access to all service elements, and health care services are not well integrated and coordinated. Critics contend that care and consumer needs do not match well. Care is often inappropriate, and services are unevenly and unequally distributed (Commonwealth Fund Commission on a High Performance Health System, 2006; Fiscella & Williams, 2008; Sultz & Young, 2004; Torrens, 2002).

CONSUMER

The consumer is the recipient of services delivered by the system. Ideally services should be planned and implemented to benefit the client. It is the consumer who is most affected by the operational efficiency or inefficiency of health care delivery.

The consumer and health care services should be the focus of the health professions. The consumer is the most vulnerable component and is the most likely to be hurt by ineffective functioning of the system. For example, health care providers might relocate or refuse certain patients (Medicaid patients) to maintain their incomes or to increase their profit margins. The consumers left behind or denied care are not the primary focus in the provider's decision process. Refer to the section in

Chapter 4 on free market failure for a discussion of how system shortcomings might have an impact on consumers.

Some critics suggest that client care is secondary to profit (Cohen & Piotrowska-Haugstetter, 2007; Feldstein, 2005; Shi & Singh, 2001). The health care system is a large business. Improving a population's health is not always the focus when planning and providing services and selecting the consumer groups to whom services will be provided. Profits and services are competing goals. Health care professionals and management personnel often derive greater benefits than the consumer by way of generous salaries, benefits, stock profits, and professional prestige (Congressional Budget Office, 1992; Krauss, 1977; Patel & Rushefsky, 2006).

DIRECT AND INDIRECT SERVICES AND PROVIDERS

In any delivery system, there are direct and indirect services and direct and indirect providers. **Direct care services** are health services delivered to an individual. Physical therapy, nursing care, and doctors' visits are examples of direct services. Direct services are provided in a variety of settings, including hospitals, public health clinics, and, in the case of home health, the home itself. The personnel who provide these types of services are considered **direct care providers.** Most health care personnel in the United States are engaged in direct care.

Indirect care services are those health services that are not personally received by the individual, although they influence health and welfare. Health planning by community agencies, monitoring and regulation of environmental hazards, and inspection of public-use facilities are examples of indirect health services. Health is certainly affected by pollution of food and water sources and by community planning decisions regulating the number of hospital beds or the type of equipment employed in these facilities. The difference is that many of us are not consciously aware of the indirect services and how they affect our health.

PUBLIC AND PRIVATE SECTORS

Direct health care services in the United States are delivered in a two-tiered system of public and private providers. The **private sector** is composed of private organizations, both for-profit businesses and nonprofit organizations. For the most part, private enterprise provides direct services of personal health care for Americans who can pay, either directly (out of pocket) or through third-party payers (private health insurance plans). Some of these providers, particularly hospitals managed by churches and other philanthropic endeavors, provide a certain number of services to community members who cannot pay.

The **public sector** consists of services provided by public funds and public organizations. Services are largely provided by some type of governmental agency. The public sector is concerned with both direct and indirect services. Involvement with direct services is an attempt to provide care for those who cannot pay and for certain other target groups for whom the government is legally required or feels compelled to provide health care, for example, veterans and American Indians. The large numbers of indirect services that are within the government's purview are there because the private sector is not interested in

providing them. Funding for public services comes from local governments and communities and state and federal agencies. Charitable organizations, although part of the private sector, might also provide limited public-sector services.

PUBLIC SECTOR: GOVERNMENT'S AUTHORITY AND ROLE IN HEALTH CARE

Each of the three levels of U.S. government assumes some of the responsibilities for health care. *Indirect services* make up a major portion of services provided by government. In keeping with a free market economy, government usually does not attempt to provide services in areas in which private enterprise satisfactorily provides care.

Various levels of government care for certain population groups not covered by private-sector services. State and local governments are more involved in direct care. Federal, state, and local governmental agencies are frequently involved in administration of a single program or basic service, such as the WIC Program or SCHIP, discussed earlier. How they are involved, or the exact role each plays, is generally the distinguishing element.

FEDERAL GOVERNMENT

The authority for the federal government's involvement is derived from the Constitution of the United States. Although it is not explicitly stated, federal authority is assumed from the charge to provide for the general welfare and from the federal role in the regulation of interstate commerce. The federal government has the power to collect and spend monies for general welfare and to regulate business and organizations that conduct operations in more than one state.

The federal role in health care has expanded, although actual implementation of programs is commonly delegated to the states. Ultimately, the federal government is responsible for protecting the health of its population.

Although all three branches of government make health-related decisions, the President and his or her staff (executive branch) and Congress (legislative branch) make the major policy decisions. These two branches set the tone for delivery of care. They dictate which groups will be served and the manner of service. Both branches are subject to political pressures that influence the decision-making process.

Once policy is decided, federal agencies are responsible for oversight and implementation. These agencies regulate and interpret health law, administer services mandated by law, and are responsible for supervision of compliance with health laws and regulations. Federal agencies are primarily involved in indirect services.

U.S. Department of Health and Human Services

The federal agency with the most health-related responsibilities is the U.S. Department of Health and Human Services (USDHHS). This department has more than 60,944 employees and a budget of $581.5 billion dollars (U.S. Bureau of the Census, 2007). Although the USDHHS is responsible for some direct services, most of its activities involve indirect care, including health planning and resource development, research, health care financing, and regulatory oversight. The USDHHS either carries out these services or delegates responsibility and funding for services to other public and private organizations. The two largest public-sector health programs, Medicare and

Medicaid, are supervised by the USDHHS. The organizational chart in Figure 3-6 illustrates some of the specific responsibilities of the USDHHS. Because the USDHHS responsibilities are varied and complex, only two offices and their functions are outlined in this chapter. Public health and political science texts can provide a more in-depth discussion of the USDHHS for those who wish to investigate this area.

The USDHHS provides both public health and welfare services. Public health functions are provided by the following agencies:

- The National Institutes of Health (NIH) funds and conducts research, including nursing research, which is financed through the National Center for Nursing Research. The NIH can be used as a referral source for clients who require experimental care.
- The Food and Drug Administration (FDA) establishes and enforces safety standards for food, drugs, and cosmetics.

FDA approval is necessary before experimental drugs can be tested and marketed in the United States.
- The Health Resource and Services Administration (HRSA) conducts health resource planning and provides access to essential health services for people who are poor or uninsured, or who live in rural and urban neighborhoods without health care services. It provides comprehensive primary and preventive services through community-based health centers (3000 sites) that serve 9 million clients each year. HRSA funds training of health personnel and provides support services for people with human immunodeficiency virus (HIV) infection/acquired immunodeficiency syndrome (AIDS).
- The Substance Abuse and Mental Health Administration coordinates and funds programs in both areas. Most programs are community based, and some are based in community health agencies.

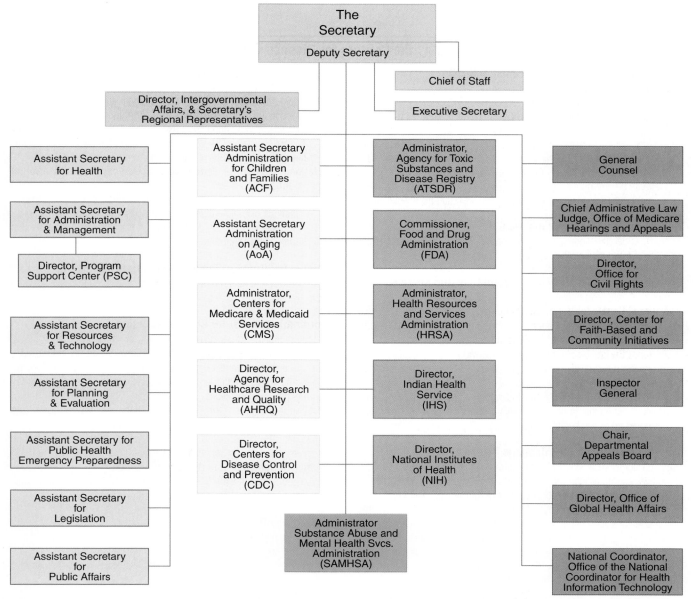

FIGURE 3-6 Organizational chart for the U.S. Department of Health and Human Services.

- The Agency for Toxic Substance and Disease Registry is responsible for preventing health-related problems associated with toxic substances.
- The Indian Health Service provides direct health care services to the American Indian and Alaskan Native populations, and oversight of health care services administered by the American Indian tribes. This agency provides care to approximately 1.5 million persons.
- The Centers for Disease Control and Prevention (CDC) is the primary source of information on communicable diseases and is a vital resource for all public health personnel. Box 3-3 details the scope of services provided by the CDC.
- The Agency for Healthcare Research and Quality is the lead agency for sponsoring and conducting research to improve the quality of health care, reduce costs, improve patient safety, and increase access to essential services.

The three other divisions of the USDHHS concentrate on providing welfare-related services:

- The Centers for Medicare and Medicaid Services (CMS), formerly the Health Care Finance Administration (HCFA), has as its primary responsibility the oversight of the Medicare and Medicaid programs, which constitute 93.5% of the federal budget for personal health care services (CMS, 2007). It also administers SCHIP. Chapter 4 provides detailed program information and explores the role of the CMS in administering these programs and ensuring the quality of the care provided to individuals served by Medicare and Medicaid.
- The Administration for Children and Families (ACF) administers the state/federal welfare programs: Temporary Assistance for Needy Families (TANF), national child support enforcement, and Head Start. It also provides funding assistance for child care, adoption, and foster care.
- The Administration on Aging (AoA) advocates for older Americans. It administers federal programs under the Older American Act, including the Meals on Wheels and home residency assistance programs.

Box 3-3   Scope of Services Provided by the Centers for Disease Control and Prevention (CDC)

Coordinating Center for Environmental Health and Injury Prevention
Includes the following agencies:

National Center for Environmental Health/Agency for Toxic Substances and Disease Registry
Provides national leadership in preventing and controlling disease and death resulting from the interactions between people and their environment.

National Center for Injury Prevention and Control
Prevents death and disability from nonoccupational injuries, including those that are unintentional and those that result from violence.

Coordinating Office for Global Health
Provides leadership, coordination, and support for the CDC's global health activities. Partners with other countries on some projects.

Coordinating Center for Health Information and Service
Includes the following agencies:

National Center for Health Statistics
Provides statistical information that will guide actions and policies to improve the health of the American people.

National Center for Public Health Informatics
Strengthens community practice of public health by building information technology.

National Center for Health Marketing
Provides leadership in health marketing science and in its application to impact public health.

Coordinating Center for Infectious Diseases
Prevents illness, disability, and death caused by infectious diseases in the United States and around the world. Includes the following departments:

National Center for Immunization and Respiratory Disease
Immunization program that brings together vaccine-preventable disease science and research, and immunization activities.

National Center for Zoonotic, Vector-borne, and Enteric Diseases
Program identifies, investigates, diagnoses, treats, and works at preventing zoonotic, vector-borne, food-borne, waterborne, mycotic, and related infections.

National Center for HIV/AIDS, Viral Hepatitis, STD, and TB Prevention
Provides national leadership in preventing and controlling human immunodeficiency virus/acquired immunodeficiency syndrome (HIV/AIDS), viral hepatitis, sexually transmitted diseases (STDs), and tuberculosis (TB). Works to develop and implement collaborative public health interventions nationwide.

National Center for Preparedness, Detection, and Control of Infectious Diseases
Works to improve preparedness for and response to new and complex infectious disease outbreaks. Lead agency to manage and coordinate response to emerging infectious diseases, and integrate and improve clinical laboratories.

National Institute for Occupational Safety and Health
Ensures safety and health of all people in the workplace through research and prevention.

Coordinating Center for Health Promotion
Includes the following departments:

National Center on Birth Defects and Development Disabilities
Provides national leadership for preventing birth defects and developmental disabilities and for improving the health and wellness of people with disabilities.

National Center for Chronic Disease Prevention and Health Promotion
Prevents premature death and disability from chronic diseases and promotes healthy personal behaviors.

Office of Genomics and Disease Prevention
Provides national leadership in fostering understanding of human genomic discoveries and how they can be used.

Office of the Director
Manages and directs the activities of the CDC; provides overall direction to, and coordination of, the scientific/medical programs of the CDC; and provides leadership, coordination, and assessment of administrative management activities.

Data from the Centers for Disease Control and Prevention, Atlanta, GA.

Office of Public Health and Science and the Surgeon General

In 1996, a reorganization of the USDHHS established all the agencies previously under the direction of the Public Health Service (PHS) as independent agencies. The Office of Public Health and Science (OPHS) contains the old administrative functions of the PHS and is responsible to the Office of the Assistant Secretary for Health (Box 3-4). The reorganization dramatically reduced the influence and position of the Surgeon General, who has little power in terms of directing health care policy. Before the reorganization, the Surgeon General had responsibility for the CDC, the FDA, the Indian Health Service, and the NIH, and other departments. After the reorganization the Surgeon General's only real administrative responsibility was the U.S. Public Health Service Commissioned Corps. A subsequent reorganization also removed that responsibility from the Office of the Surgeon General. Now he or she serves in an advisory and educational capacity on public health matters but has no authority to make health care policy.

Several recent Surgeons General have attempted to enhance their impact on health policy by publicizing selected health issues. This probably played a role in the reorganization decision. C. Everett Koop, for example, emphasized public awareness of AIDS, and Antonia Novello highlighted the effects of substance abuse, especially the effects of alcohol and tobacco on adolescents. Joycelyn Elders was the subject of extensive criticism concerning her efforts to address adolescent sexual behavior. She was forced to resign. President Clinton and Congress were unable to agree on a successor, and the office functioned with an acting Surgeon General from 1993 to 1998. Richard Carmona served as Surgeon General from 2002 to 2006 during the presidency of George W. Bush. He testified before Congress that his efforts to address health concerns such as inequality of health care, global health problems, and the health status of prisoners in U.S. correctional facilities were suppressed by political appointees at the USDHHS (Lee & Kaufman, 2007). Dr. Carmona also testified that he resisted efforts to include content that was primarily political rather than scientifically supported positions on health issues as well as efforts to eliminate content on health issues not supported by the administration. He contended that content that was suppressed included the issues identified earlier in this paragraph as well as the mediocre performance of abstinence-only programs supported by the Bush administration. Dr. Carmona was not nominated for a second term, and the post of Surgeon General remains vacant at this time.

Other Federal Agencies

Several other federal agencies provide health-related services. Box 3-5 lists the most important of these and some of their health care responsibilities. Note that most provide indirect services that play an important role in the health and welfare of the population. Imagine the potential for outbreaks of food poisoning if there were no inspection of the food, meat, and poultry produced for public consumption. The current rash of environmental problems, such as air and water pollution, toxic dumps, and food pollutants, point to the need for continued, vigilant health monitoring.

Some federal agencies, including the *Department of Veterans Affairs (VA)* and the *Department of Defense (DOD)*, provide direct health care to specific populations. The VA is an independent agency that reports directly to the President. It is responsible for providing direct health care to certain groups of military veterans, especially those who have service-connected injuries, receive veterans' pensions, are 65 years or older, and/ or are medically indigent. Therefore, the VA serves as a source of care for veterans who have exhausted other health care resources.

The VA operates hospitals that provide inpatient and outpatient medical, surgical, and psychiatric services. It also operates satellite and independent clinics and offers limited nursing home and residential facilities. The VA is a large direct care system with 157 hospitals, 850 community-based clinics, 42 domiciles, and 206 veterans centers (nursing home units) (U.S. Department of Veterans Affairs, 2004). The VA served 5.5. million beneficiaries in 2006 (U.S. Department of Veterans Affairs, 2006).

The DOD provides both direct and indirect care to 9.2 million active-duty military members and their dependents (Smith, 2006). The war in Iraq has stressed the ability of both the DOD and the VA to provide care to wounded active and retired military personnel. Walter Reed Hospital in Washington, DC, was the main focus of media reports related to health care service deficits. However, there is concern that the entire military health care system is overburdened and underfunded, which will severely compromise the ability to care for all military personnel and their families in the years to come.

The DOD provides indirect care for family members of military personnel and retirees through the TRICARE (formerly CHAMPUS) insurance program. The DOD operates hospitals and clinics in the United States as well as overseas and provides limited care to retired career military personnel and their dependents based on availability of resources.

Public/community health is an emphasis in the DOD, which assumes responsibility for the health of all persons living on military bases. Environmental regulation (of food, water, and so forth), preventive health practices, and health promotion activities are public health services provided by the DOD.

Box 3-4 Office of Public Health and Science (OPHS)

The following programs and offices are part of the Office of Public Health and Science, which reports to the Assistant Secretary for Health:

Advisory Committee on Blood Safety and Accountability
Commissioned Corps of the U.S. Public Health Service
National Vaccine Program Office (NVPO)
Office of Disease Prevention and Health Promotion (ODPHP)
Office of HIV/AIDS Policy (OHAP)
Office for Human Research Protections (OHRP)
Office of Minority Health (OMH)
Office of Population Affairs (OPA)
Office of Research Integrity (ORI)
Office of the Surgeon General (OSG)
Office on Women's Health (OWH)
Medical Reserve Corps
Presidential Advisory Council on HIV/AIDS
President's Council on Physical Fitness and Sports (PCPFS)
Regional Health Administrators (RHAs)

AIDS, Acquired immunodeficiency syndrome; *HIV,* human immunodeficiency virus.

BOX 3-5   Sample Listing of Other Federal Agencies Involved in Health Matters (not Part of U.S. Department of Health and Human Services)

Department of Agriculture
- Develops dietary guidelines for national nutritional policy.
- Does research and provides prevention data in areas of improved crop and animal protection.
- National School Lunch Program enforces food safety regulations; grades meats and other foods.
- Administers the Food Stamp Program.

Department of Defense
- Provides direct and indirect medical services to military members and their families.
- Provides environmental health services to military communities.

Department of Housing and Urban Development
- Provides mortgage insurance for hospitals and long-term care facilities.
- Constructs rural hospitals and neighborhood clinics.

Department of Justice
- Operates facilities for the health care of federal prisoners.

Department of Labor
- Occupational Safety and Health Administration provides technical assistance and enforces health and safety standards in the workplace.
- Mine Safety and Health Administration inspects mines and enforces health and safety standards.

Environmental Protection Agency
- Controls air and water quality and pollution standards.
- Oversees solid waste and toxic substances disposal.
- Regulates pesticides.
- Oversees radiation hazard control.
- Oversees noise abatement.

National Science Foundation
- Provides money for health research.

U.S. Department of Veterans Affairs
- Provides health care for military veterans.

STATE GOVERNMENTS

States derive their authority to govern from the Constitution, which reserved for the states all power not specifically given to the federal government. States play a broad role in health care. They finance care of the poor and disabled, primarily through the Medicaid program; operate state mental hospitals; ensure quality of service through licensure and regulation of health practitioners and facilities; and attempt to control health care costs and regulate insurance companies (Sparer, 2005; Sultz & Young, 2004). States play the major role in directing and supervising public health activities for their citizens, including disease control, sanitation, and environmental oversight.

Because state governments have diverse organizational structures, there is no single way in which health care services are organized and supplied by the states. Health care concerns are spread throughout various state agencies.

The State Health Agency

Each state has a state health agency that is the principal agency for health care services for that state. Roles and responsibilities of state health agencies vary. Some have vast authority over most health care issues, whereas others share power with a number of other agencies or organizations. Figure 3-7 presents a hypothetical state health agency with considerable authority. Most states provide the listed health services either through state health agencies or through other state agencies. In states where the state health agency is the state health department, the director might hold the title of health officer or health commissioner.

According to the Association of State and Territorial Health Officers (ASTHO), most state health agencies are actively involved in the following areas: (1) personal health, (2) community health, (3) environmental health, (4) health resources, (5) health education, (6) health planning and policy development, (7) enforcement of public health laws, (8) laboratory services, (9) general administration and services, and (10) funding to local health departments not allocated to program areas. The service areas are linked to the 10 core functions of public health (Association of State and Territorial Directors of Nursing, 2002). Chapter 29 expands on core functions and services in public health agencies. Most direct care is aimed at poor and high-risk groups. Local health departments may share in providing some of these services if directed to do so by the state authority.

Other Health-Related State Activities

Green and Anderson (1982) have identified approximately 36 state agencies outside the state health agency that have health-related responsibilities. Departments of education are responsible for school health programs and health education policy. Licensing of health professionals is usually the purview of the state board of licensing and examination for that specific profession. Vocational rehabilitation, occupational health, health planning, and selected environmental health responsibilities might be found outside the scope of the state health agency.

The National Commission on Community Health Services (1967) recommended consolidation of all official health services into a single agency to streamline bureaucracy, reduce duplication of efforts, and potentially cut costs. Now, more than 40 years later, there has been little progress toward implementing this recommendation, and it is not likely that we will see substantial consolidation of health-related services in the near future. As a result, the states' health care responsibilities, including environmental health, are still divided over an extensive and bewildering number of departments, commissions, agencies, and boards.

LOCAL GOVERNMENTS

Local governments are created by the state government, which delegates authority to the local level. The local unit can be a city, village, township, county, or special district. State legislatures

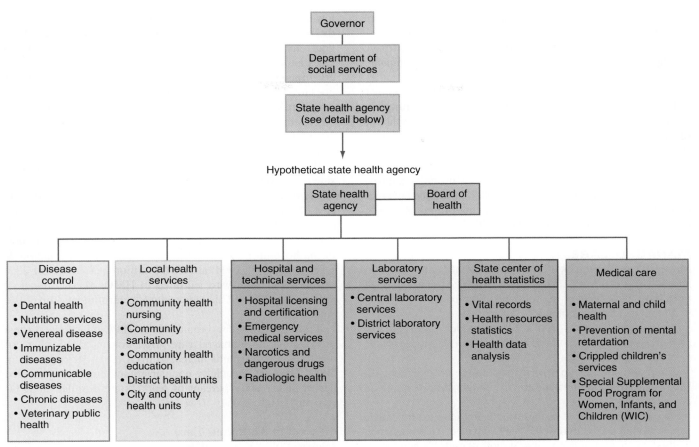

FIGURE 3-7 Hypothetical state superagency incorporating the health department.

determine the responsibilities and roles of local units, including the definition of the unit's role in health care.

The local governments perform many of the direct personal services. Maternal and child health programs are examples of such endeavors. The WIC Program and SCHIP are programs in which authority is shared. Most of the responsibility for health care at the local level resides in the local health department. Some local health departments provide ambulatory health services for poor persons, especially in areas where other providers limit service to this group (Milio, 2002; National Association of County and City Health Officials [NACCHO], 2006). Funding of local health departments is shared by local, state, and federal governments. Federal funding is usually in the form of grants for specific programs (Sultz & Young, 2004). Most of the burden for operating local health departments is assumed by local governments (Milio, 2002; NACCHO, 2006).

Like state governments, local units do not consolidate all health care services in the local health department. Many variants of organizational structure exist. Mental health and environmental health services, such as waste disposal, air pollution, and water-quality control, are commonly found under the auspices of other local agencies. School health programs might be the responsibility of the local school district rather than the local health department. Communities that operate general public hospitals and other such facilities frequently have separate organizational and funding structures for those facilities.

PRIVATE-SECTOR ROLE IN HEALTH CARE DELIVERY

Private-sector health care concentrates primarily on providing health services to individuals and families. The private sector is composed of both for-profit and nonprofit organizations, although most are for profit.

FOR-PROFIT PROVIDERS AND ORGANIZATIONS

For-profit providers and organizations are business arrangements that provide services for a payment. For-profit providers concentrate on direct care and services. Providers, for example, include health professionals (physicians, nurses, dentists, and others), nursing homes and hospitals, drugstores and medical supply companies, and pharmaceutical companies. They range in size from small enterprises, such as physicians in solo practice, to moderate-sized businesses, such as independent hospitals, to large conglomerates such as managed care organizations and health insurance companies.

ROLE OF INSURANCE AND OTHER THIRD-PARTY PAYERS

Health insurance companies pay for an individual's health care in return for a prepayment or premium. Blue Cross (for hospital fees) and Blue Shield (for doctor fees) were among the first prepaid health insurance plans. These two plans were nonprofit and remain largely so today. They are included in the discussion of for-profit organizations because they are not charitable organizations and charge a fee for services. There were 40 million members by 1950 (Anderson, 1985). After Blue Cross/Blue Shield proved insurance to be a viable method for financing health care services, commercial insurance companies began to offer competing plans.

The financing of health care by the insurance company rather than by the individual is called **third-party reimbursement**. The federal and state governments also assume the role of a third-party reimburser when they pay health care providers through Medicare and Medicaid. By the 1960s, health insurance plans had become one of the largest payers of hospital and physician charges (see Chapter 4). Currently, approximately 84.3% of the population has health insurance coverage, either through their employers, government programs, or self-purchase (U.S. Bureau of the Census, 2007).

MANAGED CARE

Managed care combines the two functions of health insurance and delivery of health care services. Managed care organizations have all or most of the following features:

- Prepayment arrangements
- Negotiated discounts from service providers and suppliers
- Agreements for preauthorizations for certain procedures
- Audit of performance

There are several types of managed care arrangements. In Box 3-6, various models and their distinguishing features are described.

The common thread in these managed care arrangements is restrictions on the traditional fee-for-service reimbursement method, with contracts binding on both the plan's health care providers and the consumers. The goals of managed care are to lower costs and ensure that maximum value is received from the resources used to produce and deliver health care. These goals are achieved by improving efficiency of delivered services and influencing the behavior of providers and consumers through rewards and penalties. For example, if a consumer goes to a health provider not covered by the plan, he or she will pay more out of pocket than if an in-plan provider were used.

Health maintenance organizations (HMOs) are the oldest model of managed care and the most restrictive on consumer choice. They limit an individual's choice of provider to those with HMO contracts. If a client uses providers outside the organization, in most cases the client will pay a large copayment, or the client might not be compensated for the cost of care. Most cost savings with HMOs come from efforts to reduce hospitalization rates among members. HMO members have fewer hospital admissions and spend fewer days in the hospital per episode of hospitalization (Harrington & Estes, 2008b). In 2004, almost 64 million individuals, or 23% of the population, were enrolled in HMOs (U.S. Bureau of the Census, 2007). This represented an enrollment drop of 9% since 2002.

Preferred provider organizations (PPOs) are the fastest growing of the managed care arrangements. Their share of health plan participants increased from 1% in 1986 to 40% in 2000. They are especially popular among employer-provided health plans. Sixty percent of workers are enrolled in PPOs (Kaiser/HRET, 2006).

Growth in Managed Care

Managed care is expanding primarily because organizations have demonstrated that services can be provided at a lower

---

Box 3-6   Types of Managed Care Organizations

Health Maintenance Organizations (HMOs)

Health maintenance organizations are networks or groups of providers who agree to provide certain basic health services for a single yearly fee (capitation). The consumer pays the same amount for coverage regardless of the amount and type of services provided. There are five HMO models differentiated by the method used to engage physicians and other health providers in terms of organization and payment:

Staff: Providers are salaried employees.

Group: Providers are a single multispecialty group under contract to provide services to HMO clients. Services might be delivered in HMO facilities or in clinics operated by the provider group.

Network: Providers are two or more independent groups under contract to provide services to HMO members.

Independent practice association (IPA): Contracts are with solo providers (physicians and small single-specialty group practices). There is a large panel of participating providers.

Mixed: HMO contracts with more than one type of provider. There might be salaried providers, single-practice physicians, and large groups under contract. Clients select a single provider method for their health care needs.

Preferred Provider Organizations (PPOs)

Preferred provider organizations have a looser organizational structure and are a more recent development. They contract with a network of providers (doctors, hospitals, and others) to provide service at a discounted rate to members. There is a fixed premium (insurance cost). Members might, in addition, be expected to pay a portion of the cost of selected services. Clients may use non-PPO providers, but they must pay more out of pocket to do so.

Point of Service (POS)

Point-of-service plans are a hybrid of the PPO concept. These are networks for providers. The consumer selects a primary care physician from network providers to act as his or her primary care physician. The physician acts as a gatekeeper who determines the consumer's need for specialized health care services and referrals. Consumers need the gatekeeper's permission to seek other services, and they will incur additional expense if they do not get the primary physician's approval before seeking other care.

Health Care Networks

There are corporations with a consolidated set of facilities and services for which consumers or employers pay a specific monthly fee. The services offered are intended to be comprehensive, and consumers are expected to receive all care within the network or from providers arranged by the network. A network includes the following components: a major hospital, several smaller hospitals, a long-term care facility, a rehabilitation center, a home health agency, and a subacute care center. Examples of health networks are Helix Health Care System and MedAtlantic Health Care.

Data from the Centers for Disease Control and Prevention, Atlanta, GA.

cost with managed care than with other types of health care provider arrangements. Refer to Chapter 4 for a discussion of how costs are affected by these health care service options. Managed care models are especially popular with employers because they reduce the employers' cost of providing health care benefits to employees. In 2006, 80% of employed persons were insured through a managed care plan (Kaiser/HRET, 2006).

VOLUNTARY COMPONENT OF THE PRIVATE SECTOR

Voluntary agencies have long been a part of the U.S. health care system. What exactly is a voluntary agency? All private-sector organizations, whether for-profit or nonprofit, are voluntary to some extent. They all originate through some sort of private initiative and are not compelled by government sanction to organize or to provide health care services. In more common usage, the term *voluntary,* with respect to health care agencies, usually applies to nonprofit agencies.

There are many hundreds of voluntary nonprofit agencies—thousands if voluntary nonprofit hospitals are included. This section focuses on nonhospital-type voluntary agencies involved in health care.

Goals and Types of Voluntary Agencies

Voluntary agencies engage in a variety of health-related activities. The classic work by Gunn and Platt (1945) identified the basic functions of voluntary agencies, which are still valid today. These basic functions are summarized in two basic concepts:
1. Creativity
   * Efforts to address unmet health needs
   * Efforts to improve or design new methods to meet recognized health needs
   * Efforts to plan and coordinate health activities to avoid overlap and conflict between public and private initiatives

2. Advocacy
   * Promotion of health legislation to benefit the public interest
   * Promotion of public health programs and defense against political interference or funding reductions
   * Provision of health education to the public and support for professional education

An agency might concentrate on one function or be involved in a number of different functions, depending on its stated mission.

There are several types of health-related voluntary agencies. The most common are agencies supported by contributions from the general public (e.g., the American Heart Association), philanthropic trusts (e.g., the Robert Wood Johnson Foundation), and health professional organizations (e.g., the American Public Health Association). The largest group and the most familiar to the general public are agencies that receive their support from citizen donations and fundraising campaigns. Box 3-7 provides examples of each type of voluntary agency.

Specialized agencies usually rely on public donations from a large number of contributors. Most attempt some type of fundraising campaign, including mail or media, door-to-door solicitations, and telethons. So many organizations have made public appeals for support that a number of charities have banded together in a united appeal process. The United Way and Community Chest efforts are an attempt to limit requests for contributions and to consolidate efforts.

Distinctions from Other Types of Organizations

Voluntary agencies have operational freedoms that other types of organizations do not. They are less constrained by laws and regulations and can move quickly to initiate new programs or change existing ones. They enhance creativity in care and are often the initiator of new programs, research, or services to underserved groups. Although voluntary organizations contribute to health care, they play a very small role in the delivery of services to the nation's population. If charitable giving is

---

BOX 3-7   Types of Voluntary Agencies

Agencies Supported by Private Funds
The goals of publicly supported organizations vary greatly, but many are clearly health related. Most have very specific purposes. Some examples are the following:
* Agencies that concentrate on a specific illness, disease, or body organ (e.g., American Heart Association, American Diabetes Association, American Cancer Society)
* Agencies concerned with providing services to specific target groups, such as children, elderly persons, or homeless persons (e.g., National Society for Crippled Children, National Council on Aging)
* Hospice organizations that target terminally ill clients and their families
* Agencies that concentrate on a certain type of health-related service or phase of health (e.g., Planned Parenthood Federation of America, National Safety Council, Visiting Nurse Association)

Foundations and Private Philanthropies
Foundations are established and funded by private donations. These philanthropic organizations are involved in a number of health-related areas, including basic research, professional education, international health,

and assistance to health departments located primarily in rural or isolated areas. The Robert Wood Johnson Foundation, the Milbank Memorial Fund, the Rockefeller Foundation, the W. K. Kellogg Foundation, and the Carnegie Foundation are a few of the philanthropic organizations with a primary interest in health care. Community Resources for Practice at the end of the chapter provides information on how to find out about these organizations and their special interests.

Professional Organizations
Professional organizations are funded by membership dues. Professional organizations are concerned with health issues, especially those involving the well-being of their members. They do not provide direct health care services. Activities include the following:
* Providing continuing education
* Establishing and improving standards and qualifications for professional practice
* Encouraging research
* Safeguarding the independence and interests of the professional membership by lobbying

used as an indirect measure of impact, then their efforts provide a mere 1.1% of the total health care budget (AAFRC Trust for Philanthropy, 2005; CMS, 2007).

PUBLIC AND PRIVATE HEALTH CARE SECTORS BEFORE 1965

Before 1965, there was a two-tiered system of health care delivery in the United States. People who could afford it paid for health care either out of pocket or through health insurance programs. People who could not afford to pay or lacked health insurance relied on the charity of individual health practitioners, organizations, or limited government funded care.

PROVIDERS OF HEALTH CARE

Initially, physicians provided care in the home and office, and nursing care was supplied by family members and visiting nurses in the home. As other types of health professionals appeared (pharmacists, dentists, podiatrists, radiologists), they set up practice using a similar business model of reimbursement. The greatest exception was nursing. Nurses were employed by other health professionals or providers, primarily physicians and hospitals. Most nurses did not engage in independent practice.

Over time, hospitals replaced the family as the principal caregivers for seriously ill persons. In 1960, most general hospitals were nonprofit community hospitals, primarily serving paying clients. Publicly owned hospitals provided health care for most nonpaying persons. The state and local governments assumed the responsibility for most of the public health activities directed at citizens and communities as well as the bulk of inpatient psychiatric care for the poor mentally ill.

FOCUS OF CARE: PRIVATE SECTOR

An individual-centered focus on acute illness is the historical method of health care delivery in the United States. Physician practice and institutional health facilities depended on the treatment of persons with acute problems. An individualized, acute care focus in health care services meant that most of the energy was spent at the level of **secondary prevention** (treating illness) and **tertiary prevention** (eliminating or reducing the long-term effects of an illness or disability). This emphasis is evidenced by the growth of hospitals, clinics, and other facilities and services with an acute care and disability focus.

FOCUS OF CARE: PUBLIC SECTOR

Community health officials and policies emphasized primary prevention, which was aimed at avoiding accidents, illnesses, and diseases before they occurred. By the 1960s, public health efforts had significantly reduced the dangers of many life-threatening health problems. Sanitation, food inspection, and other environmental controls, combined with immunization efforts, ameliorated the more common hazards for a large percentage of the population. Lower mortality rates were accepted as the norm. Funding support and public interest for primary prevention activities ebbed.

In response to a lack of interest in population-centered health services, public health practitioners redirected their interest to blocks of people or target groups and families. Public health concentrated on reducing the risks of illness and death from specific diseases among family members and target groups. As examples, maternal/child health services and sexually transmitted disease clinics were services provided. Population-based efforts, although never really halted, were deemphasized during this period.

PUBLIC AND PRIVATE SECTORS, 1965 TO 1992

The year 1965 is commonly viewed as a turning point in U.S. health care delivery services. In the 1960s, two issues became of paramount importance: (1) public recognition that access and quality of care were disproportionate, particularly with respect to poor and elderly individuals, and (2) rising health care costs. Attempts to solve these two problems resulted in implementation of a number of strategies.

MEDICARE AND MEDICAID

In 1965, federal legislation was aimed at facilitating access to health services and reducing or eliminating the two-tiered system of health care. Medicare (for the elderly) and Medicaid (for the poor) were created. Chapter 4 provides a detailed discussion of these programs and cost-containment efforts. Providers who had avoided the elderly and poor were encouraged to treat them, because payment for service was now guaranteed. As providers willingly mingled middle-class, privately insured patients with government-insured patients, the boundaries of the two-tiered health care system began to blur.

COST CONCERN AND CONTAINMENT EFFORTS

Cost became an issue of increasing concern even as access and equity of care were being addressed. Personal health care expenditures had steadily increased since before World War II. This concern led to initial attempts at cost cutting. The driving force for cost saving was third-party payers (government and insurance companies), employers, and unions. These large organizations were immediately and directly affected by escalating costs (Califano, 1986; Feldstein, 2005).

In the beginning, the general public and providers of care were not as concerned with cost. Insurance served as insulation from the actual cost of care. The direct effect of out-of-pocket medical expenses was a greater concern. Health care providers were essentially satisfied because they received adequate compensation from the insurance companies.

The enactment of Medicare and Medicaid legislation opened the way for federal efforts at cost containment. The USDHHS had oversight of both programs and directed the HCFA, now the CMS, to initiate efforts at containing costs. Subsequent amendments to these two acts expanded the authority of the HCFA to contain costs. Hospitals were the area in which increasing costs were especially dramatic and were the focus of the greatest effort at cost containment. According to the HCFA, overall expenditures on hospital care rose from $8.09 billion to $305.3 billion between 1960 and 1992. A substantial portion of that increase was the result of improvements in treatment and technology. Cost-containment measures slowed the growth of hospital costs compared with other health care services. For example, reducing a patient's hospital length of stay had a dramatic impact on reducing hospital costs (Sultz & Young, 2004).

EFFORTS AT HEALTH PLANNING

Throughout the late 1960s and the 1970s, Congress initiated efforts aimed at increasing the level of health planning for the country. **Website Resource 3A** offers a brief synopsis of the two most important laws that culminated in the inception of health systems agencies (HSAs). The HSAs and other health planning agencies were charged with assessing the health status of populations in their areas, identifying specific health needs, developing plans to ensure adequate services and treatment of expected health problems, and strengthening preventive measures to reduce the incidence of disease.

Opposition to health planning boards was strong. Especially resistant were **vested interests,** groups whose professional practices or finances might be affected by the decisions of the boards. For example, the American Hospital Association (AHA) and the American Medical Association (AMA) both opposed these measures (Pickett & Hanlon, 1990). With the advent of the Reagan administration, government support eroded. President Reagan was philosophically opposed to health planning because it set limits on the "free market" delivery system. Funding for HSAs was eliminated by the 1982 budget, which effectively dampened the move toward national health planning (Patel & Rushefsky, 2006). Many states have maintained some of the oversight and review functions, transferring these activities to other agencies.

COMPETING FOCUSES OF CARE: PREVENTION OR CURE

During these years, two competing concepts of care fought for supremacy. The debate was between curative, illness-oriented (secondary and tertiary) care and preventive (primary) care.

Consumer and Professional Support for Prevention Focus

Public health personnel had long supported a proactive approach, emphasizing preventive health practices. It was not until cost became a significant concern that public opinion shifted again, to a more historical public health focus on planning and delivering health care (Fleury et al., 1996; Walker, 1992). Several experimental programs proved to be cost effective. A few large employers implemented fitness and health-teaching programs. These innovations resulted in an improvement in health status and a reduction in illness and sick days. Ultimately, they saved employers money by reducing sick pay benefits and lowering health insurance claims (Califano, 1986; Reed, 1991).

Coupled with employer efforts, an awakening of consumer interest in health status and health care services occurred. Consumer groups became active in monitoring and questioning standard medical practice, as well as espousing consumer responsibility for health-seeking behaviors (Illich, 1977).

Employees and labor unions drew public attention to the link between occupational exposures and hazards and certain illnesses and injuries. Their efforts helped the push toward laws intended to improve working conditions. Safety measures to eliminate or reduce illness and injury received broad support (Pickett & Hanlon, 1990; Roemer, 1991).

Comparison of Health Status Indicators

Information about models of care in other developed countries became more available to consumers, health professionals, sociologists, and economists (see Chapter 5). Instead of concentrating on physical care, political activists, economists, and sociologists argued that it would be more efficient to correct poverty, because poor health was significantly associated with a deprived standard of living (Blum, 1981; Brown, 2001; McKeown, 1976). They pointed to evidence from developing countries that showed a direct correlation between improvements in health status of the population and improved economic status.

Comparisons of standard measures of health in developed countries indicated that the U.S. performance was mediocre. People began to question this country's emphasis on acute care. Milio (1981, 1983) and others argued that health status should not be measured in terms of presence or absence of disease or high or low death rates. In general, healthy people have a better quality of life than people who are not healthy. The aim should be to encourage health and maintain as many people as possible in a disease-free state. It is more cost effective to place emphasis on prevention rather than on care or treatment of illness (Leviton & Rhodes, 2005; Lewis, 2001). A strong preventive component that would be directed toward eliminating or postponing illness for as long as possible is necessary to truly improve the health status of the population. Former Governor Dick Lamm of Colorado offered a "Ten Commandments" proposal for improving the health care system. One of these was "Honor not only thy doctor and thy hospital, but thy public health nurse and thy sewage disposal plant worker" (Lamm, 1990, p. 126).

Health Planning and the Relationship to Prevention

During the 1960s and 1970s, support grew for increasing the emphasis on prevention rather than illness care. Local and regional planning agencies, such as the HSAs, were involved in planning efforts. As an example of regional planning, a health plan for cardiac disease would include both an adequate supply of cardiac hospital beds (curative, secondary prevention) *and* aggressive health teaching aimed at reducing the population's risk of developing heart disease (preventive, primary prevention).

The focus on prevention-related activities also increased at the federal level. Growing research evidence supported the idea that preventive measures were less costly than treatment of specific illnesses. National goals were developed that were intended to improve the health status of the population. Action plans were devised to meet these health goals. Most actions were preventive and aimed at reducing risks within specific age groups (U.S. Public Health Service, 1979). For example, an immunization strategy targeted communicable childhood diseases, hepatitis among health care workers, and flu in elderly persons.

In the 1980s, the efforts at health planning and emphasis on prevention stalled. A political and philosophic shift at the federal level resulted in substantial funding cuts for public health and preventive health planning efforts (Shonick, 1995). Efforts to revive the emphasis on public health and preventive focus in the 1990s had little success.

EMPHASIS ON STATE CONTROL AND ADMINISTRATION OF HEALTH PROGRAMS

President Reagan came into office determined to limit the federal role of government (Shonick, 1995). The Reagan administration oversaw severe cuts in federal funding for public health and developed a block grant system of state administration for most remaining health and welfare programs (Patel & Rushefsky, 2006).

States resisted these efforts, caught in a bind between federally mandated service requirements and shrinking federal funds (Congressional Budget Office, 1992; Harrington & Pellow, 2001). The Omnibus Budget Reconciliation Act (OBRA) of 1981, which created block grants and state oversight, also reduced federal funding by 25% (Kronenfeld, 1997). States had to choose between eliminating or reducing benefits and increasing state budgets to continue coverage at the current level (Patel & Rushefsky, 2006). Chapter 4 provides a more detailed discussion of funding impacts on state budgets. Currently, the state-administered block grant system is still in effect, and funding remains a major concern.

RISING NUMBER OF UNINSURED

In the 1980s and 1990s, there was a steady rise in the number of people without health insurance (Harrington & Pellow, 2001). Strict criteria for eligibility in government insurance programs and the rising cost of private health insurance are the main causes (see Chapter 4). The uninsured are primarily poor and members of minority groups. Their uninsured status places them at greater risk of poor health. Chapter 21 describes the impact of poverty and lack of health insurance on health status.

The nation continues to grapple with health coverage problems and has enacted incremental legislation to improve access for certain groups. For example, SCHIP provides health insurance for children whose parents have limited income but are not eligible for Medicaid. Other efforts include increasing health insurance portability for workers who change employers and expansion of health benefits for the nation's veterans.

PUBLIC AND PRIVATE SECTORS TODAY

Evolution continues as the health care system reacts to changes and pressures from providers and consumers. Issues arising in the 1980s and early 1990s have continued to affect practice today. Escalating costs, cost shifting, tensions between health professions, and a fragmented structure have been instrumental in variously impeding or expanding access to services, as well as dictating the level of services available for selected groups within the population. Managed care organizations have prospered, with dramatic increases in the population they serve, at the expense of more traditional types of service programs.

CONTINUING SHIFT IN FEDERAL AND STATE RELATIONSHIPS

Federal efforts to reduce services and responsibilities and to shift duties to the states continue. States still must meet federally established criteria for health-related programs. Federal minimum standards for air and water quality and Medicaid services, for example, both have an impact on public health. In both areas, federal regulations must be met by the states, even if it means that states incur additional expenses. State and federal officials continue to pressure each other to assume a greater share of the health care burden.

Federal retrenchment and the financial hardships at the state and federal levels have led to a weakening of public health

agencies at all levels (Leviton & Rhodes, 2005). State and local health departments have suffered severe funding cuts, which has resulted in reductions in staff (including public health nurses), reductions in worker benefits, stagnating and/or stationary salary scales that have not kept pace with inflation, reductions in the amount and type of direct care provided to risk groups, and imposition of fees for services once provided without charge (Sultz & Young, 2004; Walker, 1992). Remaining staff operates under increasing stress and pressure to produce. It is ironic that at a time of increasing emphasis on health promotion and disease prevention, which is the very essence of community health practice, the survival of some public health agencies is doubtful (Brown, 2001).

POWER CONFLICTS WITHIN THE SYSTEM

Change is not always beneficial to all concerned; therefore, some resistance and conflict can be expected. Cost increases, growing consumer awareness, and competing philosophies about the nature of health care delivery have produced some changes that have created conflict among various participants (providers and consumers) as they struggle to gain or maintain power. Funding and regulatory conflicts between federal and state/local governments have been discussed. Many other power-related conflicts exist.

Insurance companies, physicians, and state regulatory bodies struggle over treatment and cost issues. Malpractice frequently pits administration, physicians, nurses, other health care workers, and lawyers against one another as they struggle over issues of cost, liability, and jurisdiction. As consumer groups attempt to gain a greater voice in the delivery and organization of health care services, many of those already involved in the decision-making process work to retard or dilute the influence of consumer groups. In the health care industry, power struggles have intensified and can be expected to continue as attempts to resolve the budget crisis continue.

Treatment Decisions: Multiple Players and the Impact on Physician Practice

Health insurance providers and managed care organizations have expanded their roles in both practice and cost areas, including determining treatment modalities, necessity of medical supplies and diagnostic tools, and appropriate time frames for treatment. Hospitals, in turn, pressed with ever-tightening budget restraints, have initiated additional curbs on physician practice (Rice & Kominski, 2001). Physicians have vigorously resisted outside influences in practice decisions, pointing to the need for professional autonomy to ensure optimal client care. Nevertheless, insurance plans, managed care providers, and hospitals have gradually assumed influence over practice decisions. Some physicians have reacted to managed care's attempts to impact practice by becoming financial partners in regional physician-owned and -operated managed care organizations or physician-hospital care networks, a form of integrated system. Both of these operate in direct competition with other types of managed care arrangements (Sultz & Young, 2004). Physicians have also organized labor unions in an attempt to counter unilateral decisions made by managed care that impact practice behavior. There are five multistate physician unions, one sanctioned by the AMA (Geyman, 2002).

Nursing Concerns

Competing interests hamper nurses' struggles toward greater respect and autonomy. Direct reimbursement has created conflict with physician groups. New legislation has increased third-party reimbursement for nurse practitioners and some other advanced practice nurses, especially in the Medicare and Medicaid programs. The AMA opposes direct reimbursement for nurses. Nurse staffing and supervision decisions have been undermined by the increased use of unlicensed assistive personnel.

These conflicts can be expected to continue because, as nursing increases its voice and power, others must share in the decision-making process. A nursing voice on a hospital or home care board, for instance, means that someone else is displaced or his or her influence is diluted by the addition of a new member. It is crucial that nurses increase their presence in the policy-making arena to protect their practice environment and influence delivery and service decisions (Unruh & Spetz, 2007).

As nurses' wages increase, administrators must find ways to meet these salary concessions. Wage increases were historically passed on to the consumer, but current budgetary constraints do not always allow that possibility. Even in the midst of a nursing shortage, nursing salaries have not increased as much as could be expected (Feldstein, 2005; Unruh & Fottler, 2008). Administrators must make shifts in budgets to accommodate nursing gains. Building or maintenance projects, investments in new equipment, travel budgets, administrators' compensation packages, and wage or benefit increases for other health care professionals are affected by nursing salary gains. Whenever possible, administrators, especially hospital administers, have resisted salary increases in favor of sign-on bonuses, recruitment of newly graduated nurses, and substitution of unlicensed assistive personnel.

Nurses have become more politically active, speaking out on the impact cost cutting has on quality of care. The Joint Commission on Accreditation of Healthcare Organizations (JCAHO; now known as the Joint Commission) reported that 24% of adverse events were related to low nurse staff levels (JCAHO, 2005). Other studies showing adverse results of higher nurse/client ratios are well publicized (Aiken, 2007; Rothberg et al., 2008; Schnelle et al., 2008). The ANA has developed a Nursing Report Card for Acute Care, a set of nursing-sensitive quality indicators for immediate use in collecting data linking staffing, skill mix, and patient outcomes (ANA, 1999). It is important that nurses use these indicators and insist that they become part of quality studies conducted by others.

Shared Decision Making

Historically, physicians have assumed the major role in making decisions about client care and treatment. They have also had the most influence on policy decisions affecting health care (Feldstein, 2005; Sultz & Young, 2004). A large number of well-educated health professionals now demand a greater share in the decision-making process. Physicians account for only 16.5% of all educated medical professionals (U.S. Department of Labor, Bureau of Labor Statistics, 2006; see Table 3-1). Although physicians have resisted efforts at power sharing, other health professionals have gained a voice in shaping health policy and services. President Clinton's Health Reform Task Force made a point to consult nurse leaders and professional nursing organizations. Nurses have also been involved at the state level in planning boards for health care services, for example, the Oregon Health Plan and MinnesotaCare. Health professionals will continue to jockey for influence during the term of the current president and the terms of succeeding presidents.

SPECIALIZATION AND FRAGMENTATION

More than 12.3 million people are employed in the health care industry, which has seen a rapid increase in the number of specialized workers (U.S. Bureau of the Census, 2007, p. 406). Technologic advances have led to increasingly more complex care requirements. This has fueled demand for specialization. It takes special skills to operate a magnetic resonance imaging or computed tomography scanner, or to prepare and maintain a heart-lung bypass machine. Add to this the myriad types of care and treatment options available, and it is easy to see how specialization in health care has become so widespread. Nurses and physicians have moved from general practice into specialty areas. Specialization is often viewed as more prestigious than general practice. Specialty and geographic imbalances still exist in the distribution of physicians (Sultz & Young, 2004). There are disagreements as to whether there will be an oversupply of physicians in the near future and whether the ratio of primary care doctors to specialists is in balance or whether there is a surplus of specialists and a shortage of primary care doctors (Brewer, 2005; Feldstein, 2005). Up to this point, specialization has not been problematic for nursing. Federal estimates of future needs point to a continuing demand for graduate nurses prepared as nurse practitioners and clinical specialists, including community health specialists. The Quad Council of Public Health Nursing Organizations (2007) predicts a continued shortage into the future, with some states reporting that 20% of positions are currently vacant.

Fragmentation remains a major feature of our health care system. In 1975, Roemer and colleagues identified the following as the most important problems associated with fragmented health care: poor access to care, gaps and inequities, inadequate prevention efforts, discontinuous and inappropriate care, poor responsiveness to consumer needs, inefficient use of scarce resources, ineffective planning and evaluation, escalating costs, inadequate quality controls, and fragmented policies. Although some attempts have been made to address these issues, they remain largely the same over 30 years later (Sultz & Young, 2004).

Subspecialization of professions enhances the problem of fragmented care for individuals, because specialists tend to concentrate on their specialties rather than take a holistic care view. It is easy to conceive of one person's being seen by two or three specialists without coordination of overall care. For example, a nurse might have a patient who is taking medication prescribed by two or three physicians. Without coordination, danger exists that medications might be counterproductive or even life threatening in combination. Multiple agency involvement in a single patient's care compounds the problem of professional subspecialization. Consider some of the resources that might be needed to provide quality care to a stroke patient after hospital discharge: the primary doctor, a physician specialist, a nursing service, physical therapy and other rehabilitative services, respite workers to relieve family caregivers, Meals on Wheels, telephone monitoring, various assistive devices, home remodeling to accommodate physical deficits, and senior daycare. Most communities still have no coordination in overseeing services for their citizens. Patients or their families are often expected to coordinate services. Many miss available resources because they lack the skill and information necessary to plan for care.

QUALITY-OF-CARE CONCERNS

There is a real concern that emphasis on cost containment has been detrimental to the delivery of health care services. The question being asked is: *Are cost-cutting decisions affecting access and quality of care?* The Institute of Medicine estimates that between 44,000 and 98,000 people die each year as a result of medical errors (Geyman, 2002). An extensive review of health records across the country conducted by McGlynn

and colleagues (2003) indicated that 45% of patients do not receive the recommended preventive care; 46% do not receive the recommended acute care; and 44% do not receive the recommended chronic care. The Commonwealth Fund reported that the United States had more medically related errors and ranked last on safe patient care compared with five other developed countries (Davis et al., 2007). A number of legislative efforts have attempted to allay concerns about the quality of health and ease access to care for selected risk groups. Box 3-8 lists some of the most relevant legislation and some pending efforts as well.

The extent to which cost containment impacts the receipt of recommended care, the quality of care provided, and the access to care is still under investigation. The federal government

---

Box 3-8   Recently Enacted and Proposed Health Reform Measures

Health Insurance Portability and Accountability Act (HIPAA) of 1996—Federal Law
- Limits insurance exclusions for preexisting conditions.
- Requires insurers to renew coverage for consumers; may not drop coverage due to illness history.
- Allows portability of health insurance from job to job.
- Allows access to insurance coverage for small employers.
- Confidentiality provisions took effect in 2003; allow individuals more control over records, require providers to safeguard records, and guarantee the individual access to his or her personal records.

Maternity Length of Stay—State Law
- Requires insurers to cover hospital maternity stays in accordance with medical criteria; most allow 24- to 48-hour hospital stay after an uncomplicated delivery.

Mandated Grievance Procedures—State Law
- Requires a quick review process when services are denied by managed care and other insurers.
- Covers denied access to specialists, failure to pay for medical services.
- Reduces the ability of insurers to take punitive action against the patient, doctor, or other medical workers who provide information to patients with respect to care alternatives.

Any Willing Provider—State Law
- Requires health plans to admit any provider who accepts the plan's terms and payment rates.

Other Specific Service Requirements—State Law
- Limits same-day discharge for mastectomies.
- Prudent layperson decision reimbursement—insurers must pay for emergency department care if symptoms would lead a prudent layperson to seek care.

Mental Health Parity Act of 1996—Federal Law
- Requires employers and health insurers to provide the same benefits for mental health (if they offer a mental health benefit) as they do for other types of health benefits; intended to prevent employers from limiting mental health benefits. Annual renewal requirement means that the provisions can be discontinued at any time simply by not renewing the legislation. Also does not mandate insurers/employers to offer mental health benefits, just dictates what they must do if these are offered.

Patient Safety Act—Federal Proposal
- Requires all health care institutions to collect and provide to the public information on staffing, skill mix, and patient outcomes; supported by the American Nurses Association.

Patient Care Mechanism—Federal Law
- Balanced Budget Act of 1997—federal law allows states to care for Medicaid patients via managed care plans.

Health Insurance Pools—State Law
- Twenty states have health insurance cooperatives. These pools help small employers provide health care by pooling their money with that of other small companies, which gives them greater flexibility to negotiate lower prices.

SCHIP—State Children's Health Insurance Program—Federal Law
- Series of incremental access provisions that extended health care coverage to low-income children and prenatal care and delivery to pregnant women.

Medicare Prescription Drug, Improvement, and Modernization Act of 2003
- Provides a prescription drug program (which started in 2006). The program provides partial cost reimbursement for drugs based on income and limits set by the act.
- Provides some prevention measures; for example, physical examinations and screening for heart disease and diabetes for all *new* Medicare enrollees.
- Requires changes to Medicare structures and payment systems starting in 2006 (additional funds for rural physicians and hospitals) and 2010 (encourages private competition by health insurance companies with Medicare subsidized by $12 billion of federal money).
- For additional information, see Table 4-2 (pages 96–97) and **Website Resource 4A.**

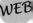

Patient Bill of Rights—Federal Proposal—Languished in Congress from 1992 to 2004
- Defines basic services and patient rights for consumers covered in any type of health insurance plan.

Universal Health Coverage—State Law
- Provides health care access to all residents: currently exists in Massachusetts, Vermont, Maine, and Oregon.

collects quality data from Medicare and managed care organizations. Some of the sources of these quality data are listed in Box 3-9. At the present time, most states have some regulations with reporting criteria for both private source and Medicaid managed care plans (Patel & Rushefsky, 1999).

Reporting of some data is voluntary; reporting of other data is mandatory and is tied to provider compensation. The coupling of payment to participation in data reporting has been expanding. For example, Medicare, Medicaid, and some employer-provided health insurance plans will only insure with managed care plans that participate in the evaluation process.

Quality-of-care issues are not limited to managed care. Other health care providers are also required to make annual reports. For example, hospitals are required to publish data on the number of hospital deaths and their readmission rates. In keeping with ongoing concerns about the quality of health care in the United States, the Agency for Healthcare Research and Quality is required by Congress to report annually on the nation's quality of health care and disparities in care delivery (Kelly et al., 2008). The Agency for Healthcare Research and Quality released the first set of reports in 2003. There is also concern about the quality of services available to the elderly with chronic and disabling conditions. Harrington (2007) reports that cost containment has been the overwhelming concern in long-term care services during the past 20 years. Cost of services, rather than quality of care, has dictated decision making.

Detailed comparisons between managed and nonmanaged or fee-for-service care is a new area of investigation. So far, the results are mixed. Some studies of satisfaction show that enrollees are equally satisfied in both plans. Other studies show that managed care consumers are not as satisfied as fee-for-service consumers (Pulcini & Hart, 2007a; Schur et al., 2004). With respect to specific medical conditions, the results are similarly mixed. Garret and Zucherman (2008) examined U.S. counties that required all Medicaid patients to be enrollment in managed care. They reported that adults in mandatory managed care had a lower number of emergency department visits but this was not offset by an increased use of ambulatory and preventive care. One Medicare outcomes study found that early detection of colorectal cancer was greater in fee-for-service and non-group HMOs than in other managed care organizations (Lee-Feldstein et al., 2002). One study of breast cancer patients found no difference in time to detection or patient outcome when managed care and fee-for-service plans were compared (Lee-Feldstein et al., 2000). Another study found that HMOs patients were more likely to get mammograms than fee-for-service patients (American Association of Health Plans, 2006). A study of managed care mental health services for children found that managed care reduced the cost of services compared with fee-for-services programs (Catalano et al., 2000). Women in mandatory Medicaid managed care were found to have 13% fewer Papanicolaou tests and breast examinations than women in fee-for-service programs (Garrett & Zucherman, 2008). The authors expressed concern that although managed care controlled costs, prevention efforts were not improved.

As part of a new effort to "pay for performance," the CMS announced that Medicare will no longer pay hospitals for treatment of preventable medical complications, including hospital-acquired infections, injuries from falls, reactions to transfusions of the wrong blood type, air embolisms, bedsores developed in the hospital, and foreign objects left in patients during surgery. Medicare policy does not allow hospitals to independently bill patients for treatment of these mistakes.

Comprehensive evaluations of quality issues are necessary. Consumers and employers need to be made aware of and to use comparison data in making decisions about health plans and

---

Box 3-9   Sources for Quality Data

HEDIS—Health Employer Data and Information Set
(Developed by the National Committee on Quality Assurance [NCQA])
- Accreditation service; voluntary for all managed care plans.
- Data on all types of insurance plans.
- Employers can use the data to help decide which health plan to offer their employees.
- HOS*—Medicare Health Outcomes Survey, part of HEDIS data. Medicare+Choice is required to collect and review data on seniors every 2 years. Can track health status over time if seniors stay in managed care.

OASIS*—Standardized Outcome and Assessment Information Set for Home Care
A measure of patient functional, behavioral, social, and clinical status; data are reported to state agencies for use in the nursing home certification process.

FIM*—Functional Independence Measures
Data measures collected to incorporate into a larger patient assessment tool; used to determine the amount of prospective payment by Medicare to inpatient rehabilitative facilities.

Joint Commission (formerly known as Joint Commission on Accreditation of Health Care Organizations)*
Hospital data required as part of the accreditation process includes quality outcome measures, such as number of hospital deaths, readmission rates.

Comprehensive Data Collection Programs—Voluntary
Pilot programs designed to improve health status of the frail elderly and other high-risk groups by coordinating inpatient/outpatient services and collecting outcome measures.
- PACE—Program for the All-Inclusive Care of the Elderly
- SHMOII—Social Health Maintenance Organization Model II

Centers for Medicare and Medicaid Services Website†
- HOS—10 quality measures on all Medicare-participating nursing homes
- HHAs—11 quality measures on home health agencies
- NCQA—HEDIS reports

Data from Clauser, S. B., & Berman, A. S. (2003). Significance of functional status data for payment and quality. *Health Care Financing Review, 24*(3), 1-11; and Carter, G. M., Relles, D. A., Ridgeway, G. K., et al. (2003). Measuring function for Medicare inpatient rehabilitation payment. *Health Care Financing Review, 24*(3), 25-43.
*Participation required for Medicare payment.
†Website can be accessed through the **WebLinks** section of the book's website at *http://evolve.elsevier.com/Maurer/community/*.

providers. Quality data are becoming more readily available to the consumer via the Internet and print media. The Community Resources for Practice section at the end of the chapter provides a list of foundations with websites for consumer use that can be accessed through the Evolve website. Nurses need to expand their involvement in quality care issues. There are several ways nurses can assist with quality concerns:

- Consumer education: provide information on health service and access rights
- Legislation and regulation: ensure quality of care as an integral part of health care delivery
- Research: design, implement, and publish the results of quality-related research

STRATEGIES EMPLOYED TO ADDRESS PROBLEMS

Since the early 1970s, attempts have been made to address specific problems within the system. Efforts have been aimed at improving efficiency, coordinating planning, and controlling costs. Some have been more successful than others. Following is a brief discussion of the most important strategies. Chapter 4 provides a more detailed discussion of selected cost-cutting strategies.

Decrease Costs

Major effort has been applied to seeking solutions to the cost issue. Hospital expenses seemed a logical place to initiate reforms because hospitals accounted for approximately 50% of all personal health care expenditures in 1980. By 2005, hospitals accounted for only 37.7% of health care expenditures (CMS, 2007).

Shorten Hospital Stays and Increase Home Health Care. The primary efforts at reducing hospital Medicare costs were federal actions. Prospective payment and diagnosis-related groups were imposed on hospitals that cared for Medicare patients. These reforms were an attempt to encourage hospitals to curb costs (see Chapter 4).

The net effect of federal reform has been a reduction in the average length of hospital stay for Medicare patients and an increased demand for home health and other community care services. The number of transfers to after-hospital care facilities has doubled. Home health care and other community agencies, such as public health departments, were and remain affected by the increased demand for community-related services (Sultz & Young, 2004).

Managed/Coordinated Care Techniques. The intent of coordinated care strategies is to include a mechanism for reviewing care before and during treatment to reduce costs and eliminate the use of unnecessary services. Coordinated or managed care applies to other strategies aimed at controlling costs as well as managed care organizations. Third-party payers usually develop these. Some of the current techniques include the requirement for prior approval for hospital admissions and for second opinions for surgery and other costly treatment options, controls on the use of specialists, and case management of care provided to high-cost patients.

Economists are concerned that the cost savings associated with all types of managed care techniques are limited. They contend that the savings benefits of managed care have now been realized (Mechanic, 2008). Without substantial new reform measures limiting access and services, the health care budget will increase and consume an ever-larger share of the gross domestic product (Feldstein, 2005; Patel & Rushefsky, 2006).

Generic Medication Substitution, Drug Co-Payments, and Pharmacy Choice Limitations. Insurance plans that pay the pharmacy directly for medications have specified that generic drugs be used whenever possible. Other plans simply put a cap on the amount reimbursed to the patient in an effort to encourage the use of generics. There is also a widespread effort to educate consumers and health professionals about the cost savings associated with generic drugs.

Co-payments for drugs have increased from $2 to $5, $10, $20, or more. Patients are often expected to pay substantially more if they want or need nongeneric drugs. Some insurance plans that provided a drug plan free to enrollees are now charging a monthly fee for the drug plan. Some plans require patients with chronic conditions to receive their medications by mail from large processing centers under contract to the insurance provider.

Reduce Waste of Equipment. Because of the emphasis on budget reduction, institutions have been more vigorous in attempts to encourage judicious use of disposable equipment. Some institutions have formalized their cost-benefit reviews to make more fiscally sound equipment decisions. A number of nurseries have returned to cloth diapers because they cost less than disposables. Inventory reduction, which reduces stored supplies, cuts back on the amount of supplies on hand. Although this practice is effective, supply shortages can arise if unexpected events occur to disrupt the supply pipeline. Health facility managers are employing more rigorous review procedures in the decision-making process concerned with new equipment and costly new technologies. These actions were first encouraged by health planning legislation that attempted to reduce duplication of services. Now, because of tight budget restraints, administrators are continuing the practice.

Emphasize Managed Care

Today managed care is the largest provider of health care services in the country. Eighty percent of employees covered in employer health insurance plans are enrolled in managed care (Kaiser/HRET, 2006). Federal and state efforts at cost reduction have expanded managed care to vulnerable populations covered by Medicaid and Medicare programs. In 2004, 61% of the Medicaid population was enrolled in managed care models (CMS, 2005). Managed care is not a popular option for seniors. In 2006, about 13% of Medicare enrollees used Medicare Advantage, the managed care option (Kaiser Family Foundation, 2006). There was an effort in 2003 to tie the prescription drug plan (Medicare D) to mandatory enrollment in Medicare managed care. That effort failed and is not part of the prescription drug law passed by Congress. There is every indication that managed care will continue to expand its reach in the health services market to populations currently served by fee-for-service providers.

Increase Productivity of Health Professionals

One method to reduce costs is judicious use of skilled workers. To that end, techniques that increase the efficiency of the skilled workforce and the use of substitute personnel are common.

Increase Patient Ratios and Use of Unlicensed Assistive Personnel. Increased patient ratios and use of unlicensed assistive personnel have been especially dramatic within the hospital environment. Nurses report increasing workloads, redistribution of labor, and an ever-increasing reliance on unskilled labor to reduce the number of registered nurses per unit (Unruh & Fottler, 2008). Evidence is surfacing to indicate that these changes have had serious impact on morale, patient care, and patient outcomes (Aiken, 2007; Person et al., 2004). Although in some circumstances restructuring of the work environment can both improve productivity and maintain quality of service, this does not appear to be the case with the current hospital changes.

Use More Nurse Practitioners and Other Physician Extenders. Nurse practitioners and physician assistants are considered effective in certain settings. For health managers, economics is the major motivator. Nurse practitioners cost less than physicians, their care is of similar quality, and consumers are pleased with their service (Diers & Price, 2007; Pulcini & Hart, 2007b). Nurse practitioners are particularly effective in managing chronic problems and increasing patient compliance with mediation regimens, appointment schedules, and behavioral changes (Sultz & Young, 2001). The Medicare and Medicaid programs took the lead in expanded the use of nurse practitioners (see Chapter 4). As emphasis shifts toward noninstitutional services, nurse practitioners are expected to assume responsibility for the care of a large portion of the elderly and persons with a medically stable chronic illness or disability.

The trend toward expanded use of nurse practitioners could be reversed by an oversupply of physicians. As the supply of doctors increases, the potential exists that physician groups might attempt to reduce the supply or limit the practice of nonphysician practitioners. Physician assistants may be more vulnerable to such a possibility because their practice is more dependent on physician sponsorship.

Increase Accountability of Provider Services

Oversight of services and costs is becoming tighter. Itemized bills are required and are carefully scrutinized by consumers and third-party payers. Both government and private insurers have instituted mechanisms to review patient service records for appropriateness of services and costs. Utilization review studies indicate that these mechanisms are cost effective (Rice & Kominski, 2001). Nurses are often employed as reviewers because their expertise is an asset to the insurers.

The government has increased efforts to scrutinize billing costs to identify billing fraud and abuse. The CMS is at the forefront of that effort. Recently the CMS announced fraud charges against a South Florida infusion therapy company accused of falsely billing $170 million for services it did not provide to Medicare patients (Larkin & Marcus, 2007).

Reverse Aborted Implementation of Health Care Planning

As previously discussed, health planning gradually evolved from a voluntary into a mandatory process with stringent criteria. Public Law 93–641, as fully implemented, operated a short period of time. The program produced modest successes in terms of cost containment by retarding the rate of increase in specific health care costs. It also allowed greater local participation in the decision-making process (Patel & Rushefsky, 2006).

Promote Continuity of Care and Case Management

Ensuring that people get what they need to maintain or improve their health status requires the creation of some method of coordinating all necessary services. This is especially important in a system noted for fragmented care. The use of case managers has proved to be effective. Pilot studies sponsored by the USDHHS have shown that the use of case managers to coordinate services to elderly clients has been beneficial. Clients received all necessary services, and the need for institutional care, the most costly service method, was delayed, which benefited the entire system. Community nurses make excellent case managers because they are already familiar with many community resources and the referral process. Case management has been a responsibility of community health nurses since the profession's inception. With the increase of managed care Medicare and Medicaid enrollees, there will be an added demand for nurses to play case management roles.

Increase Patient Cost Sharing

All insurance plans have raised consumer costs for health plans—even HMOs, which have historically had less patient cost sharing than other plans. Cost sharing comes in the form of increasing premiums, adding or increasing co-payments, and raising the deductible paid by consumers before the insurance plan pays anything (Patel & Rushefsky, 2006). Increasing patient cost share reduces the employer's insurance cost and increases the profits for insurance companies and their shareholders (Harrington & Estes, 2008b; Hollister & Estes, 2008).

A NATIONAL HEALTH CARE SYSTEM?

Reform efforts have had little impact on cost and have proved unsuccessful at reaching underserved populations. In *Nursing's Agenda for Health Care Reform* (ANA, 1992), the ANA strongly advocated a national health care plan with **universal coverage,** health insurance coverage for everyone. The ANA supported universal access to care with community-based primary care, illness prevention, and health promotion initiatives. In 1993, the United States seemed prepared to implement some type of national health care, but vigorous opposition derailed the attempt (Navarro, 2008). Despite this failure, the health care system has seen significant changes in payment structure and health care delivery in both the private and public sectors. Managed care organizations of every type have proliferated.

Although cost saving was a primary concern in 1993, quality of care is now becoming a focus (Kelly et al., 2008). The large number of uninsured is a major concern. Legislative and regulatory efforts are aimed at protecting consumers' rights and improving access for selected populations. Incremental rather than dramatic change is the current policy. There is a question whether further significant cost savings can be achieved under the present circumstances (Geyman, 2008; Mechanic, 2008). Economists believe that most of the cost savings associated with shifting populations into managed care have been realized. The current question is: *Can managed care provide care to all and still be profitable?* Some believe managed care organizations will self-destruct when they cease to demonstrate additional cost savings. Piecemeal legislative corrections of health provider/insurer decisions are cumbersome and unworkable. At a minimum, some expanded public oversight will be needed. Light (2008) argues that fundamental reform and universal health care coverage are the keys to good-quality health care. He has identified nine benchmarks for fairness in a health care system. They are the following:

- Good public health and basics
- Democratic accountability and empowerment
- Universal access—coverage and participation
- Equitable financing—by ability to pay
- Comprehensive and uniform benefits
- Universal access—minimization of nonfinancial barriers
- Value for money—clinical efficacy
- Fair and efficient costs
- Patient autonomy and choice

Perhaps it is time to look again at proposals for national health care systems. There are two types of national health care systems: a single-payer system and an all-payer system. They are outlined in Table 3-2 and discussed in the following sections.

SINGLE-PAYER SYSTEM

In a single-payer system, the government is the sole funder of health care. All citizens are covered, and private health insurance is unnecessary. The monies to finance care come from tax revenues. Centralized control of costs and utilization of services are elements of such systems. Fixed fees are assigned for all health services. Administration can be either contained at the federal level or allocated to the states.

ALL-PAYER SYSTEM

An all-payer system is one in which health care is financed by a number of sources, public and private. A wide variety of proposals fall into this category. Each has its own structure, but some common elements exist. Although all citizens would be covered, control would be more decentralized. Public financing would be from tax revenues; private financing, through insurance and out-of-pocket payments. Theoretically, there would be some minimum standard of service that must be offered to all citizens, and providers would be free to add more. Costs and utilization of service would be less centralized and more difficult to manage. *Nursing's Agenda for Health Care Reform* (ANA, 1992) takes the position that an all-payer system is the one most likely to work for U.S. health care reform. Currently, the ANA continues to advocate for universal coverage.

No health care system is without problems. Each new proposal has advantages and disadvantages. As the country searches for an alternative delivery system, it is imperative to examine and debate all plans, including the current model. Criticisms of each should not be taken at face value but investigated for validity and relevance.

STATES AND UNIVERSAL COVERAGE

In the absence of a federal effort at universal coverage, many states have taken action. Three states—Massachusetts, Vermont, and Oregon—have mandated universal health coverage. Other states have passed laws authorizing state government to investigate the costs of universal care, or to increase insurance coverage for selected vulnerable populations, or to mandate employer-provided health insurance. Box 3-10 lists the states considering coverage and those with active political coalitions advocating universal coverage. State progress toward universal health care might be tempered by the current state budget crises.

INTEGRATED DELIVERY SYSTEMS: THE PRESENT REALITY

Consolidation of health care delivery services into larger and larger health networks will continue. These voluntary mergers of health facilities and providers create networks that reduce the provider options available to consumers. Some of the networks are controlled directly by third-party payers. Sultz and Young (2004) note that managed care organizations continue to merge into managed care conglomerates. Consolidation and expansion is continuing, and it is expected that in the near future a single network will either dominate or monopolize a geographic area and assume responsibility for the health status of the regional population (Burns & Pauley, 2002; Kreitzer, 2007; Sultz & Young, 2004). If that happens, regulatory oversight will become inevitable to protect consumer interests. If change occurs as predicted, the final structure will resemble the managed competition model proposed by President Clinton's Health Task Force, complete with governmental oversight.

VESTED INTERESTS

There is an inevitable tension between various interest groups, for example, purchasers, consumers, practitioners, health plans, and shareholders of for-profit corporations (Navarro, 2008; Patel & Rushefsky, 2006). These competing segments are concerned about how change will affect their interests. Any change has its critics. Among the most vocal are those who have a vested interest in maintaining the status quo. In health care, the providers have a lot at stake. Any change will have an impact on practice, and some could reduce profits. The goal of each provider group is to minimize impact on its area of special interest. For example, the AMA opposes legislation expanding the scope of practice for nurse practitioners and direct reimbursement for their services (Feldstein, 2005). To that end, groups might engage in efforts to advance proposals

---

TABLE 3-2   National Health Care System Proposals

	Insurer	Coverage	Finance	Payment
Single-payer system	Government	Universal	Combination of taxes (e.g., income and sales)	Fees set by government
All-payer system	Mix of insurers, government, and private organizations	Universal, but there might be some differences in type of care	Combination of taxes and private monies (e.g., employer insurance and out of pocket)	Fees can be set by government for all or only for special groups

Box 3-10   Status of State Efforts toward Universal Care

States with Universal Coverage

Massachusetts, Vermont; pending in 2009 or 2010: Maine, Oregon

States with Legislation Introduced, Pending, or Under Study

California, Connecticut, Florida, Hawaii, Illinois, Indiana, Kansas, Kentucky, Maryland, Minnesota, Missouri, New Hampshire, New York, North Carolina, Pennsylvania, Texas, Wisconsin

States Where Legislation Was Considered and Vetoed by the Governor or Not Passed by the Legislature

Montana, Missouri, Washington

Data from National Conference of State Legislatures. (2008). *Health reform bills 2007-2008.* Retrieved January 25, 2008 from *http://www.ncsl.org/programs/health/universalhealth2007. htm*; and National Conference of State Legislatures. (2006). *Universal coverage bills, 2006.* Retrieved May 11, 2007 from *http://www.ncsl.org/programs/health/universal-health06.htm* and *http://www.ncsl.org/programs/health/universal/health2007htm.*

with little or no impact on their own operations and defeat or drastically alter those with more stringent controls.

Perhaps because they have the most to lose, the biggest players in the debate over health care reform have been the drug and insurance companies, the AMA, and the hospital industry (Kennedy, 1990). Each works to advance favorable proposals and to defeat plans that have an impact on its own independence or profit. Insurance companies are especially concerned about the single-payer system, although some physician groups and hospitals are also opposed.

A consortium of physicians, Physicians for a National Health Plan, support universal coverage. The American Medical Student Association (AMSA) is actively working to promote universal health care (AMSA, 2007).

Nursing and public health have traditionally been more active in supporting consumer rights and universal access to health care. The ANA supported Medicare and Medicaid long before those in other disciplines did. Both the ANA and the American Public Health Association have been active in support of a national health care system. However, because no profession is completely altruistic, nursing, too, is concerned about protecting its interests (Patel & Rushefsky, 2006).

Several strategies exist to influence the political decision-making process: one is to contribute funds to support the election of sympathetic politicians in an effort to influence policy and regulation of health care. The health industry contributed $307 million to the 2006 federal candidates. Those funds came from a few organizations, including the ANA. The ANA shares represented 0.2% of the total (Table 3-3). Lobbying is another way to advance an agenda and is not as easy to track as campaign contributions. As the debate on national health care continues, pay particular attention to news accounts of lobbying activity. Look for each organization's budget for lobbying activities, and scan newspapers and television for organization-sponsored advertisements about health care plans.

Influencing the President, any health-related task force, and Congress is an accepted part of the political process. Nurses need to become more astute in evaluating the impact of personal interests on any organization's position on specific delivery plans and on the information about those plans they supply to the general public. Nurses need to become very active in the political process and to make their voices heard or risk being excluded.

CHALLENGES FOR THE FUTURE

The health care system is in a state of turbulent change. Public health practitioners have long advocated universal access to health care. Cost concerns point toward retrenchment in funding and service. At the same time, the concept of health as a right has gained in popularity. The latter two issues have engendered concern about what direction to take. Supporters of the right to health care want expanded services. Supporters of funding reduction seem devoted to service cuts. Change in either direction is vigorously opposed by the other group. We could be headed toward either inertia or stalemate, or a time of collective community in which we tackle the problem with creativity and drive. The challenge is to find a way to cut or maintain cost levels and to simultaneously ensure a minimum standard of health for the entire population. The current structure is evolving to meet that expectation. Major changes to the Medicare program in 2003 and the addition of more uninsured children to SCHIP in subsequent years have continued that evolution. A philosophic shift toward a more community-directed health promotion focus and away from an illness-oriented focus would make that goal more viable. To provide a higher quality of care, competing interests need to form a coalition rather than to concentrate on protecting vested interests.

TABLE 3-3 Campaign Contributions by Health Care Organization and Industry PACs for 2006 Federal Campaign	
Group	**Contribution ($)**
Pharmaceutical/health products	172,178,724
American Medical Association PACs	19,880,000
American Hospital Association	17,415,135
American Nurses Association	587,238
Hospitals/hospital systems/nursing home organizations	4,028,877
Health services/health maintenance organizations	33,162,158

Total data from the Federal Election Commission; compiled by the Center for Responsive Politics. Retrieved June 1, 2007 from *http://www.opensecrets.org/Lobbyists/indus. Asp?lNd=H&format=print.*

PACs, Political action committees.

KEY IDEAS

1. The U.S. health care system is a fragmented, noncentralized arrangement consisting of multiple public and private providers.
2. The cost of health care is paid by a similar system of multiple sources.
3. Community/public health nurses need to know both how the health care system is structured and how it operates, because it has a significant impact on nursing practice and determines who has access to services and what types of services are available.
4. Although the United States has the most advanced medical technology, qualified personnel, and abundant resources in the world, it does not lead in health status compared with other developed countries, and on some specific indicators (e.g., infant mortality), it compares poorly.
5. Acute care, rather than disease prevention or health promotion, has been the major focus of the health care delivery system in the United States.
6. Recognition is growing of the importance of disease prevention as an effective means of improving health status.
7. The crisis in federal, state, and local government budgets has severely decreased the ability of states and local governments to deliver public health services.
8. Cost-containment strategies have been only marginally successful, slowing the rate of increase rather than reducing the cost of care.
9. Cost-containment measures and recognition of the importance of community care will continue to increase the demand for community health services, including community health nursing.
10. Health care is at a crossroads. Incremental change is the current model. Many players influence the decision-making process. Vested interests are intent on tailoring change to their advantage.
11. To improve the health status of the country, any decision about the evolving structure of our health care system must ensure a reasonable standard of care for all citizens.

LEARNING BY EXPERIENCE AND REFLECTION

1. Develop your vision of the ideal health care system. List some of the characteristics that constitute such a system. What would be the goal or goals of your ideal system?
2. Think about how you would go about implementing your ideal system. Consider some of the problems you are likely to encounter. Identify individuals, groups, and organizations with a vested interest in the present system. How might you expect them to react to your proposal?
3. From your current practice, identify a chronically ill individual and explore his or her thoughts on the present system.

Explore his or her concerns about health care: how needs are being met, expectations of how the illness will affect life in the future, and ideas on what (if anything) should be changed about the current method of care delivery.
4. Investigate current health-related issues in your community. Arrange an interview, in person or by phone, with a legislator who represents your community in the state legislature or with a staff member. Explore health-related issues, find out his or her position, and lobby for your position on the issue or issues.
5. Discover which agencies in your state are responsible for the public health of citizens. Is there centralized or decentralized management of state responsibilities? Determine some key indicators of health. Compare your state's indicators with those of surrounding states. How does your state fare?
6. You are a community/public health nurse in the public health department of Coty, a town of approximately 25,000 population on the outskirts of a major metropolitan city. Your health department provides primary obstetric care to certain prenatal populations. You notice that among your clients the infant mortality rate is higher than the national average. The director of public health has authorized you to explore the problem and design a plan that will reduce the infant mortality rate in your area.
   a. How would you start to locate information that might be helpful to your study? Determine if resources for prenatal care are available, accessible, acceptable, adequate, and effective.
   b. What other health issues could have an impact on your problem? Are the surrounding areas having similar problems, or is your town unique?
   c. What about the local providers of care? What would their concerns be with an intervention plan? If they are opposed, how might you structure your plans to reduce opposition?
   d. What types of issues would be essential in constructing an evaluation plan? Can you anticipate potential barriers to an effective evaluation plan?

COMMUNITY RESOURCES FOR PRACTICE

Following is a list of foundations involved with health care issues. Information about each organization is found on its website, which can be accessed through the **WebLinks** section of this book's website at *http://evolve.elsevier.com/Maurer/community/*.

Carnegie Corporation of New York: Interested in education, including health education
Kaiser Family Foundation: Interested in health issues, including access, insurance, and other policy concerns
Milbank Memorial Fund: Interested in health care and health statistics
Robert Wood Johnson Foundation: Interested in ambulatory care and health personnel
Rockefeller Foundation: Interested in health issues
W. K. Kellogg Foundation: Interested in health delivery and education

STUDY AIDS   http://evolve.elsevier.com/Maurer/community/

Visit the Evolve website for this book to find the following study and assessment materials:

- Quiz
- Web Scenario
- Critical Thinking Questions and Answers for Case Studies
- Care Plans
- *Healthy People* Updates
- Glossary

WEBSITE RESOURCES

The following item supplements the chapter's topics and is also found on the Evolve site:

WEB   3A: Federal Health Planning Efforts

REFERENCES

AAFRC Trust for Philanthropy. (2005). *Giving USA, 2004*. Indianapolis IN: Author.

Aiken, L. H. (2007). Nurse staffing impact on organizational outcomes. In D. J. Mason, J. K. Leavitt, & M. W. Chaffee (Eds.), *Policy and politics in nursing and health care* (5th ed.; pp. 550-559). St. Louis: Saunders.

American Association of Health Plans. (2006). *Health care quality: Utilization of health services*. Retrieved May 11, 2007 from *http://ahip.org/content/default.aspx?bc=41/331/361*.

American Medical Association. (2004). *Physician characteristics and distribution in the U.S., 2003*. Chicago: Author.

American Medical Student Association. (2007). *Position on universal coverage*. Retrieved August 16, 2007 from *http://amsa.org*.

American Nurses Association. (1992). *Nursing's agenda for health care reform: Executive summary*. Kansas City, MO: Author.

American Nurses Association. (1999). *Nursing-Sensitive Quality Indicators for Acute Care Settings and ANA's Safety and Quality Initiative*. Silver Spring, MD: Author.

Anderson, O. W. (1985). *Health services in the United States: A growth enterprise since 1875*. Ann Arbor, MI: Health Administration Press.

Association of State and Territorial Directors of Nursing. (2002). *Public health nursing: A partner for healthy populations*. Washington, DC: American Nurses Association.

Blum, H. (1981). *Planning for health* (2nd ed.). New York: Human Sciences Press.

Blumenthal, D. (2004). New stream from an old cauldron: The physician-supply debate. *New England Journal of Medicine, 350*(17), 1780-1787.

Brewer, C. S. (2005). The health care workplace. In A. R. Kovner & S. Jonas (Eds.) *Health care delivery in the United States* (pp. 297-323). New York: Springer.

Brown, E. R. (2001). Public policies to extend health care. In R. M. Andersen, T. H. Rice, & G. F. Kominski (Eds.), *Changing the U.S. health care system: Key issues in health services, policy, and management* (2nd ed., pp. 31-58). San Francisco: Jossey-Bass.

Burns, L. R., & Pauly, M. V. (2002). Integrated delivery network: A detour on the road to integrated health care. *Health Affairs, 21*(4), 128-134.

Califano, J. A., Jr. (1986). *America's health care revolution: Who lives? Who dies? Who pays?* New York: Random House.

Carter, G. M., Relles, D. A., Ridgeway, G. K., et al. (2003). Measuring function for Medicare inpatient rehabilitation payment. *Health Care Financing Review, 24*(3), 25-43.

Catalano, R., Libby, A., Snowden, L., et al. (2000). The effect of capitated financing on mental health services for children and youth: The Colorado experience. *American Journal of Public Health, 90*(12), 1861-1865.

Centers for Medicare and Medicaid Services. (2005). *Medicaid managed care penetration rates by state as of December 31, 2004*. Retrieved August 16, 2007 from *http://www.cms.hhs.gov/Medicaid/managedcare/mmcpr04.pdf*.

Centers for Medicare and Medicaid Services. (2007). *National health expenditures: Selected calendar years 1960-2005*. Retrieved August 20, 2007 from *http://www.cms.hhs.gov/NationalHealthExpendData/downloads/tables.pdf*.

Center on Policy Attitudes. (2000). *Americans on health policy*. Retrieved September 9, 2003 from *http://policyattitudes.org/OnlineReports/Healthcare/exec_sum.html*.

Clauser, S. B., & Berman, A. S. (2003). Significance of functional status data for payment and quality. *Health Care Financing Review, 24*(3), 1-11.

Cohen, S. S., & Piotrowska-Haugstetter, M. (2007). A primer on political philosophy. In D. J. Mason, J. K. Leavitt, & M. W. Chaffee (Eds.), *Policy and politics in nursing and health care* (pp. 63-74). St. Louis: Saunders.

Commonwealth Fund Commission on a High Performance Health System. (2006). *Why not the best? Results from a national scorecard on U.S. health system performance*. New York: Author.

Congressional Budget Office. (1992). *Economic implications of rising health care costs* (CBO study). Washington, DC: U.S. Government Printing Office.

Davis, K., Schoen, C., Schoenbaum, S. C., et al. (2007). *Mirror, mirror on the wall: An international update on the comparative performance of American health care*. The Commonwealth Fund. Retrieved January 29, 2007 from *http://www.commonwealthfund.org/publications/publications_show.htm?doc_id=482678*.

Diers, D., & Price, L. (2007). Research as a political and policy tool. In D. J. Mason, J. K. Leavitt, & M. W. Chafee (Eds.), *Policy and politics in nursing and health care* (5th ed.; pp. 195-207). St. Louis: Saunders.

Federal Election Commission; compiled by the Center for Responsive Politics. Retrieved June 1, 2007 from *http://www.opensecrets.org/Lobbyists/indus.Asp?INd=H=print*.

Feldstein, P. J. (2005). *Health care economics* (6th ed.). Clifton Park, NY: Delmar.

Fiscella, K., & Williams, D. R. (2008). Health disparities based on socioeconomic inequities: Implications for urban health care. In C. Harrington & C. L. Estes, (Eds.), *Health policy: Crisis and reform in the U.S. health care delivery system* (5th ed.; pp. 49-60). Sudbury, MA: Jones & Bartlett.

Fleury, J., Peter, M. A., & Thomas, J. (1996). Health promotion across the continuum: Challenges for the future of cardiovascular nursing. *Journal of Cardiovascular Nursing, 11*(1), 14-26.

Flint, S. S. (1997). Insuring children: The next step. *Health Affairs, 16*(4), 79-81.

Garrett, B., & Zucherman, S. (2008). National estimates of the effects of mandatory Medicaid managed care programs on health care access and use, 1997-1999. In C. Harrington & C. L. Estes (Eds.), *Health policy: Crisis and reform in the U.S. health care delivery system* (5th ed.; pp. 332-344). Sudbury, MA: Jones & Bartlett.

Gebbie, K. M. (2007). Could a national health system work in the United States? In D. J. Mason, J. K. Leavitt, & M. W. Chaffee (Eds.), *Policy and politics in nursing and health care* (5th ed.; pp. 282-286). St. Louis: Saunders.

Geyman, J. P. (2002). *Health care in America: Can our ailing system be healed?* Boston: Butterworth-Heinemann.

Geyman, J. P. (2008). Myths as barriers to health care reform in the United States. In C. Harrington & C. L. Estes, *Health policy: Crisis and reform in the U.S. health care delivery system* (5th ed.; pp. 407-413). Sudbury, MA: Jones & Bartlett.

Gingrich, N. (2002). *Designing a twenty-first century health and healthcare system*. Washington, DC: Gingrich Group.

Gold, M. (1999). The changing U.S. Health Care System: Challenges for responsible public policy. *Milbank Quarterly, 77*, 3-37.

Green, L. W., & Anderson, C. L. (1982). *Community health* (4th ed.). St. Louis: Mosby.

Gunn, S. M., & Platt, P. S. (1945). *Voluntary health agencies: An interpretative study*. New York: Ronald Press.

Harrington, C. (2007). The politics of long-term care. In D. L. Mason, J. K. Leavitt, & M. W. Chaffee (Eds.), *Policy and politics in nursing and health care* (5th ed.; pp. 295-303). St. Louis: Saunders.

Harrington, C., & Estes, C. L. (2008a). Health care delivery system issues. In C. Harrington

& C. L. Estes (Eds.), *Health policy: Crisis and reform in the U.S. health care delivery system* (5th ed.; pp. 153-158). Sudbury, MA: Jones & Bartlett.

Harrington, C., & Estes, C. L. (2008b). The economics of health care. In C. Harrington & C. L. Estes (Eds.), *Health policy: Crisis and reform in the U.S. health care delivery system* (5th ed.; pp. 249-254). Sudbury, MA: Jones & Bartlett.

Harrington, C., & Pellow, D. (2001). The uninsured and their health, micro-level issues. In C. Harrington & C. L. Estes (Eds.), *Health policy: Crisis and reform in the U.S. health care delivery system* (3rd ed.; pp. 56-64). Boston: Jones & Bartlett.

Health Resources and Services Administration. (2006). *The registered nurse population: National sample survey of registered nurses March 2004: Preliminary findings*. Washington DC: U.S. Department of Health and Human Services, HRSA.

Hogberg, D. (2006, July). Don't fall prey to propaganda: Life expectancy and infant mortality are unreliable measures for comparing the U.S. health care system to others. *National Policy Analysis*, No. 547.

Hollister, B., & Estes, C. L. (2008). The economic and health security of today's young women. In C. Harrington & C. L. Estes (Eds.), *Health policy: Crisis and reform in the U.S. health care delivery system* (5th ed.; pp. 123-133). Sudbury, MA: Jones & Bartlett.

Hospice Association of America. (2007). *Hospice facts and statistics*. Washington DC: Author.

Illich, I. (1977). *Medical nemesis: The expropriation of health*. Toronto: Bantam Books.

Joint Commission on Accreditation of Healthcare Organizations. (2005). *Health care at the crossroads: Strategies for addressing the evolving nursing crisis*. Oak Brook Terrace, IL: Author.

Kaiser Family Foundation. (2006). *The growth of private plans in Medicare at a glance*. Retrieved January 23, 2008 from *http://www.kff.org/Medicare/7473.cfm*.

Kaiser/HRET. (2006). *Employer benefits 2006: Annual survey*. Menlo Park, CA: Kaiser Family Foundation/Health Research and Education Trust. Retrieved January 23, 2008.

Kelly, E., Moy, E., Stryer, D., et al. (2008). The national healthcare quality and disparities reports: An overview. In C. Harrington & C. L. Estes (Eds.), *Health policy: Crisis and reform in the U.S. health care delivery system* (5th ed.; pp. 215-220). Sudbury, MA: Jones & Bartlett.

Kennedy, E. M. (1990). The politics of health. In P. R. Lee & C. L. Estes (Eds.), *The nation's health* (3rd ed.; pp. 121-122). Boston, MA: Jones & Bartlett.

Kover, A. R., & Knickman, J. R. (2005). Overview: The state of health care delivery in the United States. In A. R. Kovner & J. R. Knickman (Eds.), *Jonas and Kovner's health care delivery in the United States* (8th ed.; pp. 1-2). New York: Springer.

Krauss, E.A. (1977). *Illness: Political sociology of health and medical care*. New York: Elsevier.

Kreitzer, M. J. (2007). Successes and struggles in complementary health care. In D. J. Mason, J. K. Leavitt, M. W. Chaffee (Eds.), *Policy and politics in nursing and health care* (5th ed.; pp. 336-344). St. Louis: Saunders.

Kronenfeld, J. J. (1997). *The changing federal role in U.S. health care policy*. Westport, CT: Praeger.

Lamm, R. D. (1990). The ten commandments of health care. In P. R. Lee & C. L. Estes (Eds.), *The nation's health* (3rd ed.; pp. 124-133). Boston: Jones & Bartlett.

Larkin, C., & Marcus, A. (2007, August 21). Firm charged with Medicare fraud. *Washington Post*, p. D2.

Lee, C., & Kaufman, M. (2007, July 29). Appointee blocked health report: Surgeon General's draft report rejected for not being political. *Washington Post*, pp. A-1, A-5.

Lee-Feldstein, A., Feldstein, P. J., Buchmueller, T., et al. (2000). The relationship of HMOs, health insurance, and delivery systems to breast cancer outcomes. *Medical Care*, 38(7), 705-718.

Lee-Feldstein, A., Feldstein, P. J., Buchmueller, T. (2002). Health care factors related to stage at diagnosis and survival among Medicare patients with colorectal cancer. *Medical Care*, 40(5), 359-361.

Leviton, L. C., & Rhodes, S. D. (2005). Public health: Policy, practice, and perceptions. In A. R. Kovner & J. R. Knickman (Eds.), *Health care delivery in the United States* (8th ed.; pp. 90-129). New York: Springer Publications.

Lewis, C. (2001). The role of prevention. In R. M. Andersen, T. H. Rice, & G. F. Kominski (Eds.), *Changing the U.S. health care system: Key issues in health services, policy, and management* (pp. 436-456). San Francisco: Jossey-Bass.

Light, D. W. (2008). Improving medical practice and the economy through universal health insurance. In C. Harrington & C. L. Estes (Eds.), *Health policy: Crisis and reform in the U.S. health care delivery system* (5th ed.; pp. 433-436). Sudbury, MA: Jones & Bartlett.

Lindblom, C. E. (1953). *Politics, economics, and welfare*. New York: Harper Press.

McGlynn, E. A., Asch, S. M., Adams, J., et al. (2003). The quality of health care delivered to adults in the United States. *New England Journal of Medicine*, 348(26), 2635-2645.

McKeown, T. (1976). *The role of Medicare: Dream, mirage, or nemesis?* London: Nutfield Provincial Hospitals Trust.

McKinsey and Company. (2007). *Accounting for the cost of health care in the United States*. Retrieved February 15, 2007 from *http://www.mckinsey.com/mgi/reports/pdfs/healthcare/MGI-US-HC-fallreport.pdf*.

Mechanic, D. (2008). The rise and fall of managed care. In C. Harrington & C. L. Estes (Eds.), *Health policy: Crisis and reform in the U.S. health care delivery system* (5th ed.; pp. 345-352). Sudbury, MA: Jones & Bartlett.

MedPac. (2006). *A data book: Healthcare spending and the Medicare program*. Washington DC: U.S. Government Printing Office.

Merrill, J. C. (1994). *The road to health care reform: Designing a system that works*. New York: Plenum Press.

Milio, N. (1981). *Promoting health through public policy*. Philadelphia: F. A. Davis.

Milio, N. (1983). *Primary care and the public's health*. Lexington, KY: Lexington Books.

Milio, N. (2002). *Facing managed care, lean government, and health disparities*. Ann Arbor: University of Michigan Press.

National Association of County and City Health Officials. (2006). *2005 National profile of local health departments*. Washington DC: Author.

National Commission on Community Health Services. (1967). *Health administration and organization in the decade ahead*. Cambridge, MA: Harvard University Press.

National Conference of State Legislatures. (2006). *Universal coverage bills, 2006*. Retrieved May 11, 2007 from *http://www.ncsl.org/programs/health/universalhealth06.htm* and *http://www.ncsl.org/programs/health/universalhealth2007.htm*.

National Conference of State Legislatures. (2008). *Health reform bills 2007-2008*. Retrieved January 25, 2008 from *http://www.ncsl.org/programs/health/universalhealth2007.htm*.

Navarro, V. (1995). Why Congress did not enact health care reform. *Journal of Health Politics, Policy, and Law*, 20(2), 455-461.

Navarro, V. (2008). Why Congress did not enact health care reform. In C. Harrington & C. L. Estes (Eds.), *Health policy: Crisis and reform in the U.S. health care delivery system* (5th ed.; pp. 433-436). Sudbury, MA: Jones & Bartlett.

Patel, K., & Rushefsky, M. E. (1999). *Health care politics and policy in America* (2nd ed.). New York: M. E. Sharpe.

Patel, K., & Rushefsky, M. E. (2006). *Health care politics and policy in America* (3rd ed.). New York: M. E. Sharpe.

Person, S. D., Allison, J. J., Keife, C. I., et al. (2004). Nurse staffing and mortality for Medicare patients with acute myocardial infarction. *Medical Care*, 42(1), 4-12.

Pew Commission urges increased action to cut U.S. physician supply. (1998, November 10). *PT Bulletin*, 10.

Pickett, G., & Hanlon, J. J. (1990). *Public health administration and practice*. St. Louis: Mosby.

Pulcini, J. A., & Hart, M. A. (2007a). Financing health care in the United States. In D. J. Mason, J. K. Leavitt, & M. W. Chaffee (Eds.), *Policy and politics in nursing and health care* (5th ed.; pp. 384-408). St. Louis: Saunders.

Pulcini, J. A., & Hart, M. A. (2007b). Politics of advanced practice nursing. In D. J. Mason, J. K. Leavitt, & M. W. Chaffee (Eds.), *Policy and politics in nursing and health care* (5th ed.; pp. 568-573). St. Louis: Saunders.

Quad Council of Public Health Nursing Organizations. (2007). *The public health nursing shortage: A threat to the public's health.* Retrieved August 22, 2007 from *http://www.astdn.org.*

Reed, G. B. (1991). On-site health-monitoring program keeps "lifestyle" diseases in check. *Occupational Health and Safety, 60*(10), 56, 59-62.

Reinhardt, U. E. (1986). Rationing the health care surplus. *Nurse Economics, 4*(May/June), 101-108.

Rice, T. H., & Kominski, G. F. (2001). Containing health care costs. In R. M. Andersen, T. H. Rice, & G. F. Kominski (Eds.), *Changing the U.S. health care system: Key issues in health services, policy, and management* (2nd ed.; pp. 82-99). San Francisco: Jossey-Bass.

Roberts, M., & Rhoades, J. A. (2007, June). *The uninsured in America, first half of 2006: Estimates for the U.S. civilian noninstututionalized population under age 65* (Statistical Brief #171). Rockville, MD: Agency for Healthcare Research and Quality.

Rodwin, V. G. (2005). A comparative analysis of health systems among wealthy nations. In A. R Kovner & J. R. Knickman (Eds.), *Jonas and Kovner's health care delivery in the U.S.* (8th ed.; pp. 162-211). New York: Springer.

Roemer, M. I. (1991). *National health care systems of the world.* New York: Oxford University Press.

Roemer, R., Kramer, C., & Frink, J. E. (1975). *Planning urban health service: From jungle to system.* New York: Springer.

Rothberg, M. B., Abraham, I., Lindenauer, P. K., et al. (2008). Improving nurse-to patient staffing ratios as a cost-effective safety intervention. In C. Harrington & C. L. Estes (Eds.), *Health policy: Crisis and reform in the U.S. health care delivery system* (5th ed.; pp. 226-231). Sudbury, MA: Jones & Bartlett.

Schnelle, J. F., Simmons, S. F., Harrington, C., et al. (2008). Relationship of nursing home staffing to quality of care. In C. Harrington & C. L. Estes (Eds.), *Health policy: Crisis and reform in the U.S. health care delivery system* (5th ed.; pp. 238-248). Sudbury, MA: Jones & Bartlett.

Schur, C. L., Beck, M. L., & Yegian, J. M. (2004). Public perceptions of cost containment strategies: Mixed signals for managed care. *Health Affairs, 23*(suppl 2), W4-516-525.

Shi, L., & Singh, D. A. (2001). *Healthcare delivery in America.* Gaithersburg, MD: Aspen.

Shonick, W. (1995). *Government and health services: Government's role in the development of U.S. Health Services 1930-1980.* Oxford, England: Oxford University Press.

Smith, S. D. (2006). *Military transforming use of medical records.* American Forces Press Service. Retrieved August 8, 2007 from *http://www. defenselink.mil/news/NewsArtile.aspx?ID=1600.*

Sparer, M. S. (2005). The role of government in U.S. health care. In A. R. Kovner & J. R. Knickman (Eds.), *Health care delivery in the United States* (8th ed.; pp. 131-161). New York: Springer.

Sultz, H. A., & Young, K. M. (2001). *Health care USA: Understanding its organization and delivery* (3rd ed.). Gaithersburg, MD: Aspen.

Sultz, H. A., & Young, K. M. (2004). *Health care USA: Understanding its organization and delivery* (4th ed.). Sudbury MA: Jones & Bartlett.

Torrens, P. R. (2002). Overview of the organization of health services in the United States. In S. J. Williams & P. R. Torrens (Eds.), *Introduction to health services* (6th ed.; pp. 18-46). West Albany, NY: Delmar.

Unruh, L., & Spetz, J. (2007). A primer on health economics. In D. J. Mason, J. K. Leavitt, & M. W. Chaffee (Eds.), *Policy and politics in nursing and health care* (5th ed.; pp. 363-375). St. Louis: Saunders.

Unruh, L. Y., & Fottler, M. D. (2008). Projections and trends in RN supply: What do they tell us about the nursing shortage? In C. Harrington & C. L. Estes (Eds.), *Health policy: Crisis and reform in the U.S. health care delivery system* (5th ed.; pp. 198-206). Sudbury, MA: Jones & Bartlett.

U.S. Bureau of the Census. (2007). *Statistical abstract of the United States: The national data book* (126th ed.). Washington, DC: U.S. Government Printing Office.

U.S. Department of Health and Human Services, Health Resources and Services Administration, Bureau of Health Professionals, Division of Nursing. (2006). *National sample survey of registered nurses, 2004.* Washington DC: U.S. Government Printing Office.

U.S. Department of Labor, Bureau of Labor Statistics. (2006). *Occupational outlook handbook 2006-2007 edition.* Washington, DC: U.S. Government Printing Office.

U.S. Department of Veterans Affairs. (2004). *Who we are: Performance and accountability report, FY2004.* Washington DC: Author.

U.S. Department of Veterans Affairs. (2006, November 15). *Fiscal year 2006 performance and accountability report.* Washington DC: Author.

U.S. Public Health Service. (1979). *Healthy people: The Surgeon General's Report on Health Promotion and Disease Prevention* (DHEW Publication No. 7955071). Washington, DC: Office of Assistant Secretary for Health and Surgeon General.

Walker, B. (1992). The future of public health. *Public Health Policy Forum, 82*(1), 21-23.

White House Domestic Policy Council. (1993). *The President's health security plan.* New York: Times Books.

Wilensky, H. L. (1975). *Welfare state and equality: Structural and ideological roots of public expenditures.* Berkeley: University of California Press.

World Health Organization. (2007). *World health statistics, 2007.* Geneva, Switzerland: Author.

Suggested Readings—General

Andersen, R. M., Rice, T. M., & Kominski, G. F. (2001). *Changing the U.S. health care system: Key issues in health services, policy, and management* (2nd ed.). San Francisco: Jossey-Bass.

Feldstein, P. J. (2005). *Health care economics* (6th ed.). Clifton Park, NY: Delmar.

Inglehart, J. K. (1992). The American health care system: Managed care. *New England Journal of Medicine, 327,* 742-747.

Suggested Readings—Select Topics

United States Health Care System

Davis, K., Schoen, C., Schoenbaum, S. C., et al. (2007). *Mirror, mirror on the wall: An international update on the comparative performance of American health care.* The Commonwealth Fund. Retrieved January 29, 2007 from *http://www.commonwealthfund.org/publications/publications_show. htm?doc_id=482678.*

Kovner, A. R., & Knickman, J. R. (Eds.). *Jonas and Kovner's health care delivery in the United States* (8th ed.). New York: Springer.

Health Care System Reform and Comparison of National Health Care Systems

Harrington, C., & Estes, C. L. (Eds.). (2008). *Health policy: Crisis and reform in the U.S. delivery system* (5th ed.). Sudbury, MA: Jones & Bartlett.

McGlynn, E. A. (2004). There is no perfect health system. *Health Affairs, 23*(3), 100-102.

Physicians for a National Health Program. (2007). *Snapshots of health systems in 16 countries.* Retrieved February 28, 2007 from *http://www. pnhp.org/facts/international_health_systems. php?page=all.*

Sultz, H. A., & Young, K. M. (2004). *Health care USA: Understanding its organization and delivery* (4th ed.). Sudbury MA: Jones & Bartlett.

Current and Future Status of Public Health

Hinman, A. R. (1990). 1889 to 1989: A century of health and disease. *Public Health Reports, 105,* 374-380.

Institute of Medicine. (2003). *The future of the public's health in the twenty-first century.* Washington, DC: National Academy Press.

4

Financing of Health Care: Context for Community/Public Health Nursing

Frances A. Maurer

FOCUS QUESTIONS

What sources provide funding for health care in this country?

What has been the general pattern of expenditures for health care?

Are there groups who are at greater risk for diminished or no access to health care services?

How have Medicare and Medicaid affected health care delivery to the populations they serve?

What methods have been used to attempt cost containment in health care?

Has cost containment affected services? If so, in what ways?

How can nurses influence the costs and delivery of health care services?

CHAPTER OUTLINES

KEY TERMS

Today's nurses need to have a clear understanding of the finance mechanisms of the health care system. In the past, such topics were not considered relevant to the practice of nursing and were also considered irrelevant to the planning and distribution of good nursing care. The expectation was that people should be provided with the best and most appropriate nursing care and medical treatments regardless of their ability to pay.

Although universal access to care is admirable, it has never been a reality in this country. Debate rages about potential rationing of health care, but health care is already rationed by the ability to pay. A person's financial status affects the quality and quantity of care she or he receives. Current events have served to highlight that problem to health care providers, the public at large, and individual consumers.

RELEVANCE OF HEALTH CARE FINANCING TO COMMUNITY/ PUBLIC HEALTH NURSING PRACTICE

Why is the financing of health care services important to the community health nurse? Why not just continue providing appropriate care to a caseload or community and leave others to worry about the financial costs and how to meet them? For one thing, nurses will find that nursing practice, to some extent, is shaped by those financial constructs. If a community health nurse is providing home visits to a client newly diagnosed with diabetes, the number of home visits allowed is limited by the government agency or private insurance company that finances the visits. A nurse assigned to provide skilled nursing care in the home to an individual (e.g., dressing changes) might find that the person requires other services, such as nutritional health teaching or medication monitoring. These services might not be covered by the payer, especially if they are not related to the specific medical condition for which the visits are made. If, while on a home visit, a community health nurse discovers that other household members need or would benefit from nursing care, these members might not be covered by the insurance company, or, if they are covered, treatment of the problem identified might not be considered a reimbursable service by the payer.

Why should community health nurses care whether needed services are paid for? Why not just provide the service while in the home? Although occasionally this solution is possible, more often, time constraints will not allow the nurse to do this. The nurse's employing agency is reimbursed only for specific services provided to patients. Therefore, the agency will set a nurse's patient load for the day based on a reasonable time to perform those designated services. Nurses who routinely provide additional services to patients or care for other household members might fall behind in the agency's caseload expectation. Nurses may not be covered in case of a malpractice claim because the additional service was not first sanctioned by the agency. Therefore, the community health nurse faces a dilemma: How to reconcile the ideals of good nursing care with the realities dictated by circumstances, the nurse's employer, and the financial reimbursement system.

RELATIVE MAGNITUDE OF HEALTH SPENDING IN THE UNITED STATES

Since 1965, national expenditures on health care have risen steadily and are a serious concern. Yearly costs have risen from $12.7 billion in 1950 to $1988 billion in 2005 (Figure 4-1). Of even greater concern than escalating costs is the growth of health care as a portion of the national budget. Health care continues to increase its share of the **gross domestic product (GDP)** in comparison with other expenditures. The GDP is a monetary measure of the production of a country. Health care currently outstrips the combined costs of both defense and education (Figure 4-2).

The increasing proportion of the GDP (16%) devoted to health care means that individuals and families spend more on health care and have less to spend on food, clothing, housing, schooling, leisure, and other needs or interests. The personal cost of health care—what each American spends on health care services and products such as insurance premiums, medications, and physician and hospital services—has doubled every decade. The average yearly cost for every American was $5598 in 2005 (Centers for Medicare and Medicaid Services [CMS], 2007c). By the year 2016, it is estimated that health care costs will average $12,782.20 per year for each person in the country (Poisal et al., 2007).

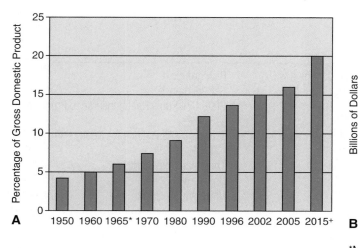

A

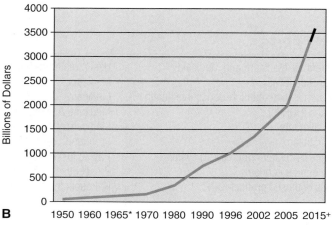

B

*Medicare and Medicaid programs begin   +Projected costs

FIGURE 4-1 Health care costs for selected years, 1950-2015. (Data from Health Care Finance Administration, Office of the Actuary, and Office of National Estimates.)

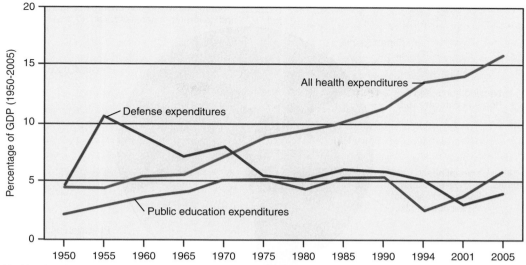

FIGURE 4-2 Health, education, and defense spending. *GDP*, Gross domestic product. (Data from Augenblick, J. [2001]. *The status of school financing today*. Denver: Educational Commission of the States. Garamone, J. *Historical context important when considering budget requests*. Retrieved April 2, 2008 from http://www.defenselink.mil/news/newsarticle.aspx?id=2966; Levit, K., Smith, C., Cowan, C., et al. [2003]. Trends in U.S. healthcare spending 2001. Health Affairs, *22*[10], 154-164; Centers for Medicare and Medicaid Services [2007]. Table 1: National health expenditures aggregate, per capita amounts, percent distribution, and average annual percent growth, by source of funds: Selected calendar years 1960-2005. Retrieved May 30, 2007 from http://www.cms.hhs.gov/NationalHealthExpendData/downloads/tables.pdf; U.S. Bureau of the Census. [2007]. Statistical abstract of the United States: The national data book [126th ed.]. Table 490: National defense outlays and veterans benefits: 1960 to 2007. Washington DC: U.S. Government Printing Office; and World Bank. [2007]. World development indicators on line. Government expenditures: Public education expenditure as a percent of GDP. Washington DC: World Bank.)

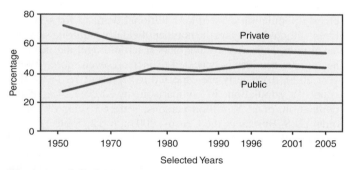

FIGURE 4-3 Public and private shares of health care costs. (Data from Centers for Medicare and Medicaid Services.)

PRIVATE- AND PUBLIC-SECTOR SHARES OF HEALTH EXPENSES

Governments at all levels provided 45.4% of the total health care costs in 2005 (Figure 4-3). Two large programs, Medicare and Medicaid, account for 37.3% of the country's entire health expenses (CMS, 2007c). In 1965, before Medicare and Medicaid, the federal share of health care expenses was roughly equal to the combined state and local contributions. By 1970, the federal share had doubled. In 2005, the federal government paid approximately 76% of public-sector costs, and state and local governments paid 24% (CMS, 2007c).

In 1965, the private sector accounted for 74% of all health care expenses. By 1975, after Medicare and Medicaid were well established, the private-sector share dropped to 57.5%. Today, the private-sector share of expenditures remains relatively stable at 54.6%. The pattern of health expenditures is a reflection of age and social risk factors. Health care services provided to risk groups cost more than care provided to more healthy individuals. **Risk groups** are groups with a likelihood of accidents or illness because of low income or inability to easily access health care services. As social health programs make access and care available to these risk groups (e.g., the elderly and the poor), these expenses escalate.

PRIORITIES IN HEALTH CARE EXPENDITURES

By far, the largest amount of money is spent on personal health care and very little on public health. In Figure 4-4, expenditures for 2005 are broken down by type and source of funding. Personal health care services accounted for all but 16.3% of the entire health budget (CMS, 2007c). Hospital care is the most costly category, and physicians' and clinical services are the second highest cost area.

Public health, research, and construction together account for a mere 9.2% of the entire budget. Public health activities are subsidized wholly by the public sector. State and local governments bear the major costs of providing these services. Public health's share of funding has remained relatively stable since the early 1970s. Government, especially the federal government, bears the major responsibility for research. Most of these funds are used or distributed by the National Institutes of Health. The private-sector invests much of the construction funds for building projects.

COST INCREASES AFFECT THE ENTIRE ECONOMY: YOU AND ME

Health care expenditures are particularly significant in the economy, because they are so extensive. As health care expands its share of the country's GDP, other industries lose ground. For example, for every 1% increase in GDP of health care, there is a corresponding 1% loss in revenues to other industries. Eventually, everyone is affected by increases in health costs. Government agencies must pay for increases in services that they are pledged to provide. Government expenses are ultimately the responsibility of the taxpayer. As federal and state health care costs have escalated, the increased expense has been passed on to individual taxpayers via

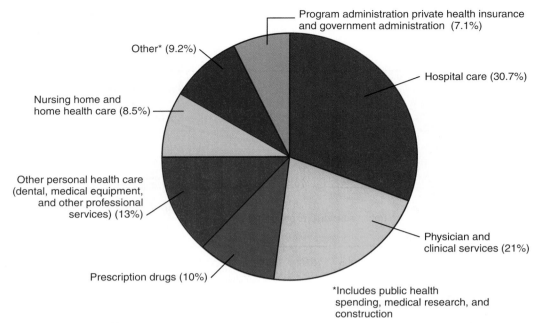

FIGURE 4-4 Where U.S. health care dollars were spent in 2005. (Data from Centers for Medicare and Medicaid Services, Office of the Actuary, National Health Statistics Group. [2007]. Table 2: National health expenditures aggregate amounts and average annual percent change, by type of expenditure: Selected calendar years 1960-2005. Retrieved August 20, 2007 from *http://www.cms.hhs.gov/NationalHealthExpendData/downloads/tables.pdf*.)

income and other taxes. Insurance companies pass on increases in expenses to employers. Employers, in turn, usually pass on the extra costs to their employees by increasing the employees' share of health insurance contributions. Those without health insurance pay *out of pocket,* which refers to personal and direct payment for health care. No one escapes increases in the cost of health care services.

REASONS FOR THE INCREASE IN HEALTH CARE COSTS

There are three basic factors responsible for escalating costs. The first is inflation. Inflation as a generic factor affects the costs of all types of goods and services and has played a significant role in cost increases. Between 1950 and 1990, there were several periods of heavy inflation. The net effect was a dramatic increase in the cost of basic goods and services, such as food, fuel, electricity, telephone, construction, labor, and insurance. As inflation increases prices, the health care industry's costs for these goods and services are also increased, and these higher expenses are passed on to the consumer. Inflation helps to explain increases in the overall monetary expenditures for health care, but does little to explain health care increases in the share of the GDP. These are more closely related to other factors (Bodenheimer, 2008; McKinsey & Company, 2007):

- Growth in the number of elderly in the population
- Use of advanced technology
- Growth of specialties in medical care
- Reimbursement mechanisms and administrative costs
- Burden of uninsured and underinsured populations

Increased demand for services is primarily the result of federal programs (Medicare and Medicaid) and an aging population. Before these programs were instituted, cost was a rationing factor for poor and elderly persons in need of care. Medicare and Medicaid reduced the access barrier and created a greater demand for health care among groups for which it

was previously restricted. At the same time, the growth of the elderly population created an additional demand for services. Even without Medicare, the number of elderly requiring services has grown, and, as baby boomers reach old age, the need for health care services is expected to increase even more. By the year 2020, the elderly are expected to represent 16.5% of this country's population. In comparison, in 2005, 12.4% of the population, or 36.8 million persons, were 65 years of age or older (U.S. Bureau of the Census, 2007a, p. 12, Table 11).

Technologic advances in medicine have been enormous and expensive (Emanuel et al., 2007). Development costs of new procedures, drugs, and equipment are high, and new technologies generally require more skilled technicians and professional operators. Advances in medical treatment have also created an increased demand for services, because refinements frequently increase the number of patients who can be successfully treated. Sultz and Young (2004) substantiate the impact of new technology on rising health care costs. They suggest that better planning could reduce some of these costs and rescue utilization. Torrens (2002) suggests that more stringent research is needed to determine whether higher-cost technologies are more beneficial and cost effective. Shi and Singh (2001) contend that technology's impact on cost is a mixed bag. Some procedures cost more, whereas others reduce costs over time. For example, computed tomography scans cost more than radiographs, but they have reduced the need for exploratory surgery.

GROUPS AT RISK FOR INCREASED COSTS AND FEWER SERVICES

To further complicate matters, as health care costs have escalated, government and private industry have made efforts to contain expenditures. These efforts have resulted in actions that have either limited access to health care or reduced available services to certain segments of the population. Three specific groups have been particularly hard hit by escalating costs and reductions in services: the elderly, poor children, and a growing population of medically indigent individuals. The medically indigent are those who do not have health insurance coverage, do not qualify for government health care assistance, and are unable to pay health care costs on their own.

In 2005, 49.3% of the aged were 75 years or older (U.S. Bureau of the Census, 2007a, p. 12, Table 11). The elderly, especially frail elderly persons, are at increased risk for disability, chronic disease, and need for expanded health services. As will be seen, the services they receive under Medicare are limited and require co-payments.

Children in low-income families are another risk group. The percentage of children below the poverty level rose from 17.9% in 1980 to a high of 22% by 1993 (Lewit et al., 1997; U.S. Bureau of the Census, 2002a). During that same time, the social service and health care assistance programs designed to assist them were, in many instances, cut back (Pepper Commission, 1990). By 1993, a growing economy increased employment opportunities, and the State Children's Health Insurance Program (SCHIP) contributed to increased access to health insurance and a decline in the number of poor children. Currently, one of every six children (12.9 million) lives in poverty and one of every 10 children is uninsured (U.S. Bureau of the Census, 2006).

In 2006, approximately 50.4 million persons were medically indigent (Roberts & Rhoades, 2007). Those in this group are **uninsured,** with no health insurance, including government-sponsored medical insurance. They are the "working poor." Their income makes them ineligible for government assistance but is not sufficient for them to purchase their own health care or insurance.

The uninsured and underinsured contribute to escalating health care costs because those individuals delay seeking care in a timely manner for acute and chronic conditions, and forgo or delay preventive care. The result of these behaviors is increased severity of illness, more complications of illness, and greater use of emergency rooms (Institute of Medicine [IOM], 2007), actions that increase the eventual cost of treatment. Chapter 21 provides a more detailed discussion of the impact of poverty and lack of health insurance on health status.

HEALTH CARE FINANCING MECHANISMS

Currently, health care financing is very complex. Services are paid for by a variety of sources and methods rather than a single funding source (Figure 4-5). Health insurance is a voluntary arrangement developed and managed by commercial insurance companies, Blue Cross and Blue Shield, and managed care organizations. Employers provide insurance for many of their workers. Health care for the poor is provided by local, state, and federal funding, primarily through Medicaid. State and local health departments provide some direct services, most of them concentrated in the area of preventive health services (well-baby clinics, family planning, immunizations). Senior citizens are usually covered under the Medicare program, and some might also have additional insurance to supplement Medicare coverage. The federal government provides directly funded care to a variety of groups, including military personnel and their families, armed services veterans, and American Indians. Individuals might also pay for health care services directly.

Insurance and government-funded programs are examples of **third-party payment,** in which a third party (i.e., someone

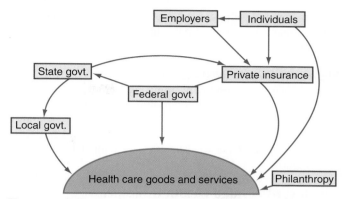

FIGURE 4-5 Funding sources for health care goods and services.

other than the recipient of care) directly pays for all or part of the health services provided. The third party might be a private insurance company or the government. Frequently, the client has no idea of the exact costs of the services provided and sometimes never sees the bills.

SELF-PAYMENT

Self-payment, or **self-insurance,** is a method by which a person or a family essentially assumes the financial cost of all medical services. This was the most common method of purchasing services before the 1930s. Currently, however, it is the least common method of payment, primarily because individuals are very wary of the financial burden posed by chronic or catastrophic illness. Today, self-payment costs are usually **co-payments** (a consumer share of the cost for a particular service) and **deductibles** (the amount a consumer must pay up front before insurance assumes any cost for services). Additional out-of-pocket costs are for services not provided by insurance plans. Private out-of-pocket costs make up 12.5% of the total expenditures for health care (Figure 4-6).

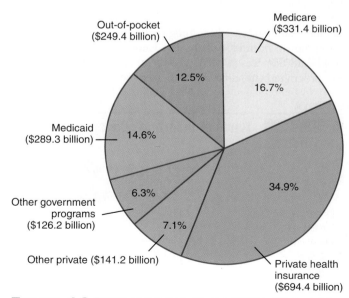

FIGURE 4-6 Funding sources for health care (2005) in billions of dollars (total = $1987.7 billion). The category "Other private" includes industrial health services, nonpatient revenues, and privately financed construction. (Data from Centers for Medicare and Medicaid Services, Office of the Actuary, National Health Statistics Group.)

The percentage of self-payment expenditures have doubled since 1996 as managed care and other insurance providers increase the co-payments and deductibles required by their policies.

HEALTH CARE INSURANCE

Health insurance gradually replaced self-payment. Since 1970, it has been the most common means of paying medical costs. Private health insurance premiums and health insurance payments for health services accounted for $694.4 billion in 2005, or 34.9% of the total health care budget for that year (CMS, 2007c).

Employer-Provided Health Insurance

The most common form of health insurance is employer-provided insurance, in which employees and their families are covered through employers (Table 4-1). Usually, the employer pays some or all of the cost of insurance for workers. Employer-provided health care insurance is an expected (but not universal) benefit for employees. This type of coverage appears to be eroding (Figure 4-7). By 2007, more than 41% of workers were not covered (Kaiser/HRET, 2007). Employees of small companies are less likely to have employer-sponsored health insurance. Only 45% of firms with 10 or fewer employees offer health insurance plans, whereas almost all companies with 100 or more employees do so (Kaiser/HRET, 2007).

Employers' costs of contributions have risen over the years as premium costs have increased. Employers paid on average $1767 in premiums for a single employee in 1981 and $3785 in 2007 (Kaiser/HRET, 2007). Premiums increased 23% between 2005 and 2007 (Kaiser/HRET, 2007). Rising costs have forced employers to reexamine the cost of offering health insurance benefits. Hefty insurance costs are directly related to decreases in the number of employer-offered plans during the same period.

As employer costs have continued to increase, more and more cost-containment strategies have been initiated. Chrysler Corporation, for example, expecting more than $1 billion in health care costs by 1991, pioneered the introduction of managed care programs for its employee health plans. Cost-containment strategies are becoming routine in employer-provided group health insurance plans. The **Centers for Medicare and Medicaid Services (CMS),** the federal agency in charge of the two programs in its name, reports that employer cost-containment

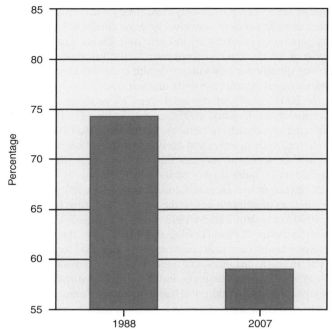

FIGURE 4-7 Percentages of employees with employer-sponsored health insurance for selected years. (Data from Kaiser/HRET [2007]. *Employer health benefits 2007 survey.* Menlo Park, CA: Kaiser Family Foundation.)

strategies include reimbursement for generic-only prescriptions; increasing reliance on second opinions for surgery; provisions for preadmission testing to eliminate the greater costs incurred for these hospitalization services; and increased reliance on outpatient surgery. **Health maintenance organizations (HMOs),** the most tightly controlled health insurance and service providers, and other managed care plans (preferred provider organizations [PPOs], and point-of-service plans) are offered to employees as an alternative or exclusive health plan. By 2007, almost 92% of employees in employer-sponsored plans were in managed care (Kaiser/HRET, 2007).

Recently employers have started to offer **consumer-directed high-deductible health plans (HDHPs)** as a means to control their health insurance costs. These plans are called *consumer directed* because the health care consumer decides how to use the money in the account. There are two types of HDHPs. One type is an HDHP with a health reimbursement option in which employees pay a high initial deductible and the employee is reimbursed for portions of the health costs in excess of the deductible by a health insurance plan usually provided by the employer. The second type of HDHP plan is a health savings account. In this plan an employer usually pays a certain amount into a health account and the employee has the option of adding more. The employee usually picks the insurance plan or opts just to pay for health care costs from the health savings account.

In HDHPs, the employee's deductible costs range from $1000 to $5000 per single employee and as much as $2000 to $11,000 for family coverage. HDHPs are best suited for young healthy individuals and their families (Straight, 2007). Many employees, however, do not have an option because that may be the sole plan offered by the employer. HDHPs accounted for only 5% of employer offered health plans in 2007, but their popularity with employers is growing (Kaiser/HRET, 2007).

TABLE 4-1 Types of Insurance Coverage for Individuals		

	Enrolled, *n*	
Type	Millions	%
Employment based	174.8	59.5
Medicare	40.2	13.7
Medicaid	38.1	13.0
Military*	11.2	3.8
Inidividual	26.8	9.1
Uninsured	46.6	15.9

Data from U.S. Bureau of the Census. (2006). *Income, poverty, and health insurance in the United States: 2005* (Current Populations Reports, P60-231). Washington DC: U.S. Department of Commerce, Economics and Statistics Administration.
*Includes CHAMPUS, TRICARE, and CHAMPVA.

Employers have also become more involved in their benefits programs, increasing self-funding of health benefits, using non-insurance program administrators to monitor costs, and requiring employees to shoulder more of the cost of health insurance. Some employers have eliminated family coverage or made the employee premiums so high that lower-wage employees cannot afford family coverage. On average, employees are required to pay 16% of the premium cost for individuals and 28% of the premium cost for a family plan (Figure 4-8). The employee share of health premiums and cost sharing (deductibles and per-episode costs) has increased as employers have reduced their contributions to health plans. This action by employers places additional families at risk for poor access to health care. The average annual premium for an employee with family coverage is $3281; deductibles average another $1359 for PPOs and $340 for hospital costs (Kaiser/HRET, 2007).

The current political debate centers on whether health insurance coverage should be mandated for all firms with employees. Most small business leaders are opposed to employer-mandated health insurance, claiming the net effect would be a loss of jobs, increasing costs to consumers, and some business failures. Proponents argue that it is sound business practice to provide coverage because it will attract a more stable workforce. There have been some moves in the direction of employer-mandated health insurance for workers, and several states have passed legislation requiring such benefits (Davis & Schoen, 2003; Krisberg, 2007). Massachusetts, for example, has enacted expanded coverage for all citizens. Employers have the option of providing health insurance or paying into a state insurance pool (Lee, 2007a). Pennsylvania, California, Oregon, and Vermont have enacted similar plans (Health Care Financing and Organization, 2007; Krisberg, 2007).

Other Health Insurance Options

There are several non–employer-related methods of purchasing health insurance. **Medicare** is a government insurance program designed primarily for use by older Americans. Medicare will be addressed later in this chapter. In addition, individuals can purchase health insurance on their own.

Privately Purchased Health Insurance

Approximately 8.5 million individuals have **private insurance** and purchase their own health insurance (Collins et al., 2008). Most do not have access to a sponsored insurance program. Individuals are more likely to purchase private health insurance if they have an adequate income and relatively regular employment. Twenty percent of the self-employed and 17% of farm workers are self-insured.

Most noninsured families have low incomes (Figure 4-9). For these families, cost is the deterrent. Unlike with employer-provided health insurance, the **premium** cost (the price charged by the insurance carrier) is paid totally by the individual. Where not regulated by state laws, premiums for an individual cost $3000 or more (Collins et al., 2008). Family coverage costs even more. For low-income and marginally middle-income individuals, these premium costs are unaffordable. For example, Collins and colleagues (2008) report that 43% of people whose income was 200% or less of the poverty level found it very difficult to find affordable health insurance.

Private health insurers can more easily discriminate based on the characteristics of the individual than can group insurers. Insurers charge higher premiums for persons living in urban environments, smokers, older persons, and females (compared with males in the same age group) and for those with preexisting conditions. Unless state laws prohibit it, insurers can deny insurance coverage to individual applicants. Denial rates average approximately 33% of applicants in states with no guaranteed coverage guidelines. In response to insurance selection practices, and in an effort to make privately purchased health coverage feasible for more individuals, approximately half of

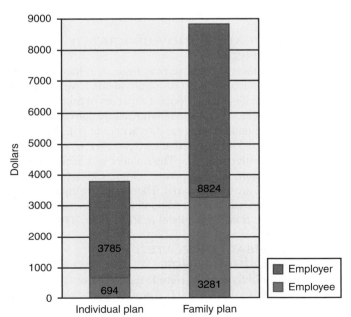

FIGURE 4-8 Average annual costs of employee/employer premiums, 2007. (Data from Kaiser/HRET. [2007]. *Employee health benefits 2007 survey.* Menlo Park, CA: Kaiser Family Foundation.)

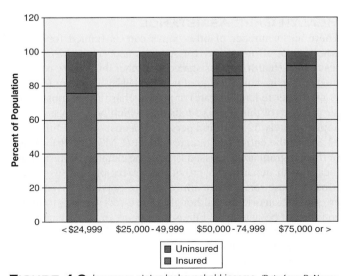

FIGURE 4-9 Insurance status by household income. (Data from DeNavas-Walt, C., Proctor, B. D., & Smith, J. [2007]. *Income, poverty, and health insurance coverage in the United States: 2006* [U.S. Census Bureau, Current Populations Reports, P60-233]. Washington DC: U.S. Department of Commerce, Economics and Statistics Administration, U.S. Bureau of the Census.)

the states have attempted reforms. These efforts include the following:

- High-risk insurance pools for otherwise uninsurable individuals
- Establishment of an insurer of last resort, usually Blue Cross/Blue Shield
- Guaranteed issuance of insurance to all who apply
- Guaranteed renewal of insurance to all
- Limits on deniability due to preexisting conditions
- Premiums rating restrictions

Thirty states operate high-risk pools for persons who must self-insure (Chollet, 2002). Although state laws have improved access for some individuals, only those states that have mandated premium restrictions have made private insurance more feasible for low-income individuals. State reforms are limited by state jurisdictions. If an insurance carrier decides the conditions cause too great an expense, it can choose not to operate in that state and is then not bound by that state's regulations.

INSURANCE PORTABILITY

The Health Insurance Portability and Accountability Act (HIPAA) passed by the federal government in 1996 has made limited efforts to improve access to health insurance for individuals. The law guarantees access to private insurance for individuals who have just left a qualified group insurance plan, requires the renewal of insurance coverage, and authorizes federally tax exempt medical savings accounts that can be used to pay health insurance premiums for self-employed individuals. The federal reforms do not address affordability of premiums or allow medical savings accounts or tax-exempt premiums for other groups, such as the unemployed or the employed with no employer health insurance plan.

Gabel and colleagues (2003) reported that the health portability act has reduced insurance providers' use of preexisting conditions to deny coverage. The act does not limit the amount an insurer can charge. Substantial premium costs have undercut the intent of the portability act. Many individuals simply cannot afford to purchase coverage (Patel & Rushefsky, 2006).

HEALTH CARE ASSISTANCE

There are a number of other ways care is funded for people who cannot afford to pay for services and do not have health insurance. Health care assistance is another third-party payment mechanism in which payment is provided by a government program (either federal or state) or private charity. The most familiar program of this type is Medicaid, which provides service to approximately 52.4 million persons at a cost of $235 billion, or 11.8% of the entire health care budget (CMS, 2007b). Details of this program are discussed later in the chapter. Both state and local health departments provide a variety of health services. Most of these services are aimed at poor populations, and most are prevention oriented, although some direct services to ill persons might be available. Funds to support these services are a mix of federal, state, and local monies (see Chapter 29).

Private charity provides a variety of services to the needy. Nonprofit organizations usually target special health needs or special risk groups. Philanthropic gifts to hospitals assist with payments for persons without insurance, and many health care providers offer some free care. Spontaneous fundraisers meet expensive special needs, such as liver or heart transplantation for certain individuals. It is difficult to quantify the actual dollars provided by charitable organizations and events for direct health services to individuals. Philanthropic activities accounted for 1.1% of the total health budget in 2005, or approximately $21.85 billion (CMS, 2007c; see Chapter 3). That amount includes both direct care to individuals and contributions to research and facilities development. It is safe to say that charitable contributions make up a minuscule portion of the health care budget.

LACK OF HEALTH INSURANCE

More than 50.4 million persons are not covered by health insurance or assistance of any kind and are unable to pay for health care services on their own (Roberts & Rhoades, 2007). Others are without health insurance at some time during a calendar year. Most of the uninsured are the working poor—workers attempting to provide a living for themselves and their dependents at low-paying jobs with few benefits. They and their dependents make up an estimated 72% of the medically indigent (Kaiser Commission on Medicaid and the Uninsured, 2007). In 2006, 27.6 million workers were uninsured, most of whom (80%) were full-time workers (DeNavas-Walt et al., 2007). The remainder of the uninsured are individuals who are currently unemployed or uninsurable and others who fall outside the eligibility requirements for Medicare or Medicaid (e.g., some of the homeless, some elderly, and children).

Many of the uninsured work in a service industry, such as food or janitorial service. Those jobs require few skills and little education, offer fewer benefits, and are generally low paying. Service-type jobs are increasing, which places more workers at risk. By 2004, there were 22.7 million service jobs, an increase of 8.8 million from 1983 (U.S. Bureau of the Census, 2002b, p. 383; 2007b, Table 603). Most of those employed in service positions receive no health insurance benefits. When the uninsured need health care, they are limited in their options. They must pay at the time of service or find a health care provider who is willing to defer payment. Many delay seeking care, hoping they will improve on their own.

UNDERINSURANCE AND ASSOCIATED FINANCIAL RISK

In addition to those with no medical insurance, there are millions who are underinsured. These individuals have insurance plans that require large out-of-pocket expenses or limit coverage of catastrophic illnesses. Workers who change jobs and cannot afford insurance under the portability act are at risk. Medicare enrollees are at risk because Medicare pays for less than 50% of their total health care costs. The number of underinsured is difficult to measure. Estimates vary. Some estimates indicate that 26% to 34% are underinsured. Those who are underinsured risk less access to health care and poorer health because of their insurance status (IOM, 2007; Patel & Rushefsky, 2006).

LEVEL OF HEALTH RELATED TO MEDICAL INSURANCE

The medically indigent (uninsured) have greater health risks (Geyman, 2008; Inglehart, 2002). These families have a harder time acquiring the basic necessities of food, clothing, shelter, and transportation, and medical needs force them to make hard choices regarding exactly what services they can afford. Studies show that the uninsured include a larger number of people in fair to poor health, with a greater incidence of chronic illness and early death (IOM, 2007). They are less likely to seek care early, make fewer visits to physicians, and are less likely to be hospitalized than are insured individuals (Patel & Rushefsky, 2006). Because they delay care, their health problems are usually more severe when they do seek care (Sultz & Young, 2004). The uninsured overuse hospital emergency departments because they have no personal health care provider (Kaiser Commission, 2007). The cost of such care is assumed either by the hospital or by government programs. Emergency department care is a more costly form of service than care at clinics or physicians' offices. The American Hospital Association (AHA) reports that the cost of uncompensated care in hospitals has doubled every 5 years. The estimated costs of uncompensated care (for hospitals and other providers) is between $31.2 and $40.7 billion dollars (AHA, 2007; Hadley & Holahan, 2004).

UNINSURED CHILDREN: A SPECIAL CONCERN (THE SCHIP PROGRAM)

Although there are fewer uninsured children than uninsured adults in most states, they are an aggregate of special concern to health professionals. The cost of providing access and treatment to children is low, and the long-term benefits to health care costs are high. Untreated illnesses and lack of preventive services create or exacerbate health problems that persist throughout life. Treatment of the chronic conditions that result is far more costly than the services that could have prevented such problems.

The number of uninsured children has declined since the passage of the **State Children's Health Insurance Program (SCHIP)** in 1997. SCHIP expands health insurance coverage to low-income, uninsured children who are not already covered by other types of assistance programs. It is funded by federal grants to participating states, which design and administer the program. Before 1997, approximately 25% of children were not covered by any insurance program, including Medicaid. Since the inception of SCHIP, the percentage of children without health benefits has declined to 11.7% (DeNavas-Walt et al., 2007).

Some states have expanded SCHIP coverage to children in families with incomes above 200% of the poverty level and to vulnerable adults. The federal government has had differences with the states regarding this expansion of services. The federal government's position is that these families are substituting publically funded health insurance for private health insurance. One recent study refutes that claim. In an investigation in 2002 of children newly enrolled in SCHIP, only 14% of parents reported that they had access to private insurance, and half of those parents (7%) reported that the insurance costs were unaffordable (Sommers et al., 2007).

PUBLICLY FUNDED PROGRAMS FOR HEALTH CARE SERVICES

Medicare and Medicaid are the two programs that provide a major portion of health care services to populations that have been identified as having greater need (elderly persons) or having fewer resources (the poor) than the majority. Specific costs and benefits change periodically. Rather than concentrating on current benefits, this discussion focuses on exploring each program's basic purpose, evolution, and beneficiaries.

A brief comparison of covered and excluded services for each program is given, and examples and costs are used to illustrate points under discussion. This information is important to community health nurses because many of their clients are covered by these programs. Nurses need to know what services clients can expect if they are enrolled in these programs.

MEDICARE

Medicare was created in 1965. It was an attempt to ensure that adequate medical care would be available to the aged and some chronically ill persons and that the price of such services would not be so prohibitive that individuals would have to forego basic care. It has significantly improved access to health services for eligible persons, and it has helped reduce the number of elderly in poverty.

Medicare is federally funded and is financed by a tax on wages. Every citizen who is currently working provides a portion of her or his salary to the Medicare program. Employers and employees contribute an equal percentage of wages to fund Medicare. The contribution levels for both employer and employee have risen, so that both pay 1.45% of the worker's salary into the Medicare Insurance Fund. The costs, for both workers and employers, have risen. Medicare's budget increased from $4.7 billion in 1967, the first full year of operation, to $336 billion in 2005, a 7150% increase (CMS, 2007b).

Medicare has evolved into an important source of income for health care providers. It furnishes more than 28% of total income to hospitals and 21% of all income to physicians (CMS, 2007b). Physicians in certain medical specialties commonly exceed the 21% average Medicare income level. These include thoracic surgeons, internists, and radiologists.

Beneficiaries

The primary beneficiaries of Medicare are the elderly who have contributed to the system during their working life or the spouses of contributors. In 1972, Congress extended coverage to persons under age 65 years with long-term disabilities or end-stage renal disease. In 2006 there were 42.5 million persons receiving Medicare benefits, 33.5 million of whom were seniors and 7 million of whom were disabled persons (Kaiser Family Foundation, 2007).

Benefits

Medicare is divided into four parts: Part A is hospital insurance, Part B is supplementary medical insurance, and part D covers prescription drugs. All contributors are covered by Part A. Part B and Part D are voluntary and are limited to those who choose to participate and pay a premium deducted from their Social Security checks. Part C is Medicare managed care. Most Medicare recipients (95%) opt to participate in Part B coverage. Part D, which began in 2003, has a 53% participation rate (Kaiser Family Foundation, 2007). The cost of premiums has steadily increased, and voluntary contributions currently pay for only 25% of the total cost of Part B benefits; the rest is financed by the federal government. Benefits under Part A, Part B, and Part D are listed in Table 4-2.

Criticisms

Several major concerns have been raised about the program structure. Most criticisms have to do with institutional bias, service restrictions, and equity.

TABLE 4-2   **Medicare Benefits**

Medicare (Part A): Hospital Insurance—Covered Services for 2008

Services	Benefit	Medicare Pays	You Pay
Hospitalization: Semiprivate room and board, general nursing, and miscellaneous hospital services and supplies (Medicare payments based on benefit periods)	First 60 days 61st to 90th day 91st day* and beyond	All but $1024 All but $256/day All but $512/day	$1024 $256/day $512/day All costs
Skilled nursing facility care: Semiprivate room and board, general nursing, skilled nursing and rehabilitative services, and other services and suppliest[†] (Medicare payments based on benefit periods)	First 20 days Additional 80 days Beyond 100 days	100% of approved amount All but $128/day Nothing	Nothing $128/day All costs
Home health care: Part-time or intermittent skilled care, home health aide services, durable medical equipment and supplies, and other services	Unlimited as long as client meets Medicare conditions	100% of approved amount; 80% of approved amount for durable medical equipment	Nothing for services; 20% of approved amount for durable medical equipment
Hospice care: Pain relief, symptom management, and support services for the terminally ill	For as long as physician certifies need	All but limited costs for outpatient drugs and inpatient respite care	Limited costs sharing for outpatient drugs and inpatient respite care
Blood	Unlimited, if medically necessary	80% of cost after first three pints per calendar year	For first three pints[‡]; 20% of additional pints

Medicare (Part B): Hospital Insurance—Covered Services for 2008

Services	Benefit	Medicare Pays	You Pay
Medical expenses: Physicians' services; inpatient and outpatient medical and surgical services and supplies; physical, occupational, and speech therapy; diagnostic tests; and durable medical equipment and other services	Unlimited, if medically necessary	80% of approved amount (after $135 deductible); 50% of approved amount for outpatient mental health services	$135 deductible,[§] plus 20% of approved amount and limited charges above approved amount[¶] plus 50% for outpatient mental health services
Clinical laboratory services: Blood tests, biopsies, urinalyses, and more	Unlimited, if medically necessary	Generally 100% of approved amount	Nothing for services
Home health care: Part-time or intermittent skilled care, home health aide services, durable medical equipment and supplies, and other services	Unlimited for as long as client meets conditions for benefits	100% of approved amount; 80% of approved amount for durable medical equipment	Nothing for services; 20% of approved amount for durable medical equipment
Outpatient hospital treatment: Services for the diagnosis or treatment of illness or injury	Unlimited, if medically necessary	Medicare payment to hospital based on hospital cost after co-payment by recipient	Co-payment amount varies (after $135 deductible)
Blood	Unlimited, if medically necessary	80% of approved amount (after $135 deductible and starting with 4th pint)	First 3 pints plus 20% of approved amount for additional pints (after $135 deductible)[||]
Preventive Services: for example, mammogram, Pap and pelvic examinations, prostrate screening, immunizations (pneumococcal pneumonia, flu, hepatitis B)	As outlined in *Medicare Handbook*	80% of approved amount All costs for pneumonia and flu immunizations	Usually 20% of approved amount. Nothing for flu and pneumonia immunization. All costs of shingles vaccine

TABLE 4-2   Medicare Benefits—cont'd

Medicare Prescription Drug Coverage (Part D)

Services	Benefit	Insurance Co-Payment	You Pay
Prescription drugs provided through private insurance companies For additional information, see **Website Resource 4A** on the book's Evolve website.	Varied	Varied	Varied

JEB

2008 Part A monthly premium. None for most beneficiaries; persons who did not contribute during employment years might purchase by paying a premium.
2008 Part B monthly premiums: $96.40 (premium might be higher if you enroll late or have income over $82,000).
*This 60-reserve-days benefit might be used only once in a lifetime.
†Neither Medicare nor private Medigap insurance will pay for most nursing home care.
‡Blood paid for or replaced under Part B Medicare during the calendar year does not have to be paid for or replaced under Part A.
§Once client has had $135 of expenses for covered services in 2008, the Part B deductible does not apply to any further covered services received for the rest of the year.
¶Federal law limits charges for physician services.
‖Blood paid for or replaced under Part A Medicare during the calendar year does not have to be paid for or replaced under Part B.
From *Medicare and you.* (2008). Washington, DC: U.S. Department of Health and Human Services, Centers for Medicare and Medicaid Services.

Institutional Bias: Change from Inpatient to Outpatient. The Medicare payment structure previously was heavily weighted in favor of hospital care. Similar services provided in outpatient settings were not covered, which resulted in a substantial rise in the rate of hospitalization of elderly persons.

More recently, as a result of the need for cost-cutting measures, hospitals received permission to expand services provided by more cost-effective outpatient clinics. Outpatient clinics are less labor intensive, take up little space, and cost less to operate than inpatient services. For example, outpatient clinics can operate with fewer employees, are not staffed 24 hours a day, and require less high-technology equipment than inpatient units. The use of hospital outpatient services grew by 57% between 1990 and 1998 (Levit et al., 2003), and continued growth is expected. Between 1982 and 2001, hospital outpatient revenues increased 35%, whereas inpatient revenues grew by only 3.5% (Gourevitch et al., 2005). Other types of outpatient services, such as freestanding emergency care centers and preferred provider organizations, are also expected to grow (see Chapter 3).

Limited Access and Unequal Burden of Risk. Cost sharing is a requirement of the Medicare program. In addition to the Part B payment, recipients must pay a portion of the expenses of the services that they use. Critics charge that co-payments, especially for hospital care, have escalated until they are a major hardship for a large percentage of the covered population. Medicare pays less than half (45%) of recipients' health care costs (Kaiser Family Foundation, 2007).

Co-payments were instituted to save the government money and to encourage judicious use of services. Numerous studies support co-payments as a method that tends to reduce usage. There is an inverse relationship between services used and the rate of co-payment: a 20% or 25% co-payment significantly reduces the use of services (Butler, 1997; Congressional Budget Office, 1992a; Inglehart, 2002). In other words, as the personal cost declines, people seek more health care, and as personal cost increases, people curtail the use of services.

Critics of cost sharing charge that it discourages people from receiving necessary medical care or encourages them to postpone care until the condition becomes more severe or even life threatening. Although there are few data from controlled studies to support this argument, it is known that people who are

living on small amounts of money tend to be sicker when they seek care and require more extensive care as a result (Collins et al., 2008; Feder et al., 2001; Geyman, 2008). It would appear logical to assume that the same condition holds true with persons whose co-payment levels are relatively high with respect to their incomes. Data to support or deny this position would be extremely useful when planning changes to the system.

Equity. A major concern with cost sharing is the question of equity. Medicare is a program in which everyone, regardless of circumstances and finances, essentially pays the same amount or cost for similar benefits. Therefore, greater cost burdens are placed on the poor because their out-of-pocket expenses reflect a larger proportion of their incomes than the costs of persons with larger incomes. This disproportionate cost is illustrated in Figure 4-10. If three patients are hospitalized for the same number of days, with the same problem, and receive the same treatment, their costs (Medicare co-payments and deductibles) are essentially the same, but the impact on their finances is not. As income goes up, the impact of health care expenses is less. The greatest burden is to Mr. A., who has the lowest income. Partially in response to this concern, the Medicare program initiated a means-tested premium for Part B in 2007. Premiums for people with incomes above $82,000 ($164,000 for a couple) cost more than premiums for those with incomes below that level (CMS, 2008).

Protection from Financial Hardship

Medicare does not protect the individual from financial destitution, the primary reason for creation of the program. Currently, the cost of co-payments and restrictions on coverage make it very difficult for many persons who face a major illness, particularly a long illness, to afford the health care services they need.

The chronically ill can easily have several hospital stays because of complications and deteriorating health status. While in the hospital, a person can expect to see the primary physician and one or two specialists and to undergo radiography and other diagnostic examinations. With co-payments and deductibles for covered services and no ceiling on potential expenses, it is easy to see that a chronically ill person could quickly accrue a bill of several thousand dollars. Health care costs take over half the income of older low-income women in poor health (Maxwell et al., 2001).

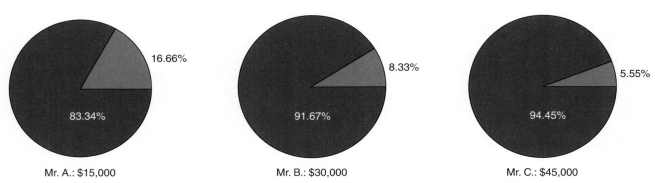

FIGURE 4-10 Percentage of income needed for health care for three individuals with different incomes and similar health care needs. All three persons have $1500 out-of-pocket expenses in deductibles and co-payments for Parts A and B Medicare benefits.

Often the elderly are faced with the prospect of "spending down" to qualify for another health coverage program—Medicaid. Spending down is the process whereby a person must first exhaust most assets to pay medical bills. When the person's assets are nearly gone, she or he will qualify for medical assistance care under Medicaid, the program that provides care to the poor.

Medigap Insurance

To insure against devastating financial loss, most elderly persons (approximately 64%) have some additional health care insurance from private companies (CMS, 2007b). "Medigap" policies are intended to reimburse out-of-pocket costs for Medicare-covered services. In addition, some pay for services not covered by Medicare. In 1990, Congress directed the National Association of Insurance Commissioners to standardize Medigap policies because of fraud, abusive sales tactics, and problems with benefit comparisons. Because of confusion, many elderly had purchased two or more policies with duplicate benefits (Advocates for Senior Alert, 1990). This group developed 10 standardized plans (Figure 4-11). Each Medigap insurance provider must offer the basic policy (A) and may choose to offer any or all of

Basic Benefits: (Included in ALL Medigap Plans A through J)

- Inpatient Hospital Care: Covers the Part A coinsurance and the cost of 365 extra days after Medicare coverage ends.
- Medical Costs: Covers the Part B coinsurance (generally 20% of the Medicare-approved amount) or copayments for hospital outpatient services.
- Blood: Covers the first three pints of blood each year.

A	B	C	D	E	F*	G	H	I	J*
Basic Benefits	Basic Benefits	Basic Benefits	Basic Benefits	Basic Benefits	Basic Benefits	Basic Benefits	Basic Benefits	Basic Benefits	Basic Benefits
		Skilled Nursing Facility Coinsurance	Skilled Nursing Facility Coinsurance	Skilled Nursing Facility Coinsurance	Skilled Nursing Facility Coinsurance	Skilled Nursing Facility Coinsurance	Skilled Nursing Facility Coinsurance	Skilled Nursing Facility Coinsurance	Skilled Nursing Facility Coinsurance
	Medicare Part A Deductible	Medicare Part A Deductible	Medicare Part A Deductible	Medicare Part A Deductible	Medicare Part A Deductible	Medicare Part A Deductible	Medicare Part A Deductible	Medicare Part A Deductible	Medicare Part A Deductible
		Medicare Part B Deductible			Medicare Part B Deductible				Medicare Part B Deductible
					Medicare Part B Excess Charges (100%)	Medicare Part B Excess Charges (80%)		Medicare Part B Excess Charges (100%)	Medicare Part B Excess Charges (100%)
		Foreign Travel Emergency	Foreign Travel Emergency	Foreign Travel Emergency	Foreign Travel Emergency	Foreign Travel Emergency	Foreign Travel Emergency	Foreign Travel Emergency	Foreign Travel Emergency
			At-Home Recovery			At-Home Recovery		At-Home Recovery	At-Home Recovery
				Preventive Care (not covered by Medicare)					Preventive Care (not covered by Medicare)

*Medigap Plans F and J also offer a high-deductible option. You must pay the first $1860 (deductible in 2007) in Medigap-covered costs before the Medigap policy pays anything. You must also pay a separate deductible for foreign travel emergency ($250 per year).
Note: Medigap K and L provide for different cost sharing. Seniors must pay $4140 or $2070 out of pocker before benefits kick in. Both policies cover similar services.

FIGURE 4-11 Ten standard Medigap insurance policies. (Data from Centers for Medicare and Medicaid Services. [2007]. *Choosing a Medigap policy: A guide to health insurance for people with Medicare.* Baltimore MD: Author.)

the remaining plans (B through L). These new insurance plans eased comparison of costs and benefits for the elderly.

The need for Medigap insurance places the poor elderly at the greatest financial risk. Although 67% of Medicare recipients carry extra coverage, 33% do not, usually because they cannot afford coverage. Some of these people might be eligible for Medicaid because of low income. Premiums for Medigap insurance are expensive, ranging from $1085 to $2665 or more per person per year (Fox et al., 2003). With increasing premium costs, more elderly can be expected to be unable to afford coverage. For example, an elderly couple living on a fixed income of $20,000 per year would pay 10% to 20% of their total income in Medigap premiums alone. In addition, they would pay the medical cost of Part B Medicare premiums and a 20% co-payment on any medical services needed.

Services not Covered
Medicare has only recently covered prescription drugs for enrollees on a voluntary basis. A common misconception is that Medicare includes long-term nursing home care. These benefits are severely restricted. Skilled nursing home care is limited to 100 days per year with mandatory deductibles (see Table 4-2).
Nursing Home Care. Custodial nursing home care, the type of care required by most elderly nursing home residents, is not covered by Medicare or by many private insurance plans. The average annual cost of nursing home care per patient varies by geographic region but now is estimated to be between $52,000 and $85,000 (American Association of Retired Persons, 2007; MetLife, 2002), an amount that can rapidly deplete personal savings. In fact, many nursing home residents meet the income means test for Medicaid coverage. Approximately 34% of the costs of nursing home care are paid by the individual or private health insurance, 44% by Medicaid, and 15.7% by Medicare or private insurance (CMS, 2007c).

> Mrs. Jones had Alzheimer's disease and required custodial nursing care for 2 years before her death. The cost of 2 years of care was $80,000. The Jones family had to spend down, using $15,000 of their savings, before Medicaid paid for nursing care.

As the incidence of chronic illness increases with age, the probability of nursing home admission also increases. The lifetime risk of needing institutional care is about 44%. Two of every five elders can expect to stay in an extended-care facility, either as an intermediate step between hospital and home, or at the end of life (Merlis, 2003). This important and common need, one of considerable concern for elder individuals, is not covered by Medicare. Other services and benefits that are not covered are outlined in Box 4-1. The most burdensome of these are prescription gap coverage, deductibles, and co-payments, especially for the elderly with chronic illnesses and disabilities. In 2008, the Part A hospitalization deductible increased to $1024, and the monthly cost of Part B coverage increased to $96.40, or $1156.80 per person per year.
Prescription Drugs. Until 2006, Medicare did not provide prescription drug coverage except as part of the Medicare+Choice program. Because only a small percentage of seniors participate in the managed care program, most paid for prescription drugs out of pocket. The costs of drugs are rising. About 16% of out-of-pocket costs in health care are attributed to drug costs (CMS, 2007b). Because the elderly consume a larger number

---

Box 4-1 **Medical Services not Covered or Limited under the Medicare Program**
• No coverage for long-term care (custodial care over an extended period in the home, a custodial nursing home, or a residential care facility)
• Limited coverage for nursing home care (only for a skilled nursing home for limited periods of time)
• Part A and Part B deductible and co-payment obligations
• Limited prescription drug coverage (see Box 3-8)
• No coverage for dental, eye, ear, and foot care, including eyeglasses, hearing aids, and dentures
• Limited coverage for home health services; does not cover unlimited nursing care or custodial care, Meals on Wheels or other food service programs, or homemaker services
• No coverage for routine physical examination
• No coverage for diabetic supplies, such as insulin and syringes, unless used with an insulin pump

of prescription drugs, they are at special risk with no prescription insurance and rising drug costs. The elderly live in families in which health expenditures, including prescription drugs, account for 10% to 40% of total income (Sambamoorthi et al., 2003; Selden & Banthin, 2003). About 25% of seniors without supplemental drug coverage report skipping doses to make medication last longer (Safran et al., 2002).

> Mr. and Mrs. Smith have an annual income of $30,000. Both have chronic medical conditions. Mr. Smith has a heart condition that requires prescription drugs costing $1788 per year. Mrs. Smith has Parkinson's disease and pays another $2240 a year for medication. The total cost of their medications is $4018 per year. In addition, they pay $1408 in premiums for Medicare Part B coverage and $2700 per year in Medigap insurance. These medical expenses total $8126 per year, or approximately 27% of their annual income. Physician office visits, laboratory bills, and other medical costs, excluding hospitalization, if necessary, would be in addition to these expenses.

The elderly often do not comply with prescribed medication therapy because the costs are more than their limited budgets can handle.

Attempts at Program Change
Efforts to alter Medicare services, providers, and payment mechanisms have been and continue to be made.
Early Efforts at Medicare Reform: Easing Consumer Cost Concerns for Prescription Drugs and Catastrophic Illness. In 1988, Congress attempted to improve Medicare coverage by easing the cost burden on patients with chronic and catastrophic illnesses and adding a prescription drug plan. This comprehensive reform package was repealed because of opposition from senior groups concerned with the additional costs. Congress did act to reduce the financial concerns of married couples. In 1990, a separate amendment was passed providing some relief from catastrophic expenses. Some joint financial assets held by a married couple were protected. The Medicare and Medicaid programs would provide services for the ill partner, and the healthier spouse was allowed to retain limited assets (the family home and some income).

Physician Reimbursement Mechanism. In 1997, Congress considered a bill allowing physicians more flexibility in their payment structures. Doctors who contract directly with the patient and do not accept Medicare assignment would not be subject to Medicare restrictions. They could charge whatever they chose for their services, vacillating between Medicare and client payments at will. Under the current system, physicians may not charge more than 15% above the Medicare-approved price, even if they do not participate in the Medicare program.

Physicians who treat Medicare patients must accept the Medicare-approved price, and many are unsatisfied with that level of compensation. The American Medical Association (AMA) reports that 45% of physicians indicate they limit the number of new Medicare patients they will care for because of Medicare compensation levels (Nelson, 2006).

Medicare Managed Care Plan

Established in 1997, **Medicare+Choice** encouraged the use of managed care arrangements by persons with Medicare insurance. The providers received a predetermined fee and agreed to provide benefits at least equal to the current Medicare package. Managed care organizations that participated in Medicare+Choice initially received incentive payments to enroll seniors (Sultz & Young, 2004).

Benefits of Managed Care. Enrollment in a managed care organization meant that Medicare recipients did not have to purchase Medigap insurance but had to accept the health service restrictions of their plan. Some seniors found this arrangement beneficial because they did not have to struggle with the Medicare and/or Medigap paperwork and because Medigap insurance was costly for many (Gold & Mittler, 2001).

Declining Enrollment in Managed Care. Medicare+Choice was not popular with Medicare participants. Peak enrollment was approximately 5.5 million people (15% of eligible participants) (Hileman et al., 2002; Zarabozo, 2002). After initial gains in the late 1990s, the number of participants and providers declined. The decline in health care providers was the result of government funding cuts that reduced payments. The disenrollment of participants was both voluntary, due to dissatisfaction, and involuntary, due to provider discontinuance of service. Between 1998 and 2002, 2.3 million enrollees were terminated from Medicare+Choice as providers withdrew from the program (Pizer & Frakt, 2002). Only half of those disenrolled were able to find coverage with another managed care plan.

Recent Changes to Medicare Coverage: Effects of the 2003 Medicare Reform Act

In 2003, Congress passed amendments to the Medicare program, making substantial changes to covered services including establishment of a prescription drug plan (see Box 3-8) and reinventing Medicare managed care. The 2003 reforms did not expand coverage in other areas of concern to seniors (e.g., extended home health care or nursing home coverage).

Medicare Part D: Prescription Drugs. A drug coverage plan became part of Medicare with the 2003 reforms. The costs of this new plan will not be known for some time, because the major changes are to be phased in between 2006 and 2010. Cost estimates are substantial—$400 to $534 billion over the next decade (Zaneski, 2004). Seniors enrolled in the plan pay a base premium of $27.93 per month or $335.16 per year (CMS, 2008).

A substantial concern with Part D is the coverage gap or "doughnut hole." If a senior's drug costs exceed a certain amount, then the individual pays the full cost of medications between that amount and the end of the gap. In 2007, the gap started at $2400 and ended at $3850 (out-of-pocket personal drug costs of $1450, in addition to monthly premium costs) (CMS, 2007c).

Gap coverage and the large number of and options in drug plans have created confusion among seniors. Cubanski and Neuman (2007) reported that many seniors were unaware of the coverage gap. Some Medicare Part D policies and those available through Medicare managed care cover the gap amount. These policies are more expensive, approximately twice the cost of the base plan (Cubanski & Neuman, 2007). Approximately 13% of seniors participating in Medicare Part D reached the coverage gap in 2006 (Lee & Levine, 2006).

Medicare Part C: Medicare Advantage. The **Medicare Advantage** managed care program, established in 2003, replaced Medicare+Choice. It is intended to increase enrollment in Medicare managed care. In 2006, 16% of seniors were enrolled in Medicare Advantage (Kaiser Family Foundation, 2008). To encourage managed care plans to participate in Medicare Advantage, Congress offered financial incentives to those plans. In 2005 that incentive was $800 per enrollee or 11% more than the cost of similar benefits in Medicare (Kaiser Family Foundation, 2008). In effect, Congress created a competition with the original Medicare program and provided cost incentives to managed care plans that participated.

Medicare Advantage is promoted as easier to navigate than Medicare and as a plan that can save seniors money. Initial research does not support that claim. Biles and colleagues (2008) found that seniors in good health did save on out-of-pocket health expenses (premiums for Part B, D, Medigap insurance, and deductibles) when enrolled in Medicare Advantage. They also reported that 22% of Medicare Advantage plans cost seniors in poor health more than the out-of-pocket costs of health care premiums (including Medigap insurance) and deductibles.

Because the program is relatively new, problems are just beginning to surface. There are a large number of participating managed care organizations, each of which offers a variety of insurance plan choices with different premium costs. This has created confusion similar to the problems encountered when Medigap insurance was first offered (Salganik, 2006). Medicare recipients are locked into a managed care plan for a full year, which makes it impossible for seniors to change plans if they discover problems with their plan selection. Insurance agents marketing managed care plans to seniors have used deceptive practices to enroll consumers and have misrepresented benefits available in those plans. Thirty-nine states have reported abuses (Williamson & Lee, 2007). In response, seven insurance companies temporarily suspended marketing of plans to seniors (Lee, 2007b). Further evaluation of the existing program is needed. Perhaps there will be additional changes to the program as problems become manifest.

At the present time, Medicare remains a program with limited coverage, and it is a program with increasing cost liabilities for the consumer. The current concern is whether Medicare can address the needs of the chronically ill in a more comprehensive fashion, and, if so, at what cost to the individual and the nation.

MEDICAID

Medicaid, created in correlation with Medicare in 1965, is a grant program designed to provide medical assistance to the poor. It is funded by both federal and state governments. Medicaid has done a moderately competent job of providing care to limited segments of poor pregnant women and young children but has been less successful in caring for the aged poor, the disabled, and adults and children who are not covered under the pregnant women and children programs. Medicaid provides benefits to approximately 50% of those below the poverty level.

The individual states administer the program. Overall, the federal government pays approximately 50% of the Medicaid budget, but the specific allotment for each state varies from 50% to 76.8%, depending on criteria set by the federal government. Poorer states receive a greater share from the federal government. For example, Mississippi receives the full 76.8% federal share, whereas Alaska receives 59.8% federal funding. Medicaid is financed by income tax revenues at the federal level and by general tax revenues at the state level, with some contributions from local municipalities.

Like Medicare costs, Medicaid costs have risen dramatically (Figure 4-12). In 1968, the program cost approximately $3.45 billion in both federal and state contributions; in 2005, costs were $300.7 billion. By the year 2016, Medicaid costs are expected to be $677 billion (CMS, 2006). Medicaid expenditures represent an increasing burden on state budgets. In fact, expenses have often outpaced the rate of growth in state revenues, which has created a major concern for state administrators.

Beneficiaries

The number of persons that Medicaid serves has varied. In 1983, the number of persons receiving benefits was approximately 21.5 million, the same number as in 1979. Because the number of persons in poverty grew by approximately 10 million during that same time period, the net effect was that approximately 55% fewer poor were covered by the program (Sorkin, 1986). During recessions, the number of people eligible for Medicaid usually increases. In 2003, Medicaid enrolled 55.2 million people in the program (CMS, 2007b). Past and current studies indicate that many more people who are not enrolled in the program are also in need (Berk & Schur, 2001; General Accounting Office [GAO], 1996; IOM, 2007; Kaiser Commission, 2004a).

Mandated and Optional Recipients

The states are required by the federal government to provide services to certain groups and have the option of providing benefits to others (Box 4-2). The states have some control over the number of state residents covered under federally mandated programs. The states can establish most of the eligibility criteria, such as income and asset ceilings, as well as other criteria. Most states provide Medicaid coverage for families with children on welfare, known as **Temporary Assistance for Needy Families (TANF)** (formerly Aid to Families with Dependent Children [AFDC]). However, not all poor families qualify for TANF and Medicaid. See Chapter 21 for a more detailed discussion of TANF, poverty, and the relations of poverty to health status.

In addition to beneficiaries mandated by the federal government, states may extend care to other groups, for whom care may or may not be funded by federal matching funds. Many states offer optional programs. Thirty-five states cover medically needy families, but income and asset ceilings vary (CMS, 2005b). Some families might find that their incomes are too high to qualify initially, but extensive medical expenditures will reduce their assets to qualifying levels. Fifteen states chose not to extend coverage to medically needy families through optional programs.

From time to time, the federal government mandates coverage for certain at-risk populations. This was done in 1984, 1985, 1986, 1989, 1990, 1993, and 1997 as a result of increased concern over the uneven coverage criteria for pregnant women and children. Medicaid coverage was extended in all states, first to pregnant women and to children younger than 5 years in two-parent homes that met TANF and AFDC income eligibility standards. Gradually, benefits were extended to the following:

- All pregnant women and children younger than 6 years at or below 133% of the federal poverty level
- Families who meet the TANF requirements
- All children aged 6 through 19 years in families with income below the poverty level
- Caretakers, relatives, or legal guardians who take care of children under age 18, (age 19 if still in school)
- Selected Supplemental Security Income (SSI) recipients
- Individuals and couples living in medical institutions with monthly incomes up to 300% above SSI standards (CMS, 2005a; Dotson, 2002; GAO, 1995).

The result has been an expansion of the Medicaid program to certain populations using the federal poverty level as a criterion. This has reduced some of the uneven application of the TANF various state standards for Medicaid eligibility.

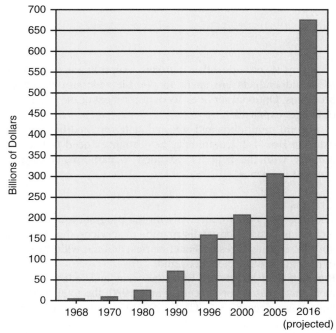

FIGURE 4-12 Medicaid costs for selected years, 1968-2005, in billions of dtollars. (Data from Centers for Medicare and Medicaid Services.)

Box 4-2   Medicaid Beneficiaries and Services

Medicaid Recipients

Federally Mandated Recipients
- All persons in federal aid programs, including Supplemental Security Income (SSI) and Temporary Assistance for Needy Families (TANF)*
- Pregnant women and children under 6 years of age with a family income below 133% of the poverty level
- Recipients of adoption assistance and foster care who are under Title IV-E of the Social Security Act
- Children aged 18 years and younger, born after September 30, 1983, with a family income below the poverty level
- Selected financially devastated persons

Federally Optional Recipients
- Certain medically needy families with incomes above the TANF limits
- Elderly, blind, or disabled adults who do not qualify for income assistance (welfare)
- Certain tuberculosis-infected persons (financial limit), for tuberculosis drugs and ambulatory care only
- Low-income children included in the State Children's Health Insurance Program (SCHIP)
- Infants younger than 1 year of age and pregnant women not covered under mandatory rules whose income is no more than 185% of the poverty level (states determine their cutoff percentage)
- Children under 21 years of age who meet the TANF income and resource requirements
- Recipients of state supplemental income payments
- Individuals in waived home and community-based settings who would be eligible if institutionalized (e.g., mentally ill)
- Institutionalized individuals eligible under special income levels (amount set by each state)

Major Benefits under Medicaid

Federally Required
- Inpatient and outpatient hospital care
- Prenatal and postpartum care
- Physician services
- Diagnostic services (laboratory tests, radiography)
- Skilled nursing facility services for persons 21 years or older
- Vaccines for children's program
- Home health care for persons eligible for skilled nursing services
- Family planning services and suppliers
- Nurse-midwife services
- Rural health clinic services and federally qualified health center (FQHC) services
- Certified family or pediatric nurse practitioner services
- Medical and surgical dentist services
- Early and periodic screening, diagnosis, and treatment (EPSDT) for people under 21 years of age

State-Determined Optional Services
- Diagnostic services
- Prescription drugs
- Dental care, eyeglasses, podiatry, optometry
- Rehabilitation and physical therapy
- Physician-directed clinic services
- Mental health rehabilitation or stabilization
- Transportation
- Residential intermediate care facilities for the mentally retarded (ICF-MR)
- Nursing facility services for people under 21 years of age
- Hospice care and case management
- Prosthetic devices
- Home and community-based care to certain persons with chronic impairments

Data from Centers for Medicare and Medicaid Services (CMS). (2002). *Medicare and Medicaid statistical supplement 2001.* Health Care Financing Review. Baltimore, MD: Author; CMS. (2005). *Medicaid at-a-glance 2005: A Medicaid information source.* Baltimore, MD: Department of Health and Human Services, Centers for Medicare and Medicaid Services, Center for Medicaid and State Operations.
Note: Covered services are provided to those groups with federally required coverage. Mandated services to optional groups are less comprehensive.
*Before August 1996, TANF was called *Aid to Families with Dependent Children (AFDC)*.

Cost savings were the reason for extending coverage. Providing for prenatal and pediatric care to these populations cost significantly less than providing treatment for problems that would have resulted without care. Still, the program expansions were limited. Nonpregnant females are not covered and are therefore still subject to their state's established criteria.

The following needy groups are excluded from Medicaid benefits altogether:
- Single persons and childless couples not aged or disabled
- Most two-parent families
- Families with a father who works at a low-paying job unless they have very low incomes as determined by state TANF criteria
- Legal aliens who entered the United States on or after August 22, 1996, who are barred for 5 years (CMS, 2005a; Hoffman et al., 2001).

Benefits
Medicaid benefits vary greatly depending on the state. States must provide federally mandated minimum services but are

at liberty to provide other services. Approximately 50% of Medicaid budgets are spent to provide federally mandated programs. Optional services account for most of the remainder of budget expenses.

Federal minimums and selected state optional benefits are listed in Box 4-2. Community health nurses need to become familiar with the benefits extended to participants in their states of residence.

Criticisms
The most important concerns with the program are related to increasing costs, unequal distribution of services, the impact of cost-cutting measures on beneficiaries, and the wide variation in benefits and recipients covered.

Program Cost Increases. Both the states and federal government have reason for concern. Since 1980, the total Medicaid budget has risen 82.3% (CMS, 2007b). Increases in program costs have occurred at both the federal and state levels. In 2005, both state and federal costs rose 9.1% (Patel & Rushefsky, 2006). Medicaid costs represent a greater share of state budgets than of the federal budget. In addition, state Medicaid costs have risen at three to five times the rate of increases in state revenues (Kaiser Commission, 2005). The percentage of state and local budgets consumed by Medicaid costs rose from 14% in 1987 to 22.9% in 2005, or $137 billion (National Association of State Budget Officers, 2006).

States must also contend with federal actions that have effectively reduced the expected federal share of the Medicaid budget. In 1981, as part of the Reagan administration's cost-cutting measure known as the Omnibus Budget Reconciliation Act, federal Medicaid grants to the states were reduced 11.5%. Federal actions allowed states more administrative discretion but also imposed new service directives that increased state Medicaid costs (Patel & Rushefsky, 2006). The federal Medicaid contribution is recalculated annually, so states risk a reduction of federal funds each year.

Unequal Distribution of Services to Beneficiaries. A relatively small group of people account for most of the costs in the Medicaid program. The elderly, blind, and disabled—25% of the beneficiaries—use 69.6% of the Medicaid budget (Figure 4-13). Medicaid pays for more than half of nursing home patient-days (Grogan & Patashnik, 2003). The average annual Medicaid costs are four to seven times higher for the aged and disabled than for children and their parents. Faced with expanding numbers of aged and disabled participants, the program has become increasingly inefficient at serving the very people for whom Medicaid was originally intended.

Variable Program Qualifications among States. Eligibility standards for Medicaid are primarily state determined (Patel & Rushefsky, 2006). There is wide variation in the services offered and recipients covered. Because states have discretion over the services and groups they can elect to cover, benefits are uneven and not comparable from state to state. Refer to Box 4-2

for optional coverage of groups and benefits. States expanded coverage to another 6.3 million in 2003 (CMS, 2005b).

States also determine the income level for eligibility (Patel & Rushefsky, 2006). Each state has its own ceiling on income and allowable personal assets based on a percentage of the federal poverty level (e.g., 100% of the poverty level, 50%, and so on). If the federal poverty level for a family of four is $20,516 (in 2006), a state with a ceiling of 50% of the poverty level will provide benefits to a family if the family's income is $10,258 or less per year; if their income is $10,300, they are ineligible in that state. However, the same family might very well be covered in other states with higher ceilings. Figure 4-14 shows how one family might be affected by different state ceilings. It is estimated that Medicaid benefits do not reach 33% to 50% of the population below the poverty level because of variations in state eligibility rules.

Solving this type of inequity requires federal action. The solution is mandated uniform federal standards for eligibility and services. Each state would be expected to provide the same services to all who meet the federal standard of income need. One of the main difficulties in enacting such requirements is that the federal government would effectively dictate service populations and mandatory services without necessarily increasing its share of each state's Medicaid budget. The net result would be an even greater burden on state budgets than is presently the case.

Federal and State Cost-Containment Effects on Beneficiaries. Cost cutting has resulted in dropping some needy individuals or some necessary services to needy individuals. Changing the eligibility requirements—for example, barring noncitizens from benefits for 5 years from the date of immigration—has been the major method used to reduce the number of eligible recipients. Starting in 2001, states have experienced budget deficits that necessitated making cuts in Medicaid reimbursement or tightening eligibility requirements (Patel & Rushefsky, 2006). For example, in Missouri 89,000 individuals were dropped from Medicaid and 370,000 others had benefit cuts, and Tennessee had to cut recipients in TennCare (a Medicaid managed care program) (Gardner et al., 2007).

Lowering the income ceiling for Medicaid qualification has the effect of restricting the number of persons who can qualify for the program (Rowland, 2008). Follow-up studies of dropped populations indicate that when services are terminated, there is a general worsening of health status, less satisfaction with health care, and increased inability to obtain other sources of care compared with persons not terminated from programs (Coburn & McDonald, 1992; Cohen et al., 1996; GAO, 1996; Halfon & Newacheck, 1993; Long et al., 2008). The long-term effects of restricting access can be costly, because people are sicker and require more intense treatment by the time they obtain care.

Most other methods of cost containment involve attempts to reduce the cost of services to the state and federal government. One method employed is cost sharing or co-payments. Although co-payments and deductibles in this program do not approach the costs in other co-payment programs (e.g., Medicare), they generally tend to have the same effect. People who can least afford it pay the most in terms of relative cost. It is important for community health nurses to understand the economic burdens health care can impose and the impact cost can play on an individual's ability to access and utilize health care services.

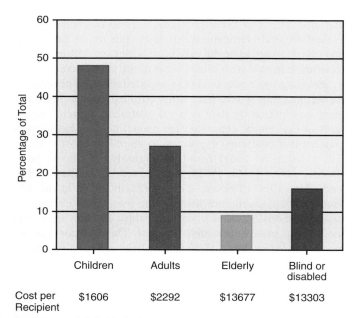

FIGURE 4-13 Medicaid cost of serving the disabled and elderly compared with serving children and other adults. (Data from Centers for Medicare and Medicaid Services. [2007]. *An overview of the US health care system chart book.* Baltimore, MD: Author.)

	Children	Adults	Elderly	Blind or disabled
Cost per Recipient	$1606	$2292	$13677	$13303

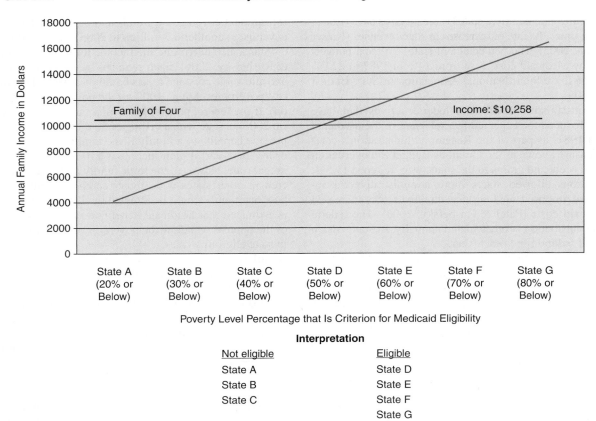

FIGURE 4-14 Income as a percentage of the poverty level as a criterion for Medicaid eligibility in selected states. In states *A, B,* and *C,* the hypothetical family is not eligible; in states *D, E, F,* and *G,* the family is eligible.

Controlling the amount paid for a service by establishing set fees for services is another means of cost containment. Set fee schedules have resulted in an effort by some providers to limit service to Medicaid populations. For example, some physicians refuse to treat Medicaid patients or place a limit on the number of such patients they will accept in their practices (Dovey et al., 2003; Hunt & Knickman, 2005). The willingness of physicians to accept Medicaid patients is tied to the level of payment received: lowering the fee any further will reduce access for a larger number of poor patients.

Another method of cost containment is to limit the choices or dictate the providers of service. The result of limited choice is that Medicaid recipients can be told where to go to obtain certain services and can be denied service if they do not comply with these restrictions. Some might argue that such limits deny patients the ability to seek compatible providers and, in some cases, might place an unnecessary or impossible burden on patients in terms of time and transportation. Nevertheless, there is a very real probability that more services will be controlled by such programs as states grapple with increases in their health care budgets.

Medicaid Managed Care

Since 1993, the federal government has allowed states waivers to expand managed care to Medicaid populations. States can either require or allow Medicaid recipients to use managed care programs. All 50 states have received waivers and have managed care programs for their Medicaid benefits patients (Pulcini & Hart, 2007a; Rowland, 2008). Approximately 61% of all beneficiaries are enrolled in managed care plans (CMS, 2007b).

Some states see managed care as a means of expanding Medicaid services to populations not historically covered by benefits. For example, 1.1 million in Florida and 500,000 in Tennessee are now covered. Other states, such as Oregon, Rhode Island, Maryland, Massachusetts, and Oklahoma, have also experimented with expanded coverage to targeted populations. Although these programs are too new for detailed evaluation, early indications are that states might have actually saved money in health care costs. Gold and Mittler (2000) reported that, at least initially, most of the states saved money by enrolling more people. Those enrolled received health care earlier than they would have if not enrolled, and earlier treatment was less costly than delayed treatment. Current projections of the cost of expansion are budget neutral, but there is concern that continued expansion to more low-income, high-risk populations could result in increasing Medicaid costs (Boben, 2000; GAO, 1995). Garrett and Zuckerman (2008) studied the effect of managed care on Medicaid recipients and found that managed care lowered the number of emergency department visits, some visits to health care providers, and the rates of use of preventive services. This is a cost saving, but there are few data on how these changes have affected the health status of Medicaid recipients.

Current Concerns Regarding the Medicaid Program

Efforts at Medicaid cost containment continue, and coverage is sporadic based on state requirements. In addition, in fiscally difficult years states cut coverage and services to needy populations and in fiscally good years they expand coverage. For example, in 2004, 19 states cut services and 12 states expanded services.

In 2005, 9 states cut services and 14 states expanded services (Kaiser Commission, 2004b). As a result, vulnerable populations see-saw back and forth between health coverage and no coverage.

The federal government is anxious to reduce its share of Medicaid costs and has proposed changes to the funding mechanism. These changes include outright reduction in funding to the states and a reorganization of Medicaid into a federal block grant program (O'Brien, 2008; Patel & Rushefsky, 2006). These efforts, if successful, will limit enrollment and reduce services to additional vulnerable groups. State governors are leery of such efforts, fearing the result would be additional burdens on state Medicaid budgets.

TRENDS IN REIMBURSEMENT

Cost concerns have stimulated changes in the reimbursement structure and delivery of services. These changes are expected to continue and evolve in the future as efforts at cost containment intensify. Reimbursement mechanisms have significant implications for community nursing, because they affect the types of services nurses can provide and have a direct influence on the scope of independent practice.

PROSPECTIVE AND RETROSPECTIVE REIMBURSEMENT: WHO WINS?

The two payment systems for health care services are retrospective and prospective. With **retrospective payment,** service is provided and then payment is after the fact. A patient goes to her or his physician for a sore throat, is seen and treated, and then is billed for the service. Retrospective payment is a cost-based reimbursement system. Retrospective payment essentially allows individuals and institutions to recover all costs of care. Retrospective payment provides no incentive for efficient management of health services. Alternative services that might be as effective and cost less need not be considered. With retrospective payment, the patient or third-party payer assumes all the risk of higher costs. The hospital, physician, or other providers of service bear no financial risks.

Prospective payment compensates the provider on a *case* basis for health services. The facility or provider can expect only a predetermined amount, regardless of the amount of time, energy, and service involved in providing care. Such a payment structure encourages efficiency; there is an incentive to use effective and cost-efficient alternatives.

Prospective payment is a method of placing limits on the increasing costs of medical services and encouraging efficient management techniques. Any provider who reduces the cost of supplying service below the reimbursement price cuts operating losses and/or makes a profit. As an extra incentive, the provider is allowed to keep all money the provider is paid, even if the costs for that service are less than the reimbursement schedule. Prospective payment has become the most popular form of payment system.

The **diagnosis-related group (DRG) system** is a major prospective payment system initiated by the federal Medicare program. It consists of a predetermined fee structure for services provided by hospitals for a list of over 468 diagnoses (Patel & Rushefsky, 2006). The length of stay and costs reimbursed for each diagnosis are preset. For example, a patient who is admitted with a stroke and no complications would be expected to stay in the hospital several days and then be transferred to a rehabilitation facility. If the hospital can treat and discharge the patient earlier than the prescribed length of stay, the hospital makes more profit. If the hospital needs to keep the patient longer, the hospital makes less profit. There are procedures for waivers and appeals if the patient required extra services and hospital days.

The DRG system has been expanded to other service areas by the federal government. Physicians, ambulatory clinics, dentists, and nursing homes are some of the service providers who are affected. As long as the interest in reducing the cost of service persists, expansion of the DRG system is a real possibility.

Managed care can also be viewed as a type of prospective payment system. HMO, PPO, and POS providers care for an individual for a predetermined premium or price (see Chapter 3). Because these types of service provision have proven to be cost effective in delivery of care, their popularity continues to increase. Most employers include managed care plans in their health plan offerings. Federal and most state employees have these options. Some employers have limited employees exclusively to managed care plans. The Medicare and Medicaid programs are increasing their reliance on managed care systems.

MANAGED CARE, NATIONAL MANAGED CARE COMPANIES, AND INTEGRATED HEALTH SYSTEMS

A number of trends have been identified in the managed care market. There is a movement toward allowing consumers more choices in service decisions. More and more people are enrolled in managed care; at the same time, the number of managed care organizations is diminishing. Concerns about access and quality of care have lead to a growing effort to study these issues in the managed care environment.

Consumer Choice

Consumer choice is dictating a trend away from HMOs, a more restrictive model, and toward PPOs and POSs, more permissive models (Kaiser/HRET, 2007). With permissive models, patients have greater choice. They may designate a primary care physician. They are also allowed more flexibility in seeking out-of-network providers and services.

Consolidation: Empires and Integrated Systems

The movement is toward bigger and larger managed care organizations. Most of the larger companies are for-profit and have continued to grow through consolidation of smaller managed care organizations. Sultz and Young (2004) refer to this trend as a move toward managed care empires. Some experts predict that in the next 5 years, consolidation will reduce the number to only three to five large national companies. Others contest that claim. Mechanic (2008) asserts that managed care organizations that restrict consumer choices and physician autonomy will decline. He believes managed care will continue to evolve into forms that address costs, practice rationing of services, and reduce restrictions on consumer choices but at the same time require greater financial contributions and cost sharing by the health care consumer.

Integrated systems are also a growing trend. Integrated systems are large organizations that own or control a complete range of health care facilities and provide service to a large population of consumers, for example, Kaiser Permanente and the Department of Veterans Affairs. Their goal is to provide all health care services required by their enrollees. Services include inpatient and outpatient care; prescription drugs; ambulatory services; home health care; case management; physical therapy; diagnostic and laboratory services; and rehabilitative and custodial care facilities.

Integrated systems save money by controlling the type of services provided to their enrollees. The aim is to employ case management to oversee comprehensive medical services and save money without sacrificing quality of care.

Quality Versus Cost: A Concern

Managed care has been successful in reducing costs of care in selected areas. Between 1990 and 1996, managed care saved an estimated $116 to $180 billion in health care services (Patel & Rushefsky, 1999). During that same period, employers saved approximately 11% in premium costs. Since that time, the cost savings for managed care has slowed, and Medicare managed care has shown negligible savings.

One of the reasons for the initial cost savings was that managed care organizations were able to pick their customers, pre-selecting out those who were likely to require the most costly services. This process is known as "creaming" or skimming the best customers off the top. Since then, large employers have taken measures to eliminate the practice. Medicare+Choice disallowed such practices at the beginning of the program. Whether Medicare Advantage will continue to do so remains to be seen.

Quality of care has been a continuing concern in the managed care market. Anecdotal evidence provides specific examples of limited access to specialists or services (Patel & Rushefsky, 1999; Roemer, 2001). It is also much harder to hold a managed care organization responsible for adverse effects that result from denial of care or service. Federal regulations, upheld in court trials, limit malpractice suits against managed care organizations (Patel & Rushefsky, 2006). For example, a New Orleans court ruled that a company could not be sued for damages by a woman whose fetus died after the company refused her hospitalization for her high-risk pregnancy. In another case, a St. Louis court disallowed a suit against a company after it refused to approve heart surgery recommended by the patient's doctor. The patient died (Patel & Rushefsky, 1999). In the early 2000s the courts seemed to ease limits on legal action against managed care organizations, but in 2004 the Supreme Court found in favor of Aetna (a managed care organization) in a suit brought by a health care client (Patel & Rushefsky, 2006).

There have been several unsuccessful efforts at the federal level to pass legislation allowing malpractice suits against managed care organizations. The industry has vigorously defended the status quo. As a reaction to the lack of federal legislation and other quality issues, 47 states have enacted legislation regulating some practices in managed care organizations (Patel & Rushefsky, 2006). For example, the state of Maryland mandates that pregnant women cannot be discharged from hospitals on the day of delivery and that patients cannot be charged for emergency department visits that "any prudent layperson" would consider necessary.

RATIONING OF HEALTH CARE

Not everyone in this country has access to health care services. Cost-containment measures that increase out-of-pocket expenses and make health insurance unattainable for some have the effect of rationing health care. Those who cannot afford care, or are not included in the specialized health/welfare programs, do without. As the health care system proceeds to expand cost-containment measures, it is helpful to visit the issues of cost and access.

Care and Cost in a Free Market Environment

The U.S. economic system is biased toward a strong capitalistic or **free market economy.** This means that, in general, business has traditionally been allowed to operate independently, without much governmental interference. That same inclination has been followed in the system or market providing health care services. The private sector plays a substantial role in the delivery of health care, and private providers are free to set the price for health care services.

In a free market, not everyone can purchase services. As the price of services goes up, the number of consumers who can participate or purchase health care goes down. In a free market economy, the price of a product determines how much will be produced (supply) and consumed (demand). In the health care system, products include all types of care (either services or goods), such as physician office visits, nursing care, dental care, medications, diagnostic tests, and prosthetics.

Figure 4-15 shows how price influences both the production (supply) and the consumption (demand) of a specific good (in this case, Pill A). Notice that a pharmaceutical company is willing to make (supply) many more Pill As if they can charge a price of 70 cents per pill. The consumer is more willing or able to afford Pill A (demand) if the price is 10 cents per pill. A price in

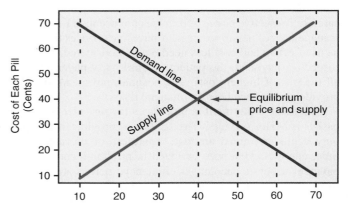

FIGURE 4-15 How price influences supply and demand of pill A. The supply line shows that, as the price of an item increases, production and, therefore, the amount of goods produced increases. When the price is high, the producer is willing to make larger quantities, and as the price falls, the producer makes fewer pills. The demand line demonstrates how price affects the consumer's demand for pill A. The higher the price, the less the demand. When the free market operates effectively, competition forces a balance between the amount supplied and the amount demanded. The price of goods produced at that point is called the *equilibrium price,* 40¢ per pill in this case. If the price were higher, the producer would be willing to supply a greater quantity, but the consumer would not be willing (or would be unable) to purchase that quantity, and there would be an oversupply. If the cost were lower, the consumer would be willing to buy a greater quantity, but the producer would not be willing (or able) to produce the quantity in demand at that price, and there would be a shortage.

the middle is where the consumer and manufacturer compromise, dictating both price (40 cents per pill) and supply.

Health Care as a Right or Privilege

If one believes that health care is a privilege based on the ability to pay, then there is no problem with providing care via the free market system. Those who can afford services receive them, and those who cannot do without. Despite its free market leaning, the United States feels that some measure of care should be considered the right of its citizens. The government has assumed responsibility for financing health care for selected aggregates of the population—namely, the elderly and the very poor. The government has, in effect, become the guarantor of last resort for specific risk groups.

Under these conditions, a true market economy for health care does not exist, and, some would argue, with good reason. The increasing concern regarding the U.S. health care system is the lack of access for many for whom the government is not a guarantor of last resort. The question of universal coverage is again in the news.

Chapter 3 provides a more detailed discussion of the issues surrounding lack of access and universal coverage. The American Nurses Association (ANA) supports development of a system of **universal coverage,** or health care for all (ANA, 1991, 2007; Trossman, 2003). Whatever your personal position on this issue, it is useful to explore the extent of access and services and their impact on the health status of risk groups. You will be in a better position to evaluate the impact of specific remedies as they are considered and debated.

IMPACT OF MALPRACTICE AND HEALTH INSURANCE ON PROVIDERS AND CONSUMERS

There are growing concerns that the cost of malpractice insurance might affect consumer services. In response to the current malpractice insurance crisis, the U.S Congress is considering legislation to limit malpractice claims. There is also some evidence that restrictions in a client's health insurance policy might influence a physician's decision to prescribe appropriate care.

Malpractice Insurance Costs: Physicians, Hospitals, and Access to Care

The cost of physician coverage for malpractice insurance has increased substantially in the United States, and some companies have discontinued offering malpractice insurance (Thorpe, 2004). In 2003 the median increase in malpractice premiums ranged from 15% to 30% depending on the state and practice area (Patel & Rushefsky, 2006). In 2005, for example, obstetricians/gynecologists paid $141,760 in health insurance premiums in the state of Nevada (Berntsen, 2005). Physicians have responded to malpractice costs by going bare (doing without insurance), leaving professional practice, or becoming hospital employees.

Not all states will allow physicians to practice without malpractice insurance. Some states, such as Massachusetts, Kansas, and Wisconsin, require a minimal level of coverage. Some states, such as Pennsylvania, require more extensive coverage. Some doctors have altered their practice to cut insurance costs. They have discontinued riskier procedures or eliminated emergency department visits, and some have stopped all hospital practice (GAO, 2003).

As an alternative to carrying personal liability insurance, some doctors have changed employment status from private practice to salaried positions. This is an ongoing trend among physicians. The employer, usually a hospital, becomes responsible for malpractice coverage. In these instances, the burden of insurance premiums switches from physician to hospital.

Hospitals have been experiencing an increase in their customary insurance premiums. Now, those hospitals are seeing additional increases in premiums related to their expanding physician staff. Some hospitals report that coverage costs have doubled in 1 year (Glabman, 2003). Hospitals have responded to this crisis by going bare, reducing the maximum values on their policies, raising their deductible levels, and forming offshore insurance companies. The offshore companies do not have to conform to state insurance laws.

The impact of current malpractice insurance costs on total health care costs is not known. Although malpractice costs are high, they are a relatively small percentage of total health costs. In past malpractice crises, studies show a limited impact on the health care budget. The Congressional Budget Office (1992a, 1992b) reported that malpractice premiums make up only 1% of the total health care budget. During the current crisis, the GAO (2003) has not been able to determine any appreciable impact on the health care budget.

There is concern that patient access to physicians and hospital services might be limited because of the malpractice crisis. The GAO report (2003) studied nine states affected by the current crisis. The report found no widespread access problems at this time. It reported some reduction in access for emergency surgery and infant deliveries predominantly in rural areas. These access problems were sporadic and correlated with the difficulty of recruiting and keeping physicians in those areas.

Impact of Insurance on Practice

Health insurance issues might affect the quality and quantity of health care services. Some contend that expenses are incurred by the practice of defensive medicine. *Defensive medicine* means that providers employ certain strategies solely to reduce their risk of being sued. Several studies (Congressional Budget Office, 1992b; GAO, 2003) suggest that the costs of defensive medicine are highly exaggerated. It found that most testing and procedures are done to reduce the uncertainty of medical diagnosis, and these would continue with or without the risk of lawsuits.

Another concern is whether a patient's insurance coverage or lack thereof influences physician decisions related to the health care services they prescribe. Wynia and colleagues (2003) report that a third of doctors do not offer pertinent services to patients because their insurance companies do not cover the service. Moreover, the trend appears to be increasing.

EXPANDED INSURANCE COVERAGE: BENEFITS AND RISK GROUPS

Gradually, over the past 30 years, the United States has moved to expand health benefits and health insurance to targeted groups: women and children, the elderly, the disabled, and low-income families above the poverty level. Medicaid has expanded into low-income populations it had previously excluded. Medicare has expanded the categories of disabled persons it serves. States, through Medicaid and other programs, have acted to include more lower-wage workers and their families in health insurance programs. The federal government has moved to protect workers from lack of insurance due to employment changes or preexisting health problems.

In the future, we can expect to see continued *incremental* change as insurance coverage is extended to more people and health benefits are expanded. Managed care will play a pre-eminent role in these changes. States will address the problem of low-income workers by expanding the Medicaid program, requiring employers to provide coverage, and expanding high-risk pools to lower insurance costs. The federal government has passed a prescription drug benefit, Medicare D, for senior citizens. It has been suggested that Medicare can be adjusted to allow workers without insurance and early retirees to buy into the plan (Davis & Schoen, 2003).

As people and benefits are added, we can expect to see greater restrictions on individual choices to cut costs. For example, prescription drugs will be limited to generics, and managed care might become the only employer-provided health insurance option. These changes will be accompanied by greater cost sharing for health care services. Co-payments and deductibles will rise as the government and employers seek to limit their share of health care costs. Medicare and private health insurance could change from a defined benefit to a defined contribution plan. The government or employer will contribute a fixed amount into the consumer's account. It will be up to the consumer to decide how to spend it (Park et al., 2003; Pulcini & Hart, 2007a). If health care costs are greater than the amount deposited, the additional costs will be borne by the consumer.

REIMBURSEMENT FOR COMMUNITY/PUBLIC HEALTH NURSING SERVICES

In the near future, the role of nursing in community settings can be expected to expand in all three areas of primary, secondary, and tertiary prevention. Currently, trends are heavily weighted toward expanded reimbursement for secondary and tertiary community nursing services. Although most nurses will still be employed in hospital settings, the number of nurses involved in providing care for the ill and disabled in the community will increase. The overriding reason for these expanding opportunities is cost. The strategies for cost containment already mentioned, coupled with a number of other factors, are responsible for the growth in community-based services. Some of these other factors are as follows:

- The DRG system has resulted in a reduction in the average length of hospital stay. Patients are discharged earlier and more frequently require nursing service in the home (Rice & Komenski, 2001; Sultz & Young, 2004).
- The financial cost of institutional care is greater than the cost of providing support services in the home and community. As a result, the government and insurance payers are expanding their coverage of community support services as a substitute for or as a means of delaying institutional care (Harrington, 2007; Kitchener et al., 2005).
- The aging of the U.S. population makes it probable that there will be a larger population of chronically ill elderly who require care, which thus expands the market for community services (Harrington, 2007).
- The search for less costly labor substitutes will enhance the use of nursing services to provide additional care in the community (Brewer, 2005; Sochalski, 2002; Sultz & Young, 2004).
- Care provided by nurses in independent practice settings demonstrates high levels of quality and patient satisfaction (Diers & Price, 2007; Pulcini & Hart, 2007b).

The last factor has generated conflict. Traditionally, physicians and the AMA have resisted direct third-party payment for nursing services (Diers & Price, 2007). The ANA believes that nurses should have the opportunity to be compensated for care by third-party insurers. Every effort to expand third-party reimbursement for nursing services has met with resistance. There is also some resistance to expanding nursing payments by private and public third-party payers. In 1997, Congress passed legislation providing Medicare reimbursement for nurse practitioners and clinical nurse specialists, regardless of geographic location.

Restriction on reimbursement has resulted in restricted practice areas for nursing. Although nothing prevents nurses from providing service for a fee in the community, the market for such services will remain constricted as long as consumers must personally bear the cost of such services. Allowing third-party reimbursement for independent nursing services will dramatically increase the demand for such services. Thirty-two states have passed legislation authorizing reimbursement to nurse practitioners from private and commercial insurers (ANA, 2007). The key to passage of such legislation lies in obtaining the support of third-party payers and prominent community leaders. As cost-cutting measures become more prevalent, the possibility of such support becomes more likely.

Federal and state governments have played a major role in expanding third-party reimbursement for nurses, especially in government-financed health programs (Pulcini & Hart, 2007b). Federal employee insurance plans are authorized to make direct payment to nurse practitioners and clinical nurse specialists. The federal government supports community health centers. They act as a safety net, providing services to geriatric populations and to rural and urban underserved populations. They enhance health, prevent or delay more intensive care, and are cost effective. These centers serve more than 10 million persons each year, 66% of whom are below the poverty level. These projects aim at increasing independent nursing practice in the community. Community health centers receive direct payment for nursing services. Currently there are more than 1000 such centers (Sardell, 2007). Some centers are funded by the Department of Health and Human Services; others, by a variety of state, local, and private sources. If funding continues, these types of service centers are expected to increase in popularity.

THE NURSE'S ROLE IN HEALTH CARE FINANCING

Nurses are not accustomed to considering themselves part of the decision process involved in financing and reimbursement for health care services. Nursing practice has only relatively recently begun to emphasize this aspect of delivering care. Nurses generally become aware of the impact of finances through their own personal or professional experiences. In community health practice, it is more likely that nurses are aware of the financial concerns related to delivery of care, because there is longer involvement with clients and an emphasis on the psychosocial and family issues related to care.

There are a number of ways nurses can initiate or facilitate care for clients in the community setting. Only a few are discussed here. Once nurses are sensitive to the link between finances and acquisition of services, they will be able to devise additional strategies.

REFERRING CLIENTS FOR BENEFITS AND SERVICES

Client referral is the simplest of nursing actions and one that can provide great benefit and financial relief to clients. Often, it is just a matter of matching clients to existing programs for which they qualify. However, to do so, nurses will need baseline data on their local community services (i.e., local, state, and federal benefit programs) and on the insurance coverage of respective clients. This does not mean that nurses must become experts in program criteria, application processes, and benefit packages, but they should become aware of existing programs, the types of clients who are generally served by those programs, and the name and phone number of the initial contact for such programs.

Some of the major state and federal benefit programs have been discussed in this chapter, along with some general criteria for eligibility. This information will allow you to screen potential program-client matches. Remember that the selection criteria change from time to time, so your actions should not be directed toward narrowly applying selection criteria. Your role is to identify potential client-program matches, interpreting eligibility criteria broadly and leaving the reimbursing agency to do a more stringent investigation.

There are many community programs and resources that have not been listed or examined in this chapter. Each community health nurse will, in the course of her or his practice, devise her or his own community resources list and become familiar with the services that such resources can provide. It takes 3 to 6 months for a community health nurse to devise a basic list of community resources that includes both widely known programs and those that are unique to the individual community. As the community health nurse becomes more proficient in her or his practice, the list of references and resources will grow. The information a nurse supplies to clients can reduce or eliminate some of the financial burdens imposed by illness, as well as secure access for primary care, health promotion, and health protection (e.g., immunizations).

ADVOCATING FOR CLIENTS IN APPEAL PROCESSES

Clients might apply for help and find that they have been denied service. Although most agencies should take time to inform clients of their options, many clients might be confused about their rights of appeal and the reason for denial. There are a number of ways nurses can advocate for their clients in the appeal process.

First, ascertain the reason for denial of the claim. Frequently, inadequate information was supplied to the agencies. If this is the case, helping the client to complete the application correctly might be all the action needed. Other ways nurses can be advocates include exploring the appeals method, personally contacting personnel within the agency to verify information or provide additional data, and enlisting the services of other experts who might assist the client in the process.

IDENTIFYING ALTERNATIVE SOURCES OF PAYMENT

A variety of service sources is available, especially within urban communities. If one program or agency has denied benefits to the client, other sources should be sought. As a nurse becomes proficient in identifying possible resources, she or he will become more expert at locating other potential service resources.

PROVIDING DOCUMENTATION TO ENSURE REIMBURSEMENT

Agencies and programs have become increasingly insistent on adequate documentation of services. Programs continually monitor claims for benefits to ensure that they meet selected standards. When documentation is not in a format acceptable to the agency, there is a risk that nursing services will not be covered. Even if the provided nursing services are considered reimbursable by the program, nurses should document in a way that makes clear to the agency that the specified service has been provided.

Inadequate or incomplete documentation of provided services has implications for both employers and clients. Agencies must provide correct paperwork to recoup their costs for services. Similarly, a nurse's client might incur unexpected out-of-pocket expenses because she or he has to pay for covered services that should have been reimbursed by the insurance company. Complete and accurate nursing records reduce these risks.

COLLECTING DATA TO EVALUATE THE IMPACT OF REIMBURSEMENT MECHANISMS

As noted earlier, there are consequences of the reimbursement structure. Some of these are intended; others are unintentional. Health care professionals are concerned that there might be additional unintended consequences of the DRG system. The DRG system encourages hospitals to reduce a patient's length of stay. Longer stays are not profitable for hospitals. Health professionals are concerned that patients are being discharged in a sicker state and in need of more skilled community services than was previously the case. There is an ongoing debate with respect to whether early discharge translates into poorer outcomes.

Community nurses who provide care to the elderly and other patients after hospital discharge are an invaluable source of data to assist with risk assessment of early discharges. As this and other reimbursement mechanisms change and service practices are altered, nurses have a unique opportunity to collect data regarding the implications of such mechanisms and practices for health and health care delivery practice in the community.

LOBBYING FOR LEGISLATIVE AND ADMINISTRATIVE CHANGES

One of the most effective ways to affect health care delivery and reimbursement is through political action, an avenue on which the nursing profession continues to concentrate more attention.

One in every 10 women voters is a registered nurse; thus, the potential for political influence is enormous. Nurses can influence legislation in several ways. As individuals, they can become more involved in the process by identifying their state and federal representatives and contacting them on important health issues. Nurses can become active in their affiliated party or in campaigns for individuals who represent or support their views of health care needs. Thus, nurses can be an effective force in putting health care issues on the public agenda.

It is imperative that nurses become involved in the decision-making processes related to delivery of health care services and reimbursement. Nursing practice is affected by such issues. Moreover, community health nurses and other public health professionals have always demonstrated concern for the social implications of health care delivery, particularly the issues of equity and accessibility of care.

As a member of the nursing profession, you can support your representative organization's position on health care issues. You might want to become active in nursing organizations and help set the agenda of health concerns addressed by your profession. The ANA developed a policy statement, *Nursing's Blueprint for Managed Care* (Trossman, 1998). The blueprint is designed to spearhead the nursing community's role in shaping managed care. The support of every nurse will be crucial to nursing's success at using the political process to address health goals.

KEY IDEAS

1. The practice of nursing in community and hospital settings can be limited or directed by the cost of delivering health care services.
2. Nurses need to know about the financing system of health care to understand its impact on individual clients and their health status.
3. Health care in the United States is costly and is rationed by the ability to pay.
4. Certain groups are at greater risk of limited access to health care services because of cost. The three groups at greatest risk are the elderly, the medically indigent, and poor children.
5. Health care is financed by a variety of options (i.e., self-payment, health insurance, and health assistance programs). Medicare is a government-operated health insurance program. Medicaid and SCHIP are government-operated health assistance programs.
6. Employers have attempted to curb their costs by placing restrictions on the types of services covered under their health insurance plans, by limiting their employees' plan options, by negotiating with health care providers for reduced fees, and by increasing the employees' share of health insurance premiums.
7. Medicare and Medicaid costs are a growing problem in government budgets, and these programs provide limited health care services to certain populations. Medicaid provides health care services to less than 50% of the population below the poverty level.
8. Poverty is linked to poor health, limited access to health care services, and delay in seeking such services. Cost-containment measures that result in less access are not cost productive. Acute and delayed care is ultimately more costly than preventive services and immediate treatment.
9. Managed care has become the most common form of health care delivery for both public- and private-sector health markets.
10. Health care costs, universal access to care, and the quality of health care are ongoing, often competing concerns in health care delivery in the United States.

LEARNING BY EXPERIENCE AND REFLECTION

1. Develop your ideas for the "ideal" method to finance health care delivery in this country. How similar to or different from the present system for financing health care is your method?
2. Identify groups that are affected by the way health care is delivered and paid for in this country. How might each of these vested interests be affected by your "ideal" method of financing health care? For those who would be affected by the change (if any), consider how you might present your position to convince them to support your proposal.
3. Interview senior citizens. What kind of experiences have they had with health care services? Do they have any chronic conditions that require sustained medical care? Discover how much and what kinds of their medical bills Medicare pays. Ask if they would be willing to tell you their out-of-pocket expenses for medical care, including deductibles and co-payments under Medicare. Consider how these expenses might affect their ability to purchase other necessities, such as food, shelter, and clothing, and how much is left to purchase incidentals and leisure treats.
4. Find out your state's cap for Medicaid eligibility for a family of three. What percentage of the current poverty level is your state's eligibility cap—30%, 50%, 70%, or some other percentage? Plan a 1-month budget for a family of three for minimally adequate food, clothing, and safe shelter. Include the cost of a telephone, electricity, and fuel. Compare your state's Medicaid cap for this fictional family with your monthly budget. Is the capped income more or less than your expected monthly costs? If less, consider what you might be willing to forgo paying for or purchasing. What if you had additional expenses, including medical costs? How would you restructure your budget to meet these unexpected expenses? Is this achievable?
5. Review your current health insurance status. If you have coverage, who provides this coverage? If your health care is employer provided, what are your premiums, and what is the cost to your employer? Are there limits to your benefits? If so, what kind? Do you have a co-payment and/or deductible? If so, how much are they? Does your insurance plan provide a catastrophic health benefit?

STUDY AIDS   http://evolve.elsevier.com/Maurer/community/

Visit the Evolve website for this book to find the following study and assessment materials:

- Quiz
- Web Scenario
- Critical Thinking Questions and Answers for Case Studies
- Care Plans
- *Healthy People* Updates
- Glossary

REFERENCES

Advocates for Senior Alert. (1990). *The Medigap mess.* Washington, DC: Author.

American Association of Retired Persons. (2007). Long-term care: What you don't know could cost you. *AARP Bulletin, 48*(1), 33.

American Hospital Association. (2007, October). *Uncompensated hospital care cost fact sheet.* Retrieved January 25, 2008 from *http://www.aha.org/aha/content/2007/pdf/07-uncompensated-care.pdf.*

American Nurses Association. (1991). *Nursing's agenda for health care reform* (PR1291). Kansas City, MO: Author.

American Nurses Association. (2007). *Access to health coverage. Position statement.* Retrieved May 16, 2008 from *http://www.nursingworld.org/MainMenu/Categories/ANAPoliticalPower/Federal/LEGIS/HealthCoverage.aspx.*

Augenblick, J. (2001). *The status of school financing today.* Denver: Educational Commission of the States.

Berk, M. L., & Schur, C. L. (2001). Access to care: How much difference does Medicaid make? In C. Harrington & C. L. Estes (Eds.), *Health policy: Crisis and reform in the U.S. health care delivery system* (3rd ed.; pp. 276-283). Boston: Jones & Bartlett.

Berntsen, K. J. (2005). Looking beyond tort reform toward safer healthcare systems. *Journal of Nursing Quality, 20*(1), 9-12.

Biles, B., Nickolas, L. H., & Guterman, S. (2008). Medicare beneficiary out-of-pocket costs: Are Medicare Advantage plans a better deal? In C. Harrington & C. L. Estes (Eds.), *Health policy: Crisis and reform in the U.S. health care delivery system* (5th ed.; pp. 336-344). Sudbury, MA: Jones & Bartlett.

Boben, P. J. (2000). Medicaid reform in the 1990s. *Health Care Financing Review, 22*(2), 1-5.

Bodenheimer, T. (2008). High and rising health care costs. Part 3: The role of health care providers. In C. Harrington & C. L. Estes (Eds.), *Health policy and nursing: Crisis and reform in the U.S. health care delivery system* (5th ed.; pp. 275-280). Sudbury, MA: Jones & Bartlett.

Brewer, C. S. (2005). The health care workforce. In A. R. Koverner & J. R. Knickman (Eds.), *Jonas and Kovner's health care delivery in the United States* (8th ed.; pp. 418-463). New York: Springer.

Butler, R. N. (1997). On behalf of older women: Another reason to protect Medicare and Medicaid. In C. Harrington & C. L. Estes (Eds.), *Health policy and nursing: Crisis and reform in the U.S. health care delivery system* (2nd ed.; pp. 327-331). Sudbury, MA: Jones & Bartlett.

Centers for Medicare and Medicaid Services (CMS). (2002). *Medicare and Medicaid statistical supplement 2001.* Health Care Financing Review. Baltimore, MD: Author

Centers for Medicare and Medicaid Services. (2005a). *Medicaid at a glance 2005: A Medicaid information source.* Baltimore, MD: Author.

Centers for Medicare and Medicaid Services. (2005b). *2005 CMS statistics.* Washington DC: U.S. Department of Health and Human Services.

Centers for Medicare and Medicaid Services. (2006). Table 3: National health expenditures: Aggregate and per capita amounts, percent distribution, and annual percent change by source of funds: Calendar years 2001-2016. Retrieved November 1, 2007 from *http://www.cms.hhs.gov/NationalHealthExpendData/downloads/proj2006.pdf.*

Centers for Medicare and Medicaid Services. (2007a). *Choosing a Medigap policy: A guide to health insurance for people with Medicare.* Baltimore MD: Author.

Centers for Medicare and Medicaid Services. (2007b). *An overview of the U.S. Health care system chart book, January 31, 2007.* Baltimore, MD: Centers for Medicare and Medicaid Services, Office of the Assistant Secretary for Planning and Evaluation.

Centers for Medicare and Medicaid Services. (2007c). Table 1: National health expenditures aggregate, per capita amounts, percent distribution, and average annual percent growth, by source of funds: Selected calendar years 1960-2005. Retrieved August 20, 2007 from *http://www.cms.hhs.gov/NationalHealthExpendData/downloads/tables.pdf.*

Centers for Medicare and Medicaid Services. (2008). *Medicare and you 2008.* Baltimore, MD: Author.

Chollet, D. (2002). Expanding individual health insurance coverage: Are high-risk pools the answer? *Health Affairs*, Supplement Web Exclusives, W349-352.

Coburn, A. F., & McDonald, T. P. (1992). The effects of variations in AFDC and Medicaid eligibility on prenatal care use. *Social Science and Medicine, 35*(8), 1055-1063.

Cohen, L. A., Manski, R. J., & Hooper, F. J. (1996). Does the elimination of Medicaid reimbursement affect the frequency of emergency department dental visits? *Journal of the American Dental Association, 127*(5), 605-609.

Collins, S.R., Kriss, J.L., Davis, K., et al. (2008). Squeezed: Why rising exposure to health care costs threatens the health and financial well-being of American families. In C. Harrington & C. L. Estes (Eds.), *Health policy: Crisis and reform in the U.S. health care delivery system* (5th ed.; pp. 286-289). Sudbury, MA: Jones & Bartlett.

Congressional Budget Office. (1992a). *Staff memorandum: Factors contributing to the growth of the Medicare program.* Washington, DC: U.S. Government Printing Office.

Congressional Budget Office. (1992b). *Economic implications of rising health care costs.* Washington, DC: U.S. Government Printing Office.

Cubanski, J., & Neuman, P. (2007, January-February). Status report on Medicare Part D enrollment in 2006: Analysis of plan-specific market share and coverage. *Health Affairs Web Supplement, 26*(1), W1-12. Retrieved April 1, 2008 from *http://content.healthaffairs.org.*

Davis, K., & Schoen, C. (2003). Creating consensus on coverage choices. *Health Affairs*, Web Exclusive, W3-199-211. Retrieved April 1, 2008 from *http://content.healthaffairs.org.*

DeNavas-Walt, C., Proctor, B. D., & Smith, J. (2007). *Income, poverty, and health insurance coverage in the United States: 2006* (U.S. Census Bureau, Current Populations Reports, P60-233). Washington DC: U.S. Department of Commerce, Economics and Statistics Administration, U.S. Bureau of the Census.

Diers, D., & Price, L. (2007). Research as a political and policy tool. In D. J. Mason, J. K. Leavitt, & M. W. Chaffee (Eds.), *Policy and politics in nursing and health care* (5th ed.; pp. 195-207). St. Louis: Saunders.

Dotson, J. A. W. (2002). Squeezing the turnip: Equitable distributions of funding to provide maternal and child health services in rural America. *Nursing Leadership Forum, 7*(11), 16-19.

Dovey, S., Weitzman, M., Fryer, G., et al. (2003). The ecology of medical care for children in the United States. *Pediatrics, 111*(5, Pt 1), 1024-1029.

Emanuel, E. J., Fuchs, V. R., & Garber, A. M. (2007). Essential elements of technology and outcomes assessment initiative. *Journal of the American Medical Association, 298*(11), 1323-1325.

Feder, J., Uccello, C., & O'Brien, E. (2001). The differences different approaches make: Comparing proposals to expand health insurance. In C. Harrington & C. L. Estes (Eds.), *Health policy: Crisis and reform in the U.S. health care delivery system* (3rd ed.; pp. 298-313). Sudbury, MA: Jones & Bartlett.

Fox, F. D., Snyder, R. C., & Rice, T. (2003). Medigap reform legislation of 1990: A 10-year review. *Health Care Financing Review, 24*(3), 121-137.

Gabel, J. R., Jensen, G. A., & Hawkins, S. (2003). Self-insurance in times of growing and retreating managed care. *Health Affairs, 22*(2), 202-210.

Garamone, J. Historical context important when considering budget requests. Retrieved April 2, 2008 from *http://www.defenselink.mil/news/newsarticle.aspx?id=2966.*

Gardner, D. B., Wakefield, M. K., & Gardner, B. G. (2007). Contemporary issues in government. In D. J. Mason, J. K. Leavitt, & M. W. Chaffee (Eds.), *Policy and politics in nursing and health care* (5th ed.; pp. 622-646). St. Louis: Saunders.

Garrett, B., & Zuckerman, S. (2008). National estimates of the effects of mandatory Medicaid managed care programs on health care access and use, 1997-1999. In C. Harrington & C. L. Estes (Eds.), *Health policy: Crisis and reform in the U.S. health care delivery system* (5th ed.; pp. 332-335). Sudbury, MA: Jones & Bartlett.

General Accounting Office. (1995). *Medicaid spending pressures drive states toward program reinvention* (GAO/HEHS-95-122). Washington, DC: U. S. Government Printing Office.

General Accounting Office. (1996). *Health insurance for children: Private insurance continues to deteriorate* (GAO/HEHS-96-129). Washington, DC: U.S. Government Printing Office.

General Accounting Office. (2003). *Medical malpractice: Implications of rising premiums on access to health care* (GAO-03-836). Washington, DC: U.S. Government Printing Office.

Geyman, J. P. (2008). Myths as barriers to health care reform in the United States. In C. Harrington & C. L. Estes (Eds.), *Health policy: Crisis and reform in the U.S. health care delivery system* (5th ed.; pp. 407-413). Sudbury, MA: Jones & Bartlett.

Glabman, M. (2003). Bare bones: As the cost of malpractice insurance skyrockets, doctors, hospitals, and patients suffer. *Trustee, 56*(3), 8-13.

Gold, M., & Mittler, J. (2000). Second- generation Medicaid managed care: Can it deliver? *Health Care Financing Review, 22*(2), 29-47.

Gold, M., & Mittler, J. (2001, June). The structure of supplemental insurance for Medicare beneficiaries. *Monitoring Medicare+Choice: Operational Insights*, No. 3. Retrieved August 14, 2002 from *http://www.mathematica-mpr.com*.

Gourevitch, M. N., Caronna, C. A., & Kalkut, G. (2005). *Acute care*. In A. R. Koverner & J. R. Knickman (Eds.), *Jonas and Kovner's health care delivery in the United States* (8th ed.; pp. 212-247). New York: Springer.

Grogan, C. M., & Patashnik, E. M. (2003). Universalism within targeting: Nursing home care, the middle class, and the politics of the Medicaid program. *Social Service Review, 71*(1), 51-71.

Hadley, J., & Holahan, J. (2004). *The cost of care for the uninsured: What do we spend, who pays, and what would full coverage add to medical spending?* Washington DC: Kaiser Commission on Medicaid and the Uninsured.

Halfon, N., & Newacheck, P. W. (1993). Childhood asthma and poverty—Differential impact and utilization of health services. *Pediatrics, 9*(1), 55-61.

Harrington, C. (2007). Policy spotlight: The politics of long-term care. In D. J. Mason, J. K. Leavitt, & M. W. Chaffee (Eds.), *Policy and politics in nursing and health care* (5th ed., pp. 295-303). St. Louis: Saunders.

Health Care Financing and Organization. (2007). *Universal coverage—One state at a time*. Washington DC: Robert Wood Johnson Foundation.

Hileman, G. R., Moroz, K. E., Wrightson, C. W., et al. (2002). Medicare+Choice individual and group enrollment 2001-2002. *Health Care Financing Review, 24*(1), 145-154.

Hoffman E. D., Klees, B. S., & Curtis, C. A. (2001). Overview of the Medicare and Medicaid programs. *Health Care Financing Review*, statistical supplement, 1-20.

Hunt, K. A., & Knickman, J. R. (2005). *Financing for health care*. In A. R. Koverner & J. R. Knickman (Eds.), *Jonas and Kovner's health care delivery in the United States* (8th ed.; pp. 46-89). New York: Springer.

Inglehart, J. K. (2002). Changing health insurance trends. *New England Journal of Medicine, 347*(12), 956-962.

Institute of Medicine. (2007). *Fact sheet 5: Uninsurance facts and figures: The uninsured are sicker and die sooner*. Retrieved July 5, 2007 from *http://www.iom.edu/CMS/17645.aspx*.

Kaiser Commission on Medicaid and the Uninsured. (2004a). *The uninsured and their access to care*. Washington DC: Author.

Kaiser Commission on Medicaid and the Uninsured. (2004b). *The continuing Medicaid budget challenge: State Medicaid spending growth and cost containment in fiscal years 2004 and 2005: Results from a 50 state survey*. Washington DC: Author.

Kaiser Commission on Medicaid and the Uninsured. (2005). *Medicaid: Issues in restructuring federal financing*. Retrieved November 1, 2007 from *http://www.kff.org/about/kcmu.cfm*.

Kaiser Commission on Medicaid and the Uninsured. (2007, October). *The uninsured: A primer*. Publ. No. 7541-30. Retrieved November 1, 2007 from *http://www.kff.org*.

Kaiser Family Foundation. (2007). *Medicare at a glance*. Retrieved October 20, 2007 from *http://www.kff.org/medicare/ upload/1066-10.pdf*.

Kaiser Family Foundation. (2008). *Medicare at a glance*. In C. Harrington & C. L. Estes (Eds.), *Health policy: Crisis and reform in the U.S. health care delivery system* (5th ed.; pp. 305-310). Sudbury, MA: Jones & Bartlett.

Kaiser/HRET. (2007). *Employer health benefits 2007 annual survey*. Menlo Park, CA: Kaiser Family Foundation/Health Research and Education Trust.

Kitchener, M., Ng, T., Miller, N., et al. (2005). Medicaid home and community-based services: National program trends. *Health Affairs, 24*(1), 206-212.

Krisberg, K. (2007, March). Universal health care surging in popularity with policy- makers: States taking the lead. *The Nation's Health*. Retrieved April 1, 2008 from *http://www.apha.org/publications/tnh/archives/2007/March2007/Nation/universalhealthcare.htm*.

Lee, C. (2007a, July 1). Massachusetts begins universal health care. *Washington Post*, p. A6.

Lee, C. (2007b, June 16). Insurers to halt Medicare plan sales. *Washington Post*, p. A7.

Lee, C., & Levine, S. (2006, September 25). Millions of seniors facing Medicare "doughnut hole." *Washington Post*, p. A3.

Levit, K., Smith, C., Cowan, C., et al. (2003). Trends in U.S. health care spending, 2001. *Health Affairs, 22*(1), 154-164.

Lewit, E. M., Terman, D. L., & Behrman, R. E. (1997). Children and poverty: Analysis and recommendations. *Future of Children, 7*(2), 4-21.

Long, S. K., Coughlin, T., & King, J. (2008). How well does Medicaid work in improving access to care? In C. Harrington & C. L. Estes (Eds.), *Health policy: Crisis and reform in the U.S. health care delivery system* (5th ed.; pp. 300-304). Sudbury, MA: Jones & Bartlett.

Maxwell, S., Moon, M., & Segal, M. (2001). *Growth in Medicare and out-of-pocket spending: Impact on vulnerable beneficiaries*. New York: Commonwealth Fund.

McKinsey and Company. (2007). *Accounting for the cost of health care in the United States*. San Francisco, CA: McKinsey Global Institute.

Mechanic, D. (2008). The rise and fall of managed care. In C. Harrington & C. L. Estes (Eds.), *Health policy: Crisis and reform in the U.S. health care delivery system* (5th ed.; pp. 345-352). Sudbury, MA: Jones & Bartlett.

Medicare and you. (2008). Washington, DC: U.S. Department of Health and Human Services, Centers for Medicare and Medicaid Services.

Merlis, M. (2003). *Private long-term care insurance: Who should buy it and what should they buy?* Menlo Park, CA: Kaiser Family Foundation/ Health Research and Education Trust.

MetLife. (April 2002). *Market survey of nursing homes and home care costs*. Boston: MetLife, John Hancock Life Insurance Company.

National Association of State Budget Officers. (2006, Fall). *2005 State expenditure report*. Washington DC: Author.

Nelson, R. (2006). AJN Reports: Pay for performance. *American Journal of Nursing, 106*(12), 25-26.

O'Brien, E. (2008). Medicare and Medicaid: Trends and issues affecting access to care for low-income elders and people with disabilities. In C. Harrington & C. L. Estes (Eds.), *Health policy: Crisis and reform in the U.S. health care delivery system* (5th ed.; pp. 316-320). Sudbury, MA: Jones & Bartlett.

Patel, K., & Rushefsky, M. E. (1999). *Health care politics and policy in America* (2nd ed.). Armonk, NY: M. E. Sharpe.

Patel, K., & Rushefsky, M. E. (2006). *Health care politics and policy in America* (3rd ed.). Armonk, NY: M. E. Sharpe.

Park, E., Nathanson, M., Greenstein, R., et al. (2003). *The troubling Medicare legislation*. Washington DC: Center on Budget and Policy Priorities.

Pepper Commission. (1990). *A call for action: Final report of the Pepper Commission*. Washington, DC: U.S. Government Printing Office.

Pizer, S. D., & Frakt, A. B. (2002). Payment policy and competition in the Medicare+ Choice program. *Health Care Financing Review, 24*(1), 83-94.

Poisal, J. A., Truffer, C., Smith, S., et al. (2007). Health spending projections through 2016: Modest changes obscure Part

D's impact. *Health Affairs*, Supplement Web Exclusives, *26*, W242-253.

Pulcini, J. A., & Hart, M. A. (2007a). Financing health care in the United States. In D. J. Mason, J. K. Leavitt, & M. W. Chaffee (Eds.), *Policy and politics in nursing and health care* (5th ed.; pp. 384-408). St. Louis: Saunders.

Pulcini, J. A., & Hart, M. A. (2007b). Politics of advanced practice nursing. In D. J. Mason, J. K. Leavitt, & M. W. Chaffee (Eds.), *Policy and politics in nursing and health care* (5th ed.; pp. 568-573). St. Louis: Saunders.

Rice, T. H., & Komenski, G. F. (2001). Containing health care costs. In R. M. Andersen, T. H. Rice, & G. F. Komenski (Eds.), *Changing the U.S. health care system* (pp. 82-99). San Francisco: Jossey-Bass.

Roberts, M., & Rhoades, J. A. (2007). *The uninsured in America, first half of 2006: Estimates for the U.S. civilian noninstitutionalized population under age 65* (Statistical Brief No. 171). Rockville, MD: Agency for Healthcare Research and Quality.

Roemer, R. (2001). The continuing issues in public health and health services. In R. M. Andersen, T. H. Rice, & G. F. Komenski (Eds.), *Changing the U.S. health care system* (pp. 470-502). San Francisco: Jossey-Bass.

Rowland, D. (2008). Medicaid at forty. In C. Harrington & C. L. Estes (Eds.), *Health policy: Crisis and reform in the U.S. health care delivery system* (5th ed.; pp. 290-299). Sudbury, MA: Jones & Bartlett.

Safran, D. G., Newman, P., Schoen, C., et al. (2002, July 31). Prescription drug coverage and seniors: How well are states closing the gap? *Health Affairs*, web exclusive, W253–268.

Salganik, M. W. (2006, November 12). Drug-plan hassle redux. *Baltimore Sun*, p. C1–2.

Sambamoorthi, U., Shea, D., & Crystal, S. (2003). Total out of pocket expenditures for prescription drugs among older persons. *Gerontologist*, *43*(3), 345-359.

Sardell, A. (2007). Taking action: Community health centers: A successful strategy for improving health care access. In D. J. Mason, J. K. Leavitt, & M. W. Chaffee (Eds.), *Policy and politics in nursing and health care* (5th ed.; pp. 287-295). St. Louis: Saunders.

Selden, T. M., & Banthin, J. S. (2003). Health care expenditure burden among elderly adults; 1987 and 1996. *Medical Care, 41*(7 Suppl), III13–III23.

Shi, L., & Singh, D. A. (2001). *Healthcare in America*. Gaithersburg, MD: Aspen.

Sochalski, J. (2002). Nursing shortage redux: Turning the corner on an enduring problem. *Health Affairs, 21*(5), 151-181.

Sommers, A., Zuckerman, S., Dubay, L., et al. (2007). Substitution of SCHIP for private coverage: Results from a 2002 evaluation in ten states. *Health Affairs, 26*(2), 529-537.

Sorkin, A. L. (1986). *Health care and the changing economic environment*. Lexington, MA: Lexington Books.

Straight. S. (2007, June 10). Of sickness and of wealth: Health savings accounts make sense if you're physically and fiscally fit. *Washington Post*, pp. F1, F4.

Sultz, H. A., & Young, K. M. (2004). *Health care USA: Understanding its organization and delivery* (3rd ed.). Gaithersburg, MD: Aspen.

Thorpe, K. E. (2004, January-June). The medical malpractice "crisis": Recent trends and the impact of state tort reforms. *Health Affairs*, Web Exclusive W-4, 20-30.

Torrens, P. R. (2002). Historical evaluation and overview of health services in the U.S. In S. J. Williams & P. R. Torrens (Eds.), *Introduction to health care services* (6th ed.; pp. 2-17). West Albany, NY: Delmar.

Trossman, S. (1998). Quality managed care: A nursing perspective. *American Journal of Nursing*, *98*(6), 1-3.

Trossman, S. (2003). Health care for all: Nurses rally behind a campaign highlighting the uninsured. *American Journal of Nursing, 103*(7), 77-79.

U.S. Bureau of the Census. (2002a). *Poverty in the United States: 2001* (Current Populations Reports, P60-219). Washington DC: U.S. Department of Commerce, Economics and Statistics Administration.

U.S. Bureau of the Census. (2002b). *Statistical abstract of the United States: 2002*. Washington, DC: U.S. Government Printing Office.

U.S. Bureau of the Census. (2006). *Income, poverty, and health insurance in the United States: 2005* (Current Populations Reports, P60-231). Washington DC: U.S. Department of Commerce, Economics and Statistics Administration.

U.S. Bureau of the Census. (2007a). *Statistical abstract of the United States: The national data book* (126th ed.). Resident population by age and sex: 1980 to 2005 (p. 12, Table 11). Washington, DC: U.S. Government Printing Office.

U.S. Bureau of the Census. (2007b). *Statistical abstract of the United States: The national data book* (126th ed.). Employed civilians by occupation—States: 2004 (Table 603). Washington, DC: U.S. Government Printing Office.

Williamson, E., & Lee, C. (2007, May 16). Abuses in enrollment tactics found for private Medicare. *Washington Post*, p. A3.

World Bank. (2007). *World development indicators on line. Government expenditures: Public education expenditure as a percent of GDP*. Washington DC: World Bank.

Wynia, M. K., Van Geest, J. B., Cummins, D. S., et al. (2003). Do physicians not offer useful services because of coverage restrictions? *Health Affairs, 22*(4), 190-197.

Zaneski, D. (2004, March 24). Medicine may be insolvent by year 2019. *Baltimore Sun*, pp. 1A, 6A.

Zarabozo, C. (2002). Issues in managed care. *Health Care Financing Review, 24*(1), 1-10.

SUGGESTED READINGS

American Nurses Association. (2007). *Access to health coverage. Position statement*. Retrieved May 16, 2008 from *http://www.nursingworld. org/MainMenu/Categories/ANAPoliticalPower/ Federal/LEGIS/HealthCoverage.aspx*.

Are you really covered: Why four in ten Americans can't depend on their health insurance (2007, September). *Consumer Reports, 72*(9), 16-20.

Feldstein, P. J. (2005). *Health care economics* (6th ed.). West Albany, NY: Delmar.

Fuchs, V. R. (1996). Economic values of health care reform. *American Economic Review, 86*, 1-24.

Ginzberg, E. (1990). *The medical triangle: Physicians, politicians, and the public*. Cambridge, MA: Harvard University Press.

Harrington, C., & Estes C. L. (Eds.). (2008). *Health policy: Crisis and reform in the U.S. health care delivery system* (5th ed.). Sudbury, MA: Jones & Bartlett.

Mason, D. J., Leavitt, J. K., & Chaffee, M. W. (2007). *Policy and politics in nursing and health care* (5th ed.). St. Louis: Saunders.

Orszag, P. R. (2007). *Health care and the budget: Issues and challenges for reform. Testimony before the Committee on the Budget, United States Congress*. Washington DC: Congressional Budget Office.

Six prescriptions for change, (2008, March). *Consumers Reports, 73*(3), 14-17.

Sultz, H. A., & Young, K. M. (2004). *Health care USA: Understanding its organization and delivery* (3rd ed.). Gaithersburg, MD: Aspen.

5 International Health

Helen R. Kohler and Frances A. Maurer

FOCUS QUESTIONS

What is the concept of global health?

Why are health disparities an important global concern?

How do intergovernmental and nongovernmental organizations work to address health issues in the world?

Which countries have higher rates of deaths from malnutrition and infectious diseases?

Which countries are more concerned with chronic health conditions?

What features distinguish health care delivery systems?

Which criteria are used to compare the effectiveness of health care delivery systems?

What types of concerns are common to all forms of health care delivery systems?

How can nurses participate in the global health effort?

CHAPTER OUTLINE

Health: A Global Issue
Health Disparities among Countries
International Health Organizations
  Intergovernmental Organizations
  Voluntary Organizations
Health and Disease Worldwide
  Major Global Health Problems
  Problems Common to Developing Countries

Problems Common to Developed Countries
Health Care Delivery Systems
  Health Care Systems in Developed Countries
  Health Care Systems in Developing Countries
  Issues in Health Care Delivery Systems
New and Emerging Health Issues
  Old and New Emerging Infectious Diseases
  Environment

Tobacco Use
Terrorism and War
Mental Illness
Role of Nursing in International Health

KEY TERMS

Alma-Ata conference
Beveridge model
Bismarck model
Centers for Disease Control and Prevention (CDC)
Emerging infectious diseases
Epidemiologic transition

Global Health Council (GHC)
Globalization of health
Health disparities
Health for All
Intergovernmental organizations
Millennium Development Goals
Pan American Health Organization (PAHO)

United Nations Children's Fund (UNICEF)
U.S. Agency for International Development (USAID)
Voluntary organizations
World Bank
World Health Organization (WHO)

HEALTH: A GLOBAL ISSUE

It is a small world. There are more than 6.5 billion people living on this planet (Population Reference Bureau, 2006). At the end of the twentieth century, worldwide travel has become commonplace and rapid. In most instances, air travel has reduced transit time between countries to less than a day. People travel for business, for pleasure, and to start life anew in another country.

Because more people travel, because travel is more rapid, and because the boundaries between nations are more fluid, we need to think of health, illness, and disease from a global

perspective. Highly infectious diseases can circle the world rapidly, as the recent severe acute respiratory syndrome (SARS) epidemic illustrates (see Chapters 7 and 8). It is almost impossible to isolate a contagious disease within the country of origin. Other countries risk exposure. No nation can afford to become complacent. For example, the continued spread of human immunodeficiency virus (HIV) infection/acquired immunodeficiency syndrome (AIDS) worldwide was partially the result of complacency. Some countries were slow to recognize the threat of HIV/AIDS, others denied that the threat existed, and still others thought geographic distance from the initial epidemic protected them from the threat.

Countries with highly sophisticated medical systems are not immune to external health risks. They cannot isolate themselves from exposure risks. Developed countries are more equipped to provide highly specialized care than are poor countries. They have more sophisticated resources to treat diseases and possess more stringent surveillance and protection measures to reduce the risk of disease. However, developed countries cannot guarantee their citizens a country free from external disease sources. More than 2 million people cross national boundaries daily. It takes only a single traveler with an undetected illness to expose many people, and sometimes many countries, outside his or her native land.

HEALTH DISPARITIES AMONG COUNTRIES

The health status of populations is greatly influenced by income level and therefore varies widely among countries, as shown by the health status indicators in Table 5-1. Developed countries are richer and more economically stable. These countries can provide, in addition to other things, a better standard of health and health care for their people. Developed countries include Australia, Great Britain, Germany, and the United States, among others. Underdeveloped or developing countries are poorer, often economically unstable, and have less ability to provide health care for their people. Social disruptions and wars also affect health in negative ways. Some examples of

developing countries include Ethiopia, Honduras, Viet Nam, and Nigeria. In Nigeria, 71% of the population was living on less than $1.00 a day in 2003 (World Health Organization [WHO], 2007a). Somewhere in between are middle-income countries. These are countries that are progressing along the development spectrum but have not achieved the same standard of living as developed countries. Brazil, China, Mexico, and Turkey are examples of middle-income countries. These countries tend to provide a standard of health care that is better than that of poor countries but poorer than that of developed countries.

The health of the population in developing countries is dramatically impacted by poverty. Poorer countries have higher rates of death, disease, and disability. Children in developing countries suffer from malnutrition and premature death. Infectious diseases such as malaria, meningitis, tuberculosis, and guinea worm infestation, almost nonexistent in developed countries, are rampant in poorer nations. Life expectancy is shorter. For example, the life expectancy in Japan is 82 years; in the United States, 78 years; in China, 72 years; in Zimbabwe (experiencing social unrest and high HIV/AIDS prevalence), 42 years; and in Sierra Leone, after many years of war, just 38 years (WHO, 2007a).

Health disparities, the unequal levels of health among nations, are an ongoing concern of health professionals and world leaders. At the **Alma-Ata conference,** a Joint World Health Organization (WHO)/United Nations Children's Fund (UNICEF) International Conference on Primary Health Care held in 1978 in Alma-Ata, USSR (now Almaty, Kazakhstan)

TABLE 5-1 International Comparison of Health Indicators for Selected Countries: 2005

Country	Indicators		
	Life Expectancy at Birth	Infant Mortality Rate per 1000 Live Births	Gross National Income per Capita (in Dollars)
Low-Income Economies			
Haiti	54	83	1840
Kenya	51	78	1170
Nepal	61	56	1530
Nigeria	47	101	1040
Pakistan	61	80	2350
Sierra Leone	38	165	780
Middle-Income Economies			
Brazil	71	28	8230
China	72	23	6600
Costa Rica	78	11	9680
Indonesia	68	28	3720
Jamaica	72	17	4110
Mexico	75	22	10,030
Thailand	70	18	8440
High-Income Economies			
Australia	81	5	30,610
France	80	4	30,540
Germany	79	4	29,210
Japan	82	3	31,410
Norway	79	3	40,950
United States	78	7	41,950

Data from World Health Organization (WHO). (2007). *World health statistics 2007*. Geneva: Author.

and attended by representatives of 143 nations, the WHO renewed its goal of **Health for All** everywhere. This was a commitment to the social justice of eliminating health disparities (WHO, 1998a, 2000). As defined at the Alma-Ata conference, primary health care should encompass the following (WHO, 1978):

- Education about health problems and the means to prevent or control them (country specific)
- Improved food supply and adequate nutrition for the population
- Safe water and sanitation
- Maternal and child health care
- Immunization against infectious diseases
- Prevention and control of endemic diseases
- Adequate treatment of common diseases and injuries
- Adequate and appropriate drug supplies

The Declaration of Alma-Ata serves as a blueprint by which countries can plan improvements to health services and health status for their citizens (much as the *Healthy People 2010* goals serve as a roadmap for improving the health of the United States population). The World Health Assembly expects these efforts to be a partnership among the country's leaders, health infrastructure (organizations), communities, individual citizens, and, to some degree, other countries.

About 20 years after the Alma-Ata conference (in September of 2000) at the United Nations (UN) Millennium Summit in New York City, the largest gathering of world leaders in history (from 189 nations) adopted the UN Millennium Declaration. The global representatives present committed themselves to giving a very high priority to elimination of worldwide poverty by 2015 (WHO, 2004). The eight specific **Millennium Development Goals** are the following (Uys, 2006; WHO, 2003a):

1. Eradicate extreme poverty and hunger
2. Achieve universal primary education
3. Promote gender equality and empower women
4. Reduce child mortality
5. Improve maternal health
6. Combat HIV/AIDS, malaria, and other diseases
7. Ensure environmental sustainability
8. Develop a global partnership for development

The governments of the 22 wealthiest donor nations in the world agreed to commit 0.7% of their gross domestic product by the year 2015 toward accomplishment of the Millennium Development Goals. Figure 5-1 shows the extent to which these nations have met their commitments 5 years after the summit meeting (Concern Worldwide, 2005; UN Millennium Project, 2006).

More recently, the Pan American Health Organization and its collaborators in the Disease Control Priorities Project published the "Top 10 Best Buys" of health interventions for developing countries (Eberwine-Villagran, 2007). "Best buys" are interventions for which the money, time, and effort invested have a substantial effect on health. Some are relatively simple, whereas others require serious national or international commitment. The 10 interventions are listed in Box 5-1.

It must be remembered that the Alma-Ata Declaration of Health for All, the UN Millennium Development Goals for reducing global poverty, and the recently designated Top 10 Health Interventions of the Disease Control Priorities Project require political will and commitment, plus *predictable and sustained funding,* to be more than empty slogans.

This **globalization of health** recognizes that barriers between countries are blurring, that health issues cannot be isolated within one country, that large health disparities among countries are ultimately harmful to everyone, and that health for the world's population should be the goal of every country. The WHO has made the elimination of health disparities its primary goal (Wagstaff, 2002). Although some progress has been made, much remains to be done. Even though the global strategy of Health for All was endorsed by 143 countries at Alma-Ata in 1978, it remains a statement of aspiration, not a reality (Novelli, 2005). With respect to meeting the Millennium goals, little progress has been made during the first 6 years of the project. Former UN secretary-general Kofi Annan has observed that there is still time for achievement, but only "if we break with business as usual" and exert the sustained action required (Uys, 2006).

INTERNATIONAL HEALTH ORGANIZATIONS

Attempts to improve the level of health worldwide are a multiorganizational effort. Both intergovernmental and voluntary agencies focus on global health problems.

INTERGOVERNMENTAL ORGANIZATIONS
Intergovernmental organizations are agencies in which official representatives of various countries' governments work together to improve health status. The agency can involve many countries (multilateral agencies) or just two countries (bilateral agencies). The most well-known is the WHO.

World Health Organization
The **World Health Organization (WHO)** is a multilateral agency involving approximately 193 countries. It was founded to be "the world's health advocate" more than 50 years ago (WHO, 1998a). Although it is associated with the UN, it has its own budget and decision-making processes. Policy decisions and direction are decided by delegates of the member nations at their annual World Health Assembly held in Geneva, Switzerland. The WHO is funded by dues and voluntary contributions from member countries. For 2006 to 2007, the projected budget was $3.3 billion dollars (WHO, 2005a).

The WHO provides both technical support and health care services to member nations, with an emphasis on poorer countries. It directs and coordinates international health projects, collaborates with other organizations and agencies in health care programs, and monitors and reports on worldwide disease conditions, much like the Centers for Disease Control and Prevention does for the United States.

The WHO is leading the effort to establish international standards for medications and vaccines. One standard will ensure that the quality and dosage of medications are safe and at therapeutic levels. It also operates thousands of individual country projects, usually in conjunction with the country's health ministry, the governmental body responsible for health care. Countries receive help with health planning—for example, distribution or establishment of health care services. The WHO helps run immunization programs, build health care infrastructure, and improve sanitation levels.

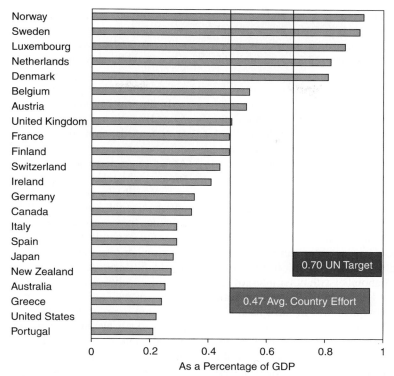

FIGURE 5-1 Government Aid to Official Development Assistance as a percentage of gross domestic product (GDP), 2005. (Data from United Nations Millennium Project. [2006]. *The 0.7% target: Net ODA [official development assistance] in 2005—as a percentage of GNI [gross national income].* Retrieved August 11, 2007 from *http://www.unmillenniumproject.org/press/action7_oecd05.htm*.)

Box 5-1 **Top Ten Best Buys of Health Interventions**

1. Vaccinate children against major childhood killers, including measles, polio, tetanus, whooping cough, and diphtheria
2. Monitor children's health (using the Integrated Management of Childhood Illness strategy) to prevent and treat childhood diseases such as pneumonia, diarrhea, and malaria
3. Levy taxes on tobacco products to increase their cost by at least one third in order to discourage smoking and reduce smoking-related diseases
4. Mount a coordinated attack on the human immunodeficiency virus (HIV) epidemic that includes promoting 100% condom use in at-risk populations; treating other sexually transmitted infections; providing antiretroviral treatment, especially for pregnant women; and offering voluntary HIV testing and counseling
5. Provide children and pregnant women with essential nutrients, including vitamin A, iron, and iodine, to prevent maternal anemia, infant deaths, and long-term health problems
6. Provide insecticide-treated bed nets in malaria-endemic areas to reduce malaria rates
7. Enforce traffic regulations and install speed bumps at dangerous intersections to reduce traffic-related injuries
8. Treat tuberculosis patients with directly observed short-course therapy to cure infected people and prevent new infections
9. Teach mothers and birth attendants to keep newborn babies warm and clean to reduce illness and death
10. Promote the use of aspirin and other inexpensive drugs to treat and prevent heart attack and stroke.

From Eberwine-Villagran, D. (2007). Best buys for public health. *Perspectives in Health*, *11*(1), 2-9.

Pan American Health Organization

The **Pan American Health Organization (PAHO)** was established in 1902 as an independent public health organization called the Pan American Sanitary Bureau. It now functions as a quasi-independent branch of the WHO. Part of PAHO's budget comes from the WHO and from other UN agencies. PAHO serves as a regional office of WHO, limited to the Americas, or Western Hemisphere. There are 25 member countries.

The primary mission of PAHO is to strengthen international and local health systems to improve the health of the population of the Americas (PAHO, 2003a). It provides expertise on disease and environmental management, supports research and scholarship efforts, and monitors diseases. The organization has a major emphasis in Latin America, an area of great need. PAHO has worked hard to provide childhood immunization and other methods of care to reduce infant mortality. For example, 19 countries participated in the Vaccine Week in the Americas campaign in 2003. In Argentina, 300,000 children between the ages of 1 and 6 years were vaccinated in June 2003 (PAHO, 2003b).

United Nations Children's Fund

The **United Nations Children's Fund (UNICEF)** (formerly the United Nations International Children's Emergency Fund) concentrates its efforts in the area of maternal and child health. It is currently working in 191 countries (UNICEF, 2007). It is an agency of the UN, from which it receives funding. In the past, UNICEF has concentrated on the control of specific communicable diseases. Although still maintaining that focus, it has expanded into the area of primary prevention. More recent efforts are geared toward ensuring fresh water and safe food supplies and providing health education for mothers of children, education for girls, and immunization programs aimed at reducing or eliminating vaccine-susceptible communicable diseases.

World Bank

The main goal of the **World Bank** is to improve the economic welfare of developing countries. To that end, the World Bank funds projects aimed at reducing poverty and eliminating threats to health. The main health-related efforts center around providing a safe environment for people—for example, safe water supply, adequate housing, proper agricultural techniques, and improved sanitation. These strategies are the classic methods for controlling the environment to reduce contamination with human and animal feces, and to eliminate pests and disease vectors to lower the risk of preventable diseases.

The World Bank funds government projects to improve a country's infrastructure. It collaborates with other intergovernmental agencies, such as the WHO, on health-related projects. It also works with voluntary organizations. In most instances, the World Bank funding mechanism offers loans to agencies and governments, rather than grants. Developing countries, which are economically unstable, sometimes have trouble repaying the loans. The World Bank provides expert consultation and advice to such governments to help stabilize their economies. Since the 1960s, loans to poorer nations have been provided at lower interest rates, and repayment is made over several decades (Basch, 1999). Loans are sometimes forgiven or eliminated for countries in severe economic crisis.

Agency for International Development

The **U.S. Agency for International Development (USAID)** is an arm of the U.S. State Department. USAID provides expertise and funding to countries that need economic development. USAID is an example of a bilateral agency in which one donor, in this case the United States, works with one recipient country. Other governments provide similar services to developing countries. Most of the USAID activities that are publicized are related to agricultural and infrastructure development. In the course of these activities, sanitation and water supplies, essential elements in increasing the level of health in populations, are also improved. In 2007, USAID was also assisting 55 countries with activities to address avian influenza, mostly by providing grants and technical assistance (USAID, 2007a).

Centers for Disease Control and Prevention

The **Centers for Disease Control and Prevention (CDC)** provides expertise in controlling and preventing disease. It directs ongoing health-related programs through the International Health Program Office. The agency is also available for consultation during emergencies, such as the 2003 SARS outbreak. In instances of disease outbreaks, experts in the field are dispatched to the country in need, consult with the country's health professionals, and provide equipment and health resources as needed to develop a comprehensive plan for disease control or elimination.

VOLUNTARY ORGANIZATIONS

A wide variety of nongovernmental **voluntary organizations** assist in the effort to improve worldwide health. These voluntary organizations are frequently referred to as nongovernmental organizations. Nongovernmental organizations are not affiliated with a particular government, although some might work in conjunction with a government agency on a specific project. Most developed countries have nongovernmental organizations that operate in health-related activities in developing countries.

In the United States, some religious groups operate health-related assistance programs for underdeveloped countries. Protestant denominations and the Catholic Church operate missions that serve selected countries (e.g., countries in Africa, Asia, and South America). The Church Rural Overseas Project, which began as an organization sending food relief to post–World War II (WWII) Europe, now provides worldwide emergency aid, long-term self-help projects, and assistance to refugees from war-torn or famine-plagued countries.

Some examples of religiously affiliated health aid organizations are Lutheran World Relief, Seventh Day Adventist World Service, American Friends Service Committee, and Catholic Relief Services. These groups operate hospitals and clinics, as well as schools. Some groups provide health-related education in an effort to increase the number of native health professionals available to communities. Church organizations provide both permanent and temporary staff for these endeavors. Catholic nuns and priests, Protestant pastors, and other religiously affiliated personnel spend years or even their whole careers in mission work. Some health professionals volunteer a year of service or do periodic work—for example, 1 month per year for special projects. Some examples of these activities are the following:

- Surgical visits for the repair of cleft lip and palates
- Immunization projects, such as measles vaccination
- Water supply projects, such as digging wells for a village or community
- Home and other construction projects, such as building a clinic facility in a community with no previous structure, or constructing or repairing a school building.

> Tanya Jensen, an operating room nurse at Cleveland General Hospital, is an active member of her church. One Sunday, Pastor Rifkin, a missionary working in Peru, spoke to the assembly about his church work. Tanya approached the pastor to ask him more about the medical problems he encountered. Pastor Rifkin mentioned that he and other missionaries had located 30 children in need of cleft lip and palate corrections. Tanya volunteered to be a member of the surgical team that the pastor was trying to organize. Four months later, Pastor Rifkin called Tanya to say he had been successful in locating a surgeon volunteer, and a mobile hospital surgery unit was temporarily donated by another church group. Tanya agreed to help. Two months later, Tanya spent 2 weeks in Peru. She and the rest of the surgical team operated and provided postoperative care for 52 children. The list of candidates grew as word about the project spread. Tanya found her time in Peru so rewarding that she has volunteered to do another trip next year.

Global Health Council

The **Global Health Council (GHC)** is one of the leading voluntary organizations focusing on global health and development. It lobbies for assistance for developing countries and educates Americans about the need for international health relief services. It serves and represents thousands of public health professionals from more than 103 countries on six continents (GHC, 2007a).

Other Service Agencies

Many organizations are involved in health service to developing countries. Some of these are foundations, privately funded philanthropic organizations, or other types of service agencies. A selection of these organizations is listed in Box 5-2. There are many more voluntary organizations engaged in improving the status of health worldwide.

HEALTH AND DISEASE WORLDWIDE

As previously noted, there is wide disparity in health status among nations. As a general rule, health status is inversely related to wealth. The poorer the country, the more likely its citizens are to experience preventable diseases and early death. In developing countries, the primary cause of death is an infectious disease. Communicable diseases are responsible for more than 40% of deaths in poor countries, but fewer than 1% of deaths in rich countries (Baum, 2002). This change in illness pattern is commonly referred to as the **epidemiologic transition.** As a country improves along the spectrum of development, life expectancy at birth increases, and the nature of illnesses changes. Illnesses related to pestilence, famine, and pandemics recede, and illnesses associated with degeneration (aging) and human-caused diseases increase.

Many infectious diseases are easily controlled or prevented by sanitation efforts and immunization programs. These types of preventive measures have been in wide use in developed countries for over a century. For this reason, people in developed countries have a better level of health, live longer, and eventually suffer and die from chronic illness. The most frequent diseases in developed countries are heart disease, cancer, and respiratory diseases (Baum, 2002).

In the twentieth century, the general trend was toward increasing life expectancy. That trend was diminished by the HIV/AIDS pandemic. The pandemic affected some countries, for example, India and parts of the African continent, more than it did others. In general, HIV/AIDS has produced more devastation in poor countries with few economic resources and inferior health care infrastructures to fight the disease. Table 5-1 illustrates the relationship between health and economic status. Countries with relatively low standards of living have high infant mortality rates and a shorter life span; for example, Sierra Leone has an infant mortality rate of 165 per 1000 live births and a life expectancy of 38 years. As a country's economic prospects improve, infant mortality rates fall, and life expectancy increases. For example, Japan has an infant mortality rate of 3 per 1000 live births and a life expectancy of 82 years.

MAJOR GLOBAL HEALTH PROBLEMS

Worldwide health problems can be divided into two categories. First are the easily preventable conditions and treatable infectious diseases. These are the types of problems common to developing countries. For the most part, these conditions are easy to fix with personnel, improvements in sanitation, and adequate funding. Other problems are more long term. Chronic conditions are more frequent in developed countries, where the easily preventable and treatable conditions have, for the most part, been eliminated or controlled. Chronic conditions, which usually affect people as they age, are more complicated to treat and require more economic resources.

Box 5-2 Sample Service Organizations

The Carter Center: Established by President Jimmy Carter and affiliated with Emory University, the Carter Center is committed to promoting human rights and improving health. Health-related projects concentrate on elimination of specific diseases that affect large numbers of people and include projects to eliminate guinea worm disease (started in 1987), lymphatic filariasis, river blindness, and schistosomiasis. It is also working to improve food production.

Doctors without Borders (Médecins sans Frontières): Founded in France in 1971, this organization provides medical care to people in more than 80 countries. It provides both health personnel and supplies to people caught in wars, refugees and displaced persons, and victims of natural disasters. It also provides long-term assistance in countries with little or no health care delivery systems, such as Sudan, Guinea, and Ethiopia. The staff is composed primarily of volunteers: doctors, nurses, and other medical professionals.

The Ford Foundation: This group provides assistance with food production and population and family planning in countries in Asia, Africa, and South America.

The Bill and Melinda Gates Foundation: Founded with an endowment of $25 billion by Bill and Melinda Gates, this organization's goal is to reduce the disease burden in developing countries. Samples of ongoing projects include prevention and treatment of human immunodeficiency virus infection, vaccine improvement, research on new vaccines, and the improvement of prenatal and infant health care.

Rotary International: Established in 1905 in Chicago, Rotary International is now a worldwide organization of business and professional leaders with 1.2 million members working in 32,000 clubs in 200 countries. It provides humanitarian services of many kinds in many countries. As its major public health project, Rotary International has committed itself to eradication of polio by helping to immunize over 2 billion children since the World Health Organization launched the Global Polio Eradication Initiative in 1988.

W. K. Kellogg Foundation: This organization develops and expands educational programs in health and agriculture. It funds the education of doctors, dentists, nurses, and technicians.

The Shriners: The Shriners are an international fraternity with members in the United States, Mexico, Canada, and Panama. They fund 25 hospitals for children that treat orthopedic conditions and burns free of charge. They also fund research in the same clinical areas, providing $24 million for research in 2002. They serve children in the United States, Canada, Mexico, and other countries.

Data retrieved October 18, 2003 from *http://www.cartercenter.org/aboutus, http://www.doctorswithoutborders.org/news,* and *http://www.gatesfoundation.org/about;* October 30, 2003, from *http://www.shriners.org/shrine/welcome.htm;* and Rotary International. (2007). *Rotary's health projects* (Fact Sheet 01/07-EN). Evanston, IL: Author.

PROBLEMS COMMON TO DEVELOPING COUNTRIES

Unsafe water is the largest contributor to illness and death in developing countries. Eighty percent of disease and death is related to the water supply (WHO, 2001a). Worldwide, more than 3 million people die each year from water-related diseases, such as diarrhea. The source of drinking water is the largest contributing factor to childhood stunting (WHO, 2007a). This section highlights some of the major health problems in poor and developing countries. These include easily treatable conditions, vector-borne diseases, and infectious diseases. The causes of death of children younger than 5 years of age shown in Figure 5-2 are found mainly in developing countries (WHO, 2005b).

Malnutrition

Malnutrition is the best global indicator of child health. Although malnutrition is a major problem for both children and adults in the developing world, children younger than age 5 are most adversely affected. In 2005, there were approximately 178 million malnourished children worldwide (WHO, 2007a). UNICEF reported that 15 million people in Africa (including 2.7 million children under the age of 5) were at risk of starvation in 2006 (UNICEF, 2006). More than half of the child deaths worldwide occur in underweight children younger than 5 years of age (WHO, 1998b, 2005b).

The best measure of malnutrition in children is growth stunting. In 2005, 32% of the children under age 5 in developing countries worldwide were stunted (short in stature for their age). The highest percentage was in Africa, where 22 of the 39 countries with the highest prevalence (40% or more) were located. Africa is the only place where child undernutrition is rising, but undernutrition continues to be most pervasive in Southeast Asia (GHC, 2007b; WHO, 2007a). Political unrest, intermittent warfare, and an increasing population contribute to the problem. Latin America, particularly South America, has the lowest rate of stunting in the developing world.

Malnutrition is a high-priority concern because it drastically affects the quality of life for millions of people. Children who are malnourished suffer growth retardation and many health and developmental problems, including the following:

- Multiple diarrheal episodes
- Increased risk of infectious diseases, such as malaria, meningitis, and pneumonia
- Premature death
- Delayed mental development and poor school performance

Poor growth in early childhood is associated with significant functional impairment in adult life. It affects a person's ability to work and impacts both the family's and country's economic prosperity (deOnis et al., 2000).

Substantial worldwide effort has led to a number of interventions, which have been somewhat successful in reducing malnutrition and starvation. Immediate food delivery to war-ravaged and famine-impacted countries provides only short-term help. Long-term activities, which are the major focus of worldwide efforts, include helping countries and their peoples with the following:

- Improvement of seed and farming techniques to produce better pest resistance and higher crop yield
- Food fortification projects to provide high-calorie foods with adequate vitamins and minerals (big bang for small food supply)
- Food supplements for the most vulnerable in the population (i.e., infants, young children, and nursing mothers)
- Education related to nutritional guidance, and family planning to space childbirth
- The usual sanitation efforts aimed at providing clean water, clean wells, and control of human and animal waste

Diarrheal Diseases

Perhaps the most heartbreaking problem is diarrhea, because it is easily controllable. Diarrhea continues to be the second leading cause of death from infectious diseases for children

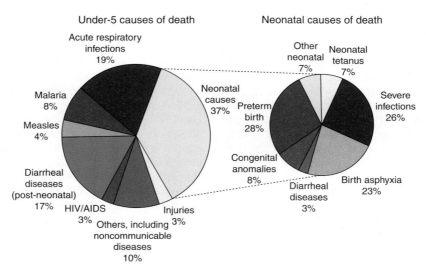

FIGURE 5-2 Causes of death of children under 5 years of age, 2000 to 2003. Totals are more than 100% due to rounding. (From World Health Organization. [2005]. *The world health report 2005: Make every mother and child count.* Geneva: Author.)

under age 5 (WHO, 2005b). Diarrhea has many causes, most associated with poor sanitation and contaminated water supplies. Cholera is one example of an illness that causes severe diarrhea. Diarrheal disease is exacerbated by poverty, lack of knowledge about the importance of personal hygiene and community sanitation, and lack of medical supplies and personnel. Reductions in mortality are the result of simple measures, including the following:

- Oral rehydration therapy to replace fluids and electrolytes (WHO/UNICEF oral rehydration salts)
- Encouragement of women to breast-feed whenever possible
- Improvements in sanitation and water supplies
- Immunizations for vaccine-preventable illnesses that produce diarrhea (e.g., measles and cholera).

The WHO has actively discouraged bottle-feeding because mothers in poor countries incorrectly used prepared formula. Canned formula was expensive, so mothers diluted the formula with water; as a result, infants were not receiving adequate nutrition. The HIV/AIDS epidemic has complicated WHO's policy against bottle-feeding. HIV-infected mothers are advised not to breast-feed their children if they have the resources and ability to properly use formula feeding. If not, exclusive breast-feeding is recommended by WHO/UNICEF/Joint United Nations Program on HIV/AIDS during only the first few months of life, followed by transition to replacement foods as soon as possible (African Network for the Care of Children Affected by AIDS, 2006; GHC, 2007b).

Human Immunodeficiency Virus/Acquired Immunodeficiency Syndrome

AIDS was first reported in 1981. By 1987, it had spread to 100 countries (Basch, 1999). By 2001, it was the leading infectious cause of death in the world, killing almost 3 million people, and by 2002 approximately 5 million people were infected with HIV, including 2 million women and 800,000 children younger than 15 years of age (WHO, 2002a; USAID, 2002). In 2006, approximately 40 million people worldwide were estimated to be infected with HIV/AIDS (WHO, 2007a). AIDS has been especially devastating in the developing world, where it is a stigma. People do not talk about it. Those with the illness do not inform their families or others at risk for acquiring the disease. Education about the spread and control of the illness is sporadic, and there are few economic resources to provide treatments commonly available in the developed world. Table 5-2 shows the prevalence of HIV in different parts of the world.

AIDS has disrupted family life, leaving many children with few adult supports. Over 1 million children die each year from AIDS, and AIDS accounted for approximately 3% of the deaths of children under age 5 in 2000 (WHO, 2007a). Many more children are orphaned. In 1998, 470,000 children in Zambia and more than 1.7 million in Uganda lost one or both parents. Sometimes whole families are ravished, leaving children without parents, grandparents, or other relatives, scavenging on their own for food and shelter.

International efforts have concentrated on primary prevention. Education about the cause and spread of the virus and advocacy of the use of condoms and other protective measures during sexual activity; improvement in the procurement,

TABLE 5-2   HIV Prevalence among Adults 15 Years of Age and Older per 100,000 Population in Selected Countries: 2005

Country	Prevalence per 100,000
Swaziland	34,457
Botswana	23,624
South Africa	16,579
Malawi	12,528
Central African Republic	9990
Kenya	6125
Nigeria	3547
Haiti	3377
Bahamas	2807
Thailand	1144
India	747
United States	508
Brazil	454
Switzerland	264
Canada	222
Greece	98
Pakistan	86
Poland	78
Norway	67

Data from World Health Organization (WHO). (2007). *World health statistics 2007.* Geneva: Author.

storage, and administration of blood; and advocacy efforts aimed at women and men who are at risk because they have multiple sexual partners are a few examples of primary prevention efforts.

Early prevention work tended to focus on Western World theories of individual change. The field has moved toward broader attention on social groups and communities of hard-to-reach populations. This move required acknowledgment that target audiences will not adopt behaviors that are not within their cultural norm (McKee et al., 2004).

Health care workers in India were faced with a growing HIV/AIDS endemic. The WHO projected that, without effective interventions, 25 million people would be living with AIDS by the year 2010. To combat the problem, health workers evaluated populations at risk. They found that in 80% of cases, sexually transmitted diseases were the result of infections contracted through sex work, either by the female sex worker or by her male patron. Condom use among sex workers was very low. Health teams developed an intervention using female sex workers to provide health teaching on disease spread and provided a ready supply of condoms. They found that using peer sex workers improved the female prostitute's willingness to listen. Female sex workers reported an 89% use in condoms and a reduction in the proportion of unprotected sexual contacts from 67% to 25% (Nagelkerke et al., 2002).

Many workplaces in Kenya are integrating HIV-related activities, especially peer education programs, into their daily operations. Employers have found that it is easier and cheaper to educate and/or treat employees than to train another person for the job vacated by someone who died from AIDS (Taravella, 2005).

Medication to maintain immune status or treat the myriad illnesses that accompany HIV infection is costly and is not available to large segments of the developing world. International groups, including WHO and UNICEF, advocate that drug companies provide medications, especially those used in the antiviral drug protocols, at low cost to poorer countries. A December 2003 initiative, the "3 by 5" prescription regime, was aimed at providing a three-in-one antiretroviral combination pill to 3 million HIV-positive people in the developing world by the year 2005 (WHO, 2003b). This attempt by the WHO was controversial because it violated pharmaceutical patents, but progress has been made. At the end of 2006, approximately 2 million people in low- and middle-income countries were receiving antiretroviral therapy. This is a 54% increase over the 1.3 million treated in 2005, which means that slightly more than one quarter (28%) of the people needing the medications now receive them. Lower prices for antiretroviral drugs have improved access, but figures are far from the target of universal coverage by 2010 (WHO, 2007b).

Voluntary counseling and testing (VCT) is a major strategy of HIV prevention and treatment programs in the community. With the help of trained counselors, people learn how to reduce their risk of infection. They can also learn their HIV status and enroll for treatment if necessary. A limited number of mobile VCT services exists, and they are helpful in getting more people tested (Kresge, 2006).

AIDS vaccine development is progressing, with 13 new trials started in eight countries in 2006. Some other trials begun in 2003 to 2005 are continuing (Kresge, 2007).

Malaria

Malaria is the most important vector-transmitted disease in the world. It is spread by the bite of the female *Anopheles* mosquito. It is endemic to most of Asia, Africa, and Latin America. An estimated 300 to 500 million cases occur annually, with over 1 million deaths each year, many in children under age 5 (BBC News, 2004). Ninety percent of cases are in sub-Saharan Africa.

Malaria has been difficult to reduce or eliminate. It is becoming resistant both to pesticides such as DDT used to control the vector mosquito and to the classic drug therapies. For example, chloroquine resistance is prevalent in much of Africa.

In 1999, the WHO introduced a reinvigorated malaria control program entitled Roll Back Malaria (WHO, 2002b). This effort is a two-part strategy aimed at reducing malaria deaths by 50% by the year 2010.

The first effort is aimed at achieving vector control by spraying for mosquitoes and larvae as well as providing community education to reduce breeding environments. For example, one WHO-sponsored study found that sponging cattle with insecticide reduced the malaria incidence by 50% in the study areas (WHO, 2001b). In Mexico, Abate, a chemical that prevents larval growth in water, is provided to community residents free of charge. Schoolchildren are given lessons about the importance of using Abate and encouraged to remind their parents to do so. An additional prevention strategy is the use of insecticide-treated bed nets, especially for children under 5 years of age.

Early detection and treatment of malaria cases is the second part of the strategy. These efforts include aggressive case finding and early treatment to reduce complications. Vaccine development is a new initiative. The CDC in Atlanta, as well as government agencies in other countries (e.g., Kenya and India) are developing and testing vaccines. A Spanish malaria expert at the University of Barcelona, working with GlaxoSmithKline Biologicals, has tested "an effective vaccine" on children in Mozambique that could be licensed by 2010 (BBC News, 2004).

Tuberculosis

Tuberculosis (TB) is a leading cause of infectious disease deaths, causing 1.55 million deaths in 2005 (WHO, 2007c). More than 8.8 million people contract TB each year (WHO, 2007c). TB is a serious health problem because the disease is becoming resistant to chemotherapy. It is highly concentrated in poorer countries with limited resources to treat the disease, and the mortality rate is high in poor countries (nearly 25%). Southeast Asia experiences approximately 3 million new cases per year, and sub-Saharan Africa has another 2.5 million cases. Although funding for treatment of TB is now quite good, reduced funding worldwide in the early 2000s for public health services exacerbated the problem of TB control.

Reduction in health services limits case finding and effective disease management. Each individual with active TB infects an average of 10 to 15 other people (WHO, 2007d). These infected individuals (nearly one third of the world's population) act as a reservoir for the bacteria. Without proper treatment, infected individuals might progress to disease, continuing the cycle by infecting others (see Chapter 8).

TB has been easily treated with medication, although effective drug therapy is not always available to many in developing countries. New drug-resistant strains of the TB organism are complicating the treatment regimen for TB. Most of these strains arose as a result of incomplete treatment or poorly supervised treatment. For this reason, the standard treatment for TB disease in the countries with the highest rates has become a short course of directly observed therapy (DOTS), in which medical supervision, drug therapy, and laboratory surveillance are combined to combat the disease. Individuals receiving DOTS are supervised as they take their medication for the entire treatment period, which can be from 6 months to 2 years. DOTS produces a cure rate of up to 95%. Globally, 89% of TB patients are being treated using DOTS (WHO, 2007c). In Peru, for example, the use of DOTS produced a 91% successful treatment rate for TB cases and a decline in the incidence of TB in Peru (WHO, 2002c).

Co-infection with HIV and the TB organism is prevalent in Africa, where approximately 314,000 new cases are identified each year (WHO, 2007c). Co-infection complicates the treatment of each illness, because each expedites the progression of the other. Currently, there may be as many as 30,000 cases of extremely drug-resistant TB worldwide, many of them in countries with a high HIV/AIDS prevalence (Krisberg, 2007a). TB is an opportunistic illness. TB takes advantage of low resistance to disease, and HIV infection weakens the immune system, thus setting a favorable stage for progression of TB in persons who are infected with the bacteria. TB is one of the leading causes of death for HIV-positive patients and accounted for 194,000 AIDS deaths worldwide in 2005 (WHO, 2007c).

Vaccine-Preventable Diseases and Integrated Management of Illness in Children

Global efforts at protecting the world's children from vaccine-preventable illnesses started with WHO's Expanded Program of Immunization. Although progress has been made, the developing world still has problems with vaccine supply, delivery, and cost. Therefore, almost 1.4 million children die each year from vaccine-preventable illnesses (WHO, 2005c). Measles is associated with the highest death rate (500,000), followed by *Haemophilus influenzae* type b infections (400,000), pertussis (300,000), and tetanus (180,000). The number of deaths does not begin to detail the extent of the problem. Although it has been improving in recent years, measles vaccine coverage in very poor countries can still be lower than 50% (WHO, 2007a). The Global Alliance for Vaccines and Immunizations was formed to combat this problem. The alliance is a public-private enterprise consisting of foundations, multigovernmental organizations, and businesses, including WHO, UNICEF, the World Bank, individual country governments, the CDC, other public health and research institutions, the Rockefeller Foundation, and the Bill and Melinda Gates Foundation. The alliance works to improve vaccination delivery for existing vaccines and to develop newer vaccines to improve protection against infections and communicable diseases. Figure 5-3 shows preparations for vaccine administration at a rural health facility.

Pneumonia, diarrhea, measles, malaria, and malnutrition, either alone or in combination, are still responsible for 7 out of 10 deaths among children in developing countries (WHO, 1998c, 2007a). To combat this combination of problems, the WHO and UNICEF developed the Integrated Management of Childhood Illness (IMCI) program. The IMCI program does the following:

- Teaches health professionals to screen for all of the potential problems at the same time and to recommend referral to first-level care facilities for seriously ill children
- Educates parents and child care workers to be alert for initial signs of illness and teaches appropriate care measures for the sick child
- Provides supportive funding to improve the availability of effective treatments in poor countries

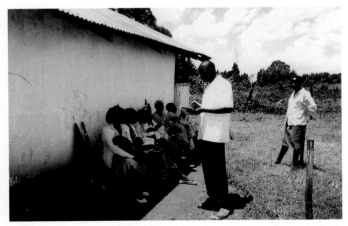

FIGURE 5-3 Effective primary health care services should be available at very simple local health facilities. Here a bachelor's-level nursing student in Kenya checks immunization records (kept by the mothers) of children brought to a rural clinic. (Copyright Helen Kohler.)

- Works toward wider immunization coverage for vaccine-susceptible illnesses
- Trains health care workers in primary care, first-level settings to effectively manage illness in infants and young children (e.g., malnutrition, dehydration, and breathing problems)

It has been estimated that if the IMCI becomes fully operational, it will save approximately 5 million children each year. Although the IMCI had been adopted in 100 countries by 2005, expansion has been slower than expected, and many children do not have the benefits of comprehensive and integrated care (WHO, 2005b).

Other Serious Health Concerns

There are many more serious health issues in the developing world. Many are preventable or easily treated. Expanding primary health care services in developing nations can have a substantial impact on these problems. Some of the more serious concerns include the following:

- Maternal mortality: Annually approximately 31 million women experience acute complications of pregnancy. Over half a million women die in childbirth each year (WHO, 2005b).
- Reproductive health: Women in developing countries have more pregnancies during their lifetimes than those in the developed world. Abortion is used as a birth control method. There are approximately 46 million abortions each year, with 68,000 resulting in maternal death (WHO, 2005b). Approximately 60% of abortions are performed under sanitary conditions; the rest are not. Unsafe abortions account for 20% of all maternal deaths.
- Refugees from famine and war: Large displacements of populations are the result of war, civil unrest, and famine. Refugees risk death, infectious disease, and ongoing malnutrition. The UN Refugee Agency (2006) estimated that there were 29 to 34 million displaced persons in 2004. The majority of displaced persons were internally displaced; that is, forced from their homes but still within their country's territorial boundary. For example, of the 6 million Sudanese who were displaced in 2004, only 8% sought refuge in other countries. The remainder stayed within Sudan's borders.
- Viral hepatitis B: More than 2 billion people, 40% of the world's population, are infected with hepatitis B, and an estimated 1 million die each year of hepatitis B and its complications (Hepatitis B Foundation, 2007). Hepatitis B vaccination is not readily available because of cost issues.
- Chronic conditions: Although a less prevalent cause of death than in developed countries, chronic diseases, especially cardiovascular disease, and cancer are important causes of death. Worldwide, diabetes affects 180 million people (WHO, 2006a). As people in developing countries adopt faulty Western lifestyles, they are prone to chronic conditions as well as infectious diseases.

Receding Health Problems

Global efforts have had success in combating some of the world's health problems. Most of these problems have been reduced or eliminated by vaccination or vector control. Smallpox, polio, guinea worm disease, and river blindness are examples of receding health problems.

Smallpox was the first success story. Vaccine provides an effective protection against smallpox. By 1940, smallpox was eliminated from Europe, North America, and Australia/New Zealand. A vigorous global effort to eradicate smallpox started in 1967. Five years later, the disease was eliminated in South America, Indonesia, and most of Africa. The last known case of smallpox was in Somalia in 1977 (Basch, 1999).

Significant progress had been made in the eradication of *polio*. This is another illness against which vaccination is effective. Polio has decreased 99% since 1988, when the Global Polio Eradication Initiative was launched. This global project was a joint effort by several private, philanthropic, and intergovernmental organizations and businesses. Rotary International and the CDC are very active in this effort. Widely endemic in 1988, polio is now found only in parts of Africa (e.g., Nigeria) and south Asia (e.g., India) (WHO, 2003c).

Although polio has been confined, outbreaks still occur. Polio vaccination is an ongoing effort. In 2002, more than 500 million children in 93 countries were immunized. In 2003, a serious lapse in vaccination programs and the resultant outbreak of polio in Nigeria led the Global Polio Eradication Initiative to spend $10 million dollars to vaccinate 15 million children in Nigeria and neighboring Ghana, Niger, Togo, and Benin.

The reduction of *guinea worm disease* is another success story. Although it is not completely eradicated, it is nearly gone. Guinea worm infestation is painful and crippling, leaving people unable to work and provide for their families. In 1986, 3.5 million people in 20 countries had guinea worm disease; by 2001, that number had been reduced to 65,000 in only nine African countries, a 98% reduction in cases (Carter Center, 2003, 2007). Sudan, Ghana, and Nigeria are the countries with most of the remaining cases.

Guinea worm disease is a vector-born illness. It is transmitted by the infected larvae of fleas, which reside in stagnant and unfiltered water. Ensuring pure water eliminates the problem. Efforts at eradication are aimed at improving the water supply and teaching villages how to protect themselves from infestations. The Carter Center (2008), along with a consortium of governments, the U.S. Peace Corps, the Japan Overseas Cooperation Volunteers, the Johnson and Johnson Company, and others are actively engaged in efforts to eliminate the remaining pockets of guinea worm disease.

Currently, *river blindness (onchocerciasis)* affects approximately 17.7 million people, about 500,000 of whom are visually impaired and 270,000 of whom are blinded (Carter Center, 2006, 2007). The condition is concentrated in Africa, Latin America, and Yemen. It is a parasitic disease transmitted by the bite of black flies. River blindness is easily treated and prevented with Mectizan (ivermectin). A significant portion of the medication distributed is donated by Merck, the Carter Center, and Lions International. About 80.5 million people have been provided with medication since 1990 (Lions International, 2007). Eradication is a two-step process: control or eradication of the vector, and provision of medical prophylaxis and treatment to at-risk populations.

PROBLEMS COMMON TO DEVELOPED COUNTRIES

People in developed countries enjoy a better standard of living than those in poorer countries, but there are still health disparities linked to income level. Poverty is a persistent causal link to poor health, even in more affluent countries. People in poverty in the developed world are, for the most part, better off

than their counterparts in poorer countries. However, they still experience a lower standard of living and poorer health status than their more affluent neighbors (see Chapter 21). Access to health care services can also be a problem for low-income individuals. This is particularly true in the United States, which does not have a national health care system (see Chapters 3, 4, and 21). As discussed later, access problems are still present, although they are not as common, in other countries with national health care systems.

Chronic Conditions

Chronic conditions, such as heart and pulmonary disease, are more common in the developed world and, along with cancer, are the leading causes of death (Table 5-3). Longer life spans allow more time for the development and progression of chronic illness. The developing world also experiences chronic conditions; however, these countries suffer a much higher burden of infectious and communicable disease than the more developed world.

One measure of chronic disease is the "Dallies," or Disability-Adjusted Life-Years (DALYs). This measure describes the number of years of healthy (disability-free) living lost because of illness or death. Approximately 46% of the DALYs lost worldwide were due to chronic conditions such as heart disease, cancer, or diabetes. The proportion of DALYs lost due to chronic illness in the developed world was twice as high, at approximately 80%. In developed countries, only 5% of DALYs lost were associated with communicable diseases or maternal, perinatal, or nutritional conditions, whereas these same conditions accounted for 40% of the disease burden in developing countries and as much as 50% to 60% of the burden in Africa (WHO, 2003a). Chapter 7 provides a discussion of some of the chronic illnesses prevalent in the United States. Because the experiences of other developed nations are similar to that of

---

TABLE 5-3   **Comparison of Top Diseases, Disabilities, and Causes of Death for Poorest and Developed Countries**

Poorest	Developed
1. Underweight	1. Tobacco
2. HIV/AIDS	2. Ischemic heart disease
3. Lower respiratory infections	3. Unipolar depressive disorder Cerebrovascular disease
4. Perinatal conditions Diarrheal diseases	4. Alcohol use disorders
5. Malaria	5. Hearing loss (adult onset)
6. Maternal conditions	6. Chronic obstructive pulmonary disease
7. Unipolar depressive disorder	7. Road accidents
8. Ischemic heart disease	8. Tracheal, bronchial, and lung cancers
9. Measles	9. Alzheimer's disease and other dementias
10. Tuberculosis	10. Self-inflicted injuries

From Murphy, E. M. (2005). *Promoting healthy behavior.* Health bulletin 2. Washington, DC: Population Reference Bureau.

the United States, these conditions are not detailed in this chapter. As developing countries improve in economic status, the mortality related to acute and infectious conditions declines, and the mortality associated with chronic conditions rises.

HEALTH CARE DELIVERY SYSTEMS

Health care delivery systems are generally based on capitalism or social welfare. In the capitalistic or entrepreneurial model, the overriding principle is minimal government involvement and reliance on private-sector providers for health care services (see Chapter 3). In the welfare models, government direction and regulation is expected. The degree of government responsibility varies. There might be total government control **(Beveridge model),** with the system funded by taxes, or a more decentralized version **(Bismarck model),** with the system funded by a combination of personal contributions and taxes.

Within these three basic models, there are many variations. Economic resources affect the type and extent of health care available in a country but are not the determining influence on the structure of health care delivery. For example, India, a developing country, has a national health care system; the United States, a very rich country, does not. Distinctions can be made between developed and developing countries with

respect to the extent and type of services a country can afford to provide to its people.

HEALTH CARE SYSTEMS IN DEVELOPED COUNTRIES

The United States is the only industrialized country with an individualized free market approach to health care (see Chapter 3). The others have developed some form of national health care systems that provide coverage to all, or nearly all, citizens (Table 5-4). Each country's system varies in its organization and delivery of care. Roemer (1991) has defined four basic types of health care delivery. He identifies the United States as the sole example of the entrepreneurial model. The United States has a very decentralized system, with very limited government planning for health care services. The government is the funder of last resort for *some* but *not all* of those who cannot afford care. Public health oversight and functions are a government responsibility, but most of the planning and public health activities are the responsibility of the individual states.

The welfare-oriented system is often referred to as the *Bismarck model,* after the German leader who first championed this system. *Most* people have medical care protection. The national government assumes responsibility for financing and planning, but organization and delivery of care are shared

TABLE 5-4   National Health Care Systems

Type	Country	Financing	Planning and Organization	Delivery of Services	Who Is Covered
Entrepreneurial	United States	Direct—out of pocket Indirect—private insurance, public sector insurance, and welfare	Decentralized Direct health care responsibility of private sector Limited public sector services, primarily public health Majority of facilities in private sector	Private sector practitioners Limited government health care workers, primarily in public health functions	Many people (14%, or 42 million) without health insurance and not eligible for programs
Welfare	Germany Belgium France Japan Canada	Indirect—Funding collected by health or sickness insurance funds or government payment (may be co-pays)	Government planning Diversified ownership Most hospitals government owned	Independent practitioners Some government health care providers	Most citizens
Comprehensive	Great Britain New Zealand Scandinavian countries Italy	Direct—government provides and pays for care through taxes (may require co-pays)	Government planning and ownership	Government organized Practitioners are salaried	All citizens
Socialist	Taiwan Spain Russia Poland Yugoslavia Cuba	Direct (may now require co-pays)	Government (highly centralized)	Government-salaried workers Limited services due to economic failures	All citizens, with priority given to workers and children due to limited resources

Data from Roemer, M. (1991). *National health care systems of the world.* NY: Oxford University Press; Espring-Anderson, G. (1990). *The three worlds of welfare capitalism.* Princeton: Princeton University Press; and Physicians for a National Health Program. (2007). *Snapshots of health systems in 16 countries.* Retrieved August 20, 2007 from *www.pnhp.org/facts/ international_health_systems.php?page=all.*

with private enterprise. Care is paid for by health insurance, which is subsidized by the government for those who have no other means. Workers in Germany, for example, have health insurance through their employers. Everyone else either has another form of insurance or is subsidized by the government. Providers usually remain in independent practice, and consumers may choose health care providers. The government owns most, but not all, hospital facilities. Australia, Canada, Germany, Japan, and France are examples of countries with welfare-oriented health care systems.

Comprehensive health care systems provide a broad scope of health care services to *all* citizens. Comprehensive systems are commonly referred to as the *Beveridge model,* after the developer of the post–WWII health system in Great Britain. Unlike in welfare systems, the government directs both the finance mechanism and the organizational structure. The national government assumes the major role in planning, organizing, financing, and delivering care to all. Most health care providers are government employees, and services are provided in government-operated health centers. Consumers have a choice of provider if the provider does not have a client overload. Most such systems allow some element of private practice by providers, but only a small percentage of citizens are served in this manner. Great Britain, New Zealand, and all of the Scandinavian nations are examples of countries with comprehensive health care systems.

Socialist systems developed in the Communist bloc countries after WWII. These systems represent the most stringent central control of health planning, funding, and services. When developed, they were successful, providing a better standard of care than was previously available to most of the population. The standard of care varied by country. Poorer socialized countries, such as Romania, were able to provide more limited services than richer countries such as Poland. Cuba, for example, follows the socialist model. Until very recently, the level of health and access to health care services in Cuba were substantially better than those in other countries in the region.

The demise of the Soviet system in the early 1990s has lead to a crisis in health care. Many of the socialist countries have experienced a deterioration in the health care structure, limited supplies, and increased mortality rates (Washington Profile, 2007). The rate of infectious diseases, such as HIV/AIDS and TB, has substantially increased (Moran & Jordaan, 2007; WHO, 2003d). A limited number of economically affluent people are able to purchase care; many go without. Now, at the beginning of the twenty-first century, the countries of Eastern Europe are still struggling to improve health care. Some of the more affluent are moving toward less restrictive comprehensive or welfare models, and some are experimenting with public-private partnerships in health care services. In these more affluent countries, the populations enjoy a better standard of health than those in the countries of the Russian federation (McKee, 2001).

Differences in Health Planning

Countries with functioning national health care systems engage in more comprehensive health planning and provide all, or almost all, citizens with comprehensive health care services. Central planning is possible because the government has the means to influence services either by providing direct care or by reimbursing the cost of care for most of its citizens.

In contrast, the United States has engaged in little central health planning. The federal government is becoming more involved in national health planning and has established national health objectives (see Chapter 1). These objectives are only guidelines, however, and do not have the force of law. Currently, those segments of the health care system not directly under federal control are free to ignore or address the objectives as they choose.

Comparison of Health Care Expenditures and Health Status Indicators

Most countries commit more public funds, provide more services, and spend less of their gross domestic product (GDP) on health care than the United States does (see Chapter 3). In most countries, health care costs are rising. The Organization for Economic Co-operation and Development (2006) reports that of 30 developed countries, all except Finland spend more of their GDP on health care today than they did in 1990. Germany had the largest increase, related in part to the increased health care demands since reunification of East and West Germany. Opponents of health care reform in the United States frequently point to the Canadian system as a reason not to provide universal coverage. Canada is often presented as having many more problems than the United States. In Table 5-5, some of the common criticisms are listed, and the validity of those concerns are explored.

Differences in expenditures of public funds would be more understandable if the U.S. system provided a better standard of health than that of other countries. That is not the case, however. The United States ranked lowest of 19 industrialized nations in both life expectancy and infant mortality. In addition the United States infant mortality rate exceeds that of other countries such as Andorra, the Czech Republic, Poland, and South Korea (WHO, 2007a). Lack of comprehensive planning for prenatal care, a characteristic not shared by countries with national health care systems, is a significant contributor to the infant mortality results (Williams, 2002).

HEALTH CARE SYSTEMS IN DEVELOPING COUNTRIES

Health care in developing and middle-income countries varies in quality and amount of care. Governments tend to provide public health services, but not at the level provided in developed countries. There is an element of a welfare-oriented approach, particularly with respect to public health functions. Responsibility for public health resides in the ministry of health. There is usually a network of local public health offices (Detels & Breslow, 2002). For example, China has a system of antiepidemic stations located throughout the country. Depending on the country, these local offices might also provide some basic primary health care to the community.

Developing countries have a mix of entrepreneurial and welfare health care systems. The wealthy can pay for health care. For the many with few economic means, there are limited national health care systems. There are both Beveridge-oriented systems (China) and Bismarck-influenced systems (India). Widespread democratization in many developing countries has led to a certain amount of decentralization of authority (Sein & Rafei, 2002). The idea of individual responsibility for health care is becoming a popular idea. The poorest countries rely on nongovernmental organizations and intergovernmental

TABLE 5-5 Canadian Health Care System: Myths and Facts

Criticism	Response	Reason
It's socialized medicine.	No	It is a social insurance plan similar to the U.S. Social Security System and Medicare. Doctors are not state employees but have private practices.
Health care is rationed.	Yes and no	There may be a wait for hospital beds, specialists, and diagnostic tests. Canadians do not have to wait to see their primary physicians. Health care is rationed through the primary physician by immediate need versus delayed need for special services, not by ability to pay. In contrast, in the U.S. system care is rationed by ability to pay (refer to Chapter 4).
There are not enough doctors.	No	The distribution of physicians is different; about 50% of physicians are primary care/family practice physicians. U.S. residents are 3% less likely to have a family doctor.
There are long waits for care.	Maybe	There is no wait for a primary care physician. Certain high-technology procedures, e.g., lithotripsy, magnetic resonance imaging, and bypass surgery, usually require some waiting. Wait time for procedures has occurred in some provinces. Hospitals operate at 95% of capacity and 1-day surgical procedures have increased (not unlike in the United States). Approximately 3.5% of Canadians have unmet health needs because of long wait times compared with 1% of U.S. residents. Overall, 7% of U.S. residents and fewer than 1% of Canadians have unmet needs because they cannot offer to pay for health care.
The quality of health care is poor.	No	Canada's infant mortality rate is lower and life span higher than in the United States. Canadians, although concerned about what cost cuts might do to services, would not trade their system for a U.S.-type delivery system. Inequality in access to health care and differences in mortality rates among income groups is far less in Canada than in the United States.
Administrative costs are greater.	No	The provider bills the government directly for all services and is paid within a month. Patients neither pay nor are billed for services. Single-payer systems are more cost efficient with regard to administrative expenses. In this country, the administrative costs for Medicare and Medicaid are only 10% of the costs of private insurance administration (see Chapter 4).
The system is troubled by escalating costs.	Yes and no	The Canadian system has experienced increasing costs and strategies have been initiated to keep costs down. Costs have remained below costs in the American system. Canada controls costs at the source; e.g., physician fees are set by negotiation between the health ministry and the physician's organization; patients do not have out-of-pocket expenses.
Physicians earn less.	Yes	Physicians in all national health systems earn less than U.S. physicians; however, their overhead with respect to administrative costs is less.

Data from Barer, M. L., & Evans, R. G. (1992). Interpreting Canada: Models, mind-sets, and myths. *Health Affairs, 11*(1), 44-61; The search for solutions: Does Canada have the right answer? (1992). *Consumer Reports, 57*(9), 579-592; McKenzie, J. F., Pinger, R. R., & Kotecki, J. E. (1999). *An introduction to community health* (3rd ed.). Boston: Jones & Bartlett; Deber, R. B. (2003). Health care reform: Lessons from Canada. *American Journal of Public Health, 93*(1), 20-24; Kunitz, S. J., & Pesis-Katz, I. (2005). Mortality of white Americans, African Americans, and Canadians: The causes and consequences for health of welfare state institutions and policies. *Melbrook Quarterly, 83*(1), 5-39; and Lasser, K. E., Himmelstein, D. U., & Woolhandler, S. (2006). Access to health care, health status, and health disparities in the United States and Canada: Results of a cross-national population-based survey. *American Journal of Public Health, 96*(7), 1300-1303.

agencies, such as WHO and UNICEF, for some or most of their health care services. Some countries are so poor that services are extremely limited. Afghanistan is an example of a country with severely limited health care services, although there have been recent improvements.

ISSUES IN HEALTH CARE DELIVERY SYSTEMS

No health care system is perfect. Some do better than others, at least in terms of comparison data such as life expectancy and infant mortality rates. To help evaluate the effectiveness of a country's health care system, the WHO (2000) identified five performance criteria. These are the following:

- Level of health of the population
- Degree of health disparities within the country's population
- Responsiveness of the health care system
- Distribution of responsiveness within the population
- Distribution of financing for health services within the population

Responsiveness refers to how well the system (administrators and service personnel) can address the concerns of the citizens and how the citizens themselves feel about the quality of and access to their health care services. Distribution of finance looks at who pays for services and how much they pay. The WHO expects a country's poor to shoulder less of the financial burden for health care than do those who are better off. Using these five benchmarks, the WHO rated France as having the best health care system among developed countries. Japan, Great Britain, and Germany all ranked higher than the United States. In 2007, Davis and colleagues conducted a comparative study of six highly developed countries and reported that the

United States ranked last among the six with reference to life expectancy, quality of care, and access to health care services. In both instances the most pressing concern with the U.S. system was the number of people without health care services, either through public- or private-sector funding.

When health care systems are examined, economics and resources, rather than organizational model, appear to be the deciding indicators of success. Nevertheless, all countries struggle to develop strategies to deal with rising health care costs, decide the types of services to make available to their populations, and determine how to fund their health care programs. In general, poor countries cannot deliver the same degree of health care services to their populations as can rich countries.

Economics alone does not account for the differences between countries. For example, the United States spends more of its GDP on health care than do other developed countries, yet the United States has poorer life expectancy and higher infant mortality than comparable countries. Mexico spends less of its GDP on health care than do poorer Latin American countries such as Nicaragua, Barbados, Bolivia, and Columbia (WHO, 2007a).

The locus of decision making and health planning might have some influence on health status but is not the overriding determining factor. For example, the central planning model used by Great Britain (Beveridge model) appears to provide good care to its population, whereas in Germany, a more decentralized method has produced satisfactory results (Hurst, 2000). The central planning model appears to help very poor countries make rapid advances in health. For example, China and Cuba made substantial initial increases in the level of health of their populations once central planning and control were instituted. However, once initial health gains have been achieved and a degree of economic prosperity begins, central planning models do not appear to function any better than other organizational models. For instance, South Korea has operated under both models and has found little difference between organizational types in terms of health status of the population (Lee, 2003).

The United States, with no national health insurance plan, has a higher percentage of persons uninsured than in other developed countries (Roberts & Rhoades, 2007). Some countries with national plans nevertheless have uninsured citizens. The numbers of uninsured in these countries is declining as incremental changes incorporate previously excluded groups. For example, Germany started with employer-provided health plans to cover workers and gradually added other groups until, by 2003, all citizens had insurance coverage (Altenstetter, 2003).

Developed and developing countries alike struggle to control costs to the system. Developed countries have controlled costs by limiting certain services, although they cover medically necessary and appropriate care (Brown, 2003). For example, home care and prescription drugs are not provided as a benefit in Canada. Dental care and eye care are covered by supplemental insurance or out-of-pocket payments in France. All the developed countries face higher expenses in treating chronic illnesses as their populations age. Beyond public health services, developing countries also struggle with costs and the types of benefits they can afford or wish to provide to their populations. Often, the result is a two-tiered health system. Limited services

provided by public employees are available to all. Extra services are paid out of pocket and provided by private sources. Such is the case in Thailand and Pakistan (Daniels et al., 2000). Sometimes health plans work only in theory, not in practice. In Pakistan, because the government is unable to provide the basic services designated by the government plan, 90% of care is delivered by private providers at extra costs to the consumers.

> Jennifer Carson, a student nurse, is doing a clinical experience practicum in Mexico as part of her community health education at Oregon State Health University. She is providing care in a clinic, where she notices that the dentist seldom has patients. One day, she asks him why he does not have many patients. Dr. Ortez tells her that the co-payment for dental services is $7 per visit. Ms. Carson does not think that is so bad, but Dr. Ortez tells her, "My patients have to choose between having their teeth cared for and buying bread for their families."

Low-income and middle-income countries face major policy decisions as they struggle with the question of how to provide health care to their people. Should it be tax funded, insurance funded, or self-funded, or funded by a combination of methods? Should there be central planning, local planning, or a combination of both? Should health professionals be government employees or self-employed entrepreneurs or a combination of both? These are the issues countries continue to struggle with as they attempt to improve health care services and the health of their peoples.

NEW AND EMERGING HEALTH ISSUES

At the turn of the twenty-first century, a number of health concerns demand particular attention. Some diseases are receding in importance, whereas others are becoming more problematic. Concerns center around old or newly emerging diseases, the deleterious effects of behavior on health, and the recognition of health risks associated with terrorism and warfare.

OLD AND NEW EMERGING INFECTIOUS DISEASES

According to Morse (1995), **emerging infectious diseases** are ones that are either old diseases that are rapidly increasing in incidence or geographic range (e.g., dengue fever) or new, previously unknown conditions (e.g., SARS). *Dengue fever* is a severe, flu-like illness that might progress to dengue hemorrhagic fever, which is life-threatening. It is a mosquito-borne infection that has increased in both scope and range, becoming endemic in more than 100 countries. Annually there are between 50 and 100 million cases in the world, and 20,000 deaths (WHO, 2007e). Yellow fever and cholera are other examples of old infectious diseases that are becoming more prevalent. HIV/AIDS is the most severe example of a newly emerging infectious disease. Other examples include Hantavirus pulmonary syndrome, Legionnaire's disease, SARS, infection with *Streptococcus* group A organisms (necrotizing or flesh-eating bacteria), and Ebola virus disease.

New infections are problematic because there is a time lag between recognition of the problem and development of effective treatments. During this lag, the disease can spread to many people and continents, with devastating results. Old diseases reemerge because of failures in control or immunization. They are problematic because new strains are often more resistant to management. As examples, the mosquito responsible for carrying malaria is becoming resistant to pesticides; control methods for dengue fever have not been able to eliminate the vector mosquito; and TB is becoming multidrug resistant.

The most recent emerging disease concern is the possible threat of a new influenza pandemic rivaling that of 1918, in which at least 20 million people died worldwide. Flu epidemics have a cyclical pattern, with large outbreaks documented in 1946, 1957, and 1968. In early 1976, the swine flu virus (which was responsible for the 1918 flu) was detected in throat swabs from four seriously ill, previously healthy, Army recruits at Fort Dix in New Jersey. Because of concern that this might be a sign that "the big one" was likely to occur soon, a swine flu vaccine was quickly made and administered to about one third of the American population before the unexpected side effect of Guillain-Barré syndrome occurred. The vaccination program was stopped in mid-December of 1976 (Neustadt & Fineberg, 1978). Fortunately, even though the time was right and the proportion of the population immunized was low, no epidemic occurred.

In 2003, SARS could have become the next global respiratory disease epidemic. However, unusual international cooperation and the readiness of WHO prevented a crisis (WHO, 2006b).

The situation with respect to avian influenza is very complex and still evolving. The H5N1 virus first appeared in sick chickens on Asian poultry farms in 2003 (Arias, 2007). This has necessitated worldwide bird surveillance and massive culling of poultry flocks since then, mainly in Far Eastern countries.

The avian flu virus is not thought to have yet made the mutation required for efficient spread from human to human. However, 322 confirmed human cases (with a case fatality rate of 61%) had been reported to WHO by August 23, 2007 (WHO, 2007f). The hardest hit countries were Indonesia and Viet Nam, which are in the Far East where people traditionally live in very close proximity to their chickens and other fowl.

It is not yet known whether the H5N1 avian influenza virus will cause a global human disease outbreak. Health officials in the United States "are united in their belief that a pandemic is likely to emerge and have been working on preparedness efforts for the past few years" (Davey, 2007, p. 57).

The CDC has developed a pandemic severity index that classifies the severity of a pandemic in terms of categories 1 through 6, similar to the tiered rating system used for hurricanes. Of concern is the belief expressed by a preeminent risk communication consultant (Sandman, 2007) that officials will have a more difficult time than a year ago convincing the public of the need to prepare for a pandemic. He argues that "teachable moments" were lost when officials focused on birds rather than on the real threat of H5N1 virus mutation.

The WHO is acting as the coordinator for the global response to human cases of H5N1 avian influenza and monitoring the threat of a pandemic. "Encouraging progress" in pandemic flu vaccine development is being made by 16 manufacturers in 10 countries (Arias, 2007).

It must be recognized that effective global surveillance for prevention or management of a pandemic is dependent on "the willingness of governments to engage in robust cooperation" by transparent reporting rather than hiding of outbreaks (Lee & Fidler, 2007, p. 217).

ENVIRONMENT

Industrialization has increased the amount of global pollution. The more affluent nations produce a disproportionately larger share of pollution. As more and more countries make economic progress, the pollution burden will increase. Health problems associated with pollution will also increase (McMichael, 2002). Developing countries have few resources to police polluters and are less inclined to do so, because pollution control is seen as a threat to economic development. For example, Mexico City is one of the most polluted cities in the world. Chapter 9 identifies some pollutants and their health effects.

When viewed broadly, the impact of the environment on health includes exposure to infectious agents, previously detailed, as well as to pollutants. The WHO (2006c) attributes 24% of the global burden of disease and 23% of deaths to environmental risk factors. McMichael (2002) cautions that we do not yet know the consequences of many environmental pollutants because of the lag time between exposure and presentation of health problems.

Two measurable global environmental changes are depletion of the ozone layer and accumulation of heat-trapping greenhouse gases. The UN Intergovernmental Panel on Climate Change (2001) reports that these two problems are directly attributable to human actions. The extent to which these changes might affect the planet is still under debate. Some of the issues associated with environmental change and pollution are the following (McMichael, 2002):

- Loss of biodiversity of plants and animals
- Increases in invasive species that choke off or consume food and water sources
- Impairment of food production because of depletion or stress—for example, overfishing
- Chemical pollution of soil, water, air, and food

Climate change and rising global temperatures due to greenhouse gas emissions could lead to serious health effects. Waterborne disease outbreaks may follow the heavy rainfalls likely to increase with continued global warming. An increase in mosquito-borne diseases could result from the increased infectiousness of mosquitos possible with just a half-degree increase in temperature. Global warming could be a tremendous public health threat unless corrective action is taken very soon (Krisberg, 2007b).

TOBACCO USE

Tobacco-related illnesses are the leading cause of premature death in industrialized countries. If current trends continue, annual worldwide tobacco-related deaths will rise "from 4.9 million in 2000 to more than 10 million by 2020, unless effective interventions take hold" (WHO, 2006d, p. 11). There are an estimated 1.3 billion smokers in the world. The incidence of tobacco use is shifting from developed to developing countries. As cigarette use has declined in the developed countries, cigarette manufacturers have greatly expanded their marketing to third world countries. About 84% of all smokers, or 900 million, live in developing and transitional countries (WHO, 2006e). If there is no change in smoking patterns, by the year 2030 approximately 70% of deaths caused by tobacco use will occur in developing countries.

Cigarette smoking is one of the largest causes of preventable deaths in the world. Reducing the incidence of smoking would go a long way toward improving the level of health in populations. For that reason, the WHO has identified smoking reduction as one of its primary health objectives. The Tobacco Free Initiative (WHO, 2001c) aims to reduce and eventually eliminate cigarette use. The Global Treaty on Tobacco Control is a first step. The treaty, passed at the 2003 World Assembly, includes the following actions:

- Endorses a global ban on tobacco advertisement and promotion to children under 18 years of age
- Places strict restrictions on advertisement and promotion to adults
- Prohibits tax-free, duty-free sales of tobacco products
- Supports adoption of price and tax measures aimed at reducing consumption
- Ends subsidies for tobacco production
- Cracks down on cigarette smuggling
- Limits exposure to second-hand smoke
- Improves product labeling and health warnings
- Encourages smoking cessation

One hundred countries have signed the treaty. Some countries have reservations about a total ban on advertising (United States, China, Japan), whereas others support the ban (New Zealand, Australia, most African states, parts of Asia).

Liability and compensation for tobacco-related illnesses were considered but were not incorporated into the current treaty (WHO, 2001c). Other efforts at tobacco control are underway. In 2001, the European Union Parliament voted to ban tobacco advertisement in print media, on the radio, and on the Internet. Tobacco advertisement was already banned on television. The WHO teamed with the CDC, the International Olympic Committee, the Fédération Internationale de Football Association, and the Fédération Internationale de l' Automobile to ban cigarettes at all sporting events (WHO, 2002d). Cigarette smoking is already banned at Olympic events. If successful, these efforts would have a substantial impact on the growing trend to limit health problems associated with tobacco use.

TERRORISM AND WAR

Health problems associated with war, civil insurrection, and terrorism appear to be escalating. No countries are immune from these threats, as the United States learned on September 11, 2001. Health professionals must deal with the health effects of conflicts and terrorism. They must also develop plans for a comprehensive public health response in the event of an incident (see Chapter 22).

The potential use of chemical and biologic agents as terror weapons is a serious concern. Both the United States and the UN have increased their preplanning efforts in this area. The CDC is the most visible public health agency involved in preplanning in the United States. Other offices of the government at all levels—federal, state, and local—are also involved in preparation. The WHO (2001d) has developed a set of strategies to assist planning. This document, titled *Public Health Response to Biological and Chemical Weapons,* advises countries to do the following:

- Improve the national surveillance system to monitor outbreaks of illness
- Improve communications and coordination of response between responsible agencies (infrastructure support, health care, and nuclear facilities, for example)

- Develop vulnerability assessments and communicate that risk to both health professionals and the public
- Prepare for handling the psychosocial consequences of deliberate terrorism
- Expedite contingency plans for a rapid and comprehensive response in the event of an incident

The immediate consequences of war and civil unrest paint a realistic picture of problems likely to occur in a terrorist attack. Health professionals responsible for the care of populations in mass-casualty incidents can examine these situations to help their preplanning preparation. Damage to sanitation, the water supply, and other critical services present an immediate health problem. The poorer the country, the longer it takes the country to recover. In 2005, parts of the U.S. East Coast, particularly Louisiana, Mississippi, and Alabama, experienced severe effects as a result of Hurricane Katrina. Electricity, potable water, and air conditioning were unavailable for days, weeks, and in some cases months. In the immediate aftermath 3 million homes or facilities were without power (National Oceanic and Atmospheric Administration, 2005). Food supplies were disrupted. Gasoline was not available because gas pumps were inoperable. Hospitals and other health care facilities were unable to function fully, which forced some to discharge patients, transport them to other facilities, or evacuate them out of the area. Communities are still struggling to recover years later. Countries that have lengthy experiences with wars and civil unrest, and with more limited resources, might take many years to recover.

Fatal injuries, infectious diseases, and disruptions in food sources are major threats in war. In 2002, more than 1.6 million people suffered fatal, intentional injuries, and 730,000 died by homicide and war (WHO, 2004). In Bosnia and Herzegovina, 250,000 people died or were listed as missing during the 3 years of conflict between 1992 and 1995 (Kinra et al., 2002). In Liberia, more than 200,000 people were killed during the 10 years of civil war (USAID, 2003a). Another 500,000 were internally displaced, compelled to leave their homes either by force or for safety. An additional 250,000 became refugees in neighboring countries. In the Darfur region of Sudan, according to 2007 media reports, at least 200,000 people have been killed and thousands more displaced during the long war there.

Immediate needs in afflicted countries center on the usual basic services of sanitation and potable water. Relief then moves on to other types of infectious disease control, attention to treatment of health problems, and the rebuilding or repair of health care facilities. For example, immediately after the defeat of the Taliban in 2001, USAID entered Afghanistan. To date, USAID (2003b, 2007b, 2008) has done the following:

- Constructed or rehabilitated 670 health clinics, birth centers, and hospitals and 3000 health posts
- Contributed $4.4 billion to development projects
- Rehabilitated or constructed 670 schools and provided 59 million textbooks
- Provided UNICEF with the funds to treat 700,000 cases of malaria
- Provided basic health services to 2 million people
- Rehabilitated 25% of the water supply in Kabul
- Continued to work on rehabilitating the water supply to Kandahar and Kunduz, cities with a combined population of 700,000.

USAID has trained almost 1000 midwives in Afghanistan. These efforts have resulted in a 20% reduction in the infant and child mortality rates and increased women's access to prenatal care by 600% (USAID, 2007c).

Beyond basic services, there are a myriad of other health issues facing health professionals in war-torn regions. Some of these are the following:

- Mass immunization needs and problems with supply of doses and personnel to administer vaccines
- Treatment of the physical and mental damages of rape
- Treatment of the effects of long-term malnutrition and dehydration, which are especially severe in children
- Reduction of the effects of exposure to depleted uranium used in some munitions
- Potential damages associated with a large cache of unexploded land mines
- The problem of child soldiers and their rehabilitation and safe reentry into society
- Reintroduction of displaced persons back to their home environments
- Long-term mental health issues associated with disasters and terrorism

This list is only a sample of the problems encountered by local and international health professionals providing care to populations caught in the midst of war and its aftermath. Global public health security will depend on international cooperation and willingness to tackle new threats (WHO, 2007g).

MENTAL ILLNESS

In 2001, the WHO devoted its annual report on world health to mental health, an area often overlooked in previous reports. The mental health of populations is important to the personal, economic, and political stability of families and societies. The WHO report (2001e) noted the following:

- Neuropsychiatric disorders account for 30% of disability worldwide.
- Some 450 million people suffer from seven common mental illnesses.
- One million people commit suicide each year, and another 20 million attempt suicide.
- Depression will be the second leading cause of the global burden of disease by 2020.

One of the detriments of increasing life spans is the risk of Alzheimer's disease. The developing world can expect an increasing rate of degenerative brain disease as health status and life spans improve. One estimate is that Africa, Asia, and Latin America can expect the number of elderly with dementia to surpass 80 million by the year 2025 (Brody, 2001). Add to that the number of people at risk for mental illness and stress-related conditions as a result of poverty, war, and terrorism, and it is clear that mental health issues will be a huge concern in the coming years.

Poor people seem to have high rates of depression and suicide. In India, for example, poor farmers had higher rates of suicide after droughts than did farmers with more economic means. In one Indian state, 82% of those committing suicide came from a disadvantaged caste that represents only 12% of the state's population (Patel, 2001). Brody (2001) reports that children in poverty are more likely to suffer from epilepsy and mental retardation than are more affluent children. In addition, children living in poverty are more often at risk for malnutrition,

exhaustive work schedules, and other abuses. These situations lead to increased stress levels.

Refugees, including children, have higher rates of mental illness. Many have experienced or witnessed physical and emotional torture. They have higher rates of posttraumatic stress syndrome and other psychiatric illnesses (Kemp & Rashbridge, 2004; WHO, 2003e). The effects of their experiences will linger long after the refugees are able to return to a stable environment.

In many countries, mental illness is a stigma. Families prefer to ignore behaviors or to expel persons who do not behave appropriately for their culture. Most countries do not have the capacity to treat mental illness. The WHO report (2001e) indicates that more than 50% of countries have only one psychiatrist per 100,000 population. More than 40% of countries have no community mental health services. Given the scope of the problem and the limited resources available, it will take years of determined effort before substantial progress can be made. The optimal mix of mental health services needed to begin making progress is shown in Figure 5-4.

ROLE OF NURSING IN INTERNATIONAL HEALTH

The work of community health nurses involves planning and providing health care services to aggregates and populations as well as direct care to individuals and families. Community health nurses have a primary health care perspective and are involved in collaborative planning with other health care professionals. Therefore, community health nurses are uniquely qualified to provide health services and leadership in international health.

Nurses can become involved in global health practice as employees of international organizations, as political activists, or as volunteers. Nurses are highly valued in international health efforts. Their expertise can enhance the volunteer programs of any international organization. Nurses, and student nurses, who are interested in international health as a career can start as volunteers. Volunteering will not only provide valuable experience, it will help the nurse determine if international health is a realistic career choice.

Nurses are employed in epidemiologic studies, communicable disease control, health planning, and the education of nurses and other health professionals. They are engaged in direct care and program administration in most intergovernmental organizations (e.g., the WHO or PAHO).

There are two nursing organizations with an emphasis on international issues. Both organizations facilitate the exchange of interests and concerns among nurses from many countries. The International Council of Nurses (ICN) is a federation of national nursing organizations. There are representatives from 120 countries. The primary goals of the ICN are the advancement of nursing as a profession and the reduction of health disparities by working for change in health policy. Sigma Theta Tau is the international honor society of nursing. This organization is dedicated to supporting nursing leadership, research, and clinical excellence. Like the ICN, Sigma Theta Tau is committed to reducing health disparities and improving health throughout the world.

One of the overriding concerns of all health professionals engaged in public health is the issue of distributive justice

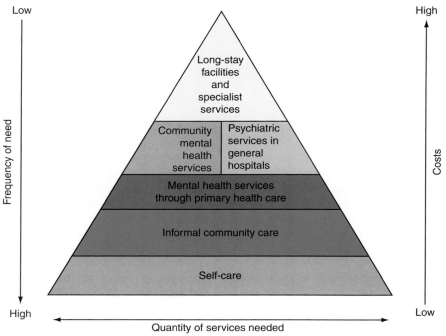

FIGURE 5-4 Optimal mix of mental health services. (From World Health Organization. [2006]. *The world health report 2006: Working together for health.* Geneva: Author.)

(see Chapter 1). Distributive justice works toward eliminating inequalities. The very real global inequalities in health and health care services should be a concern for all community health nurses. Regardless of whether their practices are in international health or at the local level, nurses can help improve global health. Volunteering, engaging in research and clinical practice, maintaining membership in international nursing groups, contributing funds to assistance projects, and engaging in the political process are all ways to help. Together, our efforts will improve the health of the world—one person, one family, one community, and one country at a time.

KEY IDEAS

1. It is in the best interest of all countries to consider health as a global priority. All nurses, whether they advocate, work, or volunteer, can contribute to the goal of world health.
2. Widespread health disparities exist among countries. Health is inversely related to economic status. Richer countries have healthier populations than poor countries.
3. Certain health interventions have been identified as "best buys"; that is, if implemented in developing countries, these actions will have a substantial positive impact on health status in these countries.
4. Intergovernmental organizations provide leadership, financing, and organizational support to assist countries in addressing their health problems.
5. There are many types of voluntary agencies working in world health. Voluntary agencies are free to concentrate on a single health issue or geographic region or to diversify to multiple health concerns and geographic regions.

6. The epidemiologic transition refers to the changing health conditions affecting populations as a country moves from poverty to prosperity.
7. The classic public health measures of sanitation, provision of safe water, and vaccination produce the most dramatic results in developing countries.
8. The problems associated with chronic diseases will increase as health improves and life spans increase throughout the world.
9. All developed countries except the United States have national health care systems dedicated to providing universal health care services to their populations. Developing and middle-income countries continue to expand health care services to their populations as their economic situations improve.
10. All countries, no matter their economic status, continue to struggle with the issues of escalating health care costs, types of health services to guarantee to their peoples, and means of funding the services they provide.
11. New infections, resistant old infections, the environment, illnesses associated with tobacco use, the health effects of war and terrorism, and the scope of mental illnesses have emerged as global health concerns.

LEARNING BY EXPERIENCE AND REFLECTION

1. Identify an international nongovernmental agency that addresses health issues. Explore its organizational structure, funding, staffing. What types of concerns does it address? Where does it concentrate its efforts? How effective has this organization been at addressing its designated health areas?
2. Perform the same exercise for an intergovernmental agency of your choice.

3. Pick a low-income, middle-income, and high-income country.
   a. What are the three leading causes of death and illness in each country?
   b. What are the infant mortality rates and life expectancy for each country?
   c. What type of health care system does each have? How is it funded?
   d. Do health disparities exist in each country? If so, which country has greater health disparity between economic groups?
   e. What has each country identified as health priorities?
4. Using the WHO (2000) criteria for evaluation of health care systems or criteria of your own design, rate how each country selected above has performed with reference to improving health and access to health care services for its population.
5. Reflect on your own health care experiences as a health care provider and as a consumer. Were your experiences positive or negative? What do you think is important in a system of health care? How would you finance such a system? How would you allocate scarce resources?

COMMUNITY RESOURCES FOR PRACTICE

Information about each of the following organizations is found on its website, which can be accessed through the **WebLinks** section of this book's website at *http://evolve.elsevier.com/Maurer/community/*.

Carter Center
Centers for Disease Control and Prevention (CDC)
Bill and Melinda Gates Foundation
Global Health Council
International Council of Nurses (ICN)
Pan American Health Organization (PAHO)
Sigma Theta Tau
United Nations Children's Fund (UNICEF)
U.S. Agency for International Development (USAID)
World Bank
World Health Organization (WHO)

STUDY AIDS   http://evolve.elsevier.com/Maurer/community/

Visit the Evolve website for this book to find the following study and assessment materials:

- Quiz
- Web Scenario
- Critical Thinking Questions and Answers for Case Studies
- Care Plans
- *Healthy People* Updates
- Glossary

REFERENCES

African Network for the Care of Children Affected by AIDS. (2006). *Handbook on paediatric AIDS in Africa* (rev. ed.). Kampala, Uganda: Makerere University.

Altenstetter, C. (2003). Insights from health care in Germany. *American Journal of Public Health*, 93(1), 38-44.

Arias, D. C. (2007). Tiered ranking system unveiled for pandemic influenza threat. *Nation's Health*, 37(3), 1, 26.

Barer, M. L., & Evans, R. G. (1992). Interpreting Canada: Models, mind-sets, and myths. *Health Affairs*, 11(1), 44-61; The search for solutions: Does Canada have the right answer? *Consumer Reports*, 57(9), 579-592.

Basch, P. F. (1999). *Textbook of international health* (2nd ed.). New York: Oxford University Press.

Baum, F. (2002). *The new public health* (2nd ed.). Victoria, Australia: Oxford University Press.

BBC News. (2004). *Hopes of malaria vaccine by 2010.* Retrieved August 12, 2007 from *http://news.bbc. co.uk/2/hi/health/3742876.stm*.

Brody, E. B. (2001). Mental health. In C. E. Koop, C. E. Pearson, & M. R. Schwarz (Eds.), *Critical issues in global health* (pp. 127-134). San Francisco: Jossey-Bass.

Brown, L. D. (2003). Comparing health systems in four countries: Lessons for the United States.

American Journal of Public Health, 93(1), 52-56.

Carter Center. (2003). *Guinea worm eradication program.* Retrieved October 18, 2003 from *http:// www.cartercenter.org/healthprograms/printdoc. asp?programID=1*.

Carter Center. (2006). *What is the magnitude of the problem?* Retrieved January 29, 2008 from *http://www.cartercenter.org/health/river_blind-ness/magnitude.html?printerfriendly=true*.

Carter Center. (2007). *Where is guinea worm disease found?* Retrieved August 11, 2007 from *http://www. cartercenter.org/health/guinea_worm/location.html*.

Carter Center. (2008). *Guinea Worm Eradication Program: How is the Carter Center involved?* Retrieved January 29, 2008 from *http://www. cartercenter.org/health/guinea_worm/center.html*.

Concern Worldwide. (2005). *Child survival.* New York: Author.

Daniels, N., Bryant, J., Castano, R. A., et al. (2000). Benchmarks of fairness for health care reform: A policy tool for developing countries. *Bulletin of the World Health Organization*, 78(6), 740-750.

Davey, V. J. (2007). Questions and answers on pandemic influenza. *American Journal of Nursing*, 107(7), 50-57.

Davis, K., Schoen, C., Schoenbaum, S. C., et al. (2007). *Mirror, mirror on the wall:*

An international update on the comparative performance of American health care. The Commonwealth Fund. Retrieved January 29, 2007 from *http://www.commonwealth-fund.org/publications/publications_show. htm?doc_id=482678*.

Deber, R. B. (2003). Health care reform: Lessons from Canada. *American Journal of Public Health*, 93(1), 20-24.

deOnis, M., Frongillo, E. A., & Blossner, M. (2000). Is malnutrition declining? An analysis of changes in levels of child malnutrition since 1980. *Bulletin of the World Health Organization*, 78(10), 1222-1233.

Detels, R., & Breslow, L. (2002). Current scope and concerns in public health. In R. Detels, J. McEwen, R. Beaglehole, et al. (Eds.), *Oxford textbook of public health: The scope of public health* (4th ed.; pp. 3-20). Oxford, England: Oxford University Press.

Eberwine-Villagran, D. (2007). Best buys for public health. *Perspectives in Health*, 11(1), 2-9.

Espring-Anderson, G. (1990). *The three worlds of welfare capitalism.* Princeton: Princeton University Press.

Global Health Council. (2007a). *Press.* Retrieved January 29, 2008 from *http://www. globalhealth. org/view_top.php3?id=182*.

Global Health Council. (2007b). *Global health council position paper on child health.* Washington, DC: Author.

Hepatitis B Foundation. (2007). *General information: FAQ.* Retrieved January 29, 2008 from *http://www.hepb.org/patients/general_ information.htm.*

Hurst, J. (2000). Challenges for health systems in member countries of the Organisation for Economic Co-operation and Development. *Bulletin of the World Health Organization, 78*(6), 751-760.

Kemp, C., & Rashbridge, L. (2004). *Refugee and immigrant health: A handbook for health professionals.* Cambridge, England: Cambridge University Press.

Kinra, S., Black, M. E., Mondic, S., et al. (2002). Impact of the Bosnian conflict on the health of women and children. *Bulletin of the World Health Organization, 80*(1), 75-76.

Kresge, K. J. (2006). *Couples voluntary counseling and testing.* New York: International AIDS Vaccine Initiative.

Kresge, K. J. (2007). AIDS vaccine trials. *AIDS Vaccine Bulletin, 5*(1), 1.

Krisberg, K. (2007a). Drug-resistant TB becoming more commonplace globally. *Nation's Health, 37*(6), 1, 20.

Krisberg, K. (2007b). Climate change predicted to have dire effects on health. *Nation's Health, 37*(3), 1, 12.

Kunitz, S. J., & Pesis-Katz, I. (2005). Mortality of white Americans, African Americans, and Canadians: The causes and consequences for health of welfare state institutions and policies. *Melbrook Quarterly, 83*(1), 5-39.

Lasser, K. E., Himmelstein, D. U., & Woolhandler, S. (2006). Access to health care, health status, and health disparities in the United States and Canada: Results of a cross-national population-based survey. *American Journal of Public Health, 96*(7), 1300-1303.

Lee, J. C. (2003). Health care reform in South Korea: Success or failure? *American Journal of Public Health, 93*(1), 48-51.

Lee, K., & Fidler, D. (2007). Avian and pandemic influenza: Progress and problems with global health governance. *Global Public Health, 2*(3), 215-234.

Lions International. (2007). *The SightFirst program.* Retrieved September 5, 2007 from *http://www.lions-csfii.org/live/content/sightfirst_program.shtml.*

McKee, M. (2001). The health consequences of the collapse of the Soviet Union. In D. Leon & G. Walt (Eds.), *Poverty inequality and health: An international perspective* (pp. 17-36). Oxford, England: Oxford University Press.

McKee, N., Bertrand, J. T., & Becker-Benton, A. (2004). *Strategic communication in the HIV/ AIDS epidemic.* New Delhi: Sage.

McKenzie, J. F., Pinger, R. R., & Kotecki, J. E. (1999). *An introduction to community health* (3rd ed.). Boston: Jones & Bartlett.

McMichael, A. J. (2002). The environment. In R. Detels, J. McEwen, R. Beaglehole, et al. (Eds.), *Oxford textbook of public health: The scope of public health* (4th ed.; pp. 195-214). Oxford, England: Oxford University Press.

Moran, D., & Jordaan, J. A. (2007). HIV/AIDS in Russia: Determinants of regional prevalence. *International Journal of Health Geographics, 6*(22), 1-23.

Morse, S. S. (1995). Factors in the emergence of infectious diseases. *Emerging Infectious Diseases, 1*, 7-15.

Murphy, E. M. (2005). *Promoting healthy behavior.* Health Bulletin 2. Washington, DC: Population Reference Bureau.

Nagelkerke, N., Jha, P., deVlas, S. D., et al. (2002). Modeling HIV/AIDS epidemics in Botswana and India: Impact of interventions to prevent transmission. *Bulletin of the World Health Organization, 80*(2), 89-96.

National Oceanic and Atmospheric Administration. (2005). *Climate of 2005: Summary of Hurricane Katrina.* Retrieved June 24, 2007 from *http://www.ncdc.noaa.gov/oa/climate/research/2005/katrina.html.*

Neustadt, R. E., & Fineberg, H. V. (1978). *The swine flu affair.* Washington, DC: U.S. Department of Health, Education and Welfare.

Novelli, W. D. (2005). Managing health, health care, and aging. In W. H. Foege, N. Daulaire, R. E. Black, et al. (Eds.), *Global health leadership and management* (pp. 37-51). San Francisco: Jossey-Bass.

Organization for Economic Co-operation and Development. (2006). *Rising health costs put pressure on public finances.* Paris: Author.

Pan American Health Organization. (2003a). *What is PAHO?* Retrieved October 18, 2003 from *http://www.paho.org/english/paho/what-paho.htm.*

Pan American Health Organization. (2003b, June). Vaccine week in the Americas: A gesture of love. *PAHO Today,* Special Edition. Retrieved October 18, 2003 from *http://www.paho.org/ english/DD/ pin/ptoday_vaccination.htm.*

Patel, V. (2001). Poverty, inequality, and mental health in developing countries. In D. Leon, & G. Walt (Eds.), *Poverty inequality and health: An international perspective* (pp. 39-62). Oxford, England: Oxford University Press.

Physicians for a National Health Program. (2007). *Snapshots of health systems in 16 countries.* Retrieved August 20, 2007 from *http://www.pnhp.org/facts/international_health_systems. php?page=all.*

Population Reference Bureau. (2006). *2006 world population sheet.* Washington, DC: Author.

Roberts, M., & Rhoades, J. A. (2007). *The uninsured in American, first half of 2006: Estimates for the U.S. civilian noninstitutionalized population under age 65* (Statistical Brief No. 171). Rockville, MD: Agency for Healthcare Research and Quality.

Roemer, M. (1991). *National health care systems of the world.* New York: Oxford University Press.

Rotary International. (2007). *Rotary's health projects* (Fact Sheet 01/07-EN). Evanston, IL: Author.

Sandman, P. (2007, Spring). The two faces of pandemic risk communication. *Advances from the University of Minnesota School of Public Health,* p. 9.

Sein, T., & Rafei, U. M. (2002). The history and development of public health in developing countries. In R. Detels, J. McEwen, R. Beaglehole, et al. (Eds.), *Oxford textbook of public health: The scope of public health* (4th ed.). Oxford, England: Oxford University Press.

Taravella, S. (2005). *The Kenyan workplace: A strong tool for HIV prevention and treatment.* Arlington, VA: Family Health International.

United Nations Children's Fund. (2006). *With the horn of Africa on the brink of famine, need for drought relief grows.* Retrieved January 29, 2008 from *http://www.unicef.org/emerg/27402_33193. html?q=preintme.*

United Nations Children's Fund. (2007). *About UNICEF: Who we are.* Retrieved January 28, 2008 from *http://www.unicef.org/about/who/ index_introduction.html?q=printme.*

United Nations Intergovernmental Panel on Climate Change. (2001). *Climate change 2001: The scientific basis.* Oxford, England: Oxford University Press.

United Nations Millennium Project. (2006). *The 0.7% target: Net ODA [official development assistance] in 2005—as a percentage of GNI [gross national income].* Retrieved August 11, 2007 from *http:// www.unmillenniumproject.org/press/action 7_oecd05.htm.*

United Nations Refugee Agency. (2006). *The state of the world's refugees 2006—Chapter 7: Internally displaced persons: Introduction.* Retrieved September 5, 2007 from *http://www.unhcr.org/cgi-bin/texis/vtx/print?tbl=PUBL&id=4444d3cc11.*

U.S. Agency for International Development. (2002). *Report on the global HIV/AIDS epidemic 2002.* Retrieved August 23, 2003 from *http://www.aids. org/barcelona/presskit/ barcelona%20report/contents_html.html.*

U.S. Agency for International Development. (2003a). *Liberia—Complex emergency* (Situation Report No. 33). Washington, DC: Author.

U.S. Agency for International Development. (2003b). *Improving health—USAID Afghanistan.* Retrieved October 27, 2003 from *http:// www.usaid.gov/location/ASIA_near_east/afghanistan/health.html.*

U.S. Agency for International Development. (2007a, May 24). *Avian influenza. Program update.* Washington, DC: Author.

U.S. Agency for International Development. (2007b). *USAID/Afghanistan: Outgoing USAID director announces completion of over 1000 development projects since July 2006.* Retrieved September 6, 2007 from *http://afghanistan. usaid.gov/en/Article.159.aspx.*

U.S. Agency for International Development. (2007c). *USAID/Afghanistan: Overview.*

Retrieved September 6, 2007 from *http://usaid. gov/locations/asia_near_east/countries/ afghanistan*.

U.S. Agency for International Development. (2008). *Afghanistan*. Retrieved January 29, 2008 from *http://www.usaid.gov/locations/Asia_near_East/ countries/Afghanistan*.

Uys, L. A. (2006). Encouraging service through collaboration: Development of nursing and midwifery in Africa [Electronic version]. *Reflections on Nursing Leadership, 32*(4),1-7.

Wagstaff, A. (2002). Poverty and health sector inequalities. *Bulletin of the World Health Organization, 80*(2), 97-105.

Washington Profile. (2007). *Russia profile: Health and demography in the post-Soviet space,* September 3-4. Retrieved September 5, 2007 from *http://www.washprofile.org*.

Williams, S. J. (2002). Patterns of illness and disease and access to health care. In S. J. Williams & P. R. Torrens (Eds.), *Introduction to health care services* (6th ed.; pp. 61-90). Clifton Park, NY: Delmar.

World Health Organization. (1978). *Primary health care: Report of the International Conference on Primary Health Care, Alma-Ata*. Geneva: Author.

World Health Organization. (1998a). *Health for all in the twenty-first century*. Geneva: Author.

World Health Organization. (1998b). *World health report 1998: Life in the twenty-first century: A vision for all*. Geneva: Author.

World Health Organization. (1998c). *Reducing mortality from major killers of children* (Fact Sheet No. 178). Geneva: Author.

World Health Organization. (2000). *World health report 2000: Health systems: Improving performance*. Geneva: Author.

World Health Organization. (2001a). Water and health, hand-in-hand for a day. *Bulletin of the World Health Organization, 79*(5), 486.

World Health Organization. (2001b). Sponging cattle with insecticide halves malaria incidence in study. *Bulletin of the World Health Organization, 79*(8), 797.

World Health Organization. (2001c). Countries split over tobacco treaty. *Bulletin of the World Health Organization, 79*(7), 690.

World Health Organization. (2001d). *Public health response to biological and chemical weapons*. Retrieved October 23, 2003 from *http://www. who.int/emc/pdfs/BIOWEAPONS_exec_ sum.2pdf*.

World Health Organization. (2001e). *World health report 2001: Mental health: New understanding, new hope*. Geneva: Author.

World Health Organization. (2002a). *Deaths by cause, sex, and mortality stratum in WHO regions, estimates for 2001*. Retrieved October 23, 2003 from *http://www.who.int/entity/who/2002/en/annex_ table2.xls*.

World Health Organization. (2002b). *What is roll back malaria?* Retrieved October 23, 2003 from *http://www.who.int/inf-fs/un/ Informationsheet02. pdf*.

World Health Organization. (2002c, August). *Tuberculosis* (revised) (Fact Sheet No. 104). Geneva: Author.

World Health Organization. (2002d). WHO attacks tobacco sponsorship of sports. *Bulletin of the World Health Organization, 80*(1), 80-81.

World Health Organization. (2003a). *World health report 2003: Shaping the future*. Geneva: Author.

World Health Organization. (2003b). *Two diseases—One patient: Report of the Third Working Group Meeting, Monteaux*. Geneva: Author.

World Health Organization. (2003c). *Poliomyelitis* (Fact Sheet No. 114). Geneva: Author.

World Health Organization. (2003d). *Introduction to managing TB at the raion level*. Geneva: Author.

World Health Organization. (2003e). *Mental health in emergencies: Mental and social aspects of health of populations exposed to extreme stress*. Geneva: Author.

World Health Organization. (2004). *World health report 2004: Changing history*. Geneva: Author.

World Health Organization. (2005a). *WHO programme budget 2006-2007: Orientations for implementation in the African region*. Retrieved September 5, 2007 from *http://www.afro.who.int/ rc55/documents/afr_rc55_7_pb_2006-2007.pdf*.

World Health Organization. (2005b). *World health report 2005: Make every mother and child count*. Geneva: Author.

World Health Organization. (2005c, March). *Immunization against diseases of public health importance: The benefits of immunization*. (Fact Sheet No. 288). Geneva: Author.

World Health Organization. (2006a, September). *Diabetes: What is diabetes?* (Fact Sheet No. 312). Geneva: Author.

World Health Organization. (2006b). *World health report 2006: Working together for health*. Geneva: Author.

World Health Organization. (2006c). *Preventing disease through healthy environments: Towards an estimate of the environmental burden of disease*. Geneva: Author.

World Health Organization. (2006d). *World health statistics 2006: Part 1. Ten statistical highlights in global public health*. Geneva: Author.

World Health Organization. (2006e). *Facts and figures about tobacco. First Conference of the Parties to the WHO Framework Convention on Tobacco Control, 6-17 February 2006*. Geneva: Author.

World Health Organization. (2007a). *World health statistics 2007*. Geneva: Author.

World Health Organization. (2007b). *Access to HIV treatment improves*. Retrieved August 29, 2007 from *http://health.netscape.com/story/2007/04/17/ who-access-to-hiv-treatment-improves*.

World Health Organization. (2007c). *WHO Report 2007: Global tuberculosis control, surveillance, planning, financing*. Geneva: Author.

World Health Organization. (2007d). *WHO Stop TB partnership: 2007 Tuberculosis facts*. Retrieved September 5, 2007 from *http://www.who.int/tb/ publications/2007/factsheet_2007.pdf*.

World Health Organization. (2007e). *Vector-borne viral infections*. Retrieved September 5, 2007 from *http://www.who.int/vaccine_research/diseases/ vector/en/print.html*.

World Health Organization. (2007f). *Cumulative number of confirmed human cases of avian influenza A/(H5N1) reported to WHO*. Retrieved August 24, 2007 from *http://www. who.int/csr/disease/avian_influenza/country/ cases_table_2007_08_23/en/index.html*.

World Health Organization. (2007g). *World health report 2007: A safer future*. Geneva: Author.

SUGGESTED READINGS

Altenstetter, C. (2003). Insights from health care in Germany. *American Journal of Public Health, 93*(1), 38-44.

Beah, I. (2007). *A long way gone: Memoirs of a boy soldier*. New York: Farrar, Straus & Giroux.

Brown, L. D. (2003). Comparing health systems in four countries: Lessons for the United States. *American Journal of Public Health, 93*(1), 52-56.

Close, W. T. (1995). *Ebola: A documentary novel of its first explosion*. New York: Ivy Books.

Deber, R. B. (2003). Health care reform: Lessons from Canada. *American Journal of Public Health, 93*(1), 20-24.

Detels, R., McEwen, J., Beaglehole, R., et al. (Eds.). (2002). *Oxford textbook of public health: The scope of public health* (4th ed.). Oxford, England: Oxford University Press.

Drexler, M. (2002). *Secret agents: The menace of emerging infection*. Washington, DC: Joseph Henry Press.

Kalipeni, E., Craddock, S., Oppong, J. R., et al. (2004). *HIV and AIDS in Africa: Beyond epidemiology*. Oxford, England: Blackwell.

Kemp, C., & Rashbridge, L. (2004). *Refugee and immigrant health: A handbook for health professionals*. Cambridge, England: Cambridge University Press.

Kolata, Gina. (1999). *Flu: The story of the great influenza pandemic of 1918 and the search for the virus that caused it*. New York: Farrar, Straus & Giroux.

Leon, D., & Walt, G. (Eds.). (2001). *Poverty, inequality, and mental health in developing countries: An international perspective*. Oxford, England: Oxford University Press.

Light, D. W. (2003). Universal health care: Lessons from the British experience. *American Journal of Public Health*, *93*(1), 25-30.

Osborn, G., & Ohmans, P. (2005). *Finding work in global health*. St. Paul, MN: Health Advocates Press.

Rodwin, V. G. (2003). The health care system under French national health insurance: Lessons for health reform in the United States. *American Journal of Public Health*, *93*(1), 31-37.

World Health Organization. (2002). *World health report 2002: Reducing risks, promoting healthy life*. Geneva: Author.

World Health Organization. (2007). *World health report 2007: A safer future*. Geneva: Author.

*Susan Wozenski**

FOCUS QUESTIONS

How are basic legal issues relevant to community/public health nursing practice?

What are the sources and purposes of public health law?

What are the responsibilities or legal duties of community/public health nurses related to public health law?

When might a community/public health nurse not be covered by the employer's professional liability insurance?

What are the responsibilities of community/public health nurses in being accountable for their own practice?

How are legal and ethical issues alike and different?

CHAPTER OUTLINE

KEY TERMS

*The author acknowledges the contribution of Penny S. Brooke to this chapter in the previous editions of the book.

PUBLIC HEALTH LAW

Public health law includes all laws that have a significant impact on the health of defined populations. These laws originate from multiple sources, including the U.S. Constitution, state constitutions, statutes, legislative rulings, governmental agency rules and regulations, judicial rulings, case law, and public policies. Public health law shapes public health practice through the numerous sources of law and disciplines of legal practice. Public health law also addresses the power and responsibility of government to protect the health of the population and defines the limits on the power of government to constrain the rights of individuals (Goodman et al., 2006).

Under the authority of the U.S. Constitution, federal public health law exists to promote the general welfare of society. Because states retain those powers not delegated to the federal government, much of public health law remains under state jurisdiction. As a result, there is significant variation among states regarding specific public health laws. Local jurisdictions, such as counties, cities, or townships, receive their authority from the state to enact public health law (Turnock, 2004).

Statutory law is enacted through the legislative branch of government. Laws of the legislative branches of the federal and state governments are called *statutes.* Similar laws of local governments are usually called *ordinances.* Statutes often authorize new health initiatives and appropriate tax funds to implement the law. Community/public health nurses can influence the political process by lobbying legislators for or against specific statutes and ordinances.

Administrative law consists of orders, rules, and regulations promulgated by the administrative branches of governments. For example, the state board of nursing is the administrative body that regulates the practice of nursing. Other examples of administrative bodies are the U.S. Department of Health and Human Services and state and local health departments. Administrative law often details the policies and procedures necessary to implement statutes. Community/public health nurses can influence the development of administrative law by initiating ideas and commenting on proposed regulations during periods for public review.

Judicial or common law is developed through federal and state court decisions. The facts and law in previously decided cases are compared with the current factual situation before the court to determine similarities and differences.

Because there are multiple layers of public health law (state, local, federal), because portions of public health law are intermingled in laws affecting other governmental operations, and because differences exist among the various state public health laws, there is some confusion as to how to interpret and enforce the laws. Recommendations to improve federal and state laws and provide clarity include the following (Turnock, 2004):

- Provide a stronger link with the overall mission and core functions of public health (see Chapter 29)
- Bring consistency to the confidentiality provisions
- Clarify the police power responsibilities in dealing with health risks and threats
- Ensure fairer, more consistent enforcement of public health laws

COMMUNITY/PUBLIC HEALTH NURSES AND PUBLIC HEALTH LAW

Official (government) health agencies often enforce laws in addition to providing health services, and nurses are often part of that enforcement process. Community/public health nurses most often work autonomously without the opportunity for on-site immediate collaboration with other nurses or members of the health care team. Nurses as professionals are accountable for the nursing judgments they make. Consumers see nurses as trustworthy experts in their field and rely on what nurses tell them. However, if a client is harmed because of a nurse's action, inaction, or incorrect advice, the nurse can be held legally accountable for the resulting injury.

Lawsuits brought against nurses most often result from action or failure to act that causes injury to patient; in many cases, they result from failure to adhere to standards of care. The number of lawsuits alleging negligence or malpractice brought against nurses has been increasing (National Practitioner Data Bank, 2005). However, lawsuits against nurses accounted for only 8% of all lawsuits in 2004, and malpractice payments involving nurses account for only 1.2% of all malpractice payments (National Practitioner Data Bank, 2004). Most claims brought against nurses involve nurses working with other practice disciplines (nurse anesthetists, nurse practitioners, obstetric nurses), not nurses in public health practice. Because of that, legal cases related to public health nursing practice are hard to find. One area that does relate to public health practice is the area of vaccine administration. Two cases have yielded conflicting decisions. In *Walker v Merck and Co.* (1986), a licensed practical nurse was deemed liable in administering a vaccination without due caution (e.g., teaching about side effects, knowing when not to administer a vaccine), whereas in *Mazur v Merck and Co.* (1992), a registered nurse was not held liable. Although such lawsuits are still rare, home health care has experienced increases in lawsuits, and suits in this area of community health practice can be expected to increase as the number of clients needing home care services increases.

Community/public health nurses not only need to understand the legal protections and rights of the public, but they also need to be able to advocate for themselves. Protection of professional practice includes avoiding compromising positions in which one is expected to practice outside the scope of nursing. The Nurse Practice Act in each state defines what is legally within the scope of nursing practice. Community/public health nurses are accountable for working within this legal framework. A copy of this statute should be available through employers, the state nurses' association, or the state board of nursing.

In this chapter, legal issues in community/public health nursing are broadly described, and the rights of the public or clients and the rights of the nurse are discussed. Laws are written to protect the rights of nurses and their clients. If nurses work within the guidelines of the law, safe care will be provided, which benefits both the client and the nurse. Federal laws and regulations apply to persons throughout the United States, whereas state and local laws apply within the respective state and local jurisdictions. It is important for nurses to be aware of the laws for which they will be held accountable in their states. For example, state or public agencies might be protected by immunity statutes, whereas private agencies might not be included in these statutory protections. Facts and legal issues of case law are used to evaluate potential liability and are constantly changing. Individual nurses are responsible for familiarizing themselves with specific laws in their states, such as the Nurse Practice Act and the state board of nursing rules and regulations. Nurses have become more mobile and might have worked in several states during their careers. Laws differ from state to state, but ignorance is no defense for the violation of a statute, rule, or regulation.

SOURCES OF LAW

All laws that govern society are designed to maintain order and to inform those who are accountable to the law of the expected behavior and of behavior that will not be allowed. Laws are written to carry out the wishes of the majority and to protect the rights of the minority. Laws and policies are made by legislators, as well as administrators, regulators, boards, and committees.

Environmental and public health issues are of special concern and interest to communities. Laws in these areas are usually enacted by the legislative and administrative bodies of individual states. Federal lawmakers provide the guidelines or the "umbrella" laws. States must abide by federal laws and must avoid enacting state statutes that conflict with federal guidelines. Both state and federal courts write case law or common law, which reflects society's current beliefs regarding what best serves public welfare. Sometimes the laws within which nurses must work lend themselves to varied interpretations. In these cases, agencies must seek the opinion of their state's attorney general.

Rules, regulations, and statutes guide the community/public health nurse and are references with which the nurse must become familiar. A specific law cannot be read in isolation; a wider scope is needed to understand the nurse's total legal responsibilities. For example, when communicable diseases are reported, both state and federal laws must be considered. Local ordinances and regulations also apply. Table 6-1 provides examples of public health law from all three levels of government that a community health nurse might encounter in caring for a family.

TABLE 6-1   Examples of Law Affecting Clients and Nursing Practice

Community Health Situation

A student nurse is asked to assess a family of five; a mother, age 36, caring for a 2-month-old infant; a 6-year-old child in school; a maternal grandmother, 65, with diabetes; and a son, 21, who works as a short-order cook. The mother receives Temporary Assistance to Needy Families (TANF) for the two youngest children. She desires to keep another youngster in her home. Neighbors have complained about the noisy dogs. The 21-year-old has been diagnosed by stool culture as being infected with *Salmonella*.

Level of Government	Sources of Applicable Law		
	Legislative Law	**Administrative Law**	**Judicial Law**
Local	Nuisances (dogs) Leash laws; requirements for rabies vaccinations	Procedure for hearings	Previous decisions regarding nuisances
State	Daycare licensing needed	Details regarding who orients mothers for daycare and what is included	
	Immunization requirements for 6-year-old	Interpretation of what constitutes "initial series" of immunizations for various ages	Court decisions regarding religious exemptions from immunizations
	Reportable diseases (Salmonella) under General Welfare; might detail that those with infectious diseases cannot handle food	Delegates authority to implement programs to protect the public's health	
	Nurse Practice Act enables students to practice	State board of nursing issues rules and regulations to allow student learners to practice nursing	
Federal	Medicare for grandmother	Forms and information necessary for clients to enroll; delegates authority to implement	Decisions regarding sexual discrimination in Social Security payments
	Medicaid for those on Temporary Assistance to Needy Families (TANF) Food stamps	States must continue to provide coverage to any family member who would have been eligible for TANF; can be cut off as a sanction if a family fails to meet its work requirements Same as Medicare for grandmother	

Courtesy of Claudia M. Smith, RN, BC, MPH, PhD, Assistant Professor, University of Maryland School of Nursing.

STATE AND LOCAL STATUTES

There are many public health statutes enacted by state legislatures that are of concern to community/public health nurses. Statutes seek to protect the rights of both the health care provider and the consumer. **Nurse Practice Acts** are broad frameworks within which the legal scope of nursing practice is defined. Many states also have statutes defining *malpractice* actions against health care providers that pertain to community health nurses. These laws have a **statute of limitations** for malpractice actions or a time frame within which a legal action must be brought. Often, the specific procedures for bringing a lawsuit against a health care provider are also defined within these malpractice statutes.

Balancing Client Rights Versus Public Health

State legislatures also enact statutes under health codes that describe laws for reporting communicable diseases, laws regarding school immunizations, and additional laws directed toward promoting health and reducing health risks in the community. An individual's right to privacy may conflict with the public health duty to protect the general public (e.g., the duty to disclose information about the public health risks of an individual's contagious disease). States have a duty to warn unless expressly forbidden by statute. For example, in a Georgia case involving a child with meningitis, a hospital was ruled liable for failure to notify persons who came in contact with the child during the contagious period. In another example, a man in California discovered that he had contracted human immunodeficiency virus (HIV) infection from his girlfriend. The court ruled that he could sue the girlfriend's doctor for failure to inform her that she had received contaminated blood, the source of the infection.

There are limits to permissible disclosures. These limits are dictated by each state's statutory and common law. For this reason, it is important for nurses to become familiar with the relevant state and local reporting and notification requirements. Some states allow health departments to engage in contact investigation and partner notification without the express permission of the infected person (Guido, 1997). For example, in the state of Georgia, one can notify a spouse, sexual partner, or child; in the state of New York, one can notify contacts if the infected person refuses to do so.

There are special circumstances surrounding the handling of contacts of persons with HIV/acquired immunodeficiency syndrome (AIDS). All clinicians are required by state law to report cases of AIDS to the local health departments. Some states require HIV infection case reporting to the health department. Most states hold the information strictly confidential, which means that health departments are not allowed to contact sexual partners or close contacts without the permission of the infected person. Some states permit the disclosure of HIV/AIDS to certain close contacts under certain conditions. It is important to be very familiar with the laws in your states pertaining to your responsibilities with reference to reporting and disclosing otherwise confidential information.

Health Records

The records required to be kept by health care providers might be described within a state's health code. State laws also usually address actions to be taken in reporting child abuse or neglect and the penalties associated with failure to report known or suspected cases of abuse. A growing number of states have enacted confidential communications protection for sexual abuse acts. Immunity from legal action is afforded to health care providers who, in good faith, report suspected abuse of a client to a legal authority. Statutes also define penalties for not reporting known cases of abuse.

Statutes affording protection for privileged communication of confidential information learned in the professional role might, but do not always, include the community/public health nurse. It is important for nurses to be aware of the protections afforded in their states to confidential nurse-client communications. If a state's statutes do not entitle nurses to a nurse-client privilege, nurses will not be able to hold all communications with clients confidential. In most states, nurse-client communications do not have the privilege of confidentiality.

Community/public health nurses must be aware of the state's laws pertaining to family privacy matters, such as abortion, distribution of contraceptives to minors, and family violence. Their clients might seek advice on these matters. Community/public health nurses might also be asked to explain a living will statute, if one exists in their state, and the uses of a durable power of attorney (see Chapter 28). Statutes that require specific behaviors, such as the procedures for pronouncing a client dead or reporting child abuse, vary among states. Practicing attorneys from each state can clarify the specific expectations of community/public health nurses in that state.

FEDERAL STATUTES

Federal statutes should be of interest to community/public health nurses. The Public Health Service and the Centers for Disease Control and Prevention (CDC) were created by Congress to coordinate the collection, sharing, and analysis of data from all of the states and the U.S. territories on certain diseases. Guidelines for dealing with legal issues pertaining to the reporting requirements, such as the importance of maintaining confidentiality, are issued by the CDC. The Occupational Safety and Health Administration (OSHA) also provides guidelines for safe and healthy work environments.

In August of 1996, Congress passed the **Health Insurance Portability and Accountability Act (HIPAA).** Enforcement of HIPAA privacy regulations began in April 2003. HIPAA provides clients with greater control over their personal health information (e.g., a client's condition, care, and payments for health care). HIPAA protects confidentiality by defining what privacy rights clients have, who should have access to client information, what constitutes the client's right to confidentiality, and what constitutes inappropriate access to health records. *Confidentiality* concerns how records should be protected, and *security* involves measures the nurse and others must take to ensure privacy and confidentiality (Frank-Stromborg & Ganschow, 2002). Providers of care must notify clients of their privacy policy and make a good faith effort to obtain a written acknowledgment of this notification. It is the nurse's responsibility to protect client confidentiality. Nurses need to understand both the federal HIPAA regulations and the state laws that are enacted to enforce those regulations, as well as any changes or updates to either of these. Employers affected by HIPAA are responsible for ensuring that the nurses they employ comply with the regulations.

Another example of a federal statute that must be understood by community/public health nurses is the Social Security Act and its amendments. In these Social Security amendments, the enactment of the Medicare and Medicaid programs is of specific interest to community health clients (see Chapter 4). Community health clients who are eligible for either Medicaid or Services for Children with Special Health Care Needs should also be made aware of the Early and Periodic Screening Diagnosis and Treatment (EPSDT) Program. These programs are discussed in detail in Chapter 27.

Without an adequate knowledge base or understanding of federally enacted programs, community health nurses might neglect to inform qualified clients of existing federal programs. Children who qualify for EPSDT are eligible to receive immunizations, eye examinations, hearing tests, and dental care. Countless previously undiagnosed conditions might be discovered and treated as a result of this early diagnosis and screening program. Other examples of federal statutory law are included in Table 6-2.

ADMINISTRATIVE RULES AND REGULATIONS

Rules and regulations are established by administrative bodies of government, such as licensing boards and regulatory agencies. Administrative bodies, including state nursing boards and health departments, are composed of experts in the field who are considered to be better prepared than the average layperson to make decisions regarding the specific rules and regulations

---

TABLE 6-2   Federal Legislation that Influences Public Health

Title	Purpose	Impact of Law
Social Security Act and Amendments		
Social Security Act of 1935 (PL 7427t), Title I: Grants to States for Old Age Assistance	To enable each state to furnish financial assistance to aged needy people.	Created Title II, Federal Old Age Benefit payment to persons over 65 years of age (Social Security); Title III, Unemployment Compensation; Title IV, Aid to Dependent Children; Title V, Maternal-Child Welfare to promote health, especially rural health of women and children; Title VI, Public Health Work to maintain public health services, including training of personnel; Title VII, the Social Security Board; Title VIII, Taxes With Respect to Employment; Title IX, tax on employers with eight or more employees; Title X, Grants to States for Aid to the Blind; Title XI, General Provisions.
Maternal and Child Health and Retardation Amendments of 1963 (PL 88156)	Amends the Social Security Act to assist states and communities in preventing and combating mental retardation.	Expanded and improved maternal and child health in Services for Children with Special Health Care Needs; provides prenatal, maternity, and infant care to combat mental retardation.
Social Security Amendments of 1965 (PL 8797), Title XIX: Grants to States for Medical Assistance Program	Provided funding to states to establish medical assistance for the needy as defined under the act.	Established a state plan to provide medical assistance to families with dependent children, the aged, the blind, and permanently and totally disabled individuals whose income and resources are insufficient to meet the costs of necessary medical care; also established rehabilitation services to assist clients in obtaining or retaining the capacity for independence or self-care.
Social Security Amendments of 1965 (PL 8797), Title XVIII: Health Insurance for the Aged (known as Medicare; Tied into Railroad Retirement Act of 1937)	Established hospital and medical insurance benefits for persons older than 65 years of age who are residents of the United States (i.e., a citizen or lawful alien who has resided continually in the United States during the preceding 5 years).	Provides specified health benefits to eligible clients. Benefits might vary from year to year; a monthly premium is paid (refer to Chapter 4).
Social Security Amendments of 1977— Health Clinic Services (PL 95210).	Authorizes reimbursement for clinic services in rural areas designated as a health manpower shortage area.	Clinics that employ physician assistants or nurse practitioners are eligible for reimbursement under Medicare or Medicaid if the client population is below 3000 or there are no physicians practicing within 5 miles of the clinic.
Public Health Services Act and Amendments		
Public Health Services Act of 1944 (PL 78410)	Created federally coordinated departments to address the public health needs of the nation; established the office of the Surgeon General and the National Institutes of Health, the Bureau of Medical Services, and the Bureau of State Services; the divisions created are administered by the Surgeon General.	Power to establish divisions was given to the Surgeon General, who serves as the administrator of the Public Health Services Act.

Continued

TABLE 6-2   **Federal Legislation that Influences Public Health—cont'd**

Title	Purpose	Impact of Law
Public Health Services Act and Amendments—cont'd		
Special Health Revenue Sharing Act of 1975 (PL 9463)	Amended the Public Health Services Act and related health laws to revise and extend the health revenue sharing program, providing comprehensive public health services; grants to state health and mental health authorities were made to assist with the cost of providing care.	Programs affected by these grants include family planning programs; community mental health center programs, including the requirements for the mental health centers; programs and centers for migrant worker health; community health centers; and miscellaneous home health services, mental health and illness of the elderly; the National Health Service Corps program; commissions on epilepsy, Huntington's disease, and hemophilia programs; assistance for nurse training and for other purposes such as the advanced nurse training and nurse practice programs, special projects, grants, and contracts.
Social Services		
Omnibus Budget Reconciliation Act of 1981, Block Grants for Social Services and Health (PL 97-35).	Created to consolidate federal assistance to states for social services into a single grant to increase the states' flexibility in using grants to achieve the goals of preventing, reducing, or eliminating dependency; achieving or maintaining self-sufficiency; or preventing or remedying neglect, abuse, and exploitation of children and adults unable to protect their own interests; to rehabilitate and reunite families and provide for community home-based care. The Maternal and Child Health Services Block Grant was created to ensure low-income persons with limited availability for health services access to quality maternal and child health services. Subtitle C block grants for social services consolidated federal assistance to the states for social services into a single grant.	Increased flexibility for states in coverage of and services for the medically needy. Human services affected by Title VI include education of the handicapped; vocational rehabilitation programs; handicapped programs and services; older Americans' domestic volunteers and senior companion programs; child abuse prevention and treatment; community services program; urban and rural special impact programs; supportive programs to Head Start; Title VIII, School Lunch and Nutrition Programs; Title IX, Health Services Facilities; rodent control; fluoridation programs; hypertension; developmental disabilities; research; health planning and maintenance; adolescent family; alcohol and drug programs; Title XXI Medicare, Medicaid, and maternal and child health reimbursement changes (changes in services and benefits); Title XXII Federal Old-Age Survivors and Disability Insurance Program newly defined benefits; Title XXIII, Aid to Families and Dependent Children (AFDC, Temporary Assistance to Needy Families [TANF])—past-due child support can be collected from federal tax refunds.
Health Centers Consolidation Act (PL 104-299) 1996	Community health centers, migrant centers, health care for the homeless, and public housing service grants are consolidated under one grant program and reauthorized through fiscal year 2001. Yearly reauthorization thereafter.	Community health centers provide comprehensive case managed primary health care to medically indigent and underserved populations. Migrant health centers provide primary care to migrant and seasonal agricultural workers and their families. Health services for the homeless provide project grants to community health centers and nonprofit coalitions, inner-city hospitals, and local public health departments to deliver primary care, substance abuse, and mental health services to homeless adults and children. Public housing service grants are awarded to community-based organizations to provide case managed ambulatory primary help and social services in clinics at or near public housing. Health centers that provide services to medically underserved populations with high incidents of infant mortality are eligible for such grants as well as health centers that have experienced a significant increase in the incidents of infant mortality. Authorizes grants to rural health centers to ensure that people living in underserved rural areas have access to health care. Grants are made for rural health outreach, network development, and telemedicine.
Health-Related Amendments to the VA/HUD FY1997 Appropriations Bill (PL 104-204), Newborns and Mother's Health Protection Act of 1996	Amends the health insurance portability and accountability act.	To prohibit insurance companies from issuing policies covering hospital stays for new mothers and babies of less than 48 hours for normal vaginal births or 96 hours for cesarean deliveries.

TABLE 6-2   Federal Legislation that Influences Public Health—cont'd

Title	Purpose	Impact of Law
Social Services—cont'd		
Mental Health Parity Act of 1996 (Spina Bifida Amendment)	Requires health insurance plans that cover mental health services to provide the same lifetime and annual limits on coverage that they provide for physical conditions. Provides veterans health benefits to children suffering from spina bifida, if at least one parent was exposed to Agent Orange in Vietnam.	If the cost of providing health coverage results in an increase of at least 1%, the law will not apply. The mental health provision does not apply to companies with 50 employees or less. Veterans' benefits will be provided to children, including medical care, rehabilitation, vocational training and education, and a cash allowance between $200 and $1200, depending on the degree of disability.
Health Insurance Portability and Accountability Act of 1996 (PL 104-191)	The act sets minimum federal standards that allow workers to maintain their insurance coverage if they lose or leave their jobs. Medical savings accounts can be established, allowing workers with high-deductible insurance plans to set up tax-deductible savings accounts to use for medical expenses; increases the amount self-employed workers can deduct from their income taxes; gives tax breaks for long-term care insurance; and allows the chronically or terminally ill to collect benefits on their life insurance policy before death without a tax penalty. Also makes it a crime to transfer personal assets to relatives and friends, nursing homes, or others in order to qualify for Medicaid.	The act does not help the unemployed who are in transition, and their families, nor does it cover mental health. Group health plans are prohibited from discriminating against workers based on their health status or medical history. Limits to 12 months the period of time by which group health plans might exclude coverage of a pre-existing medical condition, (i.e., those conditions diagnosed or treated within 6 months from enrolling in a plan). Newborns and adopted children are exempted from the 12-month waiting period for pre-existing conditions. A medical condition is covered within 30 days of birth, and adopted children are covered within 30 days of adoption or placement for adoption. Pregnancy is no longer considered a preexisting condition from the 12-month waiting period. Workers who were covered by group health plans are immediately eligible for coverage at a new job as long as the new employer provides health insurance to its employees. The new law does not restrict employers from imposing a waiting period for new employees to obtain health insurance, usually 3 months. However, during this period, the employee will be considered continuously covered. Requires insurers to offer individual coverage to people who lose or change jobs if the new employer does not offer health insurance to its employees. Guarantees the renewal of group and individual health insurance policies except in cases of fraud and nonpayment of premiums.
	Provides protection for client privacy and confidentiality of medical information. Greater security over medical records and sharing of information is required.	Hospitals and other health care organizations must designate a privacy officer, provide education on HIPAA to employees regarding security of records; adopt written privacy procedures, and obtain consent from clients for most disclosures of protected health information. A minimum amount of information necessary may only be provided under HIPAA and only those with a need to know client information may access client information without consent.
Child Abuse Prevention and Treatment Act (CAPTA) (1996 PL 104-235)	The community-based family resources program was funded in 1997. Each state has a child's trust fund that uses this money to make local grants for child abuse prevention programs. Child abuse prevention and treatment are the focus of this law.	Maintains a federal role in funding research, technical assistance, data collection, and information dissemination on child abuse treatment and prevention. A number of new protections for children, such as limiting delays and termination of parental rights, filling of false reports, and lack of public oversight of child protection, are also included. The act repeats the temporary child care and nursery's program and the McKinney Family Support Center by consolidating their activities. The act also provides the Department of Health and Human Services (DHHS) the ability to establish an office of child abuse and neglect.

Continued

TABLE 6-2   Federal Legislation that Influences Public Health—cont'd

Title	Purpose	Impact of Law
Social Services—cont'd		
The Personal Responsibility and Work Opportunity Reconciliation Act of 1996 (PL 104-193)	Transformation of the welfare system, including provisions that relate to food stamps, child nutrition, child care, children's Supplemental Security Income (SSI), child protection, child support enforcement, and immigrants. Referred to as welfare reform law, which ends 60 years of social welfare policy, completely removing many federal programs for poor families and children.	It is estimated that 2.6 million people will no longer be able to rely on the federal programs previously relied upon before this welfare reform law. Temporary Assistance to Needy Families (TANF) funding was frozen through 2002 at the amount that the states received from the federal government the prior year for AFDC, emergency assistance, and jobs. TANF abolished AFDC, jobs, and emergency assistance grants (EAG) and replaced them with TANF in a block grant to the states. Under TANF, a fixed amount of federal funds is awarded to states each year regardless of need. The states must have a plan approved by HHS to determine their own eligibility requirements and the form the benefits will take. States can transfer up to 30% of TANF funds to the child care and development block grant and to the title XX social security block grant. Children's SSI, which provides support to low-income children with severe mental or physical disabilities, received significant changes to the eligibility criteria. Children who lost their SSI benefits did not necessarily remain eligible for Medicaid, unless their family qualified on other criteria. All current and future legal immigrants are barred from receiving SSI and food stamps. Exempt immigrants include refugees, asylees, veterans, aliens on active duty, and immigrants who have worked 40 quarters. A future legal immigrants are barred from receiving TANF Medicaid, and Title XX (SSBG) for 5 years after entering the country. All federal means tests benefits and the income of their sponsor family are deemed as part of their income when eligibility determinations are being made. Illegal, or not qualified immigrants, are barred from all federal public benefits, including retirement, welfare, disability, public and assisted housing, health, post secondary education, unemployment benefits, and food assistance. Families who qualify for TANF no longer have a guaranteed legal right to child care. However, TANF prohibits states from penalizing parents of children under 6 year of age who are single and cannot find accessible child care.
Balanced Budget Act of 1997 (PL 105-33)	To expand access to health care by medicare beneficiaries.	Provides direct Medicare reimbursement to advanced practice nurses, specifically nurse practitioners (NPs) and clinical nurse specialists (CNSs) practicing in any setting.
State Children's Health Initiative Program (SCHIP) (2001)	To encourage health insurance coverage for children of needy families.	States who develop health insurance plans that provide health insurance coverage to the children of families with low incomes are provided matching federal funds to support these health plans.

Data from the U.S. Code, Congressional and Administrative News. (1935, 1937, 1944, 1963, 1965, 1975, 1977, 1981). St. Paul, MN: West Publishers; and Center for Community Change. (1996). *Less money, fewer rules, more power to the state.* The 104th Congress, Public Policy Department.
HIPAA, Health Insurance Portability and Accountability Act.

for safe practice. The authority to promulgate rules and regulations is delegated to the administrative body by the legislative branch of government, such as Congress and state legislatures (Figure 6-1).

Often the rules and regulations enacted by the administrative body are intended to provide the details for or clarification of a broader statute enacted by the legislature. As an example, the Nurse Practice Act in most states provides broad guidelines defining the scope of nursing practice. The more specific rules and regulations promulgated by the state nursing board provide necessary

details to give guidance to nurses in the state. Administrative rules and regulations cannot conflict with the statute they seek to interpret, yet the details that the rules and regulations provide can be very powerful in defining the scope of practice of nursing in the state. Regulations also provide guidelines for how to work within the health care system (e.g., how to submit an application to receive Medicare or Medicaid and even who may apply).

Administrative lawmaking, the promulgation of rules and regulations, is usually preceded by notice of the proposed rule or regulation. Those who will be affected are given an

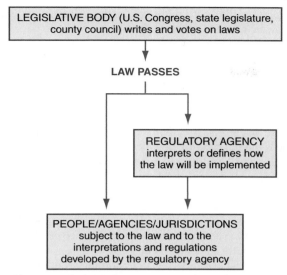

FIGURE 6-1 Relationship between laws and regulations.

opportunity to provide input. For example, because nurses are affected by the state board of nursing rules and regulations, they may provide input in writing or attend a hearing specifically held to discuss the proposed rule or regulation.

Administrative law bodies are often empowered to revoke or suspend professional licenses. Charges involving suspected violations of the Nurse Practice Act or of administrative rules or regulations, or other charges brought against a nurse related to professional practice, are heard and decided by the state board of nursing. The decision of the administrative rule–making body might be appealed to the state court system. Community health nursing issues must be understood by the administrative bodies that regulate nursing practice.

If a community/public health nurse is asked to perform a procedure that she or he believes is beyond the scope of nursing practice, the nurse or supervisor can receive clarification by requesting a declaratory ruling from the state board of nursing.

A nurse is asked to instruct school bus personnel or teachers of disabled children about replacement of an outer cannula for a tracheostomy. The nurse does not believe this is a safe and appropriate procedure. The nurse needs to consider safety factors and appropriateness of the information shared with untrained personnel (see Chapter 30). The nurse declines to instruct the personnel. The nurse's supervisor insists. The nurse should ask for a ruling from the state board of nursing.

Refusal to perform questionable duties until clarification is received should be considered reasonable and safe practice, not insubordination.

Examples of administrative rules and regulations that protect the public are those promulgated by OSHA. The occupational safety of workers is central to maintaining a healthy work force, and employers must comply with the regulations that define a safe and healthy work environment. For example, employers of health care workers are required to provide protective equipment and conduct in-service education about universal precautions to prevent the spread of HIV and hepatitis B virus.

JUDICIAL OR COMMON LAW

Common or judicial law is based on common usage, custom, and court rulings called *case precedents.* Case precedents are use-

ful for interpretation of statutory language and for comparative purposes. The facts of a current case and those of legal cases previously ruled on are evaluated for similarities and differences. The cases of most interest to community/public health nurses are those lawsuits in their states that involve circumstances very similar to the practice of community/public health nursing. For example, court decisions might provide support for exemptions from immunizations based on a person's religious beliefs. Nurses need to understand the specific facts of a case to safely assess their own situation or likelihood of liability. Cases from other states or from federal district court can also be used but do not usually carry the same weight as cases settled in the community health nurse's state.

In malpractice suits brought against community/public health nurses, an **expert witness** is called to testify to the reasonableness of the professional behavior of the nurse who is the defendant in the case. Expert witnesses focus on the recognized standard of care expected of community/public health nurses who work in the same or similar circumstances. The Case Study in this chapter, which focuses on a nurse's response to a child's asthma attack in school, demonstrates liability risks for school nurses.

Existing cases have shown that community/public health nurses must be aware of informed consent legislation in their state. Because community/public health nurses work autonomously in the field, the acquisition of informed consent might become the nurse's responsibility. Consent to treat a child must be obtained from the parent or legal guardian or custodian of the child. However, to truly provide informed consent, the client or parent must be given enough information to understand the consequences of his or her decision. For example, the significant risks and benefits of immunizations, as well as alternatives, must be disclosed to the client—or, in the case of a minor, to the parent or guardian—before consent is obtained.

Roles that the community/public health nurse assumes become legally binding duties and must be undertaken responsibly. Some community/public health nurses might be required to perform laboratory tests such as phenylketonuria (PKU) testing. Failure to adequately inform a client or guardian or performing a test improperly might lead to a liability suit. Nursing judgments, such as the assessment of an individual's condition and the documentation of signs and symptoms supporting the nursing inferences, might be critical in deciding the severity of the illness or describing adverse reactions to prescribed treatments. For example, when the nurse provides home health care to ill persons, blood pressure readings that are outside normal parameters must be reported to the physician or nurse practitioner in charge of the case. The community health nurse might be the only person who has physical contact with the community health client, and therefore communication between the health department or home care agency, physician, or other members of the health care team and the community health nurse is critical. The importance of accurate and timely communication has been tested in many legal cases involving nurses.

Community/public health nurses might find themselves involved in the process of judicial or common law in one of several roles. As a *defendant,* the nurse stands accused of causing harm to another; as an expert witness, the nurse testifies as to the standard of care in community/public health nursing; and as a **general witness,** the nurse testifies regarding the specific facts at issue in a given case. The facts of a case at trial are compared with the facts of existing case law and the testimony of witnesses. The standard in the jurisdiction is determined by previous case precedence. If the nurse is planning to rely on a previously decided case as a standard, it must be determined that the standard of care applied in that case remains current and that the current law is in good standing. Case law reflects the changes in society's views; cases might be overturned or overruled and therefore might not be safely relied on as the law in that state. Relying on the expertise of an attorney who practices in health care law is recommended when evaluating the current validity of existing cases.

Community/public health nurses currently enjoy greater autonomy than many other nurses, which makes professional accountability even more critical. Court cases relating to the practice of community/public health nursing will most likely increase as society recognizes that independent nursing judgment and autonomous decision making occur in community/public health nursing. The doctrine of **respondeat superior and vicarious liability** (i.e., being responsible for another's actions), which transfers liability from the nurse to the physician or the health department, has been replaced by individual accountability of the nurse for her or his own professional actions. Supervisory liability is one of the few instances in which vicarious liability occurs in current case law. As a supervisor of nurse's aides or licensed practical nurses in an agency, a community/public health nurse *must not* delegate tasks to these workers that are beyond the scope of their knowledge base or the legal scope of their practice. If they harm a client while providing care, the community health nurse's professional judgment when delegating such tasks will be assessed to determine whether the nurse's action was reasonable.

ATTORNEY GENERAL'S OPINIONS

In many states, the attorney general is the official legal counselor for public agencies, including health departments. Questions pertaining to the legality of procedures or the scope of nursing practice within the state can be clarified with the attorney general. The state attorney general provides both informal and formal opinions. If the legal issue is of such concern that the nurse or agency believes the liability risks are great, a formal written opinion should be requested.

The state attorney general's opinions provide guidelines based on both statutory and common law interpretations. The attorney general's office evaluates the written law, including its legislative history, and provides an opinion as to how the law should be applied. If a legal issue arises and the community/public health nurse has an attorney general's written opinion offering an interpretation of a particular issue or statute, the court will most likely view the nurse or the agency as having acted reasonably and responsibly in seeking clarification of what behavior is legal. If the nursing action conforms with the attorney general's opinion, the court will usually consider this action favorably on behalf of the nurse or agency named as a defendant in a lawsuit, when the reasonableness of the behavior is being evaluated.

The basic underlying principle is that a nurse should be able to rely on the professional advice of legal counsel. An attorney general's opinion might differ from a second opinion from the same office or an opinion from another attorney at a later date. Highly controversial issues, such as abortion and contraception for adolescents, may be influenced by political concerns and may receive differing interpretations by different individuals in the same office at different times.

CONTRACTS

A **contract** is an agreement between two persons who have the legal capacity and are competent to join into a binding agreement that is recognized under the law. Contracts protect the rights of both clients and nurses. Community/public health nurses must be aware that promises made to clients that are meant to be reassurances might be interpreted by clients as binding promises of outcomes. It is best to avoid making promises about things that are outside one's control. There are situations in community/public health nursing in which a formal contractual agreement is necessary. If one agency agrees to provide services to another agency, it is wise to have the understanding in writing. The purpose of a written contract is to provide evidence of what the parties are mutually agreeing to do.

Employment contracts are an important issue for all nurses. The customary practice in nursing has been to hire a nurse without a written contract. In this situation, the policies and procedures describing the duties and responsibilities of the community/public health nurse are often the agency's legally binding employment agreement. If an employment agreement specifies duties that are beyond the scope of nursing practice in the state, nurses must not agree to provide these services. Nurses who question whether they should perform some of the services required of them by their community health agency should bring these concerns to the attention of their supervisor and request a legal opinion about whether this practice is within the scope of nursing.

If the policies and procedures of an agency are not safe or require revisions, the community/public health nurse should request to serve on the committee that revises and reviews policies and procedures. Periodic review of policies and procedures, at least every 2 years, is sound nursing practice. The fact that an agency might require a community/public health nurse to perform a procedure will not protect the nurse as an individual if this practice is found to be outside the scope of nursing as defined by the state's Nurse Practice Act. The law will overrule any agency policy or procedure. In a Texas case, a nurse testified that she was following the physician's direction and the agency's policy. The court ruled that the state statute or Nurse Practice Act was the rule of law the nurse should be following. The fact that she relied on what the physician or her employer told her to do was an insufficient defense (*Lunsford v Board of Nurse Examiners,* 1983).

Before signing an employment or other contract, the nurse should read the contract carefully. If a person signs a contract without reading it, the court will not be sympathetic toward that person's ignorance of the agreement. With a client contract, the community/public health nurse must make certain that the terms of agreement are written out before asking the client for a signature.

CLASSIFICATION OF LAWS AND PENALTIES

Laws are enacted by state legislatures or Congress, as described previously, and specific categories of laws have associated penalties. The authorities or bodies that enforce the laws are also unique to the particular classification of the laws, whether criminal or civil.

CRIMINAL LAWS

The laws that constitute the criminal code (**criminal law**) are written for the protection of the public welfare. For this reason, when a case is brought under the criminal code, the defendant faces society or the community prosecutor instead of an individual plaintiff. Criminal cases are prosecuted by the government. The penalties attached to criminal violations are also more severe and include the possibility of incarceration. Examples of potential violations of the criminal code in community/public health nursing include the situation in which the nurse believes that her or his own judgment about the worth of a person's life is the correct one and acts to hasten the death of that person. The criminal code refers to this behavior as either murder or manslaughter. There have been cases involving nurses who saw themselves as "angels of mercy" and hastened death in hospitals and long-term care facilities.

A community/public health nurse who recklessly endangers others can be criminally prosecuted. There is some concern that states are becoming more willing to use criminal law rather than relying on state board sanctions to punish professional misconduct (Hall & Hall, 2001). For example, nurses in Denver were prosecuted for negligent homicide in the case of a fatal drug overdose in addition to facing civil prosecution for malpractice and state board sanctions. Laws relating to theft and other property violations are also found under the criminal code. Laws that prohibit abuse of children or elderly people are criminal laws written to protect these segments of the public. Most states have statutes that require nurses to report suspected child or elder abuse (see Chapter 23). In some cases, a nurse may be prosecuted for *failure* to report suspected cases of child abuse (Goldsmith, 2003).

It is not unusual to read about a nurse who has been convicted of a crime and later discover that the state board of nursing has scheduled a hearing to consider whether the nurse's license should be revoked or suspended. Certain crimes can be grounds for the loss of one's professional license if the behavior can be reasonably connected to the professional responsibilities of the nurse. Violations involving substance abuse might result in suspension of a community/public health nurse's license until proof is offered that the nurse is no longer using the substance in question. Because nurses are in a position to affect the health and safety of consumers, nurses' personal habits and behavior are linked to their professional licensure.

A conviction for a criminal violation might result in imprisonment, parole, the loss of privileges (such as a nursing license), a fine, or any combination of these penalties. If a community/public health nurse becomes aware of illegal activity in a client's home, it would be wise for the nurse to speak to the nursing supervisor to determine whether reporting the illegal activity is mandated by law. The nurse must exercise judgment regarding the threat posed to society versus the impact on the nurse-client relationship.

CIVIL LAWS

Civil laws are written to regulate the conduct between private persons or businesses. For example, malpractice laws are civil laws written to protect consumers of health care against unsafe health care practices. A private group or individual might bring a legal action for a breach of a civil law. This private group or individual is called the **plaintiff.** The person charged with violating a law or legal right is called the **defendant**. The court's ruling may result in a plan to correct the wrong between the two parties and might include a monetary payment to the wronged party, commonly known as *damages*. The penalties for most civil wrongs do not include incarceration. Some civil cases might discover violations of the criminal laws, which might then lead to criminal penalties, such as a jail term.

Civil law, under which medical or professional malpractice falls, is called **tort law**. Tort law covers both intentional and unintentional torts. An *intentional tort* is found when an outcome is planned, whereas an *unintentional tort* involves accidental or unintended behavior. In malpractice cases involving health care providers, such as community/public health nurses, no intent to harm the client is needed for the defendant to be found guilty of negligence or malpractice. **Negligence** is merely the failure to act as a reasonably prudent professional would act in a specific situation. **Malpractice** is a specific type of negligence. Failure to act as a reasonably prudent professional would act constitutes malpractice if the inaction results in harm to the patient. To be found guilty of negligence or malpractice, a nurse must have accepted a duty to the client, the breach of which has injured the client. The commissions or omissions of the nurse must have *directly* caused the injury. If a nurse unintentionally harms a client, a malpractice or negligence case under the civil statutes would be the most likely result. If a community/public health nurse intentionally plans an injurious outcome, a criminal case could result, which might then lead to criminal penalties, such as a jail term.

There might be both civil and criminal components to a case when behavior violates laws that govern the practice of any licensed professional. A violation of both civil and criminal statutes in community/public health nursing might occur when a state's Nurse Practice Act defines or restricts some functions of the nurse in a way that requires them to be performed under the directions of a physician or other licensed professional, such as a pharmacist. To act as a professional, explicit legal authority must exist. Standing or written orders, such as for medication administration, give the nurse authorization to act if the behavior is dependent on the directions of another licensed professional. Custom or usual practice will not substitute for the specific authority required by law. A violation of a professional practice act might be prosecuted as a crime, even if no actual harm occurs to a client.

If a community/public health nurse does not have a standing order for a particular medication but knows the routine and orders the medication from a pharmacy, the nurse could be both civilly and criminally liable for this action. Even if the nurse attempts and fails to reach the physician to obtain permission, this action is illegal. The nurse has violated the Medical Practice Act, practiced outside the scope of the Nurse Practice Act, and fraudulently and criminally ordered medication without a license to do so. If the client is harmed by the nurse's action, a civil suit can be brought by the client against the nurse for the injury or damages caused by the nurse's negligence. Therefore, one action can lead to both civil and criminal liability. The Medical Practice Act gives physicians, not nurses, the authority to diagnose disease and prescribe medication. However, in an increasing number of states, some advanced practice nurses are now licensed to prescribe medications.

A nurse must also be judicious in the information provided to clients. In one case, a nurse was charged with interfering with the physician-patient relationship when the nurse provided information to the patient that was outside the physician's prescribed treatment plan (*Tuma v Board of Nursing*, 1979). On a patient's request, the nurse discussed alternative treatments for cancer with a hospitalized woman who was about to start chemotherapy. When the woman stopped chemotherapy, the son told the physician about the conversation, and the physician brought charges against the nurse (Kelly & Joel, 1995). The Idaho Board of Nurses suspended the nurse's license for 6 months for unprofessional conduct. The Idaho Supreme Court eventually ruled that she could not be found guilty of unprofessional conduct because the state's Nurse Practice Act did not define unprofessional conduct (Kelly & Joel, 1995). The nurse's behavior itself was not addressed by the court.

The common areas for malpractice in nursing are the following (Croke, 2003; Cutrona, 2001):
- Failure to ensure patient safety
- Improper treatment or negligent performance of a treatment
- Inadequate assessment and intervention in monitoring situational changes
- Medication errors
- Failure to conform to agency protocols, policies, and procedures

PURPOSES AND APPLICATION OF PUBLIC HEALTH LAW

Public health laws are written for several purposes, including protecting the public's health, advocating for persons or vulnerable groups who otherwise might not be served, regulating health care delivery and financing, and regulating the professional accountability of health care providers.

PROTECTING THE PUBLIC'S HEALTH

One of the main purposes of laws that apply to community/public health nursing is to protect the public. Examples of existing laws that protect the public are mentioned here, and these laws are discussed in more detail in relevant chapters (e.g., Chapter 8). Protection of the public health occasionally must override the personal rights of individuals. For example, immunizations help to protect groups of people, as well as the individual, from illness. Some people might not desire to be immunized, but the good of the group must take priority in most cases (see *Ethics in Practice* box in Chapter 27).

Involuntary and emergency psychiatric admissions laws are written to protect not only the public but also people who are a danger to themselves. The standards and procedure for involuntarily committing a client to a hospital must be understood and acted upon in a timely manner. The nurse might be called on to provide evidence of the necessity of involuntary hospitalization of a client for the client's own safety and protection or the safety and protection of the family or neighbors. Emergency psychiatric admissions against the client's will are time limited. State statutes usually identify the procedure for such admissions. The nurse must consider the need to protect the client's autonomy when evaluating the need to initiate an involuntary hospitalization.

A growing number of laws focus on dangerous products. These laws seek to protect the public by imposing liability on the product's manufacturers. Producers of products are held to a high standard in an effort to protect the public from dangerous products. Environmental hazards and laws relating to occupational safety are discussed in Chapter 9.

ADVOCATING FOR RIGHTS

A second purpose of public health law is protecting the rights of groups of people. In Chapter 23, the rights of vulnerable children and elders are discussed. Examples of federal laws that are written to protect special groups are laws addressing the rights and needs of children with disabilities in school (see Chapters 27 and 30), laws protecting adults with disabilities (see Chapter 26), and occupational health and safety laws protecting workers (see Chapter 9). Many occupational health and safety laws focus on environmental hazards. Some laws are written to protect both the public and specified members of society. For example, as stated earlier, laws that require parents to immunize their children protect both the child and the general public.

Other examples of federal laws enacted to protect the rights of groups of people include the Civil Rights Acts of 1964 and 1965 and the **Americans with Disabilities Act (ADA)** of 1990. The rights of all people to move freely throughout our country and to be treated equally and without discrimination in the provision of services or employment are protected by the **Civil Rights Acts.** If a community health agency has a limited supply of needed vaccines and decides to reserve these limited resources for only white male clients, a civil right's violation has occurred. Such a policy would discriminate against all persons of other races as well as against white females. The ADA and its amendments protect people who have disabilities from discrimination based on their disabilities.

REGULATING HEALTH CARE DELIVERY AND FINANCING

Another purpose of public health law is to regulate or provide health care delivery and financing. The federal government has greatly affected society by regulating health care delivery and health care financing. The Social Security Act of 1935 and its 1965 amendments created both Medicare and Medicaid programs (see Chapter 4).

The **Public Health Services Act** and its amendments were promulgated through a federal regulatory statute. The Public Health Service was created to collect and analyze data on selected diseases from all of the states and territories of the United States. Efforts to control or regulate the control and spread of disease are organized by both the Public Health Service and the CDC. The 1975 amendments of the Public Health Services Act also provided grant funding to states for various categories or "blocks" of public health services (see Table 6-2). This funding is often called *block grant funding*.

Public health law includes appropriations for populations at risk. These populations might include vulnerable groups of persons who have been identified as needing special protection or groups with specific health care problems. Amendments to the Social Security Act of 1963 addressed specific needs of maternal and child health, as well as mental retardation planning. The Social Security Amendments of 1977 and the Rural Health Clinic Amendments are directed toward specific populations in rural communities. The Omnibus Budget Reconciliation Act of 1981 created block grants for both maternal and child health, and social services (see Table 6-2).

REGULATING PROFESSIONAL ACCOUNTABILITY

Public health laws not only are intended to protect the health of our communities, advocate for public rights and needs, and regulate health care standards and financing but also serve to regulate the professional accountability of health care providers.

Accountability means being answerable for one's professional judgment and actions within a realm of authority (Turnock, 2004). Community/public health nurses are held accountable for upholding public health laws and regulations. Whether a community/public health nurse is working for a state, federal, or private agency, a general understanding of the appropriate and applicable laws is needed. For specific interpretations of these laws as they apply to nursing practice or clients' rights, the advice and counsel of the agency's attorney is recommended. Professional accountability is further defined in policy manuals, accrediting body guidelines, and standards and ethical codes of professional organizations (see Chapter 1).

LEGAL RESPONSIBILITIES OF COMMUNITY/PUBLIC HEALTH NURSES

The duties of all nurses are legally binding responsibilities for which the nurse is accountable. In addition, the community/public health nurse has many responsibilities that are unique to a practice focused on public health.

PRACTICE WITHIN THE SCOPE OF THE LAW

As stated earlier, community/public health nurses must practice within the scope of the Nurse Practice Act and all relevant statutes and administrative rulings and relevant civil and criminal law. Community/public health nurses must also carefully follow the rules for reimbursable services under Medicaid and Medicare. Clients must be screened for financial eligibility, and the signature of the client must be witnessed after the client's rights and the legal contract for services are explained.

The community/public health nurse must honor the contracts made with clients. Contracts might include both written and implied agreements between the client and the nurse. If a contract cannot be honored, written documentation in the nursing notes should state the reason why, and the client should be notified (Cutrona, 2001). If the client unilaterally ends the relationship either explicitly or by consistently not keeping appointments with the nurse, this should also be documented. The community/public health nurse or a designate should contact the client if the nurse must cancel an appointment, a clinic visit, or other service. The client should also be notified about any substitutions of personnel.

The nurse might be charged with abandonment if follow-through on contracted care is not completed. **Abandonment** is the unilateral termination of a professional relationship without affording the client reasonable notice and alternative health care services. Planning for the client's discharge from services prevents abandonment. The client or family should be given adequate notice and should be informed about resources for any necessary continuing care (Cutrona, 2001). After the

client's written permission is obtained, a copy of the health records, including the nursing plan of care, should be transferred to another provider.

Refusal to work mandatory overtime places nurses at risk of liability for abandonment, because client safety might be compromised. Nurses report increasing use of mandatory overtime as employers attempt to cope with the current nursing shortage. To protect nurses, California enacted legislation in 2001 prohibiting mandatory overtime. Illinois, Minnesota, Maryland, New Jersey, New York, Oregon, and Washington have similar legislation, and many other states have similar bills pending (Service Employees International Union, 2007).

INFORMED CONSENT

Informed consent means that clients understand the risks and benefits of potential treatment alternatives before they voluntarily consent to them. Clients must have adequate information, explained in an understandable way, to make informed decisions. In obtaining informed consent for a medical procedure, the community/public health nurse's role might be limited to witnessing the client's signature, while the treating physician explains medical treatment information (Mahlmeister, 2008). However, in public health nursing practice, the nurse often explains the scope of services and witnesses the client's signature. Permission to obtain or transfer medical records is one example of informed consent (Figure 6-2).

Many nursing procedures are performed with implied consent. Implied consent occurs when the nursing procedure is explained to the client and the client's actions, such as exposing an injection site, indicate a willingness to proceed. A good rule to follow in deciding whether to rely on implied consent or to require a written form is the following: the more intrusive the procedure, the greater the likelihood that requiring a written and signed consent form will be in the client's and nurse's best interest. If a procedure is performed against the client's will or without consent, charges of *assault* (the threat of touching) and *battery* (the actual touching of the client) can be brought against the nurse.

Informed consent might be especially difficult to receive if the nurse is involving the client in research, because all the potential risks might not be known in many cases. Informed consent should be obtained by the researcher, who can also explain the benefits of the research.

Community/public health nurses might be asked to witness the signing of forms related to nursing services as well as to non–health-related matters (e.g., wills). Witnessing a signature means that the witness is stating that the individual signed voluntarily, understood the document, and intended his or her signature to mean agreement with the contents of the document. "Witnessing to signature only" means that the witness has seen another person sign his or her name. This might be written in when witnessing a signature on a non–health-related document, such as a will. All forms signed by the client, parent, or guardian, and the date each form was signed, should be listed on the health care record.

REFUSAL OF CARE AND LIMITS OF CARE

An issue of growing concern is the client's right to refuse treatment. If a community/public health nurse is unaware that the client has created a living will, a special directive, or a durable power of attorney that specifically states that certain procedures, such as resuscitation, are not desired, the nurse might act without

Name_____

H.D. No. _____

Service Unit_____

CONSENT TO OBTAIN OR RELEASE
CLIENT MEDICAL RECORD INFORMATION

☐ Male

_____ ,   ☐ Female, born _____ , residing at
Client full name   Date of birth

_____   _____   _____   _____
Address of client   City   State   Zip Code

hereby requests that the following information   _____
                                                                          Specific information requested

_____

be disclosed by   _____
                              Name of person, program and/or organization receiving information

_____   _____   _____   _____
Address   City   State   Zip Code

TO: _____
          Name of person, program and/or organization receiving information

_____   _____   _____   _____
Address   City   State   Zip Code

solely for the purpose of   _____
                                          (Be specific)

to apply both now and in the future. This consent expires on   _____
                                                                                          Date, event or condition

---

I voluntarily consent for Prince George's County Health Department, Cheverly, Md., to obtain or release medical record information for the purposes stated above.

I understand that this consent can be revoked by me in writing at any time. I understand that this information may not be redisclosed without my permission.

Signed (check one):   ☐ Client
                                    ☐ Legal Guardian   _____   _____
                                                                       Signature   Date

---

Explained by: _____   _____
                          Health care provider or representative   Date

_____   _____
Title   Phone number

FIGURE 6-2 Consent to obtain or release client medical record information. (Courtesy Prince George's County Health Department, Cheverly, Maryland.)

the client's consent and in a manner that is not in the client's proclaimed best interest. A client can deny consent to treatment or withdraw previously granted consent at any time. Even a verbal withdrawal of consent is valid and must be communicated immediately to members of the health care team. Documentation of the refusal or withdrawal of consent is also important.

PRIVACY

The legal right of the client to maintain privacy and confidentiality in the nurse-client relationship must also be protected (Mahlmeister, 2008). Because community/public health nurses often deal with clients who have special privacy concerns (e.g., minors who desire contraceptives; clients with sexually transmitted diseases), nurses should be cautious when leaving telephone messages for clients. The nurse should leave her or his name and a short message that does not provide specific information about the nature of the call or identify the type of care facility (e.g., sexually transmitted disease clinic, maternity/family planning clinic). If a transfer of information regarding a client is requested, the community health nurse must obtain a signed release form from the client before transferring this information.

Release forms should identify exactly what information is allowed to be released, to whom, and the duration of the time for which the release is being granted (see Figure 6-2). Such releases are very common in community/public health nursing, because the nurse is often the case manager who coordinates care among a variety of health care and social services providers and agencies. A relatively new area of concern is the sharing of medical information among health care agencies, utilization reviewers, and health insurers facilitated by computer-generated data banks (Monarch, 2002). In community health, agencies and nurses must provide as much protection as possible for clients' confidential records.

In some jurisdictions, the communications between a nurse and client enjoy a statutory legal privilege that protects the privacy of this communication. Not all states or jurisdictions have enacted statutes that attach this legal privilege to nurse-client communications. A *legal privilege* is a legislatively created protection that the nurse will not be forced to disclose confidential communications with a client. If a legal privilege does not exist in a state, the nurse can be called on to disclose conversations with the client. A legal privilege does exist between a lawyer and his or her client and is intended to encourage the client to be totally truthful about his or her participation in the events at issue in the case. There might be instances in which even statutorily created legal privileges do not apply. For instance, most child and elder abuse reporting laws require that the nurse disclose reasonable suspicions of abuse. Nurses should be aware of any state legal privileges for nurse-client communications where they practice.

STANDING ORDERS

Some agencies use standing orders. Community/public health nurses need to protect themselves by ensuring that standing orders are regularly reviewed and updated as well as by having the physician sign the standing order that is acted upon by the nurse. The community health nurse must be especially cautious to clarify orders when following verbal or standing orders.

Verbal orders can be a source of risk to the community/public health nurse. The dangers of miscommunication are greatly heightened when communication is verbal. The likelihood of a client's being injured increases when the nurse allows verbal order giving to become a pattern within the agency. When a verbal order has been acted upon by the nurse and a client is injured, there is no written evidence of what the physician ordered. The nurse will have difficulty demonstrating that the doctor's verbal order was followed accurately.

Written confirmation of verbal orders must be received as soon as reasonably possible. In practice, community/public health nurses often write the orders they verbally receive and mail them to the physician along with a self-addressed envelope. The physician is requested to verify and sign the orders and mail them back to the community health nurse.

CLIENT EDUCATION

Caring for the client in home, clinic, school, and other community settings always includes the duty to teach the client. Community-based teaching might include both preventive and self-care information. Community/public health nurses must remember that the client's ability to understand what is being taught is of utmost importance. If the client does not speak English, the nurse might need the assistance of an interpreter. If the nurse is not sure whether the client is capable of understanding the instructions, it is important to involve a family member or other persons who will be involved in providing the client's ongoing health care. If the client is a child, the parents or guardian should be fully informed about how to perform the care that the community health nurse is teaching. It is a good idea to have the client explain or demonstrate to the nurse his or her understanding or perception of what the nurse has explained. In this way, the nurse can be sure that the client understands the nurse's directions (see Chapter 20).

Alla Orhan, a home health nurse, was assigned to ensure that Mr. Fredplay, a client with newly diagnosed diabetes, understood how to inject his insulin. She arrived at his home at the appointed time to find that he had not done his early morning insulin injection. She asked Mr. Fredplay what he had been taught in the hospital and how many injections he had done. He replied that the hospital nurse had drawn up insulin into one syringe and then helped him to inject himself. He said that he was not sure how much insulin to draw up; the nurse had told him something about swabbing the top of the bottle with alcohol, but he couldn't remember how to inject and was scared to do the injection. Because he was 3 hours overdue for his injection, Ms. Orhan drew up and administered his insulin. She demonstrated the correct procedure as she did so. After she administered the medication, she had Mr. Fredplay repeat the instructions back to her, and wrote the instructions down in his presence so he would have a "cheat sheet" to which he could refer when he was alone. She also had him draw up the solution several times and practice injecting into an apple until he was sure of his technique. She then made arrangements to come to his home at 7:30 AM the next morning to watch him repeat the injection.

It is also important that the community/public health nurse teach the client *accurately*. If the nurse needs references to provide correct information, she or he should postpone answering a question until the information is gathered. It is essential that the information taught be accurate and up to date. If the nurse is unsure about how to answer a question asked by the client, it is not unprofessional to tell the client that she or he will check and get back to the client with accurate information. It does not destroy a nurse's credibility to admit that she or he is not a walking textbook; it is far more important to provide a correct response to the client.

DOCUMENTATION

It is important for the community/public health nurse to be consistent in recording the care provided to clients. Thorough, accurate, and timely recording demonstrates quality of care, helps ensure reimbursement for services, and reduces the risk of lawsuits (Higgenbotham, 2001). Information regarding client visits and care should be documented as soon as possible after the care. When providing care in the home, the nurse might need to record some immediate, brief notes that are then used as the basis for more thorough documentation in the client's health record when the nurse returns to the agency.

Documentation is important not only as a means of communicating with other health care providers who might be working with a client but also as the ongoing written memory of the nurse. If the client later develops a problem, accurate and timely documentation of the care provided will supply the nurse with a record of what *has* or *has not* been done for the client and why (Frank-Stromborg & Christensen, 2001). Documentation also provides an ongoing history for future health care providers to determine what care has been provided for the client and what still needs to be done. The nurse's records are usually a part of the client's health care history. In documentation, as in all other community/public health nursing procedures, it is important to comply with the employer's policies and procedures. If a lawsuit ensues, the documentation kept by the nurse will be reviewed to establish the reasonableness of the care provided by the nurse. Therefore, accurate and up-to-date recording is essential. It is difficult, if not impossible, to remember later everything done for every client if thorough recording is not completed at the time of care delivery. The records of the community/public health nurse can be subpoenaed in a trial to determine whether the nurse caused harm to the client.

AGENCY POLICIES

Community/public health nurses must be informed about their employers' written policies and procedures. Deviations from policies and procedures can often become common practice in an agency, but this does not make these practices legally sound, and they might be viewed as substandard care (Hall & Hall, 2001). If employer policies and procedures do not comply with reasonable nursing care or have not undergone periodic review, it is important for nurses to be involved in changing them to conform to safe practice. Nurses can actively participate in policy making committees to provide input regarding safe nursing care within the scope of the state's Nurse Practice Act. It is important to ensure that the employer's policies and procedures do not require practice outside the scope of the nursing license.

The employing agency's policies and procedures are standards against which the community/public health nurse's behavior will be measured if a lawsuit is brought. Therefore, it is important for the nurse to follow the agency's policies and procedures once the nurse is assured that these policies and procedures are legally sound. If the nurse has questions about the legality of any policies or procedures, she or he should consult the agency's attorney. Shortcuts or ignorance about the standards set by an employer can increase the nurse's risk of a malpractice suit.

PUBLIC HEALTH LAW ENFORCEMENT

Community/public health nurses also have the legal responsibility to enforce laws, especially laws enacted to protect the public health. Public health nurses might be hired by local, state, or federal authorities that have enacted rules and regulations requiring specific enforcement of laws in areas such as infection control and reportable events.

Nurse's Role and Public Health Law

State public health codes define the duty to report communicable diseases. Community/public health nurses are often involved in investigating and treating communicable disease, performing contact investigations, and filing follow-up reports to state and local health departments and the CDC. Other conditions that are reportable by all community/public health nurses under law include suspected abuse and neglect of children, elderly persons, or persons being cared for by others (Mahlmeister, 2008). Selected immunizations are required by law for school attendance (Marchand, 2001). It is usually the school nurse who reviews health records for compliance with mandatory immunization.

Nurse as Agent of Employer

A community/public health nurse is an agent of her or his employer. The legal meaning of **agent**, in this sense, is that the nurse, as an employee, represents the employer and has the delegated authority to carry out the purposes of the employer. For example, if a nurse is working for a state health department, the nurse is an agent of the state. The legal liability and responsibilities of the community/public health nurse vary depending on the employer. The hiring agency's policies and procedures statements, as well as the employee manual, should inform the nurse of any special duties or responsibilities. Examples of public settings in which community/public health nurses work are public schools, health departments, and federal employee health programs. Community/public health nurses might also be found working in private schools, clinics, or organizations such as Planned Parenthood.

Community/public health nurses hired by a public agency might also be required to enforce laws for licensing and inspection of daycare facilities and nursing homes, such as insuring that licensed facilities comply with regulations aimed at providing a safe environment for clients of daycare or long-term care facilities. Laws are constantly being enacted and revised. To be of the greatest assistance to their clients, community/public health nurses must be aware of the laws related to their practice, knowledgeable about changes in existing law, and prepared to enforce state laws.

REFERRALS AND ADVOCACY

Nurses need to be familiar with the laws that have been enacted to protect their clients' rights and with the legislated services their clients are likely to be eligible to receive. The community/public health nurse is often placed in the position of serving as the client's advocate. Advocating for patients is a special duty of nurses, and one that is recognized as such in the American Nurses Association (ANA) *Code of Ethics*. State laws may impose on nurses a duty to act as a client advocate. One state with such laws is California (Markus, 2006). As an advocate, the nurse should be able to identify available community resources and assist clients in pursuing the rights that are legally afforded them. For example, the community/public health nurse might become aware that a client is being unduly harassed by a creditor and might be able to help by directing the client to a consumer protection agency that can assist the client in resolving his or her financial difficulties. Providing referrals to available community resources is a valuable responsibility of the community/public health nurse.

The nurse should be familiar with the legal aid services available for low-income clients. Providing referrals to appropriate legal services is a community/public nursing function. These services ensure that all of the public's rights are protected. People who could not otherwise afford legal services can be represented by legal aid staff. Federal cutbacks in funding have forced legal aid offices to limit the number and prioritize the types of cases they handle. This has reduced available legal services for low-income clients.

SPECIAL AND VULNERABLE POPULATIONS

Laws related to special populations affect the community/public health nurse's clients. Such laws have been enacted specifically to protect the rights of persons with disabilities, foster children, elderly persons, and the abused. Access to health care might be the client's greatest problem. Laws written to protect the uninsured, persons who reside illegally in the United States, the homeless, and migrant workers should be explored by the community/public health nurse. Laws related to housing and the rights of the renter or tenant are also important to understand. Many state legislatures have enacted laws to protect families from eviction under certain circumstances.

FAMILY LAW

The community/public health nurse very often will deal with laws considered to be family law. Issues of guardianship or the legal right and power to decide for another might arise, and it is important for the community/public health nurse to understand how to advise clients on how to acquire guardianship and the obligations that go along with being a guardian. If the nurse is obtaining consent for a procedure to be performed on a minor or on a person who is incompetent, the guardian must sign the consent form for treatment. In the case of a divorced couple, the spouse who has been awarded custody of the children is the legal guardian of those children and the person from whom consent must be obtained.

Determining who has the right to consent to treatment for minors is a growing problem in health care. When the parents are divorced or children do not live with their parents the legal process of consent becomes complicated. All health care providers, including nurses, need to determine whether the person giving consent is legally entitled to do so (Holloway, 2001).

> Alice Gomez, a community/public health nurse, is doing a contact investigation of tuberculosis. She visits the Morales family because Sara Morales, a 10-year-old girl, is a close school contact of an individual with active disease. At home with Sara are her aunt Alicia, her cousin Maria, and her grandmother Alva. Ms. Gomez wants to do a screening purified protein derivative (PPD) test for tuberculosis and is granted permission to do so by Sara's aunt. The aunt tells Ms. Gomez that she is Sara's legal guardian. After the home visit, Ms. Gomez finds out that Sara's actual guardian is her mother Consuela, who lives in the household but was not present during her visit.

Issues surrounding family privacy and reproductive rights are also very relevant. Not only are there federal legislation and court rulings, but many state legislatures and courts have created laws affecting the legality of providing information about contraception to minors (see Chapter 24). It is important for the community/public health nurse to be aware of the abortion laws in the state in which the nurse is practicing. The U.S. Supreme Court decisions have encouraged states to handle the abortion issue, within certain guidelines, in a manner that reflects their own community standards. The community/public health nurse must understand her or his own state's standards to advise and correctly inform community health clients.

Parental Consent

The legal age of consent in most states is 18 years of age, although four states have ages ranging from 19 to 21 years. Some minors are considered emancipated; that is, they have legal independence from parents or guardian. In general, persons under 18 years of age who are married or in the military are emancipated. In addition, teenagers who are pregnant or have a child, are self-supporting, or are living apart from their parents are considered independent in some states.

Parental consent is generally required before a minor receives medical treatment, but exceptions are becoming widespread (Table 6-3). Many states permit minors to consent to

TABLE 6-3   State Consent Laws for Unmarried Minors

	Contraceptive Services	Prenatal Care Services	STIs
Total allow consent	26	33	51*
Total require parental consent or notice or have other restrictions	21	3	0
Total no specific law	4	15	0
	Abortion Services	Medical Care for Child	Place Child for Adoption
Total allow consent	3	31	29
Total require parental consent or notice or have other restrictions	42	0	10
Total no specific law	6	20	12

Data from Alan Guttmacher Institute. (2007). *State policies in brief: An overview of minors' consent law.* New York: Author. Retrieved September 25, 2007 from *http://www.guttmacher. org/statecenter/spibs/spib_OMCL.pdf.*
* Includes the District of Columbia.

contraceptive services. Parental consent is not always needed for the teen to seek diagnosis and treatment of a sexually transmitted disease. Prenatal care and delivery services can be accessed by minors in many states without parental consent. The majority of states mandate parental involvement in a minor's decision to obtain an abortion (Alan Guttmacher Institute, 2007). Minors who are parents have the authority to make all decisions regarding their infants. A juvenile may even relinquish her baby for adoption without her parents' consent in most states. In addition to rights related to reproductive issues, adolescents are afforded other consent rights by states. Most states permit minors to seek medical care and counseling. Many states grant minors confidential access to outpatient mental health services. Some states allow a minor to marry without parental consent when the minor is expecting a child, and some states allow teenagers to drop out of high school without their parents' permission.

Parental Refusal to Seek Medical Care for Minors

Sometimes community/public health nurses are aware of situations in which parents of a sick child do not seek medical care. Frequently, these cases are tied to child abuse or neglect issues. In such circumstances, the nurse should follow the prescribed procedure for reporting the abuse or neglect (see Chapter 23). Parents might be reluctant to seek care if they lack health insurance coverage. In these cases, the nurse can refer the family to an emergency clinic or to appropriate social services to obtain treatment and work out payment options.

A community/public health nurse might come in contact with parents who refuse to seek medical treatment for children for religious reasons. For example, Jehovah's Witnesses do not consent to blood transfusions, and Christian Scientists do not accept some medical interventions, such as chemotherapy for cancer. In most instances, the severity of the illness dictates whether courts will overrule parental decisions. In life-threatening situations, the court is more likely to overrule a parent's religious objections to treatment (*Nurse's Legal Handbook*, 2002). Nurses must know the laws in their states.

More than 40 states have exemptions from civil child neglect laws for parents who do not believe in taking children to doctors, and a few states have exemptions from criminal law (Asser & Swan, 1998). In states with such parental exemptions, it is legally difficult to force parents to accept medical care for their children. Nurses need to consult with supervisors and legal counsel to ensure that their actions are legally and professionally responsible. Although these situations are rare, Asser and Swan (1998) report that at least 172 deaths of children from easily treatable conditions occurred over the 20-year period ending in 1995.

END OF LIFE/SELF-DETERMINATION

With the movement toward shorter hospital stays and discharge of persons to home for long-term care of terminal illnesses, a growing area of discussion between community health nurses and their clients involves the clients' wishes as they plan for death. Most states have enacted living will statutes that define how clients may let their wishes be known when death is imminent. Clients must have the capacity to create a living will or, in other terms, must be deemed competent to make these important decisions for themselves. However, many living will statutes apply only to terminally ill clients.

Persons might assign a **medical durable power of attorney** to a trusted person, who then becomes empowered to act as a surrogate decision maker if the client becomes incompetent or is unable to make his or her desires known to health care providers. Laws support the idea that clients should have the right to make choices and give consent for treatment. Community health nurses can be most supportive of their clients by informing them of their rights and of possible ways to formally document their wishes that care be provided or withheld under certain circumstances. Specific directives will be the most clear and convincing evidence of a client's wishes. The competent client's wishes should always be followed when legally possible. Even when a client has created a living will or special directive, family members might object to the client's decision to deny treatment. The community health nurse's role, as client advocate, can become more complicated when the client's family interferes. The law specifically protects a person's right to refuse treatment, but in reality, the family is not always in support of their loved one's choosing to refuse lifesaving medical procedures. The community health nurse needs to stay in close communication with the client's physician and the family members to support the client in ultimately maintaining the right to consent or to deny consent to treatment.

The *Client Self-Determination Act of 1992* requires that facilities that receive federal funding (including hospitals, nursing homes, home health agencies, hospices, and prepaid health care organizations) inquire whether clients being admitted to their services have executed a living will or special directive (see Chapter 28).

ENVIRONMENTAL PROTECTION

Nurses can also encourage their clients to pursue their rights and to protect themselves through laws relating to environmental hazards. Laws related to the use of seat belts and infant car seats should be discussed with clients. Other environmental hazard laws include those pertaining to chemical use or waste disposal (see Chapter 9). Food preparation laws apply where food is being prepared for service to the public. Community/public health nurses can help clients avoid unexpected barriers to employment by helping them become aware of their rights, responsibilities, and liabilities as food handlers. Laws related to sanitation and other environmental issues are often carried out by local and state health departments. A growing number of states are developing separate divisions to address the environmental hazard laws that are increasingly being legislated.

NURSE LOBBYING

The practice of a community/public health nurse is greatly affected by legal responsibilities. Nurses should become actively involved and lobby through the legislative and administrative processes. Nurses serve as client advocates when they lobby for improved health care. A **lobbyist** informs decision makers and educates others who need to understand community health care issues. Nurses are informed providers of care who can serve as experts in teaching lawmakers and policy makers about the needs of the community and specific clients.

The American Public Health Association and the ANA lobby on behalf of public health and nursing issues. These two organizations also provide information to their members about upcoming legislation and its impact on health and nursing. N-Stat (Nurses Strategic Action Team), a program of the ANA, provides up-to-date action alerts to nurse members on pending federal legislation. Nurses can use this information to communicate their positions to their legislators. Box 6-1 outlines an effective approach nurses can use to interact with their elected legislators.

HOW TO FIND OUT ABOUT LAWS

Because laws have important ramifications for community/public health nursing practice, nurses must be informed. There are a number of information sources regarding laws affecting nursing practice. If a nurse is employed by a community health agency, the attorney who represents the agency should be the nurse's legal advisor. The agency's attorney will be able to direct the nurse to written health codes and local or state health department policies that are written to conform to existing state laws. Agency protocols often dictate the appropriate channels of communication. Nurses should consult first with their supervisor or health officer regarding questions or concerns about existing policies or procedures before consulting the agency's attorney.

BOX 6-1 Tips for Visits to Legislators

1. Call ahead to make an appointment to meet with the legislator. If the legislator is unavailable, ask to meet with the staff person who handles health issues.
2. Be prepared. Know the background of the legislator and the history of the bill or issue you are discussing. Contact the government relations staff at your professional nursing organization to let them know about the visit. They might be able to provide important information about the issue, the political climate, your legislator's previous record on this issue, and the overall lobbying strategy on this issue.
3. At the beginning of the visit, introduce yourself and state what you want to discuss. Specify the issues and bills.
4. Ask the legislator what his or her position is on the issue or bill.
5. Many legislators and staff might not be familiar with nursing practice or legislative concerns. Be prepared to discuss them in basic terms. If possible, be prepared with facts about nursing practice in your state or district.
6. Ask if he or she has heard from others who support this issue or bill. Ask what the supporters are saying.
7. Ask if he or she has heard from opponents. Ask who the opponents are and what their arguments are.
8. Offer to provide additional information if you do not have data at hand, but do not make promises you cannot keep. It is better to admit you do not know than to promise and not deliver or to convey erroneous information.
9. Follow up with a thank you note and share your reflections on the visit.
10. Keep a written record of your visit. Notify government relations staff of your professional nursing organization so that they can follow up with the legislator.
11. Spend more time with your legislators, even if their positions are not in agreement with yours. You might lessen the intensity of their positions and maintain contact for subsequent issues.
12. Invite legislators to meet you and your colleagues at your work site to help expand their understanding of nursing and health care issues.

From Reinhard, S. C., & Cohen, S. S. (1993). Lobbying policy makers: Individual and collective strategies. In D. Mason, S. Talbott, & J. Leavitt (Eds.). *Policy and politics for nurses: Action and change in the workplace, government, organizations, and community* (2nd ed.; p. 493). Philadelphia: Saunders.

Law schools or the state attorney general's office generally provide excellent law library resources. The law librarian can be a great resource person to assist the nurse in locating the sources and references to review. Legal aid services and state offices of consumer affairs can also be helpful to the nurse and the community health client. Computerized search systems, such as Lexis, Scorpio, and FindLaw, provide information about resources such as books and journal articles, as well as current case law and legislation.

There is a growing body of literature developed by advocacy groups concerned about the public's health and welfare. Community/public health nurses must continue to update their knowledge of health-related laws and become familiar with updated materials on developing trends in health care law. Numerous continuing education programs related to community/public health nursing and the legal aspects of nursing are available in many communities. Attendance at these continuing education programs is highly recommended. Because laws continually change with societal trends, it is not safe to rely on outdated information related to health care law. Professional associations and the media often provide initial information about current or potential changes in laws that affect a community/public health nurse's practice.

STANDARDS OF CARE

The standard of care defines the legal responsibility of the community/public health nurse. It serves as the measuring rod of what appropriate professional nursing care should include. There are both internal, self-set standards of care and externally created standards by which professional behavior is evaluated.

DEFINITION OF A STANDARD OF CARE

A **standard of care** is defined by the courts as the care that a reasonably prudent community/public health nurse would provide under similar circumstances. If the nurse has an advanced nursing degree, a higher standard of competence is expected. The standard of care is also related to what is called the *locality rule.* Specific geographic areas or similar communities (rural or urban) are compared when setting the standards for nursing care.

INTERNAL AND EXTERNAL STANDARDS

The professional behavior of a community/public health nurse is measured against both internal and external standards of reasonableness. *Internal standards* include policies and procedures and might be viewed as self-set standards of the employing agency. The community/public health nurse's job description is an internal standard within which the nurse must work. If the nurse's job description requires the nurse to practice outside the scope of nursing, the Nurse Practice Act takes priority over this internal standard. Courts review these internal standards to evaluate whether they are in accord with what professionals in the field have determined is desired performance. Hospital or agency rules are admissible as evidence of standards of care in the community. Another internal standard used to evaluate the reasonableness of nursing practice is the nursing care plan. If the nurse outlines a care plan for a client and then deviates from this plan, the court might determine that the nurse strayed from a reasonable standard of care. Nursing care plans are the most direct evidence of nursing care judgment.

With national accreditation of most agencies and an increasingly mobile society, a national standard for nursing care has also been developed.

External standards of the reasonableness of the care provided by a community/public health nurse are determined by reviewing the nurse's actions in relation to the Nurse Practice Act or the rules and regulations of the state board of nursing. Other external standards that courts use in evaluating the reasonableness of nursing care include the guidelines submitted by accrediting agencies and professional associations, national standards such as the CDC's universal precautions, well-established standards of care, and the nursing theories of recognized authorities. It is a common court procedure to introduce authorities in the field to verify the standard of care (see Chapter 1).

ROLE OF THE EXPERT WITNESS

The standard of care serves as a means of comparing what a reasonably prudent nurse would reasonably do with what the defendant in a court case actually did. In a legal case involving professional behavior, an expert witness is required to explain to the jury or judge what reasonable community/public health nursing behavior entails. The practice of professionals, such as nurses, is deemed to be "beyond the ken" of the average person. This means that nurses' professional behavior is not commonly understood and is a very specific body of knowledge that must be explained to the average juror and judge.

The expert witness in a case must be truly qualified as an expert in the area of nursing in the case being decided (Mahlmeister, 2008). The expert witness must be certified by the court as having the credentials and the knowledge to provide the court with an accurate and up-to-date evaluation of prudent community/public health nursing. Once the expert is recognized by the court, the expert's opinion or testimony is given no greater weight than the testimony of any other witness. Although juries might be influenced by the credentials and the expertise of an expert witness and might tend to give the testimony more weight than that of other witnesses, the rules of the court do not demand this.

Both parties to a suit are allowed to introduce expert witnesses and testimony. Often, the differing opinions of experts serve to reduce the credibility or impact of both experts' testimony. Plaintiffs, defendants, or their attorneys seek to find an expert who agrees with their views of the behavior of the nurse. For example, if a plaintiff's attorney hires an expert to evaluate a case and that expert returns an opinion that the defendant nurse acted reasonably and prudently as expected of a community/public health nurse, the plaintiff's attorney will not introduce this expert's testimony at the time of trial.

A community/public health nurse who is being sued deserves to have the nursing care she or he provided analyzed by a community/public health nurse who operates in a comparable setting. If the nurse holds a master's or doctoral degree, the expert witness most likely will also be required to have comparable educational preparation. A specialist is held to the standard of care for a member of the given specialty. Therefore, a higher standard of care will be applied to community/public health nurses holding advanced degrees. Nurses are also held accountable for the knowledge they should have gained in their education, as well as for the materials presented in continuing education programs they attend.

Standards of care change with the growing body of knowledge and expectations of what care community/public health nurses will provide. The ANA standards of care for community/public health nurses are discussed in Chapter 1. Community/public health nurses must attend community education programs to stay abreast of current trends in practice. The courts will not evaluate the actions of a nurse who received a degree 20 years previously by the standards of care taught in the nursing curriculum at that time. Examples of changes in the standards of care include the community/public health nurse's involvement in abortion and contraception advice and the care needed to treat communicable diseases, such as hepatitis and AIDS.

QUALITY AND RISK MANAGEMENT

Nurses can reduce the possibility that they will be financially and emotionally devastated by a lawsuit by using quality management information to identify and reduce risks, and thereby prevent injury to clients. Quality management involves learning from past experiences and avoiding known risks to clients. Evaluating provided care and the outcomes of care produces an assessment of quality. Risk management is a component of quality management and serves to indicate where special attention might be needed both to minimize risks and to improve quality of care. The responsibility for ensuring quality care rests with the individual provider, as well as with the employer. A nurse who comes to work overly tired automatically increases the need for risk management. The nurse's role is too important to the client's well-being for the nurse to attempt to provide services while functioning with diminished capacity, regardless of the reason. The employer's policies and procedures should also provide for a safe level of care. If the nurse does not follow these guidelines and protocols, the client can be placed at risk. For example, the nurse in an immunization clinic must always inquire about a client's allergies before administering a vaccine to avoid the risk of an allergic reaction. In one home care case, a nurse failed to follow agency protocol to monitor antibiotic blood levels twice weekly when administering intravenous gentamicin. The client suffered inner ear damage, and the nurse was held accountable (Eskreis, 1998).

CONTINUING EDUCATION

From a legal standpoint, one of the best ways for the nurse to maintain quality assurance in community/public health practice is by keeping updated on new theories and evidence-based advances in client care. The standards of care are based on the most recent information, not on what a nurse learned in a nursing program. Nurses are also accountable for having knowledge of and functioning within the laws of the country and the states in which they practice. The fact that a nurse does not realize that she or he is breaking the law is not a sound defense. Ignorance of the law does not protect nurses from legal liability.

INCIDENT REPORTS

Incident reports are a means of risk management or quality assurance. They should be the community health care agency's internal source for identifying real and potential risks. They can be used to alter existing patterns of care and can even provide the basis for rewriting policies and procedures to ensure a high quality of care. An example of an incident that would need to be reported by a community/public health nurse is giving the wrong vaccine to a client. This incident might encourage better labeling of vaccines and improvements in clarifying the client's identity before proceeding with any procedure.

Incident reports should be written carefully in compliance with an agency's procedures for reporting actual or potential harm to a client. Because public policy desires to encourage practices that reduce the risks for harm, incident reports have traditionally been protected from use in lawsuits against health care providers. However, a newer trend is developing in which incident reports are available as evidence. It is therefore important that the statements in incident reports describing the occurrence be made in nonaccusatory terms. Nurses should describe the event in factual terms without pointing fingers at certain persons or assigning blame for the injuries that resulted. It is always safest to document facts rather than opinions. As with all documentation, incident reports should be truthful and should be submitted in a timely fashion, and nurses should follow the agency's policy when filing an incident report.

An incident report is an internal risk management document. If reference is made to its existence in the client record, however, a plaintiff's attorney might then have access to the report. A growing number of jurisdictions are allowing incident reports to become "discoverable" (Mahlmeister, 2008). This means that if an incident report is subpoenaed, it must be shared with the opposing side.

TIMELY DOCUMENTATION AND COMMUNICATION

The nurse's notes are a risk management and quality assurance tool not only for the employer but also for the individual nurse. A nurse's documentation can serve as proof that the nurse acted reasonably and safely. As discussed earlier, documentation should be accurate and thorough, and performed in a timely manner. If care is not documented in a timely manner, other health care providers might perform their services for clients based on inaccurate or incomplete information. It is also important that nurses, as members of the health care team, communicate verbally in a timely manner with other team members. When the potential for a lawsuit is being evaluated, the nurse's notes are very often the first record to be reviewed by the plaintiff's legal counsel. If the nurse's credibility seems questionable based on these documents, a greater risk of liability exists for the nurse (Eskreis, 1998).

PROFESSIONAL LIABILITY INSURANCE

Professional liability insurance might be considered a means of risk management. Liability insurance will not prevent the nurse from being sued but will rather serve as a safety net to protect the nurse's personal resources and ability to be defended against a lawsuit. Many nurses rely on their employer's professional liability insurance policy as their total coverage. If the employer and the nurse find themselves in the position of having a conflict of interest (e.g., the nurse did not follow the agency's policy and procedures), it is likely that the nurse will be less protected by the policy than the employer. It is recommended that nurses carry their own personal professional liability insurance in addition to that provided by their employers. A professional liability policy is a contract between the insured professional and the insurance company. If nurses carry their own liability coverage, they are buying the protection of the insurance company, provided they comply with all of the conditions of the policy.

When the nurse is selecting a professional liability policy, it is suggested that the nurse seek an occurrence policy rather than a claims-made policy. An **occurrence policy** provides protection if the incident occurs while the nurse is insured by the policy. Under a **claims-made policy,** not only does the incident have to occur while the nurse is insured by the company, but the policy also has to be in force at the time the plaintiff brings suit against the nurse. Statutes of limitations in various jurisdictions limit the time under which a plaintiff may bring suit against a health care provider. If the statute of limitations is 2 years, the nurse could be sued by a client who has not been seen for 2 years. Therefore, under a claims-made policy, the nurse would have to continuously maintain the same policy or buy tail coverage from the insurance company. **Tail coverage** extends the policy's protection beyond the term of the policy and can be very expensive.

Community/public health nurses might be asked to provide assistance that is not within the scope of their employment and, therefore, is not within the coverage of the employer's liability insurance. Although the nurse might be covered by the employer during travel between visits to clients, automobile trips to and from work are not within the scope of employer insurance. Another risk involves transporting clients in the nurse's automobile. If an accident occurs and the client is injured, the fact that the nurse is driving the client in the capacity of an employed professional affects the relationship defined and might diminish the nurse's protection. If the nurse is participating in a health screening clinic that is sponsored by an agency other than the nurse's employer, the employer's liability insurance likely does not cover the nurse when the nurse is acting in that capacity. The nurse's membership on community boards, if she or he is not acting as a representative of the employer, and any private nursing business also is not covered under an employer's liability insurance policy.

PROFESSIONAL INVOLVEMENT

Professional involvement in organizations or on committees that define the standards of care for community/public health nursing is another means of risk management. Nurses also benefit their profession when they participate on community boards. Nursing input is very valuable when future planning or current community issues are being discussed. Nurses must be willing to represent nursing and client perspectives regarding community needs and future directions. Membership in professional nursing organizations, such as the ANA, the National League for Nursing, and state nursing associations, is also important. The viewpoint of nurses becomes more powerful when nurses work together to create an organized and cohesive profession.

ETHICS AND LAW

Ethical and legal issues are closely related to other areas of concern for nurses. Legal and ethical issues surround the right to choose how one will live while dying and who should have the right to make decisions regarding the treatment plan. Because nurses work in a society that is based on laws, they must help to change laws that do not reflect nurses' ethical values. *Ethical issues* reflect moral ideas of right and wrong, whereas *laws* deal with the regulation of social behavior. Laws are passed to protect society as a whole or segments of the population that need special protection. The ethical implications of these laws are related to legal responsibilities in community/public health nursing. The community/public health nurse's moral beliefs and values regarding the rights of family members to deal with privacy matters, including contraception and abortion, coexist with legal responsibilities for nurses.

Abuse in society is an ethical issue that imposes direct legal responsibilities on nursing practice. The reporting laws of most states mandate that a health professional who becomes aware of abuse must disclose this information to the proper authorities. The community/public health nurse must be careful to document factual and accurate information to prepare such a report. It is important to avoid including hearsay evidence (reports from others) in one's reports.

Ethical decision making can be very difficult and emotionally charged. Decision makers with differing values attempt to be fair to the people involved while determining what is considered wrong or right or where the duties, obligations, and responsibilities lie. Consensus is not easily achieved. When an ethical issue becomes important to society, laws are usually passed that provide guidance about how society has determined nurses must respond. Because ethical issues are highly emotionally charged, the legal system does not intervene until there is a clear mandate from society to make a decision. Current court decisions on the client's right to refuse or terminate life-saving treatment are examples of how one ethical issue—the right to die—has become a legal issue with implications for nursing care delivery.

The managed care environment is often disproportionately focused on cost savings and profit margins. As an example, the public outcry regarding premature discharge of newly delivered mothers has resulted in legal protections that ensure newborns adequate time in the hospital to be observed and screened for PKU before being sent home. The issue was not just the length of hospitalization but also the quality of postpartum care that was provided. Without an opportunity to observe and assess the mother and her newborn, community/public health nurses were very likely to confront problems that were not detected in the hospital before the mother and newborn were discharged.

The managed care environment is now virtually the entire health care system in which nurses work. A nurse does not have to be employed by a health maintenance organization to see his or her practice change markedly. Capitation, shifting financial incentives, and efforts to shift care from intensive inpatient services to other settings such as community-based and extended care facilities, affect virtually every nurse and every client. Ethics requires that practitioners review all appropriate services with their clients. In a recent national survey, 31% of physicians indicated that in some situations they had not offered their patients appropriate services because of perceived coverage limitations (Wynia et al., 2003). The ANA, specialty nursing groups, other health care providers, and consumer protection groups have combined efforts to ensure that restrictions in health care plans do not adversely affect clients. Of particular concern are whistle blower protection, elimination of financial incentives to delay or deny health care services, and hospital length-of-stay issues. Mental health parity legislation (see Chapters 25 and 33) and

managed care's ongoing immunity from malpractice suits are current concerns (Bloche, 2004). There is an ongoing effort at both the federal and state levels to limit managed care's immunity from prosecution for medical errors or for denial of services.

A nurse's right to speak out on issues in health care delivery is sometimes protected by whistle blower laws, which vary from state to state (Markus, 2006). In one instance, a nurse, Linda Carl, was fired in retaliation for reporting that her employer's treatment facilities were not in compliance with state regulations. She sued for damages. A Texas court awarded her a judgment of $1.16 million (Monarch, 2002). In another case, the National Labor Relations Board provided some protection for whistle blowers, ruling that nurse Barry Adams had been illegally fired for speaking out against unsafe nursing care (NLRB judge rules for Massachusetts nurse, 1998). The nurses in both cases were supported by the respective regional chapters of the ANA. Although both nurses were successful, they experienced job loss, loss of seniority, stress, and a protracted legal battle. Both verdicts were appealed by the employers. In the current health care environment, nurses can expect to encounter many more such situations that have both ethical and legal ramifications. Most states do not have whistle blower protection. Fifteen states have passed protective legislation for health care workers who report quality of care and client safety concerns (Monarch, 2002).

Whereas ethics is influenced by attitudes, values, and beliefs that determine what is right, wrong, or fair, laws generally address only what is wrong in a particular society. It is not always possible or desirable to attempt to translate ethical principles into legal terms. Laws might restrict or protect personal freedoms. Ethics is a broader, more universal concept than law, which is narrower and deals with the system of compliance in a given society. As advocates, nurses might provide a bridge between ethics and law. Justice, or the principles of fairness and equity, is needed in law and in ethics.

KEY IDEAS

1. Community/public health nurses need a clear understanding of the laws that govern their nursing practice, including criminal law, civil law, and family law.

2. Most environmental and public health laws are enacted at the state level but must conform to broad directives in federal legislation.

3. Administrative bodies are responsible for formulating the rules and regulations that clarify and interpret the intent of legislation. The state board of nursing is an example of an administrative body that interprets the legislative intent of the state's Nurse Practice Act.

4. Nurses interested in affecting or changing laws must understand the importance of lobbying administrative agencies as well as legislative representatives.

5. Community/public health nurses might incur both criminal and civil sanctions for acts performed in the course of their nursing practice. Civil malpractice is the most common action. Criminal prosecution is usually reserved for egregious acts, such as mercy killing.

6. All community/public health nurses have a duty to be knowledgeable about and practice within the scope of their states' Nurse Practice Acts. They should be clear

about their responsibilities related to physician orders (both standing and verbal), documentation of services, and the relationship between their employing agencies' policies and their professional responsibilities.

7. Nurses must be aware of client rights, including the right to informed consent, the right to privacy, and the right to select or reject health care services as well as determine the limits of health care services received.

8. Nurses whose practice includes vulnerable populations, such as persons with disabilities, children, elderly persons,

and victims of abuse, have a duty to understand the law regarding their professional responsibilities and the rights of their clients.

9. The legal yardstick against which any nurse's professional competence is judged is the standard of care, or what a reasonably prudent nurse would do in a similar situation.

10. Community/public health nurses should be vigilant in monitoring and influencing laws that affect their professional practice and the health of individuals, families, and communities.

CASE STUDY   Understanding a Nurse's Legal Responsibilities

In a case involving a community/public health nurse, the court determined that the nurse was negligent in failing to properly assess the seriousness of a schoolchild's asthma attack.

The child came to the school nurse's office seeking help. The nurse gave another child's inhaler to the student and sent her back to class but soon learned her classmates were still concerned that she needed help. The nurse assessed the student and determined that neither an ambulance, supplemental oxygen, not a wheelchair was needed for the student to travel to her physician's office. Within minutes, the student collapsed and stopped breathing; she died following a brief comatose period.

The plaintiff presented expert testimony from a registered nurse and an asthma specialist. Their opinions were that the defendant nurse deviated from the standard of care in the community for school nursing and directly caused the student's death. Three experts testified on the defendant's behalf that the nurse did not deviate from the standard of care nor cause the death of the student.

The jury concluded that the nurse was negligent and ordered the defendant to pay the child's family $142,289. The nurse's failure to provide the needed care in a timely fashion was found by the court to be directly related to the child's death. The nurse had also violated the school district's policy by not calling the student's parents.

The court found that the school nurse has a higher duty of care than a hospital nurse to make an assessment of the need for emergency medical services. The nurse was not expected to provide medical care, but rather to determine the need for emergency care. The nurse's action also fell below the required standard of reasonable

judgment by authorizing the use of another student's asthma inhaler (*Schlussler v Independent School District*, 1989).

Several nursing actions might have helped the community health nurse in this case to provide safe, appropriate care in these circumstances:

- Better physical assessment skills might have enabled the nurse to determine the severity of the student's signs and symptoms and to conclude that, without available medication, emergency care was appropriate.
- The nurse might have consulted with other nurses and physicians to develop written criteria to determine when emergency care is needed in selected circumstances.
- The nurse might have followed the basic standard of care and laws governing prescription medications by not giving the student someone else's medication.
- The nurse might have monitored the student for a longer period of time, recognized that the asthma attack was not abating, and then called for emergency services.
- The nurse might have followed school policy and informed the parents of the student's illness, in which case the parents might have come to the school in time to initiate a request for emergency services.
- The nurse might have created a health form to be completed by parents and, for those students with chronic illnesses, requested orders from the students' physicians regarding individualized treatment.

 See **Critical Thinking Questions** for this Case Study on the book's website.

LEARNING BY EXPERIENCE AND REFLECTION

1. Review your state's procedure for enacting laws. Contact your state legislature for a copy of the process or visit your local library for the information. Information may also be found online.

2. Identify your district representatives to your state legislature. Find out if any of them serve on committees that help to determine public health or professional practice legislation. If so, call or write, asking them for copies of the current issues before their committee and their position on those issues.

3. Contact your state board of nursing; check its websites. Ask about pending hearings regarding a rule, regulation, or disciplinary matter. If possible, attend hearings that are relevant to your practice. If you are not able to attend, ask the board to send you information on a proposed change or new rule or regulation. Review the proposal and try to identify what impact it would have on your practice.

4. Courtrooms are open to the public. Attend a trial or hearing as an observer of the legal process. Ask a court clerk if there are any health-related cases on the court schedule. If so, attending the trial will give you some idea of how a health-related matter is handled within the court system.

5. Read the local newspaper. Identify a health-related issue that is under consideration by either the legislature or an administrative agency. Follow the progress of the debate or hearings via the news. Try to identify the various interested parties and their positions on the issue. Write, call, or visit your legislator or the administrative agency and express your views on the issue.

6. Contact your state nurses' association and obtain a list of issues that are critical to nursing. Determine your associa-

tion's position on the issues and its rationale for that position. Ask how your nursing organization lobbies for its positions with the legislature and administrative agencies.

7. Obtain a copy of your state's Nurse Practice Act and *read it*.

8. Review the policy and procedure manual from a community/public health nursing agency. Identify forms that must be signed by clients to receive services, transfer medical records, and authorize reimbursement.

STUDY AIDS   http://evolve.elsevier.com/Maurer/community/

Visit the Evolve website for this book to find the following study and assessment materials:

- Quiz
- Web Scenario
- Critical Thinking Questions and Answers for Case Studies

- Care Plans
- *Healthy People* Updates
- Glossary

REFERENCES

Alan Guttmacher Institute. (2007). *State policies in brief: An overview of minors' consent law.* New York: Author. Retrieved September 25, 2007 from *http://www.guttmacher.org/statecenter/spibs/spib_OMCL.pdf.*

Asser, S., & Swan, R. (1998). Child fatalities from "religion motivated" medical neglect. *Pediatrics, 101*(4), 625-629.

Bloche, M. G. (2004). Back to the 90s—The Supreme Court immunizes managed care. *New England Journal of Medicine, 351*(13), 1277-1279.

Center for Community Change. (1996). *Less money, fewer rules, more power to the state.* The 104th Congress, Public Policy Department.

Croke, E. M. (2003). Nurses, negligence, and malpractice: An analysis based on more than 250 cases against nurses. *American Journal of Nursing, 103*(9), 54-63.

Cutrona, A. K. (2001). Home health nursing. In M. E. O'Keefe (Ed.), *Nursing practice and the law: Avoiding malpractice and other legal risks* (pp. 317-335). Philadelphia: F. A. Davis.

Eskreis, T. R. (1998). Seven common legal pitfalls in nursing. *American Journal of Nursing, 98*(4), 34-40.

Frank-Stromborg, M., & Christensen, A. (2001). Nurse documentation: Not done or worse, done the wrong way—Part II. *Oncology Nursing Forum, 28*(5), 841-846.

Frank-Stromborg, M., & Ganschow, J. R. (2002). How HIPAA will change your practice. *Journal of Nursing, 32*(9), 54-57.

Goldsmith, J. (2003). Negligent nurse or scapegoat? *American Journal of Nursing, 103*(6), 23.

Goodman, R. A., Moulton, A., Matthews, G., (2006). Law and public health at CDC. *MMWR Morb Mortal Wkly Rep, 55*(suppl 2), 29-33.

Guido, G. W. (1997). *Legal issues in nursing* (2nd ed.). Norwalk, CT: Appleton & Lange.

Hall, J. K., & Hall, D. (2001). Negligence specific to nursing. In M. E. O'Keefe (Ed.), *Nursing practice and the law: Avoiding malpractice and other legal risks* (pp. 132-149). Philadelphia: F. A. Davis.

Higgenbotham, E. L. (2001). Documentation. In M. E. O'Keefe (Ed.), *Nursing practice and the law: Avoiding malpractice and other legal risks* (pp. 163-174). Philadelphia: F. A. Davis.

Holloway, R. (2001). Patient rights. In M. E. O'Keefe (Ed.), *Nursing practice and the law: Avoiding malpractice and other legal risks* (pp. 189-198). Philadelphia: F. A. Davis.

Kelly, L., & Joel, L. A. (1995). *Dimensions of professional nursing* (7th ed.). New York: McGraw-Hill.

Lunsford v Board of Nurse Examiners, 648 S.W. 2d 391 (Tex. App. 1983).

Mahlmeister, L. R. (2008). Legal issues in nursing and health care. In B. Cherry & S. R. Jacob (Eds.), *Contemporary nursing: Issues, trends, and management* (4th ed.). St. Louis: Mosby.

Marchand, D. V. (2001). American jurisprudence. In M. E. O'Keefe (Ed.), *Nursing practice and the law: Avoiding malpractice and other legal risks* (pp. 3-22). Philadelphia: F. A. Davis.

Markus, K. (2006). The nurse as patient advocate: Is there a conflict of interest? In P. S. Crown & S. Moorhead (Eds.), *Current issues in nursing* (7th ed.). St. Louis: Mosby.

Mazur v Merck and Co., 964 F. 2d 1348, 1992.

Monarch, K. (2002). *Nursing and the law: Trends and issues.* Washington DC: American Nurses Association.

National Practitioner Data Bank. (2004). *2004 Annual Report.* Retrieved November 13, 2007 from *http://www.npdb-hipdb.hrsa.gov/pubs/stats/2004_NPDB_Annual_Report.pdf.*

National Practitioner Data Bank. (2005). *2005 Annual report.* Retrieved September 17, 2007 from *http://www.npdb-hipdb.hrsa.gov/pubs/stats/2005_NPDB_Annual_Report.pdf.*

NLRB judge rules for Massachusetts nurse in whistle-blowing case. (1998). *American Nurse, 30*(1), 7.

Nurse's legal handbook (4th ed.). (2002). Philadelphia, PA: Springhouse Corporation.

Reinhard, S. C., & Cohen, S. S. (1993). Lobbying policy makers: Individual and collective strategies. In D. Mason, S. Talbott, & J. Leavitt (Eds.). *Policy and politics for nurses: Action and change in the workplace, government, organizations, and community* (2nd ed.; p. 493). Philadelphia: Saunders.

Schlussler v Independent School District, 1989. No. 200, et al. Case number MM89-14V. Minnesota Case Reports.

Service Employees International Union. (2007). *State legislation to limit mandatory overtime* (SEIU Fact sheet). Retrieved September 21, 2007 from *http://www.seiu.org/health/hosp/mandatory_overtime2/mot_factsheet.cfm.*

Tuma v Board of Nursing, 593 P. 2nd 711 (ID, 1979).

Turnock, B. J. (2004). *Public health: What it is and how it works* (3rd ed.). Sudbury, MA: Jones & Bartlett.

Walker v Merck and Co., 648 F. Supp. 931, 1986.

Wynia, M. K., VanGeest, J., Cummins, D. S., et al. (2003). Do physicians not offer useful services because of coverage restrictions? *Health Affairs, 22*(4), 190-197.

SUGGESTED READINGS

Aiken, T. D. (Ed.). (2004). *Legal, ethical and political issues in nursing*. Philadelphia: F. A. Davis.

American Nurses Association. (2001). *Code of ethics for nurses with interpretive statements*. Washington, DC: Author.

Badzek, L., & Gross, L. (1999). Confidentiality and privacy: At the forefront for nurses. *American Journal of Nursing, 99*(6), 52, 54.

Badzek, L., Leslie, N., & Richert, B. (1998). Legal considerations at the end-of-life. *Journal of Nursing Law, 5*(2), 51-63.

Brent, N. J. (2001). *Nurses and the law: A guide to principles of applications* (2nd ed.). Philadelphia: Saunders.

Killion, S. (1993). Case commentary—*Bass v. Barksdale*: Implications for public health and home care nurses. *Public Health Nursing, 10*(2), 129-133.

Kjervik, D., & Badzek, L. (1998). Legal considerations at the end-of-life. *AANA Journal, 25*, 593-597.

Marrelli, T. M. (2000). *Nursing documentation handbook* (3rd ed.). St. Louis: Mosby.

O'Keefe, M. E. (2001). *Nursing practice and the law: Avoiding malpractice and other legal risks*. Philadelphia: F. A. Davis.

Tucker, S. M., Canobbio, M. M., Wells, H. G., et al. (2000). *Patient care standards—Collaborative planning and nursing interventions* (7th ed.). St. Louis: Mosby.

Core Concepts for the Practice of Community/Public Health Nursing

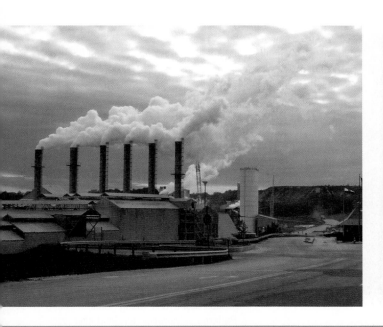

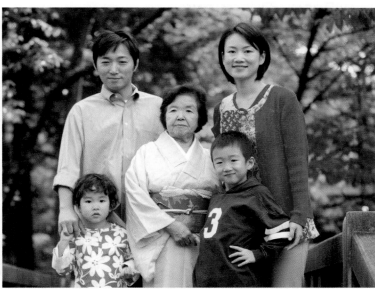

Epidemiology: Unraveling the Mysteries of Disease and Health

*Gina Castelnovo Rowe**

FOCUS QUESTIONS

What is epidemiology?

How does the diagnosis of the health status of a population differ from an assessment of a family or an individual?

What statistical measures are used in epidemiology?

How are data used in determining the health status of a community?

How are epidemiologic concepts and methods, such as incidence and prevalence or knowledge of the natural history of a disease, used

in assessing health, planning programs, and evaluating the quality of health care delivery?

What is known from epidemiologic data about the overall health of the American population and aggregates?

How is epidemiologic information used to frame or focus health-related research?

CHAPTER OUTLINE

KEY TERMS

Analytic studies
Case-control
Cohort
Correlation
Descriptive studies
Epidemics
Epidemiology
Experimental trial

Health information systems
Incidence
Morbidity
Mortality
Pandemics
Prevalence
Primary prevention
Rate

Ratio
Records
Secondary prevention
Surveillance
Surveys
Tertiary prevention
Vital statistics

*The author acknowledges the contribution of Anita J. Tarzian for her work on this chapter in the previous edition of the book.

"Too Much Heart Surgery?" "Where Do We Stand in the Fight against Cancer?" "What Doctors Don't Know about Women: NIH Tries to Close the Gender Gap in Research." "Baby Boomers Enter Their Fifties." "Decline of Birth Rate in United States." "Evaluation of Health: Haves and Have Nots." "Increasing Global Burden of AIDS."

What is the source of the information that produces these headlines? Who collects it? How is the information used in nursing and health care? Understanding health problems, conditions related to health, and ways to improve the well-being of a population requires a systematic approach to gathering factual information. This chapter does the following:

- Presents an overview of basic formulas and methods of epidemiologic investigation
- Explores how epidemiology helps identify the impact of environment, heredity, and personal behaviors and relate these factors to the health status of individuals and groups
- Identifies the most important health issues for all age groups in the United States

The last objective is a critical first step in assessing the health needs of populations, aggregates, and target groups.

Epidemiology is the discipline that provides the structure for systematically studying the distribution and determinants of health, disease, and conditions related to health status. Epidemiologic concepts are used to understand and explain how and why health and illness occur as they do in human populations. Nursing and medical science employ these concepts to help guide clinical practice and influence health outcomes. For example, the Healthy Babies Program, which includes home visiting by a nurse during an infant's first year, was established to decrease infant mortality and promote health.

Florence Nightingale, the first nurse epidemiologist, pioneered the use of statistics to improve public health. During the Crimean War, Nightingale collected data and systemized record-keeping practices to improve hospital conditions. She invented pie charts and other graphical illustrations to depict mortality rates and show how improvements in sanitary conditions would lead to a decrease in deaths. By focusing on health and disease trends among populations, Nightingale saved or improved the lives of countless individuals, the ultimate goal of epidemiology.

INTERESTS OF POPULATION-BASED DATA

In community health nursing, the community or the total population under investigation replaces the individual as the focus of concern and study. Nursing at the community level extends the boundaries of practice beyond those that are traditionally associated with caregiving activities. The thinking and decision making that a community health nurse uses to define the health status of a community are markedly different from those used in assessing individual clients or families. Applying the nursing process to the entire community is complex and generally requires educational preparation at the graduate level.

The concepts and methods employed in assessing health status that affect program planning in health care, as well as analysis and applications of epidemiologic data, form the basis of this chapter. An in-depth understanding of statistics is not required to understand epidemiology. Computation of the simple formulas used in this chapter requires only basic mathematical skills: addition, subtraction, multiplication, and division.

A FEW STATISTICS

Rate, ratio, incidence, and *prevalence* are common terms used to help describe illness and disease among population groups.

Rates and Ratios

A **rate** is a statistic used to describe an event or characteristic. In epidemiology a rate is used to make comparisons among populations or to compare a subgroup of the population (specific rate) with the total population. The numerator of a rate is the actual number of events, and the denominator is the total population at risk. In epidemiology the rate is usually converted to a standard base denominator—such as 1000, 10,000, or 100,000—to permit comparisons between various population groups (Box 7-1). A rate description includes time, person/population, and place specifications (e.g., the number per year [time] in uninsured children [population] in a specific city [place]).

Using standard base rates makes comparing the magnitude of an event (e.g., illness, death) in different population groups easier. For example, if city A had 125 teenage pregnancies in an at-risk population group of 120,602 female teenagers (14 to 19 years old), the rate of teenage pregnancies in city A could be expressed as 125 per 120,602. If city B had 492 teenage pregnancies in an at-risk population of 194,301 female teenagers, the rate of teenage pregnancies in city B would be 492 per 194,301 (see Box 7-1). Comparison of these two rates is difficult because

---

BOX 7-1   Rates and Ratios

A. Rates

1. A rate is:

$$\frac{\text{Number of events}}{\text{Population at risk}} \times 100,000 \text{ (or another standard base number)}$$

Example:
City A's teen pregnancy specific rate is arrived at by:

$$\frac{125 \text{ (number of pregnancies)}}{120,602 \text{ (population at risk)}} \text{ or } \frac{125}{120,602}$$

2. In epidemiology, this rate is converted to a common base such as 100,000, which is accomplished by multiplying the specific rate by the common base:

$$\frac{125}{120,602} \times 100,000 = 103 \text{ or } 103 \text{ teenage pregnancies per } 100,000 \text{ adolescents 14 to 19 years old}$$

Example:
Converting city B's specific rate of 492/194,301 to a common base of 100,000:

$$\frac{492}{194,301} \times 100,000 = 253 \text{ or } 253 \text{ teenage pregnancies per } 100,000 \text{ adolescents 14 to 19 years old}$$

B. Ratios

Ratios are expressed on a common base. Thus, the ratio of city A to city B is 103 to 253, which is expressed as 103:253. Dividing 253 by 103 equals 2.4563, or a ratio of 1:2.4563, which is expressed as approximately 1:2.5.

no common reference point exists. However, if the denominators of these two rates were converted to a common at-risk population of 100,000, city A's rate would be 103 per 100,000, and city B's rate would be 253 per 100,000. Common base rates permit accurate comparisons and are much easier to understand.

Health statistics are sometimes reported as a **ratio,** which is simply the comparison of one number with another. A ratio is often used to compare one at-risk population with another. Ratios are usually simplified by reducing the numbers so that the smallest number becomes 1. To use the example of cities A and B, the ratio of teenage pregnancies in city A to those in city B would be 103 (city A) to 253 (city B), or 103:253, which can be reduced to approximately 1:2.5; in other words, city B has approximately 2.5 times as many teenage pregnancies per 100,000 female teenagers aged 14 to 19 years as does city A.

Suppose you were told that more homicides occurred in Los Angeles than in Washington, DC. How would you compare the rates, rather than just the numbers? Would you need to know the total population at risk for each city? In 2006 there were 480 homicides in Los Angeles, a city of 3,879,455 people, and 169 in Washington, DC, a city of 581,530 people. The murder rate for Los Angeles was 12.37 per 100,000 population compared with 29.06 per 100,000 population in Washington, DC (Federal Bureau of Investigation, 2007a, 2007b). The murder rate for Washington, DC was more than two times higher than that for Los Angeles.

Measures of Morbidity and Mortality

Statistics on **mortality** (death rates) and **morbidity** (illness rates) are collected routinely and used to describe the frequency of death or disease for a given time, place, and group of persons. Morbidity statistics also include measures related to specific symptoms of a disease, days lost from work, and number of clinic visits. In the United States, the law requires that death records be kept; they are tabulated by the National Center for Health Statistics and help determine trends in the United States.

Incidence and Prevalence Rates

Incidence refers to the rate at which a specific disease develops in a population. The incidence rate is the number of new cases of an illness or injury that occurs within a specified time. In contrast, **prevalence** measures all of the existing cases at a given point in time. Prevalence includes the new cases (incidence) plus all of the existing cases. The prevalence rate is influenced by how many people become ill and how many people recover or die (Figure 7-1).

Prevalence is important in determining measures of chronic illness in a population and is affected by factors that influence the duration of the disease. Thus prevalence rates have relevance for planning for health care services, resources, and facilities; for determining health care personnel needs; and for evaluating treatments that prolong life.

Conversely, incidence rates are used as tools for studying patterns of both acute and chronic illness. Incidence rates are important because they are a direct measure of the magnitude of new illness in a population and provide assessments about the risk associated with particular illnesses. For example, the incidence of certain childhood illnesses, such as measles, polio, and whooping cough, was drastically reduced in the United States during the twentieth century with the introduction of vaccines effective in preventing these diseases. Because they reflect only the development of a disease, incidence rates may be influenced

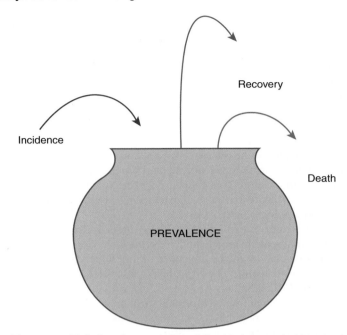

FIGURE 7-1 Prevalence pot: the relationship between incidence and prevalence. (From Morton, R. F., Hebel, J. R., & McCarter, R. J. [2001]. *A study guide to epidemiology and biostatistics* [5th ed.]. Sudbury, MA: Jones & Bartlett.)

by preventive health measures but typically remain unchanged by new medical treatment patterns. New drugs to treat type 2 diabetes mellitus can help to control blood glucose levels and prevent serious disease complications, such as heart attack, blindness, and limb amputation, but they will not affect diabetes incidence; only health promotion and disease prevention efforts targeting behavioral change in diet and exercise patterns have the potential to decrease incidence of this chronic disease.

CRUDE, ADJUSTED, AND SPECIFIC RATES

A rate can be expressed for the total population (*crude* or *adjusted* rate) or for a subgroup of the population (*specific* rate). Box 7-2 presents the formulas for frequently used mortality rates. Age-specific and age-adjusted rates are often quite helpful in making comparisons among populations.

Boca Raton, Florida, is a retirement community populated by a high proportion of persons older than 65 years of age. Orlando, Florida, also has a significant population of retirees, but the personnel of many corporate headquarters and young people who work at Disney World also live there. Comparing mortality rates in the two cities would not be justified unless the death rates of, for example, 65-year-olds and 25-year-olds are compared for each city. This comparison would be age specific. If each age-specific rate in Boca Raton were compared with the age-specific rate in a standard population, the number of deaths of people in that age group in Boca Raton would then have been adjusted to reflect the age distribution of the standard population. The same adjustment would need to be performed on data from Orlando to ensure that any differences were not the result of differences in the age distribution of the two cities. Similar adjustments can be made for gender, race, and socioeconomic class if the researcher wants to exclude the effects of these factors in making comparisons among populations.

| BOX 7-2 | **Frequently Used Mortality Rates** |

$$\text{Crude death rate} = \frac{\text{Total number of deaths during a years}}{\text{Total population at mid-year}} \times 1000$$

$$\text{Cause specific death rate} = $$
$$\frac{\text{Total number of deaths from specific cause during a years}}{\text{Total population at mid-year}} \times 1000$$

$$\text{Age-specific death rate} = $$
$$\frac{\text{Total number of deaths from a specific cause}}{\text{Total mid-year population of the given age group}} \times 1000$$

$$\text{Maternal death rate} = \frac{\text{Total number of maternal deaths}}{\text{Total number of live births}} \times 1000$$

$$\text{Infant mortality rate} = $$
$$\frac{\text{Total number of deaths of children} <1\text{year}}{\text{Total number of live births during the same year}} \times 1000$$

$$\text{Neonatal death rate} = $$
$$\frac{\text{Total number of deaths, birth to 28 days of age}}{\text{Total number of live births plus fetal deaths during year}} \times 1000$$

$$\text{Fetal death rate} = $$
$$\frac{\text{Total number of deaths during 20-28 weeks' gestation}}{\text{Total number of live births plus fetal deaths during year}} \times 1000$$

TYPES OF EPIDEMIOLOGIC INVESTIGATION

People who are engaged in epidemiologic research frequently *observe* rather than *manipulate* variables believed to influence the health of the human population. An observational methodology means that the researcher has far less control of the factors under study and that extraneous factors may not be well controlled for in the study design. Epidemiologic studies, however, do identify nonrandom patterns of health and disease and serve as the basis for determining the circumstances in which experimental studies would be beneficial. They also are of value in planning and evaluating health care services. Epidemiologic studies can be divided into three major types: descriptive, analytic, and experimental.

DESCRIPTIVE STUDIES

Descriptive studies, including prevalence and **correlation** studies, customarily *describe* the amount and distribution of disease within a population. This approach relies primarily on collection of existing data and answers the following questions:
- Who is affected (person)?
- Where is the disease distributed in the human population (place)?
- When is the disease present (time)?
- What is the overall effect of the disease (population)?

The National Health Interview Survey, sponsored by the U.S. Department of Health and Human Services (USDHHS), is administered to a random sample of individuals in the United States. Descriptive information from this survey provides demographic and health information for the nation. The results of this survey are available to the public, and researchers who are seeking to test their own hypotheses can conduct secondary analyses of this descriptive data set.

An example of a prevalence study is "Vitamin D Deficiency and Seasonal Variation in an Adult South Florida Population" (Levis, et al., 2005). At winter's end, the researchers found deficient levels of vitamin D in 38% of men and 40% of women in the study. These prevalence rates were higher than expected in a southern region, which indicated that health care providers in Florida should still consider vitamin D deficiency as a possible factor when assessing patients for osteoporosis.

An example of a correlational design is a study conducted by Ma and associates (2003) using data from the Seasonal Variation of Blood Cholesterol Study (1994 to 1998) to evaluate the relationship between eating patterns and obesity. Results indicated that the occurrence of a greater number of eating episodes per day was associated with a lower risk of obesity. In contrast, skipping breakfast was associated with increased prevalence of obesity, as was greater frequency of eating breakfast or dinner away from home. Thus, the study identified associations, or correlations, between obesity and possible contributing factors.

Descriptive studies may employ cross-sectional timing in their design, in which information on risk factors or exposures and information on outcomes or diseases is all gathered at the same time. Because data are gathered at only one point in time, it can be difficult to determine which actually occurred first, suspected risk factors or disease. Does skipping breakfast contribute to developing obesity, or do obese people tend to skip breakfast more often? Associations between variables may be noted in descriptive studies, but these are not necessarily due to cause-and-effect relationships.

ANALYTIC STUDIES

Like descriptive studies, **analytic studies** use observational methodology, but in contrast to simple descriptive designs, analytic studies begin to answer questions about cause-and-effect relationships between a potential risk factor and a specific health phenomenon or disease condition. Hypotheses, which are statements of possible relationships, are used to predict the causal association among the variables. Being able to predict risk thus points to factors that, if changed, may prevent the disease from occurring or reduce its risk. The hypotheses are tested through studies using cohort or case-control designs, and these studies may be retrospective or prospective.

Cohort studies are useful in identifying factors associated with increased risk of developing certain diseases. The Framingham Heart Study is a classic example of a prospective cohort study, which follows originally healthy people over time to observe risk factors and the development of disease. The study was begun in 1948 with funds from the National Heart Institute in Framingham, Massachusetts, to identify factors contributing to cardiovascular disease. It is still going on today in collaboration with Boston University and now includes data on three generations—the original study subjects, the offspring of the original cohort, and the generation III cohort (National Heart, Lung, and Blood Institute, 2002). Landmark findings from the Framingham Heart Study have provided information about obesity and elevated lipid levels as risk factors for atherosclerotic disease and about tobacco use, sedentary lifestyles, hypertension, and diabetes as risk factors for cardiovascular disease.

Another example of a cohort study is the Nurses' Health Study II, initiated by Dr. Walter Willett and colleagues in 1989 with funds from the National Institutes of Health. The primary goal was to gather long-term information about oral contraceptive use, diet, and lifestyle risk factors in a population of women younger than the original Nurses' Health Study cohort. Nurses between 25 and 42 years of age were included—116,686 total. Every 2 years, cohort members receive a follow-up questionnaire asking about diseases and health-related topics such as smoking, hormone use, pregnancy history, menopausal status, frequency of consumption of specific foods, and quality of life (Bertone et al., 2001).

Case-control studies are retrospective because the study begins after the health outcome has already occurred. Researchers select a group of case subjects with a known disease or health outcome and compare them to a group of control subjects who do not have the disease or health outcome. King and associates (2005) used a case-control design to investigate potential relationships between stillbirths in Nova Scotia and Eastern Ontario, Canada, and chlorine disinfection by-products found in public drinking water sources. They found that stillbirth cases were more likely than live birth controls to have been exposed to some types of these drinking water disinfection by-products (trihalomethanes) but not to others (haloacetic acids). Case-control studies are advantageous in assessing multiple exposures or risk factors for diseases or health outcomes that occur infrequently, because they can be done with smaller sample sizes than those needed to study rare or infrequent health outcomes in cohort studies.

EXPERIMENTAL TRIALS

If the evidence suggests that some relationships are appropriate for further study to confirm cause and effect, an *experimental study,* usually known as a *clinical* or **experimental trial,** may be conducted. Experimental trials always begin with carefully designed questions, hypotheses, and research protocols that specify the criteria for selection of the people (subjects) to be studied, the methods for random assignment of subjects to the experimental and control groups, the treatment procedure, the follow-up of subjects, and the details of the data analyses. In experimental studies, the researcher always manipulates variables, such as a nursing intervention or a health teaching approach, in the experimental and control groups. An example of an experimental epidemiologic study is the Physician's Health Study. In this study, 22,071 male physicians aged 40 to 84 years were randomly assigned to one of four treatment groups to study the effects of aspirin and β-carotene use on cardiovascular disease (Lloyd-Jones et al., 2001). Because of ethical concerns about not causing suffering or exacerbation of illness, experimental studies usually involve the testing of hypotheses related to disease prevention, health promotion, or, in some situations, the treatment of a specific disease.

Because community health nurses are asked to plan, implement, and evaluate health care services for specific populations, understanding epidemiologic concepts and principles is important. For example, epidemiologic investigations can evaluate the extent to which a program that is provided by nurses and designed to increase access to early prenatal care is successful in reducing prematurity and low birth weight. Epidemiologic methods may also be used to evaluate the effectiveness of primary intervention strategies and thus improve nursing practices. The trend toward outcomes research and evidence-based medicine is reflected in studies using these types of methods.

Nurse Maria Herrera worked in a community clinic in which she evaluated three children in 1 week who had confirmed lead levels above acceptable limits. Ms. Herrera partnered with the local nursing school and public health department to organize a community-wide free screening and educational intervention focused on small children. The aim of the program was to teach community members about the dangers of lead poisoning and to formulate strategies to eliminate lead exposure. During the screening, the nurses discovered that a large number of the children who tested positive for lead came from one public housing unit. The nurses enlisted public health officials in reducing the exposure threat in this housing complex.

UNDERSTANDING AGGREGATE-LEVEL DATA

A primary focus of community health nursing is the definition of health-related problems (assessment) and the posing of solutions (interventions) for populations or aggregates of people. Population-level decision making requires a different understanding from that used in direct caregiving to individuals. The questions for analysis are different. At the population level, pertinent questions might be the following:

- What are the prevalence rates of cancer among various age, gender, and racial groups?
- Which subgroups have the highest incidences of cancer?
- Who is at high risk for developing cancer?
- What programs are available for cancer prevention and early detection?
- What would be required to further reduce the risk of cancer mortality or morbidity for the entire population?

Given the focus of community health on the well-being of the community, emphasis is necessarily placed on what makes a healthy community. This includes the interrelationship between the health status of the population and the potential for healthy actions within the population, factors that influence health status, and the ability of the health care system to allocate appropriate resources and respond effectively to the needs of the population. The projected trend for health care reform and the increased prevalence of managed care delivery systems call for nurses to assume more responsibility for clients in the community. Therefore, the need for nurses to understand and practice nursing at the population level is more urgent.

In an attempt to respond effectively to these health care challenges, the USDHHS published a report establishing national health objectives for each decade. *Healthy People 2010* is the current report outlining national objectives for health promotion and disease prevention (see the *Healthy People 2010* box on page 169 and the discussion in Chapter 2). This report identifies the goals and priorities toward which health care planners and providers should work to improve the health of the U.S. population. Although the goals are directed toward healthier lives for all Americans, particular emphasis is given to special cohorts. A **cohort** is a group of people who share similar characteristics. For example, people born in the same decade represent an *age* cohort. *Healthy People 2010* has targeted certain cohort groups: newborn babies, boys and girls, adolescents and young people, women and children, and people in their later years (USDHHS, 2000).

■ HEALTHY PEOPLE 2010 ■
Quality and Years of Life Objectives

1. Decrease the total death rate to no more than 454 per 100,000 by 2010 (current baseline, 503.9; blacks, 765.7; Hispanics, 386.8; white non-Hispanics, 475.2 in 1995).
2. Reduce the death rate for adolescents and young adults (15-24 years) to no more than 81 per 100,000 by 2010 (current baseline, 95.3; blacks, 159.8; Native Americans/Alaska Natives, 134.6; Hispanics, 107.1 in 1995).
3. Reduce the death rate for adults (25-64 years) to no more than 358 per 100,000 by 2010 (current baseline, 397.3; blacks, 691.1; Asians/Pacific Islanders, 175.8; Hispanics, 288.4; whites, 365.4 in 1995).
4. Increase life expectancy to 77.3 years by 2010 (current baseline, 75.8; blacks, 69.6; whites, 76.5 in 1995).
5. Decrease years of potential life lost before age 75 to no more than 7315 per 100,000 by 2010 (current baseline, 8128.2 age-adjusted years; males—black, 20,272.8; Hispanic, 9989.4; white non-Hispanic, 9226.3; females—black 10,1179.7; Hispanic, 4378.8; white non-Hispanic, 4968.7 in 1995).

From U.S. Department of Health and Human Services. (2000). *Healthy people 2010: Understanding and improving health* (2nd ed.). Washington, DC: U.S. Government Printing Office.

CONCEPTS RELATED TO PREVENTION, HEALTH PROMOTION, AND DISEASE

Three major concepts are crucial to understanding epidemiology: the natural history of disease, the levels of prevention, and the multiple causation of disease. These concepts are an important foundation to help in planning appropriate nursing interventions for cohorts, aggregates, and populations.

NATURAL HISTORY OF DISEASE

Diseases evolve over time. Leavell and Clark (1965), in their classic description of the disease process, delineate two distinct periods: prepathogenesis and pathogenesis. The prepathogenesis period encompasses the stages of susceptibility and adaptation. During the stage of susceptibility, interactions occur among the person, the environment, and the causative agent that increase the potential for disease. This period leads to the stage of adaptation, in which changes in the body occur in response to some agent or stimulus, but these physiologic or immune system reactions are still part of a normal adaptive response. Although factors are present that increase risk during the period of prepathogenesis, *no disease exists.* For example, obesity in combination with a sedentary lifestyle and smoking increases a person's chances for developing coronary heart disease. Because some risk factors can be altered, understanding the natural history of a disease is important. Awareness of the presence of risk allows the nurse to initiate preventive measures against the disease or limit its development.

For diseases in which detection through symptoms occurs late in the disease trajectory, early detection may be possible by technologic screening procedures. In the case of breast cancer, for example, mammography can detect the disease before symptoms emerge. Many diseases, such as acute or infectious diseases, run their course, and a person experiences complete recovery. Changes resulting from chronic diseases or conditions,

however, may have long-term effects. Symptoms generally become more fixed and are less reversible as the disease continues. With advancing disease, functional changes may produce marked disability and lead to death.

Analyzing the natural history of a disease involves the use of the epidemiologic triangle (Figure 7-2). A change in any of the factors represented in this triangle (the person, the causative agent, or the environment) has the potential to change the balance of health. For the person or host, demographic characteristics, the level of health and history of prior disease, genetic predisposition, states of immunity, body defenses, and human behavior should be examined (Box 7-3). Causative agents may include biologic, physical, chemical, nutritional, genetic, or psychologic factors that have the ability to affect health and disease in the person. The environment includes anything external to the person or agent, including the presence of other persons or animals that potentially affect health and disease.

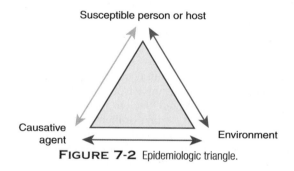

FIGURE 7-2 Epidemiologic triangle.

Box 7-3   Some Host, Agent, and Environmental Factors That Affect Health

Host Factors
Demographic characteristics: age, sex, ethnic background, race, marital status, religion, education, and economic status
Level of health: genetic risk factors, physiologic states, anatomical factors, response to stress, previous disease, nutrition, fitness
Body defenses: autoimmune system, lymphatic system
State of immunity: susceptibility versus active or passive immunity
Human behavior: diet, exercise, hygiene, substance abuse, occupation, personal and sexual contacts, use of health resources, food handling

Agent Factors (Presence or Absence)
Biologic: viruses, bacteria, and fungi and their mode of transmission, life cycle, virulence
Physical: radiation, temperature, noise
Chemical: gas, liquids, poisons, allergens

Environmental Factors
Physical properties: water, air, climate, season, weather, geology, geography, pollution
Biologic entities: animals, plants, insects, food, drugs, food source
Social and economic considerations: family, community, political organization, public policy, regulations, institutions, workplace, occupation, economic status, technology, mobility, housing population density, attitudes, customs, culture, health practices, health services

Calhoun County, Michigan, has a population of 136,000. In March 1997 a total of 153 cases of hepatitis A were reported in the county. The incidence rate for Calhoun County was 89 per 100,000, well above the national rate of 27.9 per 100,000 (Moyer et al., 1996). Of the 153 case patients, 151 were students or staff at schools in four different school districts (Centers for Disease Control and Prevention, [CDC], 1997a).

Investigation by public health officials did not identify a single event, food handler, or contaminated water supply as a source for this outbreak. However, most case clients ate lunch in schools, and further analysis revealed a strong association between illness and consumption of food items containing frozen strawberries.

The strawberries linked to this outbreak were grown in Mexico and shipped to a southern California company, where they were processed, packed, and frozen in 30-lb containers to be distributed to U.S. Department of Agriculture–sponsored school lunch programs. Whether the strawberries were contaminated in Mexico or in the processing company in California was uncertain. Further investigations continued to track the source of the contamination. Meanwhile, the CDC notified the health departments in six other states to which strawberries from the same lots as those sent to Calhoun County had been shipped. Immunoglobulin postexposure prophylaxis was offered to persons who consumed frozen strawberries from the suspected lots through school lunch programs, but only when it could be initiated within 14 days of their exposure.

Can you think of some ways that the epidemiologic concepts of *host*, *agent*, and *environment* relate to this clinical example?

MULTIPLE CAUSATION OF DISEASE

The theory of multiple causation of disease is critical to understanding epidemiologic problems. Causality is generally considered in terms of a stimulus or catalyst that produces a single effect, result, or outcome. In epidemiology the interactions of the agent, person (host), and environment are analyzed by statistical methods to determine whether a causal relationship exists between various factors and health status. Understanding these interactions and relationships is even more important and complex as one considers the natural history of noninfectious diseases, chronic conditions, and the health and well-being of a population. In these instances, multiple causes or factors are usually interacting to affect health status.

A significant number of multiple causation models in epidemiology can be found. The model of Dever (1991) recognizes input from human biology, lifestyle, environment, and the health care system in the development of a particular health condition. The Web of Causation model is a metaphoric model that has been used in epidemiology texts since the early 1960s to describe the multifactorial causes of disease (Krieger, 1994).

All the models point to the interplay of numerous factors in the presentation of a specific disease. Figure 7-3 illustrates factors associated with heart disease. Some of these factors are easily amenable to change, whereas others are not. One way to remember the categories of causes for disease is the acronym used in the *BEINGS* model of disease causes. These categories include the following:
- (B) Biologic factors and behavioral factors
- (E) Environmental factors
- (I) Immunologic factors

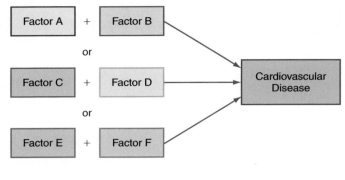

A = Work stress
B = Family history of heart disease
C = High blood cholesterol level
D = Hypertension
E = High fat diet
F = Sedentary life style

FIGURE 7-3 An example of multiple causal factors in heart disease. (Adapted from Gordis, L. [2004]. *Epidemiology* [3rd ed.]. Philadelphia: Saunders.)

- (N) Nutritional factors
- (G) Genetic factors
- (S) Services, social factors, and spiritual factors

Obviously, the factors in some of these categories are harder to change than others. For example, genetic factors remain the most difficult to manipulate, whereas nutritional factors are more easily changed.

LEVELS OF PREVENTION

Because disease occurs over time, there are many potential points at which intervention may prevent, halt, or reverse the pathologic change. A three-level model developed by Leavell and Clark (1965) based on the idea that disease evolves over time continues to be used in the conceptualization and structure of health programs (Figure 7-4).

Primary Prevention

Primary prevention is aimed at altering the susceptibility or reducing the exposure of persons who are at risk for developing a specific disease. Primary prevention includes general health promotion and specific protective measures in the prepathogenesis stage, which are designed to improve the health and well-being of the population. Nursing activities include health teaching and counseling to promote healthy living and lifestyles. Specific protective measures aimed at preventing certain risk conditions or diseases, such as immunizations, the removal of harmful environmental substances, protection from ultraviolet rays, or the proper use of car safety seats for infants and children, are also primary prevention activities. Recent advances in genetic screening have initiated a debate over its role in disease or disability prevention. Although genetic scientists hail research advances as one step on the road to ridding the world of disease and disability, others view that step more as a slippery slope. Is a child with less potential for disease or disability a *more perfect* child? If we have the technology to produce such a child (by selective abortion or gene manipulation), does the public have the right of access to this technology? What message does this send to the disabled community? From a community perspective, what other dilemmas can you imagine surfacing in relation to genetic screening?

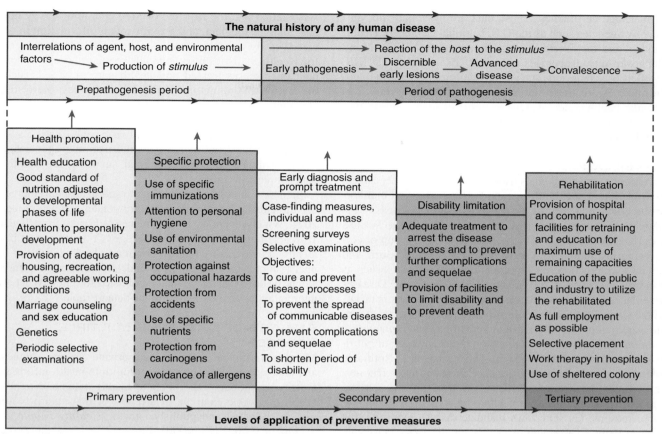

FIGURE 7-4 Levels of prevention in the natural history of disease. (Redrawn from Leavell, H. F., & Clark, E. G. [1965]. *Preventive medicine for the doctor in his community: An epidemiologic approach.* New York: McGraw-Hill.)

Secondary Prevention

Secondary prevention is aimed at early detection and prompt treatment either to cure a disease as early as possible or to slow its progression, thereby preventing disability or complications. Screening programs in which asymptomatic persons are tested to detect early stages of a disease are the most frequent form of secondary prevention. Early case finding and prompt treatment activities are directed toward preventing the transmission of communicable diseases, such as the spread of impetigo in a school. Preventing or slowing the development of a particular disease or condition and preventing complications from a disease, such as scoliosis in teenage girls, are also examples of secondary prevention.

Tertiary Prevention

Tertiary prevention is aimed at limiting existing disability in persons in the early stages of disease and at providing rehabilitation for persons who have experienced a loss of function resulting from a disease process or injury. Nursing activities include education to prevent deterioration of a person's condition, direct nursing care, and referrals to resources that can help clients minimize the loss of function.

HEALTH INFORMATION SYSTEMS

Health information is the data collected about the significant health-related events that occur over a period within a population. **Health information systems** are data collection systems for gathering health statistics and other health-related information at the population level and may include collection of vital statistics, surveillance, surveys, and records.

Data used in epidemiology are systematically collected by government agencies and private groups to measure the size and scope of health problems and factors contributing to them; to study trends and predict the future course of health problems; to identify subgroups to target for interventions; and to evaluate the outcomes of intervention programs and their costs.

Types of health information collected include vital statistics and health statistics on morbidity and disability, health behaviors, nutrition, and health care access, utilization, and costs. Data on personal, behavioral, environmental, and occupational risk factors associated with illness are collected and analyzed, and sometimes information on related political and economic issues that affect health is also collected.

Much epidemiologic information is now available on the Internet, for example, the home pages of the U.S. Bureau of the Census and the CDC. These two websites also contain many helpful links to other websites. (See the resource list at the end of the chapter and this book's website for additional information.)

VITAL STATISTICS

A major source of information about a population comes from the vital statistics that are recorded about them. **Vital statistics** is the term used for the data collected from the ongoing registration of *vital* events, such as death certificates, birth certificates, and marriage certificates. These data are systematically collected by agencies such as the U.S. National Center for Health Statistics and the World Health Organization (WHO). Many other governmental agencies within the CDC and the USDHHS, as well as private groups such as the Children's Defense Fund, also make use of these statistics and issue reports related to particular health concerns. One example of such a publication is the *Morbidity and Mortality Weekly Report (MMWR)* published by the CDC.

SURVEILLANCE

Surveillance is the ongoing systematic collection, analysis, and dissemination of health information for the purpose of monitoring and containing specific, primarily contagious, diseases. An example of a surveillance and response system is the WHO's Global Outbreak Alert and Response Network, a group of collaborating institutions formed to rapidly identify, confirm, and respond to internationally important disease outbreaks, such as avian influenza (WHO, 2007). The National Notifiable Diseases Surveillance System in the United States is operated by the CDC and the Council of State and Territorial Epidemiologists to provide weekly reports *(MMWR)* and annual reports *(Summary of Notifiable Diseases, United States)* on the occurrence of notifiable diseases, a list of which is provided in Chapter 8. Notifiable disease reports are received from all U.S. states and territories, but morbidity data from surveillance efforts are not as accurate as mortality data collected by vital statistics registration, for several reasons: (1) state laws mandate disease reporting, but reporting to the CDC is voluntary; (2) not all cases receive care and not all treated cases are reported; and (3) the completeness of reporting varies. Noninfectious chronic diseases, such as diabetes, arthritis, and asthma, are not notifiable. The CDC does coordinate other surveillance systems, such as the Pregnancy Risk Assessment Monitoring System and the Behavioral Risk Factors Surveillance System. These surveillance systems are also ongoing, but data are collected only periodically, and only from samples. In 1973, the National Cancer Institute (NCI) established the Surveillance, Epidemiology, and End Results (SEER) Program to provide data on cancer incidence and track patients diagnosed with cancer. SEER contracts with 18 population-based local and state registries that submit cancer data covering approximately 26% of the U.S. population twice a year (NCI, 2007).

SURVEYS

Because ongoing national surveillance systems result in incomplete data on morbidity and disability, the CDC's National Center for Health Statistics, the National Institutes of Health, and other agencies periodically conduct a number of large-scale, representative **surveys** on samples of the total population. Examples include the National Health and Nutrition Examination Survey (NHANES) and the National Household Survey on Drug Abuse. Surveys use random samples drawn from multiple geographic areas. NHANES, first conducted in the early 1960s, focuses on chronic disease prevalence and related biophysical measures. A segment on nutrition was added in 1971.

RECORDS

Hospital **records,** such as patient charts, are no longer often used except when local data are being gathered, because national and state organizations such as the American Hospital Association and the Institute of Medicine now survey hospitals, analyze the data, and provide much information in organized, easily available formats. The CDC's National Center for Health Statistics also conducts regular surveys to collect data on diseases treated and health care provided, such as the National Ambulatory Medical Care Survey, the National Hospital Discharge Survey, and the National Nursing Home Survey.

Other organizations that routinely use health statistics, such as local health departments, regional planning agencies, and other local and state governmental agencies, are additional data sources.

Table 7-1 shows the breakdown of visits to hospital emergency departments by leading diagnoses for gender and age groups in 2004. Which diagnosis is seen more commonly in girls under 15 years of age than in boys of this age? (You are correct if you identified pyrexia of unknown origin as a leading cause of hospital visits for girls but not boys under 15 years.) Are there any diagnoses listed for boys that are not listed for girls? What other interpretations are possible from the data in Table 7-1?

ANALYSIS OF DATA FROM MULTIPLE SOURCES

Many government agencies and private groups synthesize and analyze the data collected by multiple health information systems to produce reports about health status and trends in health care. One example of a report of this nature is information collected and published in the *Healthy People 2010* document (USDHHS, 2000). Figure 7-5 shows the percentage of adults by age and race or ethnic background who have diabetes. Older adults are more likely to have diabetes than are younger adults. Use Figure 7-5 to compare the risk of diabetes across four ethnic groups. Which group has the highest risk of diabetes? Which group has the lowest risk? White non-Hispanics have the lowest risk. The other ethnic groups are at higher risk, somewhat influenced by age. Native Americans have the highest risk through age 59 years. In later life, black non-Hispanics and Mexican Americans catch up to or exceed the Native American group.

In the United States, approximately 21 million people (7% of the total population) have diabetes, either diagnosed or undiagnosed (CDC, 2005). Primary prevention aimed at reducing health risks and increasing healthy behaviors to reduce the incidence of diabetes not only would be beneficial for the health of individuals but also would decrease the nation's health care costs. Nurses using incidence data can target intervention to high-risk groups. In the case of diabetes, all of the higher-risk groups should be targeted.

DEMOGRAPHIC DATA

Age, sex, race, ethnicity, social class, occupation, and marital status are demographic characteristics that are frequently used when describing human populations. These factors contribute to variations in health status, health-related behaviors, and use of health care services.

Major demographic findings, reported by the U.S. Bureau of the Census, provide specific information that describes the population. This information is collected every 10 years in the national census. In addition to the overall profiles of the population, many specific reports are issued each year, for example,

TABLE 7-1   Visits to Hospital Emergency Departments by Diagnosis: 2004

Leading Diagnosis	Number (1000)	Rate/1000 Persons	Leading Diagnosis	Number (1000)	Rate/1000 Persons
Men			**Women**		
All ages	50,320	357	**All ages**	59,896	406
Under 15 years	12,262	394	**Under 15 years**	10,681	360
Otitis media	928	30	Acute upper respiratory infections	813	27
Acute upper respiratory infections	907	29	Otitis media	809	27
Contusions with intact skin surfaces	674	22	Pyrexia of unknown origin	533	18
Open wound, excluding head	666	21	Contusions with intact skin surfaces	441	15
Open wound of the head	642	21	Open wound of head	360	12
15-44 years	21,553	353	**15-44 years**	28,483	462
Open wound, excluding head	1412	23	Abdominal pain	1654	27
Contusions with intact skin surfaces	1128	18	Complications of pregancy, childbirth, & the puerperium	1216	20
Spinal disorders	754	12	Contusions with intact skin surfaces	1188	19
Sprains and strains of neck and back	751	12	Chest pain	934	15
Chest pain	745	12	Spinal disorders	850	14
45-64 years	10,134	297	**45-64 years**	11,372	315
Chest pain	736	22	Chest pain	773	21
Open wound, excluding head	463	14	Abdominal pain	620	17
Spinal disorders	450	13	Spinal disorders	448	12
Abdominal pain	420	12	Contusions with intact skin surfaces	442	12
Contusions with intact skin surfaces	302	9	Rheumatism, excluding back	299	8
65 years and older	6372	433	**65 years and older**	9360	469
Chest pain	375	26	Chest pain	529	27
Heart disease, excluding ischemic	292	20	Heart disease, excluding ischemic	520	26
Abdominal pain	216	15	Contusions with intact skin surfaces	394	20
Pneumonia	200	14	Abdominal pain	350	18
Syncope and collapse	192	13	Fractures, excluding lower limb	340	17

Source: U.S. Bureau of the Census. (2007). *Statistical abstract of the United States, 2007: The national data book* (126th ed.). Washington, DC: U.S. Government Printing Office.

age, gender, marital status, and educational level reports. A report of national population trends and projections might include information about the overall population, as well as information about the number of women of childbearing age, the baby boom generation (born between 1946 and 1964), and growth resulting from net immigration. Such a report may also include data related to the trends of the population younger than 25 years, such as preschool children, and those older than 65 years, as well as life expectancy for those with a given birth year. Community health nurses will find this information useful in planning health care services and anticipating the needs of target groups in the population.

Community health nurses in Miami-Dade County, Florida, wanted to provide an adult daycare program for persons with mild to moderate dementia or Alzheimer's disease. To apply for a funding grant, the nurses needed to estimate the number of persons in the community who might access the daycare program. National and local statistics were used to determine the following:

- The number of persons over age 65 in the community
- The number of such persons living alone
- The prevalence of mild to moderate dementia in this age group
- The number of persons age 65 and older with incomes below the poverty level

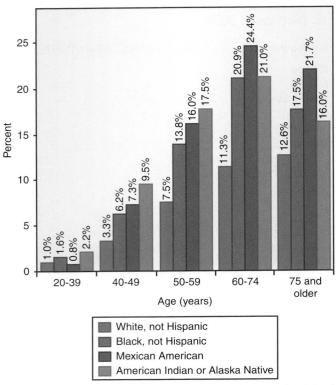

FIGURE 7-5 Percentage of adults with diabetes by age and racial and ethnic background. (Redrawn from U.S. Department of Health and Human Services. [2000]. *Healthy People 2010: Understanding and improving health* [2nd ed.]. Washington, DC: U.S. Government Printing Office.)

From this information, the nurses were able to identify and survey eligible persons in the community to determine if a need for such a program existed. In the course of their survey, the group found that the Latino seniors and their families might be hesitant to make use of such services because of a cultural expectation that people should take care of their own. When the grant was written, strategies to encourage Latino family caregivers to take advantage of respite care were incorporated into the proposal. The plan was funded, and the program attracted an average daily attendance of 23 persons. Caregivers and attendees expressed appreciation for the program.

AGING POPULATION

The number of elderly persons is expected to increase at a moderate rate until 2010 (Figure 7-6). At that point the age group 65 years and older will accelerate because of the aging baby boom generation. The number of elderly persons in the population is important information for community health nurses and other health care planners, because this age cohort requires more health care services.

Although the overall growth of the population is expected to slow and possibly stop around 2045, the average life span continues to rise. The real and projected gains in life expectancy are presented in Figure 7-7. An interesting exercise is to compare the age profile of the population of the United States with that of an underdeveloped country, such as the Dominican Republic (Figure 7-8). The Dominican Republic profile more closely resembles a right triangle, with significantly more children and young adults (under the age of 35 years). The proportion of older

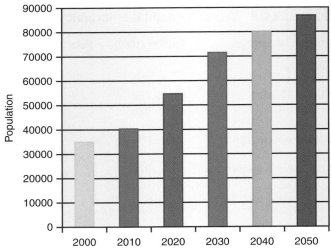

FIGURE 7-6 Projections of the elderly population in the United States (65 years and older) in thousands. (Compiled from U.S. Bureau of the Census. [2004]. *U.S. interim projections by age, sex, race, and Hispanic origin.* Retrieved July 27, 2007 from *http://www.census.gov/ipc/www/usinterimproj/;* and U.S. Bureau of the Census. [2007]. *Statistical abstract of the United States, 2007: The national data book* [126th ed.]. Washington, DC: U.S. Government Printing Office.)

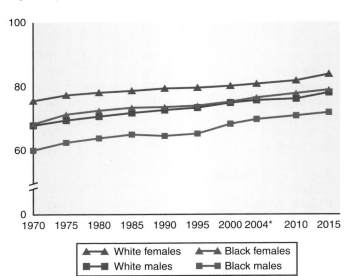

FIGURE 7-7 Life expectancy at birth for black and white men and women: 1970 to 2010. (Redrawn from U.S. Bureau of the Census. [2007]. *Statistical abstract of the United States, 2007: The national data book* [126th ed.]. Washington, DC: U.S. Government Printing Office.) *Preliminary data for 2004.

people (over 55 years) is small. The United States distribution is not as triangular, with less dramatic differences in age distributions. What might account for these different age distributions?

GENDER, RACE, AND LIFE EXPECTANCY

The first of two broad goals of *Healthy People 2010* is to increase the quality of life, as well as the years of healthy life, for the nation's population (see the *Healthy People 2010* box on page 169).To that end, *Healthy People 2010* has committed to ending the discrepancies in morbidity and mortality found between the sexes and racial and ethnic groups (USDHHS, 2000).

The information presented in Figure 7-7 has been expanded to a table that allows comparisons of projected gains in average life expectancy between two groups (Table 7-2). Closely analyze the table and make hypotheses as to the difference in net gain.

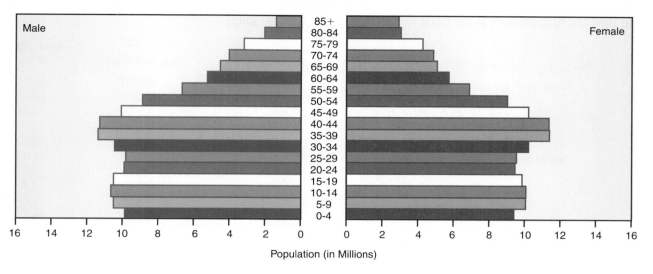

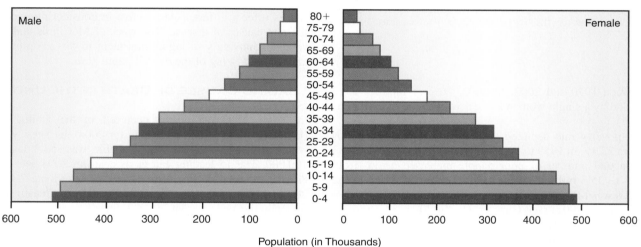

FIGURE 7-8 Distribution (in percentage) of the populations of the United States and the Dominican Republic by age and sex, 2000. (Redrawn from U.S. Bureau of the Census. [2001]. *International database.* Washington, DC: U.S. Government Printing Office; and U.S. Bureau of the Census. [2000]. *International database.* Retrieved from *http://www.census.gov/cgi-bin/ipc/idbpyrs.pl?cty_US&out_s&ymax_250 and http://www.census.gov/cgi-bin/ipc/idbpyrs.pl?cty_DR&out_s&ymax_250.*)

What might be some possible reasons that women live longer than men?

Give thought to what is presented in Table 7-2. Which groups are expected to experience the highest net gain by 2010? Notice that black men and black women are expected to make the most gain, compared to years of life in 1970. Now make some guesses as to possible reasons for the higher gains for both black men and black women.

- What might be a social reason for the difference? What is known about the relationship between socioeconomic status and health status?
- What reason related to health risk behavior might account for the difference? What is known about health screening patterns among the black population?
- What health service barrier might contribute to the difference? Who have been the primary subjects of health care research?

For a more detailed discussion of race and ethnicity and health variables, refer to Chapter 10.

DEPARTMENT OF COMMERCE HEALTH-RELATED STUDIES

U.S. Department of Commerce studies determine which areas of the country are growing the fastest and which states are projected to have inhabitants with the highest median age. The department publishes other records, including information on city and urban growth and decline, households and families, marital status and living arrangements, fertility among women, percentage of women in the labor force, labor force and occupations, poverty, unemployment, and race and ethnicity. For example:

- The Hispanic population is growing more rapidly than the non-Hispanic population in the United States. Estimates are that by 2015, 16.6% of the U.S. population will be Hispanic (U.S. Bureau of the Census, 2007).
- The proportion of families headed by married couples has declined for whites, blacks, and persons of Hispanic origin

TABLE 7-2   Real and Projected Gains in Years of Life for Men and Women from 1970

	2003	2010 (Projected)	2003	2010 (Projected)
	All Men		All Women	
	74.8	75.6	80.1	81.4
1970	−67.1	−67.1	−74.7	−74.7
Gain in years	7.7	8.5	5.4	6.7
	White Men		White Women	
	75.3	76.1	80.5	81.8
1970	−68.0	−68.0	−75.6	−75.6
Gain in years	7.3	8.1	4.9	6.2
	Black Men		Black Women	
	69.0	70.9	76.1	77.8
1970	−60.0	−60.0	−68.3	−68.3
Gain in years	9.0	10.9	7.8	9.5

Data from U.S. Bureau of the Census. (2007). *Statistical abstract of the United States, 2007: The national data book* (126th ed.). Washington, DC: U.S. Government Printing Office.

TABLE 7-3   Actual Causes of Death in the United States: 2000

Cause	Estimated Number	Percentage of Total Deaths
Tobacco	435,000	18.1
Diet/activity patterns	400,000	16.6
Alcohol	85,000	3.5
Microbial agents	75,000	3.1
Toxic agents	55,000	2.3
Motor vehicles	43,000	1.8
Firearms	29,000	1.2
Sexual behavior	20,000	0.8
Illicit drug use	17,000	0.7
Total	**1,159,000**	**48.2**

Compiled from Centers for Disease Control and Prevention. (2004). Fact sheet: Physical inactivity and poor nutrition catching up to tobacco as actual causes of death. Retrieved July 18, 2007 from *http://www.cdc.gov/nccdphp/factsheets/death_causes2000.htm*.

between 1970 and 2003. In 2003, 26% of families were headed by a single woman and 6% by a single man (Fields, 2004).

- The poverty rate declined dramatically during the 1960s (from 22.4% in 1959 to 12.1% in 1969). From 1978 to 1983 the actual number of poor people increased again (from 24.5 to 35.3 million, or by 44%). The poverty rate in the 1990s was higher than at any time since the 1970s (Proctor & Dalaker, 2002) (see Chapter 21). In 2005, 38.2 million Americans (13.3%) had incomes below the poverty level (Webster & Bishaw, 2006).

MAJOR CAUSES OF DEATH

The leading causes of death are frequently the focus of epidemiologic study; however, the bigger challenge lies in understanding the factors that contribute to the development of the disease, or death, or both. In 2000, the CDC updated estimates of the actual causes of death, using methodology first described by McGinnis and Foege (1993, 1999). These researchers argued that major external (nongenetic) factors are responsible for approximately one half of the deaths in the United States (Table 7-3) and advocated for change in the way that causes of death are reported. For example, when a person who smoked for 45 years dies of lung cancer, they would list the cause of death as cigarette smoking, not cancer. This method would emphasize the modifiable (lifestyle, behavioral, and environmental) causes of death, thus focusing attention and health resources on disease prevention rather than treatment. Clearly, the public health burden imposed by causes such as tobacco use, diet and activity patterns, alcohol use, firearms, sexual behavior, motor vehicle accidents, and illicit use of drugs will guide and shape future health policy priorities, including public health nursing priorities. These actual

causes offer a different perspective in considering quality of life and causes of disease. The work of McGinnis and Foege validates nursing's strong commitment to disease prevention and the well-being of the overall population.

LEADING CAUSES OF DEATH IN THE UNITED STATES: TRENDS

In 2004, 2,397,615 deaths occurred in the United States (USDHHS, 2006). The death rate for 2004, the latest year for which comparable statistics are available, was 853.3 deaths per 100,000. The 15 leading causes of death in 2004 account for 83% of the total deaths in the United States (Table 7-4). The 2004 ranking of the first five leading causes of death remain basically the same as that in 1992. Starting with deaths occurring in 1999, the United States began using the tenth revision of the International Classification of Diseases, which affected the categorization of deaths due to respiratory diseases (the fourth leading cause) and primary hypertension and hypertensive renal disease. Diabetes moved from the seventh to the sixth leading cause of death in 2004, surpassing influenza and pneumonia. In 2004, homicide (the tenth cause in 1992) slipped to number 15; suicide (the ninth cause in 1992) dropped to number 11; influenza and pneumonia dropped from sixth to eighth; and human immunodeficiency virus (HIV) infection (the eighth cause in 1992) dropped out of the top 15 causes of death. Deaths from Alzheimer's and Parkinson's diseases appeared in the ranking of leading causes in 2004 at numbers 7 and 14, respectively. When the 1992 and 2004 data are compared, it appears that the United States has made some progress in reducing influenza, pneumonia, and HIV deaths and deaths by suicide and homicide. In the meantime, deaths resulting from chronic diseases (diabetes, Alzheimer's and Parkinson's diseases, and nephritis, nephrotic syndrome, and nephrosis) and from septicemia have risen.

Heart Disease and Stroke

In 2004, over 800,000 Americans died of diseases of the heart and stroke. Over 300 risk factors have been associated with cardiovascular disease, but in developed countries, over a third of cardiovascular disease can be attributed to five major risk

TABLE 7-4   Deaths and Death Rates for 1992 and 2004 for the 15 Leading Causes of Death: United States

Rank (2004)	Cause of Death (ICD-9)	Death Rate 1992	Death Rate 2004	No. of Deaths
	All causes	853.3	800.8	2,397,615
1	Diseases of heart	282.5	217.0	652,486
2	Malignant neoplasms	204.3	185.8	553,888
3	Cerebrovascular diseases	56.3	50.0	150,074
4	Chronic lower respiratory tract diseases	—	41.1	121,987
5	Accidents	33.8	37.7	112,012
6	Diabetes mellitus	19.7	24.5	73,138
7	Alzheimer's disease	—	21.8	65,965
8	Pneumonia and influenza	29.8	19.8	59,664
9	Nephritis, nephrotic syndrome, and nephrosis	8.8	14.2	42,480
10	Septicemia	7.8	11.2	33,373
11	Suicide	11.7	10.9	32,439
12	Chronic liver disease and cirrhosis	9.7	9.0	27,013
13	Essential (primary) hypertension and hypertensive renal disease	—	7.7	23,076
14	Parkinson's disease	—	6.1	17,989
15	Homicide	10.4	5.9	17,357

Adapted from U.S. Bureau of the Census. (2001). *Statistical abstract of the United States* (120th ed.), Table 105. Washington, DC: U.S. Government Printing Office; National Center for Health Statistics, *Vital statistics of the United States,* annual, and *National Vital Statistics Report* (formerly *Monthly Vital Statistics Report*), and unpublished data; and Minino, A. M., Heron, M., Murphy, S. L., et al. (2006). *Deaths: Final data for 2004.* Health E-stats. Retrieved July 27, 2007 from *http://www.cdc.gov/nchs/products/pubs/pubd/hestats/finaldeaths04/finaldeaths04.htm.*

Data are based on a continuous file of records received from the states. Rates are age-adjusted rates per 100,000 U.S. standard population.
ICD, International Classification of Diseases.

factors: (1) tobacco use, (2) alcohol use, (3) high blood pressure, (4) high cholesterol level, and (5) obesity (WHO, 2004). Other modifiable risk factors include lack of physical activity, a diet low in fruits and vegetables and high in saturated fat, and diabetes mellitus. High levels of total cholesterol, low-density lipoprotein cholesterol, and triglycerides, and low levels of high-density lipoprotein cholesterol increase risk for both coronary heart disease and stroke. Nonmodifiable risk factors include advancing age and family history. Men have higher rates of coronary heart disease than premenopausal women, but rates for women after menopause become similar to those for men, and risk for stroke is comparable in women and men. Other risk factors include psychosocial stress and low socioeconomic status.

Cancer

About 10.1 million Americans who were alive in 2002 had a history of cancer, but over half of these were diagnosed 5 or more years earlier and were considered *cured* (generally defined as being symptom free for 5 years after treatment); others still have cancer diagnoses and are being treated (American Cancer Society [ACS], 2006). For some types of cancer, a person is considered cured after a shorter period, but for other forms follow-up may be required for a longer time.

In 2006, the ACS expected approximately 1 million cases of basal and squamous cell skin cancer and 1,399,790 cases of other new cancers to be diagnosed, and about 565,000 deaths from cancer (over 1500 per day) (ACS, 2006). According to the ACS, the cancer mortality rate in the United States has risen steadily since the mid-1940s. Major increases have occurred in both male and female death rates due to lung cancer, whereas rates for cancer at other sites have declined or leveled off (Figures 7-9 and 7-10). By 1990, lung cancer had surpassed breast cancer as the leading cause of cancer death in women.

In 2006, more than 6 out of 10 persons (65%) diagnosed with cancer were expected to survive for the *relative* 5-year time frame after treatment. This number represents a gain from 1 in 5 (20%) in the 1930s and 1 in 3 (30%) in the 1960s. The improved survival rate is used to document progress in early detection and treatment.

The importance of prevention should not be underestimated. Research suggests that "screening examinations by a health care professional can result in the detection of cancers of the breast, colon, rectum, cervix, prostate, testis, oral cavity, and skin at earlier stages, when treatment is more likely to be successful" (ACS, 2003, p. 1). Individuals with these cancers represent over one half of clients with recent cancer diagnoses, of whom 80% are expected to survive 5 years. With early detection, the survival rate can increase to over 95%. Many skin cancers can be prevented with protection from ultraviolet radiation in sunlight (both ultraviolet A and ultraviolet B rays), and cancer from cigarette smoking and heavy alcohol use can be completely prevented. The ACS estimates that cigarette smoking causes approximately 30% of cancer deaths and a total of 440,000 premature deaths annually, mostly from lung and other cancers, ischemic heart disease, stroke, and chronic obstructive lung disease. Health-related economic losses associated with cigarette smoking amount to an estimated $157 billion annually (American Lung Association, 2004).

Human Immunodeficiency Virus Disease

Acquired immunodeficiency syndrome (AIDS) was first reported in the United States in June 1981. By 1987, there were

Age-Adjusted Cancer Death Rates,* Females by Site, United States, 1930-2003

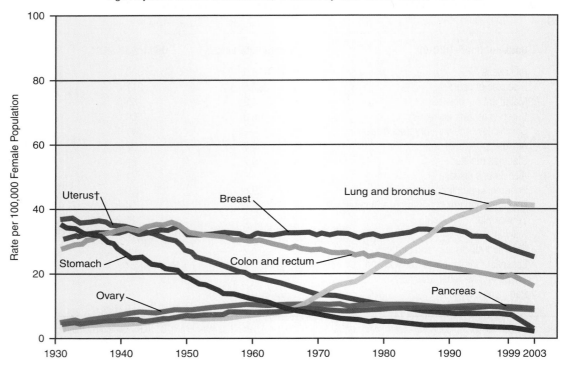

*Per 100,000, age-adjusted to the 2000 US standard population. †Uterus cancer death rates are for uterine cervix and uterine corpus combined.
Note: Due to changes in ICD coding, numerator information has changed over time. Rates for cancers of the liver, lung and bronchus, colon and rectum, and ovary are affected by these coding changes.

FIGURE 7-9 Age-adjusted cancer death rates for women by cancer site, United States, 1930 to 2003. (From U.S. Mortality Public Use Data Tapes 1960-1999, U.S. Mortality Volumes 1930-1959, Centers for Disease Control and Prevention [CDC], National Center for Health Statistics, 2002; and U.S. Cancer Statistics Working Group. [2006]. *United States cancer statistics: 2003 incidence and mortality.* Atlanta: U.S. Department of Health and Human Services, CDC, and National Cancer Institute.)

50,000 reported cases of AIDS. That number reached 206,396 by December 31, 1991, and the cumulative total through 2004 was 908,905 persons with AIDS reported to the CDC by state and local health departments (U.S. Bureau of the Census, 2007, Table 177).

Although homosexual and bisexual men and intravenous drug users account for the majority of AIDS deaths, people of all types and ages die of AIDS. Those who have received a blood transfusion or blood product, children born to mothers with HIV disease, and persons who contracted HIV infection from heterosexual contact are also represented in the death rates. Better screening of blood donors and donated blood since HIV transmission through blood products was recognized has largely checked the increase in AIDS cases from blood product contamination.

The expanded surveillance case definition of AIDS in 1993 substantially increased the number of reported AIDS cases. Laboratory-initiated reporting accounted for 39% of reported cases in 1993 and 57% of cases in 1996 (CDC, 1997b). The introduction of triple-drug combination antiretroviral therapy in 1996 is thought to be largely responsible for the 26% reduction in the death rate from AIDS in 1996. HIV/AIDS dropped from the first to the second leading cause of death for persons aged 25 to 44 in 1996, to the fifth leading cause of death in 1998, and to the sixth leading cause of death in this age group in 2004 (U.S. Bureau of the Census, 2007).

Education for prevention of HIV disease is critical for reducing the incidence of AIDS. Persons engaging in unprotected sexual contact with multiple sexual partners are at increased risk for HIV infection. To be safer, men and women need to know the drug and sexual histories of their sexual partners *and* take adequate precautions. Knowledge alone does not ensure adequate protection. The CDC (1997b) reported that almost half of women infected in 1996 knew their partners' HIV status and still did not take precautions.

Table 7-5 shows selected characteristics of persons living with AIDS in 1994 and from 2000 to 2004. Use the table to answer the following questions:
• What can you say about the rate of increase in heterosexual exposure for men and women?
• What can you say about the numbers of persons living with AIDS based on race or ethnicity?

Answers to the preceding questions are as follows: Although this table does not give rate information, you can see that the increase in AIDS cases from heterosexual contact is dramatic—from 23,034 men and women in 1994 to 95,270 in 2004. Women appear to be more vulnerable to contracting HIV from heterosexual contact. Throughout the 1980s and 1990s, there were more whites than persons of other racial or ethnic groups living with AIDS, but in 2000, the number of blacks living with AIDS surpassed the number of whites, and this number continued to increase by an additional 35% between

Age-Adjusted Cancer Death Rates,* Males by Site, United States, 1930-2003

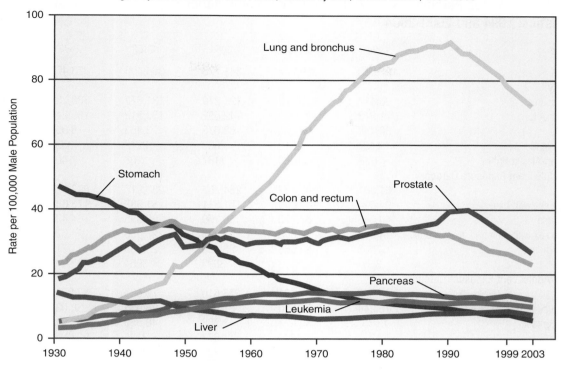

*Per 100,000, age-adjusted to the 2000 US standard population.
Note: Due to changes in ICD coding, numerator information has changed over time. Rates for cancers of the liver, lung and bronchus, colon and rectum are affected by these coding changes.

FIGURE 7-10 Age-adjusted cancer death rates for men by cancer site, United States, 1930 to 2003. (From U.S. Mortality Public Use Data Tapes 1960-1999, U.S. Mortality Volumes 1930-1959, Centers for Disease Control and Prevention [CDC], National Center for Health Statistics, 2002; and U.S. Cancer Statistics Working Group. [2006]. *United States cancer statistics: 2003 incidence and mortality.* Atlanta: U.S. Department of Health and Human Services, CDC, and National Cancer Institute.)

2000 and 2004. The number of Hispanics living with AIDS has also more than doubled since 1994. Minority groups also carry a heavier burden from AIDS in terms of the percentage of the total population affected.

Accidents and Unintentional Injuries

In the United States, unintentional injuries are a cause of death, but these injuries are largely preventable (Table 7-6). Considerable progress has been made in reducing deaths by motor vehicle accidents by using a multiphased incremental strategy. The plan included legislative, educational, and public service efforts (see Chapter 16). Legislation was passed mandating seat belt use, use of child safety seats, and the judicious use of alcohol by drivers (CDC, 2003a). Other actions included media public education advertisements promoting the use of child safety seats and discouraging alcohol use when driving. Private agencies sponsored loaner seat programs in which parents who were unable to afford car seats were loaned age-appropriate seats.

Drowning and fires are the other most frequent causes of injury-related deaths. Alcohol use is associated with 40% of residential fire deaths.

Emerging Infectious Diseases: Viral Epidemics

Some researchers point to airborne virus–caused **epidemics** (outbreaks of infection affecting a larger number of people

than would be expected, all at the same time) and **pandemics** (outbreaks affecting extremely high numbers of people, usually in many countries) as the major health threat of this century. Epidemics of viral diseases, such as avian influenza and severe acute respiratory syndrome (SARS), are particularly problematic because they are difficult to treat. SARS, a respiratory illness first reported in Asia in February 2003, spread worldwide and tested the global response to an epidemiologic health crisis. Most of the U.S. cases occurred in travelers returning from other parts of the world. The CDC listed only 177 reported cases and no SARS-related deaths in 2003 (CDC, 2003b). But SARS is a reminder that community health personnel will need to be especially vigilant and quick to identify any new epidemic in the future.

Organizations such as the WHO and the CDC are working together to monitor cases of avian influenza in Southeast Asia and to establish procedures to contain the spread of such potentially contagious diseases. Because more health care is being delivered in community health care settings rather than in acute care hospitals, the Public Health Service updated its *Guideline for Isolation Precautions: Preventing Transmission of Infectious Agents in Healthcare Settings* in 2007 to incorporate recommendations that can be applied in home, ambulatory and long-term care settings, and to address emerging infectious diseases and renewed interest in multidrug-resistant organisms (Siegel et al., 2007).

TABLE 7-5　Estimated Persons Living with Acquired Immunodeficiency Syndrome by Selected Characteristics: 1994 and 2000-2004

Characteristic	1994	2000	2001	2002	2003	2004
Total	197,060	320,177	341,773	364,496	388,477	415,193
Race/Ethnicity						
White, non-Hispanic	86,417	119,420	125,279	131,672	138,238	145,935
Black, non-Hispanic	71,818	132,090	142,552	153,512	165,246	178,233
Hispanic	36,448	63,894	68,673	73,463	78,557	84,001
Asian/Pacific Islander	1457	2612	2893	3242	3638	4045
Native American/Alaska Native	668	1099	1187	1288	1404	1506
Male Adult/Adolescent Exposure Category						
Male total	161,081	248,726	264,267	280,917	298,272	317,698
Men who have sex with men	94,694	142,069	151,511	161,937	173,086	185,326
Injecting drug use	40,046	57,778	60,150	62,335	64,432	67,091
Men who have sex with men and inject drugs	14,884	22,603	23,293	23,953	24,627	25,367
Heterosexual contact	7903	22,568	25,480	28,738	32,071	35,671
Other	3554	3708	3833	3954	4057	4242
Female Adult/Adolescent Exposure Category						
Female total	32,702	67,601	73,610	79,639	86,262	93,566
Injection drug use	16,244	26,656	27,924	28,955	30,033	31,472
Heterosexual contact	15,131	39,121	43,708	48,559	53,947	59,599
Other*	1327	1824	1977	2125	2282	2494
Pediatric[†] exposure category	3277	3848	3895	3939	3941	3927

Source: Centers for Disease Control and Prevention. (2007). *HIV/AIDS Surveillance report*, annual; U.S. Bureau of the Census. (2007). *Statistical abstract of the United States, 2007*. (126th ed,). Washington, DC: U.S. Government Printing office.
*Includes hemophilia, blood transfusion, perinatal, and risk not reported or not identified.
[†]Less than 13 years of age.

TABLE 7-6　Deaths and Death Rates from Accidents by Type: 1980-2003

Type of Accident	Deaths (Number)					Rate per 100,000 Population				
	1980	1990	2000	2001	2003	1980	1990	2000	2001	2003
Total	105,798	91,983	97,900	101,537	109,277	46.7	37.0	34.8	35.7	37.6
Motor vehicle traffic	53,1172	46,814	43,354	43,788	43,340	23.5	18.8	15.7	15.4	14.9
Other land transport	N/A	N/A	1,492	1,493	1,544	N/A	N/A	0.5	0.5	0.5
Other transport (water, air, space)	2923	1864	1,903	4,435	1,317	N/A	N/A	0.7	1.6	0.5
Accidental falls	13,294	12,313	13,322	15,019	17,229	5.9	5.0	4.8	5.3	5.9
Accidental drowing	6043	3979	3,482	3,281	3,306	2.7	1.6	1.3	1.2	1.1
Smoke, fire and flames	5822	4175	3,377	3,309	3,369	2.6	1.7	1.2	1.2	1.2
Firearms, unintentional	1667	1175	776	802	730	0.7	0.5	0.3	0.3	0.3
Accidental poisoning	4331	5803	12,757	14,078	19,457	N/A	N/A	4.6	4.9	6.7
Complications of medical and surgical care	2282	2669	3,059	3,021	2,855	1.0	1.1	1.1	1.1	0.9

Effective with deaths occuring in 1999, the United States began using the Tenth Revision of the *International Classification of Diseases (ICD)*. For earlier years, causes of death were classified according to the revisions then in use (e.g., the Ninth Revision for 1979-1998).
Source: U.S National Center for Health Statistics, *National vital statistics reports* and *Vital statistics of the United States*, annual; U.S. Bureau of the Census. (2007). *Statistical abstract of the United States*, 2007 (126th ed.). Washington, DC: U.S. Government Printing Office.

HEALTH PROFILES OR STATUS AND THE LIFE CYCLE

Certain health risks and behavior patterns are associated with selected age groups. A brief overview of health risks, morbidity, and mortality information especially pertinent to selected age groups is presented here.

PATTERNS OF MORTALITY AND MORBIDITY DURING PREGNANCY AND INFANCY

The health status of the infant cannot be separated from that of the mother. Prenatal problems and problems that are present in the period immediately following birth are discussed together.

The infant mortality rate, because of its sensitivity, is one of the most widely used statistics in evaluating the overall improvement in health in the United States. It is also used in making comparisons with other countries (see Chapter 5). Traditionally, the high rate of infant mortality has been viewed as an indicator of unmet health needs and unfavorable environmental conditions. The infant mortality rate has steadily declined, dropping from 29.2 per 1000 live births in 1950 to 6.9 per 1000 live births in 2003 (U.S. Bureau of the Census, 2007). In 2003, 28,025 actual infant deaths occurred. Although the infant death rate for the United States has improved, it is still higher than that of other industrial countries (see Chapter 3).

The disparity in the death rates between minority and majority populations is quite large. For white infants, the mortality rate was 5.7 per 1000 live births (570 per 100,000) compared with 14 per 1000 live births for black infants (U.S. Bureau of the Census, 2007). Figure 7-11 compares infant deaths by cause of death for 1980 and 2004. Examine this graph to compare the changes in the leading causes of infant death between 1980 and 2004. Four causes account for more than 50% of all infant deaths: congenital anomalies, conditions related to short gestation and low birth weight, sudden infant death syndrome, and maternal complications. Between 1980 and 2004, deaths due to congenital anomalies decreased but deaths due to short gestation and low birth weight and maternal complications increased as a percentage of total infant mortality. Changes over time in the classification of infant deaths make it difficult to compare the percentage of deaths due to respiratory distress and/or sudden infant death syndrome.

Low birth weight is associated with several preventable causes, including lack of prenatal care, maternal infection, maternal smoking, maternal use of alcohol and drugs, poor maternal nutrition, and pregnancy before the age of 18 years. Lower socioeconomic and educational levels are also often associated with low birth weight (see Chapter 21). An expectant mother who receives no prenatal care is three times more likely to give birth to a low-birth-weight infant. Poor prenatal care is compounded by poverty and is one reason why *Healthy People 2010* emphasizes improvements in prenatal care and targets high-risk groups (adolescents and poor women) for concentrated intervention.

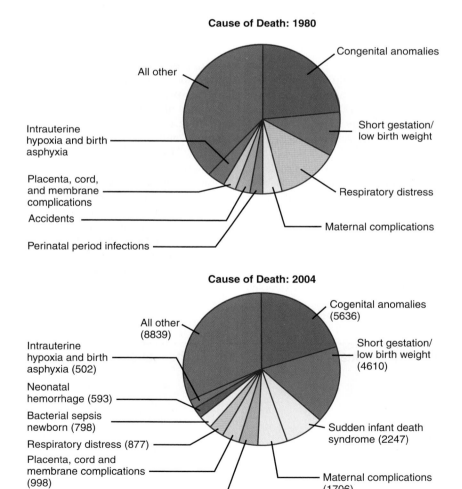

FIGURE 7-11 Causes of infant mortality: comparison of 1980 and 2004 (deaths of infants under 1 year old per 1000 live births; excludes deaths of nonresidents of the United States; 1980 deaths classified according to the ninth revision of the International Classification of Diseases [ICD], and 2004 deaths classified according to the tenth revision of the ICD). (Data from National Center for Health Statistics. [2004]. *Deaths: Preliminary data for 2004, tables for E-stat.* Retrieved July 27, 2007 from *http://www.cdc.gov/nchs/data/hestat/preliminarydeaths04_tables.pdf;* and National Center for Health Statistics, *Vital Statistics of the United States,* annual, *Monthly Vital Statistics Reports,* and unpublished data.)

PATTERNS OF MORTALITY AND MORBIDITY IN CHILDHOOD

Because of public health measures, the rate of childhood deaths in the United States has dramatically declined since the mid-1950s. Infectious diseases such as polio, diphtheria, scarlet fever, measles, pneumonia, and whooping cough have been virtually eliminated in this country through immunizations. Worldwide, millions of children still die each year from vaccine-preventable diseases or ineffective treatment of infectious diseases (see Chapter 5).

Deaths in Childhood

The leading causes of death in children are presented in Table 7-7. From 1977 to 1989 the significant drop in the childhood death rate (23%) was attributed mostly to the mandatory use of motor vehicle safety restraints for young children in all 50 states and the increased use of seat belts. Since then, properly used safety seats and air bags have decreased childhood deaths. Nonetheless, 40% of unintentional injuries result from motor vehicle accidents (see Table 7-6), which are the leading cause of death in children in the United States. In 2005, 1451 deaths in children 14 years and younger were caused by motor vehicle accidents. Almost half of children who died did not have safety restraints, and 25% of motor vehicle–related child fatalities involved a drinking driver (CDC, 2007).

Illness in Childhood

Infectious diseases such as recurrent tonsillitis, recurrent ear infections, mononucleosis, hepatitis, meningitis, bladder or urinary tract infections, diarrhea or colitis, rheumatic fever, and pneumonia remain an important morbidity problem in childhood. In addition, in 1993 and 2001, the American Academy of Pediatrics (AAP) identified *new childhood morbidities* that should be addressed, including behavioral and mood problems, learning disabilities and other school-related problems, violence, drug and alcohol use/abuse, and the behavioral effects of media exposure (AAP, 2001).

Childhood obesity is one example of morbidity that is of increasing concern. The number of children and adolescents who are overweight was relatively stable from the 1960s to 1980. However, as tracked by successive NHANES studies, the prevalence of overweight children and adolescents nearly doubled between 1980 and 1995. Results from the 2003 and 2004 NHANES (NHANES V) indicate that 18.8% of children aged 6 to 11 years and 17.4% of adolescents aged 12 to 19 years are overweight—up from 15% in 1999. The CDC (2006) implicated poor diet and lack of exercise as causes, which is consistent with a national trend across age groups (Figure 7-12).

Healthy development in childhood is a primary concern. Developmental problems and chronic physical conditions are on the rise in this age group, and children living in poverty are at higher risk. Hearing and speech impairment, lead poisoning, and emotional and learning disorders are significant issues. Prevention efforts aimed at establishing healthy parenting priorities, improving environmental conditions, and promoting healthy habits can improve the health profiles of children in all of these problem areas.

PATTERNS OF MORTALITY AND MORBIDITY IN ADOLESCENTS AND YOUNG ADULTS

For individuals between 15 and 24 years of age, unintentional injuries, most of which involve motor vehicles, are responsible for about 45.5% of deaths (Figure 7-13). Alcohol is involved in 40% of fatal accidents (National Highway Transportation and Safety Administration, 2005). Mortality rates for adolescents and young adults are rising again after declining in the early 1980s, when raising the minimum drinking age resulted in fewer motor vehicle accident–related deaths. The upward trend in mortality that began in the mid-1980s is believed to be related in part to the increase in the speed limit on rural interstate highways and inconsistent use of seat belts.

Take a moment to review the pie graph. What are the second and third most common causes of death in this age group? Homicide is the second leading cause of death in this age group and the leading cause of death for black boys and young men. The rate for black men aged 15 to 24 years was over seven times the rate for white men in this age group in 2004, and the discrepancy is just under a sevenfold difference when homicide rates for black and white men of all ages are compared (CDC, 2006). Race is not as important a risk factor, however, when socioeconomic characteristics are taken into account. Suicide is the third leading cause of death in this age group.

TABLE 7-7   **Leading Causes of Death in Children: 2003 (in Thousands)**

Rank	Cause	Total	1-4 Years	5-14 Years
1	Unintentional Injury	4335	1717	2618
2	Malignant neoplasms	1468	392	1076
3	Congenital anomalies	927	541	386
4	Homicide	700	376	324
5	Diseases of heart	450	186	264
6	Suicide	250	—	250
7	Pneumonia and influenza	310	163	147
8	Chronic lower respiratory	173	55	118
9	Septicemia	162	85	77
10	Certain conditions originating in the perinatal period	98	99	19

Source: U.S. National Center for Health Statistics, *Vital Statistics of the United States*, annual; and unpublished data; and U.S. Census Bureau. (2007). *Statistical abstract of the United States, 2007* (126th ed.). Washington, DC: U.S. Government Printing Office.

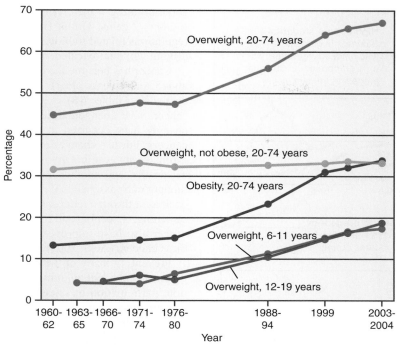

FIGURE 7-12 Overweight and obesity trends among U.S. children and adults, 1960 to 2004. (From National Health Examination Survey and National Health and Nutrition Examination Survey; and Centers for Disease Control and Prevention, National Center for Health Statistics. [2006]. *Health, United States, 2006, with chartbook on trends in the health of Americans.* Washington, DC: U.S. Government Printing Office.)

Are the causes of death different for men and women in this age group? Figure 7-13 does not differentiate the sexes. Go to this book's website or go directly to the website for the National Center for Health Statistics to answer this question.

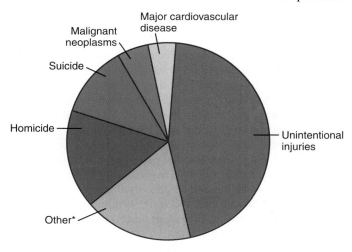

*Other includes congenital malformations, deformations, and chromosomal abnormalities; chronic lower respiratory disease; HIV; septicemia, diabetes mellitus, influenza and pneumonia, and preumonitis due to solids and liquids.

FIGURE 7-13 Causes of death among adolescents and young adults aged 15 to 24 years, 2003. *"Other" includes congenital malformations, deformations, and chromosomal abnormalities; chronic lower respiratory tract disease; human immunodeficiency virus infection; septicemia; diabetes mellitus; influenza and pneumonia; and pneumonitis due to solids and liquids. (Data from Centers for Disease Control and Prevention, National Center for Health Statistics. [2006]. Leading causes of death and number of deaths, according to age: United States. In *Health, United States, 2006, with chartbook on trends in the health of Americans.* Washington, DC: U.S. Government Printing Office.)

The data show that women of all races have relatively lower suicide rates than do men (CDC, 2006).

Other major health problems of this age group, such as cancer and heart disease, are overshadowed by unintentional injuries, homicide, and suicide. However, during this period, young people develop habits that have importance for health in later years. Lifestyle patterns related to nutrition, physical fitness and exercise, cigarette smoking and drug use, safety, and sexual conduct emerge during this period and help determine the rate of future chronic illness as this cohort ages. For example, substance use and abuse, often initiated in young adulthood, persists until other health concerns arise. About 90% of adults who smoke started by age 21, and one third of these adults had become smokers by their fourteenth birthday (American Lung Association, 2004). Even though the overall percentage of people who smoke has declined from 48% in 1965 to 23% of men and 19% of women in 2004, these numbers are still significant (Figure 7-14). Educational level is a predictive factor for smoking. In 2004, adults with less than 12 years of education were almost three times as likely to smoke as those with a bachelor's degree or higher (CDC, 2006). Between 1991-1993 and 2003-2005, binge drinking in high school students decreased moderately in males but remained relatively constant in females, and marijuana use increased markedly in both male and female ninth- to twelfth-graders. In 2005, among eleventh- and twelfth-graders 33% of males and 27% of females reported binge drinking in the previous 30 days, and 25% of males and 19% of females reported marijuana use in the previous 30 days (CDC, 2006). Alcohol and drug use continue to be significant problems and are major contributors to accidents and violence.

Unintended pregnancies and sexually transmitted diseases present health risks in this population. Estimates indicate

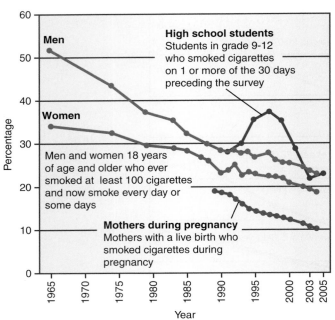

FIGURE 7-14 Smoking patterns among men, women, high school students, and mothers during pregnancy: United States, 1965 to 2005. (Redrawn from Centers for Disease Control and Prevention, National Centers for Health Statistics. [2006]. Leading causes of death and number of deaths, according to age: United States. In *Health, United States, 2006, with chartbook on trends in the health of Americans.* Washington, DC: U.S. Government Printing Office.)

that over 60% of men and women have engaged in sexual intercourse before age 20 years (Moeher et al., 2005). Over 80% of all teenage mothers did not intend to become pregnant (CDC, 2006). Chapter 24 addresses adolescent sexual activity, pregnancy, and their relationship to health and economic status.

Prevention through health education and role modeling is important for this age group. However, education alone does not bring about the desired changes in behavior. Motivational counseling and adequate support, especially for high-risk groups, is necessary to further reduce the health and social risks of alcohol and drug abuse, school failure, delinquency, violence, and unwanted pregnancy, and the risk of development of future chronic disease.

PATTERNS OF MORTALITY AND MORBIDITY IN ADULTS

Nearly all of the major health problems faced by people between 25 and 65 years of age are preventable, totally or in part, through lifestyle or environmental changes. Personal responsibility for maintaining health is paramount. For example, the dramatic decline in heart disease, strokes, and, to a lesser extent, accidents in this age group since 1970 is associated with reduced cigarette smoking, lower blood cholesterol levels, increased control of high blood pressure, decreased alcohol consumption, increased (mandatory) seat belt use, lower speed limits, and the availability of air bags in automobiles (USDHHS, 2002). The public's awareness of the relationship between risk and health has influenced social norms. Reduced public acceptance of risks related to smoking has been the impetus for establishment of antismoking laws and creation of smoke-free work environments. Increased concern

about drinking while driving has launched movements such as Mothers Against Drunk Drivers and has resulted in tougher regulations related to blood alcohol levels, stiffer penalties for driving while intoxicated, and raising of the drinking age.

Cancer has become the leading cause of death for individuals 45 to 64 years of age as deaths from heart disease have decreased (Table 7-8). Although overall mortality rates for cancer have changed little since the mid-1950s, significant changes have occurred in some age groups and for selected cancers. Further changes are believed possible. For example, estimates suggest that smoking is responsible for 30% of cancer deaths, and another one third (such as colon cancer) are thought to be associated with diet. Both of these cancers can be decreased through reduction of risky behaviors and aggressive screening. Screening and early diagnosis of breast and cervical cancer also have improved the survival rates of women with these cancers (ACS, 2003).

Preventing many of the chronic diseases affecting this age group is dependent on individual actions, including risk reduction, participation in screening efforts, and prompt attention to signs and symptoms to ensure early diagnosis and treatment. All health care providers are challenged to empower individuals to develop or modify lifestyle patterns that maintain health and prevent disease. Individual responsibility is not the only factor affecting health. The environment, workplace standards, socioeconomic status, media images, educational level, and access to information and health care are all powerful influences that affect adult behavior and choices that support health.

PATTERNS OF MORTALITY AND MORBIDITY IN OLDER ADULTS

The proportion of persons older than 65 years will continue to increase, with the over-85 cohort showing the most rapid growth. Individuals reaching 65 years of age now can expect to live into their early eighties. The substantive question facing these individuals, however, is not so much the question of living as the question of the quality of their remaining years of life. Even in this age group, increasing evidence suggests that some lifestyle changes can result in major health and quality-of-life benefits. The outcomes of the top three causes of death—heart disease, cancer, and stroke (Table 7-9)—can still be altered. For example, older smokers who quit smoking increase their life expectancy, reduce the risks associated with heart disease, and improve circulation and respiratory functioning. Eating a nutritionally balanced diet, reducing weight, and decreasing sodium intake can reduce the risk of heart disease and promote the maintenance of elder health.

Chronic neurologic, musculoskeletal, and other problems such as arthritis and osteoporosis, visual and hearing impairments, incontinence, digestive conditions, and dementia are all concerns of this age group. Because of the impact of illness on day-to-day living, disease prevention and preservation of function are desirable. Pain can affect function and is often undermanaged in older adults (Ebersole et al., 2004).

A key to physiologic decline is lack of physical activity (Figure 7-15). A large portion of this age group (40% to 60%) reports no participation in leisure-time physical activity. Fewer than one third report participating in some leisure-time activity, such as walking or gardening, and fewer than one fourth report regular leisure-time activity (CDC, 2006). Regular physical

TABLE 7–8   Deaths and Death Rates for the 10 Leading Causes of Death in Specified Age Groups: United States, Preliminary 2004*

Rank	Cause of Death[†]	No.	Rate
Aged 25 to 44 years			
	All causes	124,376	147.8
1	Unintentional injury	28,273	33.6
2	Malignant neoplasms (cancer)	18,263	21.7
3	Diseases of heart	15,744	18.7
4	Suicide	11,403	13.6
5	Homicide	7192	8.5
6	Human immunodeficiency virus disease	6312	7.5
7	Chronic liver disease and cirrhosis	3035	3.6
8	Cerebrovascular diseases	2893	3.4
9	Diabetes mellitus	2568	3.1
10	Influenza and pneumonia	1204	1.4
Aged 45 to 64 years			
	All causes	439,003	621.0
1	Malignant neoplasms	145,293	205.5
2	Diseases of heart	100,037	141.5
3	Unintentional injury	25,307	35.8
4	Diabetes mellitus	16,252	23.0
5	Cerebrovascular diseases	16,051	22.7
6	Chronic lower respiratory tract diseases	15,324	21.7
7	Chronic liver disease and cirrhosis	13,784	19.5
8	Suicide	10,622	15.0
9	Nephritis, nephritic syndrome, and nephrosis	6006	8.5
10	Septicemia	5955	8.4

*Data are based on a continuous file of records received from the states. Rates are per 100,000 population in the specified group. Figures are based on weighted data rounded to the nearest individual, so categories may not add to totals.
[†]Based on the International Classification of Diseases, tenth revision (1992).
From National Center for Health Statistics. *Vital statistics of the United States,* annual, and unpublished data; and U.S. Bureau of the Census. (2007). *Statistical abstract of the United States, 2007* (126th ed.), Washington, DC: U.S. Government Printing Office; and Minino, A. M., Heron, M., Murphy, S. L., & Kochanek, K. D. (2006). Deaths: Final data for 2004. *Health E-Stats.* Retrieved July 26, 2007 from *http://www.cdc.gov/nchs/products/pubs/pubd/hestats/finaldeaths04/finaldeaths04.htm.*

TABLE 7–9   Leading Causes of Death of Adults 65 Years and Older, 2003

Rank	Cause	No.	Rate
	All causes	1,804,373	5023.4
1	Diseases of the heart	563,390	1568.5
2	Malignant neoplasms (cancer)	388,911	1082.7
3	Cerebrovascular diseases	138,134	384.6
4	Chronic lower respiratory tract diseases	109,139	303.8
5	Alzheimer's disease	62,814	174.9
6	Pneumonia and Influenza	57,670	160.6
7	Diabetes mellitus	54,919	152.9
8	Nephritis, nephrotic syndrome, and nephrosis	35,254	98.1
9	Unintentional injury	34,335	95.6
10	Septicemia	26,445	73.6

Data are based on a continuous file of records received from the states. Rates are per 100,000 population in the specified group. Figures are based on weighted data rounded to the nearest individual, so categories may not add to totals.
Data from Heron, M. P., & Smith, B. L. (2007). Deaths: Leading causes for 2003. *National Vital Statistics Reports,* 55(10), 1-91.

activity and exercise are associated with reduced incidence of coronary heart disease, hypertension, non–insulin-dependent diabetes, colon cancer, depression, and anxiety (Ebersole et al., 2004; National Institute on Aging, 2002). All of these chronic diseases are concerns of the age group older than 65 years.

Primary health services for this age group include counseling for promotion and maintenance of healthy behaviors and prevention of life-limiting and life-threatening conditions. Control of hypertension, management of other chronic conditions, and aggressive screening for skin, breast, cervical, and

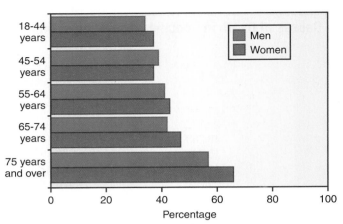

FIGURE 7-15 Adults not engaging in leisure-time physical activity by age and sex: United States, 2004. (Redrawn from Centers for Disease Control and Prevention, National Center for Health Statistics. [2006]. Leading causes of death and number of deaths, according to age: United States. In *Health, United States, 2006, with chartbook on trends in the health of Americans.* Washington, DC: U.S. Government Printing Office.)

prostate cancer are important health service issues. Because the rate of death from pneumonia and influenza increases in this age group, pneumococcal and influenza vaccination is encouraged.

Life changes in this age group frequently threaten the individual's functional independence. Retirement, changes in family and social roles, illness, disability, loss of spouse and close friends, and changing support networks place the individual at risk for bereavement, loneliness, and low self-esteem—all associated with social isolation and depression (refer to Chapter 28).

Caregiver availability and caregiver burden are issues that will need to be addressed in the coming decades. Approximately two thirds of older persons live in family settings (American Association of Retired Persons, 2000). As the number of elderly persons increases, the number of traditional family caregivers (wives, daughters, and daughters-in-law) available to provide care is expected to decline. Fewer marriages, smaller family size, increased workforce participation by women, and delayed childbearing all serve to limit the number of available family caregivers (Wackerbarths & Johnson, 2002).

HEALTH PROFILES OR STATUS OF POPULATIONS AT HIGH RISK

Improvement in the overall health of Americans requires special attention to improvement in the health of persons who are at especially high risk. Understanding the differences between the total population and these higher-risk populations is one way to begin to address the gap in the health status and health care services of these groups. In considering the groups included in this section, two caveats are important. First, data systems for collecting information at the national and state levels are, in many cases, quite limited. Second, the population subgroups are extremely heterogeneous, which makes generalizations about an entire cohort inappropriate unless they are reassessed at the local level. The data presented are intended to help identify broad risk groups and not to stereotype behavior of the particular groups (see Chapter 10).

PATTERNS OF MORTALITY AND MORBIDITY IN PERSONS WITH LOW INCOMES

Those with low socioeconomic status include family groups or individuals who are unemployed, underemployed, or in low-wage jobs, as well as many single-parent families who live in substandard housing and have an educational achievement rate below that of the general population.

Poverty increases health risks in many ways. The death rates of poor persons are approximately twice the rates of persons above the poverty level. The incidences of disease are significantly higher. Poverty also increases the risk of infant mortality, as noted earlier in this chapter. Chapter 21 details the impact of poverty on health status and health behaviors.

Changing the health effects of income-related disparities is a challenging task. Although a difficult and time-consuming endeavor, it is well worth the effort. The rewards will include lower health costs and improved health status of the U.S. population (see Chapters 3, 4, and 21).

PATTERNS OF MORTALITY AND MORBIDITY AMONG MINORITIES

The term *minority* refers to a group of individuals who share a common ethnicity or ancestry (characteristic) and who represent a smaller proportion of the population than the largest represented group. Predominant minority populations in the United States are African Americans, Hispanics, Asians, Pacific Islanders, Native Americans, and Alaska Natives (see Chapter 10). These categories, however, are oversimplifications of the diversity within each racial or ethnic group. Great diversity can be found between and among racial and ethnic groups, including diversity in characteristics associated with health status, such as lifestyle patterns, genetic influences, socioeconomic status, and health risks.

Gathering health-related information about racial and ethnic groups is confounded by the large number of diverse data sources (Figure 7-16). Each data source collects specific pieces of information, some for all racial and ethnic categories, others for only

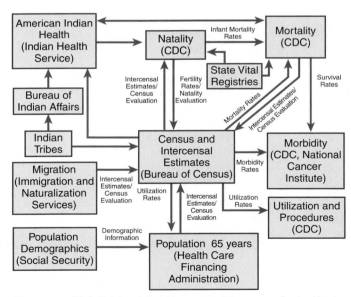

FIGURE 7-16 Interrelationship among data sources for health statistics on United States race and ethnic population. (Redrawn from Centers for Disease Control and Prevention. [1993, June 25]. *Morbidity and Mortality Weekly Report, 42,* 2.)

white, black, and Hispanic categories. Other variables correlated with health status, for example, educational attainment or socioeconomic status, are not always collected in these surveys. This lack of data makes determining the degree to which health status is influenced by race and ethnicity alone more difficult. Collection of racial and ethnic information has been initiated at various times. Continuous collection of health data has been carried out the longest for black and white racial groups. Most of the national data on African Americans is collected under the racial description of "black," and these studies are reported using that designation. For the minority groups for which comparable information exists, the data indicate greater rates of health problems and death (Table 7-10). Reducing health disparities and improving the health status of minority populations is a primary goal of the *Healthy People 2010* national health objectives.

African Americans

Many health risks of African Americans are associated with poverty. In 2004, 24.7% of blacks were below the poverty level, compared with 8.6% of non-Hispanic whites (USDHHS, 2006). Although it is improving, life expectancy for blacks lags behind that of the total population. The leading causes of death associated with chronic conditions are the same as those for the majority of the overall population. Heart disease, cancer, and stroke are the three leading causes of death for both blacks and whites; however, blacks do not live as long with these conditions. After adjustment for normal life expectancy, only 53% of blacks diagnosed with cancer reached the 5-year postdiagnosis mark compared with 64% of whites between 1992 and 1998 (ACS, 2003). Blacks, particularly young black men and boys, are more likely to die from homicide and legal intervention. In 2004 the homicide rate for black men was 35.1 compared with 5.3 for white men. For men between 15 and 24 years of age, the rates were 77.6 for blacks and 10.2 for whites (CDC, 2006). Blacks also have higher rates of unintentional injury and diabetes. Diabetes is almost 30% more frequent among blacks; black women, especially those who are overweight, are at highest risk.

Both blacks and Hispanics are at greater risk of contracting AIDS and sexually transmitted diseases. Other health-related indicators, such as rates of low birth weight, infant mortality and morbidity, and adolescent pregnancy, also show striking disparities when blacks are compared with other groups in the total population (see Chapter 24). *Differences decrease dramatically for most diseases when death rates are adjusted for income level.* This indicates that socioeconomic class, rather than race, is the primary contributing factor for the disparities in health status. Caregiver bias may also influence care and treatment options (Johnson et al., 2004; Smedley et al., 2003).

Health care–seeking behaviors of the African American population are apparently different from those of the white population. Some of the difference is related to problems of access. More African Americans than whites do not receive adequate routine and preventive health care services. Blacks make less frequent visits to physicians. Black mothers are twice as likely not to receive prenatal care until the last trimester of pregnancy, and more African Americans receive medical care from clinics and emergency rooms (Baldwin, 2003; USDHHS, 2006). Changing the patterns of access to and delivery of health services is a major challenge if the frequency and severity of complications from illness are to be reduced. Health care reform in the early 1990s intended to address the disparity in services. After federal efforts at health care reform failed, many states initiated their own attempts to address health care access barriers for uninsured and underserved populations.

Hispanic Americans

Hispanic Americans constitute the largest and fastest-growing minority group. This group is young (median age is less than 26 years, compared with 35 years for the total population) and has a high birth rate.

Hispanics are the second poorest minority group, and their health status reflects the influences of poverty. This group also includes a small but significant migrant farm worker population, which requires special attention. Hispanics actually have less access to health care and preventive health care services than do other groups, because more of them do not have health insurance (see Chapter 21). Language is another barrier to obtaining care.

As in the total population, the two leading causes of death in Hispanics are heart disease and cancer; however, the death rates associated with these diseases are higher than for non-Hispanics. Death rates for unintentional injuries, homicides, chronic liver disease and cirrhosis, and AIDS are higher than those for whites, whereas death rates for suicide, stroke, and chronic obstructive pulmonary disease are lower than those for whites. Alcohol

TABLE 7-10 Rates for Racial and Social Groups for Selected Health Behaviors: 2003

Health Measure	American Indian or Alaska Native	Asian or Pacific Islander	Black Non-Hispanic	Hispanic	White Non-Hispanic	Total
Diseases of heart death rate*	87.2	77.0	202.8	70.9	251.7	235.6
Unintentional Injury death rate*	50.6	14.9	32.4	26.1	39.5	37.6
Infant mortality rate†	8.73	4.83	13.60	5.65	5.70	6.84
Percentage low birth weight	7.4	7.8	13.6	6.7	7.1	8.0
Tuberculosis case rate*	8.2	Asian: 29.6‡ Native Hawaiian or other Pacific Islander: 16.4‡	11.7	10.3	1.4	5.1

*Incidence/100,000 population.
†Deaths/1000 live births.
‡Asian and Native Hawaiian or Pacific Islander races first reported in 2003.
Data from National Center for Health Statistics. (2006). *Health, United States, 2006*, Hyattsville, MD: USDHHS; National Center for Health Statistics. *Vital statistics of the United States*, annual, and unpublished data; and U.S. Bureau of the Census. (2007). *Statistical abstract of the United States, 2007* (126th ed.). Washington, DC: U.S. Government Printing Office.

consumption is a major health risk, especially among Hispanic adolescents, who report higher rates of episodic heavy drinking and current alcohol use (Grunbaum et al, 2004). The cultural, and therefore the health, profile of this group is diverse. For example, Mexican Americans have a low rate of cerebrovascular disease, whereas the opposite is true for Puerto Ricans living in New York City. Cuban Americans are high users of prenatal services, but Mexican Americans and Puerto Ricans are not.

Asians and Pacific Islanders

Because health data are often collected using black and white racial categories, and because the number of Asians and Pacific Islanders is relatively small, finding consistent health status reports on this minority group is difficult. Moreover, in 2003, the CDC began reporting some types of data separately for Asians and Native Hawaiians or other Pacific Islanders. In areas with a significant concentration of this minority group, local studies are used to identify health status and health risks.

As with other minority groups, socioeconomic status and degree of acculturation tend to influence the health status within this cohort. The risk of cancer is approximately the same as that for the general population but is higher in selected subgroups for certain types of cancer. For example, Native Hawaiian women have a higher rate of breast cancer, Southeast Asian men have a higher rate of lung cancer, and Asian and Pacific Islanders in general have a liver cancer rate three times higher than that of the white population (ACS, 2006). For individuals who get cancer, the risk of death is greater. The 5-year survival rate for Asians and Pacific Islanders is lower than that for whites (ACS, 2006).

Asian and Pacific Islander immigrants are at serious risk for two infectious diseases: tuberculosis and hepatitis B. Among Southeast Asian immigrants, the incidence of tuberculosis is 40 times higher than that in the general population. Higher rates of hepatitis B place Asian immigrants at greater risk of serious side effects, such as chronic liver disease, cirrhosis, and liver cancer (ACS, 2003).

Native Americans, Aleuts, and Eskimos

Native Americans suffer from a variety of illnesses that can be prevented or ameliorated by early diagnosis and treatment. Many of the health problems in this group are exacerbated by poverty and substance abuse. Detailed data have been collected for Native Americans, who have much higher rates of alcoholism and related problems such as accidents, homicides, and suicides (Figure 7-17). An estimated 75% of unintentional injuries and 54% of motor vehicle accidents in this group are alcohol related (Shalala et al., 2000). As a result, Native Americans are at greater risk of early death than are members of the general population.

Rates of heart disease and cancer are lower among Native Americans, perhaps because these are generally diseases of older age. Cirrhosis and diabetes are two chronic conditions that affect Native Americans at a higher rate than the general population. Diabetes is so common that, in many tribes, 20% of members have the disease. In 2003 the Native American age-adjusted death rate for diabetes was almost two times the all-races rate (USDHHS, 2006). Native American children are at risk for many of the health problems associated with higher levels of poverty.

Many of the health problems of Native Americans, particularly tuberculosis, diabetes, and pneumonia, can be reduced or

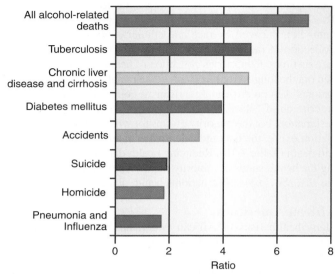

Ratio of American Indian/Alaska Native Selected Age-Adjusted Death Rates (1996-1998) to U.S. All-Races (1997)

FIGURE 7-17 Ratio between Native American age-adjusted death rates for selected causes in 1994 to 1996 and death rates for the U.S. all-races population in 1997. (Data from Thompson, T. G., Grim, C. W., Hartz, G. J., et al. [2001]. *Trends in Indian health: 2000-2001.* Rockville, MD: Indian Health Service.) In 1996 to 1998, the Indian (Indian Health Service) age-adjusted death rates for the above causes were considerably higher than those for the U.S. all-races population in 1997. These Indian rates have been adjusted for miscoding of Indian race on death certificates.

eliminated by early diagnosis and treatment. Some problems can be reduced or eliminated by changing patterns of behavior. Public health officials and Native American leaders are engaged in health projects aimed at reducing risky behaviors, improving lifestyle habits, and facilitating access and provision of services for Native American populations.

CONTINUING ISSUES

The nation continues to struggle with the effects of chronic illness, both at the human level in terms of suffering and at the national level in terms of economic loss. Minority populations are at greater risk, experiencing chronic illness at an earlier age and having higher rates of early death compared with the general population. An important goal of *Healthy People 2010* is eliminating health disparities among racial and ethnic groups.

The advent of new contagious diseases (e.g., HIV/AIDS, SARS), the antigenic variations in older known contagious diseases, and the continuing presence of preventable diseases have revealed that humanity and science do not have the means to completely control or prevent infectious diseases. Newly emerging and highly treatment-resistant diseases are expected to become significant issues in the near future. Nursing and society must work in concert with environmental and medical science to prevent and cure infectious and chronic diseases. Using epidemiology-based research, the science of nursing must be ready to provide strategies for disease prevention and health promotion. Community health nurses will need to make continuing efforts to explore factors that affect human health behaviors, lifestyles, and participation in activities that reduce diseases for populations, aggregates, and target groups.

KEY IDEAS

1. Epidemiology is the study of the health status of human populations.
2. Epidemiologists and nurse researchers use descriptive, analytic, and experimental research methods to study causative factors of illness, disability, and premature death; to describe the natural history of disease; to identify populations at risk for poor health; and to determine the effectiveness of screening, health education, and treatment measures.
3. Epidemiology is helpful to community/public health nurses for describing the health status of a population and the factors that contribute to its well-being, for targeting aggregates at risk of specific health conditions, and for evaluating the effectiveness of nursing interventions in populations.
4. Rates and ratios are statistics used to describe births, deaths, and incidences and prevalences of disease and disability in populations.
5. The natural history of a disease is influenced by characteristics of the people (host), agents (biologic, chemical, and physical), and environment that make up the epidemiologic triangle.
6. Age, sex, race, social class, occupation, and marital status are demographic characteristics frequently used when describing human populations. These factors contribute to variations in health status, health-related behaviors, and use of health care services.
7. Much of the disparity in the health status of minority populations is linked to poverty.
8. Community/public health nursing involves attending to the health status of multiple subpopulations as well as of the total population.
9. Health care services and programs are aimed at three levels of prevention: primary, secondary, and tertiary.
10. Understanding the multiple factors that contribute to illness, injury, and premature death is necessary but not adequate for improving the health status of the U.S. population. A key challenge for community and public health nurses is to use knowledge of risk factors to shape health policy priorities and to influence positively the health profile of the people they serve.

LEARNING BY EXPERIENCE AND REFLECTION

1. Obtain a copy of your local health department's annual report. See whether you can identify prevalent health needs and problems in your local community.
2. What are the five leading causes of death in your community? Are these mortality data similar to or different from the national mortality data?
3. Do special cohort groups have higher rates of morbidity or mortality than others do in your community? If so, what types of health problems contribute to the higher rates?
4. Do higher or lower rates of infectious disease exist in your community than in your state and in the United States?
5. As a community/public health nurse, how would you prepare a plan to reduce health problems identified in activity 3 or 4 in this section? Whose support would you need to enroll to implement such a plan? How would you go about acquiring community support for your plan?

COMMUNITY RESOURCES FOR PRACTICE

Data on health care providers with occupationally acquired HIV infection are published in the CDC's *HIV/AIDS Surveillance Report*. Free copies are available from the CDC National AIDS Clearinghouse, PO Box 6003, Rockville, MD 20849-6003; telephone (800) 458-5231. This report can also be downloaded from the Internet at *http://www.cdc.gov.*

Information about each of the following organizations is found on its website, which can be accessed through the **WebLinks** section of this book's website at *http://evolve.elsevier.com/Maurer/community/*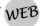

American Cancer Society
American Lung Association
American Public Health Association
Association of Schools of Public Health
Environmental Protection Agency
National Institutes of Health
U.S. Bureau of the Census
World Health Organization

STUDY AIDS   http://evolve.elsevier.com/Maurer/community/

Visit the Evolve website for this book to find the following study and assessment materials:

- Quiz
- Web Scenario
- Critical Thinking Questions and Answers for Case Studies

- Care Plans
- *Healthy People* Updates
- Glossary

REFERENCES

American Academy of Pediatrics. (2001). The new morbidity revisited: A renewed commitment to the psychosocial aspects of pediatric care. *Pediatrics, 108*(5), 1227-1230.

American Association of Retired Persons. (2000). *A profile of older Americans 1999.* Retrieved July 26, 2007 from *http://www.aarp.org/.*

American Cancer Society. (2003). *Cancer facts and figures: 2003.* Retrieved July 26, 2007 from *http://www.cancer.org/downloads/STT/CAFF2003PWSecured.pdf.*

American Cancer Society. (2006). *Cancer facts and figures: 2006.* Retrieved July 26, 2007

from *http://www.cancer.org/downloads/STT/CAFF2006PWSecured.pdf.*

American Lung Association. (2004). *Smoking overview.* Retrieved July 16, 2007 from *http://www.lungusa.org/site/apps/s/conent.asp?c=dvLUK900E&b= 34706&ct=66968.*

American Lung Association. (2007). *Search Lung USA*. Retrieved January 30, 2008 from *http://www.lungusa.org/site/apps.s. content. asp?c=duLUK9OOE&b=3470b&ct=66721*.

Baldwin, D. M. (2003). Disparities in health and health care: Focusing efforts to eliminate unequal burdens. *Online Journal of Issues in Nursing, 8*(1). Retrieved July 17, 2007 from *http://nursingworld.org/MainMenuCategories/ANAMarketplace/ANAPeriodicals/OJIN/TableofContents/Volume82003/Num1Jan31_2003/DisparitiesinHealthandHealthCare.aspx*.

Bertone, E. R., Willett, W. C., Rosner, B. A., et al. (2001). Nurses'Health Study. Prospective study of recreational physical activity and ovarian cancer. *Journal of the National Cancer Institute, 93*(12), 942-948.

Centers for Disease Control and Prevention. (1993, June 25). *Morbidity and Mortality Weekly Report, 42*, 2.

Centers for Disease Control and Prevention. (1997a). Hepatitis A associated with consumption of frozen strawberries: Michigan, March. *Morbidity and Mortality Weekly Report, 46*(13), 288-289.

Centers for Disease Control and Prevention. (1997b). *HIV/AIDS surveillance report* (year-end ed.). Atlanta: Author.

Centers for Disease Control and Prevention. (2003a). *Child passenger safety: Fact sheet*. Retrieved July 26, 2007 from *http://www.cdc.gov/ncipc/factsheets/childpas.htm*.

Centers for Disease Control and Prevention. (2003b). *Basic information about SARS* (Fact sheet). Retrieved July 27, 2007 from *http://www.cdc.gov/ncidod/sars/factsheet.htm*.

Centers for Disease Control and Prevention. (2004). *Fact sheet: Physical inactivity and poor nutrition catching up to tobacco as actual causes of death*. Retrieved July 18, 2007 from *http://www.cdc.gov/nccdphp/factsheets/death_causes2000.htm*.

Centers for Disease Control and Prevention. (2005). *National diabetes fact sheet*. Retrieved July 26, 2007 from *http://www.cdc.gov/diabetes/pubs/estimates05.htm#prev*.

Centers for Disease Control and Prevention. (2006). *Health, United States, 2006, with chartbook on trends in the health of Americans*. Hyattsville, MD: U.S. Department of Health and Human Services, Centers for Disease Control and Prevention, National Center for Health Statistics.

Centers for Disease Control and Prevention. (2007). *Child passenger safety*. Retrieved July 26, 2007 from *http://www.cdc.gov/ncipc/factsheets/child-pas.htm*.

Dever, G. E. A. (1991). *Community health analysis: Development of global awareness at the local level* (2nd ed.). Gaithersburg, MD: Aspen.

Ebersole, P., Hess, P., & Luggen, A. S. (2004). *Toward healthy aging: Human needs and nursing response* (6th ed.). St. Louis: Mosby.

Federal Bureau of Investigation. (2007a). *California: Offenses known to law enforcement*. Retrieved January 30, 2008 from *http://www.fbi.gov/ucr/cius2006/data/table_08_ca.html*.

Federal Bureau of Investigation. (2007b). *District of Columbia: Offenses known to law enforcement*. Retrieved January 30, 2008 from *http://www.fbi.gov/ucr/cius2006/data/table_08_dc.html*.

Fields, J. (2004). *Current population reports, America's families and living arrangements: 2003*. Retrieved July 28, 2007 from *http://www.census2010.gov/prod/2004pubs/p20_533.pdf*.

Gordis, L. (2004). *Epidemiology* (3rd ed.). Philadelphia: Saunders.

Grunbaum, J.A., Kann, L., Kinchen, S., et al. (2004). Youth risk behavior surveillance—United States, 2003. Retrieved January 30, 2008 from *Morbidity and Mortality Weekly Reports Surveillance Summaries, 53*(SS02), 1-96.

Heron, M., & Smith, B. L. (2007). Deaths: Leading causes for 2003. *National Vital Statistics Reports: From the Centers for Disease Control and Prevention, National Center for Health Statistics, National Vital Statistics System, 55*(10).

Johnson, R. L., Saha, S., Arbelaez, J. J., et al. (2004). Racial and ethnic differences in patient perceptions of bias and cultural competence in health care. *Journal of General Internal Medicine, 19*(2), 101-110.

King, W. D., Dodds, L., Allen, A. C., et al. (2005). Haloacetic acids in drinking water and risk for stillbirth. *Occupational and Environmental Medicine, 62*(2), 124-127.

Krieger, N. (1994). Epidemiology and the web of causation: Has anyone seen the spider? *Social Science and Medicine, 39*(7), 887-903.

Leavell, H. R., & Clark, E. G. (1965). *Preventive medicine for the doctor in his community: An epidemiological approach*. New York: McGraw-Hill.

Levis, S., Gomez, A., Jimenez, C., et al. (2005). Vitamin D deficiency and seasonal variation in an adult south Florida population. *Journal of Clinical Endocrinology and Metabolism, 90*(3), 1557-1562.

Lloyd-Jones, D. M., O'Donnell, C. J., D'Agostino, R. B., et al. (2001). Applicability of cholesterol-lowering primary prevention trials to a general population: The Framingham Heart Study. *Archives of Internal Medicine, 161*(7), 949-954.

Ma, Y., Bertone, E. R., Stanke, E. J., et al. (2003). Association between eating patterns and obesity in a free-living U.S. adult population. *American Journal of Epidemiology, 158*(1), 85-92.

McGinnis, J. M., & Foege, W. H. (1993). Actual causes of death in the United States. *Journal of the American Medical Association, 270*, 2207-2212.

McGinnis, J. M., & Foege, W. H. (1999). Mortality and morbidity attributable to use of addictive substances in the United States. *Proceedings of the Association of American Physicians, 111*(2), 109-118.

Minino, A. M., Heron, M., Murphy, S. L. et al. (2006). Deaths: Final data for 2004. *Health E-stats*. Retrieved July 26, 2007 from *http://www.cdc.gov/nchs/products/pubs/pubd/hestats/finaldeaths04/finaldeaths04.htm*.

Moeher, W., Chandra, A., & Jones, J. (2005). *Sexual behavior and selected health measures: Men and women 15-44 years of age, United States, 2002*. Advanced Data from Vital and Health Statistics. Retrieved July 26, 2007 from *http://www.cdc.gov/nchs/products/pubs/pubd/ad/361-370/ad362.htm*.

Morton, R. F., Hebel, J. R., & McCarter, R. J. (2001). *A study guide to epidemiology and biostatistics* (5th ed.). Sudbury, MA: Jones & Bartlett.

Moyer, L., Warwick, M., & Mahoney, F. J. (1996). Prevention of hepatitis A virus infection. *American Family Physician, 54*(1), 107-114.

National Center for Health Statistics. (2006). *Health, United States*, 2006. Hyattsville, MD: USDHHS.

National Cancer Institute. (2007). *Surveillance, epidemiology, and end results*. Retrieved July 26, 2007 from *http:/www.seer.cancer.gov/*.

National Center for Health Statistics. (Annual). *Vital statistics of the United States*.

National Heart, Lung, and Blood Institute. (2002). *Framingham Heart Study: 50 years of research success*. Retrieved July 26, 2007 from *http://www.nhlbi.nih.gov/about/framingham/*.

National Highway Transportation and Safety Administration. (2005). *Alcohol-related crashes and fatalitie*s. Washington, DC: National Highway Transportation and Safety Administration, National Center for Statistics and Analysis.

National Institute on Aging. (2002). *It's never too late to start* (Exercise pamphlet). Retrieved July 27, 2007 from *http://www.nia.nih.gov/news/pr/2002*.

Proctor, B. D., & Dalaker, J. (2002). *Poverty in the United States: 2001*. Retrieved July 26, 2007 from *http://www.census.gov/prod/2002pubs/p60-219.pdf*.

Shalala, D. E., Trujillo, M. H., Hartz, G. J., et al. (2000). *Trends in Indian health 1998-1999*. Retrieved July 26, 2007 from *http://www.ihs.gov/PublicInfo/Publications/trends98/trends98.asp*.

Siegel, J. D., Rhinehart, E., Jackson, M., et al. (2007). *Guideline for isolation precautions: Preventing transmission of infectious agents in healthcare settings*. Atlanta: U.S. Department of Health and Human Services, Public Health Service, Centers for Disease Control and Prevention.

Smedley, B. D., Stith, A. Y., & Nelson, A. R. (Eds.). (2003). *Unequal treatment: Confronting racial and ethnic disparities in health care*. Washington, DC: National Academy Press. Retrieved July 26, 2007 from *http://www.nap.edu/catalog/10260.html*.

Thompson, T. G., Grim, C. W., Hartz, G. J., et al. (2001). *Trends in Indian Health: 2000-2001*. Rockville, MD: Indian Health Service. Retrieved July 26, 2007 from *http://www.ihs.gov/NonMedicalPrograms/HIS_Stats/Trends00.asp*.

U.S. Bureau of the Census. (2001a). *International database*. Washington, DC: U.S. Government Printing Office.

U.S. Bureau of the Census. (2001b). *Statistical abstract of the United States* (120th ed.), Table 105. Washington, DC: U.S. Government Printing Office.

U.S. Bureau of the Census. (2004). *U.S. interim projections by age, sex, race, and Hispanic origin.* Retrieved July 27, 2007 from *http://www.census. gov/ipc/www/usinterimpro/.*

U.S. Bureau of the Census. (2007). *Statistical abstract of the United States, 2007: The national data book* (126th ed.). Washington, DC: U.S. Government Printing Office.

U.S. Cancer Working Group. (2006). *United States cancer statistics: 2003 incidence and mortality.* Atlanta: U.S. Department of Health and Human Services, Centers for Disease Control and Prevention, and National Cancer Institute.

U.S. Department of Health and Human Services. (2000). *Healthy People 2010: Understanding and improving health.* Washington, DC: U. S. Government Printing Office. Retrieved July 26, 2007 from *http://www.healthypeople. gov/document/.*

U.S. Department of Health and Human Services. (2002). *Health, United States, 2002.* Washington, DC: U.S. Government Printing Office.

U.S. Department of Health and Human Services. (2006). *Health, United States, 2006.* Washington, DC: U.S. Government Printing Office.

Wackerbarths, B., & Johnson, M. M. S. (2002). Essential information and support needs of family caregivers. *Patient Education and Counseling, 47*(2), 95-100.

Webster, B. H., & Bishaw, A. (2006). *Income, earnings and poverty data from the 2005 American community survey* (American Community Survey Reports). Retrieved July 26, 2007 from *http://www.census. gov/prod/2006pubs/acs-02.pdf.*

World Health Organization. (2004). *The atlas of heart disease and stroke.* Retrieved July 26, 2007 from *http://www.who. int/cardiovascular_diseases/resources/atlas/en/.*

World Health Organization. (2007). *Global outbreak alert and response network.* Retrieved July 26, 2007 from *http://www.who. int/csr/outbreaknetwork/en/.*

SUGGESTED READINGS

Coughlin, S. S., & Beauchamp, T. L. (1996). *Ethics and epidemiology.* Oxford, England: Oxford University Press.

Gerstman, B. B. (1998). *Epidemiology kept simple. An introduction to classic and modern epidemiology.* New York: Wiley-Liss.

U.S. Department of Health and Human Services. (2000). *Healthy People 2010: Understanding and improving health.* Washington, DC: U. S. Government Printing Office. Retrieved July 26, 2007 from *http://www.healthypeople. gov/document/.*

U.S. Department of Health and Human Services. (2006). *Health, United States, 2006.* Washington, DC: U.S. Government Printing Office.

8 Communicable Diseases

Frances A. Maurer

FOCUS QUESTIONS

What methods have been used historically to safeguard populations against communicable diseases?

What are the elements of a communicable disease, and how do they interact?

How do boards of health demonstrate responsibilities for controlling the spread of communicable diseases?

Why are the concepts of epidemiology appropriate to use for preventing and controlling communicable diseases?

What are the implications for the nursing process in caring for individuals and families with communicable diseases?

Where can nurses and clients obtain information about support resources for coping with communicable diseases?

CHAPTER OUTLINE

KEY TERMS

Agent	Invasiveness	Resistance
Artificial immunity	Natural immunity	Sources of contamination
Bioterrorism	Nosocomial infections	Vector
Host	Pathogenicity	Virulence
Infective dose	Reservoirs	

COMMUNICABLE DISEASES AND CONTROL

Communicable diseases occur in every country, in every urban and rural area, and in every neighborhood, from the very rich to the very poor. Nurses who provide quality care in combating communicable diseases must have a basic understanding of epidemi-

ology, infection control, microbiology, medicine, public health, and nursing. Furthermore, the community nurse must have knowledge of the legal system, which mandates prevention and control of communicable diseases locally, nationally, and worldwide. Nurses must also have knowledge of effective support systems that can be used by individuals, families, and communities.

The public health community faces new challenges. The resurgence of old diseases, such as measles and tuberculosis (TB); the appearance of drug-resistant bacteria such as methicillin-resistant *Staphylococcus;* and the emergence of new diseases, such as severe acute respiratory syndrome (SARS), human immunodeficiency virus (HIV) infection and acquired immunodeficiency syndrome (AIDS), and Ebola virus disease, require health professionals to be alert, conscientious monitors of the public health. The potential for **bioterrorism,** the use of disease-producing agents as weapons, is also a growing concern of public health agencies.

Communicable disease control involves controlling environmental elements and personal behaviors that facilitate the spread of disease. The knowledge of how to control disease has been acquired through centuries of whimsical practice, lucky guesses, serendipitous observation, and strict scientific inquiry. The most dramatic controls have been achieved by establishing public hygiene measures. A brief historic review of attempts at disease control provides the community health nurse with an appreciation of the efforts needed to reach the level of disease control we have today.

DISEASE CONTROL: BIBLICAL TIMES TO THE PRESENT

Communicable diseases such as smallpox and leprosy existed even before the birth of Christ. Plague raged intermittently throughout Europe and China during the thirteenth and fourteenth centuries, decimating the population. In the fourteenth century, physicians first formulated a theory to explain the communicable disease process. Although it was not completely accurate, this and subsequent trial-and-error efforts helped physicians develop sound principles for communicable disease control (Box 8-1). Today, quarantine, sanitary precautions, and travel restrictions remain methods of communicable disease control.

As the relationship between disease-producing microorganisms and factors that are beneficial to their growth became more apparent, control measures became more specific. Sanitary regulation of the environment and isolation of infected individuals became accepted strategies. These control measures were widely enforced. Streets were cleaned, the throwing of garbage into rivers and streets was discouraged, standing water was drained, and infected individuals were isolated. In America, quarantine laws became acceptable in the mid-1800s.

EARLY STATE AND FEDERAL EFFORTS AT DISEASE CONTROL

In 1869, the first state health department was established in Massachusetts; health departments in other states soon followed. By 1901 all but five states had some type of board of health. The Massachusetts health department controlled communicable diseases by regulating sanitary conditions and by building water and sewage systems. As boards of health developed, they began to realize the importance of accurate statistics for tracking and controlling communicable diseases. Statistics provided a way to identify trends, incidence, and effective treatment.

Communicable disease control at the federal level was almost nonexistent until the 1800s. In 1872, the Marine Hospital Service, the forerunner of the Public Health Service, was founded by an act of Congress. At approximately the same time, the American Public Health Association was established. The American Public Health Association provided a forum for physicians and other public health workers to set standards of care. In 1878 the

| BOX 8-1 | Early Efforts at Disease Control |

- **Fourteenth century**—Physicians developed theory of communicable disease process:
  - Disease spreads through contact with an infected person or article.
  - Environmental factors such as waste, garbage, and stagnant water also facilitate or spread disease.
  - Unhealthy persons such as the weak, malnourished, or those with poor hygiene are at greater risk of disease.
  - Weather conditions and a person's moral life influence the spread of disease (Risse, 1988).
- **Mid-seventeenth to eighteenth century**—Plague in Venice in 1656 led to development of quarantine measures: ships quarantined, overland trade suspended, public gatherings forbidden, schools closed, streets cleaned, sick confined to pest houses. Observation of the relationship between cowpox and higher immunity to smallpox started efforts to use the cowpox virus to control the spread of smallpox and led to development of smallpox vaccination.
- **Nineteenth century**—Role of the vector in disease transmission was still unknown. Theory of miasma developed, which blamed communicable disease on bad air and spontaneous generation of infectious agents. Although not completely accurate, this theory lead to public health measures that worked. These measures included eliminating garbage, refuse, and animal remains, as well as draining stagnant water.
- **1800s**—European cholera epidemic occurred. Physicians reexamined prevailing theories and discounted slow development of putrid air and idea that only immoral affected by disease. Sanitary conditions helped, but did not completely control the cholera epidemic.
- **1900s**—Swift progress was made. Microorganisms were identified as the cause of specific diseases (diphtheria, tuberculosis, pneumonia, and typhoid fever) (Dowling, 1977). Jacob Henle developed scientific criteria to link organism to specific disease: (1) identify organism, (2) isolate it, and (3) use the organism to generate disease. This approach remains a basic principle used by public health personnel to investigate new diseases and illnesses.

Quarantine Act was passed, granting the federal government the power to impose quarantine. In 1912, the Marine Hospital Service officially became the Public Health Service (PHS), and states were held responsible for reporting statistics to the federal government via the PHS (Miller, 2002; Mullan, 1989).

Federal support for research assistance in communicable disease control led to several important actions. In 1930, the Ransdell Act established the National Institutes of Health (NIH), which continues to be the major source of research for the PHS. In 1946, the Communicable Disease Center, currently known as the Centers for Disease Control and Prevention (CDC), was established. The CDC's original mandate was control of infectious diseases. Over the years, however, the scope of the CDC has expanded to include noninfectious diseases and environmental issues. The CDC is responsible for collecting morbidity and mortality statistics on reportable infectious diseases.

The 1970s were a decade of health reform and legislation. The needs of migrant workers were supported, and vaccines were made available to the poor. Funding for the NIH was increased, and a national effort began to decrease the incidence of cancer, heart attacks, and strokes. In the 1980s the important role of the PHS was underscored by the advent of HIV infection. The need for HIV infection prevention and education efforts, the issue of confidential or anonymous testing and counseling, the need for contact tracing and notification, and the care of infected individuals in hospitals and in the community have served to emphasize the need for a public health response to communicable diseases.

Today public health officials face many challenges, including the need for a quick response to a bioterrorism attack (see Chapter 22); the potential for rapid spread of infectious diseases due to the ease of travel between countries; and the rise of new and drug-resistant diseases. The public health community must meet these challenges in spite of limited funding for public health programs.

SUCCESSES IN COMMUNICABLE DISEASE CONTROL

Public health practices have initiated community protection measures such as creating safer environmental conditions and providing treatments and vaccine as soon as they become available. Water quality regulations, sewage regulations, and food-handling regulations have decreased the incidence of enteric diseases. Currently, water is chlorinated, milk is pasteurized, preservatives are added to foods, and safe sewage plants are built. Antibiotics help reduce the spread of communicable diseases (e.g., rheumatic fever, TB, syphilis) by lessening the time during which infected persons are contagious.

Vaccine development and immunization programs eliminated smallpox and have dramatically decreased the incidence of childhood diseases such as measles, mumps, pertussis, polio, and rubella. In 1977 a national campaign, the Childhood Immunization Initiative, resulted in massive immunizations of young children. Unfortunately, a reduced emphasis on public health at the national level, with corresponding funding cuts, diminished the impact of this early immunization effort (Jekel et al., 2007). When the public becomes complacent, some diseases resurface or new ones emerge to affect the health of populations.

CONTEMPORARY ISSUES IN COMMUNICABLE DISEASE

Despite significant success in communicable disease control since the 1940s, these diseases are still among the leading causes of death in the United States. Infectious diseases account for 25% of all doctor visits. When considered as a group, three infectious diseases—pneumonia, influenza, and HIV infection—constituted the fourth leading cause of death in the United States in 2003 (U.S. Department of Health and Human Services [USDHHS], 2006a). The public health community is especially concerned about a resurgence in the incidence of vaccine-preventable childhood illnesses (e.g., measles), TB, sexually transmitted diseases, and hepatitis and the emergence of new diseases, the most prominent of which are HIV infection, SARS, and West Nile virus infection (Table 8-1). The objectives of *Healthy People 2010* (USDHHS, 2000) have targeted all of these communicable diseases for special attention to significantly reduce their impact on the American people (refer to the *Healthy People 2010* box on page 195).

TABLE 8-1   Frequency of Notifiable Diseases over Time

Disease	Number of Cases							
	1930	1940	1950	1960	1970	1980	1990	2005
AIDS							41,595*	41,120
Chlamydia (first report 1995)								976,445
Legionellosis						475*	1370	2301*
Lyme disease								23,305
Measles (rubeola)	419,465	291,162	319,124	441,703	47,351	13,506	27,786	66
Mumps	NA	NA	NA	NA	104,953	8576	5292	314
Pertussis	166,914	183,866	120,718	14,809	4249	1730	4570	25,616
Poliomyelitis	9220	9804	33,300	3190	33	9	7	0**
Rabies, animal	3002	7210	7901	3567	3224	6421	4826	5915
Rabies, human	59	41	18	2	3	0	1	2
Rheumatic fever	NA	NA	NA	9022	3227	432	108	‡
Rubella (German measles)	NA	NA	NA	NA	56,552	3904	1125	11
SARS								0
Smallpox	48,907	2795		Last documented case in the United States was in 1949				
Syphilis	213,309	472,900	217,558	122,538	91,382	68,382	134,255	33,278
Tuberculosis	124,940	102,984	217,742	122,538	91,382	68,832	134,255	14,097
Typhoid fever	27,201	9809	2484	816	346	510	552	324
Varicella								32,242***
West Nile virus								3830¶

Data from Centers for Disease Control and Prevention. (1979). *Annual summary and summary of notifiable diseases*—1990, 2002, 2007. Atlanta: CDC.
*New emerging reportable disease.
†Includes indigenous and imported.
‡No longer requires mandatory notification.
¶Not a reportable communicable disease at present, West Nile virus cases reported in 2006, no current cases of SARS.
**One case of vaccine-related polio.
***Added back to list in 2003.
NA, Not available; *SARS*, severe acute respiratory syndrome.

■ HEALTHY PEOPLE 2010 ■
Health Status Objectives

1. Reduce annual incidence of AIDS cases among adolescents and adults to no more than 1 per 100,000 population (baseline: 19.5 per 100,000 in 1998).
2. Reduce the number of new cases of HIV/AIDS diagnosed among adolescents and adults (no current baseline).
3. Reduce the incidence of gonorrhea to no more than 19 cases per 100,000 people (baseline: 122 in 1997).
4. Reduce the proportion of adolescents and young adults (15 to 24 years of age) with *Chlamydia trachomatis* infections to no more than 3%.

Select Population	Chlamydia: 1997 Baseline (Family Planning) Female Percentage	Chlamydia: 1997 Baseline (Sexually Transmitted Disease Clinic) Female Percentage	Male Percentage
African American	11.1	15.2	18.5
Native American, Alaska Native	6.3	13.1	12.6
Asian, Pacific Islander	4.7	12.0	16.6
Hispanic	5.2	14.0	18.5
White	3.1	9.2	11.5

5. Eliminate sustained domestic transmission of primary and secondary syphilis to fewer than 0.2 cases per 100,000 (baseline: 3.2 per 100,000 in 1997).
6. Reduce to 14% the number of adults 20 to 29 years of age with HSV-2 infection (baseline: 17% in 1988-1994).
7. Reduce the percentage of women 15 to 44 years of age who have ever required treatment for PID to no more than 5% (baseline: 8% in 1995).
8. Reduce or eliminate indigenous cases of vaccine-preventable disease.

Disease	2010 Target Goal	1998 Baseline
Measles	0	74
Mumps	0	666
Pertussis (children under 7 years of age)	2000	3417
Polio (wild-type virus)	0	0
Varicella (chickenpox)	223,000	2,228,000

9. Reduce hepatitis A cases to an incidence of no more than 4.3 per 100,000.

Select Population	1997 Baseline per 100,000
African American	26.9
Native American, Alaska Native	77.4
Asian, Pacific Islander	19.6
Hispanic	78.3
White	29.9

10. Reduce hepatitis B cases among adults 25 to 39 years of age to 5.2 per 100,000 population (baseline: 20.5 per 100,000 in 1997).
11. Reduce by 75% hepatitis B cases in high-risk groups.

Risk Group	2010 Target Goal for Number of Cases	1997 Baseline for Number of Cases
Injection drug users	1784	7135
Heterosexually active persons	1223	15,021
Men who have sex with men	1302	5209
Occupationally exposed workers	60	239

12. Reduce newly acquired hepatitis C cases to an incidence of no more than 1 per 100,000 (baseline: 2.5 per 100,000 in 1997).
13. Reduce tuberculosis to an incidence of no more than 1 per 100,000 (baseline: 6.8 per 100,000 in 1998).

From U.S. Department of Health and Human Services. (2000). *Healthy People 2010: Understanding and improving health* (2nd ed.). Washington, DC: U.S. Government Printing Office; and U.S. Department of Health and Human Services. (2006). *Healthy People 2010: Midcourse review.* Washington, DC: U.S. Government Printing Office.
AIDS, Acquired immunodeficiency syndrome; *HIV,* human immunodeficiency virus; *HSV-2,* herpes simplex virus type 2; *PID,* pelvic inflammatory disease.

VACCINE FAILURE AND LAPSED IMMUNIZATIONS

The resurgence of certain communicable diseases has been the result of lapses in control measures and the diminished effect of vaccines over time.

Childhood Immunizations: Measles, Mumps, and Pertussis

When immunization efforts were relaxed in the 1980s, young people became more susceptible to certain vaccine-preventable diseases. The most apparent proof of these lapsed immunization practices was the increase in measles cases in the late 1980s and early 1990s. Between 1989 and 1991, some 55,000 new cases were reported. Investigations of the resurgence of measles in high school and college populations revealed that the vaccine did not provide lifelong immunity. In 2005, half of all measles cases were linked to a single unvaccinated source case, and most of those affected were underimmunized (CDC, 2006a). One to two booster doses are now recommended for continued protection against measles (CDC, 2005a). Measles outbreaks continue to occur in unvaccinated children and adults (CDC, 2007a).

As with measles, mumps outbreaks have occurred among highly vaccinated populations. The risk of mumps has shifted from young children to older children, adolescents, and young adults and is usually associated with vaccine failure over time. The two-dose schedule of measles, mumps, and rubella vaccine adopted in 1989 led to a 95% decline in the incidence of mumps (CDC, 2001a). A resurgence of mumps among adolescents and young adults who had received the recommended two doses has led to the recommendation of a third dose for those at high risk (CDC, 2006b).

Pertussis outbreaks have occurred in undervaccinated populations. In 2004 and 2005, 345 cases of pertussis were reported among Amish preschool-age children in Delaware (CDC, 2006c). Vaccination rates among the Amish are low, although vaccination is not prohibited by their religion.

Public health has renewed the emphasis on childhood immunization as evidenced in *Healthy People 2010* and its predecessor, *Healthy People 2000*. To evaluate the degree of immunization coverage, the National Immunization Program at the CDC renewed the effort for a population-based immunization registry. Registries at the state and local levels are being expanded to track each child's immunization status. This information is necessary to ensure protection of the population from vaccine-preventable diseases and to identify children who are at risk when exposed to disease. A *Healthy People 2010* objective is to have 95% of children under 6 years of age enrolled in the immunization registry by 2010. In 2004, 56% of children were enrolled (CDC, 2006d).

Significant progress has been made in inoculating young children. By 2002, 95% of school-aged children in kindergarten and first grade had had all the recommended vaccinations (CDC, 2006e). Ninety percent vaccination of susceptible groups provides substantial protection against a recurrent epidemic. Monitoring of vaccination status for entry into school and day-care identifies children at risk. In Washington DC, for example, a review of immunization status by school nurses determined that 50% of children needed one or more vaccinations to meet the district's school entry requirement (CDC, 2003a). Stringent surveillance has increased the complete immunization rate to over 90% of all DC students (CDC, 2006d).

Failure to Implement Recommended Vaccinations: Pneumococcal Pneumonia and Influenza

Several episodes of pneumonia outbreaks in chronic care facilities in Massachusetts, Maryland, and Oklahoma in 1995 and 1996 were determined to be the result of failure to vaccinate at-risk populations with pneumococcal pneumonia vaccine. Investigation revealed that fewer than 5% of these institutions' populations were immunized. The death rate at the three institutions ranged from 20% to 28% of infected seniors (CDC, 1997a)—a preventable tragedy.

Pneumococcal disease and influenza account for over 36,000 deaths each year (CDC, 2006f). The majority of these deaths (90%) occur in people over the age of 65. Influenza immunization rates are approximately 53% in this age group. Pneumococcal vaccination rates in older adults have improved but are still low (51%) (CDC, 2006f). Nurses should make an effort to ensure that both vaccinations are routinely administered in hospitals, nursing homes, congregate settings, and other community settings that serve the older adult population.

Vaccine-Transmitted Disease: Polio

Since the introduction of polio vaccine, the United States has eliminated poliomyelitis transmitted from infected persons with the disease. Public health personnel still need to be vigilant to reduce the risk of importing poliovirus from other countries where it is still indigenous.

Acquisition of polio in association with administration of the live polio vaccine is rare. Persons who are at risk for developing vaccine-related polio are newly immunized individuals, close contacts, or immunosuppressed persons. One case of vaccine-acquired paralytic poliomyelitis (VAPP) was reported in the United States in 2005 (CDC, 2006g). To reduce the risk of VAPP, the CDC recommended a sequential vaccination series starting with inactivated poliovirus followed by live or activated oral polio vaccine. This new method cut the risk of VAPP in half.

DRUG-RESISTANT DISEASES

One trend of special concern to public health practitioners is the increase in drug-resistant strains of organisms that cause communicable diseases. After years of successful treatment, cases of gonorrhea, TB, pneumonia, and syphilis are on the rise. These increases are the result of less success with standard antibiotic therapies. Examples of drug-resistant organisms are the following:

- *Neisseria gonorrhoeae*—resistant to fluoroquinolone; cases found in Hawaii and Los Angeles (CDC, 2002a)
- *Candida albicans* (vulvovaginitis)—resistant to fluconazole (MacNeil et al., 2003)
- *Staphylococcus aureus*—commonly resistant to methicillin and now becoming resistant to vancomycin, the last currently known drug treatment choice (CDC, 2006h, 2006i)
- *Salmonella*—a new strain, serotype typhimurium, is resistant to ampicillin, chloramphenicol, streptomycin, sulfonamides, and tetracycline; strain is common in the United Kingdom and has surfaced in the United States (CDC, 1997b)
- *Shigella sonnei* (gastroenteritis)—resistant to ampicillin and trimethoprim-sulfamethoxazole; cases found in daycare centers in Kansas, Kentucky, and Missouri (CDC, 2006j)

Drug-resistant communicable diseases are a special concern not only because they are more complicated to treat but also because the delay in control increases the risk of infection for every person, including health care workers. Community health nurses must be alert to screen high-risk groups (Box 8-2), be aware of current treatments, and be able to identify the signs of drug-resistant infection in clients. In addition, community health professionals must take an active role in educating practitioners and the public alike concerning the prudent use of antimicrobial drugs to reduce the emergence of drug-resistant strains.

TUBERCULOSIS: DIFFICULT TO CONTROL

Nearly one third of the world's population is infected with TB. It is a leading infectious cause of death worldwide, causing more than 2 million deaths each year (CDC, 2007b; Ziv et al., 2004). Persons infected with the TB organism but without overt disease are asymptomatic and are not contagious to others. If infection progresses to TB disease, individuals will have symptoms and become contagious. A person who has a compromised immune system, practices poor nutrition, lives in poverty, or has other diseases is at greater risk of progressing from TB infection to TB disease (see Chapter 21). People who live in or emigrate from countries in which TB is indigenous are at greater risk of having been infected (see Chapter 5). Without prophylactic treatment for the infection, individuals have a 5% to 15%

Box 8-2 Groups at Greater Risk for Contracting Disease

Tuberculosis
- Individuals with human immunodeficiency virus infection
- Prisoners and homeless persons
- Poor urban individuals
- Minorities (Native Americans and Alaska Natives, Asians, Pacific Islanders, African Americans, Hispanics)
- Health care workers

Sexually Transmitted Diseases
- Adolescents
- Young adults
- Persons with multiple sex partners
- Persons engaging in drug-related activities
- Prostitutes
- Minority groups (African Americans and Hispanics)

Hepatitis
- Persons with poor personal hygiene or living in poor conditions (overcrowded or unsanitary conditions)
- Persons who emigrate from areas where hepatitis B virus infection is common (Africa, Asia, South America)
- Travelers to areas where hepatitis is endemic
- Intravenous drug users
- Persons with multiple sex partners
- Alaska Natives
- Health care workers

Human Immunodeficiency Virus Infection
- Persons with multiple sex partners
- Intravenous drug users
- Prostitutes
- Minority groups (African Americans and Hispanics)
- Bisexual and homosexual males

---

chance of progressing to disease. HIV-infected individuals are at special risk. The number of persons with the dual diagnosis of HIV and TB has increased dramatically, with 10% to 15% of all TB cases also having HIV (CDC, 2007c).

The risk of acquiring TB infection or disease is relatively low in the United States. Immigrants from countries in which TB is indigenous are at greater risk because they are more likely to have been exposed and infected in their country of origin (CDC, 2006k). Control of TB has been less successful among foreign-born individuals than among native-born Americans. Figure 8-1 illustrates the problem. As cases of TB disease among native-born Americans have declined, the incidence among foreign-born persons has increased. Today, public health agencies have renewed efforts to identify and treat foreign-born individuals. Closing the gap between TB rates among foreign-born and native-born Americans is a national health objective and a goal of the CDC.

In the United States, effective TB treatment and case finding led to dramatically fewer new cases each year by the 1980s. That decline reversed as a result of lax surveillance, program funding cuts, and an upsurge of susceptible risk groups (CDC, 1997c). By the early 1990s, improved funding and the reinstitution of tighter TB case supervision resulted in a decline in new cases by 3.8% per year (CDC, 2006k). One of the most effective treatment methods is directly observed therapy. Directly observed therapy involves having community health nurses or other trained personnel observe the ingestion of each dose of prescribed drug by individuals diagnosed with TB (Coberly & Chaisson, 2007; Jekel et al., 2007). Health personnel may observe therapy at clinic visits, during home visits, or at the individual's work site.

Partially as a result of lax control measures, multidrug-resistant TB (MDR-TB) strains developed as TB clients became less compliant with their drug therapy. These strains are a public health concern because they require longer, more costly treatment. MDR-TB is often fatal; the cure rate is lower, approximately 50% to 60%, even with intensive treatment and follow-up (Coberly & Chaisson, 2007; Hutchinson et al., 2003). Outbreaks of MDR-TB have occurred in institutional settings, including prisons and nursing homes. Today a new strain causing extensively drug-resistant TB (XDR-TB) has developed. This organism is resistant to almost all the drugs commonly used to treat TB (CDC, 2006l). As a result, the mortality for XDR-TB is very high. Although MDR-TB and XDR-TB are a serious problem worldwide (see Chapter 5), they are rare in the United States, accounting for fewer than 2% of new TB cases.

SEXUALLY TRANSMITTED DISEASES

The incidence of sexually transmitted disease (STD) is estimated at more than 19 million new cases per year (USDHHS, 2006b). The three most common diseases are chlamydia, human papillomavirus (HPV) infection, and trichomoniasis. HPV infection and trichomoniasis are not reportable communicable diseases. Chlamydia became a reportable disease in 1995. Approximately 1 million new cases of chlamydia and 6.2 million new cases of HPV infection occur each year (CDC, 2007d, 2007e). Because most people with STDs are asymptomatic or have mild symptoms, many are untreated. For example, up to 85% of women and 50% of men with chlamydia are asymptomatic (CDC, 2007d; USDHHS, 2000).

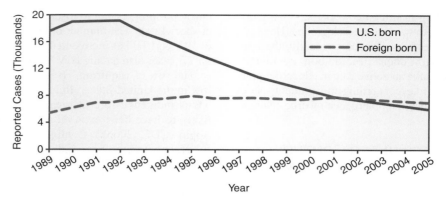

The number of tuberculosis cases among foreign born persons in the United States increased from 5411 (23% of the total number) in 1989 to 7656 (55% of the total number) in 2005.

FIGURE 8-1 Tuberculosis cases among U.S.-born and foreign-born persons by year—United States, 1989 to 2005. (From Centers for Disease Control and Prevention [CDC]. [2001]. Summary of notifiable diseases—United States, 2001. *Morbidity and Mortality Weekly Report, 50*[53], 1-108. Published May 2, 2003 for 2001; and CDC. [2006]. Trends in tuberculosis—United States, 2005. *Morbidity and Mortality Weekly Report, 55*[11], 305-308.)

The cost of treatment is high and is compounded when drug-resistant strains develop. The medical cost of treatment for STDs exceeds $13 billion each year (USDHHS, 2006b).

Individuals with untreated STDs are **reservoirs,** sources of infection for new sexual partners. Nationwide, the estimated reservoir of those with STDs includes 45 million (20% of the population) with genital herpes infection and approximately 20 million with HPV infection (CDC, 2007d; USDHHS, 2000).

Gonorrhea rates in the United States remain the highest in the developed world. Drug-resistant strains of both syphilis and gonorrhea have developed that require more prolonged and costly treatment. Some STDs (e.g., herpes infection) have no cure and require lifelong monitoring to control. The rise in STDs is related to the development of drug-resistant strains and the increased incidence of sexual activity in certain aggregates within the population.

Persons at greater risk include adolescents and young adults, drug addicts, persons with multiple sex partners, and prostitutes (Kaiser Family Foundation, 2006; Zenilman, 2007). The greatest risk is to individuals who engage in unprotected sexual activity. Adolescents are particularly vulnerable because they tend to ignore the consequences of unprotected sex (CDC, 2006m). Prostitutes who have unprotected sex have the highest risk of transmitting and acquiring an STD. Ethnic and racial minorities, especially Native Americans and Alaska Natives, Asian and Pacific Islanders, and Hispanics, are at greater risk of STDs than the general population (USDHHS, 2000). The CDC suggests that the higher risk among certain minorities may be related to other associated risk factors, such as lower socioeconomic status, reduced access to health care, limited health-seeking behaviors, increased risk of illicit drug use, and residence in communities with higher prevalence rates.

Public health efforts to reduce STDs should stress primary prevention to reduce the incidence of STDs and the long-term effects (e.g., chronic illness, sterility, cancer) associated with certain STDs. New evidence suggests that some of these prevention efforts have helped. STD rates are declining, especially among target population subgroups, such as adolescents, African Americans, and Hispanics. Adolescents are becoming more responsible in their sexual behaviors, postponing the age of first intercourse and using condoms more consistently during sexual activity (see Chapter 24). Nonetheless, the rates are too high.

There is a vaccine against HPV that protects against both cervical cancers and genital warts caused by the HPV virus (USDHHS, 2006b). It is recommended for administration to young girls (12 years and older). There is considerable debate about the appropriate target groups and administration of HPV vaccine. In 2007, the state of Texas mandated this vaccine for age-appropriate girls. That ruling met with much resistance, and Texas rescinded the mandatory requirement for HPV vaccination of school-aged girls.

HEPATITIS

Hepatitis A, B, C, D, and E are caused by different microorganisms. Hepatitis can be transmitted by fecal-oral contamination, sexual intercourse, and injection. Hepatitis is a reportable disease. The CDC reports that one in every three persons in the United States is infected with hepatitis A, B, or C (CDC, 2006n).

Hepatitis A and hepatitis B are the two most common forms of hepatitis. Hepatitis A virus (HAV) is transmitted by the fecal-oral route, and thus nonhygienic living conditions place people at risk. Sanitary control measures reduce the spread of HAV. Some HAV outbreaks have been traced to infected food handlers serving the public (e.g., in restaurants). In 2003, over 555 people in seven states contracted HAV as a result of eating at a single Mexican restaurant in Pennsylvania (CDC, 2003b). Sanitary control measures reduce the spread of HAV.

Hepatitis B virus (HBV) and hepatitis C virus (HCV) are passed from one person to another in blood and body fluids through sexual relations and shared needles, toothbrushes, and razors. The CDC estimates that approximately 60,000 people are infected with HBV each year (CDC, 2006n). In 2005 the reported case rate for hepatitis B was 1.8 per 100,000, a drop of 80% since 1990 (CDC, 2007a). Although hepatitis B is more common, hepatitis C is emerging as a leading cause of chronic liver disease and cirrhosis in the United States. Approximately 26,000 persons acquire HCV each year, and an estimated 3.2 million Americans are chronically infected with HCV

(CDC, 2006n). HBV and HCV infections are largely the result of needle sharing and sexual relations with infected persons (Webber, 2005). Groups at particular risk include those with multiple sex partners, intravenous drug users, travelers to and emigrants from HBV-endemic countries, health care workers and others exposed to blood and blood products in their work (e.g., police and institutional staff), hemophiliacs, and men who engage in homosexual intercourse. Infection with HBV and other blood-borne pathogens is an occupational risk for health care workers. Health professionals are at much greater risk of acquiring work-related HBV than of acquiring work-related HIV/AIDS. Even so, only 239 cases of work-related HBV transmission were reported in 1997 (USDHHS, 2006b). Scrupulous adherence to universal precautions greatly reduces the risk to health care workers. Likewise, homosexual men who employ safer sex practices have also reduced their risk.

Hepatitis-infected individuals can become carriers for life. The very young have the greatest risk of acquiring carrier status. About 90% of infants infected with HBV at birth will become carriers, whereas the risk for young adults is less than 10% (Robinson, 2000). Screening pregnant women for infection and treatment substantially reduces the risk of HBV transmission to infants.

Vaccines against both HAV and HBV are available. HBV vaccine is recommended for all children and adults, with particular emphasis on at-risk adults. HBV vaccination of infants and adolescents has dramatically reduced the number of new cases in persons under 19 years of age (down 75%), and the number of new cases is expected to continue to decline in these age groups. HAV vaccine is currently recommended for all children 1 year of age or older and for at-risk populations such as travelers to HAV-endemic countries or geographic areas of high concentration in the United States (CDC, 2007e). No vaccine is currently available against HCV.

HUMAN IMMUNODEFICIENCY VIRUS INFECTION

Worldwide, there are 40.3 million adults and children infected and living with HIV and AIDS (Joint United Nations Programme on HIV/AIDS, 2005). The number of Americans living with HIV/AIDS has reached 1.1 million (CDC, 2006o). By the end of 2004, more than 522,723 people had died of AIDS (CDC, 2006o). Initially, the estimated number of persons living with HIV infection was not reliable, because HIV surveillance was not mandatory. Most states have now implemented HIV surveillance reports. As a result, the prevalence estimates of HIV cases are more reliable, totaling approximately 1.2 million in the United States (CDC, 2006p). Nonetheless, these HIV surveillance reports may not reflect the true number of HIV-positive persons, because many people do not want to know their HIV status and are not tested, while others use widely available home testing kits and do not share their HIV status with at-risk intimate partners. An estimated 27% of HIV-infected persons are unaware of their HIV status (CDC, 2006o).

Because AIDS-related care is long term and extensive, the cost of treatment is high. The lifetime costs of treatment for one person with HIV or AIDS is now more than $155,000 (CDC, 2007f). Although no cure for AIDS is available, recently established drug protocols have increased the time people survive with the disease, which has also increased the cost of care. HIV infection was the second leading cause of death among persons aged 25 to 44 years in 1995 but had dropped to the sixth cause of death by 2003 (Nelson et al., 2007; USDHHS, 2006a). HIV/AIDS remains the leading cause of death for African Americans in this age group.

HIV prevention efforts and the widespread use of antiretroviral therapies have had an impact on the progression of HIV infection to AIDS. Starting in 1996, the incidence of AIDS began to decline. At the same time, the prevalence or number of people living with AIDS increased because of more effective treatment.

Because AIDS is a disease that weakens the individual's body defense system, people with AIDS experience many different symptoms or conditions. For diagnostic purposes, the CDC has developed a listing of conditions that are diagnostic of AIDS. This list is found in **Website Resource 8A.** A significant number of communicable diseases are among these, including candidiasis, herpes infection, TB, and pneumonia. The diagnostic categories for AIDS are similar for children but include conditions commonly seen in HIV-infected children (CDC, 1994a).

The groups at special risk for acquiring HIV infection are similar to those at risk for HBV infection. Most diagnosed AIDS clients are men (71%) and homosexual or bisexual (60%). Table 8-2 indicates that the growth in newly diagnosed AIDS cases is occurring among heterosexual and intravenous drug–using women, heterosexual men, and men who engage in sexual activity with other men. Since 1991, there has been an 80% decline in perinatally acquired HIV/AIDS. Only 57

TABLE 8-2   Estimated New Cases* of HIV/AIDS among Persons Aged 13 Years or Older by Sex and Exposure Category, 2004

Exposure Category	2004 Number	2004 Percentage	Percentage Change from 2001-2005
Men			
MSM[1]	68,434	60	+15
IDU[2]	17,540	16	−2 (same)
MSM-IDU	5723	5	−1
Heterosexual	19,209	16	+9
Other**	705	.06	−.04
Total	112,106	70	−5
Women			
IDU	9665	21	+13
Heterosexual	34,204	71	+59
Other**	746	1.6	+.6
Total	45,146	30	+8
Overall Total	157,252	100	

Adapted from *Morbidity & Mortality Weekly Reprt, 46*(37), 863-870; Centers for Disease Control and Prevention. (2001). *HIV/AIDS Surveillance Report, 13*(2), 37. *Morbidity & Mortality Weekly Report*, 2006, 55(05) 121-125. Racial/Ethnic disparities in Dignoses of HIV/AIDS 33 Statos, 2001–2004.

*Estimates are presented rounded to the nearest 10 because they do not represent exact counts of persons with AIDS by exposure category but are estimates that are approximately 1 ± 3% of the true value.

**Risk not reported or identified.

[1]Men who have sex with men.

[2]Injecting drug users.

babies were born HIV positive in 2003 (USDHHS 2006b). The decline in HIV-positive babies is attributed to the successful attempt to identify potentially infected pregnant women and the use of antiretroviral mediations to reduce perinatal transmission. Adolescent AIDS cases doubled between 1988 and 1995. African Americans and Hispanics are at eight to nine times greater risk than whites and other racial and ethnic groups. AIDS prevention strategies must be geared toward all who engage in risky behaviors, because an effective vaccine is not available.

A long time delay exists between HIV infection and the development of AIDS; in fact, the average latency period is 10 years (Webber, 2005). Because of this time delay, aggregates among the more recently determined high-risk groups are often unaware of or dismiss their danger, for example, sexually active adolescents and homosexual men. After years of steadily decreasing numbers, a second-wave epidemic is emerging among young men who engage in homosexual activity (CDC, 2006p). Because many of their compatriots do not have noticeable symptoms, ignoring the problem is easy for both adolescents and young homosexual men. These new cases of HIV-positive individuals will result in an increasing number of AIDS cases in these groups as late as 10 to 15 years from now. Public education campaigns should be directed toward increasing awareness in these risk groups.

Timely access to care is important. Many HIV-infected persons are not identified until they are diagnosed with AIDS. To ensure that HIV-infected persons benefit from the latest antiretroviral treatment, early diagnosis is crucial. HIV counseling and testing programs in health care settings must improve the process of identifying of persons at risk as well as counseling and screening efforts. People frequently have a number of STDs at the same time. For example, approximately 20% to 50% of men and women identified as HIV positive are coinfected with either chlamydia or gonorrhea (Steiner et al., 2003). Screening for other STDs should be part of the protocol for any screening programs.

NEWLY EMERGING AND REEMERGING DISEASES

A significant number of health problems have raised public concern in recent years. Some of these are newly emerging illnesses and some are preexisting problems that surge in incidence from time to time. A few examples are given in the following sections.

Norwalk-like Virus Infection

Periodic outbreaks of gastroenteritis caused by Norwalk-like viruses (NLVs) or Noroviruses have occurred over the years. The latest outbreaks have occurred on cruise ships and in other areas (Figure 8-2). These viruses are transmitted through contaminated food and water and account for the vast majority of cases of nonbacterial gastroenteritis (CDC, 2006q). NLVs are highly infectious. In addition to the usual **sources of contamination** (vehicles of transmission), in epidemic situations person-to-person contact, droplets, and contaminated environmental objects such as doorknobs, utensils, and bed linens can transmit the viruses.

Control of NLV is a two-part process. Primary prevention efforts reduce the risk of initial contamination by ensuring safe food and water (see page 227). Preventing subsequent

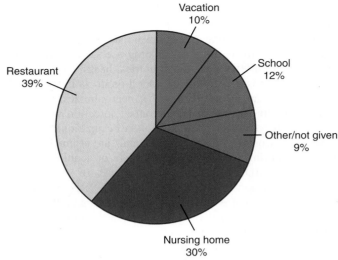

FIGURE 8-2 Settings for 348 outbreaks of Norwalk-like viruses reported to the Centers for Disease Control and Prevention (CDC), 1996 to 2000. (Data from CDC. [2001]. Norwalk-like viruses: Public health consequences and outbreak management. *Morbidity and Mortality Weekly Report, Recommendations and Reports, 50*[RR-9], 18.)

person-to-person transmission of NLV via fecal-oral and airborne routes, especially in institutional settings, is important. Prevention requires frequent hand washing with soap and water, use of masks by personnel who clean contaminated areas, careful handling of bed linens, and cleaning of surfaces with a germicidal product (e.g., 10% household bleach). Cruise ships or camps may be shut down to be cleaned.

Nancy A. is a nurse who is assigned to do communicable disease investigation at the CDC in Atlanta. In October, Nancy and other team members were assigned to investigate an outbreak of acute gastroenteritis (AGE) on a cruise ship. The ship was on a 7-day cruise of the Caribbean, with 2318 passengers and 988 crew members. The ship returned to port, and the CDC team proceeded to board and investigate the problem.

The team used personal interviews and written questionnaires to gather information. They found that, during the voyage, 2% of the crew and 260 (12%) of the passengers reported illness to the ship health personnel. The questionnaire that was distributed revealed that 21% of the crew and passengers met the criteria for AGE. Fecal samples demonstrated the presence of Norovirus. The team recommended, and ship personnel completed, a thorough cleaning and disinfecting before new passengers were allowed to board.

The ship sailed the same day after the cleaning effort. New cases of AGE emerged among the second set of passengers and crew. The ship returned to port early. The CDC team recommended a more aggressive cleaning and sanitation strategy. This work was completed in 1 week. The ship was cleared to resume cruises. No new cases of AGE emerged on the subsequent cruise (CDC, 2002b).

Hantavirus Pulmonary Syndrome: A New Infection

Hantavirus produces Hantavirus pulmonary syndrome. Approximately 438 cases in 32 states have been reported since the virus was first identified in 1993. The significant fatality rate (30% to 40%) is the reason for public health concern (CDC, 2006r). Death is the result of noncardiogenic pulmonary edema and cardiovascular collapse. Infection occurs through exposure to aerosol secretions and excretions from one specific rodent species confined to the American continents (Figure 8-3). Persons living in close contact with rodent byproducts are at greatest risk. Most cases of Hantavirus are among poor individuals, many living in dirt-floor homes, and among ardent backpackers. A nurse was responsible for making the connection between the presence of rodents and the risk of becoming infected with Hantavirus during epidemiologic investigations on Southwestern Native American reservations.

Lyme Disease

Lyme disease is the most common vector-borne disease in the United States. The **vector** (carrier of infection) is a tick infested with a spirochete. The infected ticks are carried by deer and rodents. Between 1991 and 2005 the number of cases of Lyme disease doubled. In 2005, 23,395 cases of Lyme disease were reported (Figure 8-4). Efforts to prevent Lyme disease emphasize the following (CDC, 2002c):

- Reduction of the tick population
- Avoidance of tick-infested habitats
- Use of insect repellents
- Prompt removal of attached ticks

A vaccine, LYMErix, was licensed in 1998 but was removed from the market in February 2002. Insect control remains the primary method of controlling Lyme disease.

West Nile Virus Infection

West Nile virus (WNV) has become an increasing problem in the United States, spreading over a wide geographic area and infecting more people each year. By 2002, WNV was considered an epidemic. Because of this, the CDC provides surveillance, even though WNV is not on the list of diseases for which reporting is mandatory.

WNV is a vector-borne virus spread by infected mosquitoes. The virus has been found in wild birds, chickens, horses, dogs, and squirrels, as well as humans. During 2006, 3830 human

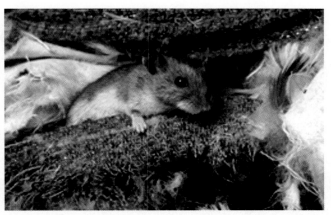

FIGURE 8-3 Deer mouse nesting in furniture, a source of the Hantavirus. (Retrieved from http://www.cdc.gov/ncidod/hanta/hps/noframes/infstprx/infprx2.htm.)

cases were reported (CDC, 2006s). WNV started in 1999 in the New England area and by 2006 had spread to all but two states (Figure 8-5). WNV infection is serious because 35% of people with the infection develop meningoencephalitis. Public health surveillance of the number of dead birds and an aggressive mosquito-control program are the primary methods used to reduce risk to the population.

Avian Influenza

Since 2003 there have been numerous outbreaks of avian flu among poultry in many Asian countries (CDC, 2006t). Cross-species transmission of the virus has occurred. In 2004, 17 people in Thailand developed influenza after exposure to infected poultry. Although few people have been infected with avian flu, it is of concern because of its potential to affect large populations. This strain is closely related to the influenza virus responsible for the epidemic that killed millions of people during World War I (Kay, 2005). As a result, the WHO, CDC, and health

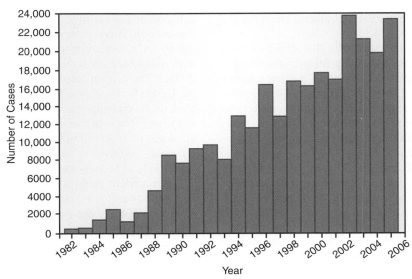

FIGURE 8-4 Numbers of cases of Lyme disease, by year—United States, 1982 to 2005. (Redrawn from Centers for Disease Control and Prevention [CDC]. [2002]. Lyme disease—United States, 2000. *Morbidity and Mortality Weekly Report, 51*[2], 29-31; and CDC [2003, 2004, 2005, 2006, 2007]. Summary of notifiable diseases—United States [selected years]. *Morbidity and Mortality Weekly Report, 50*[53], 1-108; *51*[53], 1-84; *52*[54], 1-85; *53*[53], 1-79; *54*[53], 2-92.)

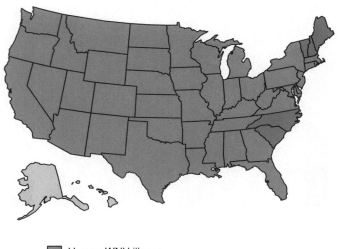

Human WNV illness
Nonhuman WNV infection only
No WNV virus

FIGURE 8-5 Areas reporting West Nile virus (WNV) activity—United States, 2006. (Redrawn from Centers for Disease Control and Prevention. [2006]. West Nile virus activity—United States, January 1-November 7, 2006. *Morbidity and Mortality Weekly Report, 55*[44], 1204-1205.)

departments in many countries employ vigilant surveillance to control infected poultry and prevent the spread to humans. There have been no cases of avian flu in the United States.

INFLUENCES OF MODERN LIFESTYLE AND TECHNOLOGY

Some current trends in communicable diseases can be attributed to modernization and new technology. Industrialization and the crowding of a large number of people into the relatively small space of a city provide fertile ground for an increase in certain diseases. Crowding threatens sanitary and other environmental conditions. In hard economic times, more families are forced to move in with relatives, which produces more crowded conditions, or they move to housing that is affordable but frequently less safe, with environmental hazards and more crime.

Daycare arrangements and facilities for children have increased as rising numbers of mothers (or primary caregivers) enter the workforce. Between 8 and 11 million children are now in daycare (CDC, 1994b; U.S. Bureau of the Census, 2005). These children are at greater risk of enteric infections (hepatitis A, cryptosporidiosis), respiratory tract infections, and middle ear infections. Infected children, in turn, are infecting other household members.

The greater mobility of individuals and groups has facilitated the transmission of diseases that would not otherwise cross natural boundaries, such as oceans or mountains. Each year, more and more people travel between countries. The spread of HIV infection can be traced to international and intracountry travel. For example, within Africa, cases of HIV infection are heavily concentrated along travel routes (rivers and roads) from one country to another. HIV infection has also been traced to transoceanic travel as travelers infected elsewhere return to their home countries. The spread of the SARS epidemic is another example.

In February 2003, China notified the WHO that a SARS of unknown origin was present in six different regions in the country, having started in approximately November 2002. In February 2003, a man who had traveled to China was hospitalized in Vietnam with similar symptoms. Health care providers at the Vietnam hospital also developed the same illness. The man initially treated in Vietnam was transferred to a hospital in Hong Kong, where he died. By that time, Hong Kong had a cluster of similar cases linked to another traveler to China. By mid-March 2003, the WHO had reports of 264 individuals from 11 countries with suspected or probable SARS (CDC, 2003c). By mid-June 2003 a total of 8465 SARS cases were identified in 29 countries, with a 9.5% mortality rate.

Examples of traveler-related illness episodes in the United States include 75 cases of SARS in 2003, cholera in California, a new form of leishmaniasis among troops returning from the Persian Gulf conflict, and 96 cases of dengue fever in 2005 (CDC, 1994b, 2003d, 2006u). Thirty-six percent of the cases of measles in the United States are brought in from other countries (CDC, 2006a). Almost all cases of malaria (1190 in 2004) have been brought in from Africa, Asia, and Central America (CDC, 2006v). Plague in New York City, pertussis in North Carolina, and yellow fever in Texas are other examples of diseases brought in from abroad (CDC, 2002e, 2002d, 2003e).

World commerce increases the possibility of transporting infected products from one country to another. The live-animal market has been a source of infection and is the reason many countries have strict animal quarantine standards. Even so, monkeys, reptiles, and birds shipped between countries have been identified as sources of illness. Monkeypox outbreaks in the United States have been traced to U.S.-raised prairie dogs and Gambian giant rats imported from Ghana via Texas (CDC, 2003f). All of the infected animals eventually ended up with a single distributor in Illinois.

Several disease outbreaks have been associated with food shipments. The United States has strict guidelines for food shipped into this country, but lapses and outright disregard of these standards occur. For example, an outbreak of hepatitis A in Michigan was traced to improper processing of imported Mexican strawberries by a California importer (CDC, 1997d). Raw meat infected with roundworms was the source of recent trichinellosis (CDC, 2003g). The contaminated meat products were manufactured in the United States, Egypt, Vietnam, and Yugoslavia. In 2007, pet food ingredients imported from China were linked to the death and severe illness of many household pets, and the United States Food and Drug Administration issued a warning about potential poisonous additives in toothpaste imported from China (China rejects U.S. alert on toothpaste, 2007).

Even modern medical interventions increase the possibility of rapidly transmitting communicable diseases. Hickman catheters threaded into the jugular vein to provide easy access for drug administration and diagnostic procedures, central venous pressure catheters, and other intravenous lines provide a route for infectious organisms. Intubation devices, intracranial pressure monitors, and respiratory nebulizers are all sources of **nosocomial infections.** Nosocomial infections may account for 15% of hospital deaths (that is, deaths from infections acquired in the hospital).

One new disease, legionellosis, is reported under the National Notifiable Disease Surveillance System (NNDSS). Legionellosis flourishes as a result of new technology, with the causative organism thriving in damp, moist areas such as heating and air conditioning ventilation systems. Legionellosis was first identified during an epidemiologic investigation of an outbreak of illness among veterans attending an American Legion Convention in the early 1980s. Periodic outbreaks have occurred ever since, although careful maintenance of ventilation systems reduces the probability of infection.

ISSUES OF POPULATION SAFETY VERSUS INDIVIDUAL RIGHTS

Throughout history, governments and public health officials have struggled with the problem of balancing individual rights with the right of the community to be protected from infection. As a general rule, the safety of populations has taken precedence over individual rights. To reduce the risk of exposure in populations, individual rights have been curtailed or revoked. For example:

- Lepers were forced to wear bells to warn others of their passing or were quarantined in separate communities.
- Cities required individuals to dispose of their sewage in approved privies.
- People who polluted water sources were imprisoned.
- Plague victims were isolated in their homes or removed to central infected houses.
- During epidemics, the names of infected individuals were published.

Similar strategies were used in other epidemics, including the measles epidemics early in the twentieth century. Failure to comply with regulations was punishable by civil penalties such as fines or by more drastic measures such as imprisonment or execution (Risse, 1988). For example:

- During World War I, prostitutes were confined in central locations and treated to reduce the spread of venereal disease epidemics.
- The first widespread immunization program mandated that children be vaccinated against typhoid (Risse, 1988).
- In the 1914 and 1919 polio epidemics, physicians and nurses made house-to-house searches to identify all infected persons. Infected children were removed to hospitals, and the remaining family members were quarantined until they became noninfectious. Parents were unable to leave their homes to bury their child if the child died in the hospital.

Today the issue of individual rights versus community protection is an ongoing concern. Workplace safety is one important issue. Carriers of hepatitis A are restricted from certain jobs, such as food handling. The CDC recommends that HIV-infected health care workers be selectively assigned to duties so as not to place other health care workers or clients at risk. The CDC recommends that persons at risk for HIV infection not give blood and that they change risky sexual and intravenous drug practices. This issue is especially pertinent today in light of the potential use of infectious disease agents as bioweapons (see Chapter 22).

An important area in which individual rights clash with public safety involves the right of people to continue to knowingly place others at risk. Two salient contemporary examples of this problem are the following:

- What should be done with a client with TB who refuses to follow the treatment regimen?
- What should be done with an HIV-infected individual who continues to share needles or engage in unprotected sex after diagnosis?

Many states have laws to enforce treatment or isolation of persons with known communicable diseases. Most public health practitioners prefer to enroll the client in the treatment regimen by using education, encouragement, and careful monitoring of compliance. If these measures fail, however, individuals may be restrained in hospitals or institutions for a course of therapy until they can no longer infect others and the disease is contained (see the *Ethics in Practice* box).

The problem of HIV-infected persons who continue risky behaviors is more difficult. How would one go about monitoring what people are doing in their private lives? Should one even try? Health care workers have been struggling with this dilemma for quite some time. HIV/AIDS has no cure. If one were to confine these clients, for how long would one do so? For life? At the present time, only a few AIDS clients have been confined against their will because of their refusal to protect others against infection. In some cases, individuals with HIV infection or AIDS have been criminally prosecuted for knowingly placing others at risk, either through unprotected sex or deliberate injury such as biting or scratching.

Many individuals in the public health sector have argued for some time that HIV/AIDS should not be singled out for special treatment and that public health supersedes the individual's right of privacy. Several states have begun screening newborns for HIV infection without the specific permission of their mothers. The PHS revised its guidelines to recommend the voluntary screening of all pregnant women (CDC, 2001b). In 1997 the Council of State and Territorial Epidemiologists recommended that all states require health care providers and laboratories to report HIV cases by name to enable standard public health follow-up and contact investigations. The Association of State and Territorial Health Officers has endorsed these recommendations and has developed an HIV/AIDS surveillance policy in consultation with the CDC (CDC, 1997e).

ROLE OF THE NURSE IN COMMUNICABLE DISEASE CONTROL

Historically, nursing has been an integral part of disease control. Individuals with communicable diseases have always needed reliable nursing care. Initially, nursing was provided by members of religious orders, who were often the only help available during epidemics. In 1883, communicable disease nursing was based primarily on the premise of preventing the spread of disease through cleanliness and fresh air. Aronson (1978, p. 15) recalls the safety precautions for nurses making home visits:

> Before leaving the client's house, the nurse was required to wash her hands with carbolic soap and rinse her mouth with a fresh potassium permanganate solution. It was very important for the nurse ... to do the disinfection because ... people were very slow to learn.

In addition to caring for the sick, teaching hygiene to families was a major responsibility of community nurses and is still a primary focus in the current control of communicable diseases today.

ETHICS IN PRACTICE

Tension between Individual and Societal Rights

Gail A. DeLuca Havens, PhD, RN

Codes of ethics can be thought of as moral codes. Moral commitments "to adhere to the ideals and moral norms of the profession," such as maintaining competency in practice, are expressed in the American Nurses Association (ANA) *Code of Ethics for Nurses* (2001, p. 5) and are made by individuals when they become nurses. The fundamental concept underlying the *Code of Ethics for Nurses* is respect for persons. Certain principles growing out of this concept guide nurses' decision making. These include fostering self-determination, doing good, avoiding harm, being truthful, respecting privileged information, keeping promises, and treating people fairly. In their moral decision-making hierarchy, Beauchamp and Childress (2001) refer to principles and rules as action guides. Principles are the more global and basic conceptions that justify the rules.

When ethical principles are being considered, it is important to remember that individuals are *interdependent* members of a community. The nurse will encounter situations in which the tension between individual liberty and the need to preserve the health and well-being of the community creates an ethical dilemma in practice. For instance, the nurse promises, as expressed by the principle of fidelity in the ANA *Code,* to maintain client confidentiality. However, such a promise is not absolute when innocent parties are in direct jeopardy (e.g., threatened with being killed) (ANA, 2001). This particular kind of dilemma is made even more troublesome for the nurse who is attempting to deal with two opposing or contradictory promises. For example, the implicit promise of the nurse to maintain client confidentiality, as expressed in the ANA *Code,* may contradict the nurse's obligation to obey a law that requires reporting a particular situation (ANA, 2001). The nurse also has an ethical responsibility to respect the client and promote self-determination. Consider the following situation.

Kay is a community health nurse who has been employed by a home health agency for more than 10 years. Several of her clients live in a homeless shelter and have been referred to her agency for follow-up tuberculosis treatment after hospital discharge. Today she is making her first visit to Paolo, a 33-year-old Hispanic man discharged after treatment in the hospital for acute, infectious tuberculosis. Kay explains that her agency, along with the city's health department, helps persons with tuberculosis continue to take their medication as prescribed until they are cured. Kay asks Paolo how he is feeling this morning. He replies that he is tired; he did not sleep well this first night in a place not familiar to him. After she completes Paolo's admission history and physical examination, Kay tells him that she, or a nurse substituting for her, will be visiting Paolo daily for 2 weeks to observe him taking his medication and then twice weekly for at least 6 months. Paolo protests that he is not a child and that he can be depended on to take his medication as prescribed. Kay explains that the current standard of care is that everyone in the community being treated for tuberculosis receive directly observed medication therapy. It will help him remember to continue to take medication as prescribed, particularly when he begins to feel better. Stopping the medication makes the treatment he received in the hospital ineffective. When medication is stopped, often the tuberculosis becomes infectious again. In addition, not completing treatment increases the likelihood that he will develop a

type of tuberculosis that is resistant to medication therapy (Centers for Disease Control and Prevention [CDC], 2003a). He could be very ill again. The city has an obligation to protect its residents from becoming infected with tuberculosis. Kay tells Paolo that she will be communicating with health department personnel because they are the ones who referred him to her.

Paolo agrees, reluctantly, to cooperate in therapy. He asks how long it will take to be cured. Kay knows that the response to therapy varies, but most persons can be cured within 9 months (CDC, 2003b). Kay explains that 6 months of medication has been prescribed to cure his tuberculosis. Before Kay leaves, Paolo takes his first dose of medication, and they establish a schedule for his observed daily self-administration. Paolo's treatment continues as planned over the next several months. He gains strength and eventually finds a job. Returning to work requires that his medication regimen be modified. Paolo has no trouble adapting it to his more demanding schedule. Several weeks pass with this new arrangement until, one evening, Paolo does not appear. Kay leaves a message for him to call her, but does not hear from him. When Paolo fails to appear again the following evening, Kay returns to the shelter. Eventually, Kay learns that Paolo has not been complying with his prescribed medication regimen. He does not deny it and tells Kay that, because he has been taking medication for more than 3 months and feels better, he believes that he is cured of his tuberculosis and no longer needs therapy.

How should Kay respond? Should she respect Paolo's right to self-determination by not interfering with the decisions he has made? What if Paolo were to be harmed by this noninterference? What if others were to be harmed? Does Kay's obligation to Paolo to maintain confidentiality remain even when his behavior might compromise the health and well-being of others? Under what circumstances might a nurse place the health and well-being of members of a community before those of an individual client?

In this situation, because Paolo is an adult who is responsible for his own health, Kay could simply disregard the fact that Paolo has not been adhering to his prescribed medication regimen. However, she would not be helping Paolo to protect himself or others. Another strategy that Kay might employ would be to engage Paolo in problem solving to further explore his reasons for not complying with the medication regimen. Uncovering reasons for noncompliance often results in identifying ways to avoid it. One of the strategies recommended for directly observed therapy is for the nurse to adopt a nonjudgmental attitude toward clients, acknowledging that individuals often will not be 100% compliant with medication regimens. Kay could acknowledge that, because Paolo is feeling better, it is understandable that he is not taking his medication as prescribed. However, she also ought to remind him that he places himself at great risk for getting very sick again and developing drug-resistant tuberculosis by not following his medication regimen. This course of action might also be an opportunity to foster Paolo's self-determination, to maintain the confidential nature of his care, and to strengthen the client–nurse relationship.

However, adopting this strategy does jeopardize Paolo's health and the health of the people with whom Paolo comes in contact.

Kay does not know whether Paolo's tuberculosis is infectious. Kay initiates tuberculosis screening for the people with whom Paolo has been in contact and creates an opportunity for Paolo to have his tuberculosis reevaluated. This action ought to diminish the potential for harm from active tuberculosis to Paolo and to others with whom he has been in contact. Because Kay's authority has been delegated to her by the health department, she can communicate with the health department without legally violating confidentiality. Kay is aware that many states require quarantine of individuals who do not successfully complete a medication regimen for tuberculosis. To protect the public, a community health nurse can recommend that formal action be taken to ensure that a person complies with treatment. In this instance, quarantine means that individuals can be hospitalized or incarcerated for treatment of tuberculosis against their will.

As a third strategy, Kay can follow the established protocol to initiate quarantine, reporting Paolo's lack of compliance with medication therapy to the appropriate people. However, this breaches the confidential nature of the client-nurse relationship and compromises the trust and mutual respect that have been established between Paolo and Kay. The ANA *Code* (2001) alerts nurses to the reality of suspending individual rights but warns that this ought to "be consid-

ered a serious deviation from the standard of care" (p. 9). Usually a nurse does not select the third alternative until the second alternative has proven ineffective. How might Paolo be affected by this experience? How might Kay be affected by this experience? Which alternative would you choose?

REFERENCES

American Nurses Association. (2001). *Code of ethics for nurses with interpretive statements*. Washington, DC: Author.

Beauchamp, T. L., & Childress, J. F. (2001). *Principles of biomedical ethics* (5th ed.). New York: Oxford University Press.

Centers for Disease Control and Prevention. (2003a, June 20). Treatment of tuberculosis: American Thoracic Society, CDC, and Infectious Disease Society of America. *Morbidity and Mortality Weekly Report, Recommendations and Reports, 52*(RR-11), 1-80. Retrieved May 22, 2007, from *http://www.cdc.gov/mmwr/PDF/rr/rr5211.pdf*.

Centers for Disease Control and Prevention. (2003b). *Treatment of drug-susceptible tuberculosis disease in persons not infected with HIV* [Fact sheet]. Retrieved May 22, 2007, from *http://www.cdc.gov/tb/pubs/tbfactsheets/treatmentHIVnegative.htm*.

Nurses have developed a new specialty—infection control. Most of the time, infection control nurses are employed in hospitals or in large institutional settings. These nurses are concerned primarily with protecting staff and clients from communicable and infectious organisms by developing and monitoring infectious control practices and educating staff and clients.

Community health nurses play a major role in contact investigation for reportable communicable diseases. Sometimes other health personnel may also be engaged in contact investigation. Community health nurses interview infected persons to help identify contacts placed at risk by exposure to infected individuals. Community nurses also perform home visits to monitor persons under treatment and ensure compliance with the accepted treatment protocol (e.g., the TB observed therapy strategy). Nurses employed in special settings may also engage in epidemiologic investigations of new diseases or outbreaks of recognized illnesses, for example, Hantavirus disease in the Southwest and food poisoning outbreaks such as a *Salmonella*-caused episode in four states that resulted from the consumption of unpasteurized milk. Chapter 7 provides additional information about epidemiologic investigation.

Bridget Smith, a nurse with the Ohio Department of Health, was assigned to a team investigating the suspected food poisoning and hospitalization of two children. The children were diagnosed with *Salmonella enterica* infection. The cause was suspected to be raw (unpasteurized) milk. The milk came from a popular dairy and restaurant. During the next 45 days, the health department received reports on 94 other potential cases. As the number of potential cases increased, the department issued a regional public health alert. The health team performed case finding by screening the dairy workers, interviewing customers of the restaurant, and obtaining specimens (food and stool) for analysis. The team verified that a total of 62 people had illness consistent with *Salmonella* infection (40 customers and family members and 16 dairy workers).

Testing of the food samples uncovered *Salmonella* in the raw milk, cream, and butter purchased by customers. Four barn workers had positive test results. The barn workers milked the cows, bottled the milk, and made ice cream. The health department reviewed the findings and ordered the dairy to cease selling raw milk products. The team recommended that dairy workers increase their hand washing, replace some of their equipment and utensils, and improve the cleaning procedure in the dairy. No additional cases of *Salmonella* infection appeared (CDC, 2003h).

EPIDEMIOLOGY APPLIED TO COMMUNICABLE DISEASE CONTROL

Epidemiology began as the study of communicable diseases affecting large populations (see Chapter 7). Although the scope of epidemiology has expanded to include noncommunicable diseases and other health-related issues, epidemiologic principles are still the backbone of communicable disease control.

EPIDEMIOLOGIC PRINCIPLES AND METHODS

Preventing communicable diseases begins with knowledge about the links in the chain of infection. The relationships and interactions among the infectious **agent** (causative microorganism), the **host** (human or animal incubating the agent), and the environment—that is, the components of the epidemiologic triangle—are important. Communicable disease control depends on discovering the weak link in the triangle and developing measures that attack and reduce or eliminate that threat. Control efforts include prevention activities and efforts to reduce the seriousness of an illness as measured by the severity, the length of illness, the cost of treatment, the short- and long-term effects, and the risk of death.

COMMUNICABLE DISEASE INVESTIGATION

In accordance with epidemiologic principles, communicable disease investigation involves five steps: identifying the disease, isolating the causative agent, determining the method of transmission, establishing the susceptibility of the populations at risk, and estimating the impact on the population. With this knowledge, public health officials can plan an effective intervention program. The community health nurse contributes to the investigation effort at every level. The nurse in direct client care may be the first to identify the onset of a communicable disease, to determine new victims and their relationship to known victims (contact cases), and to discover patterns in the spread of the communicable disease. The role of the community health nurse has broadened beyond direct care. Nurses are currently involved with other health care professionals in population-focused investigation and intervention program design.

CAUSATIVE AGENT

Factors associated with the agents causing infectious diseases include pathogenicity, infective dose, physical characteristics, organism specificity, and antigenic variations. **Pathogenicity,** or seriousness, encompasses **invasiveness** and **virulence,** terms used to assess the strength of the agent in victims. Highly virulent (stronger) organisms cause greater morbidity and mortality. For example, some influenza viruses are more virulent than others. Although influenza A and B are similar, the symptoms of influenza A are usually more severe, last longer, and require more frequent hospitalization than the symptoms of influenza B (Bridges et al., 2003). The degree of invasiveness (spread) is important, because highly invasive organisms have an opportunity to affect more body systems. For example, the bacterium causing gonorrhea is usually confined to the genitourinary region. However, the spirochete that causes syphilis invades many different tissues, including the brain, which results in more diverse symptoms.

The amount of agent needed to produce illness **(infective dose)** varies. Some agents are highly infectious; others are less so. For example, a disease such as chickenpox is highly infectious. Many people become infected even when exposed to relatively small amounts of chickenpox virus. Agents that are less infectious, such as TB, require host exposure to larger numbers of TB bacilli for longer periods for transmission of disease.

Transmission ability is also influenced by the agent's host requirements (agent specificity) and its ability to vary its genetic structure (mutate). Some agents are highly particular about hosts. For example, the smallpox virus can infect only humans. Agents that are limited in the hosts they can infect are considered highly specific.

The ability of some agents to alter their genetic structure also poses problems for control efforts, because the **resistance** (ability to resist a medication) of different strains may make treatment less effective. For example, many variants of the organism causing gonorrhea are resistant to penicillin. In recent years, *Staphylococcus aureus* infection has become difficult to treat because some strains are resistant to methicillin and other drugs (CDC, 2006h, 2006i).

MEANS OF TRANSMISSION

The frequency of transmission of an infectious disease depends on the opportunities present for organism transport from its source to a new host. Transmission can occur through direct or indirect contact (Figure 8-6). Direct contact includes physical contact with an infected individual, animal, or other carrier, or with large droplets (greater than 5 μm) that travel very short distances (less than 1 m). Indirect contact involves passive transmission by something other than the source, usually an object that has been in direct contact with the source (e.g., contaminated water, air, dust, dressings, instruments, body secretions, small droplets traveling longer distances, vectors). For example, *Salmonella* bacteria can be transmitted directly (through person-to-person contact by the oral-fecal route) or indirectly (by way of food contaminated with infected feces). Knowledge about transmission methods allows community health nurses to reduce the risk of transmission to communities through health education and assurance of good aseptic technique.

CHARACTERISTICS OF THE HOST

Individuals possess defense mechanisms to combat or impede transmission of communicable disease agents. These defense mechanisms include tears, skin, mucus, saliva, and the cilia (hairs) in the nose. Nose hair, for example, traps organisms transmitted by breathing and reduces an agent's chance of reaching a vulnerable body site. Even when defense mechanisms are compromised, health care professionals can assist in reducing the chance of infection. For example, *Staphylococcus* bacteria enter the body through a break in the skin barrier. Even when a wound breaks the skin barrier, good aseptic technique will reduce the risk of staphylococcal infection.

Immunity, either natural or artificially created, is another host characteristic useful in combating communicable disease. The immune system can halt symptoms by stopping the infection process before symptoms develop. Immunity is one example of primary prevention. **Natural immunity** occurs when the individual has been infected with the disease and develops immunity because of the body's antigen-antibody response to the infection. Before the advent of vaccines, mothers deliberately exposed their children to others with mumps or measles, purposely infecting them, because it was widely believed at the time that the illness would be less serious in young children than in those infected as adolescents or adults.

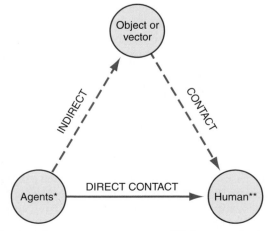

*Number of agents
Characteristics of agents
Pathogenicity

**Defense mechanisms
Immunity
Personal characteristics

FIGURE 8-6 Transmission of communicable disease.

Artificial immunity is developed through vaccination rather than through exposure to a communicable disease. Artificial immunity can be active or passive. Active immunity is a result of vaccination with live, killed, or attenuated organisms or a toxoid of the agent. Live vaccines usually produce immunity that lasts for long periods but may not be advisable for certain individuals. For example, pregnant women and immunocompromised individuals should not be vaccinated with live antigen (e.g., polio vaccine). With the shorter-acting vaccines using toxoid or attenuated, absorbed, and killed toxins (e.g., tetanus toxoid), boosters are needed to keep antibody levels high enough to be effective. Most people can use these vaccines.

Passive immunity can also be used to prevent infection. This type of immunity is derived from either antitoxins or antibodies (immunoglobulins), such as those transmitted from a mother to a fetus. This immunization is temporary and will have to be repeated with each exposure. Immunoglobulin should not be given with live vaccines of measles, mumps, or rubella because the expected antibody response is decreased when the two are given together.

ENVIRONMENT

Altering the environment to reduce conditions that favor the spread of infectious agents is a very effective means of communicable disease control. Temperature, humidity, radiation, pressure, and ventilation can all be used to decrease the transmission of infectious diseases. For example, organisms that thrive in heat can be exposed to cold, those that grow best in humidity can be controlled in a climate with little humidity, and so on.

Crowding, famine, and the mobility of people increase the possibility of spreading infections. Crowding is a problem because it provides agents with many potential victims rather than only a few. In a famine, humans are weakened by poor nutrition and other health problems and are less able to resist an infectious disease. A starving population has many more susceptible hosts than would be the case with a well-nourished population. Finally, mobility increases the likelihood that agents are carried to other environments. The most obvious way to combat such a spread is quarantine. Countries routinely close borders when threatened by severe communicable diseases. During the 1950s, the primary method of reducing the spread of polio was home quarantine. SARS is a recent example of an infectious disease leading to a closed-border quarantine.

AGENT-HOST-ENVIRONMENT AND FAVORABLE CONDITIONS

A basic knowledge of the impact of environment, host, agent, and the interrelated features in disease transmission is essential for community health nurses. Nurses must have the skill to assess households and communities for favorable environments, susceptible hosts, and likelihood of viable agents. In addition, nurses must have the expertise to advise families and communities regarding the strategies necessary to make the environment less habitable, reduce host susceptibility, and reduce or eliminate the agent source. In some instances, interventions can be directed at only one factor; in others, all three may be altered to improve community resistance to infection. For example, needles contaminated with HIV-infected blood can transmit HIV. A weak bleach solution will

kill the virus, altering the environment and reducing the risk to a potential host (Figure 8-7). HIV can also be transmitted by sexual contact with an HIV-infected person. Using barrier method precautions during sexual contact (dental dam, condoms, or nonoxynol-9 spermicidal jelly) will contain or kill the virus. Diseases that are spread through contaminated water or food are controlled by boiling or treating the water (chlorination) and by storing, preparing, and serving foods using sanitary techniques. For example, meats, poultry, vegetables, and fruits are inspected for infestation and approved for use only when they are free from contaminants and safe for human consumption.

TRENDS IN COMMUNICABLE DISEASE

The study of diseases over time provides valuable information for public health planners. Trends are studied so that community health needs can be anticipated and intervention strategies preplanned. Trends are also useful in examining the impact of intervention programs. If programs are effective and efficient, they can be used again and again with modifications that consider physical, psychologic, sociologic, and economic changes in the population. Variations in disease frequency can be examined to identify regular trends and episodic occurrences (Merrill & Timmreck, 2006). Regular trends include expected seasonal and yearly variations. For example, hay fever occurs during the fall and spring seasons, and upper respiratory tract infections are common in the winter. An episodic occurrence is a sudden change in the rate of transmission or an epidemic. For example, a large number of community residents may suddenly contract food poisoning, or a countrywide measles epidemic may occur.

Trends can also be observed over longer periods. At the beginning of this chapter, a historic review provided evidence of change in the characteristics, spread, and treatment of communicable diseases over centuries. A more detailed examination of U.S. data shows a clear picture of communicable disease trends since the 1950s (see Table 8-1). As public health measures become more effective in controlling certain communicable diseases, other diseases, new diseases, or mutant strains of known diseases become more prominent.

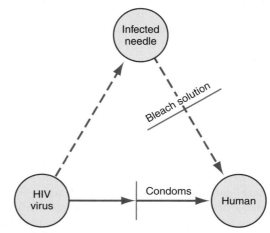

FIGURE 8-7 Breaking the chain of infection in human immunodeficiency virus infection (HIV) and acquired immunodeficiency syndrome.

RESEARCH AND RESEARCH ORGANIZATIONS

The first methodic studies of communicable disease were conducted in 1913. In these studies, scientists explored the effects of water quality and pollution, and the resulting information helped in the design of community interventions to control the spread of disease through contaminated water. Surveys and contact investigation strategies were refined. Several organizations are committed to researching the characteristics and transmission patterns of communicable diseases. The two most important research centers devoted to the study of the incidence of communicable diseases, treatment for diseases, and trends in diseases are the CDC and the WHO.

The U.S. CDC, based in Atlanta, receives reports from local and state health departments and publishes a yearly summary of communicable diseases in the *Morbidity and Mortality Weekly Report.* Whenever an unusual outbreak of disease occurs, the CDC sends scientific teams to the location of the outbreak to assist local authorities. The CDC is equipped with modern computer and telecommunication technologies to track data and coordinate monitoring efforts.

The WHO supervises research into communicable diseases worldwide (see Chapter 5). The WHO monitored the smallpox epidemic and vaccination efforts; in fact, smallpox eradication is credited to the coordinated efforts of the WHO (Barquet & Domingo, 1997). The WHO is currently coordinating worldwide immunization efforts.

The WHO adapts solutions from one part of the world for use in similar situations in other areas. Researchers continue to study interventions in health care, adapting successful interventions to different cultures and discarding unsuccessful ones. For example, vasectomy as a birth control measure is acceptable in some cultures but unacceptable in others. The WHO's goal is to make health services available in every country and dramatically reduce the rates of communicable diseases. Community health nurses are an integral part of the WHO's intervention and research initiatives. Health practitioners, many of them nurses working on site, are able to provide accurate, realistic, reliable data to assist this mighty effort.

HIGH-RISK POPULATIONS AND HEALTH CARE WORKERS

High-risk populations need special attention, from prevention through treatment and recovery. Donnelly and DePauw (2004, p. 3079) call these individuals *compromised hosts,* which they define as 'individual[s] who [have] one or more defects in the body's natural defense mechanisms.' These defects in defense are significant enough that the individual is rendered predisposed to severe, often life-threatening infection.

The age, sex, genetic makeup, and general well-being of the host can contribute to or decrease the resistance to infectious diseases. Generally infants, young children, and elderly individuals (especially those who are undernourished or have a chronic illness) have a lower resistance to infection. The severity of illness in these groups is also greater. Preschool children are at special risk because they spend a lot of time in groups and do not have fully developed immune systems. Many older adults have diminished immunity from underlying medical problems or an impaired nutritional status (Wilks et al., 2003). Older adults' skin is fragile and easily broken, and they may have been exposed for longer periods to environmental hazards. Consequently, the risks for urinary tract infections, infectious diarrhea, and upper respiratory tract infections such as TB and pneumonia are increased. Community health nurses who understand these factors can develop nursing strategies to increase resistance and generate more efficient defense mechanisms in clients at particular risk.

Immunosuppressed clients are also at risk for contracting communicable diseases. People undergoing immunosuppressive therapy after bone marrow or organ transplantation or therapy for acute lymphocytic leukemia risk infection from multiple organisms. Other conditions that may cause a defect in the cellular immunity of a person are Hodgkin's disease and HIV infection. Cancerous conditions such as acute leukemia, myeloma, hairy cell leukemia, and brain tumors predispose clients to reduced resistance to diseases. Clients with spinal cord injuries are susceptible to urinary tract infections and skin infections.

Intravenous drug abusers are at risk because drug abuse can directly cause infection. An infected needle left by one person and shared by another will transmit infection. There may be indirect causes for the increase of infections in intravenous drug abusers as well. Many drug abusers are poorly nourished, live in substandard conditions with poor sanitation, and are more often exposed to others who carry communicable diseases.

Health care workers are considered a risk group because their work environment places them in proximity to numerous infectious organisms. Hepatitis B and HIV infection can both be transmitted when health care workers are exposed to blood, semen, or vaginal secretions. The resurgence of TB and other drug-resistant infections creates another occupational hazard. Time delays during diagnosis or until treatment is effective place health care workers at risk. Correct and consistent infection control measures are absolutely necessary to provide optimal protection in both inpatient and community settings. Community health nurses should be especially vigilant to maintain safe technique during home and clinic interactions. The Occupational Safety and Health Administration (OSHA) standards issued in 2001 require that safer injection devices be adopted and that records be kept of all sharp injuries. Implementation involves the use of needle-shielding or needle-free syringes in all situations (CDC, 2006w).

ROLE OF BOARDS OF HEALTH

LEGISLATIVE MANDATE

Local boards of health are charged with maintaining the health of the community. Boards provide direct services to individuals, gather data from these individuals and families, collate the data, report the data to state and local agencies, and maintain records for research purposes. Local boards carry out the legislative mandates of both the state and federal governments. The costs for carrying out the mandates are usually shared by all three levels of government. The CDC offers financial assistance for many programs aimed at control of infectious diseases.

ENVIRONMENTAL CONTROL

The primary responsibility for environmental oversight and prevention of associated health problems rests with the health department. Jekel and colleagues (2007) list some of the responsibilities related to water, food, and sewage controls. The water supply is protected by chlorinating and fluoridating municipal water supplies, testing private and public drinking water for contaminants, regulating the digging of wells, and limiting or restricting construction in watershed districts. The health department protects food supplies through surveillance of restaurants, grocery stores, and markets. These departments check for proper food storage, preparation, and service and monitor the health of persons serving and preparing the food. If any food processing or packaging plants are within the jurisdiction, these are scrutinized as well. Sewage disposal and treatment are controlled. Public swimming pools and beaches are inspected frequently to ascertain the safety of water and facilities. Most local boards of health either have direct control or work closely with the public agency that mandates construction codes for public and private buildings.

REPORTABLE DISEASES OVERSIGHT

The CDC tracks national statistics for and trends in communicable diseases through the NNDSS, which maintains regular surveillance of all disease for which reporting is mandatory, as well as other diseases of interest or concern (Box 8-3). For example, reporting is not mandatory for either SARS or monkeypox, but both are monitored and tracked by the CDC. The CDC also issues guidelines and recommendations on the prevention and treatment of specific diseases. An excellent source for this information is the *Morbidity and Mortality Weekly Report* published by the CDC. This publication is a valuable resource for community health nurses because it provides information on specific diseases and public health problems and supplies epidemiologic data on reportable diseases, as well as other communicable diseases and public health concerns such as HPV infection and adolescent homicide.

State public health departments have the legal responsibility for controlling communicable diseases and reporting notifiable communicable diseases to the CDC. Most of the reporting to the CDC is done electronically. Figure 8-8 is a pertussis report form showing the type of information filed with the CDC. The state health departments issue reporting directions and treatment recommendations to local health departments, and those departments gather information about communicable diseases from health care providers in their regions.

Direct diagnosis and treatment, counseling, contact tracing, and follow-up are done by local health departments. Community health nurses perform many of these services.

In addition to collecting information on all notifiable communicable diseases, states may investigate other health concerns at their discretion. Throughout the United States, approximately 90 diseases are reportable through the health department surveillance systems. Surveillance data help the CDC and individual states decide which health concerns should have priority.

Many communicable diseases show seasonal fluctuations or uneven geographic distributions or higher incidences in selected risk groups; others have cycles during which they are more or less severe. Surveillance data reveal these trends. Appropriate strategies can then be planned to prevent or reduce the impact of these diseases. Surveillance also assists in identifying the most effective control methods. For example, the CDC was able to identify a resurgence of measles among adolescents and young adults. Researchers found that the combined measles-mumps-rubella vaccine was less long acting than was previously thought. New immunization standards were developed to include a booster dose around age 11 or 12 years.

IMMUNIZATIONS AND VACCINES: OVERSIGHT AND RECOMMENDATIONS

Immunization is the most effective primary prevention method for controlling communicable diseases in populations. Vaccines are not presently available for all communicable diseases. Immunization is important not only for children, but also for older adults, the chronically ill, and other individuals who are at increased risk (e.g., health care workers). Figures 8-9 and 8-10 provide lists of recommended immunizations and suggested target groups. **Website Resource 8B** contains a list of conditions that are contraindications to vaccine administration. **Website Resource 8C** provides guidance about situations in which the normal vaccination schedule for adults might be changed or contraindicated.

State and local health departments provide immunization clinics and free immunizations to selected populations and oversee vaccine distribution and safety. Local health departments have the responsibility to report specific vaccine-related information to the U.S. Department of Health and Human Services in compliance with the National Childhood Vaccine Injury Act. All health care providers who administer a vaccine must record the serial number of the vial, the name of the company, and any adverse reactions to the vaccine. **Website Resource 8D** provides a sample state vaccine report form. If the vaccine is privately purchased, the report goes through the local board of health to the U.S. Food and Drug Administration; if it is publicly purchased, reporting is done directly to the CDC.

In the early 1980s a significant number of severe reactions to the pertussis vaccine (i.e., psychomotor limitations, paralysis) generated concern that parents were not receiving adequate information about the risks associated with vaccines. As a result, in 1986, Congress passed the National Childhood Vaccine Injury Act, or Child Injury Act. This law requires that a parent's signature be obtained before a child is immunized to testify that the parent has been informed of the risks associated with administration of the vaccine and establishes (1) a reporting system for tracking all vaccine doses and (2) a fund to assist children with adverse reactions to the vaccine (see **Website Resource 8D**). To receive compensation for vaccine reactions, the affected person must have an injury of at least 6 months' duration and at least $1000 in expenses directly related to the injury.

PROTECTION OF INTERNATIONAL TRAVELERS

Local boards of health serve the public by acting as a conduit of information on health-related matters for international travelers. These boards provide information on country-specific immunization requirements and strategies to protect a traveler's health while in another country. The Office of Overseas Travel at the CDC supplies most of the travel-related information to local and state units; for example, information on water and food safety, sanitary conditions, sanctions or penalties for illegal drug use, and necessary steps to ensure travelers that they are in compliance with the laws regulating legal medication use in foreign countries. In most countries, travelers must carry documentation on prescription drugs. Community health nurses in local health departments can assist travelers in collecting information pertinent to their travel plans.

Box 8-3   Nationally Notifiable Infectious Diseases—United States, 2007

Revised to include the addition of "novel influenza A virus infections."

- Acquired immunodeficiency syndrome (AIDS)
- Anthrax
- Arboviral neuroinvasive and nonneuroinvasive diseases
  - California serogroup virus disease
  - Eastern equine encephalitis virus disease
  - Powassan virus disease
  - St. Louis encephalitis virus disease
  - West Nile virus disease
  - Western equine encephalitis virus disease
- Botulism
  - Botulism, food-borne
  - Botulism, infant
  - Botulism, other (wound and unspecified)
- Brucellosis
- Chancroid
- *Chlamydia trachomatis,* genital infections
- Cholera
- Coccidioidomycosis
- Cryptosporidiosis
- Cyclosporiasis
- Diphtheria
- Ehrlichiosis*
  - Ehrlichiosis, human granulocytic
  - Ehrlichiosis, human monocytic
  - Ehrlichiosis, human, other or unspecified agent
- Giardiasis*
- Gonorrhea
- *Haemophilus influenzae,* invasive disease*
- Hansen's disease (leprosy)
- Hantavirus pulmonary syndrome
- Hemolytic uremic syndrome, postdiarrheal
- Hepatitis, viral, acute
  - Hepatitis A, acute
  - Hepatitis B, acute
  - Hepatitis B virus, perinatal infection
  - Hepatitis C, acute
- Hepatitis, viral, chronic
  - Chronic hepatitis B
  - Hepatitis C virus infection (past or present)
- Human immunodeficiency virus (HIV) infection
  - HIV infection, adult (13 years or older)
  - HIV infection, pediatric (younger than 13 years)
- Influenza-associated pediatric mortality
- Legionellosis
- Listeriosis
- Lyme disease
- Malaria
- Measles

- Meningococcal disease
- Mumps
- Novel influenza A virus infections
- Pertussis
- Plague
- Poliomyelitis, paralytic
- Poliovirus infection, nonparalytic[†]
- Psittacosis
- Q fever*
- Rabies
  - Rabies, animal
  - Rabies, human
- Rocky Mountain spotted fever
- Rubella
- Rubella, congenital syndrome
- Salmonellosis
- Severe acute respiratory syndrome–associated Coronavirus (SARS-CoV) disease[‡]
- Shiga toxin–producing *Escherichia coli* (STEC)
- Shigellosis
- Smallpox[§]
- Streptococcal disease, invasive, group A
- Streptococcal toxic shock syndrome
- *Streptococcus pneumoniae,* drug resistant, invasive disease
- *Streptococcus pneumoniae,* invasive disease in children younger than 5 years
- Syphilis
  - Syphilis, primary
  - Syphilis, secondary
  - Syphilis, latent
  - Syphilis, early latent
  - Syphilis, late latent
  - Syphilis, latent, unknown duration
  - Neurosyphilis
  - Syphilis, late, nonneurologic
  - Syphilitic stillbirth
- Syphilis, congenital
- Tetanus
- Toxic shock syndrome (other than streptococcal)
- Trichinellosis (trichinosis)
- Tuberculosis
- Tularemia*
- Typhoid fever
- Vancomycin-intermediate *Staphylococcus aureus* (VISA)*
- Vancomycin-resistant *Staphylococcus aureus* (VRSA)*
- Varicella (morbidity)
- Varicella (deaths only)
- Vibriosis[†]
- Yellow fever

From Centers for Disease Control and Prevention. (2007). *Nationally notifiable infectious diseases: United States, 2007.* Retrieved June 3, 2007 from *http://www.dcd.gov/epo/dphsi/phs/infdis2007.htm.*

*New to list since 1997.
[†]New to list in 2007.
[‡]New to list since 2003.
[§]Added back to list since 2003.

Patient	Name (last, first, M.I.)								Hospital Record No.	
	Parents' names	Mother						Father		
	Address			City		County	State	Zip Code		Telephone No.
Reporting Physician/ Nurse/Hosp/ Clinic	Name			Address						Telephone No.
Investigator	Name						Telephone No.			

- - - - - - - - - - (Identifying information above should not be sent to CDC) - - - - - - - - - -

PERTUSSIS CASE INVESTIGATION
NOTE: This form has two pages

State Case ID _____

A. Case Demographics and Information

	County	State	Zip Code

City ☐☐☐☐☐☐☐☐☐☐☐☐☐☐☐☐☐☐☐   County ☐☐☐   State ☐☐   Zip Code ☐☐☐☐☐

Date of Birth ☐☐ ☐☐ ☐☐   m m d d y y

*Age ☐☐ (99 Unknown)

Age type ☐
- 0–(0-120 Yrs.)   3–(0-28 Days)
- 1–(0-11 Mos.)   4–Age group
- 2–(0-52 Wks.)   9–Age unknown

*Race ☐
- N Native Amer/Alaskan Native   W White
- A Asian/Pacific Islander   O Other
- B African American   U Unknown

Ethnicity ☐
- H Hispanic
- N Not Hispanic
- U Unknown

Sex ☐
- M Male
- F Female
- U Unknown

*Outbreak Associated ☐
(Leave blank unless case affiliated with outbreak and want to note outbreak name/number)

Imported ☐
- 1–Indigenous (acquired in USA reporting state)
- 2–International (acquired outside USA)
- 3–Out of state (acquired in USA outside reporting state)
- 9–Unknown

Event name Pertussis   **Disease code** 40.00   **Case count** (For individual record) 1

Date of report ☐☐ ☐☐ ☐☐ m m d d y y

Comments _____
(Other data)

Case status ☐
- 1–Confirmed   4–Ruled out
- 2–Probable   9–Unknown
- 3–Suspected

B. CLINICAL DATA

Cough ☐
- Y Yes
- N No
- U Unknown

Cough onset date ☐☐ ☐☐ ☐☐ m m d d y y

*Paroxysmal cough ☐
- Y Yes
- N No
- U Unknown

*Whoop ☐
- Y Yes
- N No
- U Unknown

*Posttussive vomiting ☐
- Y Yes
- N No
- U Unknown

*Apnea ☐
- Y Yes
- N No
- U Unknown

*Final interview date ☐☐ ☐☐ ☐☐ m m d d y y

*Cough at final interview ☐
- Y Yes
- N No
- U Unknown

*Duration of cough at final interview ☐☐☐ days (range 1-150; 999 Unknown)

*Was CDC clinical case definition met? ☐
- Y Yes
- N No
(refer to last page for case definition)

C. COMPLICATIONS

*Chest X-ray for pneumonia? ☐
- P–Positive   X–Not done
- N–Negative   U–Unknown

*Seizures due to pertussis? ☐
- Y Yes
- N No
- U Unknown

*Acute encephalopathy due to pertussis? ☐
- Y Yes
- N No
- U Unknown

*Hospitalized due to pertussis? ☐
- Y Yes
- N No
- U Unknown

If yes, hospitalized (range 1-998; 999 Unknown) ☐☐☐

*Died? ☐
- Y Yes
- N No
- U Unknown

D. TREATMENT

Were antibiotics given? ☐
- Y Yes
- N No
- U Unknown

First antibiotic received ☐
- 1–Erythromycin (incl. Pediazole, Ilosone)
- 2–Co-trimoxazole (Bactrim/Septra)
- 3–Clarithromycin/azithromycin
- 4–Tetracycline/doxycycline
- 5–Amoxicillin/penicillin/ampicillin/Augmentin/Ceclor/cefixime
- 6–Other
- 9–Unknown

Date first antibiotic started ☐☐ ☐☐ ☐☐ m m d d y y

Number of days first antibiotic actually taken (range 0-98; 99 Unknown) ☐☐ Days

Second antibiotic received ☐
- 1–Erythromycin (incl. Pediazole, Ilosone)
- 2–Co-trimoxazole (Bactrim/Septra)
- 3–Clarithromycin/azithromycin
- 4–Tetracycline/doxycycline
- 5–Amoxicillin/penicillin/ampicillin/Augmentin/Ceclor/cefixime
- 6–Other
- 9–Unknown

Date started second antibiotic ☐☐ ☐☐ ☐☐ m m d d y y

Number of days second antibiotic actually taken (range 0-98; 99 Unknown) ☐☐ Days

FIGURE 8-8 Pertussis report form. (Courtesy Department of Health and Mental Hygiene, Baltimore, MD.)

Continued

E. LABORATORY

Was laboratory testing for pertussis done?

	Y Yes
	N No
	U Unknown

Culture — Date Specimen Collected [m m / d d / y y] Result [ ]

DFA — Date Specimen Collected [m m / d d / y y] Result [ ]

PCR — Date Specimen Collected [m m / d d / y y] Result [ ]

Serology (1st specimen) — Date Specimen Collected [m m / d d / y y] Result [ ]

Serology (2nd specimen) — Date Specimen Collected [m m / d d / y y] Result [ ]

Result codes

P–Positive	X–Not done
N–Negative	S–Parapertussis
I–Indeterminate	U–Unknown
E–Pending	

Is case laboratory-confirmed?

	Y Yes
	N No
	U Unknown

Note: Serology result is based on either single sample or combined result from acute and convalescent samples

F. VACCINE HISTORY (Complete only for children <15 years)

Has the child ever received any doses of diphtheria, tetanus and/or pertussis-containing vaccines?

	Y Yes
	N No
	U Unknown

What was the date of the last pertussis-containing vaccine prior to illness onset?

[m m / d d / y y]

Immunization History

	Vaccination Date	Vaccine Type	Vaccine Manufacturer		Vaccination Date	Vaccine Type	Vaccine Manufacturer
A.	[m m / d d / y y]	[ ]	[ ]	E.	[m m / d d / y y]	[ ]	[ ]
B.	[m m / d d / y y]	[ ]	[ ]	F.	[m m / d d / y y]	[ ]	[ ]
C.	[m m / d d / y y]	[ ]	[ ]	G.	[m m / d d / y y]	[ ]	[ ]

Type code

W	DTP Whole Cell
A	DTaP
D	DT or Td
T	DTP-Hib Tetramune
P	Pertussis only
O	Other
U	Unknown

Manufacturer codes

C	Connaught
L	Lederle
M	Massachusetts Health Department
I	Michigan Health Department
O	Other
U	Unknown

Number of doses of pertussis-containing vaccine prior vaccine to illness onset

[ ] (Range 0-6; 9=Unknown)

If the child is not vaccinated with ≥ 3 doses of pertussis, what is the reason

[ ]

1	Religious exemption	5	Parental refusal
2	Medical containdication	6	Age <7 months
3	Philosophical exemption	7	Other
4	Previous pertussis confirmed by culture or MD	8	Missed OPPTY
		9	Unknown

G. EPIDEMIOLOGIC INFORMATION

Date pertussis case first reported to a health department

[m m / d d / y y]

Date case investigation started

[m m / d d / y y]

*Epi-linked?

	Y Yes
	N No
	U Unknown

*Outbreak related?

	Y Yes
	N No
	U Unknown

If yes, outbreak name _____
(Name of outbreak this case is associated with)

Transmission setting
(Where did this case acquire pertussis?)

[ ]

1	Day Care	9	Unknown
2	School	10	College
3	Doctor's Office	11	Military
4	Hospital Ward	12	Correctional Facility
5	Hospital ER	13	Church
6	Hospital Outpatient Clinic	14	International Travel
7	Home	15	Other
8	Work		

Setting
(outside household) of further documented spread from this case
(Setting outside household in which secondary transmission of pertussis from this case occurred)

[ ]

1	Day Care	9	Unknown
2	School	10	College
3	Doctor's Office	11	Military
4	Hospital Ward	12	Correctional Facility
5	Hospital ER	13	Church
6	Hospital Outpatient Clinic	14	International Travel
7	>1 Setting outside of household	15	Other
8	Work	16	No documented spread outside household

Number of contacts in any setting for whom antibiotics were recommended
(home, school, day care, etc.)

[ ] (range 0-998; 999 Unknown)

* Required data to be added to NETSS CDC database

• Enter into or update MERSS and send hard copy to Center for Immunization after completion

FIGURE 8-8, CONT'D

Vaccine ▼ Age ►	Birth	1 month	2 months	4 months	6 months	12 months	15 months	18 months	24 months	4–6 years	11–12 years	13–14 years	15 years	16–18 years
Hepatitis B[1]	HepB	HepB	HepB[1]		HepB						HepB Series			
Diphtheria, Tetanus, Pertussis[2]			DTaP	DTaP	DTaP		DTaP			DTaP	Tdap	Tdap		
Haemophilus influenzae type b[3]			Hib	Hib	Hib[3]	Hib								
Inactivated Poliovirus			IPV	IPV		IPV				IPV				
Measles, Mumps, Rubella[4]						MMR				MMR		MMR		
Varicella[5]						Varicella					Varicella			
Meningococcal[6]									MPSV4		MCV4		MCV4 / MCV4	
Pneumococcal[7]			PCV	PCV	PCV	PCV			PCV		PPV			
Influenza[8]					Influenza (yearly)					Influenza (yearly)				
Hepatitis A[9]						HepA series				HepA series				

This schedule indicates the recommended ages for routine administration of currently licensed childhood vaccines, as of December 1, 2005, for children through age 18 years. Any dose not administered at the recommended age should be administered at any subsequent visit, when indicated and feasible. ■ Indicates age groups that warrant special effort to administer those vaccines not previously administered. Additional vaccines might be licensed and recommended during the year. Licensed combination vaccines may be used whenever any components of the combination are indicated and other components of the vaccine are not contraindicated and if approved by the Food and Drug Administration for that dose of the series. Providers should consult respective Advisory Committee on Immunization Practices (ACIP) statements for detailed recommendations. Clinically significant adverse events that follow vaccination should be reported through the Vaccine Adverse Event Reporting System (VAERS). Guidance about how to obtain and complete a VAERS form is available at http://www.vaers.hhs.gov or by telephone, 800-822-7967.

☐ Range of recommended ages   ▦ Catch-up immunization   ☐ Assessment at age 11–12 years

1. **Hepatitis B vaccine (HepB). AT BIRTH:** All newborns should receive monovalent HepB soon after birth and before hospital discharge. Infants born to mothers who are hepatitis B surface antigen (HBsAg)-positive should receive HepB and 0.5 mL of hepatitis B immune globulin (HBIG) within 12 hours of birth. Infants born to mothers whose HBsAg status is unknown should receive HepB within 12 hours of birth. The mother should have blood drawn as soon as possible to determine her HBsAg status; if HBsAg-positive, the infant should receive HBIG as soon as possible (no later than age 1 week). For infants born to HBsAg-negative mothers, the birth dose can be delayed in rare circumstances but only if a physician's order to withhold the vaccine and a copy of the mother's original HBsAg-negative laboratory report are documented in the infant's medical record. **FOLLOWING THE BIRTH DOSE:** The HepB series should be completed with either monovalent HepB or a combination vaccine containing HepB. The second dose should be administered at age 1–2 months. The final dose should be administered at age ≥24 weeks. Administering four doses of HepB is permissible (e.g., when combination vaccines are administered after the birth dose); however, if monovalent HepB is used, a dose at age 4 months is not needed. Infants born to HBsAg-positive mothers should be tested for HBsAg and antibody to HBsAg after completion of the HepB series at age 9–18 months (generally at the next well-child visit after completion of the vaccine series).

2. **Diphtheria and tetanus toxoids and acellular pertussis vaccine (DTaP).** The fourth dose of DTaP may be administered as early as age 12 months, provided 6 months have elapsed since the third dose and the child is unlikely to return at age 15–18 months. The final dose in the series should be administered at age ≥4 years. Tetanus toxoid, reduced diphtheria toxoid, and acellular pertussis vaccine (Tdap adolescent preparation) is recommended at age 11–12 years for those who have completed the recommended childhood DTP/DTaP vaccination series and have not received a tetanus and diphtheria toxoids (Td) booster dose. Adolescents aged 13–18 years who missed the age 11–12-year Td/Tdap booster dose should also receive a single dose of Tdap if they have completed the recommended childhood DTP/DTaP vaccination series. Subsequent Td boosters are recommended every 10 years.

3. **Haemophilus influenzae type b conjugate vaccine (Hib).** Three Hib conjugate vaccines are licensed for infant use. If PRP-OMP (PedvaxHIB® or ComVax® [Merck]) is administered at ages 2 and 4 months, a dose at age 6 months is not required. DTaP/Hib combination products should not be used for primary immunization in infants at age 2, 4, or 6 months but may be used as boosters after any Hib vaccine. The final dose in the series should be administered at age ≥12 months.

4. **Measles, mumps, and rubella vaccine (MMR).** The second dose of MMR is recommended routinely at age 4–6 years but may be administered during any visit, provided at least 4 weeks have elapsed since the first dose and both doses are administered at or after age 12 months. Children who have not previously received the second dose should complete the schedule by age 11–12 years.

5. **Varicella vaccine.** Varicella vaccine is recommended at any visit at or after age 12 months for susceptible children (i.e., those who lack a reliable history of varicella). Susceptible persons aged ≥13 years should receive 2 doses administered at least 4 weeks apart.

6. **Meningococcal vaccine (MCV4).** Meningococcal conjugate vaccine (MCV4) should be administered to all children at age 11–12 years as well as to unvaccinated adolescents at high school entry (age 15 years). Other adolescents who wish to decrease their risk for meningococcal disease may also be vaccinated. All college freshmen living in dormitories should also be vaccinated, preferably with MCV4, although **meningococcal polysaccharide vaccine (MPSV4)** is an acceptable alternative. Vaccination against invasive meningococcal disease is recommended for children and adolescents aged ≥2 years with terminal complement deficiencies or anatomic or functional asplenia and for certain other high risk groups (see MMWR 2005;54[No. RR-7]); use MPSV4 for children aged 2–10 years and MCV4 for older children, although MPSV4 is an acceptable alternative.

7. **Pneumococcal vaccine.** The heptavalent pneumococcal conjugate vaccine (PCV) is recommended for all children aged 2–23 months and for certain children aged 24–59 months. The final dose in the series should be administered at age ≥12 months. Pneumococcal polysaccharide vaccine (PPV) is recommended in addition to PCV for certain high-risk groups. See MMWR 2000;49(No. RR-9).

8. **Influenza vaccine.** Influenza vaccine is recommended annually for children aged ≥6 months with certain risk factors (including, but not limited to, asthma, cardiac disease, sickle cell disease, human immunodeficiency virus infection, diabetes, and conditions that can compromise respiratory function or handling of respiratory secretions or that can increase the risk for aspiration), health-care workers, and other persons (including household members) in close contact with persons in groups at high risk (see MMWR 2005;54[No. RR-8]). In addition, healthy children aged 6–23 months and close contacts of healthy children aged 0–5 months are recommended to receive influenza vaccine because children in this age group are at substantially increased risk for influenza-related hospitalizations. For healthy, nonpregnant persons aged 5–49 years, the intranasally administered, live, attenuated influenza vaccine (LAIV) is an acceptable alternative to the intramuscular trivalent inactivated influenza vaccine (TIV). See MMWR 2005;54(No. RR-8). Children receiving TIV should be administered an age-appropriate dosage (0.25 mL for children aged 6–35 months or 0.5 mL for children aged ≥3 years). Children aged ≤8 years who are receiving influenza vaccine for the first time should receive 2 doses (separated by at least 4 weeks for TIV and at least 6 weeks for LAIV).

9. **Hepatitis A vaccine (HepA).** HepA is recommended for all children at age 1 year (i.e., 12–23 months). The 2 doses in the series should be administered at least 6 months apart. States, counties, and communities with existing HepA vaccination programs for children aged 2–18 years are encouraged to maintain these programs. In these areas, new efforts focused on routine vaccination of children aged 1 year should enhance, not replace, ongoing programs directed at a broader population of children. HepA is also recommended for certain high risk groups (see MMWR 1999;48[No. RR-12]).

The Childhood and Adolescent Immunization Schedule is approved by the Advisory Committee on Immunization Practices (http://www.cdc.gov/nip/acip), the American Academy of Pediatrics (http://www.aap.org), and the American Academy of Family Physicians (http://www.aafp.org).

FIGURE 8-9 Recommended child and adolescent immunization schedule by vaccine and age. (From Centers for Disease Control and Prevention. [2006]. Recommended childhood and adolescent immunization schedule—United States, 2006. *Morbidity and Mortality Weekly Report, 54*[52], Q1-Q4.)

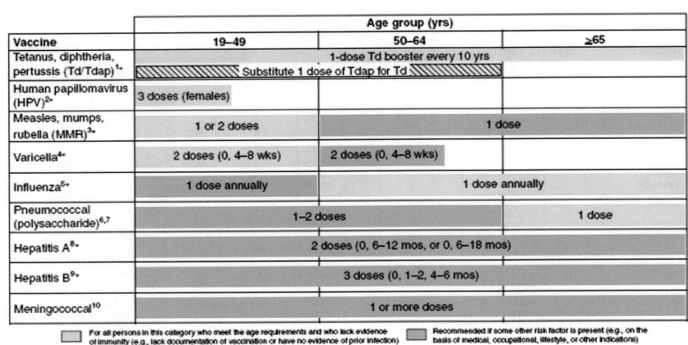

Vaccine	Age group (yrs)		
	19–49	50–64	≥65
Tetanus, diphtheria, pertussis (Td/Tdap)[1]*	1-dose Td booster every 10 yrs		
	Substitute 1 dose of Tdap for Td		
Human papillomavirus (HPV)[2]*	3 doses (females)		
Measles, mumps, rubella (MMR)[3]*	1 or 2 doses	1 dose	
Varicella[4]*	2 doses (0, 4–8 wks)	2 doses (0, 4–8 wks)	
Influenza[5]*	1 dose annually	1 dose annually	
Pneumococcal (polysaccharide)[6,7]	1–2 doses		1 dose
Hepatitis A[8]*	2 doses (0, 6–12 mos, or 0, 6–18 mos)		
Hepatitis B[9]*	3 doses (0, 1–2, 4–6 mos)		
Meningococcal[10]	1 or more doses		

☐ For all persons in this category who meet the age requirements and who lack evidence of immunity (e.g., lack documentation of vaccination or have no evidence of prior infection)

☐ Recommended if some other risk factor is present (e.g., on the basis of medical, occupational, lifestyle, or other indications)

* Covered by the Vaccine Injury Compensation Program.
NOTE: These recommendations must be read along with the footnotes, which can be found on pages Q2–Q4 of this schedule.

This schedule indicates the recommended age groups and medical indications for routine administration of currently licensed vaccines for persons aged 19 years, as of October 1, 2006. Licensed combination vaccines may be used whenever any components of the combination are indicated and when the vaccine's other components are not contraindicated. For detailed recommendations on all vaccines including those used primarily for travelers or that are issued during the year, consult the manufacturers' package inserts and the complete statements from the Advisory Committee on Immunization Practices (http://www.cdc.gov/nip/publications/acip-list.htm).

Report all clinically significant postvaccination reactions to the Vaccine Adverse Event Reporting System (VAERS). Reporting forms and instructions on filing a VAERS report are available at http://www.vaers.hhs.gov or by telephone, 800-822-7967.

Information on how to file a Vaccine Injury Compensation Program claim is available at http://www.hrsa.gov/vaccinecompensation or by telephone, 800-338-2382. To file a claim for vaccine injury, contact the U.S. Court of Federal Claims, 717 Madison Place, N.W., Washington, D.C. 20005, telephone, 202-357-6400.

Additional information about the vaccines in this schedule and contraindications for vaccination is also available at http://www.cdc.gov/nip or from the CDC-INFO Contact Center at 800-CDC-INFO (800-232-4636) in English and Spanish, 24 hours a day, 7 days a week.

See **Website Resources 8B** and **8C** for footnotes, contraindications, and recommended immunization schedules for special populations.

Approved by the Advisory Committee on Immunization Practices,
the American College of Obstetricians and Gynecologists, the American Academy of Family Physicians
and the American College of Physicians

FIGURE 8-10 Recommended adult immunization schedule, by vaccine and age group. (From Centers for Disease Control and Prevention. [2006]. Recommended adult immunizations, schedule—United States, October 2006–September 2007. *Morbidity and Mortality Weekly Report, 55*[40], Q1-Q4).

NURSING CARE IN THE CONTROL OF COMMUNICABLE DISEASES

Community health nurses may focus their energies on population groups or on individuals and their family members. In either case, their ultimate goal is the same: protecting populations from the spread of communicable diseases. To be effective, community health nurses must be familiar with basic information about communicable diseases, including causative organisms, incubation period, mode of transmission, symptoms, protective measures, and the necessary treatments. This information is critical to planning care aimed at preventing transmission of infectious diseases or ameliorating the symptoms of persons who have

acquired a disease. Basic information about a number of specific diseases is given in Table 8-3. The diseases are arranged according to five general routes of infection: respiratory, integumentary, gastrointestinal, serum, and sexually transmitted. Some diseases can be transmitted through more than one route. For example, HIV infection and hepatitis are discussed under blood-borne diseases, but both are also transmitted through sexual contact, and hepatitis can be transmitted through the fecal-oral (gastrointestinal) route as well. Table 8-3 presents only a brief overview of selected communicable diseases. For more complete information, refer to the Heymann text, *Control of Communicable Diseases Manual* (2004), published by the American Public Health Association.

TABLE 8-3 Communicable Diseases, Community Health Concerns, and Treatment (Compiled by Gayle Hofland)

Disease (Causative Agent)	Symptoms	Mode of Transmission	Complications and Community Health Concerns	Treatment or Nursing Management
Respiratory Route				
Chickenpox (*Varicella zoster* virus)	*Prodromal:* low-grade fever, headache, listlessness. *2nd:* pruritic rash which has three phases; macular, papular, and vesicular, which scab and crust over. Rash usually on scalp and trunk (where *most* concentrated) but can spread to entire body and mucous membranes such as the mouth with appearance as shallow white ulcers. *Fetal effects:* rare congenital symptoms (Congenital Varicella Syndrome) of low birth weight, extremity atrophy, scarring of skin, eye and neurologic abnormalities.	Very contagious, person-to-person direct contact with respiratory secretions or contact with airborne respiratory droplets. Indirect contact via soiled articles infected from lesions or discharge from skin lesions, vesicle discharges, or nasal or pharyngeal secretions. *Incubation period:* 10-21 days. *Communicable:* 1-2 days before and until lesions are crusted over.	Seasonal with increased incidence in late winter and early spring. Older adults and immunocompromised may develop shingles with virus reactivation. A shingles vaccine has been developed for people over the age of 60 who have not had shingles. *Complications:* secondary bacterial infections of skin caused by itching and scratching. *Others:* encephalitis, pneumonia, death.	Isolation at home until lesions are crusted over. *Supportive:* rest, relief of itching and prevention of bacterial skin infection (clean and dry skin, short nails or mitts to prevent scratching, calamine lotion, tepid oatmeal baths, antihistamines), antipyretics (non-aspirin due to the association with Reye's syndrome). Antivirals are considered for the immunocompromised and those at risk for severe disease to decrease symptoms. *Prevention:* Vaccine immunization, education. Those at risk for serious disease and the immunosuppressed should receive immune globulin or varicella zoster immune globulin with exposure to prevent disease.
Diphtheria (*Corynebacterium* diphtheriae)	Flu-like symptoms with sore throat, fever, swelling of cervical lymph nodes and larynx with potential respiratory distress. Characterized by formation of gray tenacious membrane on tonsils and pharyngeal walls.	Person-to-person direct contact with airborne respiratory droplets or indirect contact with contaminated articles. *Incubation period:* 2-5 days. *Communicable:* variable, as long as 4 weeks without antibiotics.	Asymptomatic carrier state possible; should be treated with antibiotics. *Complications:* respiratory obstruction, suffocation (especially in children under 5 years). With toxin release in the blood; myocarditis, neuritis.	Hospitalization, antitoxin (immediately on diagnosis), antibiotics. Isolation (until two negative throat cultures). Respiratory support; oxygen, humidification. *Prevention:* vaccine immunization. Contacts of diphtheria should receive prophylactic antibiotics.
Meningococcal meningitis (*Neisseria meningitides*) (bacteria)	Flu-like symptoms; fever, headache, stiff neck, nausea, vomiting, photophobia, lethargy. Rapid progression of disease may be fatal.	Direct contact with respiratory secretions (i.e., kissing, coughing) *Incubation period:* 2-10 days	Increased risk seen with close and prolonged contact (i.e., first-year college students living in dormitories, military recruits) and in travel to areas with high meningococcal disease. Medical emergency, early diagnosis and treatment is essential to prevent complications. *Complications:* permanent hearing loss, mental retardation, loss of phalanges or limbs, death.	Hospitalization, antibiotics. droplet precautions. *Prevention:* vaccine Immunization. Close contacts of disease should receive prophylactic antibiotics.
Pertussis or Whooping cough (*Bordetella pertussis*) (bacteria)	*1st: catarrhal stage:* symptoms of upper respiratory infection. *2nd: paroxysmal stage:* numerous rapid coughs	Direct contact with respiratory secretions or rarely by indirect contact with contaminated articles.	Incidence has increased gradually since the 1980s. Infants younger than 1 year are most severely affected with asphyxia possible.	Respiratory isolation, antibiotics, hospitalization with oxygen, humidification, fluids, nasotracheal suctioning.

Continued

TABLE 8-3   **Communicable Diseases, Community Health Concerns, and Treatment—cont'd**

Disease (Causative Agent)	Symptoms	Mode of Transmission	Complications and Community Health Concerns	Treatment or Nursing Management
Respiratory Route—cont'd				
Pertussis or Whooping cough—cont'd	followed by high-pitched inspiratory "whoop." Vomiting, small scleral and conjunctival hemorrhages caused by severe coughing.	*Incubation period:* Usually 7-10 days. *Communicable:* very contagious from early catarrhal stage to 2 weeks after onset.	*Complications:* otitis media, pneumonia, seizures, encephalopathy, death.	*Prevention:* vaccine immunization. Close contacts of pertussis should receive antibiotic prophylaxis.
Rubella and German measles (rubella virus, rubivirus)— "three day measles"	*Prodromal:* low-grade fever, malaise, sore throat, coryza, cough. *2nd:* fine red maculopapular rash begins on face and scalp with spread down to body and limbs lasting 1-3 days. Occipital lymph node enlargement, arthralgia, arthritis. *Fetal infection:* congenital rubella syndrome most common in first trimester exposure; deafness (most common symptom), cataracts, heart defects, microcephaly, mental retardation, spontaneous abortion, premature delivery, fetal death.	Direct or indirect contact with respiratory droplets or nasopharyngeal secretions. Transmission to fetus during active maternal infection. Infants with congenital rubella syndrome may shed virus from body secretions for up to a year. *Incubation period:* 14-21 days. *Communicable:* 7 days before to 5-7 days after rash appears. Moderately contagious.	Mild self-limiting disease except to fetus. To prevent congenital rubella syndrome, women of childbearing years should be immunized before pregnancy and delay pregnancy for 3 months after immunization. Alternately, women can be vaccinated immediately after delivery.	Isolation at home until rash disappears. *Supportive:* rest, fluids, cool mist vaporizer, analgesics (avoid aspirin due to the association with Reye's syndrome). *Prevention:* vaccine immunization. Pregnant women should avoid contact with persons with rubella.
Rubeola and measles (rubeola virus, paramyxovirus— "red or hard measles," "9 day measles")	*Prodromal:* cold-like symptoms, cough, and high fever (103°-105° F), malaise. Conjunctivitis, photophobia. Koplik spots in the mouth (bluish-white and very fine) that disappear with rash onset. 2nd: red maculopapular rash begins in hairline with face down distribution covering most of the body.	Person-to-person direct contact with saliva or airborne respiratory droplets. *Incubation period:* 7-14 days. *Communicable:* 4 days before to 4 days after rash. Highly contagious. Permanent immunity is acquired after disease.	*Complications:* otitis media, pneumonia, encephalitis. Measles during pregnancy can cause miscarriage, premature labor, and low birth weight infant. Generally MMR vaccine is contraindicated in immunosuppression, however, persons who are HIV positive and asymptomatic should be considered for the vaccine because the illness could be fatal.	Isolation at home until 5 days after rash disappears. *Supportive:* rest, fluids, tepid baths, cool mist vaporizer. Comfort by dimming the lights, washing eyes with warm saline water. Analgesics (avoid aspirin due to the association with Reye's syndrome). *Prevention:* vaccine immunization. Avoid vaccination during pregnancy and delay pregnancy for 3 months after vaccination. Immunoglobulin given within 5 days after exposure to lessen effects of disease.
Mumps (mumps virus) (paramyxovirus)	*Prodromal:* low-grade fever, headache, anorexia, myalgia. *2nd:* pain and swelling of parotid or other salivary glands (unilateral or bilateral), earache, pain with chewing.	Airborne or person-to-person direct contact with saliva and respiratory droplets. More commonly a childhood disease. *Incubation period:* 14-18 days. *Communicable:* 3 days before to 9 days after the onset of symptoms. Permanent immunity is usually acquired after contracting the disease.	*Complications:* sensorineural deafness, meningitis, encephalitis. Orchitis after puberty, but sterility is rare. Potential for spontaneous abortion if woman is infected in early pregnancy.	Isolation, no less than 9 days after beginning of swelling, until swelling subsides. *Supportive:* rest until swelling subsides. Cool or warm compresses, warm salt water gargles, fluids, soft bland diet, avoid citrus fruits to decrease pain. Analgesics (avoid aspirin due to the association with Reye's syndrome). *Prevention:* vaccine immunization (delay pregnancy for 3 months after vaccination).

TABLE 8-3 Communicable Diseases, Community Health Concerns, and Treatment—cont'd

Disease (Causative Agent)	Symptoms	Mode of Transmission	Complications and Community Health Concerns	Treatment or Nursing Management
Respiratory Route—cont'd				
Tuberculosis (TB) (*Mycobacterium tuberculosis*)	Latent TB: no symptoms; immune system keeps TB infection inactive with no spread to others. Positive skin test, normal chest x-ray and sputum culture. TB disease: low-grade fever, weight loss, listlessness, night sweats, respiratory congestion, cough, hemoptysis. Positive skin test, may have abnormal chest x-ray and/or sputum culture. Sites other than the lungs may be infected (extrapulmonary TB disease); if so, symptoms will be specific to the site (i.e., meninges, joints, bladder, lymphatic system).	Inhalation of respiratory droplets containing bacteria. *Communicable:* until after several weeks of appropriate treatment for active TB disease.	Latent TB can become active with weakened immune system. Risk factors for active TB include poverty, poor health, immigrant status, HIV positive status, the very young and old age. Globally, the immergence of extensively drug resistant and multi-drug resistant TB is a concern, especially for those with weakened immune systems. *Complications:* pulmonary tissue damage and necrosis, respiratory failure.	Persons infected (without active disease) are treated prophylactically with antitubercular medications. Multiple drug therapy, isolation, rest, respiratory supportive care for persons with active disease. *Prevention:* Better living conditions, proper nutrition, and positive health practices (cover nose and mouth when coughing). Bacille Calmette-Guérin vaccine (BCG) given in some other countries.
Influenza (influenza virus) "Flu"	Respiratory symptoms such as runny or stuffy nose, dry cough, sore throat. May be accompanied by headache, fever (usually high), body aches, fatigue.	Inhalation of respiratory droplet spread from nose and mouth. Less often spread via contact with soiled surface and then touching nose or mouth. *Incubation period:* 1-4 days. *Communicable:* day before symptoms and extends for 1 week after symptoms.	Very infectious, most common in the fall and winter months. People age 65 and older, those with chronic medical conditions, young children and pregnant women are most likely to have complications of the flu. *Complications:* pneumonia, dehydration, bronchitis, sinus and ear infections, death.	*Supportive:* rest, liquids, oxygen as needed, analgesics, antipyretics, (avoid aspirin due to the association with Reye's syndrome). Antivirals given within 2 days of illness can decrease duration of illness. *Prevention:* good health habits, rest, proper diet, hand hygiene. Yearly influenza vaccination (especially high risk patients and health care workers of high-risk patients). Pneumococcal vaccination is also recommended.
Mononucleosis (Epstein-Barr virus) "kissing disease"	Fever, fatigue, enlarged lymph nodes (especially cervical lymph nodes), sore throat, malaise. At times enlarged liver and spleen.	Direct contact with oral secretions. Common disease of older children and adolescents. *Incubation period:* 4-6 weeks.	Usually self-limiting disease and resolves in several weeks. Often associated with strep infections thus a throat culture may also be performed. *Complications:* potential for splenic rupture.	*Supportive:* maintain adequate rest, prevent fatigue, fluids, warm saline gargles, analgesics, antipyretics, (avoid aspirin due to the association with Reye's syndrome). Avoid activity that may cause blunt abdominal trauma and splenic rupture. *Prevention:* avoid transfer of saliva with someone who is currently or was recently infected with the disease.
Haemophilus-Influenzae type b (Hib) (bacterial infection)	Causes disease almost exclusively in children younger than 5 years. S/S: lower respiratory tract infection, malaise and fever. Hib can affect many organ systems and may be rapidly fatal without prompt treatment.	Spread by respiratory droplet infection and discharges from nose and throat during the infectious period. *Incubation period:* less than 10 days. *Communicable:* varies, may persist as long as	Factors that increase exposure and Hib disease include children in close contact, large household size/crowding, day-care attendance, school-aged siblings. Factors that increase susceptibility to Hib include low socioeconomic status, chronic disease states.	Hospitalization, isolation and antibiotics, analgesics, respiratory support as needed. If disease is diagnosed in a daycare setting, all parents should be notified of exposure, informed of risk, and advised regarding signs and symptoms of illness.

Continued

TABLE 8-3   Communicable Diseases, Community Health Concerns, and Treatment—cont'd

Disease (Causative Agent)	Symptoms	Mode of Transmission	Complications and Community Health Concerns	Treatment or Nursing Management
Respiratory Route—cont'd				
Haemophilus-Influenzae type b—cont'd		organism is present in the nose and throat.	*Complications:* meningitis, hearing loss, pneumonia, cellulitis, epiglottitis, septic arthritis, death.	To prevent the spread of disease, the antibiotic rifampin may be recommended for household and daycare contacts not immunized for Haemophilus. *Prevention:* vaccine immunization.
Erythema Infectiosum (fifth disease) (parvovirus B19)	Mild viral illness begins with a mild cold then three stages of skin eruptions: *1st:* "slapped cheek" appearance *2nd:* maculopapular rash on the trunk and extremities, which becomes mesh-like and lacey; may itch. *3rd:* periodic rash fading with eruptions (recurs with heat, exposure to sun) may appear for weeks to months.	Communicable by respiratory droplet infection (i.e., sharing drinking cups or utensils). *Incubation period:* 4-14 days. *Communicable:* most infectious before rash presents.	Community outbreaks are common, most frequently in the winter and spring. The highest incidence is seen in school-age children between 5 and 15 years. *Complications:* rare risk of fetal injury and fetal loss to non-immune, pregnant women. May cause serious illness in immunocompromised and persons with sickle cell anemia.	Usually a mild disease. Symptomatic treatment. Affected children do not have to be excluded from child care or school because children are unlikely to be contagious after the rash has become manifest. *Prevention:* hand-washing. Do not share eating utensils.
Scarlet fever (Group A streptococci)	*1st:* characterized by fever, pharyngitis (intensely red or edematous with purulent yellow exudate on tonsils), "strawberry tongue" (whitish coating with red, swollen papillae). *2nd:* rash with sandpaper feel most often seen on neck and chest; dark red skin creases. Rash blanches with pressure. Skin desquamation (especially tips of fingers/toes) after fever subsides.	Spread by respiratory droplets or direct contact with infected secretions, rarely by indirect contact through objects. *Incubation period:* 2-7 days. *Communicable:* 10-21 days before and during clinical illness or until 1 day after antibiotic therapy begins.	Symptomatic contacts are cultured. *Complications:* otitis media, rheumatic fever, glomerulonephritis.	Antibiotics *Supportive:* warm saline gargles, cool mist vaporizer. Encourage fluids, soft diet. Sucking on candy may relieve discomfort of sore throat. *Prevention:* hand-washing. Keep drinking glasses and utensils separate from others.
Severe-Acute Respiratory Syndrome (SARS) (coronavirus)	Variable S/S. Prodromal: high fever, chills, headache, malaise. Respiratory disease, from mild to severe symptoms: Cough, dyspnea, hypoxemia, pneumonia, respiratory distress syndrome, death.	Person-to-person direct contact with respiratory secretions. Potential spread by indirect contact with objects contaminated with infectious droplets. *Incubation period:* 2-7 days. *Communicable:* unknown; however, is most likely infectious when S/S are present.	Most cases of SARS have occurred among travelers in areas of the world affected by SARS. Persons with SARS should limit out of home contacts for 10 days after symptoms are gone. Close contacts to SARS should monitor for symptoms, if present, limit public activities and seek medical evaluation.	Isolation, antibiotics, antivirals, steroids. *Supportive:* respiratory support, hydration. *Prevention:* respiratory and contact precautions (hand washing, avoid sharing eating utensils, towels, bedding, etc. with SARS patient)
Integumentary Route				
Impetigo (group A streptococcal or staphylococcal bacteria)	Skin blisters usually found in the corners of the mouth near the edge of nose. Blisters break and form yellow crusts that resolve with little or no scarring; blisters may be itchy, and scratching may occur.	Direct contact with lesions or secretions. Scratching spreads the disease to other areas of the body. Indirect contact with secretions via towels, clothing, and linens that have touched infected skin.	Any break in the skin may allow bacterial entry. Most common in hot, humid climates and summer months which disrupt the normal flora of skin. Most problematic in children. Infected children should be kept home until not	Topical antibiotics after removal of crusts by washing lesions with warm, soapy water (cover affected areas to prevent spread). Wash all clothing and linens in hot water. Oral antibiotics in severe cases. *Prevention:* keep skin clean. Educate on hand-washing and

TABLE 8-3   **Communicable Diseases, Community Health Concerns, and Treatment—cont'd**

Disease (Causative Agent)	Symptoms	Mode of Transmission	Complications and Community Health Concerns	Treatment or Nursing Management
Integumentary Route—cont'd				
Impetigo—cont'd		*Incubation period:* 4-10 days. *Communicable:* very contagious as long as lesions are present.	contagious (usually 24 hours after treatment has begun). *Complications:* cellulitis; acute glomerulonepritis in preschool age children.	use of separate towels and washcloths.
Pediculosis (parasitic lice)	Lice and eggs (nits) may be present in scalp hair or pubic hair or on the body. Itching and other signs of skin irritation, such as pin-sized blood spots, a rash, or swollen glands, may be present.	Direct or indirect transfer of adult lice or nits (eggs) via body contact or contact with personal items that are infected with the parasites. Head lice—live 3 days without a blood meal. Body lice—live 10 days without a blood meal. Pubic lice—live 1-2 days without a blood meal.	Nuisance disease. Occurs without regard to socioeconomic status but seen more in overcrowding where sanitation and hygiene are poor. *Complications:* sores caused by scratching.	Lice are treated with medicated pediculicide shampoos or topical medication. Nits (eggs) should be removed from scalp hair with a fine-toothed comb. To prevent re-infestation with lice: wash and dry all affected garments (clothing, linens, towels) on hot settings, dry clean or remove from body blood contact, vacuum floors and furniture, wash combs and brushes. *Prevention:* educate not to borrow combs, hats, and so forth. Bathing, clean clothes, and hand-washing to prevent transfer of eggs.
Scabies (parasitic mite)	Skin rash (small raised red bumps), itching which is most intense at night. Mite burrows, just below the skin, appear as gray or white tracts; may be especially evident in skin folds on wrists, finger webs, belt line, elbows, knees, armpits and genitals.	Direct person-to-person contact or possible transmission on clothing and bed linens. *Communicable:* as long as eggs or mites are alive. Mites do not live more than 2-3 days away from the human body.	High incidence seen in cases of overcrowding and among household contacts where there is frequent skin-to-skin contact. Sexual partners and persons with prolonged direct skin-to-skin contact with infested person should be treated. *Complications:* sores caused by scratching, which may become infected. Symptoms may persist for several weeks after the mites have been killed.	Topical scabicide application from the chin down as directed; a second treatment may be necessary. Bedding and clothing used by an infested person must be thoroughly cleaned or removed from body contact for at least 3 days. *Prevention:* educate to change clothing daily; launder with hot water and dryer.
Tetanus (lockjaw) (*Clostridium tetani*) (bacteria)	Descending, progressive pattern of tonic spasms. The first sign is jaw stiffness (lock jaw) followed by stiffness of the neck, difficulty swallowing, rigid respiratory muscles, generalized body stiffness, tonic spasms of skeletal muscles, and opisthotonos.	Wound contamination by soil containing Clostridium tetani bacteria from animal and human feces. *Incubation period:* usually 8 days	Neonatal tetanus (more common in undeveloped countries) is caused by contamination of umbilical cord of an infant born to unimmunized mother. *Complications:* spasms may interfere with ventilation and cause fractures of the spine and long bones, as well as death. Prognosis is improved with early identification and treatment, recovery may take several months.	Hospitalization, antitoxins, sedatives, muscle relaxants, antibiotics, wound debridement. Minimize environmental stimuli to decrease spasms. Maintain patent airway and adequate ventilation. *Prevention:* vaccine immunization. Tetanus immune globulin or tetanus antitoxin with unclean, major wounds and uncertain immunization status.

Continued

TABLE 8-3   Communicable Diseases, Community Health Concerns, and Treatment—cont'd

Disease (Causative Agent)	Symptoms	Mode of Transmission	Complications and Community Health Concerns	Treatment or Nursing Management
Gastrointestinal Route				
Poliomyelitis	Three patterns of infection are possible: 1. Asymptomatic. 2. Non-paralytic: flu-like symptoms, muscle weakness and stiffness. 3. Paralytic: paralysis which may affect any muscle group, including limbs and respiratory muscles.	Direct contact of virus with the mouth, predominately spread through the feces (fecal-oral transmission). Humans are the only natural host and reservoir of the virus. *Incubation period:* 6-20 days. *Communicable:* 7-10 days before and after onset of symptoms.	Crowded living conditions and poor sanitation promote spread. *Complications:* permanent paralysis; disability and deformities. Post-polio syndrome with symptoms of fatigue, muscle pain, weakness, or paralysis may be experienced 30-40 years after the initial paralytic polio infection.	Isolation with enteric precautions. *Supportive:* rest, respiratory support as needed. Physical therapy, positioning or range of motion to prevent contractures. *Prevention:* vaccine immunization. Sanitation to prevent fecal-oral transmission.
Salmonellosis (bacteria)	Sudden onset of acute gastroenteritis with abdominal cramps, diarrhea, nausea, fever, and sometimes vomiting and dehydration. Stools may be loose for days-months after acute episode.	Direct via person-to-person oral-fecal contact or indirectly by ingestion of food contaminated with feces containing *Salmonella.* *Incubation period:* 12-72 hours. *Communicable:* during the entire period of infection (may be as long as several months after symptoms disappear).	Infections more frequent in warm weather (summer months). Uncooked eggs, poultry, raw milk, and meats are usual sources which harbor bacteria. Some pets and reptiles (i.e., turtles, snakes) may harbor infection. *Complications:* infection can spread to bloodstream and cause death in people with weakened immune systems, the elderly and infants.	Fluids and enteric isolation. Antibiotics for severe symptoms. *Prevention:* hand-washing after toileting and touching pets, before food preparation and eating. Exclude persons who are infected from food handling. Refrigerate foods; wrap fresh meats in plastic to avoid blood contamination of other foods; discard cracked or dirty eggs. Cook foods thoroughly.
Shigellosis (bacteria)	Stomach cramps, diarrhea (may contain blood), fever, nausea, and dehydration. Usually resolves in 5-7 days.	Direct person-to-person by fecal-oral route or indirect transfer to the mouth by contaminated foods, toys, or contaminated water. *Incubation period:* usually 1-3 days. *Communicable:* as long as organism is present in stools; may be one month or more.	Infants and children who are not potty trained are more often infected because of poor hygiene. Seasonal, more common in warm weather. *Complications:* high fever and seizures in children under 2 years of age with severe infection.	*Supportive:* fluids. Antibiotics for severe symptoms. *Prevention:* hand-washing, careful personal hygiene, dispose of diapers properly; exclude those infected from food handling. *Prevention with travel to developing countries:* drink only bottled water. Eat cooked, hot foods and peel fruits yourself.
Pinworms (intestinal worms)	Anal itching. With heavy infection, loss of appetite and difficulty sleeping.	Transmitted via ingestion of eggs of the worms, either directly via hands and fingernails or indirectly through transfer of eggs to food, water, or articles (such as toys) to the mouth. *Communicable:* pinworm eggs can live up to 2 weeks on objects.	Infestation in school and daycare settings is common. It is not necessary to screen asymptomatic children, but children should be examined if symptoms occur. *Diagnosis:* cellophane tape application to anal area early in the morning to confirm egg deposits.	Treat with prescription or over-the-counter anthelmintic medications in two-step treatment with second treatment 2 weeks after first. Bathe and change underwear every morning; wash night clothes and sheets after treatments. Discourage anal itching to prevent re-infection. *Prevention:* teach hygiene to prevent fecal-oral transmission.

TABLE 8-3   Communicable Diseases, Community Health Concerns, and Treatment—cont'd

Disease (Causative Agent)	Symptoms	Mode of Transmission	Complications and Community Health Concerns	Treatment or Nursing Management
Gastrointestinal Route—cont'd				
Rotavirus	Vomiting, diarrhea, fever, abdominal pain.	Direct fecal-oral transmission or indirect transmission by ingestion of contaminated water or food. *Incubation period:* 1-3 days *Communicable:* very contagious.	Leading cause of gastroenteritis in infants and young children. Children with diarrhea should be excluded from daycare until symptom free. *Complications:* severe dehydration can cause death.	Self-limiting disease in healthy persons. *Supportive:* fluids; enteric precautions. *Prevention:* vaccine immunization. Hand-washing.
Toxoplasmosis *(Toxo-plasma gondii)* (parasite)	Most persons have no symptoms or only mild symptoms (enlarged lymph nodes, muscle aches and pains). *Fetal infection:* may result in spontaneous abortion, stillbirth, or varied complications after birth.	Most commonly by ingestion of food and water contaminated by the feces of cats or ingestion of the parasite via uncooked or undercooked meat. Transplacental infection when the mother has a primary infection. Immunosuppression may reactivate a prior infection.	Toxoplasmosis screening may be done for those at risk of serious disease; pregnant women and those with a weakened immune system. *Complications:* immunosuppressed and AIDS patients may develop life-threatening disseminated visceral disease (encephalitis, myocarditis, etc.). Complications of fetal infection include blindness, encephalitis, hydrocephalus, and mental retardation.	Usually self-limited; treatment not needed with healthy, nonpregnant persons. Pregnant and immunosuppressed individuals are treated with anti-infective drugs. *Prevention:* wear gloves while gardening. Wash hands after outdoor activities, care of cat litter box and contact with raw meat. Cook all meats thoroughly and wash all surfaces that have contact with raw meat.
Hepatitis A (hepatitis A virus)—"viral or infectious hepatitis"	Rapid onset of symptoms; nausea, vomiting, abdominal cramps, jaundice, dark-colored urine, and clay-colored stools. May be asymptomatic.	Person-to-person by fecal-oral route and can be transmitted during oral sexual activity. Also spread by ingestion of contaminated food, milk, undercooked shellfish, and water. *Incubation period:* time of exposure to symptom onset; 15-50 days (28 day average).	Very contagious and spreads rapidly. Common in day-care centers, among illicit and intravenous drug users and men who have sex with men. Outbreaks have been linked to ingestion of seafood from polluted water. *Complications:* rarely, acute liver failure.	Self-limiting disease. Enteric precautions. Supportive care. *Prevention:* good hand-washing and screening of food handlers. Vaccine immunization. Immune serum globulin when exposure has been identified. *Prevention with travel to developing countries:* drink only bottled water. Eat cooked, hot foods and peel fruits yourself.
Serum Route				
Hepatitis B (HBV) (hepatitis B virus) (serum hepatitis)	General gastrointestinal symptoms or no symptoms. Liver deterioration, if present, is noted by markedly enlarged and tender liver, dark urine, light stool, jaundiced eyes. HBV infection can be self limited or chronic. Acute infection usually runs a 3-4 week course but symptoms may last up to 6 months.	Exposure to infected blood (e.g., via wounds, intravenous drug use) and by intimate sexual contact with contaminated human secretions (semen, cervical secretions, saliva). In health care workers, exposure to infected blood is often via	Health care workers, persons with multiple sex partners, injection drug users, infants of infected mothers, household contacts of infected persons, and hemodialysis patients are at increased risk of disease. Chronic carriers can transmit disease to others. The greatest risk for acquiring chronic carrier status is the	Symptomatic treatment of acute hepatitis (i.e., rest, nutrition, fluids). *Prevention:* vaccine immunization. Condoms during sexual intercourse may decrease risk of infection. Hepatitis B immune globulin and vaccine post exposure for the unvaccinated. Chronic carriers of HBV must not share razors,

Continued

TABLE 8-3   Communicable Diseases, Community Health Concerns, and Treatment—cont'd

Disease (Causative Agent)	Symptoms	Mode of Transmission	Complications and Community Health Concerns	Treatment or Nursing Management
Serum Route—cont'd				
Hepatitis B—cont'd		accidental needle puncture. Can be passed from mother to newborn at birth. *Incubation period:* 1-6 months.	very young (90% of infants infected with HBV at birth will be carriers). *Complications:* chronic hepatitis, cirrhosis, liver cancer, death.	toothbrushes, or any objects contaminated with blood.
Human immunodeficiency virus (HIV)	*Initial infection:* Asymptomatic or non-specific symptoms (decreased appetite, weight loss, fever, night sweats, diarrhea, tiredness, swollen lymph nodes). *2nd:* symptoms of immune compromise; opportunistic infections and cancers that allow for the diagnosis of AIDS (i.e., Kaposi's sarcoma, *Pneumocystitis jiroveic* pneumonia, Toxoplasma gondii, Candidiasis, *Cryptococcus,* Cytomegalovirus, Herpes simplex, others). Death.	Contact with infected body secretions (semen or vaginal secretions during sexual intercourse; parenteral exposure of blood and blood products; perinatal or transplacental transmission; breast milk). *Incubation period:* a few days to a few weeks after initial infection. Potentially 10 years or more before AIDS.	Increased risk of HIV with other sexually transmitted diseases resulting from skin breaks. At risk: men who have sex with men, injection or intravenous drug users who share equipment, heterosexuals with numerous partners, unprotected sex with someone at risk for HIV, infants born to HIV mothers. Persons positive for HIV infection may be asymptomatic for years and may unknowingly engage in risky behavior, putting others at risk.	Antiretroviral treatment to slow the decline of immune system function. Treatment for altered immune system depends on specific presenting opportunistic illness or disease. *Prevention:* education about safe sexual and personal habits. Condoms to decrease risk of exposure. Do not share needles, syringes, or injection equipment. Needle exchange programs. Immediate antiretroviral treatment post exposure. Efforts at vaccine development continue.
Sexually Transmitted Route				
Herpes (herpes simplex virus; HSV-1; HSV-2)	S/S: 2-12 days after exposure or may be no symptoms. *Prodromal S/S:* burning or "prickly" sensation. *2nd:* clusters of small blisters that rupture and cause painful ulcers. Symptoms may include fever, painful intercourse, painful urination, and swollen and tender groin glands. *Fetal effects:* abortion, preterm labor. Birth canal exposure—blindness, brain damage, or death.	Direct contact with oral and genital secretions. Mother-to-infant transmission at birth. Both HSV-1 and HSV-2 viruses can cause genital herpes. HSV-1 is most commonly an infection of the mouth and lips, "fever blisters", "cold sores". *Incubation period:* 1-26 days. *Communicable:* most contagious from time sores are present until they heal and scabs fall off. Transmission can occur during asymptomatic periods when lesions are not present.	Virus stays dormant in body and successive eruptions occur commonly as a result of stress or other illnesses. Recurrence tends to become less severe and fewer over the years and in some, stops recurring. *Complications:* uncommon but include encephalitis, meningitis.	Incurable. Antivirals are given to control symptoms and suppress recurrent episodes. *Symptomatic:* sitz bath, analgesics, antipyretics. Pouring water on perineum while voiding may decrease pain with urination. Keep lesions clean and dry (i.e., well-ventilated clothing). *Prevention:* avoid touching active blisters, hand washing. Sexual abstinence. Condom use can decrease risk of infection. Cesarean section birth for maternal prodromal symptoms or active herpes to prevent neonatal herpes.
Cytomegalovirus (CMV)	Usually asymptomatic. If symptomatic, resembles mononucleosis (fever, sore throat, fatigue, swollen glands). *Fetal effects:* Usually none but many include temporary enlarged liver and spleen, jaundice, to death. Permanent symptoms in newborns may not be evident	Transmitted through contact with infected body fluid (semen and vaginal secretions, blood, breast milk, urine, feces, respiratory secretions) and organ transplantation. Transplacental transmission.	Virus remains in body for life. Immunosuppressed individuals are at risk for reactivation of latent virus and frequent infectious episodes. Transmission is so common that 60% of children in day-care centers have CMV in urine or saliva (usually	Most healthy people have no symptoms. Those with serious infection are treated with antiviral medications. *Prevention:* hand-washing, personal hygiene, do not share eating utensils or drinks.

TABLE 8-3   **Communicable Diseases, Community Health Concerns, and Treatment—cont'd**

Disease (Causative Agent)	Symptoms	Mode of Transmission	Complications and Community Health Concerns	Treatment or Nursing Management
Sexually Transmitted Route—cont'd				
Cytomegalovirus (CMV)—cont'd	at birth but usually present within first years of life; low IQ, developmental disabilities, mental retardation, hearing and vision impairment.		spread by not washing hands).	
Genital warts or human papillomavirus (HPV)	Soft, pink-gray warts with "cauliflower appearance" in and around sex organs, which may or may not be painful, may or may not be visible. Warts may also be present in the anus and mouth. Infants may develop respiratory symptoms as a result of infection in the throat and mouth acquired during vaginal delivery.	Direct contact with warts; primarily sexually transmitted. Rarely passed to infants through the birth canal. *Incubation:* usually 1-3 months after contact but may be longer. *Communicable:* no cure; therefore an infected person may be contagious for life.	*Complications:* most serious complication is the link between the disease and malignancies of the cervix and genital tract. Regular pap screening is recommended. Can block opening to the vagina, urethra, rectum, or throat.	No cure. May resolve without treatment. Remove or destroy symptomatic warts: cryotherapy, laser therapy, electrocautery, surgical removal, topical or injected agents. *Prevention:* abstain from sexual contact, use condoms to decrease risk of infection. Vaccine immunization.
Gonorrhea (*Neisseria gonorrhoeae*) (bacteria)	Frequently asymptomatic infection of endocervical, vaginal, urethral, pharynx or rectum sites. Symptomatic infection: Women—pain, purulent greenish vaginal discharge, pain in the genital and pelvic areas, dysuria. Abnormal vaginal bleeding after intercourse and between periods. Men—purulent white, yellow or green discharge from the penis, dysuria, urinary frequency. Pharynx—sore throat. Rectum—mucous discharge, intense irritation. Infants born during an active case may contract conjunctivitis (ophthalmia neonatorum).	Primarily sexual contact. Mother to infant via passage through birth canal. *Incubation period:* usually 2-7 days to 3 weeks after sexual contact.	Incidence is most prevalent in young adults (15-35 yr). *Complications:* women—pelvic inflammatory disease (PID), ectopic pregnancy, premature delivery, sterility. Men—epididymitis, infertility. Rare complications; arthritis, sepsis, meningitis, endocarditis.	Antimicrobials. Antibiotics appropriate to treat *Chlamydia* (if *Chlamydia* is not ruled out) are prescribed as many people are infected with both simultaneously. Sex partners should be referred for evaluation, test, and treatment. Educate to avoid sexual intercourse until therapy is completed. *Prevention:* abstain from sexual activity. Use condoms to decrease risk of infection.
Chlamydia (*Chlamydia trachomatis*) (bacteria)	Frequently asymptomatic. Symptomatic infection: urethritis, dysuria. Women—abnormal vaginal discharge, inflammation of cervix, bleeding between periods. Men—abnormal discharge from penis. Infant effects as a result of vaginal delivery: mucous membrane infection of the eyes (conjunctivitis) and respiratory tract (pneumonia).	Primarily sexual contact (vaginal, anal, or oral sex) but infections can occur in other areas of the body if contact is made with the bacteria. Transmission to neonate by passage through the birth canal. *Incubation period:* 1-3 weeks	*Complications:* women—pelvic inflammatory disease, ectopic pregnancy, premature delivery, infertility. Men—epididymitis, sterility. Annual screening of sexually active women age 25 and younger and women with high-risk sexual behaviors is recommended. All pregnant women should be tested for *Chlamydia*.	Antibiotics. Evaluate, test, and treat sexual partners. *Chlamydia* frequently occurs with gonorrhea, therefore presumptive treatment of both infections is appropriate. Instruct to abstain from sexual intercourse until treatment is completed. *Prevention:* abstinence from sexual contact, use condoms to decrease risk of infection.

Continued

TABLE 8-3   Communicable Diseases, Community Health Concerns, and Treatment—cont'd

Disease (Causative Agent)	Symptoms	Mode of Transmission	Complications and Community Health Concerns	Treatment or Nursing Management
Sexually Transmitted Route—cont'd				
Syphilis (*Treponema pallidum*) (bacteria)	Disease stages if left untreated. *Primary stage:* chancre sore at site of infection (genital, rectum, lips); usually painless with contagious fluid. *Secondary stage:* occurs 3-6 weeks later; may have fever, sore throat, body rash (especially soles of feet and palms of hands), sores (mucous patches that are highly infectious), inflamed eyes, patchy hair loss. *Latent stage:* signs and symptoms disappear but infection remains in the body. *Tertiary stage:* destruction of body organs (brain, skeleton, heart, and large blood vessels) via lesions called gummas. Fetal infection, "congenital syphilis": abortion, stillbirth, skeletal deformities, organ defects.	Primary transmission occurs via contact with mucocutaneous syphilis lesions during vaginal, anal, or oral sex. Mother to fetus transmission during pregnancy. *Incubation period:* approximately 3 weeks. *Communicable:* infectious to others in the primary and secondary stages, rare after first year of infection.	Incidence is increasing, especially among young adults. *Complications:* blindness, brain damage, dementia, paralysis, heart disease, death.	Parenteral penicillin; if individual is allergic to penicillin, other antibiotics are given. *Prevention:* abstinence from sexual activity, use of condoms can decrease the risk.
Vector Route				
West Nile virus	Frequently asymptomatic. *Mild infection:* fever, fatigue, nausea and vomiting, anorexia, headache, myalgia, rash, lymphadenopathy. *Severe infection:* encephalitis, meningitis, weakness, high fever, change in level of consciousness, seizure.	Mosquito bite from mosquito that bites both an infected bird and human. Rarely spread via intrauterine transmission, blood transfusion or organ transplantation. *Incubation period:* 3-14 days.	Most infections are mild and clinically unapparent. Severe illness more commonly associated with advanced age. Peak occurrence in late summer to early fall. Complications: permanent neurologic effects, death. Dead birds, a virus reservoir that mosquitoes feed on, may be a sign of the virus in an area.	*Supportive:* hospitalization, intravenous fluids, respiratory support, prevention of secondary infections. *Prevention:* avoid mosquito bites via repellant use, wear long-sleeves and pants and socks when outside; avoid outside hours from dusk to dawn. Eliminate and drain standing water, which is where mosquitoes breed.
Lyme disease (*Borrelia burgdorferi*) (spirochete)	Erythema migrans or bulls eye rash at site of tick bite, fever, malaise, headache, muscle aches, and arthralgia.	Bite of tick that became infected after feeding on deer affected with the spirochete. *Incubation period:* usually 7-14 days.	Peak occurrence: Late spring and summer months. Major risk factors include spending time outdoors, geography where Lyme disease is endemic, and season. *Complications:* arthritis, neurologic and cardiac disorders.	*Treatment:* antibiotics. *Prevention:* reduce exposure to tick bites; avoid walking in tall grass and brush, wear long-sleeved shirts and pants and socks, use tick repellant, carefully examine skin for ticks.

PRIMARY PREVENTION

The major thrust of community health agencies in controlling communicable diseases is primary prevention. Community health nurses play a vital role in eliminating or reducing the spread of disease by providing immunizations, prophylactic measures, and health education. Health teaching efforts are geared toward risk reduction (e.g., increasing public awareness of risky behavior, eliminating or reducing the risk of personal behaviors, and providing information for caregivers on methods to isolate and destroy bacterial or viral agents and on self-protection techniques).

Immunizations

Vaccines are the most effective way to control contagious diseases. Immunizations are available for chickenpox, measles, mumps, rubella, diphtheria, pertussis, tetanus, polio, influenza, and hepatitis A and B. Research continues on the development of vaccines for HIV, herpesvirus, and cytomegalovirus. Rabies vaccine is only selectively available to persons at high risk because of costs and side effects. Although a TB vaccine is available, it is not in common use in the United States because the rate of infection has been low and the vaccine is only moderately effective. In conjunction with the *Healthy People 2010* objectives, community health nurses should strive to increase immunization rates among all designated target groups by providing education on the need for immunization, identifying and targeting risk groups, and improving access to immunization through public and privately financed efforts. The national coverage rates exceed 90% for school-aged children (USDHHS, 2006b). The most significant progress has been made in *Haemophilus influenzae* type b and hepatitis B vaccinations.

Community health nurses educate parents of children as well as susceptible adults about the importance of immunizations and supply immunizations through clinic facilities (see the *Healthy People 2010* box on this page). When reviewing individual records, nurses should be especially diligent to ensure that vaccinations for all clients are up to date. Antibody titers can identify clients whose antibody levels have waned. Revaccination is often necessary for individuals with low antibody titers.

Elderly individuals need a tailored immunization program. By age 65, most older Americans have developed an immunity to measles (rubeola) and diphtheria, but they need to maintain their polio, tetanus, influenza, hepatitis, and pneumococcal vaccine protection. Approximately 40% of tetanus cases occur in persons over the age of 60 years (CDC, 2007a). Community health nurses need to check for outdated or nonexistent immunizations in elderly individuals and other at-risk groups. Influenza vaccines are modified each year to accommodate new strains. Unless elderly and chronically ill persons are revaccinated yearly, they may not be protected from the most recent form of influenza.

All clients should be well informed of the risks associated with each vaccine they receive. Every health care provider who administers immunizations should be aware of the responsibility to provide this information to the client or, in the case of children, to the parents.

Nurses should screen clients before administering the vaccine. The person's health status should be assessed. The individual should be asked if he or she has been ill recently or under a physician's care; if he or she has had previous reactions to medications or foods; and, if female, if she might be pregnant. In many situations, immunizations should not be given or should be delayed. These circumstances include the following:

- If any child experiences seizures after an initial dose of a vaccine series (e.g., diphtheria-pertussis-tetanus), the child should not receive the additional doses in the series.
- Immunizations probably should not be given to clients with chronic renal disease, because in such clients the ability to clear medication from the body is compromised.

■ HEALTHY PEOPLE 2010 ■
Objectives for Primary Prevention: Immunization

1. Increase immunization levels as follows:
   Achieve immunization coverage of at least 90% among children 19 to 35 months of age.

Immunization	1998 Baseline
4 doses diphtheria-tetanus-pertussis (DTP)	84%
3 doses *Haemophilus influenzae* type b (Hib)	93%
1 dose measles-mumps-rubella (MMR)	92%
3 doses hepatitis B (HB)	87%
3 doses polio	91%
1 dose varicella (chickenpox)	43%

2. Maintain immunization coverage at 95% for children in licensed daycare facilities and children in kindergarten through the first grade (baseline: 87% to 96% in 1997-1998).

3. Increase the rate of immunization coverage to 90% among adults 65 years of age or older and 60% among high-risk adults 18 to 64 years of age.

Immunization	2010 Target Goal Adults	1995 Baseline Adults
Noninstitutionalized Adults 65 Years of Age or Older		
Influenza vaccine	90%	64%
Pneumococcal vaccine	90%	46%
High-Risk Adults 18 to 64 Years of Age		
Influenza vaccine	60%	26%
Pneumococcal vaccine	60%	13%

4. Increase the proportion of young children and adolescents who receive all vaccines that have been recommended for universal administration for at least 5 years.

	2010 Target Goal	1998 Baseline
Young children of 19 to 25 months (4 DTAP, 3 polio, 1 MMR, 3 Hib, 3 HB)	80%	73%
Adolescents 13 to 19 years of age	Developmental	No baseline (0)

5. Increase to 62% the proportion of children who participate in fully operational population-based immunization registries (baseline: 21% of children under 6 years of age in 1999).

6. Increase to 55% the proportion of providers who have had systematically measured the vaccination coverage levels among children in their practice populations (baseline: 40% of public and 11% of private providers in 1997).

From U.S. Department of Health and Human Services. (2000). *Healthy People 2010: Understanding and improving health* (2nd ed.). Washington, DC: U.S. Government Printing Office: and U.S. Department of Health and Human Services. (2006). *Healthy People 2010: Midcourse review.* Washington, DC: U.S. Government Printing Office.

- Tuberculin test results may be incorrect if the test is given shortly (less than 1 month) after a live-virus vaccine is administered. Tuberculin testing should be performed simultaneously with any live vaccine administration or at least 30 days after vaccination.

Community health nurses must provide health teaching at the time of immunization. The nurse should encourage the client to remain on site for at least 15 to 20 minutes after vaccine administration to ensure that no reaction occurs. Epinephrine should be kept available so that it can be administered to reduce the effects of a reaction, if any.

Documentation is very important. Every client should be given a written record of the immunizations she or he has received, when these were administered, and possible reactions. Clinic or organization records must be comprehensive to comply with the National Vaccine Injury Compensation Act.

Prophylactic Measures

Prophylactic measures are aimed at reducing the risk of illness in persons who have already been exposed to a communicable disease. Chemoprophylactic actions include administration of vaccines, vaccine booster doses, or other medication. Prophylactic measures are not available for all communicable diseases. Community health nurses should know for which diseases risk-reduction medication is available so that they can direct persons who have been exposed to the appropriate treatment. **Website Resource 8E** provides selected prophylactic recommendations for specific communicable diseases.

Sanitation

Community health nurses must be aware of the sanitary conditions of the environment in which they and their clients live, work, and play. Some homes do not have running water or adequate sewage disposal; community health nurses may practice in neighborhoods in which this is considered normal. Community health nurses may be called into neighborhoods during a disaster when sanitation services have been suspended temporarily. For example, during riots and after hurricanes, entire neighborhoods may be without adequate, safe sanitation resources. When no adequate source of safe water and no methods of safe waste disposal or safe food preparation and storage are available, extra precautions become necessary.

Employment

Nurses have an additional need to be aware of health codes in employment situations. States and the federal government have established employment regulations that attempt to safeguard workers, and knowledge of the regulations affecting local employers is important. Nurses must play an integral role in educational, research, and practice efforts to develop and enforce these regulations.

Health care workers themselves may be at risk. Nurses, physicians, police officers, firefighters, paramedics, ambulance personnel, morticians, and persons in other similar professions are at risk for most communicable diseases, including TB, tetanus, typhoid, hepatitis B, HIV infection, and diphtheria. Many agencies require employees to receive immunizations and specialized education to protect them from communicable diseases. OSHA has directed that employees be provided with safety measures to help protect them from blood-borne pathogens. OSHA requires that employers provide health workers with yearly in-service education on infectious disease control and eliminate or minimize occupational exposure to blood-borne pathogens (Keith, 2003). An increasing number of health care facilities are offering HBV vaccine at no cost to their employees.

Travel

Community health nurses are frequently called on to advise clients traveling to other countries about protection from infectious diseases. Nurses should remind clients about differences in climate, hygiene, food preparation, water purity, and sewage management. Simple practices such as eating only fruits or vegetables that can be peeled and using bottled water for drinking and brushing the teeth are effective preventive measures. Caution about diseases that are endemic to the region and disease-specific safety precautions should be provided to travelers.

Information on mandatory immunizations is available from local health departments and the CDC. Community nurses should remind travelers to allow enough time to receive all the necessary immunizations (6 months may be needed). Many immunizations cannot be given together, and some (e.g., for hepatitis) require a series of inoculations over a set time to provide maximal protection.

Community Support Programs and Services

Nurses play an integral role in planning and implementing community support programs and services to improve the health of the nation. Many of the *Healthy People 2010* objectives can be addressed through primary prevention efforts. Nurses are involved in devising prevention programs aimed at improving environmental conditions and reducing the spread of communicable diseases. Community health nurses also participate in specific strategies to decrease the incidence of HIV infection, STDs, and other infectious diseases (see the *Healthy People 2010* box on page 227). Nurses can educate the community on the importance of being tested for HIV and HBV; they can instruct individuals and families on methods of preventing and transmitting STDs; they can enlighten communities on the importance of immunizations for children, adults, and elderly individuals; and they can take part in community efforts to improve sanitation measures.

PREVENTION RELATED TO MODE OF TRANSMISSION

Health education on preventive measures can be taught to family members and significant others who are at risk or are in direct contact with infected persons. Community health nurses can tailor general precautions to the specific route of transmission.

Respiratory Route

For diseases spread by the respiratory route, action should be geared toward reducing the risk of contact with droplets to eliminate spread. In light of the risk that pneumonia, TB, and other respiratory conditions pose to persons who are exposed, containing respiratory secretions is vital. Affected persons should be instructed to sneeze and cough into tissues and dispose of them in a receptacle. Although most pathogens die when exposed to heat, light, and air, frequent hand-washing will further reduce the threat of passing viable organisms from the hand to other persons.

■ HEALTHY PEOPLE 2010 ■
Objectives to Reduce Risk for STDs and HIV/AIDS

Education and Counseling

1. Increase to 90% the proportion of middle schools, junior high schools, and senior high schools that provide school health education on HIV/AIDS and STDs (baseline: 65% in 1994).
2. Increase to 25% the proportion of college and university students who receive information from their institution on each of the six priority health risk behavior areas: injuries, tobacco use, alcohol and illicit drug use, sexual behaviors that cause unintended pregnancies and STDs, dietary patterns that cause disease, and inadequate physical activity (baseline: 6% of undergraduates in 1995).
3. Increase the proportion of young adults who have received formal or informal instruction before turning 18 years of age on the following reproductive health issues: abstinence, birth control methods, HIV/AIDS, prevention of STDs through safer sex practices (baseline for formal instruction: 86% of women and 83% of men on abstinence; 70% of women and 66% of men on birth control in 2002).
4. Increase the proportion of adolescents 12 to 17 years of age who perceive great risk associated with substance abuse.

Risky Behavior	2010 Target Goal Percentage	Baseline 2002 Percentage
Consume five or more alcoholic drinks at one time	50	38
Smoke marijuana one time per month	36	32
Use cocaine one time per month	57	51

Behavior Change

1. Increase to 75% the proportion of individuals 15 to 19 years of age who have never engaged in sexual intercourse before the age of 15 (baseline: 62% of women; 57% of men 15 to 19 years of age in 1995).
2. Increase by 12% the population of adolescents who abstain from sexual intercourse or use condoms if currently sexually active (baseline: of adolescents in grades 9 to 12 in 1999, 50% report no intercourse, 27% intercourse but not in last 12 months, 58% recently sexually active and used condom at last intercourse).

Screening Programs

1. Increase to 70% the number of substance abuse treatment facilities that offer HIV and AIDS education, counseling and support (includes HIV screening) (baseline: 58% in 1997).
2. Increase to 62% the proportion of sexually active women 25 years of age or younger who are screened annually for genital *Chlamydia* infections in primary health care setting (baseline: 25% of women in managed care and 41% of women in Medicaid managed care in 2002).

From U.S. Department of Health and Human Services. (2000). *Healthy People 2010: Understanding and improving health* (2nd ed.). Washington, DC: U.tS. Government Printing Office; and U.S. Department of Health and Human Services. (2006). *Healthy People 2010: Midcourse review.* Washington, DC: U.S. Government Printing Office
AIDS, Acquired immunodeficiency syndrome; *HIV,* human immunodeficiency virus; *STD,* sexually transmitted disease.

Integumentary Route

Reducing the spread of parasites to uninfected persons depends on personal hygiene habits. Hats, combs, brushes, and other personal items should never be shared. Parasitic spread is especially difficult to control in children; hence, the recurring outbreaks of head lice in elementary schools. Scrupulous bathing and hand-washing with hot water and soap reduce the potential transfer of eggs, viruses, and bacteria. When close personal contact encourages spread, sexual contact should be avoided with the infected individual until he or she is free of parasites.

Clothing and bed linens should be washed in hot water. Sharing clothing and bedding with infected individuals should be avoided. Sealing infected linens or personal items in plastic bags for 2 weeks can also kill mites and lice.

Gastrointestinal Route

Prevention of gastrointestinal diseases is geared toward reducing the chance of transferring pathologic organisms to the mouth and digestive tract. Meticulous hand-washing after toileting or changing infant diapers and before working with food products is imperative. Fingernails should be kept short and the area under the nails cleaned regularly to eliminate this potential reservoir. For organisms that thrive in stool, isolation and careful disposal of infected stool and clean bathroom facilities are important.

Proper storage and refrigeration of foods, as well as effective food preparation and handling, are crucial. Fastidious cleaning of equipment used in food preparation is essential in both homes and institutions. Chemical treatment of the water supply, proper disposal of garbage, and sanitation of sewage completes the efforts at reducing pathogenic organisms.

Serum Route

For blood-borne diseases, efforts are directed toward reducing the risk of exposure to infected blood and blood products. Infected persons should be monitored for adequate control of body secretions, including blood and semen. Sexual contact increases the opportunity for exposure to contaminated blood, and such contact should be discontinued or barrier protection used. Needle-exchange programs are aimed at reducing the risk of infection among users of illicit intravenous drugs. Users are given sterile needles in exchange for used ones. Needle-exchange programs are controversial because some fear they will encourage the use of illicit drugs. Currently, there are 146 needle-exchange programs in the United States. In 2002 those programs exchanged 24.9 million syringes (CDC, 2005b). The number exchanged is an indicator of the extent of injected drug use in this country. Although needle-exchange programs are controversial, they seem to be effective in reducing the spread of HIV, HBV, and HBC infections (Villarreal & Fogg, 2006). Most intravenous drug users (over 70%) are infected with one or more of these diseases within 5 years of initiating drug use (Baciewicz, 2005; National Institute on Drug Abuse, 2006). Prevention efforts have now expanded to include the following:

- Vaccination against HBV
- Treatment for substance abuse
- Tailored HIV prevention counseling and testing
- Prevention of sexual transmission through education and provision of barrier birth control supplies

- Additional health care services tailored to the needs of intravenous users

Meticulous screening of the blood supply is important to reduce risk to clients who must be transfused or maintained on blood products. Efforts to improve the safety of the blood supply continue. One measure of success is the reduction in hepatitis B virus and HIV infections among individuals who must receive blood or blood products. Vaccination for hepatitis B is recommended for all risk groups, including clients who must receive blood products on a long-term basis as well as health care personnel, first responders, and police officials. Community health nurses should be careful to identify every individual at risk and encourage immunization.

Health care workers must practice universal precautions at all times. Working outside the hospital setting should not lull community health nurses into be less vigilant in using appropriate precautions. Box 8-4 provides a useful guide for teaching home safety precautions to clients and their families.

Sexually Transmitted Route

For sexually transmitted diseases, precautions essentially involve reducing sexually risky behavior. Methods include abstaining from sexual intercourse, reducing the number of sex partners, using barrier contraception during intercourse and foreplay, and avoiding sexual activity with infected persons who have not been treated or have not completed treatment. Community health nurses should concentrate their public

---

Box 8-4   Guidelines for Infection Control in the Home

Personal Cleanliness—Personal Articles

1. Hand-washing is the single most important infection control method. Hand-washing after using toilet facilities or after contact with body fluids is important. Wash hands with soap and water or antimicrobial foam or gel.
2. Do not share equipment potentially contaminated with body secretions, such as thermometers, razors, or toothbrushes.

Kitchen and Bathrooms

1. Eating utensils used by all household members must be washed with hot water and soap.
2. Kitchen counters should be cleaned with scouring powder or weak bleach solution (1:9 solution or 10% bleach and 90% water).
3. Refrigerators should be cleaned regularly with soap and water to control molds.
4. Kitchen floor should be mopped weekly or more often, if necessary. Dispose of mop water by pouring down toilet and disinfecting toilet with bleach solution.
5. Toilet, bathtub, shower, and bathroom floor should be cleaned with a freshly prepared bleach solution. If the client spills urine or has watery diarrhea that splashes onto the toilet seat, the seat must be wiped off after each spill and then cleaned with the bleach solution.
6. Clean sponges used to wash floors or clean up body fluid spills by soaking them for 5 minutes in a bleach solution. When at all possible, use paper towels rather than sponges, because they can be disposed of and do not harbor germs.

Food Preparation

1. Wash hands thoroughly before food preparation.
2. Do not lick fingers or mixing spoon while cooking.
3. Avoid unpasteurized milk to reduce risk of *Salmonella* exposure; thoroughly wash uncooked chicken; do not use cracked eggs.

Laundry and Linens

1. Clothing or linen soiled with body fluids should be stored separately in a plastic bag and should be washed separately in a washing machine using hot water, detergent, and bleach. Liquid Lysol can be used for colored laundry. (Wear disposable gloves when touching the soiled clothes or linen.) Linens not soiled by body fluids may be handled in the usual manner without special precautions.
2. Household members should not share used towels and washcloths. Other members can safely use them after they have been laundered.

Preventing Cross-Infection

1. Wear gloves when handling body fluids, linens, or other objects contaminated with body fluids. (People with exudative lesions or weeping dermatitis should refrain from caring for the client until the condition resolves.)
2. Disposable gowns or aprons may be worn to protect clothing from becoming soiled with body fluids.
3. Caregivers with a cold or influenza should wear a mask when in close personal contact with a person with acquired immunodeficiency syndrome (AIDS) to protect the client, because clients with AIDS are highly susceptible to opportunistic infections.
4. Ensure good ventilation in the living quarters.

Trash Disposal

1. Body wastes such as urine, feces, and blood should be flushed down the toilet.
2. Discard dressings, diapers, incontinent pads, or any materials soiled with body fluids and secretions in a plastic bag. Pour in a 1:9 bleach-water solution until soiled contents are soaked. Place sealed bag into another plastic bag, seal again, and place in regular trash.
3. Sharps should be discarded in a special sharps container provided by the home care agency. Transport container back to agency for disposal when container is three-fourths full. If no sharps container is available, use a metal coffee can or a puncture-proof plastic container to discard needles and sharps. When container is three-fourths full, pour 1:9 bleach-water solution over sharps material. Seal container, double-bag in plastic trash bags, and discard in the trash.*†

Sexual Practices

1. When recommended, precautions must be taken to prevent the sharing of body secretions; therefore, information about safe sex practices should be provided to the client and family members. Pamphlets and counseling are available.

Pets

1. Clean birdcages wearing gloves and mask, because birds can spread psittacosis.
2. Clean cat litter boxes wearing gloves and mask to prevent toxoplasmosis.
3. Change water in tropical fish tanks wearing gloves and mask to prevent *Mycobacterium* infection.

Adapted from Rhinehart, E., & Friedman, M. M. (1999). *Infection control in home care.* Gaithersburg, MD: Aspen; and Trotter, J. (1992). Guidelines for people with AIDS living in the community. Unpublished.
*Do not place with recyclables.
†If allowed by state law.

education efforts on these areas and aim their efforts at populations at special risk.

The majority of HIV-positive individuals acquired the infection through sexual activity (CDC, 2006p). After considerable progress was made in reducing the spread of HIV in the homosexual population, evidence suggests that the effort has stalled. Consistent use of condoms can prevent approximately one half of all sexually transmitted HIV infections and reduce the incidence of other STDs as well.

Targeting adolescents and women, the two fastest growing risk groups, is vital. Approximately 40% of U.S. adolescents engage in unprotected sexual intercourse (Kaiser Family Foundation, 2006; see Chapter 24). The spread of HIV infection in adolescents is primarily through heterosexual activity, not intravenous drug use. When planning programs for adolescents, community health nurses should try to provide a reality-based experience by encouraging clients to delay sexual activity and to act responsibly when engaging in such activity and by providing access to or information on resources for condoms. Teenaged speakers who are infected with HIV are a powerful tool for communicating the realities of ignoring the problem and should be used whenever possible.

Heterosexual women are another group at increased risk for STDs and HIV infection. Only 20% to 25% of sexually active American women have male partners who use condoms, and even in these cases, such use is sporadic (USDHHS, 2006b). Socioeconomic status impacts condom use; poor women are less likely to have male partners who use condoms. For women who are reluctant to insist on condom use or whose partners refuse to wear condoms, there is a condom designed especially for women that is recommended for both contraceptive use and STD prevention. Nurses can provide women with information on the availability and use of condoms for women, which is an effective method of barrier protection (Workowski & Levine, 2002).

SECONDARY PREVENTION

The second level of prevention includes measures directed at early detection of disease to provide early treatment, ensure treatment effectiveness, and minimize the spread of disease within the population (see the *Healthy People 2010* box on this page). Secondary prevention activities include antibiotic drug therapy, contact tracing, and follow-up of persons who are infected or exposed. The community health nurse's role in secondary prevention includes identification of cases (screening and case finding); confirmation of illness; administration or observation of administration of medication; and provision of education, oversight, and support of caregivers.

Screening Programs

Screening programs are designed to evaluate a large number of people for possible infection. Early detection can reduce complications and diminish further transmission of disease in a community. One early example is the screening of immigrants on Ellis Island between 1890 and 1920. More than 20 million people were evaluated by the Marine Hospital Service for signs and symptoms of disease. Persons who were found to be infected with a communicable disease (typhus, cholera, plague, smallpox, or yellow fever) were denied entry into the United States until they were no longer infected.

■ HEALTHY PEOPLE 2010 ■
Objectives for Secondary Prevention for Communicable Diseases

1. Increase the number of admissions to substance abuse treatment for injection drug users to 256,680 (baseline: 215,560 in 1997).
2. Increase the proportion of human immunodeficiency virus–infected adolescents and adults who receive testing, treatment, and prophylaxis consistent with current Public Health Service treatment guidelines.

Treatment-Prophylaxis	2010 Target Goal	1997 Baseline
Pneumocystis carinii pneumonia prophylaxis	95%	80%
Viral load testing	Increase	No baseline
Any antiretroviral therapy	95%	80%

3. Increase to 90% the proportion of all tuberculosis clients who complete curative therapy within 12 months (baseline: 74% in 1997).
4. Increase to at least 85% the proportion of contacts, including other high-risk persons with latent tuberculosis infection, who complete a course of treatment (baseline: 62% in 1997).

From U.S. Department of Health and Human Services. (2000). *Healthy People 2010: Understanding and improving health* (2nd ed.). Washington, DC: U.S. Government Printing Office; and U.S. Department of Health and Human Services. (2006). *Healthy People 2010: Midcourse review.* Washington, DC: U.S. Government Printing Office.

Screening for communicable diseases involves interviews, physical assessment, procurement of laboratory samples, and diagnostic testing. Screening programs for communicable diseases are most often cost effective when the screening procedure is relatively quick and inexpensive and the communicable disease is highly infectious or has the potential to inflict serious harm on the population. Screening may be done as part of employment (e.g., TB, hepatitis) or school enrollment (e.g., college requirements for a measles titer). More frequently, screening is targeted at special risk groups; for example, studies show that people often have more than one STD at a time (USDHHS, 2000). Nurse practitioners, community health nurses, and others who provide care should be aware of the need to screen for other STDs at the time a person seeks treatment for an STD (e.g., gonorrhea, chlamydia, syphilis). All TB clients should be screened for HIV infection, and all HIV clients should be screened for TB.

For most communicable diseases, screening is done for both public protection and early treatment. Because HIV infection has no cure, screening programs are more controversial. Opponents argue against screening because, once identified, infected individuals may be discriminated against in employment opportunities, health insurance plans, and other areas. Proponents argue that much is to be gained by early identification of HIV infection. HIV screening is done for the following reasons:

- To promote behavior changes
- To provide entry into clinical care
- To provide information for partner notification and education
- To protect the blood supply
- To protect the fetuses of HIV-positive women

Screening increases population protection by reducing the risk to close contacts. Although HIV screening will not facilitate a cure, it does allow HIV-infected individuals the opportunity to seek supportive care earlier and thus increase their quality of life. The CDC suggests that hospitals and clinics with a large number of HIV and AIDS cases should routinely test for infection. Screening guidelines are currently under revision and are expected to include additional recommendations for routine screening (USDHHS, 2006b).

HIV/AIDS screening is still voluntary and confidential and should include a pretest and posttest counseling session. Clients who test positive are referred for further services, but all clients are counseled about risky behaviors and safer sex practices. Resources for counseling and teaching clients with HIV or AIDS are available by calling the special toll-free PHS telephone number listed in Community Resources for Practice at the end of the chapter. The CDC recommends HIV screening for pregnant women and newborn babies (USDHHS, 2006b). Many states require screening of infants at birth because early identification of HIV-positive infants allows for immediate treatment and consistent follow-up.

Mandatory Versus Voluntary Screening for Human Immunodeficiency Virus.
In 1999 the Institute of Medicine recommended voluntary HIV testing of all pregnant women. In response to this recommendation, the CDC developed screening guidelines for all populations, including pregnant women (CDC, 2001b, 2001c). The CDC guidelines, currently under revision, recommend voluntary screening for all pregnant women. Approximately 25 states have laws or regulations covering HIV testing for pregnant women. Some states mandate testing; others recommend testing. Many states require HIV testing of all newborns.

States have mandated screening for certain other risk groups and professions. For example, some states require HIV screening as a condition of employment for health care workers or police officers. Because the rate of HIV infection is nearly five times higher in prisoners than in the general population, 16 states and the federal prison system require HIV testing for all prisoners (Braithwaite & Arriola, 2003). The CDC recommends mandatory testing of all new inmates and periodic voluntary testing of inmates during incarceration (CDC, 2006x). As noted earlier, mandatory testing is controversial. The American Public Health Association and the WHO oppose mandatory testing. Proponents argue that mandatory testing identifies more HIV-positive persons than does voluntary testing (Braithwaite & Arriola, 2003).

Anonymous, Blind, or Confidential Testing.
In addition to undergoing routine testing, people can be screened for communicable diseases in anonymous, blind, or confidential programs. These three methods are normally used when screening for communicable diseases that carry a degree of public censure or stigma. Blind screening involves testing samples drawn for other purposes and stripped of identification (e.g., screening of hospitalized patients who have blood drawn for routine admission blood work). The purpose is to get an accurate estimate of the incidence of communicable disease in the population. Blind studies can provide valuable information about patterns but do not allow for treatment, because samples are not traceable to the person who provided the sample.

Anonymous testing allows people to register for screening under an identifier code or number, and confidential testing registers people by name. In both cases, test results are available only to the client. Anonymous testing is offered as a strategy to increase people's willingness to come for testing. Provision of anonymous testing may increase the number of persons willing to be tested for HIV infection. The CDC recommends the use of name-based patient testing, and that recommendation has been adopted by 45 state and local health departments (USDHHS, 2006b).

Screening procedures for HIV and AIDS have been altered to better achieve a decrease in risky behavior. At first, anonymous and confidential testing results were supplied over the telephone. Currently, however, most programs require individuals who are tested to pick up the results (even when negative) in person to provide an additional opportunity to counsel clients on risk factors, risky behaviors, and safer sex precautions. Community health nurses and others involved in HIV screening programs should be aware that some people become depressed after learning of their HIV-positive status. Individuals newly diagnosed with HIV infection should be referred for counseling and support services.

Case Finding and Contact Tracing.
The purpose of case finding is to identify every case of disease and to provide swift treatment for new cases. Community health nurses often function as case finders. Searching for potential cases begins by identifying individuals with the most intimate contact (level I) and proceeds to those with less close contact (levels II and III) (Figure 8-11). For most communicable diseases, if no cases are discovered among the level I contacts, proceeding to level II is unnecessary. For example, when screening schoolchildren for cases of head lice, the nurse would first screen the grade in which the contact case was found and any grades that contain family members of that child. If these grades are free of lice, screening the rest of the school serves little purpose. Nurses should consider the cost effectiveness of health screening and save resources for necessary services.

All sexual partners should be identified when performing contact tracing for STDs and HIV. People will occasionally have multiple sex partners whom they consider casual acquaintances rather than close partners. For contact tracing, all sexual partners are level I contacts. Case finding requires patience and sensitivity on the part of the investigator. Some communicable diseases, particularly STDs and HIV infection, may be a source of embarrassment for the infected individuals. If the nurse is not accepting and caring during the interviews, clients may not

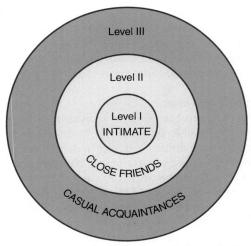

FIGURE 8-11 Priority of case-finding contacts.

cooperate, which reduces the chance of locating potential cases. Box 8-5 provides a number of golden rules that interviewers may find useful when conducting contact tracing interviews.

Specimen Collection

Community health nurses are often expected to obtain specimens from clients, prepare the specimens for transport to the laboratory, and receive the results. Accurate laboratory results depend on correct collection, storage, and transport of specimens. The nurse should take care to follow laboratory directions exactly (e.g., refrigerate the sample, if so directed). Laboratories require that accurate information accompany the specimen to assist in the identification of the infectious agent. In addition, nurses need to be safety conscious, because specimen collection can be dangerous if the nurse is careless. All nurses must consistently follow appropriate infection control measures, including universal precautions (see Chapter 31).

Community health nurses should be familiar with the usual time frame for receiving the results of each test. Bacterial culture results are usually available in a short time because most bacteria grow in hours. *Mycobacterium* organisms (i.e., TB agent) may take longer (sometimes weeks). Nurses should counsel clients about the expected arrival time for the results to help reduce some of the wait-time anxiety.

Comfort Measures

Most communicable diseases are treated at home, not in the hospital. In addition to care and treatment regimens applicable to specific diseases, the nurse can teach general symptomatic comfort and care measures to caregivers.

In general, rest, adequate nutrition and hydration, and fever control are important. Adequate hydration is essential and may be problematic in children and older adults. The nurse should instruct caregivers to be alert for signs of poor hydration (e.g., poor skin turgor, depressed fontanels in infants). Intravenous

fluid replacement may be necessary, especially if gastrointestinal upsets are severe, as may be the case in salmonellosis or shigellosis. Aspirin or acetaminophen can be used to reduce fever. High fevers are common in children and may require water sponge baths for cooling. Aspirin should be avoided in children because of the link to Reye's syndrome.

Skin disruptions such as blisters and body rashes require scrupulous hygiene to reduce the risk of infection. Scratching can exacerbate the problem and, in certain conditions, may spread the disease. Some relief from itching may be gained by bathing in tepid water with cornstarch or oatmeal. Children can sleep with cotton gloves on to reduce the risk of scratching in their sleep. Genital eruptions from STDs should be kept clean and as dry as possible. A hair dryer on a low heat setting can be used to ensure that wet skin and skinfolds are completely dry. Wearing of loose clothing and cotton underwear can help to speed healing.

Compliance with the prescribed medication regimen is essential. Failure to follow through with the complete medication regimen is thought to be one important reason for the increasing number of drug-resistant organisms. Compliance can be particularly problematic when therapy is long term, as in TB, for which clients are required to remain on medication long after symptoms have resolved. Nurses can play a vital role by helping clients understand the importance of maintaining drug treatment and by providing oversight to confirm and support compliance.

Documenting resolution of a disease is the important last step in treating the illness. *Test of cure* is the term used to indicate that a treated individual has undergone repeated laboratory tests and is no longer contagious or is free of the disease. This assessment is particularly important for diseases that can linger or relapse if not completely eliminated in an individual (e.g., diphtheria, gonorrhea, chlamydia).

Legal Enforcement

Nurses must become knowledgeable not only about agency regulations for the control of communicable diseases, but also about state statutes and regulations as well as enforcement. States have different regulations concerning enforcement provisions; thus, nurses must explore the rules of the states in which they practice. Some regulations give the nurse an enforcement responsibility. For example, nurses must report the incidence of communicable disease or a violation of sanitary codes.

The law allows public health officials to compel individuals to comply with treatment if noncompliance endangers the general public. Public health officials have the authority to require compliance with treatment and the legal means to ensure compliance through forced institutionalization if all other methods fail. Incarceration is a viable but last-choice option.

Box 8-5   Golden Rules of Interviewing

1. Initial contact should be with a named source, not other household members.
2. If you must leave a telephone message, provide no information other than your name and telephone number.
3. Emphasize client confidentiality related to test results and other services.
4. Allow the contact a choice of interview location and time.
5. In cases involving drugs, do not ask for drug sources or specific drugs.
6. When tracing is performed, interviewees are not to be given the name of the initial contact, no matter how insistent they might become.
7. Incomplete information should be recorded because it may help with later contact tracing.
8. It is possible to be flexible, informal, and supportive and still get all the information required in the survey.
9. Cooperation may be encouraged by explaining the risks; adopting a 'you help us, we will help you' attitude; and leaving a business card with people reluctant to name contacts at the first interview.
10. Respect all contacts.

Modified from Poulin, C., Gyorkos, T. W., MacPhee, J., et al. (1992). Contact-tracing among injection drug users in a rural area. *Canadian Journal of Public Health, 83*(2), 106-108.

Two highly publicized cases of confinement occurred in 2007, both because of failure to comply with treatment requirements for TB disease. In Phoenix, an Eastern European man refused to wear a mask to reduce the risk of infection to others. He was confined to the prison ward of a Phoenix hospital. The first federal case of confinement in 40 years involved a U.S. citizen with XDR-TB who traveled by plane outside the United States against state health department and CDC advice. Upon his return to this county he was confined in a hospital under federal statute while undergoing treatment (Gibbs, 2007).

Community health nurses may be involved in monitoring compliance through directly observed medication administration. When clients are not compliant, nurses may be called on to initiate legal action for confinement or to serve as a witness during court proceedings. Public health laws require that clients be afforded due rights, including counsel and a hearing, when constraint measures are indicated (see Chapter 6).

Exclusion from School

Children who have a communicable disease should be kept home from school. Parents should be encouraged to keep such children at home and should notify the school nurse or daycare personnel when their child has a communicable disease. For example, chickenpox is extremely contagious, especially before the eruption of skin lesions, and no proven effective vaccine has been produced. Children with chickenpox should not return to school until the vesicles have dried as scabs.

Children are also at risk for rapid acquisition of infections caused by pests and organisms transmitted through the integumentary route. Lice and mites can rapidly infect children in daycare centers, classrooms, and summer camps. Nurses should examine all other children and adults when infection is suspected. Parents and guardians will have to be notified about the infections so they can initiate treatment efforts. Children are not usually allowed to return to school until they have been cleared to do so by a health professional. To reduce transmission, nurses can teach children not to share brushes and combs and can teach teachers and daycare workers to observe children for frequent scratching and scratch marks. The earlier the infestation can be detected, the easier it will be to prevent further spread and provide effective treatment.

TERTIARY PREVENTION

Tertiary prevention, the rehabilitation of lingering dysfunctions after illness, is not as frequently addressed in community nursing. Most communicable diseases resolve swiftly, resulting in few long-term rehabilitative needs. Several important exceptions are hepatitis, HIV infection, and some STDs, which produce long-term needs that can be classified as tertiary prevention needs. A significant number of STDs (e.g., herpes infection) have no cure and require lifelong vigilance. Other STDs (e.g., gonorrhea and HPV infection) can lead to complications, especially reproductive problems such as impaired fertility, sterility, or uterine cancer.

KEY IDEAS

1. Knowledge of the characteristics of specific infectious agents, their modes of transmission, and the susceptibility of human hosts helps in identifying ways to prevent the transmission of communicable diseases.
2. The incidence of many communicable diseases has been reduced in the United States since the 1940s as a result of environmental sanitation, immunization, antibiotic treatment, and lifestyle changes. Renewed emphasis is being placed on immunizations to prevent communicable diseases of childhood.
3. STDs and infections from HCV and HIV are rising. Multidrug-resistant forms of TB, gonorrhea, and chlamydia are emerging as a new concern.
4. Health care workers, including community and public health nurses, are at greater risk than is the general public for contracting blood-borne disease. Following universal precautions is essential.
5. All levels of government have some responsibility for preventing and controlling communicable diseases to protect the health of the public. The right of the public to be protected may take precedence over an individual's right to refuse treatment.
6. At the federal level, the CDC collects information on reportable diseases, conducts research, and recommends appropriate prevention and treatment protocols. State and local health departments have responsibilities for carrying out environmental control, identifying and reporting communicable diseases, ensuring the availability of immunizations, and ensuring that communicable diseases are treated when medically possible. Each state has its own laws governing communicable disease control.
7. Many of the *Healthy People 2010* objectives address reduction in the incidence of communicable diseases. Populations are targeted for interventions based on the epidemiology of specific communicable diseases.
8. Community and public health nurses are key health care providers in preventing and controlling communicable diseases.
9. Primary prevention includes minimizing the risk of communicable diseases, emphasizing the importance of immunizations, and screening to ensure that immunizations are up to date.
10. Secondary prevention requires community and public health nurses to screen for infected persons and to assist persons with communicable diseases in accessing appropriate medical treatment. Nurses may also be involved in the case management of persons who require treatment supervision. Contact tracing is one way of case finding.

THE NURSING PROCESS IN PRACTICE   A Client at Risk for AIDS and STDs (by Jennifer Maurer Kliphouse)

Ms. Roberts enters the health department STD clinic, where the community health nurse proceeds with the intake interview. The care at the clinic is based on the concept of case management. Personnel consist of a nurse, physician, social worker, and family planning counselor who work as a team and have weekly meetings to review cases.

During the interview, Ms. Roberts tells the nurse that she is a 33-year-old unmarried woman who suspects that she might have been exposed to the AIDS virus. Ms. Roberts reveals that she is currently sharing her apartment with her partner, Mr. Thomas. Ms. Roberts fears that she was exposed to HIV when she was 26 years old by sharing needles with a group of friends who were intravenous drug abusers. She has had six sex partners during the last 2 years. She does not use condoms. No pertinent medical or familial history is revealed. Ms. Roberts denies using intravenous drugs for more than 5 years. She tells the community health nurse that she has not had sexual contact with anyone except Mr. Thomas for 6 months.

Ms. Roberts also states that she thinks she might be pregnant. She is feeling tired all the time and has lost some weight. She has been vomiting in the morning and has noticed a yellow cervical discharge and complains of some vaginal itching. The nurse questions Ms. Roberts and finds out that her last menstrual period was 4 weeks earlier. Her vital signs are assessed and are found to be within normal limits. Ms. Roberts states that she really would like to be pregnant. She really loves Mr. Thomas, and they have talked about having a baby in the near future. The community health nurse offers Ms. Roberts voluntary HIV and hepatitis testing according to the clinic protocol. Ms. Roberts agrees to testing, and the nurse takes the blood sample, marks it, and sends it to be tested. Ms. Roberts is given an appointment to return for the test results.

The nurse goes with Ms. Roberts to see the clinic physician, who examines Ms. Roberts. During the vaginal examination, the physician notes a thick yellow cervical discharge. A sample of the secretion is obtained and sent to the laboratory. The sample will be examined and tested for chlamydia and gonorrhea organisms as a routine measure, in addition to screening for other organisms. The nurse tells Ms. Roberts that she will be notified when the test results are ready. Appointments will be made as necessary at that time. A pregnancy test is also performed. The nurse begins counseling Ms. Roberts about the routes of transmission of HIV and STDs and about safer sex practices. She counsels Ms. Roberts to encourage Mr. Thomas to use a condom with spermicide.

Ms. Roberts's pregnancy test result is positive, as is her test result for chlamydia. All the other test results (for gonorrhea, hepatitis B, and hepatitis C) are negative. Her HIV results are still pending. The nurse decides to call and tell Ms. Roberts about her test results. When the nurse calls Ms. Roberts, Ms. Roberts is very excited about the pregnancy and states that she cannot wait to tell Mr. Thomas. She does not appear to understand what the chlamydia results mean; thus the nurse decides to arrange a clinic appointment for counseling and treatment. Three days later, the results from the HIV tests come back positive.

Ms. Roberts sees the nurse for the second time. During the visit, the nurse goes over all the test results, including Ms. Roberts's HIV status. She educates Ms. Roberts about chlamydia and emphasizes the importance of treatment to reduce risk to her baby. She also reviews again Ms. Roberts's sexual history and explains that Mr. Thomas will need to be tested for chlamydia and HIV status. The nurse makes an appointment at the clinic for Ms. Roberts's first prenatal visit.

ASSESSMENT

- Conduct family assessment
- Assess family and social supports
- Assess knowledge of both partners regarding STDs, HIV infection, and AIDS, including prevention of transmission
- Assess attitude toward pregnancy

NURSING DIAGNOSES

- Deficient knowledge related to physiologic changes secondary to pregnancy, chlamydia, and HIV/AIDS as evidenced by new-onset diagnosis
- Ineffective therapeutic regimen management related to insufficient knowledge of condition, modes of transmission, consequences of repeated infections, treatment, and prevention of recurrences secondary to chlamydia infection as evidenced by lack of condom use
- Risk for infection related to lack of knowledge concerning disease transmission as evidenced by multiple sexual partners and lack of STD prevention measures
- Risk of infection transmission from mother to infant related to exposure during prenatal and perinatal periods to communicable disease via mother as evidenced by positive HIV status and positive chlamydia test result

Nursing Diagnosis	Nursing Goals	Nursing Interventions	Outcomes and Evaluation
Ineffective therapeutic regimen management related to insufficient knowledge of condition, modes of transmission, consequences of repeated infections, treatment, and prevention of recurrences secondary to chlamydia infection as evidenced by lack of condom use	Client will verbalize understanding of the pathophysiologic process of chlamydia infection, as well as of the treatment plan and modes of transmission.	The nurse provides chlamydia infection education to the client, including information about common symptoms (urethral or vaginal discharge) or lack of overt symptoms, and long-term effects (e.g., pelvic inflammatory disease) following neglect in treating the infection. The nurse also discusses the transmission modes of chlamydia, including infant exposure during birth, which can lead to neonatal conjunctivitis and blindness. The client receives prescription medication and treatment protocol counseling, with simple written instructions for personal reminders.	Ms. Roberts successfully attributes cervical discharge and vaginal itching to the chlamydia infection and indicates understanding that it is an STD. She indicates shock and disbelief that an infection that initially appears minor can lead to multiple health problems, including sterility. She also appropriately recounts verbal medication instructions and refers to the reference pamphlet when she is not exactly sure of the regimen. This indicates a successful intervention because she shows competency in using the provided reference tools.
	The client will verbalize understanding of complications related to multiple chlamydia infections.	The nurse provides free informative brochures that include photos of the effects of chlamydia infection.	When shown pictures of chlamydia infections, especially advanced cases, Ms. Roberts yells out, "I could look like THAT!?" While pictures often shock clients, they can be valuable learning and prevention tools. The colorful reaction of Ms. Roberts shows personalization and the impact of understanding possible future ramifications.

Continued

Nursing Diagnosis	Nursing Goals	Nursing Interventions	Outcomes and Evaluation
	The client will verbalize and implement proper infection control techniques.	The nurse discusses with the client previous birth control and sexual disease prevention methods, inquiring about Ms. Roberts's reasons for her past choices. Casual sexual disease prevention education follows, including the use of condoms and abstinence to reduce exposure to STDs. The nurse reviews the proper technique for condom application. Because Ms. Roberts tested positive not only for chlamydia but also for HIV, it is imperative that the nurse impress upon her the importance of condom use with current and future sexual partners. Free condoms are supplied by the clinic.	Inquiring about previous choices provides insight into Ms. Roberts's sexual disease knowledge and attitude. It also guides the nurse's discussion about future choices related to STD prevention. Unfortunately, the client's HIV status leaves only two choices for sexual encounters: abstinence or condom use. Given Ms. Roberts's history of multiple sexual partners, the nurse must ensure that she not only understands condom use but is willing to use condoms. As the client states, "Awww man, I know how to use those," the nurse requests that Ms. Roberts demonstrate proper application to ensure her knowledge.
	The client will successfully complete the treatment process.	The treatment program provides free prescription medications. A confidential STD support group meets biweekly in the neighborhood; contact information is provided to Ms. Roberts. The nurse schedules follow-up visits with Ms. Roberts to provide consistency of care and to build rapport. Finally, a retest is scheduled following completion of the medication regimen.	Ms. Roberts consents to an STD retest following completion of the medication regimen. Her chlamydia test result is negative, which suggests that the client is adhering to the treatment plan. However, Ms. Roberts will need to continue using condoms because she is HIV positive. Further counseling, support groups, and free condoms will be made available through clinic programs.

Find additional **Care Plans** for this client on the book's website.

LEARNING BY EXPERIENCE AND REFLECTION

1. Develop a position paper on the following debatable issue: should individual rights be compromised to control the spread of communicable diseases for the good of society?
2. Survey the role of boards of health in your community and state to determine how communicable diseases are prevented and controlled. What services do the boards provide?
3. Develop an educational program for pregnant adolescents to inform them about communicable diseases.
4. Explore the legal statutes in your state pertaining to control of communicable diseases.
5. Investigate the immunization criteria used in your state.
6. If possible, make arrangements through a clinical instructor to visit an STD clinic in your area and spend the day observing and assisting in nursing responsibilities.
7. Note three diseases with distinctive trends in incidence (see Table 8-3). Determine the reasons for the changes in incidence.

COMMUNITY RESOURCES FOR PRACTICE

Information about each of the following organizations is found on its website, which can be accessed through the **WebLinks** section of this book's website at *http://evolve.elsevier.com/Maurer/community/*.

American Academy of Pediatrics
American College of Obstetricians and Gynecologists
Emerging Infectious Diseases (journal)
Sexually Transmitted Diseases (journal)—American Sexually Transmitted Diseases Association
Control of Communicable Diseases Manual, published by the American Public Health Association
National Immunization Program, CDC
Division of Global Migration and Quarantine, CDC
Guide for Adult Immunization—can be downloaded from the CDC website
Travelers' Health—CDC website
National Vaccine Injury Compensation Program
Morbidity and Mortality Weekly Report (journal)
WHO Publications Centre, USA
Health and Human Services (HHS) National AIDS Hotline: telephone (800) 342-AIDS
City, county, and state boards of health and health departments: refer to the local telephone directory

STUDY AIDS   http://evolve.elsevier.com/Maurer/community/

Visit the Evolve website for this book to find the following study and assessment materials:

- Quiz
- Web Scenario
- Critical Thinking Questions and Answers for Case Studies

- Care Plans
- *Healthy People* Updates
- Glossary

WEBSITE RESOURCES

WEB

The following items supplement the chapter's topics and are also found on the Evolve site.

8A: Conditions for Case Definition in AIDS Surveillance

8B: Guide to Contraindications and Precautions to Commonly Used Vaccines

8C: Recommended Adult Immunization Schedule, by Vaccine and Medical and Other Indications

8D: Vaccine Administration: Visit Record

8E: Prophylactic Treatment Available for Communicable Disease

REFERENCES

Aronson, S. P. (1978). *Communicable disease in nursing.* New York: Medical Examining Publishing.

Baciewicz, G. J. (2005). *Injecting drug use.* Retrieved June 3, 2007 from *http://www.emedicine.com/med/topic586htm.*

Barquet, N., & Domingo, P. (1997). Smallpox: The triumph over the most terrific of the ministers of death. *Annals of Internal Medicine, 127* (8, Pt 1), 635-642.

Braithwaite, R. L., & Arriola, K. R. J. (2003). Male prisoners and HIV prevention: A call for action. *American Journal of Public Health, 93*(5), 759-763.

Bridges, C. B., Harper, S. A., Fukuda, K., et al. (2003). Prevention and control of influenza: Recommendations of the Advisory Committee on Immunization Practice. *Morbidity and Mortality Weekly Report, Recommendations and Reports, 52*(RR-8), 1-36.

Centers for Disease Control and Prevention. (1994a). 1994 Revised classification system for human immunodeficiency virus infection in children less than 13 years old. *Morbidity and Mortality Weekly Report, Recommendations and Reports, 43*(RR-12), 1-10.

Centers for Disease Control and Prevention. (1994b). Addressing emerging infectious disease threats: A prevention strategy for the United States. *Morbidity and Mortality Weekly Report, Recommendations and Reports, 43* (RR-5), 1-18.

Centers for Disease Control and Prevention. (1997a). Outbreaks of pneumococcal pneumonia among unvaccinated residents of chronic care facilities—Massachusetts, October 95, Oklahoma, February 96, Maryland May-June 96. *Morbidity and Mortality Weekly Report, 46*(3), 60-62.

Centers for Disease Control and Prevention. (1997b). Multidrug resistant *Salmonella*

serotype typhimurium—United States, 1996. *Morbidity and Mortality Weekly Report, 46*(14), 308-310.

Centers for Disease Control and Prevention. (1997c). Tuberculosis morbidity—United States, 1996. *Morbidity and Mortality Weekly Report, 46*(30), 665-670.

Centers for Disease Control and Prevention. (1997d). Hepatitis A associated with consumption of frozen strawberries—Michigan, March 1997. *Morbidity and Mortality Weekly Report, 46*(13), 288-289.

Centers for Disease Control and Prevention. (1997e). Update: Trends in AIDS incidence—United States, 1996. Public health surveillance. *Morbidity and Mortality Weekly Report, 46*(37), 863-870.

Centers for Disease Control and Prevention. (2001a). Summary of notifiable diseases—United States, 2001. *Morbidity and Mortality Weekly Report, 50*(53), 1-108. Published May 2, 2003 for 2001.

Centers for Disease Control and Prevention. (2001b). Revised recommendations for HIV screening of pregnant women. *Morbidity and Mortality Weekly Report, Recommendations and Reports, 50* (RR-19), 63-65.

Centers for Disease Control and Prevention. (2001c). Revised guidelines for HIV counseling, testing, and referral. *Morbidity and Mortality Weekly Report, Recommendations and Reports, 50*(RR-19), 1-58.

Centers for Disease Control and Prevention. (2002a). Increases in fluoroquinolone resistant Neisseria gonorrhoeae—Hawaii and California, 2001. *Morbidity and Mortality Weekly Report, 51*(44), 1041-1044.

Centers for Disease Control and Prevention. (2002b). Outbreaks of gastroenteritis associated with Noroviruses on cruise ships—United States, 2002.

Morbidity and Mortality Weekly Report, 51(49), 112-115.

Centers for Disease Control and Prevention. (2002c). Lyme disease—United States, 2000. *Morbidity and Mortality Weekly Report, 51*(2), 29-31.

Centers for Disease Control and Prevention. (2002d). Pertussis in an infant adopted from Russia—May 2002. *Morbidity and Mortality Weekly Report, 51*(18), 374-375.

Centers for Disease Control and Prevention. (2002e). Fatal yellow fever in a traveler returning from Amazonas, Brazil, 2002. *Morbidity and Mortality Weekly Report, 51*(15), 324-325.

Centers for Disease Control and Prevention. (2003a). Vaccination coverage among children entering school—United States, 2002-2003 school year. *Morbidity and Mortality Weekly Report, 52*(33), 791-793.

Centers for Disease Control and Prevention. (2003b). Hepatitis A outbreak associated with green onions at a restaurant—Monaca, Pennsylvania, 2003. *Morbidity and Mortality Weekly Report, 52*(47), 1155-1157.

Centers for Disease Control and Prevention. (2003c). Outbreaks of severe acute respiratory syndrome—worldwide, 2003. *Morbidity and Mortality Weekly Report, 52*(11), 226-228.

Centers for Disease Control and Prevention. (2003d). Update: Severe acute respiratory syndrome—United States, June 18, 2003. *Morbidity and Mortality Weekly Report, 52*(24), 570.

Centers for Disease Control and Prevention. (2003e). Imported plague—New York City, 2002. *Morbidity and Mortality Weekly Report, 52*(31), 725-728.

Centers for Disease Control and Prevention. (2003f). Multistate outbreak of monkeypox—Illinois, Indiana, and Wisconsin, 2003.

Morbidity and Mortality Weekly Report, 52(23), 537-540.

Centers for Disease Control and Prevention. (2003g). Trichinellosis surveillance—United States, 1997-2002. *Morbidity and Mortality Weekly Report, Surveillance Summaries, 52* (SS-6), 1-8.

Centers for Disease Control and Prevention. (2003h). Multistate outbreak of Salmonella serotype typhimurium infection associated with drinking unpasteurized milk—Illinois, Indiana, Ohio, and Tennessee, 2002-2003. *Morbidity and Mortality Weekly Report, 52*(26), 613-615.

Centers for Disease Control and Prevention. (2005a). Preventable measles among U.S. residents 2001-2004. *Morbidity and Mortality Weekly Report, 54*(33), 817-820.

Centers for Disease Control and Prevention. (2005b). Update: Syringe exchange programs—United States, 2002. *Morbidity and Mortality Weekly Report, 54*(27), 673-676.

Centers for Disease Control and Prevention. (2006a). Measles—United States, 2005. *Morbidity and Mortality Weekly Report, 55*(50), 1348-1351.

Centers for Disease Control and Prevention. (2006b). Brief report: Update: Mumps activity—United States, January 1-October 7, 2006. *Morbidity and Mortality Weekly Report, 55*(42), 1152-1153.

Centers for Disease Control and Prevention. (2006c). Pertussis outbreak in an Amish community—Kent County, Delaware, September 2004–February 2005. *Morbidity and Mortality Weekly Report, 55*(30), 817-821.

Centers for Disease Control and Prevention. (2006d). Immunization information systems progress—United States, 2005. *Morbidity and Mortality Weekly Report, 55*(49), 1327-1329.

Centers for Disease Control and Prevention. (2006e). Vaccination coverage among children entering school—United States, 2005-06 school year. *Morbidity and Mortality Weekly Report, 55*(41), 1124-1126.

Centers for Disease Control and Prevention. (2006f). Influenza and pneumococcal vaccination coverage among persons aged >65 years—United States, 2004-2005. *Morbidity and Mortality Weekly Report, 55*(39), 1065-1068.

Centers for Disease Control and Prevention. (2006g). Imported vaccine—Associated paralytic poliomyelitis—United States, 2005. *Morbidity and Mortality Weekly Report, 55*(04), 97-99.

Centers for Disease Control and Prevention. (2006h). Community-associated methicillin-resistant *Staphylococcus aureus* infection among healthy newborns—Chicago and Los Angeles County, 2004. *Morbidity and Mortality Weekly Report, 55*(12), 329-332.

Centers for Disease Control and Prevention. (2006i). Methicillin-resistant *Staphylococcus aureus* skin infection among tattoo recipients—Ohio, Kentucky, and Vermont, 2004-2005. *Morbidity and Mortality Weekly Report, 55*(24), 677-679.

Centers for Disease Control and Prevention. (2006j). Outbreaks of multidrug-resistant *Shigella sonnei* gastroenteritis associated with day care centers—Kansas, Kentucky, and Missouri, 2005. *Morbidity and Mortality Weekly Report, 55*(39), 1068-1071.

Centers for Disease Control and Prevention. (2006k). Trends in tuberculosis—United States, 2005. *Morbidity and Mortality Weekly Report, 55*(11), 305-308.

Centers for Disease Control and Prevention. (2006l). Emergence of *Mycobacterium tuberculosis* with extensive resistance to second-line drugs—worldwide, 2000-2004. *Morbidity and Mortality Weekly Report, 55*(11), 301-305.

Centers for Disease Control and Prevention. (2006m). Trends in HIV-related risk behaviors among high school students—United States, 1991-2005. *Morbidity and Mortality Weekly Report, 55*(31), 851-854.

Centers for Disease Control and Prevention. (2006n). Hepatitis awareness month—May 2006. *Morbidity and Mortality Weekly Report, 55*(18), 505.

Centers for Disease Control and Prevention. (2006o). Epidemiology of HIV/AIDS—United States, 1981-2005. *Morbidity and Mortality Weekly Report, 55*(21), 589-592.

Centers for Disease Control and Prevention. (2006p). Racial/ethnic disparities in diagnoses of HIV/AIDS—33 states, 2001-2004. *Morbidity and Mortality Weekly Report, 55*(05), 121-125.

Centers for Disease Control and Prevention. (2006q). Multistate outbreak of Norovirus associated with a franchise restaurant—Kent County, Michigan, May 2005. *Morbidity and Mortality Weekly Report, 55*(14), 395-397.

Centers for Disease Control and Prevention. (2006r). Hantavirus pulmonary syndrome—Five states, 2006. *Morbidity and Mortality Weekly Report, 55*(22), 627-629.

Centers for Disease Control and Prevention. (2006s). West Nile virus activity—United States, January 1–November 7, 2006. *Morbidity and Mortality Weekly Report, 55*(44), 1204-1205.

Centers for Disease Control and Prevention. (2006t). Investigation of avian influenza (H5N1) outbreak in humans—Thailand, 2004. *Morbidity and Mortality Weekly Report, 55*(Suppl 1), 3-6.

Centers for Disease Control and Prevention. (2006u). Travel-associated dengue—United States, 2005. *Morbidity and Mortality Weekly Report, 55*(25), 700-702.

Centers for Disease Control and Prevention. (2006v). Malaria in multiple family members—Chicago, Illinois, 2006. *Morbidity and Mortality Weekly Report, 55*(23), 645-648.

Centers for Disease Control and Prevention. (2006w). General recommendations on immunizations: Recommendations of the Advisory Committee on Immunization Practices (ACIP).

Morbidity and Mortality Weekly Report, Recommendations and Reports, 55(RR-15), 1-48.

Centers for Disease Control and Prevention. (2006x). HIV transmission among male inmates in a state prison system—Georgia, 1992-2005. *Morbidity and Mortality Weekly Report, 55*(15), 421-426.

Centers for Disease Control and Prevention. (2007a). Summary of notifiable diseases—United States, 2005. *Morbidity and Mortality Weekly Report, 54*(53), 2-92.

Centers for Disease Control and Prevention. (2007b). *A global perspective on tuberculosis* [Fact sheet]. Retrieved May 23, 2007 from *http://www.cdc.gov/tb/WorldTBDay/resources_global.htm.*

Centers for Disease Control and Prevention. (2007c). *The deadly intersection between TB and HIV.* Retrieved May 23, 2007 from *http://www.cdc.gov/hiv/resources/factsheets/hivtb.htm.*

Centers for Disease Control and Prevention. (2007d). *Human papillomavirus: HPV information for clinicians.* Retrieved May 23, 2007 from *http://www.cdc.gov/std/HPV/common-infection/CDC_HPV_clinicianBro_LR.pdf.*

Centers for Disease Control and Prevention. (2007e). *Epidemiology and prevention of vaccine preventable diseases: The Pink Book* (10th ed.). National Immunization Program. Washington, DC: Public Health Foundation.

Centers for Disease Control and Prevention. (2007f). Appendix C: Information on CDC's HIV/AIDS prevention budget. In *HIV/AIDS prevention strategic plan through 2005.* Retrieved May 23, 2007 from *http://www.cdc.gov/hiv/resources/reports/sps/appendix-chtm.*

Centers for Disease Control and Prevention. (2007g). *Nationally notifiable infectious diseases: United States, 2007g.* Retrieved June 3, 2007 from *http://www.dcd.gov/epo/dphsi/phs/infdis2007.htm.*

China rejects U.S. alert on toothpaste. (2007, June 4). *Baltimore Sun,* p. 6A.

Coberly, J. S., & Chaisson, R. E. (2007). Tuberculosis. In K. E. Nelson & C. A. Williams (Eds.), *Infectious disease epidemiology: Theory and practice* (2nd ed.; pp. 653-697). Sudbury, MA: Jones & Bartlett.

Donnelly, J. P., & DePauw, B. E. (2004). Infections in the immunocompromised host: General principles. In G. L. Mandell, J. E. Bennett, & R. Dolin (Eds.), *Principles and practice of infectious diseases* (6th ed.; pp. 3079-3090). New York: Churchill Livingstone.

Dowling, H. F. (1977). *Fighting infection: Conquests of the twentieth century.* Cambridge, MA: Harvard University Press.

Gibbs, N. (2007). Plague on a plane. *Time, 169*(24), 19.

Heymann, D. L. (Ed.). (2004). *Control of communicable diseases manual* (18th ed.). Washington DC: American Public Health Association.

Hutchinson, D. C., Drobinewski, F. A., & Milburn, H. J. (2003). Management of multi drug resistant tuberculosis. *Respiratory Medicine, 97*(1), 65-70.

Jekel, J. F., Katz, D. L., Elmore, J. G., et al. (2007). *Epidemiology, biostatistics and preventive medicine* (3rd ed.). Philadelphia: Saunders.

Joint United Nations Programme on HIV/AIDS. (2005). *Report on the global HIV/AIDS epidemic 2005.* Retrieved August 12, 2007 from *http://www.aids.org/barcelona/presskit/barcelona%20report/contents_html.htmin.*

Kaiser Family Foundation. (2006, September). *Sexual health statistics for teenagers and young adults in the United States.* Menlo Park, CA: Kaiser Family Foundation.

Kay, M. (2005). Influenza pandemic preparedness. *American Journal of Nursing, 105*(12), 73-74.

Keith, D. (2003). The basics of an exposure contact plan. *Journal of Perianesthesia Nursing, 18*(3), 186-195.

MacNeil, C., Weisz, J., & Carey, J. C. (2003). Clinical resistance of recurrent *Candida albicans* vulvovaginitis to fluconazole in the presence and absence of in vitro resistance. *Journal of Reproductive Medicine, 48*(2), 63-68.

Merrill, R. M., & Timmreck, T. C. (2006). *Introduction to epidemiology* (4th ed.). Sudbury, MA: Jones & Bartlett.

Miller, R. E. (2002). *Epidemiology for health promotion and disease prevention professionals.* New York: Haworth Press.

Mullan, F. (1989). *Plagues and politics: The story of the United States Public Health Service.* New York: Basic Books.

National Institute on Drug Abuse. (2006). *Assessing drug abuse within and across communities: Community epidemiology surveillance networks on drug abuse* (2nd ed.). Bethesda, MD: U.S. Department of Health and Human Services.

Nelson, K. E., Chitale, R., & Celentano, D. O. (2007). Human immunodeficiency virus infection and the acquired immune deficiency syndrome. In K. E. Nelson & C. M. Williams (Eds.), *Infectious disease epidemiology: Theory and practice* (2nd ed.; pp. 789-894). Sudbury, MA: Jones & Bartlett.

Poulin, C., Gyorkos, T. W., MacPhee, J., et al. (1992). Contact-tracing among injection drug users in a rural area. *Canadian Journal of Public Health, 83*(2), 106-108.

Rhinehart, E., & Friedman, M. M. (1999). *Infection control in home care.* Gaithersburg, MD: Aspen.

Risse, G. B. (1988). Epidemics and history: Ecological perspectives and social responses. In E. Fee & D. M. Fox (Eds.), *AIDS: The burdens of history* (pp. 36-66). Berkeley: University of California Press.

Robinson, W. S. (2000). Hepatitis B virus and hepatitis D virus. In G. L. Mandell, J. E. Bennett, & R. Dolin (Eds.), *Principles and practice of infectious diseases* (5th ed.; pp. 1652-1685). New York: Churchill Livingstone.

Steiner, K. C., Davilla, V., Kent, C. K., et al. (2003). Field delivered therapy increases treatment for chlamydia and gonorrhea. *American Journal of Public Health, 93*(6), 882-884.

Trotter, J. (1992). Guidelines for people with AIDS living in the community. Unpublished.

U.S. Bureau of the Census. (2005). Who's minding the kids? Child care arrangements: Winter 2002. *Current Population Reports,* P70-101.

U.S. Department of Health and Human Services. (2000). *Healthy people 2010: Understanding and improving health* (2nd ed.). Washington, DC: U.S. Government Printing Office.

U.S. Department of Health and Human Services. (2006a). *Health, United States, 2006.* Washington, DC: U.S. Government Printing Office.

U.S. Department of Health and Human Services. (2006b). *Healthy people 2010: Midcourse review.* Washington, DC: U.S. Government Printing Office.

Villarreal, H., & Fogg, C. (2006). Syringe-exchange programs and HIV prevention. *American Journal of Nursing, 106*(5), 58-63.

Webber, R. (2005). *Communicable disease epidemiology and control: A global perspective* (2nd ed.). Cambridge MA: CABI Publishing.

Wilks, D., Farrington, M., & Rubenstein, D. (2003). *The infectious disease manual* (2nd ed.). Boston: Blackwell.

Workowski, K. A., & Levine, W. C. (2002). Sexually transmitted diseases—Treatment guidelines, 2002. *Morbidity and Mortality Weekly Report, Recommendations and Reports, 51*(RR-6), 1-80.

Zenilman, J. M. (2007). Sexually transmitted diseases. In K. E. Nelson & C. M. Williams, *Infectious disease epidemiology: Theory and practice* (2nd ed.; pp. 963-1020). Boston: Jones & Bartlett.

Ziv, E., Daley, C. L., & Blower, S. (2004). Potential public health impact of new tuberculosis vaccines. *Emerging Infectious Diseases, 10*(9), 1529-1535.

SUGGESTED READINGS

Centers for Disease Control and Prevention. (2003). Incorporating HIV prevention into the medical care of persons living with HIV: Recommendations of CDC, the Health Resources and Services Administration, the National Institutes of Health, and the HIV Medicine Association of the Infectious Disease Society of America. *Morbidity and Mortality Weekly Report, Recommendations and Reports, 52*(RR-12), 1-24.

Centers for Disease Control and Prevention. (2003). Treatment of tuberculosis: American Thoracic Society, CDC, and Infectious Disease Society of America. *Morbidity and Mortality Weekly Report, Recommendations and Reports, 52*(RR-11), 1-80.

Centers for Disease Control and Prevention. (2005). A comprehensive immunization strategy to eliminate transmission of hepatitis B virus infection in the United States: Recommendations of the Advisory Committee on Immunization Practices (ACIP). Part I: Immunization of infants, children, and adolescents. *Morbidity and Mortality Weekly Report, Recommendations and Reports, 54*(RR-16), 1-23.

Centers for Disease Control and Prevention. (2006). A comprehensive immunization strategy to eliminate transmission of hepatitis B virus infection in the United States: Recommendations of the Advisory Committee on Immunization Practices (ACIP). Part II: Immunization of adults. *Morbidity and Mortality Weekly Report, Recommendations and Reports, 55*(RR-16), 1-25.

Cockburn, A. (1963). *The evolution and eradication of infectious diseases.* Baltimore: Johns Hopkins Press.

Cutler, J. C., & Arnold, R. C. (1988). Venereal disease control by health departments in the past: Lessons for the present. *American Journal of Public Health, 78*(4), 372-376.

Fee, E., & Fox, D. M. (1988). *AIDS: The burdens of history.* Berkeley: University of California Press.

Heymann, D.L.(Ed.). (2004). *Control of communicable diseases manual* (18th ed.). Washington DC: American Public Health Association.

Institute of Medicine. (1997). *The hidden epidemic: Confronting sexually transmitted diseases.* Washington, DC: National Academy Press.

Mandell, G. L., Bennett, J. E., & Dolin, R. (Eds.). (2004). *Principles and practice of infectious diseases* (6th ed.). New York: Churchill Livingstone.

Mullan, F. (1989). *Plagues and politics: The story of the United States Public Health Service.* New York: Basic Books.

Siegel, J. D., Rhinehart, E., Jackson, M., et al. (2007). *Guideline for isolation precautions: Preventing transmission of infectious agents in healthcare settings 2007.* Retrieved August 16, 2007 from *http://www.cdc.gov/ncidod/dhap/gl_isolation.html.*

CHAPTER 9

Environmental Health Risks: At Home, at Work, and in the Community

*Barbara Sattler**

*The chapter incorporates material written for the first three editions by Janet Primomo and Mary K. Salazar.

FOCUS QUESTIONS

What is meant by the term *environmental health?*

In what ways does the environment affect human health in the home, in the occupational setting, and in the community?

What are some of the key areas that are important to assess in the identification of household, occupational, or community environmental hazards?

What can community/public health nurses do to minimize the adverse effects of the environment on their clients' health?

What are some of the critical resources that are available to the community/public health nurse when working with clients in the home, in the occupational setting, and in the community?

CHAPTER OUTLINE

Overview of Environmental Health
Definition of Environmental Health
Historical Perspective
Nursing Involvement in Environmental Issues
Multidisciplinary Roles
Conceptual Model of Ecologic Systems
Toxicology
Sources of Environmental Hazards
Environmental Hazards at Home
Understanding "Who's in Charge"
Accessing Information and the Right to Know
Environmental Hazards in the Occupational Setting

History of Occupational Health in the United States
Environmental Hazards in the Community
Environmental Issues for the 21st Century
Air Pollution
Water and Soil Pollution
Hazardous Waste
Nanotechnology
Chemical Policies
Global Warming
Community/Public Health Nursing Responsibilities
Assessment
Surveillance

Risk Communication
Advocacy
Research
The Nurse's Responsibilities in Primary, Secondary, and Tertiary Prevention
Primary Prevention
Secondary Prevention
Tertiary Prevention
The Future of Environmental Health Nursing

KEY TERMS

Body burden
Dose response
Ecology
Environmental health
Environmental justice
Environmental Protection Agency

Exposure assessment
Hazardous waste
Household hazards
Multiple chemical sensitivity (MCS)
National Priorities List

Occupational Safety and Health Administration (OSHA)
Precautionary Principle
Right to know
Risk communication
Superfund

OVERVIEW OF ENVIRONMENTAL HEALTH

Environmental health comprises those aspects of human health, including quality of life, that are determined by physical, chemical, biologic, social, and psychologic problems in the environment. It also refers to the theory and practice of assessing, correcting, controlling, and preventing those factors in the environment that can potentially affect adversely the health of present and future generations.

In this chapter, the influence of the environment on human health is examined and the responsibilities of the community health nurse in relation to occupational and environmental health are defined. Understanding the effects of environmental factors on health and disease requires an appreciation of the complex interplay of many factors. Social, cultural, political, economic, and physical forces (chemical, radiologic, and biologic) interact with the psychologic and physiologic elements that form the foundation of human existence. In keeping with this assertion, this chapter examines a conceptual model of environmental health and uses this model to present an analysis and overview of factors affecting the connection between the environment and health. It is hoped that the discussion in this chapter will assist the reader in recognizing the environment as an important contributor to the health and well-being of individuals and populations.

DEFINITION OF ENVIRONMENTAL HEALTH

The Institute of Medicine defines environmental health as "freedom from illness or injury related to exposure to toxic agents and other environmental conditions that are potentially detrimental to human health" (Institute of Medicine, 1995, p. 15). Because of the multifactorial nature of environmental exposures and the myriad potential health effects, it is almost impossible to attribute a disease or health effects to a single exposure. Despite these difficulties, it is essential that health professionals consider the environment in relation to the health of their clients. Nursing assessments that ignore occupational and environmental risk factors may miss an important clue to a patient's or a population's health risks.

All nursing models ask us to consider the environment as a predictor of health. There are many ways in which to frame environmental health, including the following:

- Assess risks based on the medium in which they are contained (e.g., air, water, soil, food, products).
- Determine whether the health risk is from chemical (e.g., lead or pesticide), biologic (e.g., *Escherichia coli*), or radiologic (e.g., radon, UV from sun) exposure.
- Attribute the exposure to a setting or multiple settings (e.g., home, work, schools, community).
- Incorporate "host" factors, meaning the vulnerability of an individual or populations. For example, those people who are immunocompromised (e.g., human immunodeficiency virus/acquired immunodeficiency syndrome [HIV/AIDS], medically immunosuppressed) will be more sensitive to microbes in drinking or recreational water. During different developmental stages, we have different susceptibility based on our physiologic development and also based on the activities that we are likely to perform (e.g., hand-to-mouth activities of infants; work-related exposures of adults).
- Assess very specific exposures, such as the health risks that may be associated with drinking water, personal care products, or even the products that we use for patient care.

It is important to note how we begin to understand the relationship between environmental chemical exposures and their potential for harm. There are several ways in which we have historically made such discoveries, including the following:

- Humans present signs and symptoms that can be connected to a specific chemical exposure. This has most commonly occurred when workers have been occupationally exposed. In such instances, the temporal and geographic relationships to the exposures and health effects have helped to identify health hazards.
- Large, accidental releases of chemicals have befallen a community and contaminated its air or water and this has resulted in health effects. When this has occurred, we have learned about the chemicals' toxicity to humans, as well as to other species in the environment.
- In rare instances, human environmental (and occupational) epidemiologic studies have been performed and shown associations. Through such studies, we have learned about the toxic effects of chemicals.

However, the most common way in which the relationships between chemical exposures and health risks are posited is when toxicologists study the effects of chemicals on animals and we then estimate what the effects might be on humans. This estimation process is called "extrapolation." There have been over 100,000 man-made chemical compounds developed and introduced into our environment since World War II; we are most often reliant on the data that are created in animal studies to warn us about their potential toxicity to humans. For many chemicals, no toxicity data are available.

HISTORICAL PERSPECTIVE

Florence Nightingale was a great proponent of clean water and fresh air as key elements in promoting the public's health. Her practice improved the health of British soldiers in the Crimean War and reduced the high infant death rate in London. Nightingale identified the need for a clean environment with five points: pure air, pure water, efficient drainage, cleanliness, and light (Nightingale, 1860).

Some of the most significant public health success stories have resulted from eliminating environmental exposures. The greatest strides in the control of widespread disease occurred after the acceptance of the germ theory in the late 19th century (Last, 1998). Such advances in scientific knowledge about the causes of disease led to the development of sewage and water purification systems in American cities, which greatly contributed to the control of some of the worst threats to long life and good health, including typhoid, typhus, and other water-borne diseases (Newsome, 2005).

Unfortunately, former health concerns have been replaced with a whole new set of environmental concerns resulting from the effects of global warming, increasing demands by population growth, antibiotic-resistant strains of infectious diseases, and the introduction of new technology, products, and chemicals. These factors combine with lifestyle risks and stresses to create new problems (Sattler & Lipscomb, 2003). For instance, in our poorest communities, the combination of substandard housing, lack of healthy foods, poor access to health care, and higher probability of working in unhealthy jobs interact to create a multitude of health risks.

NURSING INVOLVEMENT IN ENVIRONMENTAL ISSUES

In the early 20th century, baccalaureate nursing programs included principles of public health and community hygiene in the curriculum. To protect individuals from health hazards, it was clear that nurses needed a basic understanding of environmental or community hygiene to participate in community education and the development of government-sponsored interventions. Topics covered in nursing curricula included sanitation of food and water supplies, a safe system for sewage disposal, adequate housing, the control of communicable disease, community health problems in childbearing and childhood, and the organization of public health services to maintain health (Gardner, 1936).

Today, all nurses are challenged to address some of the same environmental problems, and many new ones. The *Healthy People 2010* objectives address a great many occupational and environmental health issues (see the *Healthy People 2010* box). For example, one objective is to reduce outbreaks of water-borne disease from infectious agents and chemical poisonings; another is to reduce occupational skin disorders or diseases (including latex reactions from occupational exposures) (U.S. Department of Health and Human Services [USDHHS], 2000).

■ HEALTHY PEOPLE 2010 ■
Selected Environmental Health Objectives

Health Status Objectives

1. Reduce hospitalizations for asthma. (Target: 25 per 10,000 children younger than 5 years. Baseline: 45.6 per 10,000 children younger than 5 years; white 29.5; black 82.4 in 1998.)
2. Increase the proportion of persons with asthma who receive appropriate asthma care according to the NAEPP (National Asthma Education and Prevention Program) Guidelines (i.e., assistance with assessing and reducing exposure to environmental risk factors in their home, school, and work environments).
3. Eliminate elevated blood lead levels in children. (Target: 0. Baseline: 4.4% of children ages 1 to 6 years had blood lead levels exceeding 10 mcg/dl during 1991 to 1994.)
4. Reduce exposure of the population to pesticides (Diazinon), heavy metals (arsenic, lead, mercury), and other toxic chemicals (polychlorinated biphenyls [PCBs], dioxins, DDT), as measured by blood and urine concentrations of the substances or their metabolites.
5. Reduce water-borne disease outbreaks arising from water intended for drinking among persons served by community water systems. (Target: 2 outbreaks. Baseline: 6 outbreaks per year originated from community water systems for 1987 to 1996 average.)
6. Reduce nonfatal poisonings. (Target: 292 nonfatal poisonings per 100,000 population. Baseline: 348.4 nonfatal poisonings per 100,000 population in 1997.)

Risk Reduction Objectives

7. Reduce the global burden of disease resulting from poor water quality, sanitation, and personal and domestic hygiene. (Target: 2,135,000 deaths. Baseline: 2,668,200 deaths worldwide were attributable to these factors in 1990.)
8. Reduce the proportion of persons exposed to air that does not meet the U.S. Environmental Protection Agency's health-based standards for harmful air pollutants. (Target for carbon dioxide: 0%. Baseline: 19% in 1997.)
9. Reduce air toxic emissions to decrease the risk of adverse health effects caused by air-borne toxics. (Target: 2 million tons. Baseline: 8.1 million tons of air toxics were released into the air in 1993.)
10. Reduce the proportion of children who are regularly exposed to tobacco smoke at home. (Target: 10%. Baseline: 27% of children ages 6 years and younger lived in a household where someone smoked inside the house at least 4 days per week in 1994.)
11. Increase the proportion of persons served by community water systems who receive a supply of drinking water that meets the regulations of the Safe Drinking Water Act (SDWA). (Target: 95%. Baseline: 85% of persons served by community water systems received drinking water that met SDWA [Public Law 93-523] regulations in 1995.)
12. Reduce human exposure to organophosphate pesticides from food.
13. Minimize the risks to human health and the environment posed by hazardous sites. (Target: 98% of sites on the National Priorities List, Brownfield properties; Resource Conservation and Recovery Act facilities and leaking underground storage facilities. Baseline: 1200 sites on the National Priorities List; 2475 Resource Conservation and Recovery Act facilities; 370,000 leaking underground storage facilities; 1500 Brownfield properties in 1998.)

Service and Protection Objectives

14. Increase residences with a functioning smoke alarm on every floor. (Target: 100%. Baseline: 88% in 1998.)
15. Increase the proportion of persons living in pre-1950s housing that has been tested for the presence of lead-based paint. (Target: 50%. Baseline: 16% of persons living in homes built before 1950 in 1998 reported that their homes had been tested for the presence of lead-based paint.)
16. Increase the number of new homes constructed to be radon resistant. (Target: 2.1 million additional new homes. Baseline: 1.4 million new homes as of 1997.)
17. Increase the proportion of persons who live in homes tested for radon concentrations. (Target: 20%. Baseline: 17% of the population lived in homes in 1998 that had been tested for radon.)
18. Increase the number of states, tribes, and territories that monitor diseases that can be caused by exposure to environmental hazards.

Disease	Number of Jurisdictions	
	1997 Baseline	2010 Target
Lead poisoning	51	51
Pesticide poisoning	20	25
Mercury poisoning	14	20
Asthma	6	25

From U.S. Department of Health and Human Services. (Nov 2000). *Healthy People 2010* (2nd ed.). Retrieved August 14, 2003, from *http://www.healthypeople.gov/Publications/*.

Recently, there has been increasing interest from community activists as well as health professionals in the topic of environmental justice. The concept of **environmental justice** refers to the disproportionately high exposures of low-income and minority populations to environmental health risks, such as air pollution, hazardous waste incinerators, toxic landfills, pesticides, lead exposure, and unsafe drinking water (Brown, 1995; Bullard & Wright, 1993; Sattler & Lipscomb, 2003; Subcommittee of Environmental Justice, 1995). The higher exposure of low-income and minority populations to these environmental hazards combined with other issues associated with health disparities are important issues for nurses to address. Dr. Payne-Sturgess, a senior staff at the U.S. **Environmental Protection Agency** (EPA) has created a useful model to consider the many factors affecting environmental justice and health disparities (Figure 9-1).

Institute of Medicine Report

In the early 1990s, a group of nurses and others were convened by the National Academy of Science Institute of Medicine to assess the integration of environmental health into nursing education, practice, research, and policy/advocacy. The group authored a report in 1995 entitled *Nursing, Health, and the Environment* (Pope et al., 1995). It continues to serve as a blueprint for continuing efforts to enhance nurses' capacity to address current and emerging environmental health issues. The following competencies were recognized as essential for all nurses:

1. Basic Knowledge and Concepts

All nurses should understand the scientific principles and underpinnings of the relationship between individuals or populations and the environment (including the work environment). This understanding includes the basic mechanism and pathways of exposure to environmental health hazards, basic prevention and control strategies, the interdisciplinary nature of effective interventions, and the role of research.

2. Assessment and Referral

All nurses should be able to successfully complete an environmental health history, recognize potential environmental hazards and sentinel illnesses, and make appropriate referrals for conditions with probable environmental causes. An essential component is the ability to access and provide information to clients and communities and to locate referral sources.

3. Advocacy, Ethics, and Risk Communication

All nurses should be able to demonstrate knowledge of the role of advocacy (case and class), ethics, and risk communication in client care and community intervention with respect to the potential adverse effects of the environment on health.

4. Legislation and Regulation

All nurses should understand the policy framework and major pieces of legislation and regulations related to environmental health.

In the years since the IOM report, there has been much progress in the nursing profession regarding environmental health. Both the American Nurses Association and the American Public Health Association's Public Health Nurses' Section have adopted a set of environmental health nursing principles that are helping to guide the practice of nursing and the advocacy activities of these respective professional groups (Box 9-1).

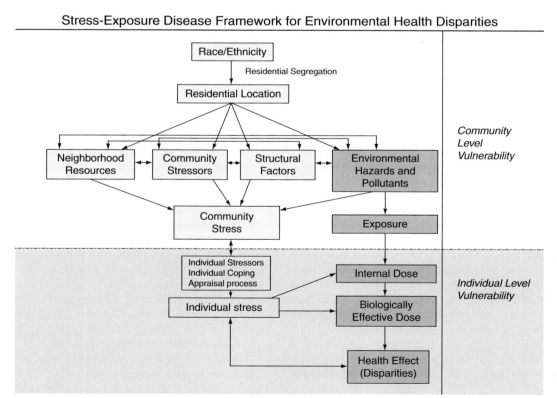

Stress-Exposure Disease Framework for Environmental Health Disparities

FIGURE 9-1 Environmental health disparities: A framework integrating psychosocial and environmental concepts. (From Gee, G., & Payne-Sturges, D. [2004]. Environmental health disparities: A framework integrating psychosocial and environmental concepts. *Environmental Health Perspectives, 112*[17], 1645-1653. Published online August 16, 2004, doi:10.1289/ehp.7074. © This is an Open Access article: verbatim copying and redistribution of this article are permitted in all media for any purpose, provided this notice is preserved along with the article's original DOI.)

Box 9-1   Environmental Health Principles for Public Health Nursing

1. Safe and sustainable environments are essential conditions for the public's health.
2. Environmental health is integral to the roles and responsibilities of *all* public health nurses.
3. *All* public health nurses should possess environmental health knowledge and skills.
4. Environmental health decisions should be grounded in sound science.
5. The *Precautionary Principle* is a fundamental tenet for all environmental health endeavors.
6. Environmental justice is a right of all populations.
7. Public awareness and community involvement are essential in environmental health decision making.
8. Communities have a right to relevant and timely information for decisions on environmental health.
9. Environmental health approaches should respect diverse values, beliefs, cultures, and circumstances.
10. Collaboration is essential to effectively protecting the health of all people from environmental harm.
11. Environmental health advocacy must be rooted in scientific integrity, honesty, respect for all persons, and social justice.
12. Environmental health research addressing the effectiveness and public health impact of nursing interventions should be conducted and disseminated.

From American Public Health Association, Public Health Nurses' Section. (2006). *Environmental health principles for public health nursing.* Washington, DC: Author. Available at *http://www.apha.org/membergroups/newsletters/sectionnewsletters/public_nur/winter06/2550.htm.*

MULTIDISCIPLINARY ROLES

Assessment, prevention, and protection in environmental health are the job of a great many disciplines. *Toxicologists* and basic scientists (e.g., geologists, biologists, neurobiologists) help to provide some of the scientific underpinnings for our understanding of how human health, ecologic health, and the environment are all interconnected and impact each other. In the applied arena, there are sanitarians (who are currently renaming themselves "environmental professionals"). *Sanitarians* often work in the public sector, especially in local health departments, and are often involved in food safety, vector control, housing-related environmental risks, and other of the environmental programs typically found in local health departments. Also in the applied arena are people who specialize in water quality, air quality, and other media-specific areas. Such specialists work in the public sector (state health departments, the Environmental Protection Agency [EPA]), and also may work in industry and in the nonprofit world, where they may help to determine the necessary environmental controls or advocate for enhanced environmental protection.

In occupational health, the area that specifically focuses on work-related health and safety issues, there are several disciplines. *Industrial hygienists* are responsible for occupational health exposures. They are trained to complete measurements for chemicals in workplace air and dust, to assess noise levels, and to address work-related temperature issues. *Occupational health nurses* work very closely with industrial hygienists and have some overlapping roles; however, nurses have the distinct role in physical assessments of the workers, maintaining health records, and other human health-specific work. Both occupational health nurses and industrial hygienists are responsible for knowing the laws and regulations regarding workplace health and safety.

Another occupational health specialty is ergonomics, the study of the interface between people and their physical environment. An *ergonomist* would address issues related to work stations and how well they "fit" the worker, in order to eliminate/reduce muscular strain or vision problems.

Nursing's role has been evolving in terms of our responsibilities in environmental health. In the state of Vermont, every political jurisdiction has an "environmental health nurse" who has been cross-trained beyond general community/public health to a wider range of environmental health issues. In the Los Angeles Health Department, a new role has been created for environmental health nurses. At the University of Maryland Medical Center a role has been created for a nurse to help lead the environmental health and sustainability work at the hospital. While these positions are still rare, it indicates a growing understanding of how important nurses' skills can be harnessed to address environmental health challenges.

More often what we are seeing is the integration of environmental health principles and practices into existing nursing work, particularly public health nursing. For example, it is quite common to have a nurse directing the lead poisoning activities within a health department or to have nurses involved in risk communication when a swimming area is compromised with pathogens. It is equally common to see school nurses involved in indoor air quality issues or concerned about the pesticides that are used on the children's playing fields.

CONCEPTUAL MODEL OF ECOLOGIC SYSTEMS

Ecology refers to the study of living things in relationship to their environment. The major impetus in the development of ecology was from the biologic sciences. As early as 1859, Darwin identified the "web of life" and recognized the highly complex set of interrelationships that were present between organisms and their environments. The word *ecology* was first used in 1868 by Haeckel, a German biologist. The term *human ecology* was coined in the 1920s in a sociologic text in an attempt to systematically apply a basic theoretic scheme of plant and animal ecology to the study of human communities (Hawley, 1950). Cultural and sociologic dimensions, as well as spatial distribution, were later included in the field of human ecology.

Ecologic systems generally have several different levels (Bronfenbrenner, 1979). The simplified version illustrated in Figure 9-2 consists of two levels. The level of system closest to the human population is the microsystem. The microsystem includes the environment immediately surrounding the person (e.g., the family and the home). The macrosystem is the larger context in which the microsystem is embedded. Culture, traditions, customs, societal norms, governmental agencies, schools, organizations, economic policies, and the physical environment constitute the macrosystem.

The basic principles of ecologic systems are similar to Commoner's laws of ecology—everything is connected to everything else and everything must go somewhere (Commoner, 1972). Because of the interrelationships and interactions among the different aspects of a system, change in any portion of a system might affect change in other parts of the system. (See Chapter 1 for a discussion of general systems theory.)

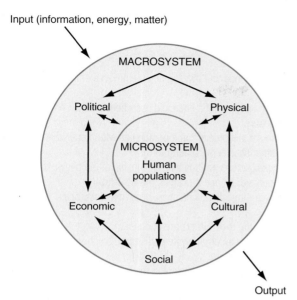

Input (information, energy, matter)

FIGURE 9-2 Simplified ecologic systems model.

In other words, systems are dynamic, and change is constant. For example, the microsystem or the family of a daycare worker might become infected with *Giardia* through an infected child at the daycare center who drank contaminated water when on a hike with the parents. The child was infected with the *Giardia* organism from the macrosystem (a mountain stream). The organism then crossed the boundaries from the macrosystem to the microsystem (the child in daycare) and infected the worker.

An ecologic system includes all the physical, social, cultural, political, and economic conditions that influence the lives of individuals, groups, and communities. As with other areas of nursing, the focus of nurses in environmental health is to promote, maintain, and support health, and specifically to explain how the environment affects well-being (Butterfield, 2002). Kleffel (1996) has proposed that nurses move toward an *ecocentric* perspective that emphasizes the linkages and interrelationships among global conditions, environmental hazards, and human health. In environmental health, particular attention is given to the identification of both positive and negative factors in the environment that might affect human beings.

The concept that everything must go somewhere is clearly demonstrated by the body burden studies that have been implemented by the Centers for Disease Control and Prevention (CDC) as part of the annual National Health and Nutrition Exam Study (NHANES). As part of the annual NHANES, the CDC is now collecting urine, blood, and breast milk samples from Americans across the country and testing them for the presence of potentially toxic chemicals that should not be in the human body. For NHANES 2003-2004, 275 chemicals were being assessed (CDC, 2005).

These chemicals do not belong in the human body. They are the result of pollutants and potentially toxic chemicals that are found in our air, water, food, soil, and products. They persist in the environment because they do not break down. They persist in the human body because we do not have an effective physiologic mechanism to excrete them and therefore they

accumulate. These chemicals include fire retardants, solvents, pesticides, and other potentially toxic substances. The list of health risks that are associated with these chemicals is long and includes neurotoxicity (e.g., learning disabilities, behavioral problems, parkinsonism); reproductive health problems (e.g., fertility, endometriosis); endocrine disruption; and carcinogenicity.

For women, body burdens of potentially toxic chemicals can be unwittingly shared with the developing fetus, as most of these chemicals cross the placenta barrier. In a 2005 study, scientists assayed the cord blood of newborns to see what potentially hazardous chemicals could be found in the blood that had been circulating in the baby immediately before birth. Many of the same industrial chemicals were found in cord blood (Houlihan et al., 2005). The evidence of our body burden of chemicals is a call to action for all nurses to integrate environmental health and precautionary principles into our professional practice. This will require us to consider how we can integrate primary and secondary prevention into our work. To do this, we will need to understand several additional concepts and learn about the resources that are available to all of us. The presence of the Web can catalyze our efforts, as the evidence that we need to underpin our decisions and practice is now often available.

TOXICOLOGY

All nursing students learn pharmacology, essentially the study of drugs. The corollary science for the study of potentially hazardous chemicals is toxiciology, sometimes referred to as the study of poisons. In the field of environmental health, we rely heavily on toxicology to inform our work. The good news for nurses is that these two sciences, pharmacology and toxicology, are very similar. Table 9-1 is a side-by-side comparison of the two.

SOURCES OF ENVIRONMENTAL HAZARDS

By its very nature, environmental health requires a public health approach to disease because environments affect many people simultaneously. An **exposure assessment** of the potential environmental hazards should be included in every health history (Sattler & Lipscomb, 2003). Box 9-2 presents questions that should be part of this assessment. The primary environments for most individuals can be divided into three broad areas: the home (Davis, 2007), the work site (Guenther & Hall, 2007; Sattler, 2003; Sattler & Hall, 2007; Shaner-McRae et al., 2007), and the community (Gilden, 2003). In the sections that follow, these environments are described. Other chapters cover related topics, such as violence (see Chapter 23).

There are a number of environmental assessment tools that can be used to supplement the basic community health assessment in order to identify environmental health threats within a community. The National Library of Medicine created *ToxTown* to help identify and address public and environmental health risks and link the information to their wealth of databases and peer-reviewed articles *(ToxTown: http://toxtown.nlm.nih.gov/)*. Note that *ToxTown* allows the viewer to choose between a town, city, farm, U.S./Mexico border community, or port, providing a great range of environmental health information.

Some basic environmental questions to ask are as follows: What is the air quality in the community? What is the water quality (both drinking water and recreational)? Are agricultural

TABLE 9-1 Comparison of Pharmacology and Toxicology

Pharmacology	Toxicology
Pharmacology is the scientific study of the origin, nature, chemistry, effects, and use of drugs.	*Toxicology* is the science that investigates the adverse effects of chemicals on health.
Dose refers to the amount of a drug absorbed from an administration.	*Dose* refers to the amount of a chemical absorbed into the body from a chemical exposure.
A drug can be administered one time, short term, or long term.	*Exposure* is the actual contact that a person has with a chemical. Exposure can be one time, short term, or long term.
A *dose-response curve* graphically represents the relationship between the dose of a drug and the response elicited.	A *dose-response curve* describes the relationship of the body's response to different amounts of an agent such as a drug or toxin.
Routes of administration include oral, intramuscular, intravenous, dermal, or topical.	*Routes of entry* are ingestion, inhalation, or dermal absorption.
With drugs there are therapeutic responses (desirable) and side effects (undesirable). Beyond the therapeutic dose, a drug may become toxic.	In toxicology, only the toxic effects are of concern. *Toxicity* is the ability of a chemical to damage an organ system, disrupt a biochemical process, or disturb an enzyme system.
Potency refers to the relative amount of drug required to produce the desired response.	The *potency* of a toxic chemical refers to the relative amount it takes to elicit a toxic effect compared with other chemicals.
Biologic monitoring is done for some drugs: clotting time is monitored in patients taking anticoagulants such as warfarin. Actual drug levels are measured for some drugs such as digoxin.	*Biologic monitoring* is done for some toxic exposures, such as blood lead levels or metabolites of chemicals such as cotinines for environmental tobacco smoke.

From Sattler, B. (1998). Environmental Health Education Center, University of Maryland School of Nursing. Used with permission.

chemicals a part of the landscape (e.g., pesticides, herbicides)? Has the land/soil been contaminated by previous or current use? Are pests a problem (e.g., mosquitoes, rodents, deer)? Is the housing stock sound and healthy? Are there major roadways in the community that may contribute to air pollution and particulate matter? Also note that a neighborhood assessment should include the positive environmental attributes that contribute to health and quality of life. Examples of questions about environmental attributes include the following: Is the community "walkable"; is it served by good public transportation; and does it have parks, green spaces, community gardens, and trees? Is there access to affordable, healthy foods and produce? For instance, does the community have access to a farmers' market during the growing season?

Box 9-2 Taking an Exposure History: I PREPARE

I—Investigate All Exposures
- Who is the population I serve, and what are my clients' exposure risks?
- What are their environmental exposure risks at home, at school, or in the community or workplace?
- Are my clients responding to usual treatments?
- Do symptoms seem unusual for my client's age or the time of year?

P—Present Work
- What is my client's daily routine at work (home or school)?
- Does my client work with chemicals? How does my client come in contact with chemicals?
- Do other members of my client's household have similar symptoms? Does my client notice any change in his or her symptoms when away from work or home?

R—Residence
- Has my client's home recently been remodeled?
- What is the source of my client's drinking water—a private well or public water systems?
- What type of heating system is in my client's home?

E—Environment
- What types of farms, landfills, industries, and factories are (or used to be) located near my client's home?

- How close to major roadways is the client's home?
- Does my client live in an urban or rural area?
- Are there polluted waterways near my client's home?

P—Past Work
- What were my client's duties in previous jobs?
- Has my client done seasonal or volunteer work? What type?

A—Activities
- What hobbies do my client and my client's family enjoy? Has anyone in the family taken up a new hobby or activity recently?
- Does my client hunt, garden, fish, or swim?
- Does my client engage in alternative or cultural health practices?

R—Resources and Referrals
- What are my sources of information and referral for my clients?
- A few examples are ATSDR, AOEC, AAOHN, OSHA, NIOSH, EPA, health departments, and poison control centers.

E—Educate
- How does my client read or receive information?
- Are there available cultural, language, or media information sources applicable to my client's needs and interests?

From Agency for Toxic Substances and Disease Registry. (2000). Available at *http://www.atsdr.cdc.gov.*

ENVIRONMENTAL HAZARDS AT HOME

There are many assessment tools that have been developed to determine environmental health risks. As a doctoral student, public health nurse Allison Davis developed a home assessment tool that she used to determine the types of environmental health risks that might be experienced by staff and residents in group homes for people with developmental disabilities (Figure 9-3). This quick and easy assessment tool can help to guide any type of home assessment. It can be used to begin to determine areas for remediation, product substitution, and general environmental health education. Table 9-2 discusses common sources of home pollution.

The National Library of Medicine has developed a helpful database of health-related information about common household products. A wide range of products are included, for example, pet care, cleaning, automotive, lawn care, and personal care prod-

ucts. The website for this information is *http://hpd.nlm.nih.gov/*. Note that the information is provided by the manufacturers.

Home Safety

For many Americans, the home is a refuge from the strains and stresses of everyday life. In addition to environmental health risks, there can also be safety risks that need to be addressed. In 2001, approximately 33,200 Americans died as a result of unintentional injuries in their homes, and another 8 million suffered disabling injuries (National Safety Council, 2003a). The leading causes of accidental death in the home are poisonings and falls (Figure 9-4). Other causes of death include fires and burns, choking and suffocation, drowning, and firearm accidents resulting from playing with or cleaning guns. The greatest number of documented accidental deaths in the home occurs in the very young (younger than 4 years of age)

Home Environmental Health and Safety Assessment Tool					
Assessment	Yes	No	N/A	Standard of Practice
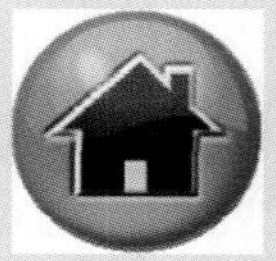 Home built before 1978	O	O	O	• Test homes built before 1978 for lead
Home tested for lead	O	O	O	
Living space in basement	O	O	O	• Maintain home to prevent chipping or peeling paint
Attached garage	O	O	O	
Home radon test	O	O	O	• Remove shoes indoors
Home radon ventilation system	O	O	O	• Test first three floors of all homes for radon
Living space in basement	O	O	O	• Do not idle car in garage
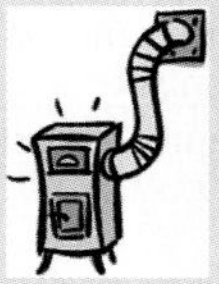 Combustion heating source	O	O	O	• Ensure proper venting of all combustion heating sources.
Gas, kerosene or propane space heater	O	O	O	• Annual assessment to ensure proper function.
Wood stove	O	O	O	
Fireplace	O	O	O	• Do not use grills or generators indoors
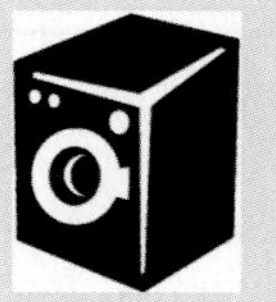 Gas dryer	O	O	O	• Gas dryers, hot water heaters, and stove need to vent outdoors
Vented	O	O	O	
Gas hot water heater	O	O	O	
Vented	O	O	O	
Gas stove	O	O	O	
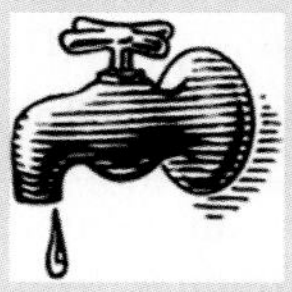 Well water	O	O	O	• Routine well testing and maintenance of private wells
Lead pipes	O	O	O	
Water tested for contaminants	O	O	O	• Review consumer confidence reports for public water supply
Known contaminants:	O	O	O	
Smoke detector	O	O	O	• Smoke detector on all floors and in bedrooms
Carbon monoxide detector	O	O	O	
Fire extinguisher	O	O	O	• Carbon monoxide detector on all levels in homes with combustion source or garage
Fire evacuation route	O	O	O	
Emergency phone numbers	O	O	O	
Disaster plan	O	O	O	
Shelter–in-place supplies	O	O	O	

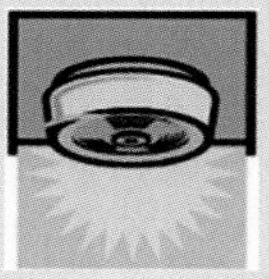

FIGURE 9-3 Home environmental health and safety assessment tool. (Copyright Del Bene Davis Home Environmental Assessment Tool, University of Maryland, Environmental Health Education Center. [March 2007]. Used with permission.)

Assessment	Yes	No	N/A	Standard of Practice
Insects in home	O	O	O	• Use of integrated pest management techniques for controlling pests
Rodents in home	O	O	O	
If yes what:_____				
Pesticide spraying in home	O	O	O	• Use least hazardous methods of pest control
If yes what / how often: _____				
Pesticide contract	O	O	O	
Frequency: _____				
Air freshener used in home	O	O	O	• Minimize use of air fresheners. Use less hazardous and irritating alternatives to control odors.
Candles	O	O	O	
Plug-ins	O	O	O	
Incense	O	O	O	
How many times per day:	O	O	O	• Use of low VOC household cleaners and green cleaning techniques
Use of strong smelling cleaners	O	O	O	
Tuna fish served in home	O	O	O	• See federal and state recommended fish consumption advisories
If yes, how often per week: _____				• Wash all fruits and vegetables before eating
Fresh fruit/vegetables used	O	O	O	
Local/organic products used	O	O	O	• Consider organic or locally grown products
Mercury thermometer in house	O	O	O	• Use non–mercury-containing medical devices
Other mercury devices	O	O	O	
Needle boxes for needles	O	O	O	• Dispose of all mercury devices and batteries per local hazard waste collection procedures
Use of traditional or cultural remedies containing mercury	O	O	O	
Smoking allowed in home	O	O	O	• Institute no smoking indoors policy
House smells like smoke	O	O	O	
Cigarette products present	O	O	O	

FIGURE 9-3, CONT'D

and the very old (older than 75 years of age). According to the National Safety Council, one home death occurs every 16 minutes, and one home injury occurs every 4 seconds (National Safety Council, 2003a). Safety campaigns to modify products and teach people how to prevent accidents are effective (McClelland et al., 1996).

Poisoning. Unintentional poisonings are a major cause of home-related deaths and accounted for more than 11,500 deaths and approximately 300,000 disabling illnesses in 2001 (National Safety Council, 2003a). Deaths from poisonings in the newborn to 4-year-old age group have fallen dramatically since 1958, in part because of the introduction of child-proof containers and educational campaigns such as "Mr. Yuk" (National Safety Council, 1991). Poisoning deaths include those from illicit drugs (such as cocaine, pain medications, cleaning substances, mushrooms, and shellfish) in addition to commonly used household poisons (e.g., pesticides, herbicides) (Davis, 2007); this helps explain the higher number of deaths in the 25- to 44-year-old age group than other

age groups. A study that examined poisoning among older adults in Massachusetts suggested that the elderly might be at higher risk than adults in younger age groups for poisoning from prescription medications (Woolf et al., 1990). A compromising health condition, medication interactions, possible dementia, and failing eyesight, problems not uncommon in the elderly, might lead to an unintentional overdose, with tragic consequences. The findings from this study indicated that men older than 70 years and women older than 60 years are at greater risk of dying as a result of accidental poisoning from medications than are younger persons.

Families can be encouraged to minimize the use of household chemicals and pesticides and to ensure safe storage when they are used. Proper ventilation should be ensured when chemicals are being used. Educating families about what to do in case of accidental poisoning is essential. Poison control centers are located in most major cities in the United States. Their telephone number can usually be found in the front of the yellow pages. If not, contact the local telephone operator. A well-trained poison

TABLE 9-2   Common Sources of Home Pollution

Agent	Description	Sources in Home
Radon	Colorless, odorless, radioactive gas from the natural breakdown (radioactive decay) of uranium; it is estimated that radon causes up to 36,000 lung cancer deaths per year	Soil or rock under the home; well water; building materials
Asbestos	Mineral fiber used extensively in building materials for insulation and as a fire retardant; asbestos should be removed by a professional if it has deteriorated; exposure to asbestos fibers can cause irreversible and often fatal lung diseases, including cancer	Sprayed-on acoustical ceilings or textured paint; pipe and furnace insulation materials; floor tiles; automobile brakes and clutches
Biologic contaminants	Include bacteria, mold and mildew, viruses, animal dander and saliva, dust mites, and pollen; these contaminants can cause infectious diseases or allergic reactions; moisture and dust levels in the home should be kept as low as possible	Mold and mildew; standing water or water-damaged materials; humidifiers; house plants; household pets; ventilation systems; household dust
Indoor combustion	Produces harmful gases (carbon monoxide, nitrogen dioxide), particles, and organic compounds (benzene); health effects range from irritation to the eyes, nose, and throat, to lung cancer; ventilation of gas appliances to the outdoors will minimize risks	Tobacco smoke; unvented kerosene or gas space heaters; unvented kitchen gas stoves; wood stoves or fireplaces; leaking exhaust flues from gas furnaces and clothes dryers; car exhaust from an attached garage
Household products	Can contain potentially harmful organic compounds; health effects vary greatly; the elimination of household chemicals through the use of nontoxic alternatives or by using only in well-ventilated rooms or outside will minimize risks	Cleaning products; paint supplies; stored fuels; hobby products; personal care products; mothballs; air fresheners; dry-cleaned clothes
Formaldehyde	Widely used chemical that is released to the air as a colorless gas; it can cause eye, nose, throat, and respiratory system irritation, headaches, nausea, and fatigue; might be a central nervous system depressant and has been shown to cause cancer in laboratory animals; remove sources of formaldehyde from the home if health effects occur	Particleboard, plywood, and fiberboard in cabinets, furniture, subflooring, and paneling; carpeting, durable-press drapes, other textiles; urea-formaldehyde insulation; glues and adhesives
Pesticides	Including insecticides, termiticides, rodenticides, and fungicides, all of which contain organic compounds; exposure to high levels of pesticides might cause damage to the liver and the central nervous system and increase cancer risks; when possible, nonchemical methods of pest control should be used; if the use of pesticides is unavoidable they should be used strictly according to the manufacturer's directions	Contaminated soil or dust that is tracked in from outside; stored pesticide containers; residue if used inside
Lead	A long-recognized harmful environmental pollutant; fetuses, infants, and children are more vulnerable to toxic effects; if the community health nurse suspects that a home has lead paint, it should be tested	Lead-based paint that is peeling, sanded, or burned; automobile exhaust; lead in drinking water; contaminated soil; food contaminated by lead from lead-based ceramic cookware or pottery; lead-related hobbies or occupations; folk remedies

control center staff, which includes pharmacists, nurses, and physicians, is available around the clock to provide information about the prevention and treatment of poisonings.

Falls. Falls are the other major cause of unintentional injuries in the home and accounted for approximately 9000 deaths in 2001; 80% of these occur in adults older than 65 years (National Safety Council, 2003a). Falls are the leading cause of unintentional injury deaths for adults older than 75 years of age (see Chapter 28). Common environmental fall hazards in the home include lack of stair rails and grab bars, tripping hazards, lack of stair railings or grab bars, unsteady furniture, poor lighting, loose electric cords and rugs, slippery surfaces, and clutter, all contributing to falls in elderly persons (CDC, 2003). Baby equipment, such as walkers, has been under scrutiny for contributing to serious falls in young children. Windows that

do not have guards are hazards for small children. Nurses can provide useful information to all family members concerning the prevention of falls in the home. For example, parents should be advised never to leave a child unattended on a diaper-changing table and to always strap children into strollers and high chairs.

Burns. Fires and burns, the third highest cause of home death, accounted for approximately 3300 deaths in 1998 (National Safety Council, 2003b). These deaths include fire-related injuries, such as smoke inhalation and asphyxiation, falls, and trauma from falling objects. Common causes of home fires include faulty electrical wiring of appliances, chimneys, and space heaters. Deaths are highest among those considered to be the most dependent: the very young and very old. One of the health protection objectives in *Healthy People 2010* (USDHHS,

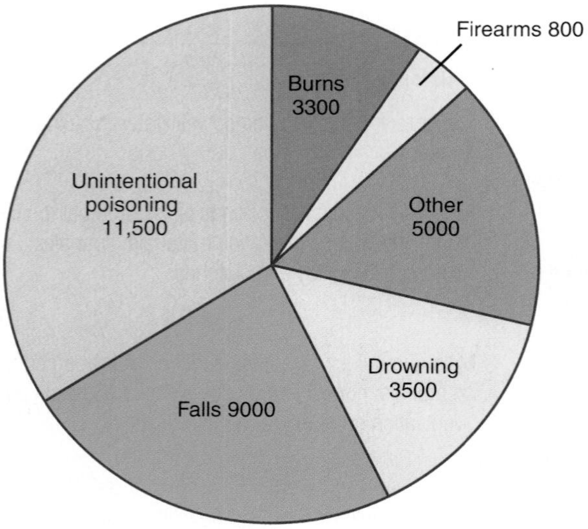

FIGURE 9-4 Causes of accidental deaths in the United States. (Data from National Safety Council. [2003]. *Report on injuries in America*. Retrieved August 31, 2003, from *http://www.nsc.org/library/rept2000htm;* and National Safety Council. [2002]. *Accident facts:* 2002 edition. Itasca, IL: Author.)

2000) is to have functional smoke detectors on each floor of all residences. By encouraging families to install smoke detectors, nurses can help prevent burn injuries and deaths.

Drowning. Drownings and near drownings are a major cause of morbidity and mortality in this country. In 2000, nearly 3500 non-boating–related deaths were reported in the United States; more than 1400 of these were children younger than 20 years. Drownings were the leading cause of injury death in toddlers (Brenner, 2003; National Center for Injury Prevention and Control, 2003). It has been estimated that for each drowning death, there are one to four near drownings that result in hospitalization. The location of drowning differs among age groups, with infants most likely to drown in bathtubs, children ages 1 to 4 years in swimming pools, and children 5 years and older in rivers, lakes, and other natural water sites (Brenner, 2003). Unfortunately, there is a disparity between African American and white children ages 5 to 19 years: the rate of drowning for African American children is 2.4 times the rate for white children. Community programs to teach parents about drowning prevention are recommended (National Safe Kids Campaign, 2003).

Firearms. Firearms accounted for 28,874 deaths in 1999 (CDC, 2001). Approximately 800 *unintentional* deaths result from firearms annually; approximately 600 of these occur while people are playing with or cleaning firearms (National Safety Council, 2002). Most firearm deaths are the result of suicides and homicides. Approximately 85% of these deaths are in males. The overall suicide rate (6.6 per 100,000) is higher than the homicide rate (5.1 per 100,000). The greatest absolute number of homicide deaths occurs in persons older than 44 years of age (almost 11,000), but the fatal firearm-related deaths per 100,000 are highest for the 15- to 24-year-old age group, and for African Americans. Nurses and other health professionals are challenged to provide education about proper gun storage to minimize firearm injuries and deaths and to address violence in school and work settings (McClelland et al., 1996). Issues related to societal violence and the availability of firearms are

complex and require communities to work together to reduce homicides and suicides (see Chapter 23).

Unintentional injuries tend to be more prevalent for families living in substandard housing because of poor construction or poor repair. However, no family is immune to home hazards.

Other Hazards in the Home

Sanitation. Hygiene and household cleanliness contribute to the maintenance of family health. A potential source of disease that is often taken for granted is the method of garbage disposal (dumping, burning, burying, or landfilling) (Morgan, 2003). Daily, each American produces approximately 4.5 pounds of solid waste, such as food scraps and paper (USDHHS, 1998). One objective of *Healthy People 2010* is to decrease this amount through waste reduction and recycling, thereby reducing contamination of water, air, and soil by solid waste (USDHHS, 2000). To maximize safety and cleanliness, garbage should be properly wrapped, and garbage cans should be kept clean and tightly closed. The increased use and disposal of disposable diapers dumps human feces, which contain numerous enteric organisms, in garbage piles and landfills (Primomo, 1990). When handled improperly, these wastes can lead to contamination of water supplies, contribute to breeding of bacteria and viruses that can be transmitted to humans via insects and rodents, and possibly serve as a reservoir for disease. Diseases that can be spread through contact with human feces include gastroenteritis and hepatitis (see Chapter 8). A detailed case study about disposable diaper use is provided in **Web Resource 9A.** Hazardous wastes are discussed later in this chapter.

Radon. Radon has been of great concern in recent years. Radon is an odorless, colorless, and tasteless radioactive gas that is the by-product of the decay of uranium; it occurs naturally in the soil (Morgan, 2003). It has been estimated that up to 36,000 lung cancer deaths per year among nonsmokers are a result of radon exposure (Lubin & Boice, 1997). Radon as a health risk has been included in the *Healthy People 2010* objectives. One objective is to increase to 20% the proportion of homes that are tested for radon. Evidence suggests that chronic exposure to radon leads to an increase of respiratory symptoms. The risk to uranium miners has been known for several years, but the recent concern has focused on the presence of radon in homes. Investigations into the effects of radon exposure in homes are continuing.

A number of factors affect exposure levels to radon, including a home's construction, its ventilation properties, the presence of cracks or openings in the foundation or walls, and the occupant's living patterns. Measuring devices to determine the level of radon can be obtained through private companies or government agencies. Certain parts of the country are more likely to have radon. Maps from the Environmental Protection Agency (EPA) (see Community Resources in Practice) show areas of high concentration. The EPA is the federal agency with the primary responsibility for protecting health and setting and enforcing standards related to environmental pollutants. If radon exposure is suspected, clients should be referred to the EPA or a company that can assess the situation.

Lead. The reduction of childhood lead poisoning is one of the most significant public health achievements in recent years.

Leaded gasoline and lead-based paint (both banned in the 1970s), including dust and chips, have long been recognized as a source of lead poisoning, particularly in young children. Other sources of lead exposure include contaminated soil; air-borne particles from steel structures, gasoline fumes, and dusts; water from lead pipes or tanks; food from ceramic-ware containers; and hobbies such as target shooting and stained glass and glazed pottery making. Despite the removal of lead from paint, gasoline, and food cans, lead persists in the paint and plumbing of many older structures, and in contaminated soil (Sanborn et al., 2002). Recent scientific data show adverse effects from lead in young children at blood levels much lower than previously considered dangerous. Blood levels greater than 10 mcg/dl are now considered harmful. The *Healthy People 2010* objectives seek to have no children with blood lead levels higher than 10 mcg/dl (USDHHS, 2000). From 1976 to 1980, the average blood lead level in children was 15 mcg/dl, and from 1991 to 1994, the average was 2.7 mcg/dl (CDC, 1997). **Website Resource 9B** provides additional information about blood levels, associated symptoms, and recommended interventions for the prevention of lead poisoning.

WEB

Lead poisonings are usually associated with older, deteriorating houses that might have leaded paint that is peeling, flaking, and chipping. In recent years, lead has been recognized as a hazard when renovating older homes. Unfortunately, families renovating older homes are often unaware that lead poisoning might be a risk for them (Agency for Toxic Substances and Disease Registry [ATSDR], 1995; Sanborn et al., 2002). Early signs of lead poisoning include disturbances in cognition, behavior, learning, attention span, and growth and development. Colic, constipation, and upper extremity weakness are signs of chronic exposure. Continued exposure leads to central nervous system symptoms (e.g., encephalopathy) and renal and hematologic effects.

Prevention of lead poisoning in young children requires community efforts to eliminate environmental exposure and to educate families about screening and prevention. The CDC recommends that because virtually all U.S. children are at risk for lead poisoning, all children should be screened (CDC, 1997). Blood lead levels are more likely to be elevated among children who are poor, non-Hispanic blacks or Mexican American, living in large metropolitan areas, or living in pre-1950s housing (CDC, 1997). Nurses working with families must identify those at risk for lead toxicity while educating children, teachers, parents, and other health care providers about how to prevent lead toxicity (Arvidson & Colledge, 1996; Davis, 2007).

At a school health fair, the Marino family learned about their health department's program to reduce lead exposure in young children. They talked with the school nurse, Alice Johnson, about their children's risks and jointly used a checklist to determine if they should test their 5-year-old twin boys for lead. The Marino's discovered their children were at risk for lead poisoning because their home was built before 1960; they were planning to remodel; they lived near an old lead smelter; and Mrs. Marino once worked in stained glass construction. The twins' blood lead levels were 10 mcg/dl, a level at which behavioral problems, impaired hearing, and diminished growth can occur. Ms. Johnson referred the Marino's to the health department for information about reducing lead

exposure. They took protective measures during their remodeling, hired a licensed contractor to remove the lead paint, and stayed with family members while the work was being done. To reduce exposures, they put mats at each entry door, removed shoes at the door, and used damp mops to clean the floors to reduce tracked-in dust and dirt that might contain lead. They emphasized thorough hand-washing and increased intake of calcium-rich and iron-rich foods. After 6 months, the boys' blood levels began to decrease.

Formaldehyde. Formaldehyde, a colorless, flammable gas, is present in a variety of household products, including carpets, draperies, paper, shampoos, and cosmetics (ATSDR, 1999). It is also used in glues for plywood and fiberboard; thus many homes have formaldehyde in their cabinetry and furniture. The most common symptoms are eye and nose irritation, respiratory symptoms, nausea, headache, and fatigue. Young children can have abdominal complaints. Formaldehyde is also a carcinogen. Less toxic products are available and should be recommended when new purchases are being made. If formaldehyde is present, increasing ventilation by opening windows and allowing fresh air to enter can help.

Carbon Monoxide. Carbon monoxide is a colorless and odorless gas that is a by-product of combustion and is an insidious poison (Blumenthal & Ruttenber, 1995). Possible sources are improperly vented furnaces, blocked flues or chimneys, and automobile exhausts, particularly when a garage is attached to a house. Exposure to carbon monoxide can cause dizziness, headache, drowsiness, nausea, or flu-like symptoms. Continued exposure might result in unconsciousness and death. Persons who have cardiovascular or respiratory diseases are particularly vulnerable to the effects of carbon monoxide. As with formaldehyde, there is an increased risk in well-insulated houses. Nurses can recommend carbon monoxide detectors to help warn of these exposures (Davis, 2007).

Environmental Tobacco Smoke. One of the most common sources of *indoor air pollution* is environmental tobacco smoke (Goldman, 2000). Since the 1960s, tobacco smoking has been recognized as a cause of lung cancer and other respiratory diseases in smokers (EPA, 1993). More recently, research has shown that environmental tobacco smoke is hazardous to nonsmokers who live or work in environments occupied by smokers. It is a major contributor to asthma exacerbations. Recent studies have found that children exposed to tobacco smoke show decreased growth; more ear and respiratory tract infections, such as pneumonia; more bronchitis; and new cases of asthma (Goldman, 2000). Secondhand tobacco smoke has carcinogenic and toxic agents that are similar to those in mainstream smoke; the EPA classifies tobacco smoke as a carcinogen.

Amanda is a 7-year-old girl with mild, persistent asthma, and her family recently moved to a new apartment. Although her asthma had been controlled with inhaled corticosteroids, Amanda's coughing, wheezing, and shortness of breath were increasingly troublesome. Her mother, Senzie Mott, referred to Amanda's asthma management plan and decided to make an appointment with her provider. During the visit, the nurse, Sandra Grember, inquired about changes at home. Amanda's mother reported the family moved recently and wondered if that might account for Amanda's symptoms. Ms. Grember asked specific questions about the home environment, including the presence of allergen-impermeable pillow and mattress covers, carpets, moisture, mold, smoking, pets, and pests, such as cockroaches and rodents. She discussed how to reduce home environmental asthma triggers and provided a brochure from the EPA. Amanda's mother welcomed the information about how to reduce asthma triggers, such as dust mites, pests, secondhand smoke, mildew, and mold. She agreed to increase her own cleaning regimen to reduce household dust and mildew, wash Amanda's bedding and stuffed animals in hot water weekly, and ask the landlord about removing the carpet that smelled of smoke and pets. A telephone follow-up was planned for 2 weeks to check on Amanda's symptoms.

Environmental tobacco smoke is also associated with sudden infant death syndrome (SIDS). According to *Healthy People 2010* (USDHHS, 2000), approximately 15 million children and adolescents were exposed to secondhand smoke in their homes in 1996. One of the *Healthy People 2010* objectives aims to reduce children's exposure to environmental tobacco smoke.

Secondhand smoke is a major problem in public places and workplaces as well. Because new homes and office buildings tend to be constructed and insulated more tightly to conserve energy, toxic allergens and toxic chemicals, such as environmental tobacco smoke, are concentrated in indoor air (Tsacoyianis, 1997). The CDC has developed an action guide for consumers to reduce secondhand smoke that includes policies to reduce smoking and exposure to environmental tobacco smoke (Box 9-3).

Implications for Nurses

Community/public health nurses are in key positions to educate families about how to promote home safety and prevent accidents and hazardous exposures, in other words primary prevention measures. Families should be informed about the hazards of secondhand smoke and be encouraged not to smoke indoors, in cars, or around children. It is important for families to know where hazardous waste disposal sites are and to discard their chemicals there rather than with their garbage and other trash. Many local solid waste or environmental health divisions provide information on how to purchase and safely store and dispose of household chemicals.

Nurses play an active role in secondary prevention or screening for environmental problems. Nurses can determine hazards that might threaten the health or safety of persons in their homes. Family history should include the occupations of household members; location, age, and physical condition of the residence, school, daycare, or work site; home remodeling activities; hobbies; use of non–lead-based ceramics for cooking or eating; source and quality of drinking water; and health of pets. A comprehensive home assessment considers the surroundings in which the home is located (Sattler & Lipscomb, 2003). For example, living in a densely populated area or one with a high noise level (e.g., near an airport) can have untoward health effects (Morgan, 2003).

The causes of health problems might be subtle and might require intensive investigative work by the nurse. For example, water contaminants might not produce a visible change in the water, and some chemicals (e.g., carbon monoxide in air) are not easily detectable. As an example of how an environmental hazard in the home can be easily overlooked, consider

BOX 9-3   Facts about Secondhand Smoke

Some of the key facts about secondhand tobacco smoke and its dangers are summarized below. Use them to inform your family and friends and to work for smoke-free policies in your community.

- Secondhand smoke (SHS) is sometimes referred to as environmental tobacco smoke (ETS), involuntary smoking, or passive smoking.
- Secondhand smoke is a mixture of the smoke emitted by the burning end of a cigarette, pipe, or cigar, and the smoke exhaled from the lungs of smokers.
- The mixture of SHS contains more than 4000 substances, more than 40 of which are known to cause cancer in humans or animals, and many of which are strong irritants.
- Secondhand smoke has been classified by the U.S. Environmental Protection Agency (EPA) as a known cause of lung cancer in humans (group A carcinogen).
- Secondhand smoke is estimated by the EPA to cause approximately 3000 lung cancer deaths in nonsmokers each year. It causes increased risk of death from heart disease and sudden infant death syndrome.
- The developing lungs of young children are severely affected by exposure to secondhand smoke because children are particularly vulnerable to secondhand smoke. This is likely due to several factors, including that children are still developing physically, have higher breathing rates than adults, and have little control over their indoor environments. Children receiving high doses of secondhand smoke, such as those with smoking mothers, run the greatest relative risk of experiencing damaging health effects.
- Children with asthma are especially at risk. The EPA estimates that exposure to secondhand smoke increases the number of episodes and severity of symptoms in 200,000 to 1,000,000 children with asthma. Moreover, secondhand smoke is a risk factor for new cases of asthma in children who have not previously exhibited asthma symptoms.
- Infants and young children whose parents smoke are among the most seriously affected by exposure to secondhand smoke, being at increased risk of lower respiratory tract infections, such as pneumonia and bronchitis. The EPA estimates that secondhand smoke is responsible for between 150,000 and 300,000 lower respiratory tract infections in infants and children under 18 months of age, resulting in between 7500 and 15,000 hospitalizations each year.

Adapted from Environmental Protection Agency. *Smoke free homes.* Available at *http://www.epa.gov/smokefree/publications.html;* and Centers for Disease Control and Prevention. *Taking action against second hand smoke: A toolkit.* Available at *http://www.cdc.gov/tobacco/ETS_Toolkit/index.htm&num.*

a study that examined the toxic effects of pesticide application for fleas (Fenske et al., 1990). The findings from this study indicated that although the concentration of the pesticide (used as directed) decreased considerably in the adult breathing zone 24 hours after application, the concentration remained high in an infant's breathing zone near the floor, in part because of its concentration in the carpet or in crevices in the floor. Furthermore, because infant skin might be more permeable to these chemicals, there is a higher risk for dermal absorption.

Community/public health nurses can address environmental health from an educational, practice, research, and/or policy/advocacy approach. For example, from an educational perspective, nurses can provide individual guidance to their pregnant patients about preparing an environmentally healthy and safe nursery by addressing potential lead-based paint risks, safety issues such as covering electrical outlets, and product selection concerns such as choosing infant toys that do not contain phthalates.

From a practice perspective, there are a number of ways in which interventions can be considered. First and foremost, a good assessment must be completed, including the elements identified previously in this chapter. Once a risk factor is identified, the nurse must determine whether the problem can be addressed at the individual level or whether a more population-based approach is needed. If a population-based approach is warranted, then the nurse will need to know whether a public agency holds some responsibility in addressing the issue. For instance, if a community is concerned about the safety of a body of recreational water, this question can be addressed most readily by the state-level department of environmental quality (or environmental protection) who are responsible for administering the elements of the Clean Water Act. If a community is concerned about the number of municipal buses that idle across from a city elementary school, then this issue might be best addressed by the transportation authority.

UNDERSTANDING "WHO'S IN CHARGE"

Understanding "who's in charge" of environmental health is a very big task and can be a very complicated one. Federal, state, and local agencies all have both distinct and overlapping roles (see Chapter 6). All branches of government can be involved: the federal legislative branch as it passes sweeping laws such as the Clean Air Act, or a specific state law that bans toxic fire-retardant materials from use in products (as recently occurred in Washington state). The executive branch includes the executive/regulatory agencies at a federal, state, and local level where they develop regulations and conduct compliance inspections to make sure that the regulations are being followed. Even the judiciary branch can be involved when it orders an emergency standard for a chemical exposure or makes a decision regarding the legality of a new regulation.

For local environmental health issues, the two most important agencies are the state department of environmental quality and the local health departments. The health departments of large cities and populated counties often have a significant environmental health division with a range of services. Some large cities (such as San Francisco) and large counties (such as Baltimore County, Maryland) have dedicated environmental protection agencies.

It is the responsibility of state-level environmental protection agencies to determine how much pollution a factory or other institution can emit into the air or water. They do this by issuing a "permit," which essentially is permission to pollute. These permits are public documents. Unfortunately, there is no cap on the number of permits that an agency can allow and consequently some communities have a large number of "permits." This can have a serious impact on air and/or water quality. Though public hearings are required as part of the permitting process, they are often *pro forma* and the mechanism by which most community members would hear about them is often inadequate.

It is the responsibility of the city or county to determine how land is to be used, and the mechanism that they use is their "zoning" laws. Land can be zoned for use as residential, commercial, light or heavy industry, or rural/farming, for example. It is through these important land use decisions that it will be determined how densely an area will be populated, whether a factory can be built next to a daycare center, or if land should be set aside for green space, for example. Zoning decisions can have a direct impact on a community's quality of life, environmental health, and their property values. No one wants a hazardous waste site to be placed in their neighborhood and yet more hazardous waste sites are located in African American neighborhoods than in white neighborhoods in the United States (Bullard & Wright, 1993). More African American residential neighborhoods are zoned for mix use than white neighborhoods, which leaves African American neighborhoods open to varied use by commercial entities and even light industry.

The expression "Smart Growth" was coined in the 1990s to describe an approach to land use decisions that maximize the use of space for public transportation, bike routes, parks, and recreational facilities, while retaining green spaces and farmlands. It also calls for development in areas that already have water, electric, sewer, and transportation infrastructures rather than creating new developments in undeveloped areas. The people who are responsible for such decisions are called "planners" and they reside in the planning offices of cities, counties (parishes, burroughs), and states. Zoning and planning decisions can have a great impact on local and area environmental quality. Public health professionals should be aware of and engaged in this decision-making.

ACCESSING INFORMATION AND THE RIGHT TO KNOW

One of the best sources for information about environmental conditions is the U.S. EPA website *(http://www.epa.gov/enviro)*. On this site, state, local, and zipcode-level information can be found. (Note that some of the information, such as emissions and effluent from factories, is reported by the regulated industry, and not actually collected or corroborated by the EPA.)

Statutes and regulations can establish the public's **"right to know"** about specific contaminants expelled into the environment. For example, all public water suppliers must test the water regularly and they must alert their customers immediately if a chemical, radiologic, or biologic contaminant, that might create a health risk, exceeds standards. Additionally, once a year the supplier has to compile a report that describes the testing that has been done, the results, and information on the source(s) of the water. These reports are technically called "Consumer Confidence Reports" and are required by law.

Another "right to know" law requires that companies that store or emit (into the air or water) 1 of 600 potentially toxic chemicals must report this to the EPA and, in turn, this information is to be accessible to the public. This is commonly known as the "community right to know" law. Another part of the same law requires that every local area (usually city/county designations) and state have an emergency planning committee. These committees are mandated to assess the chemicals that are transported, stored, or used in their area and note whether there is a potential for a leak, spill, explosion, or transportation accident and to make a plan to address such an event.

Under the Clean Air Act, there is a requirement that all companies that transport, store, or use potentially hazardous chemicals develop a set of "worst case scenarios" for things that might go wrong. These "chemical risk management plans" were originally intended for community review but since the events of 9/11, this information has been deemed confidential.

It is possible, though difficult, to gain access to this information (Afzal, 2003).

Another mechanism to access information from the government (state and federal) is through the Freedom of Information Act (FOIA). There is a single federal act that provides the mechanism for accessing information from federal agencies and then each state has its own state laws regarding how citizens can gain access to state agency information. This can be used for any sort of information, not just environmental issues.

There is still quite a bit of room for improvement regarding the public's right to know. While there are a good many things that can be found on a food label, there are some important things we do not currently have the right to know about at the point of purchase. For example, none of the following information is required to be on a food label: the use of pesticides/herbicides when growing produce; the use of genetically-modified organisms; the use of nontherapeutic antibiotics in animal feed for beef, hogs, poultry, or farmed fish; or the administration of recombinant bovine growth hormone (rBGH) to dairy cows. We can learn about certain nutritional values of our foods (e.g., calories, fats, proteins, and carbohydrates) but not about the potentially hazardous chemicals or pharmaceuticals (Huffling, 2006).

In the workplace, employees have the "right to know" about the potentially hazardous chemicals that they may be exposed to during the course of doing their jobs. Employers must label potentially hazardous chemicals/materials, maintain chemical information sheets (known as material safety data sheets [MSDS]), and train all employees about the potential health and safety risks. Most products are labeled in health care and, if you ask the person in charge of health and safety, you can usually track down a copy of a MSDS. Where most employers fall short is in the training of employees. Consider whether, as a nurse, you received formal training about the potential health risks from exposure to glutaraldehyde, ethylene oxide, or other common sterilizing agents found in health care. Did you receive information on the potential health effects associated with floor cleaning products, pesticides used in and around the hospital, or air fresheners in the rest rooms? It is the right of all workers to be trained about potential health risks and how to protect themselves through proper work practices and, if necessary, protective equipment (e.g., gloves, masks, ventilation hoods, respirators).

The Health Care Without Harm campaign, an international effort to address environmental health risks in the health care sector, published a report on the presence of chemicals that are commonly used in hospitals that are either primary asthmagens (meaning they are known or suspected of causing asthma) or asthma triggers (those chemicals that can cause an asthma event in someone who already has the diagnosis of asthma). A summary of the report has been created (Table 9-3).

ENVIRONMENTAL HAZARDS IN THE OCCUPATIONAL SETTING

Most Americans spend a substantial portion of their adult lives in work environments. These work environments are characterized by a wide range of health and safety hazards that might result in the occurrence of occupational injuries and illnesses. In 2006, private-sector employers in this country reported 3.9 million non-fatal occupational injuries and 228,000 occupational illnesses (U.S. Department of Labor, Bureau of Labor

Statistics, 2007). The true extent of the problem is unknown, because many incidents of injury and illness are not reported, and, in some cases, are not recognized as being occupationally related. An average of 137 U.S. workers die each day from work-related disease, 9000 sustain disabling injuries on the job, and 16 workers die from a work-related injury (Levy & Wegman, 2000). The following are the top occupational illnesses:

- Disorders associated with repeated trauma
- Skin diseases and disorders
- Respiratory conditions caused by toxic substances
- Disorders caused by physical agents
- Poisonings
- Dust diseases of the lungs (National Safety Council, 2002)

The immense losses resulting from occupational injury and illness affect individuals and organizations at multiple levels. The employee suffers the loss of a portion of his or her wages, might be required to bear some of the expenses related to care, and experiences the pain and suffering related to the event. The employer might suffer from a loss of productivity, high absenteeism and turnover, and low employee morale. Society pays the extra costs involved in workers' compensation through higher costs for goods and services. Society also loses the revenue from taxes that are not being paid by an unemployed person and that person's contribution to society. These facts demonstrate the significant effect that the occupational environment can have on the health and safety of communities. The *Healthy People 2010* objectives also address occupational safety and health (see the *Healthy People 2010* box on page 255).

In 1996 the National Institute for Occupational Safety and Health developed 21 research priority areas. These priorities were a result of collaboration and input from multiple sources, including employers, employees, health and safety professionals, and labor organizations. The priority areas are organized into three major categories: disease and injury, work environment and workforce, and research tools and approaches; these data are available on this book's website as **Website Resource 9C.** These listed areas are intended to guide occupational health and safety research over the next several years.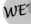

HISTORY OF OCCUPATIONAL HEALTH IN THE UNITED STATES

Attention to health and safety in the workplace is a recent phenomenon. The Industrial Revolution played a major role in the development of the field of occupational health. During the 19th century, masses of Americans, including children, worked in factories and sweatshops, on the railroads, or in the mines. They were exposed to machinery, chemicals, dusts, extremes in temperatures, backbreaking chores, and other deplorable conditions. As concerns for health and safety grew, job safety laws slowly began to be passed. **Website Resource 9D** provides a list of legislative efforts to protect workers.

Workers' compensation was a significant contribution to worker protection. It provides a partial reimbursement of lost wages and full payment for medical expenses to workers who are injured or become ill as a result of their job. There continue to be major deficiencies in the system. For example, compensation for certain occupational diseases, such as chemical sensitivity or stress-related conditions, is very limited. This is largely the result of the difficulties in establishing links between

TABLE 9-3 | **Asthma Risks Posed by Chemicals Used in Health Care Environments**

Chemical	Use in Hospitals	Asthmagen or Asthma Trigger?	How to Reduce Exposure	Safer Alternatives
Cleaners, disinfectants/sterilizers	Cleaning products, equipment sterilizers	Asthmagen and asthma trigger	Use microfiber mops, refine cleaning practices, isolate chemicals	*Products free of:* Ethylene oxide, formaldehyde, glutaraldehyde, Green Seal–approved products
Natural rubber latex	Gloves, catheters, and other hospital products	Asthmagen, possibly asthma trigger	Use nonlatex or powder-free latex gloves	Nonlatex or powder-free latex gloves
Pesticides	Indoor and outdoor areas	Asthmagen	Integrated Pest Management programs*	IPM: using nontoxic pest control methods and products
Volatile organic compounds (VOCs)	Formaldehyde: building materials, paper products, tissue fixatives	Asthmagen, possibly asthma trigger	Increase general ventilation to diffuse VOC off-gassing	Low- or no-VOC products Formaldehyde-free products
Baking flour	Kitchens and bakeries	Asthmagen and asthma trigger	Mechanical flour sprinklers, good ventilation systems, quick cleanup of spills with wet mop	Precombined dry ingredients, low-dust flour, ready-to-bake dough
Acrylics: methyl methacrylate and cyanoacrylate	Acrylic resins used in medical and dental polymers and cement	Asthmagen and asthma trigger	Isolate, enclose, and automate processes that use acrylic compounds; improve ventilation systems	*Products free of:* Methyl methacrylate Cyanoacrylate Acrylic compounds
Perfumes/fragrances	Scented cleaners, fragrance-emitting devices, people wearing perfume	Asthma trigger	Institute fragrance-free policies	Fragrance-free products
Phthalates (plasticizers)	Widespread: plastics, medical devices	Undetermined	Improve ventilation for moisture control to decrease emissions	Phthalate-free products, (both medical and office products)
Environmental tobacco smoke (ETS)	Individuals who smoke	Asthmagen and asthma trigger	Maintain a smoke-free facility and grounds	
Biologic allergens	Mold/fungus, indoor pollen, dust/dust mites, pet hair, cockroaches	Asthmagen and asthma trigger	Good housekeeping and building maintenance practices, moisture control	
Pharmaceuticals	Antibiotics, laxatives, antihypertensives, antituberculars, H_2 blockers	Asthmagen	Hoppers, ventilation hoods, personal protective equipment, respirators	Clinical substitutions if possible

This table was derived from the Health Care Without Harm report entitled *Risks to asthma posed by the indoor health care environments: A guide to identifying and reducing problematic exposures,* created 2006 by Laura Evans, MPH, and Barbara Sattler, RN, DrPH, FAAN, of the Environmental Health Education Center, University of Maryland School of Nursing. Used with permission.

*Integrated Pest Management (IPM) is a systematic approach to managing pests that provides a comprehensive framework for assessing pest problems; assessing the sources of food, water, and nesting that support growth and reproduction of pests; determining the nontoxic and least-toxic techniques and products to be employed; and evaluating success and/or need for additional considerations. For more information on IPM, see: *http://www.beyondpesticides.org.*

the disease and the work setting. Even when employees are compensated for an injury or illness, they seldom recover the full value of lost wages and expenses.

The Occupational Safety and Health (OSH) Act was created to ensure safe and healthful working conditions. The **Occupational Safety and Health Administration (OSHA),** a federal agency, administers the provisions of the OSH Act. As a result of the OSH Act, businesses and industries began to develop new occupational safety and health programs. Employers are required to adhere to specific standards. For example, OSHA wrote the Hazard Communication Standard of 1986 because of increasing concern about employee exposure to toxic substances.

The National Institute for Occupational Safety and Health (NIOSH) developed and funded the first Education and Research Centers (ERCs) across the United States. Through these centers, graduate-level education is provided for nurses, physicians, industrial hygienists, and safety managers; continuing education programs are developed; and research on occupational safety and health problems is conducted. There are a total of 15 NIOSH-funded occupational health nursing programs. A complete list of NIOSH-funded occupational health nursing programs is available on NIOSH's website. For environmental health nursing, the only graduate programs are at the University of Maryland in Baltimore and the University of Washington.

■ **HEALTHY PEOPLE 2010** ■
Occupational Safety and Health Objectives

Health Status Objectives

1. Reduce deaths from work-related injuries to no more than 3.2 per 100,000 full-time workers. (Baseline: average of 4.5 per 100,000 in 1998.)
2. Reduce the annual number of deaths with any mention of pneumoconiosis to no more than 1900 among persons ages 15 years and older. (Baseline: 2928 deaths in 1997.)
3. Reduce deaths from work-related homicides to no more than 0.4 per 100,000 workers. (Baseline: 0.5 per 100,000 in 1998.)
4. Reduce work-related injuries resulting in medical treatment, lost time from work, or restricted work activity to no more than 4.3 cases per 100 full-time workers. (Baseline: 6.2 per 100 in 1998.)

	Average Injuries per 100	Year 2010 Objective
Construction workers	8.7 (1998)	6.1
Health services' workers	7.9 (1997)	5.5
Farm, forestry, and fishing workers	7.6 (1998)	5.3
Transportation	7.9 (1997)	5.5
Mining	4.7 (1998)	3.3
Manufacturing	8.5 (1998)	6.0
Adolescent workers	4.8 (1997)	3.4

5. Reduce the injury and illness cases involving days away from work caused by overexertion or repetitive motion, including injuries caused by overexertion in lifting. (Target: 338 injuries per 100,000 full-time workers. Baseline: 675 injuries per 100,000 full-time workers in 1997.)
6. Reduce occupational skin disorders or diseases to an incidence of no more than 47 per 100,000 full-time workers. (Baseline: 67 per 100,000 in 1997.)
7. Reduce number of cases of hepatitis B in occupationally exposed workers to 62. (Baseline of 249 in 1997.)

Risk Reduction Objectives

8. Reduce new cases of work-related, noise-induced hearing loss.
9. Reduce the number of persons who have elevated blood lead concentrations from work exposures to zero. (Baseline: 93 per million persons ages 16 to 64 years had blood lead concentrations of 25 mcg/dl or greater in 1998.)
10. Increase hepatitis B vaccine coverage among occupationally exposed workers to 98%. (Baseline: 71% in 1995.)

Services and Protection Objectives

11. Increase the proportion of work sites employing 50 or more persons that provide programs to prevent or reduce employee stress. (Target: 50%. Baseline: 37% in 1992.)
12. Increase the number of office buildings that are managed using good indoor air quality practices.
13. Establish in at least 25 states a surveillance system for tracking asthma death, illness, disability, impact of occupational and environmental factors on asthma, access to medical care, and asthma management.

From U.S. Department of Health and Human Services. (2000). *Healthy People 2010 objectives.* Washington, DC: U.S. Government Printing Office.

Although there has been substantial improvement in occupational health and safety with the passage of the OSH Act, the Americans with Disabilities Act, and other mandates, a rapidly changing workplace continues to pose major challenges to occupational health and safety professionals. These changes are reflected in the organization of work, work processes, and the workers themselves. Advances in technology have increased the speed of production and the subsequent demands on workers. New chemicals, materials, and processes, with unknown health and safety effects, are constantly being developed and marketed. Many organizations are downsizing and restructuring; others are expanding their businesses across national borders. All of these changes and a trend toward outsourcing of services have resulted in an increased level of job insecurity and stress in many workplaces. According to the NIOSH (1999), job stress poses a major threat to the health of workers.

The composition of the labor force is also changing. It is projected that in the coming years, the workforce will be older and more racially diverse and will include a larger proportion of women (Lusk, 2001). All of these changes will affect how occupational health services are delivered.

Occupational Health Nursing

Occupational health is distinguishable as a subspecialty because of its environmental approach to disease and injury and its primary focus on prevention. The principal target of occupational and environmental health nursing practice is the aggregate of workers in the many occupational settings across the country. In the late 19th century, the first occupational and environmental health nurses were called *industrial nurses,* and their primary responsibility was to care for injured workers and their families. Much of their care was provided in the home, and they often took care of other family members and taught them about general sanitation and hygiene.

With the rapid expansion of industries in the early 1900s, and the passage of workers' compensation laws, the demand for industrial nurses increased dramatically. Occupational health services began to focus more on injuries to the workers in the work setting than on family-member services in the home. With the onset of World War II, the demand for industrial nurses increased. By 1942 there were more than 11,000 industrial nurses (Parker-Conrad, 2002). It is now estimated that there are more than 30,000 occupational and environmental health nurses in the United States; furthermore, many more do not describe themselves as occupational and environmental health nurses but nevertheless provide occupational health services. This latter category includes employee health nurses, infectious control nurses, and case managers.

In 1942 the American Association of Industrial Nurses (AAIN) was formed as the professional association for these nurses (Dirksen, 2006). In 1976, in keeping with the changes that were occurring within the profession, the name was changed to the American Association of Occupational Health Nurses (AAOHN), a term reflective of the broader scope of practice of the nurse in industry. As of 2003 more than 10,000 occupational and environmental health nurses were members of AAOHN.

The American Board for Occupational Health Nurses (ABOHN) is the certifying body for occupational and environmental health nurses. Currently, two credentials are available to occupational and environmental health nurses desiring to be certified as an occupational health nurse. The certified occupational health nurse (COHN) designation is offered to occupational and environmental health nurses with an associate degree or a diploma or their international equivalent. Occupational and environmental health nurses with a baccalaureate or higher degree are eligible for either the COHN or the COHN-S certification (S designates specialist). Nurses who receive the COHN or the COHN-S certifications are also qualified to apply for case management certification (COHN/CM or COHN-S/CM), which is a special area of practice for occupational and environmental health nurses.

To be certified by ABOHN, occupational and environmental health nurses must demonstrate they meet the criteria, including a minimum number of appropriate practice hours, current employment in the specialty, completion of a required number of continuing education hours in occupational health and safety, and successful completion of the board examination. As of 2003 more than 11,000 occupational and environmental health nurses completed the requirements for either a COHN or a COHN-S. Additionally, more than 900 have become certified as case managers by ABOHN (personal communication, Mary Amann, Executive Director, ABOHN, 2003).

Roles and Functions of Occupational Health Nurses. The role of the occupational and environmental health nurse has evolved and expanded in the past decade; principal functions continue to be promotion, protection, and maintenance of the health and safety of the workers. There is an expanded emphasis on wellness and lifestyle changes in addition to the reduction of risks associated with environmental exposures. The practice of this specialty involves primary, secondary, and tertiary prevention. Special skills include training in safety hazards, disaster planning, familiarity with safety equipment, and the ability to plan and implement health-education programs. Special knowledge includes an understanding of the principles of safety, toxicology, epidemiology, environmental health, and industrial hygiene. As an interdisciplinary specialty, occupational and environmental health nurses work with multiple health and safety specialists, including toxicologists, industrial hygienists, occupational physicians, safety specialists, ergonomists, and epidemiologists (Box 9-4). Occupational and environmental health nurses are also required to have up-to-date knowledge of current legal standards that affect the working population (Welker-Hood et al., 2007).

The AAOHN has developed standards of practice that enable occupational and environmental health nurses to measure the quality of the service that they deliver. Current AAOHN standards (published in 1999) define the specialty, describe the scope of practice, and provide the criteria for 11 practice standards. In addition to assessment, planning, implementation, and evaluation, the standards cover such areas of practice as resource management, professional development, research, and ethics. The standards are available through AAOHN or a local organization. In 2006 the third edition of *Core Curriculum for Occupational and Environmental Health Nurses* was published (Salazar, 2006) to provide further guidance and direction to occupational and environmental health nursing practice.

The occupational and environmental health nurse is often an independent practitioner and is frequently the only health care provider in an organization. Because management might not understand the roles and functions of occupational and

---

BOX 9-4   Description of Roles of Occupational Health and Safety Specialists
Toxicologist—Studies and describes the toxic properties of agents used in work application to which workers might be exposed.   ***Industrial hygienist***—Recognizes, evaluates, and controls toxic exposures and hazards in the work environment.   ***Occupational physician***—Focuses on prevention, detection, and treatment of work-related diseases and injuries.   ***Safety specialist***—Includes safety engineers and other safety professionals who focus on the prevention of occupational injuries and the maintenance or creation of safer workplaces and safe work practices.   ***Ergonomist***—Studies, designs, and promotes the healthy interface of humans, their tools, and their work.   ***Epidemiologist***—Studies and describes the natural history of occupational diseases and injuries in population groups.

From Levy, B. S., & Wegman, D. H. (2000). *Occupational health: Recognizing and preventing work-related disease* (4th ed.). Boston: Little, Brown.

environmental health nurses, these nurses might need to write their own job description. Whereas occupational and environmental health nurses perform according to the guidelines established by the profession and by company management, nurses often determine the priorities appropriate to a situation, establish goals and objectives, and determine the most suitable course of action. The roles of occupational and environmental health nurses vary greatly from one setting to another. Their activities might be categorized as follows: primary care provider, counselor, advocate and liaison, administrator, educator, monitor, professional member of the health team, and researcher (Box 9-5). The occupational and environmental health nurse might function in as few as one or as many as all of these roles, depending on the particular work site.

> Maria is a public health nurse in an agricultural community in eastern Washington. Some community members approached her with concerns about health problems related to pesticide exposure. Some of them had skin rashes; other people who worked with them complained of nausea, dizziness, and headaches; and some had difficulty breathing. Maria agreed to meet with all the workers who were concerned, for a health-education program. At the meeting, she provided information about pesticides, including common health problems, routes of exposure (absorption, inhalation, and ingestion), and strategies to minimize their risks. She cautioned the workers to check their clothing, because they could bring pesticides home, exposing their families. She stressed the importance of eliminating any exposure for their children, because children are prone to more severe reactions to pesticides. Maria and several other public health personnel scheduled a meeting with the Growers Association to educate their employers about safety precautions, including training of the workers to reduce their exposure risk. Because of her efforts, Maria became known as a community resource for growers, farmers, and their families about issues related to pesticides.

As with many professionals in recent years, occupational and environmental health nurses often struggle with ethical and legal dilemmas in their practice. The struggle is often precipitated by the nurse's dual responsibilities to the employer

Box 9-5 Functional Roles of Occupational and Environmental Health Nurses

Clinician—Primary responsibilities are aimed at preventing work-related and non–work-related health problems and restoring and maintaining health.

Case manager—Coordinates health and rehabilitation services for an individual worker from the onset of an injury or illness to an optimal return to work status or a satisfactory alternative.

Occupational health service coordinator—Functions as the single occupational health nurse for a business or organization.

Health-promotion specialist—Develops and manages a comprehensive, multilevel, broad-range health-promotion program that supports organizational business objectives.

Manager—Directs, administers, and evaluates an occupational and environmental health and safety service and its policies, maintaining consistency with organizational goals and objectives.

Nurse practitioner—Uses additional specialized preparation, meeting state requirements for advanced practice nursing to critically evaluate the health status of workers through health histories, physical assessment, and diagnostic tests.

Corporate director—Responsible for the total occupational and environmental health and safety program at the policy-making level.

Consultant—Serves as an advisor for developing, selecting, implementing, and evaluating occupational and environmental health and safety services.

Educator—Assumes programmatic and administrative responsibilities for curricula and/or clinical experiences in occupational and environmental health nursing.

Researcher—Identifies occupational and environmental health problems, develops researchable questions with consideration for research priorities, assesses study feasibility, and initiates and conducts research studies using all the elements of the research process.

From Dirksen, M. (2006). Occupational and environmental health nursing: An overview. In M. K. Salazar (Ed.), *Core curriculum for occupational and environmental health nursing* (3rd ed.). St. Louis: W. B. Saunders.

and the employee. It is complicated even further by the nurse's responsibility to the larger community. Legal and ethical problems seldom result in simple resolutions (see the *Ethics in Practice* box). It is incumbent upon occupational and environmental health nurses to keep abreast of laws and to develop lines of communication with other professionals with whom they can confer when difficult issues arise. Occupational and environmental health nurses must regularly read professional publications so that they are able to make decisions based on the latest available information.

Although there are often no easy answers, an underlying principle in these conflicts is the responsibility to know and to uphold the standards of the profession. Decision making must be guided by commonly held and documented standards and practices as well as by the code of ethics advanced by AAOHN. Sometimes, there is a conflict between what is legal and what is ethical. It is legal, for example, for managers or supervisors to access employee health records in certain instances. It is easy to imagine the potential for abuse of this privilege. The occupational and environmental health nurse has an ethical responsibility to protect the confidentiality of the employee. For this reason, it is crucial that written guidelines that prevent the indiscriminate use of records be established and enforced.

The AAOHN has issued two useful advisories related to confidentiality (AAOHN, 2004) and record-keeping (1996; revised 2002), which can serve as a guide to the protection of health information in the occupational setting. (AAOHN's code of ethics and interpretive statements and advisories are available on the AAOHN website; see Community Resources for Practice at the end of this chapter for access.)

Because occupational hazards are the most preventable cause of disease, disability, and death, the field of occupational health has the potential to make a major contribution to public health and the general welfare of societies. A concern of occupational health professionals is that despite the fact that most persons spend at least a third of their waking hours at work, an occupational health assessment is often an overlooked element of the health history. Even if a person does not work, she or he is likely to live with someone who does, and that, too, can have an impact on the current state of health. Retired persons might have experienced hazardous working conditions that might result in adverse effects many years after the exposure occurred.

ENVIRONMENTAL HAZARDS IN THE COMMUNITY

There are many examples of events that resulted in environmental hazards. The devastation of Hurricane Katrina and the continued health effects suffered by those who lived or worked close the September 11, 2001, ground zero site were two significant environmental health disasters. In Katrina's wake, whole communities continue to be uninhabitable and/or uninhabited. The World Trade Center events resulted in exposure to smoke, products of combustion, dust, hazardous substances, and air pollution as well as psychologic distress (CDC, 2002). Events at Three Mile Island and Love Canal illustrate classic examples of the importance and the difficulty of recognizing environmental effects on communities. Three Mile Island is a nuclear power station near Harrisburg, Pennsylvania. A leak was discovered in one of the nuclear units. Radioactive material was released into the environment. Epidemiologic studies in subsequent years determined that there was an increase in the number of cases of leukemia among persons who lived near the unit (Anderson, 1987; Smith & Fisher, 1981). The national concern precipitated by this disaster was reinforced by another nuclear accident at Chernobyl in the former Soviet Union in 1986. Recent reports indicate that this area is also seeing an upsurge in cases of leukemia among children, genetic effects, and cancer-related illnesses and deaths (Freeze, 2000).

Love Canal is a quiet residential neighborhood in New York State that was built on an old toxic waste site. Studies conducted by the EPA (Anderson, 1987) and by Love Canal homeowners in the 1970s revealed disease and genetic damage in residents that were probably connected to the release of toxic chemicals from this site. A number of studies revealed that the sludge at this site contained chemicals, including suspected carcinogens (Anderson, 1987). Eventually, many families in the Love Canal area evacuated their homes.

More incidents of a similar nature are likely (Gilden, 2003). Three Mile Island is just 1 of a multitude of nuclear power stations, and Love Canal is just 1 of approximately 44,000 potentially toxic waste disposal sites in the United States (EPA, 2007). The list of potential sources of hazards in our communities is ever increasing. Determining the precise relationship

ETHICS IN PRACTICE

The Nurse as Advocate

Gail A. DeLuca Havens, PhD, APRN, BC

Audrey is an occupational health nurse at a wallpaper manufacturing plant who is responsible for the on-the-job health and safety of all employees who are exposed to or use hazardous materials in their work. Audrey has practiced in this plant since 1985, and is an employee of a corporation that owns and operates six similar plants. She was responsible for designing, writing, and implementing the hazard communication program for the plant, thereby ensuring that the plant would be in compliance with the Occupational Safety and Health Administration (OSHA) hazard communication standard, effective in 1988.

The hazard communication program includes provisions for a material safety data sheet (MSDS) for each hazardous chemical used at the facility, labeling of hazardous chemicals, training and information for employees exposed to hazardous chemicals, and access to manufacturers' MSDSs to gain information about specific hazardous risks that might be required in the investigation and evaluation of any specific exposures (Mistretta & Endresen, 1992). Because of Audrey's efforts, plant employees have become aware of potential environmental hazards in the workplace and do not exceed recommended exposure times to maximum concentrations of hazardous materials. They report any unusual signs and symptoms so that Audrey can investigate potential hazardous sources in the workplace. Finally, they are alert for any changes in the work environment, such as poor ventilation, that might contribute to increased hazards.

This morning Audrey is meeting with Tom, the plant's general manager, to discuss the recent increase in the incidence of headaches and painful eye irritations among employees who work in one of the plant's printing areas. Audrey summarizes her findings: "Forty percent of the employees in print section E had an onset of headaches and painful eye irritations in one 24-hour period last week. In investigating, I discovered that the day before the onset of these symptoms the section had begun using a different paint pigment in one of its print runs. I reviewed the MSDS related to the pigment's ingredients and, in general, found nothing unusual. There was, however, a recommendation for use of a specific filter gauge in the ventilating system in areas in which this pigment is being used, and we are not using this filter. Employees in this section continue to experience headaches and painful eye irritation. According to the manufacturer's MSDS, no definitive long-term effects from exposure to this pigment have been confirmed. Consequently, the manufacturer's MSDS does not include any warning, but only an alert that 'continued exposure to this pigment without benefit of the recommended filtration might lead to respiratory and liver problems.'"

Tom replies, "Audrey, I, too, am concerned about the physical symptoms that employees are experiencing. I have discussed the problem with the engineering personnel and with the company's corporate and legal staffs. To accommodate the recommended filtration in the plant's ventilating system we would have to make substantial modifications to the system, at an expense the company is not in a position to incur. Because no health warnings are associated with exposure to this pigment, the company will not be making any changes to the ventilating system at this time. I trust that you will continue to be responsive to employees' symptoms, so that they

are alleviated as much as possible, without compromising the integrity of the company and your position in it."

Because of the company's decision in this matter, Audrey finds herself in the midst of a dilemma precipitated by competing obligations. On the one hand, she is responsible for the on-the-job health and safety of company employees, which includes fostering the well-being of employees while minimizing their exposure to harm. On the other hand, as an employee she has a responsibility to act in the employer's best interests as well. She also is concerned about continuing her employment. The potential for termination seemed a very real possibility judging from the general manager's reference to her position in the company. Her family depends on her salary and to be without it would jeopardize their well-being. In this particular case, to act in the employer's best interest it is likely that Audrey will not be able to act in the best interests of her fellow employees. In fact, it is possible that she could be harming them. Should Audrey act as a "responsible" employee herself, by complying with her employer's direction regarding the care of her fellow employees, or should she continue with this issue to advocate for her fellow employees?

If Audrey follows Tom's suggestion, she will avoid immediate financial expenditures for the company. This would remove a lot of the pressure, reduce her stress, and maintain the security of her position in the company and her ability to continue to support her family. As any other parent does, she has a moral obligation to attend to the safety and well-being of dependents.

However, Audrey is an occupational and environmental health nurse who must balance the rights of the employees with the responsibilities of the company, as set forth in its policies and standards (Greenberg, 2007). She has a professional obligation, according to the *Code for Nurses of the American Nurses' Association* (ANA) and the *AAOHN Code of Ethics,* to maintain the health, welfare, and safety of the client. The nurse is an advocate for the client. As such, she or he "must examine the conflicts arising between their own personal and professional values, the values and interests of others who are also responsible for client care and health care decisions...to resolve such conflicts in ways that ensure client safety, guard the client's best interests, and preserve the professional integrity of the nurse" (ANA, 2001, p.10). Advocacy is regarded as a core moral concept of nursing. Accountability is regarded as another of the profession's central moral concepts. To be accountable is to be "answerable to oneself and others for one's own actions.... Nurses are accountable for judgments made and actions taken in the course of nursing practice" (ANA, 2001, p. 16). The existing policies of the employing agency do not relieve the nurse of the accountability to act in clients' best interests.

In this situation, an appropriate course of action for Audrey would be to report her findings through the official channels established within her company for such actions. Reporting mechanisms should exist within an employment setting so that employees feel comfortable voicing concerns about particular problems within the work setting without fear of reprisal. Having voiced her concerns to the plant manager without a satisfactory response, Audrey should inform the next person in the chain of command and should inform the plant manager of her action. Although it is not always easy to bring such concerns to an employer, the nurse's accountability to the workers in this plant obligates her to take action that will serve to avoid harm to them from improper ventilation.

An alternate course for Audrey would be to not pursue the reporting of employee symptoms. Because OSHA has not classified the chemical as one requiring a warning, but only an alert, Audrey could rationalize this course of action as an acceptable one. It is a strategy that would also serve to preserve Audrey's standing in the company, which is extremely important to her position as family breadwinner. Which course of action would you pursue?

REFERENCES

American Nurses Association. (2001). *Code of ethics for nurses with interpretive statements*. Washington, DC: American Nurses Publishing.

Greenberg, M. R. (2007). Contemporary environmental and occupational health issues: More breadth and depth. *American Journal of Public Health, 97*, 395-397.

Mistretta, E., & Endresen, L. (1992). Environmental hazards in the workplace: Legal and safety considerations. *AAOHN Journal, 40*, 398-400.

between these hazards and the health outcomes in populations poses major difficulties for epidemiologists and other scientists. It takes many years, or even decades, to determine a relationship exists.

There are literally thousands of potential hazards in our environment. For the sake of clarity, these hazards are classified according to their predominant characteristics. Table 9-4 lists potential sources of hazards and the toxic effects of each class. These classifications are by no means exclusive of one another; neither are they all-inclusive. Humans are exposed to multiple risks at any given time, and yet most of us remain healthy. The human body has a tremendous capacity for self-repair. Still, there are a large number of diseases and disorders that are on the rise, and for many of them there is evidence of risk factors that are associated with the environment (e.g.,

TABLE 9-4   Examples of Environmental Hazards

Agents and Sources of Hazards	Examples of Harmful Effects
Chemical	
Insulation (formaldehyde)	Increased respiratory allergies, chemical sensitivity
Automobile exhaust (lead)	Behavior disorders, neurologic symptoms
Pesticides (polychlorinated biphenyls [PCB])	Chloracne, liver disease, headache, birth defects
Biologic and Infectious	
Water supply (*Glardia lamlia, Cryptosporidium*)	Diarrhea, bloating, malabsorption
Food (*Salmonella, Escheria coli*)	Fever, nausea, watery diarrhea
Mosquito (malaria, West Nile virus)	Chills, fever
Physical	
Physical hazards (faulty building or playground construction)	Unintentional injury or death
Noise (motor vehicles, airplanes, lawn mowers)	Hearing problems, stress, fatigue
Radiation (radon gas)	Infertility, birth defects, leukemia
Psychologic	
Natural disasters (e.g., flooding; forest fires)	Hypertension
Low economic status (unemployment, poverty)	Heart disease, ulcers
Multiple role demands (working parent)	Depression, anxiety

asthma, autism, Parkinsonism, learning disabilities, obesity, cardiovascular diseases).

The **Precautionary Principle** provides one way of doing so. The "Precautionary Principle" states that if there is some evidence about the relationship between toxic substances or environmental hazards and human health, even if scientific evidence about cause and effect is not available, precautionary measures should be taken to protect the environment and human health (Goldman, 2000). In 2003 the American Nurses Association (ANA) adopted the Precautionary Principle as a position of the ANA (Brody & Melamed, 2004). In keeping with that position, the ANA will use the precautionary approach in occupational and environmental health practice and will advocate for public policy that focuses on prevention of hazards to people and the environment.

Types of Hazards

Chemical Hazards. Chemicals come in a wide variety of forms (dusts, fumes, mists, vapors, and gases) and can affect almost every system in the body (Dirksen, 2006). Our surroundings are literally inundated with chemicals. Love Canal and the health effects of DDT (chemical name: dichlorodiphenyltrichloroethane) are disastrous examples of chemical health problems. Not only is the environment full of chemicals, but also our bodies accumulate these substances and pose a **"body burden"** of chemicals in our blood, fat, breast milk, and other tissues and body fluids (Thornton et al., 2002). Latent disease and genetic changes pose increasingly complex problems for humans.

The toxic effects of chemicals are frequently subtle, and people suffering from exposures are often misdiagnosed. The extent of biologic damage produced by a chemical depends on two things: the amount of the exposure, or its *dose,* and the *response* (**dose response**) of the person exposed. This is called a dose-response ratio. As a general rule, the higher the dose, the greater the response. However, some people have hypersensitivities or hypersusceptibilities to certain chemicals and, therefore, have a response at a much lower than expected dosage. Some individuals have "multiorgan hypersensitivity caused even by small amounts of chemical exposure that is generally considered nontoxic" for other individuals (Shinohara et al., 2004, p. 84). **Multiple chemical sensitivity (MCS)** is defined as "[1] a chronic condition [2] with symptoms that recur reproducibly [3] in response to low levels of exposure [4] to multiple unrelated chemicals and [5] improve or resolve when incitants are removed, along with a 6th criterion...requiring that symptoms occur in multiple organ systems" (Bartha et al., 1999, abstract).

It is impossible, within the limitations of this section, to describe the incalculable health effects that can result from exposure to the expansive array of common chemicals to which we are exposed on a regular basis. Think of the cleaning supplies, petroleum products, solvents, pesticides, gardening materials, medical products, building supplies, and plastic items that are a part of our day-to-day lives. It is of crucial importance to recognize chemical exposures might have profound effects on the health of individuals and our communities. As health professionals, it is our responsibility to participate in the education of community leaders and residents regarding these issues (Welker-Hood et al., 2007). An excellent resource about chemicals in the environment is the ATSDR, a federal agency whose mission is to provide health information and protect the public's health by preventing exposures to toxic substances *(http://www.atsdr.cdc.gov)*.

Biologic Hazards. Infectious disease is considered environmentally transmitted when it is spread from a common source, such as water, food, or animal vectors (Blumenthal & Ruttenber, 1995). In the past, many of the environmental health problems were related to infectious agents, such as typhoid or cholera, largely because of an inadequate understanding of sanitation and hygiene.

Despite the great advances in understanding microbes and hygiene, infectious disease continues to be a major public health problem in developing countries (see Chapter 5). Although the problems are not as great in this country, they do exist. Many rural communities are not connected to safe central water systems, and municipal water supplies can be threatened by infectious diseases, such as cryptosporidiosis, through human error or the effects of old equipment. Outbreaks of food-borne diseases, such as salmonellosis and hepatitis A, often occur. An excellent resource about infectious and communicable disease is the text entitled *Control of Communicable Diseases Manual* (18th ed.) published by the APHA (Heymann, 2004).

Vector-borne diseases might be spread by flies, mosquitoes, cockroaches, ticks, and rodents (Heymann, 2004). Two vector-borne diseases that have captured attention recently among outdoor workers are Lyme disease (tick-borne) and West Nile virus (mosquito-borne) (see Chapter 8). Workers can protect themselves against these and other vector-borne diseases by wearing long sleeves and long pants; self-checking for ticks after exposure; using insect repellents containing DEET (chemical name: *N,N*-diethyl-*m*-toluamide); and minimizing potential breeding grounds for mosquitoes.

Human feces can be a source of infectious organisms. One of the most common parasites spread in this way is roundworm, or *Ascaris lumbricoides*. Approximately 4 million persons in this country have ascariasis (Blumenthal & Ruttenber, 1995). It is particularly prevalent in warm areas that have poor sanitation. A common complication of an infestation is an intestinal obstruction caused by a bolus of worms. Nurses can emphasize the importance of hand-washing, safe drinking water supply, and adequate treatment for infected individuals to prevent the spread of disease. With increases in the population, the amount of human waste rapidly increases, as does the risk for these diseases.

Daycare settings are known to be sites where respiratory and enteric diseases, such as giardiasis, are easily transmitted among children, staff members, and families. The presence of children in diapers, combined with children's natural tendency to put objects in their mouths, contributes to the spread of infection. To prevent the spread of disease in daycare settings, a number of interventions are recommended (Schneider & Freeman, 2000):

- Proper hand-washing by staff members and children
- Exclusion or segregation of sick children
- Routine cleaning of play objects
- Separation of food-handling and diaper-changing areas and staff
- Use of sanitary diaper-changing procedures

Physical Hazards. Physical hazards in the environment include poorly designed or unsafe construction of equipment, buildings, roads, or playgrounds; improperly placed items; and general lack of attention to safety, noise, and radiation. Motor vehicles accounted for approximately 42,900 deaths in 2001 (National Safety Council, 2003a). Many more people suffered disabling injuries. In addition, there were approximately 5800 pedestrian deaths and 90,000 injuries in 2001. Vehicle safety is addressed in *Healthy People 2010* (USDHHS, 2000). One goal is to increase the use of safety belts, inflatable safety restraints, and child safety seats to 92% from a baseline of 69% in 1998. Nurses can participate in school, work site, and community educational campaigns to improve pedestrian safety and increase the use of seat belts, child seats, and helmets.

Noise. Less tangible physical hazards that have received increasing attention in recent years include noise and radiation. Although the health effects from these factors are not as readily identifiable as other physical hazards, the long-term effects from exposure can be devastating.

Noise, although often perceived as innocuous on a day-to-day basis, has been described by some as one of the most noxious and pervasive pollutants in our modern environment. The noise levels in our society have increased dramatically, and the most obvious health effect of noise is an impairment of the ability to hear. Other problems that have been associated with noise include stress-related conditions, mental illness, social maladjustment, and pathologic conditions, such as atherosclerosis and heart disease.

The amount of damage incurred by exposure to noise is directly related to the frequency and intensity of the noise and the length of exposure. The OSHA standard requires that sound levels in the workplace not exceed an average of 90 dB in an 8-hour period. However, sound levels of much lower intensity might cause gastrointestinal, cardiovascular, or neuroendocrine disturbances. There is no decibel limit for sound levels in the community or in our homes. Noise from a jet engine 25 miles away has been measured at 140 dB, a jackhammer at 100 dB, and a live performance of a rock band at 110 dB.

When a nurse becomes aware that someone is exposed to persistent sound, the first approach should be to isolate the noise if at all possible, either by using sound-absorbent material or by moving the client away from the source of noise. If these measures are not feasible, a less desirable approach is to recommend some type of hearing protection. In some cases, both approaches are used. Clients should be advised that the noise levels at concerts and discotheques might cause damage to the ear. Radio and cassette headsets might also contribute to increases in hearing loss if the volume is turned up too high.

Radiation. There are two types of radiation: ionizing and non-ionizing (Nadakavukaren, 1995). Ionizing radiation is produced when atoms disintegrate. Sources of ionizing radiation include x-ray machines, cosmic rays, uranium and other minerals, radon, nuclear power plants, television sets, and atomic fallout. Nonionizing radiation, a lower energy form of radiation, transforms energy into heat. Examples include microwaves, television and radio waves, infrared sources (e.g., welding arcs), ultraviolet rays in sun lamps or sunlight, and lasers.

Although radiation is a natural part of our environment, exposure to excessive amounts causes serious health effects. The largest source of man-made exposure to ionizing radiation is the use of x-rays. Many household products emit ionizing radiation.

The health effects from radiation are directly related to the amount of exposure. Of greatest concern is the damage that occurs to chromosomes exposed to ionizing radiation. Excessive and prolonged exposure can cause mutagenic, carcinogenic, and teratogenic effects (Levy & Wegman, 2000). Epidemiologic studies of populations exposed to high doses of radiation, such as atomic bomb survivors and clients undergoing radiation therapy, have found a much higher than expected incidence of cancer following exposure (Davis, 2007).

The effects of nonionizing radiation vary according to the source. Ultraviolet radiation causes skin cancer and is probably responsible for the increasing incidence of malignant melanoma. Infrared and ultraviolet light can cause thermal burns. Microwave radiation can cause deep thermal burns and has been associated with impaired fertility. Lasers can cause retinal damage and severe burns. Although there has been some question about the health effects of radiation from video display terminals, conclusive evidence is lacking that they are in fact harmful. Nurses can educate communities about radiation hazards. For example, school nurses can participate in primary prevention of skin cancer by teaching children to use sunscreen and to wear protective clothing.

Psychosocial Hazards. The last category of hazards is probably the most difficult to describe because it is more difficult to measure. There is little doubt, however, that psychologic factors have a profound effect on the health and well-being of our communities. Stress is just as pervasive in today's environment as the other hazards mentioned. The principal difference is that it is often much easier to determine the link between physical agents and disease than it is to identify the relationship of an illness to psychologic factors.

Environmentally induced stress is a natural by-product of our fast-paced society as well as a result of natural or man-made disasters. Many people find it difficult to keep up with rapidly changing technologic developments and feel frustrated in their efforts to do so. The latest and greatest computer today might be obsolete by tomorrow. Persons in lower socioeconomic groups suffer even more frustration, as they seem to fall further behind the mainstream of society. As the gap between rich and poor widens, the anxiety and alienation experienced by certain groups deepen. Societal stresses, such as crime, poor economic conditions, changing mores, and unemployment, affect the well-being of populations.

Many natural occurrences hasten stress. Recently, this country has experienced major and devastating earthquakes, floods, hurricanes, tornadoes, droughts, extreme heat or cold, and volcanic explosions; each has taken its toll on life and property. Concerns about the environment are becoming more prevalent. Terrorism and the aftermath of the bombing of the World Trade Center on September 11, 2001, increase the concern that our earth is being irreparably destroyed.

Stress is a manifestation of an effort to maintain a sense of order. Humans have the ability to adapt within certain parameters. When the psychologic or physical input becomes excessive, a stress response is likely to occur. If coping mechanisms are in place, the stress can actually have positive outcomes. However, if the stresses are constant, the health of the individual or the community might be severely affected. Nurses can encourage clients and community residents to discover the underlying causes of their stress and to manage their stress. Clients might be given referrals to local mental health centers to assist in managing their stress. Families can be encouraged to prepare for natural environmental disasters, such as floods and earthquakes, to minimize stress. In the event of a natural disaster, the American Red Cross and other community agencies can be called on to assist families (see Chapter 22).

ENVIRONMENTAL ISSUES FOR THE 21ST CENTURY

Healthy People 2010 provides a brief overview that serves as an introduction to the many environmental contaminants that threaten the health of our homes, communities, and world (Figure 9-5). The media for many of these pollutants are the very things that we depend on to sustain our lives: the air we breathe, the water we drink, the food we eat, and soil that is so integral to our lives. Air, water, and soil pollution not only threaten our health but also threaten our very quality of life. Numerous objectives in *Healthy People 2010* focus on environmental health issues and give direction to health professionals as they promote community health and prevent disease. Federal agencies, such as the ATSDR, CDC, NIOSH, EPA, and Housing and Urban Development (HUD), provide useful information about environmental health and safety (see Community Resources for Practice for a complete list of such resources). For example, an EPA initiative to protect the elderly is being launched to better understand and protect older adults from toxic exposures that have accumulated through their life times and exacerbate or cause chronic conditions.

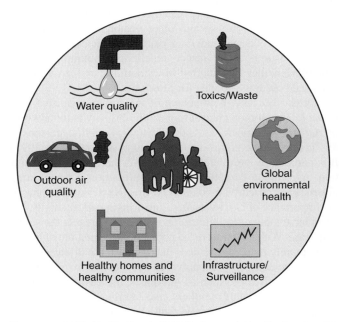

FIGURE 9-5 *Healthy People 2010:* Environmental health. (Data from U.S. Department of Health and Human Services. [Nov 2000]. *Healthy People 2010.* [2nd ed.]. Retrieved August 14, 2003, from *http://www.healthypeople.gov/Document/HTML/Volume1/08Environmental.htm&num1;_Toc490564713.)*

AIR POLLUTION

The air can become polluted from a variety of sources: manufacturing industry emissions, coal-fired power plants, automobiles and other combustion engines, wood-burning (or other fossil fuel) stoves and heating systems, forest fires, and many other sources. In the U.S., the Clean Air Act was signed into law in 1970, the same year that the EPA was established. In lieu of creating a standard for every conceivable air pollutant, a set of *"criteria pollutants"* were established that reflect critical toxicants or categories of chemicals that together create a metric for air quality. These are called the National Ambient Air Quality Standards *(http://www.epa. gov/ttn/naaqs/)*.

1. *Sulfur dioxide* is produced during combustion and industrial processes.
   - Sulfur dioxide is a major contributor to acid rain.
   - It is associated with respiratory illness, alterations in pulmonary function, aggravation of existing cardiovascular disease, and asthma.
2. *Nitrous dioxide* is produced during combustion; it affects the lungs, immune function, and asthma.
3. *Carbon monoxide* is produced during the burning of fossil fuel.
   - Carbon monoxide is produced in large amounts by motor vehicles.
   - Carbon monoxide binds very effectively with hemoglobin, precluding the binding of oxygen and resulting in anoxia; the most sensitive population are those with cardiovascular diseases.
4. *Particulate matter (PM)* consists of liquid and solid aerosols from fuel combustion, motor vehicle exhaust, high temperature industrial processes, and incineration.
   - Particulate matter includes dust, dirt, soot, smoke, and liquid droplets.
   - The lungs are a prime site for damage and exacerbation of underlying disease; the size of the particle determines the deposition in the lungs.
5. *Lead* in the aerosolized particulate matter is from industrial processes and incineration. Lead is toxic to the nervous, immune, cardiovascular, and reproductive systems, as well as damaging to heme synthesis and to the kidneys.
6. *Ozone* is an odorless, colorless gas composed of three atoms of oxygen. Ozone occurs both in the Earth's upper atmosphere and at ground level. Ozone can be good or bad, depending on where it is found. Ozone is categorized as "good" ozone or "bad" ozone.
   - "Good" ozone occurs at a layer in the stratosphere about 10 to 25 miles above the Earth and it serves to protect people from the most damaging ultraviolet (UV) rays. It has been significantly damaged by chlorofluorocarbons [CFCs].
   - "Bad" ozone is ground level ozone that is created by reaction of hydrocarbons, which include Volatile Organic Compounds (VOCs) and nitrogen oxides in the presence of sunlight.
   - VOCs are emitted from a wide range of sources: dry cleaners, cars, chemical manufacturers, paint shops, and many others.
   - The prime target organ for ozone is the lung, to which it causes damage, diminishes lung function, and sensitizes the lung to other irritants.
   - The burning of fossil fuel (e.g., in diesels, industrial boilers, and power plants) and waste incineration are two major contributors.
   - Bad, ground-level (manmade) ozone can irritate the respiratory system, aggravate asthma, reduce lung function, and inflame and damage the lung epithelium

There are a wide array of health effects associated with air pollution, including asthma and other respiratory diseases, cardiovascular diseases (including hypertension), cancer, immunologic effects, reproductive health problems (including birth defects), and neurologic problems. Air pollution standards are based on protecting the health of healthy, middle-aged white males. The standards may not be protective of more vulnerable populations, and it should be noted that adverse health effects have been found at levels below the EPA air quality standards. The elderly and those with chronic pulmonary and/or vascular diseases may be at increased risk for mortality from short-term increases in both indoor and outdoor air pollution.

Persistent bioaccumulative toxic pollutants (PBTs) become airborne during their *fate and transport* from agricultural use, industrial processes, transportation, burning waste (i.e., incineration), and energy production. *Fate and transport* refers to the process by which a pollutant moves through (and sometimes back and forth from) the air, soil, surface water, and ground water. Fate and transport also includes the residence time that the pollutant is in plants, the human body, and animals.

In May 2007, the Supreme Court ruled that the EPA must take action on greenhouse gases from motor vehicles, which resulted in an executive order from President Bush to regulate green house gas emissions from motor vehicles.

WATER AND SOIL POLLUTION

Despite advances that have been made in the purification of public water, water contamination remains a threat to some rural and suburban communities (Afzal, 2006). With a steadily increasing population creating more potential contaminants, there is a greater risk to the water supply (Figure 9-6). The three main sources of water contamination are industrial wastes, sewage, and agricultural chemicals. Many diseases have been traced to the local water supply, including cryptosporidium, hepatitis, polio, and microbes that cause gastrointestinal diseases. Antibiotic-resistant microbes, endocrine disrupters, and also human medication and medication by-products have been found in stream water. At particular risk are persons who depend on well water; however, contamination can occur in any water supply. *Healthy People 2010* includes a goal that the percentage of the population who are served by community water systems that meet Safe Drinking Water Act standards reach 95% (baseline of 85% in 1995) (USDHHS, 2000).

Soil serves as a receptacle for many of the pollutants, such as lead and arsenic, that are deposited from the air or water. Radioactive matter that disperses into the environment eventually falls to the ground and settles in the soil. Human and animal excreta are often disposed of improperly. The *Ascaris* worm mentioned earlier is commonly found in the soil. Contamination of soil by hazardous waste dumps has been an ongoing and increasing problem (Gilden, 2003). It is estimated that at least 10,000 hazardous waste dumps in the United States pose a threat to public health (Last, 1998).

The health effects of pollution are likely to remain for many years. Although there have been some efforts among activists

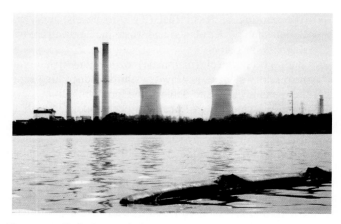

FIGURE 9-6 Oil containment boom placed in Swanson Creek, tributary to the Patuxent River, after oil spill at power-generating plant. (From National Oceanic and Atmospheric Administration, Department of Commerce. NOAA Photo Library. Available on-line at *http://www.photolib.noaa.gov/coastline/line1657.htm.*)

in this country to raise America's consciousness about some of these serious problems, much remains to be done. Health professionals need to be on the front lines in the struggle to promote healthy environments. Community health nurses are in a key position to make a difference.

HAZARDOUS WASTE

In the 1976 Resource Conservation and Recovery Act, Congress legally defined **hazardous waste** as "any discarded material that might pose a substantial threat or potential danger to human health when improperly handled." This material includes infectious wastes, agricultural and industrial by-products, radioactive substances, flammable products, and chemical agents. Hospitals today are increasingly concerned not only about the volume of waste but also about the hazardous waste they produce. Hazardous waste from hospitals, medical offices, and laboratories is tightly regulated by government agencies and must be disposed of separately from regular solid waste.

There has been an increasing urgency in recent years to respond to this important environmental issue. The Solid Waste Disposal Act of 1965, the Resource Recovery Act of 1970, the Resource Conservation and Recovery Act of 1976, and the Quiet Communities Act of 1978 were efforts to alleviate problems of hazardous waste. The Comprehensive Environment Response, Compensation, and Liability Act (CERCLA or **Superfund**) provided an organized response and funding to clean up environmental release of hazardous materials from abandoned or inactive waste sites (Blumenthal & Ruttenber, 1995). As a result of this act, a list of the most serious uncontrolled or abandoned hazardous waste sites needing remedial action was identified (called the **National Priorities List**). Although government regulation is important in the effort to control the hazards posed by wastes, it is not the final solution to the problem.

Blumenthal and Ruttenber (1995) suggest four methods of effective waste management:

- Modification of the dangerous properties of the waste so that it can be allowed to safely enter the environment
- Storage of waste in a facility that prevents its introduction into the environment

- Recycling
- Elimination of waste production

It is not uncommon to attribute many of the problems related to hazardous wastes to industries and corporations. Although industry plays a major role in the production of waste materials, the responsibility for the associated problems belongs to everyone. As a nation, we want convenient and cheap products, but we must learn how not to sacrifice the environment to satisfy this desire.

NANOTECHNOLOGY

Nanotechnology refers broadly to a field of applied science and technology whose unifying theme is the control of matter on the molecular level in scales smaller than 1 micrometer, normally 1 to 100 nanometers, and the fabrication of devices within that size range. This new technology has been applied to everything from car waxes to make-up. Because of the extremely small size of the nanocomponents, there is concern about their ability to easily penetrate deep into the human body. Nanomaterials have proved toxic to human tissue and cell cultures (Oberdörster et al., 2005). Unlike larger particles, nanomaterials may be taken up by cell mitochondria and the cell nucleus (Porter et al., 2007). Studies demonstrate the potential for nanomaterials to cause DNA mutation and induce major structural damage to mitochondria, even resulting in cell death (Geiser et al., 2005). Many more questions than answers exist at this time, and the technology is so new that no federal agency yet regulates nanotechnology.

CHEMICAL POLICIES

As the public becomes increasingly aware of the connection between the products that they commonly use in their daily lives (such as personal care products and cleaning agents) and their potential relationship to health risks, there is a growing discussion about how the chemical policies in the United States have failed to protect the public's health. In Europe, a comprehensive overhaul of their chemical policies has resulted in a new approach to product manufacturing that places the burden upon the manufacturer to prove a product is safe. This is quite different from U.S. policy, which allows products to come to market and then has little/no mechanism to withdraw them if they are discovered to be toxic. In the coming years, we can expect robust debate about our chemical policies and more products developed using "green chemistry," a new approach to chemical formulations that are inherently less toxic (Welker-Hood et al., 2007).

Sustainable Agriculture

In the United States, industrial agriculture is increasingly under scrutiny for its effects on the environment and on human health. More and more, the public is demanding food products that have been grown/produced in a more sustainable way: fair trade products, certified organic, locally-grown, without the use of nontherapeutic antibiotics, without the use of hormones, and otherwise grown in a way that promotes long-term sustainability. School districts and hospitals are using their institutional purchasing power to demand food products that have been grown sustainably from the perspective of human and ecologic health.

GLOBAL WARMING

An Inconvenient Truth, Al Gore's movie, brought global warming science into local theatres and helped to launch local, state, and national awareness and policies regarding this very critical issue. The predictions for increased storm activity, increases in temperatures, and changes that will impact food production all have the potential to create significant health needs. In addition to being strong advocates to address global warming, we also need to be prepared for the near-future, public health consequences (Afzal, 2007). "There is mounting evidence that global climate change is already effecting human health through extreme weather events, changes in air and water quality, and changes in the ecology of infectious diseases" (Afzal, 2007, p. 3).

COMMUNITY/PUBLIC HEALTH NURSING RESPONSIBILITIES

The responsibilities of the community health nurse in relation to environmental factors include assessing, monitoring, educating, advocating, and role modeling (Butterfield, 2002; Choi et al., 2006; Sattler & Lipscomb, 2003). Case studies by Clark et al. (2002), Green and Slade (2001), and Phillips (1995) provide excellent examples of the role of nursing in environmental health.

Website Resource 9E provides an extensive list of web-based resources for environmental health that can assist nurses in their practice.

ASSESSMENT

Assessment is a key component of all public health practice and involves collecting data that help to describe the population, its health status, and the health risks. In environmental health, health risks can be determined on both an individual and a population basis. Using a pneumonic tool called "I PREPARE," which was created by the Agency for Toxic Substance and Disease Registry (ATSDR, 2000, a part of the Centers for Disease Control and Prevention), nurses can add the level of environmental health knowledge when completing a history and physical examination (see Box 9-2).

Epidemiologists and others can research possible connections with environmental factors. Within communities, nurses can use surveys to determine the biggest concerns and hazards that are identified by the community. A new tool in the public health armament is the Geographic Information System (GIS) (Choi et al., 2006). This is a term that refers to a number of computer programs that can link individual data units to a geographic location so that analysis of risk factors and health outcomes can be conducted. A map can also be created that provides a visual representation of the data. For example, you could create a map that illustrates the following community data points: location of older housing stock and the location of children less than 5 years old. With these combined data, a public health nurse could then determine the best sites to which a mobile lead testing unit should be deployed.

SURVEILLANCE

While there is no federal law regarding the reporting of environmental diseases, there are health outcomes that are required to be reported in some states and are associated with environmental exposures. This includes cancer registries, birth defects registries, and blood lead level registries. Nurses can also be involved in or initiate environmental *surveillance* programs for environmental health problems, such as creating lead poisoning or birth defects registries. With registry data, clusters of problems may be noted. The federal government has begun a National Children's Longitudinal Study that will be following 100,000 children from the time the woman is pregnant through the child's 21st birthday. This study will include collection of information about exposures and health effects and will be an invaluable source of information for researchers to mine *(http://www.nationalchildrensstudy.gov/).*

RISK COMMUNICATION

In nursing, we are often engaged in communicating about health risks. We talk to parents about the risks associated with not using car seats or helmets. We talk to teenagers about the risks associated with unsafe sex. In environmental health, our risk communication often occurs in a community and usually occurs when there is already some concern about an exposure. For example, a recent transportation accident in which a tanker car released highly toxic chemicals near a residential community created many concerns for the parents and pregnant women in the community. A public health nurse might be called upon to help the community understand whether there is cause for concern and what, if anything, community members should do.

When engaging in risk communication around environmental risks, it is important to recognize that community members may be afraid and/or anxious and they may not trust someone who comes from a governmental agency. It is extremely important to listen to the community members to understand their real concerns; this means that, if a risk communication program is organized, there must be an opportunity for community members to speak. The ATSDR/Environmental Protection Agency have created guidance documents on risk communication (see *http://www.atsdr.cdc.gov/risk/evalprimer/index.html, http://www.epa.gov/superfund/community/pdfs/toolkit/37riskcom.pdf*).

ADVOCACY

Nurses are fierce defenders of the health of individuals, families, populations, and communities. Nurses can be the best advocates for institutional, legislative, and regulatory change because they are one of the most trusted professionals in society and they bring a good scientific background combined with excellent communication skills. Within our institutions, we can advocate for policies that call for integrated pest management, nontoxic cleaning products, asthma-safe products, and products that are made from recycled products. School nurses can help to develop policies about nontoxic art supplies.

In our State Houses, we can advocate for legislation that promotes clean air and water, sustainable food production, safe products, and other environmentally healthful policies. In many states, the state nurses' associations are actively engaging in environmental policy work. In Washington state the participation of the nurses' association in a statewide campaign to ban the use of toxic flame retardants from products was key to the success of the legislation. In Maryland the state nurses' association played a critical role in the passage of their state Clean Air Act that created the strongest air pollution law in the country.

At the national level, the Quad Council of Public Health Nursing has moved environmental health issues along in a number of ways. The American Nurses Association has created a pollution prevention toolkit for nurses; passed several resolutions, including one that calls for banning the use of non-therapeutic antibiotics in animal feed; and adopted a set of environmental principles. These principles are intended to guide the profession of nursing in their practice and policy work. Earlier in this chapter, Box 9-1 presents the Environmental Health Principles adopted by the Public Health Nurses' Section of the American Public Health Association.

RESEARCH

Environmental health is conducted by a range of scientific disciplines, such as clinical practitioners, epidemiologists, and toxicologists. Intervention studies have helped us to understand the best ways to eliminate or reduce environmental health risks. In the nursing literature you will find some articles on environmental health, but few of them are actual research articles. There is a huge need for nurses to engage in this area as researchers. The best single source of research on environmental health is *Environmental Health Perspectives*, which is the official peer-reviewed journal of the National Institute of Environmental Health Science (*http://www.ehponline.org/*).

THE NURSE'S RESPONSIBILITIES IN PRIMARY, SECONDARY, AND TERTIARY PREVENTION

The levels of prevention used in public health can be applied to environmental problems as a way to understand the various points of interventions (Box 9-6).

PRIMARY PREVENTION

Health promotion and illness prevention in the home, at work or school, and in the community are aimed at reducing the risk of exposure and illness. The focus of interventions is on the conditions that influence, produce, or predict health and illness in human beings. Nursing strategies are geared toward providing people with information about hazards and assisting them with modifying the origins of the problem. Individuals can also be encouraged to use protective devices, such as bicycle helmets or hearing protection, and to reduce environmental hazards by using fewer chemicals in their homes.

In the home, nurses can assess for physical hazards (e.g., asthma triggers, lead, formaldehyde, radon, chemical storage, unsafe play areas), provide education for health promotion, and facilitate and coordinate a health-promoting environment. Families should be encouraged to use community resources and obtain testing for **household hazards.** Nurses can also be role models for members of the community and advocate for changes in habits. For example, to reduce the volume of garbage produced in the United States, nurses could incorporate "trash reduction" practices into their personal shopping habits. Buying in larger quantities or bulk, purchasing items manufactured in less packaging or recyclable packaging, or using reusable products (razors, cloth diapers) rather than disposable ones are ways to reduce household trash.

Nurses who work in health care settings have an opportunity to protect the environment (see the Health Care Without Harm organization in the Community Resources for Practice at the end of the chapter). For example, health care professionals in numerous health care settings are now using many reusable products instead of disposable ones, including cloth diapers, metal wash basins, and float-type mattress pads. Nurse man-

---

Box 9-6 Prevention Interventions for Environmental/Occupational Health and Safety

Primary Prevention
- Advocate safer environmental design of products such as needles, automobiles, playground equipment, and buildings.
- Teach home safety related to falls and fire prevention, especially to families with children, older adults, and those with disabilities.
- Communicate the risks of keeping firearms in the home and review safe methods of storage if a firearm is kept at home.
- Counsel women of childbearing age regarding exposure to environmental hazards.
- Teach avoidance of ultraviolet exposure and use of sunscreen.
- Use and advocate use of environmentally preferable products, such as the least toxic cleaning supplies and chemicals.
- Advocate use of protective devices, such as earplugs for noise, seat belts, and bicycle helmets.
- Immunize occupationally exposed workers for hepatitis B.
- Develop work site health and safety programs in work settings to prevent back injuries.
- Support the development of exposure standards for toxins.
- Advocate for safe air and water.
- Support programs for waste reduction, recycling, and effective waste management in health care settings and schools.

Secondary Prevention
- Assess homes, schools, work sites, and communities for environmental hazards.
- Routinely obtain environmental and occupational health histories for individuals, counsel about hazard reduction, and refer for diagnosis and treatment.
- Screen children from 6 months to 5 years of age for blood lead levels.
- Monitor workers for levels of chemical and radiation exposure.
- Screen at-risk workers for lung disease, cancer, and hearing loss.
- Participate in data collection regarding the incidence and prevalence of injury and disability in homes, schools, and work sites.

Tertiary Prevention
- When air pollution is high, encourage limitation of outdoor activity to minimize exposure.
- Support cleanup of toxic waste sites and removal of other hazards.
- Provide appropriate nursing care at work sites or in the home for persons with chronic lung diseases and injury-related disabilities.
- Refer homeowners to approved lead abatement resources.

Compiled by Claudia M. Smith, University of Maryland.

---

agers are in strategic positions to make decisions about the types of products used and can apply the same waste reduction principles as in the home. Furthermore, nurses can pressure manufacturers to reduce the packaging in many materials used in health care settings. At the community and global levels, changes in policy are supported to reduce air, soil, and water pollution. Nurses can participate in public education and assist community members in interpretation of data about environmental risks.

SECONDARY PREVENTION

One of the critical roles of the nurse is to observe signs and symptoms of environmental exposures and assess all clients for environmental risks. For example, a toddler living in an older building who is observed eating cracking paint or playing on a dusty floor should have a blood test to screen for lead poisoning. Farm workers who are exposed to pesticides should be screened for toxins. A thorough health history of occupational and environmental exposures is essential for all individuals. The early diagnosis and treatment of environmental illness, or secondary prevention, is traditionally part of the community/public health nurse's responsibility.

In the community, nurses are involved with other health care professionals in the surveillance of health conditions that might be related to environmental and occupational exposures. For example, environmental health specialists in local and state health departments play a key role in ensuring safe water, food, and air. The reporting of disease, follow-up, and intervention are all part of surveillance of environmental and occupational disease. Sources of data include health care providers, death certificates and autopsy reports, birth certificates, disease registries, workers' compensation claims, insurance or hospital billing data, and specific environmental sampling. Nurses can participate in all the phases of data collection, analysis, interpretation, and dissemination. Nurses might be in the best position to interpret scientific findings to the community and to provide individualized and group education as needed.

TERTIARY PREVENTION

Tertiary prevention is aimed at minimizing disability and maximizing functional capacity. At this level of intervention, treatment strategies are used to assist the individual or community to adapt to changes resulting from the illness. For example, after a nuclear accident, such as that at Chernobyl, rapid evacuation of residents is imperative to minimize the exposure to radiation. Because the food and water supplies are contaminated by the radiation, it is essential to obtain new sources of food and water to limit exposure. If malignancies occur following a nuclear accident, treatment and palliative care, which are activities of tertiary prevention, are appropriate. **Risk communication** about environmental hazards with the public is also part of the nurse's role.

Nurses can stay informed of environmental issues by reading newspapers and becoming active in consumer- and health-related organizations. Being well informed is a first step in influencing the political system on environmental issues. Communicating effectively with persons in power through groups, such as the American Nurses Association (ANA), AAOHN, American Public Health Association, Health Care Without Harm, or other groups is vital (see Community Resources for Practice). Networking with others who share the same interests is highly effective as well. Because environmental health issues have complex origins and involve many professionals, an interdisciplinary approach is most effective.

THE FUTURE OF ENVIRONMENTAL HEALTH NURSING

Community/public health nurses must continue to explore environmental conditions that are potentially detrimental to human health. All community/public health nurses should recognize environmental hazards and illnesses, make appropriate referrals, educate and advocate for reduction of risks, and contribute to environmental health policy (Institute of Medicine [IOM], 1995). Chemical, physical, biologic, and

psychosocial hazards must be better understood, not only as isolated hazards but also in their complex interaction. The health effects of chronic, low-dose exposures to ubiquitous chemicals and their influence on genetic and hormonal changes need to be explored further in the 21st century (Thornton et al., 2002).

A greater focus on occupational and environmental health is being included in nursing practice, education, and research (IOM, 1995). Nurses interested in occupational and environmental health need to engage in teamwork beyond the bounds of the health care system. "Communication should extend beyond counseling individual clients and families to facilitating the exchange of information on environmental hazards and community responses" (IOM, 1995, p. 10). More occupational and environmental health content is being incorporated into nursing curricula. Minimally, every community/public health nurse should elicit environmental, home, and occupational health histories and observe for links between the environment and illness. As research reveals more about the complex interaction of hazards, continuing education in the multiple dimensions of environmental health will be essential for up-to-date community/public health nurses.

KEY IDEAS

1. The interaction of human beings with the environment (physical, political, social, economic, and cultural aspects) affects health status. The home, the workplace (or school), and the community are important sources of environmental hazards that affect health.

2. *Healthy People 2010* objectives address prevention of home injuries, reduction of worker illnesses and injuries, and reduction of human exposure to toxic agents. Hazards include chemicals, infectious agents, mechanical forces, noise, and radiation.

3. Poisonings (including drug overdoses), falls, and burns are the top three causes of unintentional injuries and deaths in homes.

4. Persons who are physically dependent, such as preschool children and the elderly, are at highest risk of preventable home injuries.

5. Chemicals such as radon, formaldehyde, carbon monoxide, and pesticides and environmental tobacco smoke in homes contribute to respiratory illnesses. Lead poisoning causes cognitive and behavioral disabilities in children, as well as other neurologic, renal, and hematologic damage.

6. Community/public health nurses provide education regarding safe home environments and assist families in identifying hazards that can be removed in the home.

7. Occupational and environmental health nursing is a branch of community/public health nursing concerned with promoting, protecting, and maintaining the health and safety of workers. Occupational and environmental health nurses can face ethical issues because of competing interests of employers and employees.

8. More disabling injuries occur in workplaces than in homes. The most frequent work-related illnesses and injuries are traumatic injuries, skin disorders, and lung diseases.

9. The Federal Hazard Communication Standard of 1986 requires employers to notify employees of exposure to toxic substances.

10. All community/public health nurses need to include occupational and environmental histories when assessing the health of individuals and their families.

11. Clean air and water; a safe, sustainable food supply; and also effective waste management and chemical policies remain critical issues for the 21st century. Community/public health nurses can advocate for collective community action to preserve natural resources.

12. Health effects of global warming, nanotechnology, and the interactions of numerous chemicals in human bodies are important areas for health research and risk communication.

LEARNING BY EXPERIENCE AND REFLECTION

1. Use the home assessment tool on your own home and compare results with fellow students; then conduct an exposure history with a fellow student using the questions in Box 9-2, "I PREPARE."

2. Describe an environmental issue in your community (such as a hazardous waste site, chemical pollutants from a plastics' manufacturer, contaminated well water, or pollution from an incinerator) and the role of the community/public health nurse in monitoring health, raising awareness, and promoting education and advocacy.

3. Spend a day with an environmental health specialist in your local health department, an occupational and environmental health nurse, or a daycare nurse consultant, or visit community agencies, such as the local poison control center. Identify the environmental hazards and the role of each professional in protecting the public from environmental hazards.

4. Outline the teaching that you would consider appropriate for the environmental health risks found in a home assessment of a client.

5. Contact an occupational or environmental health nurse in your community. Using Box 9-5 as a guide, describe the responsibilities of this nurse. See whether you can identify at least one example of primary, secondary, and tertiary prevention activities that the nurse performs.

6. Conduct an Internet search, and read information from the National Library of Medicine *ToxNet* or *ToxTown,* the Agency for Toxic Substances and Disease Registry, or the Environmental Protection Agency about lead or mercury.

COMMUNITY RESOURCES FOR PRACTICE

Information about each organization listed below is found on its website, which can be accessed through the **WebLinks** section of this book's website at *http://evolve.elsevier.com/Maurer/community/.*

Federal Agencies:
Centers for Disease Control and Prevention—National Center for Environmental Health and Agency for Toxic Substances and Disease Registry
Consumer Product Safety Commission
Department of Housing and Urban Development
Department of Energy
Environmental Protection Agency
Food and Drug Administration
National Institute for Environmental Health Sciences
National Institute for Occupational Safety and Health
Occupational Health and Safety Administration
Office on Smoking and Health

Professional Associations:
American Nurses Association—Center for Occupational and Environmental Health
American Association of Occupational Health Nurses
American Public Health Association—Public Health Nursing Section and Environmental Health Section

Nongovernmental Organizations:
American Lung Association
American Red Cross
Center for Health, Environment, and Justice
Children's Environmental Health Network
Environment and Health Forum
Environmental Defense Fund
Environmental Working Group
EnviRN (University of Maryland Environmental Health Education Center)
Health Care Without Harm
Healthy Schools Network
March of Dimes Birth Defects Foundation
National Environmental Health Association
National Safety Council
Physicians for Social Responsibility (PSR)
Poison Control Centers (look in local phone book for listing)
Sierra Club
Union of Concerned Scientists

STUDY AIDS   http://evolve.elsevier.com/Maurer/community/

Visit the Evolve website for this book to find the following study and assessment materials:

- Quiz
- Web Scenario
- Critical Thinking Questions and Answers for Case Studies
- Care Plans
- *Healthy People* Updates
- Glossary

WEBSITE RESOURCES

These items supplement the chapter's topics and are also found on the Evolve site:

- 9A: Case Study: Environmental Issues Related to Disposable Diapers and Application of the Ecological Systems Model: Disposable Diapers
- 9B: Preventing Lead Poisoning: Levels, Symptoms, and Interventions
- 9C: National Occupational Health Research Priorities
- 9D: Legislative and Other Efforts to Protect Workers
- 9E: Web-Based Resources for Environmental Health

REFERENCES

Afzal, B. (2003). Protecting the health of American communities: Access to information. *Policy, Politics, & Nursing Practice, 4*(1), 22-28.

Afzal, B. (2006). Drinking water and women's health. *Journal of Midwifery & Women's Health, 51*(1), 12-18.

Afzal, B. (2007). Global warming: A public health concern. *Online Journal in Nursing, 12*(2).

Agency for Toxic Substances and Disease Registry. (1995). Lead toxicity. *AAOHN Journal, 43*(8), 428-436.

Agency for Toxic Substances and Disease Registry. (1999). *Formaldeyhde.* ToxFAQs.™ Retrieved December 7, 2007, from *http://www.atsdr.cdc.gov/toxfaq.html.*

Agency for Toxic Substances and Disease Registry. (2000). *Taking an exposure history: I PREPARE.* Accessed September 2, 2003, at *http://www.atsdr.cdc.gov.*

American Association of Occupational Health Nurses. (1996; revised 2002). *Employee health records: Requirements, retention, and access. AAOHN Advisory.* Atlanta, GA: AAOHN Publications.

American Association of Occupational Health Nurses. (2004). *Confidentiality of employee health information. AAOHN Advisory.* Atlanta, GA: AAOHN Publications.

American Public Health Association, Public Health Nurses' Section. (2006). *Environmental health principles for public health nursing.* Washington, DC: Author. Retrieved May 6, 2008, from *http://www.apha.org/membergroups/newsletters/sectionnewsletters/public_nur/winter06/2550.htm.*

Anderson, R. (1987). Solid waste and public health. In M. Greenberg (Ed.), *Public health and the environment* (pp. 173-204). New York: Guilford.

Arvidson, C. R., & Colledge, P. (1996). Lead screening in children: The role of the school nurse. *Journal of School Nursing, 12*(3), 8-13.

Bartha, L., Baumzweiger, W., Buscher, D.S., et al. (May-June 1999). Multiple chemical sensitivity: A 1999 consensus. *Archives of Environmental Health, 54*(3), 147-149.

Blumenthal, D. S., & Ruttenber, A. J. (1995). *Introduction to environmental health* (2nd ed.). New York: Springer.

Brenner, R. A. (2003). Prevention of drowning in infants, children, and adolescents. *Pediatrics, 112*(2), 440-445.

Brody, C., & Melamed, A. (2004). The Precautionary Approach. *The American Journal of Nursing, 104*(4), 104.

Bronfenbrenner, U. (1979). *The ecology of human development.* Cambridge, MA: Harvard University Press.

Brown, P. (1995). Race, class and environmental health: A review and systematization of the literature. *Environmental Research, 69,* 15-30.

Bullard, R., & Wright, B. (1993). Environmental justice for all: Community perspectives on health and research needs. *Toxicology and Industrial Health, 9*(5), 821-841.

Butterfield, P. (2002). Upstream reflections on environmental health: An abbreviated history and framework for action. *Advances in Nursing Science, 25*(1), 32-49.

Centers for Disease Control and Prevention. (1997). *Screening young children for lead poisoning: Guidance for state and local public health officials.* Retrieved August 31, 2003, from *http://www.cdc.gov/nceh/lead/guide/guide97.htm.*

Centers for Disease Control and Prevention. (2001). Deaths: Final data for 1999. *National Vital Statistics Report, 49*(8).

Centers for Disease Control and Prevention. (2002). Impact of September 11 attacks on workers in the vicinity of the World Trade Center—New York City. *MMWR, 51,* 8-10.

Centers for Disease Control and Prevention. (2003). *Falls and hip fractures among older adults.* Retrieved August 31, 2002, from *http://www.cdc.gov/ncipc/factsheets/falls.htm.*

Centers for Disease Control and Prevention, National Center for Health Statistics. (2005). *National Health and Nutrition Examination Survey 2005-2006.* Hyattsville, MD: U.S. Department of Health and Human Services, Centers for Disease Control and Prevention. Accessed at *http://www.cdc.gov/nchs/data/nhanes/OverviewBrochureEnglish_May05.pdf.*

Choi, M., Afzal, B., & Sattler, B. (2006). Geographic information systems: A new tool for environmental health assessments. *Public Health Nursing, 23*(5), 381-391.

Clark, L., Barton, J. A., & Brown, N. J. (2002). Assessment of community contamination: A critical approach. *Public Health Nursing, 19*(5), 354-365.

Commoner, B. (1972). *The closing circle; nature, man, and technology.* New York: Bantam Books.

Davis, A. (2007). Home environmental health risks. *Online Journal in Nursing, 12*(2).

Dirksen, M. (2006). Occupational and environmental health nursing: An overview. In M. K. Salazar (Ed.), *Core curriculum for occupational and environmental health nursing* (3rd ed.). St. Louis: Saunders.

Environmental Protection Agency. *Smoke free homes.* Available at *http://www.epa.gov/smokefree/publications.html.*

Environmental Protection Agency. (1993). *Respiratory health effects of passive smoking.* Washington, DC: Author.

Environmental Protection Agency. (2007). *Superfund.* Retrieved December 7, 2007, from *http://www.epa.gov/superfund/.*

Evans, L. & Sattler, B. (2006). *Risks to asthma posed by the indoor health care environments: A guide to identifying and reducing problematic exposures.* Health Care Without Harm.

Fenske, R., Black, K., Elkner, K., et al. (1990). Potential exposure and health risks of infants following indoor residential pesticide application. *American Journal of Public Health, 80,* 689-693.

Freeze, R. A. (2000). *The environmental pendulum: A quest for the truth about toxic chemicals, human health, land environmental protection.* Berkeley and Los Angeles: University of California Press.

Gardner, M. S. (1936). *Public health nursing* (3rd ed.). New York: Macmillan.

Gee, G., & Payne-Sturges, D. (2004). Environmental health disparities: A framework integrating psychosocial and environmental concepts. *Environmental Health Perspectives, 112*(17), 1645-1653.

Geiser, M., Rothen-Rutishauser, B., Kapp, N., et al. (2005). Ultrafine particles cross cellular membranes by nonphagocytic mechanisms in lungs and in cultured cells. *Environmental Health Perspectives, 113*(11), 1555-1160.

Gilden, R. (2003). Community involvement at hazardous waste sites: A review of policies from a nursing perspective. *Policy, Politics, & Nursing Practice, 4*(1), 29-35.

Goldman, L. R. (2000). Environmental health and its relationship to occupational health. In B. S. Levy & D. H. Wegman (Eds.), *Occupational health: Recognizing and preventing work-related disease* (4th ed.). Boston: Little, Brown.

Green, P. M., & Slade, D. S. (2001). Environmental nursing diagnoses for aggregates and community. *Nursing Diagnosis, 12*(1), 5-13.

Guenther, R., & Hall, A. (2007). Healthy buildings: Impact on nurses and nursing practice. *Online Journal in Nursing, 12*(2).

Hawley, A. H. (1950). *Human ecology: A theory of community structure.* New York: Ronald Press.

Heymann, D. (Ed.). (2004). *Control of communicable diseases manual* (18th ed.). Washington, DC: American Public Health Association.

Houlihan, J., Kropp, T., Wiles, R., et al. (2005). *Body burden: The pollution in newborns.* Washington, DC: Environmental Working Group.

Huffling, K. (2006). The effects of environmental contaminants in food on women's health. *Journal of Midwifery & Women's Health, 51,* 19-25.

Institute of Medicine. (1995). *Nursing, health, and the environment: Strengthening the relationship to improve the public's health.* Washington, DC: National Academy Press.

Kleffel, D. (1996). Environmental paradigms: Moving toward an ecocentric perspective. *Advances in Nursing Science, 18*(4), 1-11.

Last, J. M. (1998). *Public health and human ecology.* Stamford, CT: Appleton & Lange.

Levy, B. S., & Wegman, D. H. (2000). Occupational health: An overview. In B. S. Levy & D. H. Wegman (Eds.), *Occupational health: Recognizing and preventing work-related disease* (4th ed.). Boston: Little, Brown.

Lubin, J. H., & Boice, J. D. (1997). Lung cancer risk from residential radon: Meta-analysis of eight epidemiological studies. *Journal of the National Cancer Institute, 89*(1), 49-57.

Lusk, S. (2001). Workers and worker populations. In M.K. Salazar (Ed.), *Core curriculum for occupational and environmental health nursing.* Philadelphia: Saunders.

McClelland, C., Thompson, P., Prete, S., et al. (1996). Assessing firearm safety in inner-city homes. *Nursing and Health Care, 17*(4), 174-178.

Morgan, M. (2003). *Environmental health.* Belmont, CA: Wadsworth/Thomson Learning.

Nadakavukaren, A. (1995). *Our global environment: A health perspective* (4th ed.). Prospect Heights, IL: Waveland Press.

National Center for Injury Prevention and Control. (2003). *Water-related injuries.* Retrieved August 31, 2003, from *http://www.cdc.gov/ncipc/factsheets/drown.htm.*

National Institute for Occupational Safety and Health. (1999). *Stress…at work* (DHHS [NIOSH] Pub. No. 99-101). Cincinnati, OH: NIOSH Publications Dissemination.

National Safe Kids Campaign. (2003). *National safe kids campaign.* Retrieved August 31, 2001, from *http://www.safekids.org/.*

National Safety Council. (1991). *Accident facts: 1991 edition.* Itasca, IL: Author.

National Safety Council. (2002). *Accident facts: 2000 edition.* Itasca, IL: Author.

National Safety Council. (2003a). *Report on injuries in America.* Retrieved August 31, 2003, from *http://www.nsc.org/library/rept2000.htm.*

National Safety Council. (2003b). Home fire prevention and preparedness. Retrieved August 31, 2003, from *http://www.nsc.org/library/facts/fires.htm.*

Newsome, S. (2005). The history of infection control: Cholera—John Snow and the beginning of epidemiology. *British Journal of Infection Control, 6*(6), 12-15.

Nightingale, F. (1860). *Notes on nursing: What it is. What it is not* (Reprinted 1992). Philadelphia: J. B. Lippincott.

Oberdörster, G., Maynard, A., Donaldson, K., et al. (2005). Principles for characterizing the potential human health effects from exposure to nanomaterials: Elements of a screening strategy. *Particle and Fibre Toxicology, 2.*

Parker-Conrad, J. E. (2002). A century of practice: Occupational Health Nursing. *AAOHN Journal, 50*(12), 537-541.

Phillips, L. (1995). Chattanooga Creek: Case study of the public health nursing role in environmental health. *Public Health Nursing, 12*(5), 335-340.

Pope, A. M., Snyder, M. A., & Mood, L. H. (Eds.). (1995). *Nursing, health, and the environment.* Washington, DC: Institute of Medicine, National Academy Press .

Porter, A., Gass, M., Muller, K., et al. (2007). Visualizing the uptake of C60 to the cytoplasm and nucleus of human monocyte-derived macrophage cells using energy-filtered transmission electron microscopy and electron tomography. *Environ Sci Technol, 41*(8), 3012-3017.

Primomo, J. (1990). Diapering decision: A community education project. *American Journal of Public Health, 80,* 743-744.

Primomo, J., Bruck, A., Greenstreet, P., et al. (1990). The high environmental cost of disposable diapers. *American Journal of Maternal/Child Nursing, 15,* 279, 282, 284.

Salazar, M. K. (Ed.). (2006). *Core curriculum for occupational and environmental health nurses* (3rd ed.). Philadelphia: Elsevier/Saunders.

Sanborn, M. D., Abelsohn, A., Campbell, M., et al. (2002). Identifying and managing adverse environmental health effects: 3. Lead exposure. *CMAJ, 166*(10), 1287-1292.

Sattler, B. (2003). The greening of health care: Environmental policy and advocacy in the health care industry. *Policy, Politics, & Nursing Practice, 4*(1), 6-13.

Sattler, B., & Hall, K. (2007). Healthy choices: Transforming our hospitals into environmentally health and safe places. *Online Journal in Nursing, 12*(2).

Sattler, B., & Lipscomb, J. (Eds.). (2003). *Environmental health and nursing practice.* New York: Springer.

Schneider, D., & Freeman, N. (2000). *Children's environmental health: Reducing risk in a dangerous world.* Washington, DC: American Public Health Association.

Shaner-McRae, H., McRae, G., & Jas, V. (2007). Environmentally safe health care agencies: Nursing's responsibility, Nightingale's legacy. *Online Journal in Nursing, 12*(2).

Shinohara, N., Mizukoshi, A., & Yanagisawa, Y. (2004). Identification of responsible volatile chemicals that induce hypersensitive reactions to multiple chemical sensitivity patients. *Journal of Exposure Analysis and Environmental Epidemiology, 14*(1), 84-91.

Smith, J., & Fisher, J. (1981). Three Mile Island: The silent disaster. *Journal of the American Medical Association, 245*(16), 1656-1659.

Subcommittee of Environmental Justice. (1995). Strategic elements for environmental justice. *Environmental Health Review, 103*(9), 796-800.

Thornton, J. W., McCally, M., & Houlihan, J. (2002). Biomonitoring of industrial pollutants: Health and policy implications of the chemical body burden. *Public Health Reports, 117,* 315-323.

Tsacoyianis, R. (1997). Indoor air pollution and sick building syndrome: A case study for the community health nurse. *Public Health Nursing, 14*(1), 58-75.

U.S. Department of Health and Human Services. (1998). *Healthy People 2010 objectives: Draft for public comment.* Washington, DC: U.S. Government Printing Office.

U.S. Department of Health and Human Services. (2000). *Healthy People 2010* (2nd ed., 2 vols.). Washington, DC: U.S. Government Printing Office. Retrieved August 31, 2003, from *http://www.healthypeople.gov/ and http://www. healthypeople.gov/Document/HTML/Volume1/08Environmental.htm.*

U.S. Department of Labor, Bureau of Labor Statistics. (2007). *Workplace illnesses and injuries in 2006. Workplace Injury and Illness Summary.* Washington, DC: U.S Department of Labor. Retrieved February 6, 2008, from *http://www.bls.gov/iif/home.*

Welker-Hood, K., Condon, M., & Wilburn, S. (2007). Regulatory, institutional, and market-based approaches towards achieving comprehensive chemical policy reform. *Online Journal in Nursing, 12*(2).

Woolf, A., Fish, S., Azzara, C., et al. (1990). Serious poisonings among older adults: A study of hospitalization and mortality rates in Massachusetts, 1983-1985. *American Journal of Public Health, 80*(7), 867-869.

SUGGESTED READINGS

American Lung Association, Environmental Protection Agency, Consumer Product Safety Commission, & American Medical Association. (1995). *Indoor air pollution: An introduction for health professionals.* Washington, DC: U.S. Government Printing Office.

American Public Health Association, American Water Works Association, Water Environment Federation. (2005). *Standard methods for examination of water and wastewater* (21st ed.). Washington, DC: American Public Health Association.

American Public Health Association and American Academy of Pediatrics Collaborative Project. (2003). *Caring for our children: National health and safety performance standards for out-of-home child care* (2nd ed.). Washington, DC: American Public Health Association.

Clark, L., Barton, J. A., & Brown, N. J. (2002). Assessment of community contamination: A critical approach. *Public Health Nursing, 19*(5), 354-365.

Davis, A. (2007). Home environmental health risks. *Online Journal in Nursing, 12*(2).

Freeze, R. A. (2000). *The environmental pendulum: A quest for the truth about toxic chemicals, human health, and environmental protection.* Berkeley and Los Angeles: University of California Press.

Garrett, L. (1994). *The coming plague: Newly emerging diseases in a world out of balance.* New York: Penguin.

Garrett, L. (2000). *Betrayal of trust: The collapse of global public health.* New York: Hyperion.

Health & the environment: Exploring critical connections. (1999). (Video). Colchester, VT: Division of Continuing Education, University of Vermont.

Keleher, K. (1995). Primary care for women: Environmental assessment of the home. *Journal of Nurse Midwifery, 40*(2), 59-64.

King, C., & Harber, P. (1998). Community environmental health concerns and the nursing process: Four environmental health nursing care plans. *AAOHN Journal, 46*(1), 20-27.

Kriebel, D., & Tickner, J. (2001). The precautionary principle and public health: Reenergizing public health through precaution. *American Journal of Public Health, 91*(9), 1351-1355.

Levine, A. (1982). *Love canal: Science, politics and people.* Lexington, MA: Lexington Books.

McClelland, C., Thompson, P., Prete, S., et al. (1996). Assessing firearm safety in inner-city homes. *Nursing and Health Care, 17*(4), 174-178.

Mistretta, E., & Endresen, L. (1992). Environmental hazards in the workplace: Legal and safety considerations. *AAOHN Journal, 40*, 398-400.

Morgan, L. (1996). Children and lead: A model of care for community health and primary care providers. *Family and Community Health, 19*(1), 42-48.

Neufer, L. (1994). The role of the community health nurse in environmental health. *Public Health Nursing, 11*(3), 155-163.

Phillips, L. (1995). Chattanooga Creek: Case study of the public health nursing role in environmental health. *Public Health Nursing, 12*(5), 335-340.

Rabe, B. (1997). The politics of environmental health. In T. Litman & L. Robins (Eds.), *Health politics and policy* (3rd ed.; pp. 381-401). Albany, NY: Delmar Publishers.

Raffensperger, C., & Tickner, J. (Eds.). (1999). *Protecting public health and the environment: Implementing the precautionary principle.* Washington, DC: Island Press.

Rogers, B. (1998). Expanding horizons: Integrating environmental health in occupational health nursing. *AAOHN Journal, 46*(1), 9-13.

Sattler, B. (2002). *Environmental health in the health care setting.* Retrieved February 6, 2008, from *http://nursingworld.org/mods/mod942/healthsetting.pdf.*

Sattler, B., Afzal, B., Condon, M., et al. (2001). *Safe workplaces and healthy learning places: Environmentally healthy schools.* Retrieved February 6, 2008, from *http://nursingworld.org/mods/archive/mod250/cesavers.htm.*

Sattler, B., Afzal, B., Condon, M., et al. (2001). *Environmentally healthy homes and communities.* Retrieved February 6, 2008, from *http://nursingworld.org/mods/mod961/961.pdf.*

Steingraber, S. (1998). *Living downstream.* New York: Vintage.

Tiedje, L., & Wood, J. (1995). Sensitizing nurses for a changing environmental health role. *Public Health Nursing, 12*(6), 359-365.

Relevance of Culture and Values for Community/Public Health Nursing

*Margaret M. Andrews**

FOCUS QUESTIONS

What are culture, race, and ethnicity?

What is the relation of culture to health and health behaviors?

How do values influence attitudes, beliefs, and behaviors related to health and illness?

What are health disparities and disparities in health care?

How do cultural differences influence cultural assessment, planning, intervention, and evaluation of care for individuals, families, and communities?

What is cultural and linguistic competence?

How are the *National Standards for Culturally and Linguistically Appropriate Health Care Standards* (CLAS) in health care used by

community/public health nurses to develop cultural and linguistic competence?

Why should community/public health nurses be concerned with being culturally competent?

What core categories should community/public health nurses explore when assessing culture?

What nursing interventions are most effective when working in culturally appropriate ways with diverse communities?

CHAPTER OUTLINE

KEY TERMS

Asylees

Cultural and linguistic competence

Cultural assessment

Cultural competence

Cultural pluralism

Cultural self-assessment

Culture

Culture-bound syndromes

Discrimination

Ethnicity

Health care disparities

Health disparities

Health literacy skill

Immigrants

Race

Racism

Refugees

Rite

Ritual

Stereotyping

Subculture

Values

---

*This chapter incorporates material written for the second edition by Frances A. Maurer and Kathryn Hopkins Kavanagh and for the third edition by Rachel W. Smith.

CULTURAL PLURALISM IN THE UNITED STATES

Cultural pluralism can be defined as mutual appreciation and understanding of the various cultures and subcultures in a society. It means that there exist cooperation between and among members of different groups and harmony in the presence of diverse lifestyles, communication patterns, religious traditions, family structures, expressions of care, and health-related beliefs and practices. With a population that exceeds 300 million, the United States is a nation of rich cultural pluralism. More than 100 million people, or one in three individuals, self-identify with one or more of the federally recognized racial and/or ethnic minority groups described in Box 10-1. Cultural pluralism can refer to a wide variety of characteristics, including religion, gender, sexual orientation, age, and related factors. The federal census data provide an overview of the types of racial and ethnic diversity found in contemporary U.S. society. Much of the community/public health nurse's practice is interconnected with population demographics, especially characteristics related to racial and ethnic trends and the socioeconomic backgrounds of individuals, families, groups, and communities.

Box 10-1   Classification Standards for Federal Data on Race and Ethnicity

- **White:** A person having origins in any of the original peoples of Europe, the Middle East, or North Africa. Included are people who indicate their race as *white* or write entries such as Irish, German, Italian, Lebanese, Near Easterner, Arab, or Polish.
- **Black or African American:** A person having origins in any of the black racial groups of Africa. Included are people who indicate their race as *black, African American,* or *Negro* or provide written entries such as African American, Afro American, Kenyan, Nigerian, or Haitian.
- **American Indian and Alaska Native:** A person having origins in any of the original peoples of North and South America (including Central America) and who maintain tribal affiliation or community attachment.
- **Asian:** A person having origins in any of the original peoples of the Far East, Southeast Asia, or the Indian subcontinent including, for example, Cambodia, China, India, Japan, Korea, Malaysia, Pakistan, the Philippine Islands, Thailand, and Vietnam. Included are *Asian Indian, Chinese, Filipino, Korean, Japanese, Vietnamese,* and *Other Asian.*
- **Native Hawaiian and Other Pacific Islander:** A person having origins in any of the original peoples of Hawaii, Guam, Samoa, or other Pacific Islands. Included are people who indicate their race as *Native Hawaiian, Guamanian* or *Chamorro, Samoan,* and *Other Pacific Islander.*
- **Some other race:** Includes all other responses not included in the *white, black* or *African American, American Indian and Alaska Native, Asian,* and *Native Hawaiian and Other Pacific Islander* race categories described above. Respondents providing write-in entries such as multiracial, mixed, interracial, Wesort, or a Hispanic or Latino group (e.g., Mexican, Puerto Rican, or Cuban) in the *Some other race* category are included here.

From U.S. Bureau of the Census. (2000). *Census of population,* Public Law 94-171. Redistricting Data File (updated every 10 years).

Figure 10-1 summarizes the current U.S. population by racial and ethnic category. The country's 198.7 million non-Hispanic whites comprise 66% of the total population and accounted for 18% of the nation's growth between 2005 and 2006. In addressing the growth among racial and ethnic minority populations, Census Bureau Director Louis Kincannon reported that there are more minority persons in this country today than there were people in the U.S. in 1910. To put this into a broader context, the U.S. minority population is larger than the total population of all but 11 countries in the world (U.S. Bureau of the Census, 2007).

Hispanics comprise the largest ethnic minority group, with 44 million people or 14.8% of the total population. Hispanics accounted for nearly one half of the national population growth during the period between 2005 and 2006. California has the largest Hispanic population of any state, followed by Texas and Florida. In New Mexico, Hispanics comprise the highest proportion of the total population (44%), followed by California and Texas (36% each). Blacks comprise the second-largest minority group with 40.2 million or 11% of the total population. The black population increased by 1.3% between 2005 and 2006. New York has the largest population of blacks of any state (3.5 million) followed by Florida and Texas. In the District of Columbia, the black population comprises 57% of the total (U.S. Bureau of the Census, 2007).

The other federally defined ethnic minority groups are Asians (14.9 million or 5% of the total population), who have the largest numbers in New York and Texas, and American Indians/Alaska Natives (4.5 million or 1.5%), many of whom reside in California, Oklahoma, Arizona, Texas, Florida, and Alaska. Native Hawaiians and other Pacific Islanders (1 million or 0.3% of the total population) are found primarily in Hawaii, California, and Washington. By the year 2030, Hispanics will represent 19% of the population, and Asians are expected to increase to 7% (U.S. Bureau of the Census, 2007). Much of the growth in the Hispanic and Asian populations is the result of immigration, and foreign-born individuals account for 11.7% of the total U.S. population.

Greater diversity in the population means that community/public health nurses are likely to come into frequent contact with members of different cultures and subcultures. The nurse's health-related cultural beliefs and values may vary significantly from those of individuals, groups, and communities different from his or her own. Bridging the racial, ethnic, and cultural divide in health poses a challenge for all nurses, especially for community/public health nurses, who provide care to diverse groups of individuals and families in community settings. *Cultural and linguistic competence* is a requisite skill for all nurses to provide culturally congruent, appropriate, and meaningful nursing and health care; avoid unnecessary misunderstandings and miscommunication; and ensure that the public receives the highest quality of community/public nursing care.

> A first-grade Vietnamese girl was sent to the school health office because the teacher noticed welts on the back of her neck. The teacher and the nurse suspected child abuse and reported the family to a social service agency. An investigation revealed that the mother had rubbed the back of the little girl's neck with a coin because the girl was not feeling well before school. Coining is a traditional form of healing practiced in

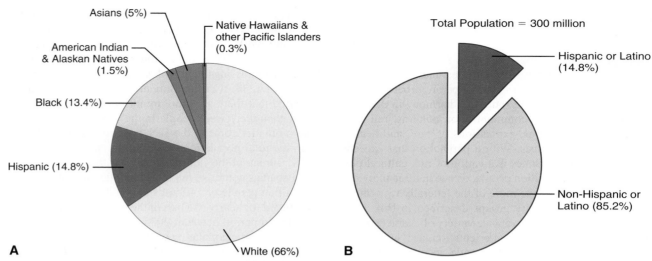

FIGURE 10-1 **A,** U.S. population by race. **B,** U.S. population by Hispanic and non-Hispanic ethnic origin. *Note:* Total is slightly higher than 100% due to rounding. (Data from U.S. Bureau of the Census. [2007, May 17]. *Minority population tops 100 million.* Retrieved July 28, 2007, from *http://www.census.gov/Press-Release/www/releases/archives/population/010048.html.*)

Southeast Asia and other parts of the world that involves vigorously rubbing the body with a coin to rid the person of the 'bad wind' that is believed to be responsible for causing illness. For those who embrace explanatory models of health and illness involving balance or harmony (e.g., yin/yang and hot/cold theories), coining is practiced for the purpose of restoring balance in the body. The resulting red welts may be mistaken for child abuse by those unfamiliar with coining as a cultural healing practice (*Transcultural nursing,* 2005).

CULTURE: WHAT IT IS

There are more than 1.8 million Web links containing definitions of **culture.** However, most anthropologists agree that culture is dynamic and refers to a group of people who have the following characteristics:

- A shared pattern of communication
- Similarities in dietary preferences and food preparation
- Common patterns of dress
- Predictable socialization patterns
- A shared sense of beliefs

According to the nurse-anthropologist Madeleine M. Leininger, who established the specialty called *transcultural nursing, culture* refers to the learned and shared beliefs, values, and life ways of a group that are generally transmitted from one generation to the next and influence people's thoughts and actions. An integral part of daily living, culture has many hidden and built-in directives and rules of behavior, beliefs, rituals, and moral-ethical decisions that give meaning and purpose to life (Leininger & McFarland, 2006). Community/public health nurses' knowledge of culture and skill in conducting comprehensive cultural assessments guide them in providing culturally competent care to people from diverse cultures.

It should be noted that there are *nonethnic cultures* such as those based on occupation or profession (e.g., culture of nursing, medicine, or the military); socioeconomic background (e.g., culture of poverty or culture of affluence); sexual orientation (gay, lesbian, or transgendered cultures); age (e.g., adolescent culture or culture of the elderly); and ability/disability (e.g., culture of the deaf/hearing impaired or culture of the blind/visually impaired). Shared life experiences (e.g., homelessness or surviving a war) are another basis for nonethnic cultures.

For community/public health nurses who provide care for diverse populations, an understanding of the concept of culture and its importance in health care is paramount. Symbols, gestures, and behaviors are often misunderstood because they have different meaning for the nurse and client. Failure to effectively communicate cross-culturally may lead to serious misunderstandings, frustration, and/or conflict between the clients and nurses. For example, an Afghani family anxiously awaits the results of the mother's clinical tests. When the nurse comes out to greet the family with the results of the tests, she smiles broadly and gives the American 'thumbs up' gesture. The family, horrified, rushes out of the office in distress. In U.S. culture, the thumbs up gesture indicates that everything is fine, but in many Middle Eastern cultures, this same gesture is considered a vulgar sign.

Culture affects the manner in which people determine who is healthy and sick; what causes health and illness; what healer(s) and intervention(s) are used to prevent and treat disease and illness; how long the person is ill; what is appropriate sick role behavior; and when the person is believed to have recovered from an illness. Culture also influences the way people receive health care information, exercise their rights and protections, and express their symptoms and health-related concerns. In some instances, biomedicine can conflict with cultural beliefs concerning health and illness. For example, although an estimated 30% of the world population has tuberculosis, in many parts of Mexico and Asia the persistent cough and night sweats associated with the disease are so prevalent that they are considered normal. Because people fail to recognize that they have a disease, they don't seek treatment. Thus, cultural beliefs can adversely affect large populations, because infected individuals unknowingly transmit the bacillus to others.

SUBCULTURES

Subcultures are groups of individuals who, although members of a larger cultural group, have shared characteristics that are not common to all members of the larger culture. The subculture is a distinguishable group. Such groups and cultural differences within the groups may be based on geography (north or south, urban or rural), economic status (poor or well off), ethnicity, and other factors. For example, persons living in Appalachia are a subcultural group based on geographic location. Differences can also be found *within* an identifiable subculture. For example, Mexican Americans, Puerto Ricans, Cubans, and Central and South Americans are all Hispanics, yet all these group have distinct subcultural patterns that distinguish them from one another. For this reason, the federal panethnic categories used in gathering census data and reporting health disparities are sometimes criticized for failing to recognize significant intragroup differences.

Persons acting in a particular social capacity or group can also be considered a subculture. These groups develop their own standards of behavior, goals, and values. The nursing profession and health system are examples of cultures or subcultures that have their own standards and beliefs, including the following (Ludwig-Beymer, 2007; Spector, 2004):

- Standardized definitions of health and illness and the importance of technology
- Health practices (immunizations, annual physical examinations, and Papanicolaou tests)
- Habits (charting, consistent use of jargon, and a systematic approach and problem-solving methodology)
- Likes (promptness, neatness and organization, and adherence)
- Dislikes (tardiness, disobedience, and disorganization)
- Customs (professional deference and adherence to the pecking order found in autocratic and bureaucratic systems, hand-washing, and certain procedures regarding birth and death)
- Rituals (performing physical examinations, carrying the community health nurse's bag when making home visits, and completing lengthy, detailed paperwork associated with new case openings)
- Expectations about pain (self-control, ability to provide detailed descriptions, and denial or downplaying of the pain they observe in others).

DIFFERENCES BETWEEN HEALTH CARE PROVIDER'S AND CLIENT'S CULTURE OR SUBCULTURE

Differences between the client's and provider's culture or subculture become apparent when clients have traditional perceptions, beliefs, and practices that differ from the nurse's practices. The community/public health nurse must be sensitive to differences among individuals that may result in practices such as coming to the clinic at unscheduled times, inability to accurately describe symptoms, failure to follow treatment plans, and lack of confidence in the medical system. A client's mistrust and lack of confidence in the health care system influence the client's acceptance of and participation in the health care planning process. Although nurses may view these behaviors as *noncompliant*, they may have a cultural basis. In one study, 51% of physicians surveyed in Los Angeles indicated that their clients do not adhere to treatment because of cultural and language barriers (Youdelman & Perkins, 2002). Some African Americans are likely to mistrust the health care system because of the Tuskegee experiments, in which 400 African American men were denied treatment for syphilis from 1932 to 1972 as part of a government study tracking the path of the disease from onset to autopsy (Bloche, 2001). Other studies reported that fewer than one half of Hispanic and Asian Americans felt confident of their ability to get needed health care (Collins et al., 2002).

VALUES

Values are preferences (or ideals) that give direction to human life by influencing beliefs and behaviors. Culture, family, personality, and life experiences contribute to the formation of values. Values make us who we are and are important in nursing because they have the potential to create barriers or facilitate communication and relationships between the nurse and his or her clients. When people interact, as nurses and clients do, their values interact. Values influence human behavior, including behavior related to health and illness; they are the foundation for acceptance and participation or rejection and repudiation of health planning and health care (Andrews & Boyle, 2008).

Differences in values and customs can be found among cultures. The culture and the society in which the individual lives or with which he or she identifies strongly influence an individual's values. Although members of a particular culture tend to share many ideas and values, differences in values exist within that culture as well. *Any assumption on the part of health providers that a given idea or custom is shared by all members of a culture can be dangerously misleading.*

The most prominent values in the United States are reflective of the dominant white, Anglo-Saxon, Protestant (WASP) cultural group. Individualism and mastery over nature are American values that permeate many aspects of health care. Privacy rights and personal freedom are based on the value of individualism. Individuals are responsible for seeking health care and cooperating with health care providers and for promoting their own health and preventing illness. Medicine attempts to control disease and distress, using such aggressive terms as *conquering* cancer and *fighting* tuberculosis. Scientific knowledge, sophisticated technologies, and a belief in intervention and mastery over problems, not a fatalistic submission to illness, are evident in health care practice. Other significant and dominant U.S. values include materialism (importance of possessions and money), reliance on technology, orientation to instant time and action, emphasis on youth, and less respect for authority and older adults.

In many of the cultures and subcultures in the United States, individualism is not a primary value. Belonging to family and community is more important. Personal privacy may not be that important; rather, sharing of information and family or group participation in the decision-making process may be of greater value. Health may or may not be a primary value. Accepting health conditions, rather than seeking interventions aimed at *curing* or *fixing* them, may be more important. The meaning of illness and differences in client-provider cultural and subcultural values may become evident during client-provider interactions.

One member of a gypsy (Roma) family became ill and was seen at a clinic. Informed of the seriousness of the problem, all members of the community came to the clinic to support the family. The nurse, unprepared to receive a large number of visitors and family members, informed the family members that they would not all be permitted to wait in the building (space, noise, and privacy of other clients were a concern). The family members became enraged, refused to leave, and insisted that they be accommodated.

Had the nurse been aware of the value placed by the gypsy (Roma) group on providing support to members in crisis, the nurse might have anticipated a large gathering and preplanned accordingly. In a situation such as this, the nurse might acknowledge the family's need for closeness and negotiate a reasonable limit on the number of people in attendance. The nurse might identify suitable accommodations for the remainder, for example, alternate some family members to the cafeteria.

Table 10-1 provides a sample list of cultural values for select cultures and identifies some implications for nurses providing health care to these populations.

RACE

The concept of race is separate from the concept of ethnicity, although the terms are often used interchangeably. **Race** has traditionally referred to a group of individuals who share common biologic features. Nonetheless, race as a valid biologic concept is under challenge, and many people have called for abandoning the race concept altogether (Fullilove, 1998; Osborne & Feit, 1992). The Human Genome Project, an extensive worldwide gene-mapping project, has determined that, although clear differences in appearance are sometime evident, no genetic differences exist among races. In other words, the minute differences among gene types are as much the result

TABLE 10-1   Cultural Values for Select Groups—Implications for Community/Public Health Nurses

Cultural Values	Health Care Implications
Anglo American Culture (Mainly U.S. Middle and Upper Classes) 1. Individualism—focus on self-reliance 2. Independence and freedom 3. Competition and achivement 4. Materialism (things and money) 5. Technology dependent 6. Instant time and actions 7. Youth and beauty 8. Equal sex rights 9. Leisure time highly valued 10. Reliance on scientific facts and numbers 11. Less respect for authority and older adults 12. Generosity in time of crisis	1. Stress alleviation by physical and emotional means 2. Personalized acts (e.g., doing special things or giving individual attention) 3. Self-reliance (individualism) by reliance on self, self-care, independence, or reliance on technology 4. Health education: desire to be given the medical facts on how to care for self
Mexican American Culture 1. Extended family valued; children highly valued 2. Traditional family is foundation of society 3. High respect for authority and older adults 4. Religion is major influence on health care practices and beliefs 5. Food is primary form of socialization 6. Traditional folk-care healers for folk illnesses 7. Belief in hot and cold theory of disease prevention	1. Succorance (direct family aid) 2. Involvement with extended family 3. Fillal love or loving; touching 4. Respect for authority 5. Mother as care decision maker 6. Protective male care 7. Acceptance of God's will 8. Use of folk-care practices 9. Healing with foods
Haitian American Culture 1. Extended family as support system 2. Religion—God's will must prevail 3. Reliance on folk foods and treatments 4. Belief in hot and cold theory 5. Male decision makers and direct caregivers 6. Reliance on native language	1. Involve family for support 2. Respect and trust 3. Succorance 4. Spiritual healing and touching 5. Use of folk food 6. Avoid evil eye and witches
African American Culture 1. Extended family networks and respect for elders 2. Religion and religious behavior valued 3. Interdependence with *blacks* for daily survival 4. Technology valued (e.g., radio, car) 5. Folk (soul) foods and folk medicine or healing models 6. Music and physical activities	1. Concern for *brothers* and *sisters* 2. Being involved 3. Giving physical presence; touching appropriately 4. Family-support and family-centered activities 5. Reliance on home remedies 6. Rely on *Jesus to save us* with prayers and songs

Continued

TABLE 10-1   Cultural Values for Select Groups—Implications for Community/Public Health Nurses—cont'd

Cultural Values	Health Care Implications
American Indian Culture	
1. Harmony with nature (land, people, environment)	1. Establishing harmony with people, the environment
2. Giving back or receiprocity with *Mother Earth*	2. Actively listening
3. Spiritual inspiration; religion as a way of life	3. Using silence *(Great Spirit)* as guidance
4. Folk healers (shamans) (the circle and four directions)	4. Rhythmic timing based on the harmony among nature, the land, and people
5. Practice culture rituals and taboos	5. Respect for folk healers, carers, and curers
6. Rhythmicity of life and nature	6. Maintaining reciprocity
7. Authority of tribal elders; respect and value for children	7. Preserving cultural rituals and taboos
8. Pride in cultural heritage and *nations*	8. Respect for elders and children
Asian and Pacific-Islander Culture	
1. Family—large extended family networks, hierarchical structure, loyalty	1. Succorance (direct family aid) and involvement with extended family
2. Devotion to tradition	2. Preserving cultural traditions
3. Many religions, including Taoism, Buddhism, Islam, and Christianity	3. Respect for authority and folk healers
4. Use of silence, nonverbal and contextual cueing	4. Hospital equals an alien place
5. Noncontact people	5. Touching inappropriate
6. Use of herbal remedies, acupuncture, moxibustion	6. Cupping (creating a vacuum in glass and placing over skin surface), bleeding (with leeches), and massage (pushing and pulling)—often used in remedies
7. Belief in *yin* and *yang*—everything in the universe contains two aspects, which are in opposition and also in unison	7. Illness is the disharmony of *yin* and *yang*
	8. Respect for elders and children

Data compiled from Andrews, M., & Boyle, J. (2003). *Transcultural concepts in nursing care* (4th ed.). Philadelphia: Lippincott, Williams & Wilkins; Lipson, J., Dibble, S., & Minarik, P. (1996). *Culture and nursing care: A pocket guide.* San Francisco: University of California, San Francisco Press; Purnell, L., & Paulanka, B. (2003), *Transcultural health care—A culturally competent approach.* Philadelphia: F. A. Davis; Spector, R. E. (2004). *Cultural Diversity in health and illness* (6th ed.). CT: Appleton-Lange.

of differences *among* members of the same race (white versus white, black versus black) as of differences *between* races (white versus black versus Asian).

Despite the scientific evidence, racial and ethnic distinctions are reflected in the formal reporting and presenting of federal health and vital statistics data. Although both terms are important determinants in collecting data and presenting health statistics, the concept of race as used by the U.S. Bureau of the Census reflects self-identification by people indicating the race or races with which they feel most closely allied, and this classification includes both racial and national-origin groups. The racial classifications that the Bureau of the Census uses adhere to the October 30, 1997, Federal Register notice entitled, 'Revisions to the Standards for the Classification of Federal Data on Race and Ethnicity,' issued by the Office of Management and Budget. These classifications are presented in Box 10-1.

ETHNICITY

Ethnicity refers to a 'shared culture and way of life, especially as reflected in language, folkways, religious and other institutional forms, material culture such as clothing and food, and cultural products such as music, literature and art' (Smedley et al., 2003, p. 523). Ethnicity provides a sense of social belonging and loyalty, and each of us belongs to an ethnic group of one kind or another. One of the most important characteristics of ethnicity is that it provides a sense of belonging or identity.

As noted earlier, *ethnicity* is commonly used interchangeably with *race,* although differences exist in the terms. Federal documents and reports delineate data by four major racial groups—American Indian, including Alaska Natives, Eskimos, and Aleuts; Asian Americans and Pacific Islanders; blacks; and whites—and by one ethnic group, Hispanics, under the combined term *racial and ethnic groups.* Hispanics create

a dilemma for census takers because they are also considered to belong to either of two racial groups. Some Hispanics are considered black, some white. Data are sometimes collected by ethnic distinction alone—Hispanic and non-Hispanic—in which case, most people of various races fall into the non-Hispanic category. Data are sometimes collected by race and ethnic groups. When this distinction is made, Hispanics are listed as an ethnic group, and members of black and white racial groups who are not Hispanic are listed as *black non-Hispanic* or *white non-Hispanic.* Collecting data by racial and ethnic categories is considered important in health care because certain groups tend to be more resistant or vulnerable to specific health problems. *The collection and value of such data for health care professionals will diminish as groups intermarry and their progeny become increasingly multiracial.*

Because the terms *race* and *ethnicity* are often used interchangeably, community/public health nurses must understand the distinctions between the terms. Nurses should avoid labeling clients by using skin markers or other features as identifiers and classifying individuals based on group association. In some instances, knowing the client's race or ethnic type is helpful in identifying individuals and groups at increased risk for certain diseases, recognizing normal and abnormal biocultural variations in the physical assessment, and evaluating clients' responses to certain medications. The most appropriate way to determine the client's racial or ethnic identity is to ask, 'How do you identify yourself?'

RACIAL AND ETHNIC HEALTH AND HEALTH CARE DISPARITIES

Disparities in health and health care exist across the spectrum of racial and ethnic groups and involve a range of health concerns (Figure 10-2). **Health disparities** are differences or

Overall picture: Adults who can seldom or never get care for illness or injury as soon as wanted, by ethnicity:

Whites **12.9%**   Blacks **18.9%**   Hispanics **25.8%**

Adults whose health providers usually listened carefully, explained things clearly, respected what they had to say and spent enough time with them, by ethnicity:

Whites **36.4%**   Blacks **26.4%**   Hispanics **27.5%**

Diabetes: Adults with diabetes who had at least one hemoglobin A1c test, a retinal eye examination and a foot exam in the past year by ethnicity:

Whites **55.1%**   Blacks **54.1%**   Hispanics **37.9%**

Cancer: Cancer deaths per 100,000 population per year for all cancers, by ethnicity:

Whites **195.6**   Blacks **242.5**   Hispanics **128.4**

Congestive heart failure: Hospitalizations for congestive heart failure per 1000 population, by race.

Whites **2.4**   Blacks **5.3**   Hispanics **insufficient data**

Mental health: People 18 or older with serious mental illness who received mental health treatment or counseling in the past year, by ethnicity in the United States:

Whites **52.8%**   Blacks **36.6%**   Hispanics **29.3%**

FIGURE 10-2 Disparity statistics for the United States. (Data from Agency for Healthcare Research and Quality. [2005]. *National healthcare disparities report.* Retrieved July 28, 2007 from http://www.ahrq.gov/qual/nhdr05/nhdr05.htm.)

inequalities in health status, including differences in life expectancy, mortality, and morbidity. Although significant progress has been made in improving life expectancy and overall indicators of health, health disparities persist. The objectives set forth in *Healthy People 2010* (U.S. Department of Health and Human Services [USDHHS], 2000) were designed to increase quality and years of healthy life and eliminate health disparities for each of the ethnic minority groups. Although significant progress has been made in reducing some health disparities, there is compelling evidence that race and ethnicity correlate with persistent and often increasing health disparities among multiple racial and ethnic minority groups at all stages of life.

Life expectancy rates are often considered reflections of the overall health of a population. Since the beginning of the twentieth century, life expectancy at birth has increased from less than 50 years to more than 76 years. Although the life expectancy at birth for blacks has more than doubled since 1900, on average, whites still can expect to live 5.4 years longer than blacks. The life expectancy for black males is 69 years, whereas white males can expect to live to 75.3 years. For black females, the life expectancy is 76.1 years, whereas white females can expect to reach 80.5 years of age. Although current life expectancy data for Hispanics and American Indians/Alaska Natives are not available, the higher incidence of diabetes and liver disease in these populations increases the likelihood that they will live fewer years (Indian Health Service, 2007; Office of Minority Health, 2007a, 2007b).

Most racial and ethnic minorities have higher infant mortality rates; higher rates of death from cancer, heart disease, diabetes, human immunodeficiency virus (HIV) infection, and acquired immunodeficiency syndrome (AIDS); more chronic and disabling diseases; and lower immunizations rates. For example,

African American, American Indian, and Puerto Rican infants have markedly higher death rates than white infants. For the past two decades there has been a widening disparity between African American and white infant death rates. African American women are more than twice as likely to die of cervical cancer as are white women and more likely to die of breast cancer than women of any other racial or ethnic group. Although heart disease and stroke are the leading causes of death for all racial and ethnic groups, death rates for heart disease are 20% higher among African American adults than among white adults, and deaths from strokes are 40% higher. American Indians and Alaska Natives are 2.6 times more likely to have diabetes, with the incidence of non–insulin dependent diabetes mellitus as high as 60% in some Indian nations. Compared with their white counterparts, African Americans are 2.0 times and Hispanics 2.9 times more likely to have been diagnosed with diabetes (Centers for Disease Control and Prevention [CDC], 2006; Indian Health Service, 2007; Office of Minority Health, 2007b; Smedley et al., 2003; USDHHS, 2001a).

Some minority populations experience problems with access to and quality of health care services. Research indicates that some minority individuals, groups, and communities receive a lower quality of health care than do nonminorities, even when insurance status, income, age, and severity of conditions are equal (American Medical Association, 2007; CDC, 2006; Office of Minority Health, 2007a, 2007b; Smedley et al., 2003).

Health care disparities may be defined as 'racial or ethnic differences in the *quality* of health care that are not due to access related factors or clinical needs, preferences, and appropriateness of intervention' (Smedley et al., 2003, pp. 3-4) (emphasis added). In populations with equal access to health care, disparities exist because of the operation of the health care system and discrimination, biases, stereotyping, and uncertainty of the clinicians (Smedley et al., 2003). African Americans have the highest incidence of end-stage renal disease but are less likely to receive renal dialysis, be referred for transplantation, or receive a kidney transplant. Hispanic and African Americans are less likely to receive evidenced-based mental health care in accordance with professional treatment guidelines, and more than one fourth of Asian Americans report experiencing difficulty in accessing specialists (CDC, 2006; Office of Minority Health, 2007b; Smedley et al., 2003; USDHHS, 2001a).

Even when conditions are comparable (e.g., comparable insurance status, educational level, income level, access to health professionals), minority members are less likely than whites to receive appropriate treatment or surgical procedures. African Americans are more likely to be diagnosed as psychotic but are less likely to be given antipsychotic medicines and more likely to be hospitalized involuntarily, to be regarded as potentially violent, and to be placed in restraints (Agency for Healthcare Research and Quality, 2005; CDC, 2006; George, 2000; Office of Minority Health, 2007b; Polyakova & Pacquiao, 2006; Smedley et al., 2003).

A wide array of factors contributes to health disparities. Patterns of segregation and discrimination, the health care environment, and specific individual health behaviors and beliefs play a role in the problem. A complex and fragmented health care environment makes receiving continuity of care difficult for people. Managed care and Medicaid managed care plans often disrupt community-based care and displace providers who are familiar with the culture and values of the ethnic community. Language barriers contribute to the problem, especially when care providers are unfamiliar with the language spoken by their clients. Geographically distant clinics and hospitals pose access problems, especially for economically stressed families without transportation. Some American Indians are required to travel more than 90 miles one way to obtain care at Indian Health Service facilities, and the wait ranges from 2 to 6 months for appointments in certain specialties, such as obstetrics/gynecology and outpatient mental health (Agency for Healthcare Research and Quality, 2005; Government Accountability Office, 2005; Indian Health Service, 2007).

ROLE OF INSURANCE IN HEALTH DISPARITIES

With 13% of the national gross domestic product (GDP) allocated to health care, the United States leads the world in health care spending. Despite this investment, nations spending substantially less sometimes have healthier populations. The U.S. performance is adversely affected by deep inequalities linked to income and health insurance coverage. The United States is the only Western industrialized nation without a universal health insurance system. Instead, the United States relies on employer-based private insurance and public coverage that fail to reach all citizens, with minority populations being at higher risk than whites for being underinsured or uninsured (see Chapter 21). Although more than one half of the U.S. population has health insurance coverage through their employers and nearly all elderly are covered through Medicare, more than one in six nonelderly Americans (45 million) lack health insurance (Figure 10-3). Lack of health insurance among vulnerable populations contributes to poorer access to health care and ultimately to health disparities. Hispanics are three times as likely to be uninsured as whites (33% versus 11%), whereas 20% of blacks are without health insurance. The cost of treatment is a major barrier to access in the United States.

More than 40% of the uninsured have no regular health care facility to go to when they are sick, and more than one third of the uninsured report that they or someone in their family went without needed care or prescription medicines because of cost (Government Accountability Office, 2005; Kaiser Family Foundation, 2007; Rowland & Hoffman, 2005; U.S. Bureau of the Census, 2003).

STRATEGIES FOR ELIMINATING HEALTH DISPARITIES

Eliminating health disparities is one of two major goals of the *Healthy People 2010* objectives. The objectives are especially focused on eliminating health disparities by 2010 in six key areas that cut across different racial and ethnic groups (CDC, 2006; Indian Health Service, 2007; Office of Minority Health, 2007b):

- Infant mortality
- Cancer
- Heart disease
- Diabetes
- HIV infection and AIDS
- Immunizations

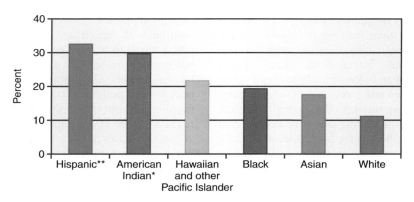

* Includes Alaskan Native.
** Hispanic may be of any race.

FIGURE 10-3 Rate of uninsured by race and ethnic group, United States, 3-year average for 2003 to 2005. (Data from U.S. Bureau of the Census. [2006]. *Current population survey: 2004 to 2006. Annual social and economic supplements.* Washington, DC: U.S. Government Printing Office.)

Federal and state governments, as well as nongovernmental health organizations, are committed to reducing health disparities in the U.S. population. **Website Resource 10A** provides a detailed list of recommended strategies to reach this goal. Community/public health nurses need to be aware of health disparities between and within racial and ethnic groups. All nurses should be aware of barriers to achieving optimal health and methods to facilitate attaining culturally competent health care for everyone. Recognizing cultural differences is a first step.

UNDERSTANDING CULTURAL DIFFERENCES

Different cultures have different views and perspectives regarding everyday concepts and normal behavior. Understanding the essential characteristics and differences that give each community its uniqueness and recognizing the different meanings of some key concepts in different cultures is useful for nurses who practice in multicultural health care settings (c.f. Andrews & Boyle, 2008; Galanti, 2004; Giger & Davidhizar, 2004; Leininger & McFarland, 2006; Purnell & Paulanka, 2003; Spector, 2004).

TIME AND SPACE
People perceive and use time in different ways: linear or circular. A *linear view* sees time as a straight line with a beginning and an end. A *circular view* sees time as a never-ending unity that repeats itself and is part of a continuous whole. Western health care providers tend to view time in a linear way, divided into segments of minutes, hours, days, weeks, and so on. We wear watches, and our watches are synchronous with those of others. Our work day begins and ends at a specific time. We keep appointments on time. Because time is money and is in limited supply, we are urged to both work and play rapidly, accurately, and smartly. We admire people who make good use of their time and control their time well.

Many people perceive time differently. They view time as circular (continuous and never ending). Time may be seen as a gift to be enjoyed rather than a limited commodity to be used. People with this view of time may not have or use a watch, may not be concerned with punctuality, and may not feel stressed to

do chores at a set time. If time is a gift to be enjoyed, practically anything may take precedence over a clinic appointment, a nurse's visit, or a day at school or work.

Individuals and groups also differ in time orientation with regard to health planning. Cultural groups with a past-time orientation, such as many Asian Americans, tend to lean toward traditional approaches to healing. Persons with a predominantly present-time orientation, such as African Americans, Native Americans, and Hispanics, may be less able to look toward the future and practice preventive health measures. Pain, dysfunction, or limitations cue the search for treatment. If these cues are absent, a present-orientated person might not appreciate the need for treatment to avoid a *future* consequence. For example, a middle-aged African American woman with hypertension may be unable to see the need for controlling blood pressure through medication to prevent a future problem, such as stroke. By contrast, the middle-class white American culture tends to be future oriented as reflected by its emphasis on punctuality, technology, and prevention. Time is structured and scheduled, including leisure time, which is often planned ahead.

Community/public health nurses and other health care professionals should be aware that clients may have a time perspective that is different from their own. Some African Americans and Mexican Americans believe that time is flexible and that activities will start on their arrival. There is no need to rush to an appointment; a delay is acceptable. If this perception is the usual one in the community, community/public health nurses should incorporate this information in planning program activities.

How human beings view and structure *space* differs among cultures in ways that are as profound and important as the differences in how they view and structure time. Space is linked with issues of territoriality, living, work and health care arrangements, touch, sound, and smell. Space as a physical boundary or territory is an important concept; just as animals protect their territory, so do humans (Giger & Davidhizar, 2004; Leininger & McFarland, 2006).

Culture determines the amount of personal space an individual requires. Some cultures are comfortable with very little distance between people; others are more comfortable with a separation of several feet. When individuals from different cultures interact, a chance exists that one will violate the other's *personal space*. Standing too close to another person can precipitate feelings of anger or fear in the person whose space is invaded. Hall (1963) identified four different relational spaces:

- *Intimate* distance ranges from 0 to 18 inches and is used when performing close physical assessments, such as eye examinations.
- *Personal* distance varies from 18 inches to 4 feet, the usual space within which communications between friends and acquaintances, as well as aspects of the physical examination, occur.
- *Social* distance is from 4 to 12 feet, the space in which small group interaction may occur.
- *Public* distance is considered anything further than 12 feet and is used in conducting workshops and community meetings.

The distance in each relational space varies widely depending on the cultural group's spatial orientation.

Some cultural groups own land and mark their plot or acreage with fences to separate it from that of their neighbors. Some cultures perceive land as belonging to everyone and to no one in particular and would not think of putting up fences. Some cultures value uniformity; others value diversity. Although the United States places great emphasis on individual freedom and creativity, many U.S. towns have covenants that restrict the individual's right to alter his or her property in any unacceptable visible way.

How people construct and use public space is an important consideration when nurses conduct community meetings. Various cultural groups perceive space as more or less formal, which can create problems among them. For example, in one nursing home, Americans of African descent used the shared lobby on each floor as formal public space and dressed accordingly. Americans of European descent, on the other hand, used the shared space informally, wearing slippers, robes, and even hair curlers.

When in clients' homes, nurses are guests, and they must be aware of how space is structured and used. Some rooms in the house may be reserved only for family and close friends, and nurses must be aware of cues regarding public and private space. In working with people from a culture that contrasts with the nurse's culture of origin, the nurse has an obligation to discover how, in general, the client's cultural group perceives and uses space and how to recognize limit-setting cues.

COMMUNICATION

Communication is an essential component of any nurse-client interaction. The effectiveness of communication depends on each party's clear understanding of the meaning of each message. The process of communication includes both verbal and nonverbal components and may be influenced by hierarchic relationships, gender, and religion.

Verbal Communication

Language is an important tool in nursing and in establishing a nurse-client relationship. The gathering of accurate information related to health care beliefs, illness, and care measures is critical. Ineffective communication may lead to misunderstandings. These misunderstandings may result in a failure to identify and access existing health services;

difficulty with appointment scheduling; inaccurate or incomplete information relevant to health status; and inappropriate follow-up and follow through with recommended treatment. Ineffective communication can result in client dissatisfaction with health care services and reluctance to return to the health care setting (c.f. Andrews & Boyle, 2008; Galanti, 2004; Giger & Davidhizar, 2004; Leininger & McFarland, 2006; Munoz & Luckman, 2005; Purnell & Paulanka, 2003; Smedley et al., 2003; Spector, 2004; Wilson-Stronks & Galvez, 2007).

Language barriers are one of the greatest obstacles to health care among culturally diverse groups. In the United States, approximately 47 million people speak a language other than English at home, and at least 39 different languages are in use (Figure 10-4). Approximately 28 million are speakers of Spanish, and of those, approximately 14 million report that they speak English less than very well (U.S. Bureau of the Census, 2005).

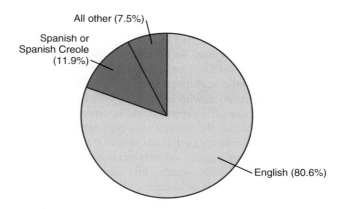

Note: Percentage distribution of persons 5 years and older. Chart below indicates Other and Spanish expanded to show specific languages spoken and frequency.

A

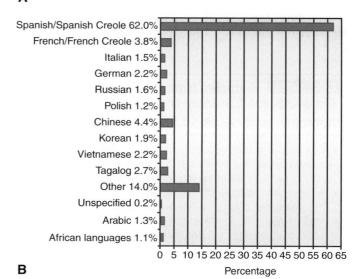

B

FIGURE 10-4 **A,** Language spoken at home, 2005; data in pie chart form. **B,** Bar graph showing data as percentage speaking Spanish and other languages. (Data from U.S. Census Bureau. [2005]. S1601: *Language spoken at home* [2005 American Community Survey]. Retrieved June 8, 2007 from *http://factfinder. census.gov/servlet/STTable?_bm=y&-geo_id=01000US&-qr_name=ACS_2005_EST_ G00_S1601&-ds_name=ACS_2005_EST_G00_*.)

Cultural and Linguistic Competence. **Cultural and linguistic competence** refers to the ability of health care providers and organizations to understand and respond to the cultural and linguistic needs of clients during the health care encounter. Laws and federal guidelines pertaining to provision of language services, means of accessing language services, and the appropriate use of language services are essential information for the community/public health nurse. In response to the need to facilitate culturally competent health care, the Office of Minority Health published *National Standards for Culturally and Linguistically Appropriate Services* (CLAS) to be implemented in health care settings (USDHHS, 2001b). These standards provide a blueprint for organizations to follow in building cultural and linguistic competence in their workforces and organizations. Box 10-2 summarizes the sections relating to direct client-provider conversations. The complete CLAS standards are available on the book's website as **Website Resource 10B.**

WEB

Linguistic competence is addressed by four of the standards. CLAS standards require health care organizations to offer language assistance services *free* to each client or consumer with limited English proficiency. Bilingual staff and interpreter service are preferred. Other options include face-to-face interpretation provided by trained staff or contract or volunteer interpreters.

Community/public health nurses must establish an effective means of communication with individuals with limited English proficiency. The use of interpreters and interpreter services is one means. However, the interpreter-client interchange may be affected by differences in dialects within the same regions; cultural, political, or religious rivalry between tribes, nations, regions, or states; and age, gender, and socioeconomic status. For example, a client and an interpreter both come from Laos; however, one is Hmong and the other is not. Because of their different tribal affiliations, each views the other with suspicion, which makes the interpretation process difficult.

Issues of status, age, sex, and privacy must be considered when selecting an interpreter. For example, in some cultures, conversations between unrelated men and women are strictly regulated or forbidden. All attempts should be made to choose interpreters with characteristics as close as possible to those of the client. If a formal interpreter is not readily available, telephone services are acceptable. Telephone services provide interpreters for most languages. The nurse and client speak into separate telephones, and the interpreter translates for each party. Accurate interpretation of client responses is critical. The CLAS standards require that organizations ensure the competence of interpreters. Family or friends should not be used as interpreters except in emergencies or at the specific request of the client. Using family members or friends provides a breach of confidentiality, and such individuals may not give an impartial interpretation of the intended message. Minor children should not be used as interpreters, even in situations in which their parents are the clients.

Community/public health nurses who routinely care for clients with English language difficulties should be prepared in advance if no interpreters are available. The best strategy is for the nurse to become proficient in the language. Another strategy is the use of a *word board* or index cards with essential words or phrases in the client's own language. For example, "Where is your pain?" or "When did it start?" Hand motions, pantomime, or simple touch may be the only available methods of communication; however, these methods are more error prone than cards or word boards.

Using a considerate approach, addressing the client by formal name, showing genuine warmth, and taking time to establish trust are important. Minorities cite the lack of time and attention given to clients by health care professionals as one of the most important reasons for their lack of trust in the health care system (Government Accountability Office, 2005; Kaiser Family Foundation, 2007). The nurse may wish to start with safer topics, use open-ended formats, and elicit opinions and beliefs to begin the dialogue. Nonverbal clues and specific behavior during conversations should be noted. The diversity of voice volume and tone used by different cultural groups should be appreciated. European Americans and African Americans may be perceived as loud and boisterous because of their voice volume. African Americans who speak black English, Gullah (a Creole blend of Elizabethan English and African languages), or other African dialects exclusively may be misunderstood as poorly educated or unintelligent (Campinha-Bacote, 1998). Gypsy language tone is normally loud and argumentative, even in normal conversation. Arab Americans tend to use an excited speech pattern that may be misunderstood as anger; a loud voice may merely indicate the importance of the message. The Chinese language is very expressive and may appear loud and abrupt to others (Chin, 1996).

Health Literacy Skills. **Health literacy skill** refers to the ability to read and understand instructions on prescription and medicine bottles, appointment slips, informed consent documents, insurance materials, and client educational materials. Health illiteracy is a frequently overlooked and underemphasized barrier to health care in racial and ethnic minority populations (Burroughs et al., 2002). An estimated 90 million American adults possess low health literacy skills. Low literacy is more frequently noted among persons of low socioeconomic status, the poorly educated, older adults, U.S-born ethnic minorities, immigrants, and persons who are disabled. Low health literacy continues to be a barrier for racial and ethnic minorities. (See Chapter 20 for ways to determine and reduce the reading level of health materials.)

BOX 10-2   Samples from the Recommended Standards for Culturally and Linguistically Appropriate Services (CLAS) in Health Care

- Clients or consumers receive from staff effective, understandable, and respectful care provided in a manner compatible with their cultural health beliefs and practices and preferred language.
- A diverse staff representative of the demographic characteristics of the service area is recruited, retained, and promoted.
- Staff receives ongoing education and training in culturally and linguistically appropriate service delivery.
- Language assistance services are offered and provided at no cost to each client or consumer with limited English proficiency.
- The competence of interpreters and bilingual staff providing language assistance is ensured.
- Easily understood client-related materials are made available and signs are posted in the languages of the commonly encountered groups.

Data from *Federal Register*, 65 (247), 80865-80879.

The CLAS standards require that organizations provide educational materials and forms in the commonly encountered languages. Community/public health nurses must ensure that materials in alternative formats are developed for individuals who cannot read or who speak nonwritten languages (e.g., sign language) and for persons with sensory, developmental, or cognitive impairments. Title VI of the Civil Rights Act of 1964 requires that all organizations that receive federal financial assistance ensure that persons with limited English proficiency have meaningful linguistic access to the health services that these organizations provide (USDHHS, 2001b).

Community/public health nurses must perform an adequate assessment of literacy skills to reduce the potential for medical errors caused by a client's language difficulties. Developing client educational materials that are *culturally congruent* with the target population and at an *appropriate reading level* is important. Many of the educational materials that are specifically targeted at minorities do not reflect the cultural values of the targeted groups, and few are written at a reading level suitable for persons with low literacy skills. *Test of Functional Health Literacy in Adults* (TOFHLA) is a tool that helps assess a client's ability to perform health-related tasks that require reading and computational skills, such as taking medications, keeping appointments, appropriately preparing for tests and procedures, and giving informed consent.

Nonverbal Communication

Nonverbal communication patterns are important to the communication process. Nonverbal communication patterns vary widely among cultures and ethnic groups. Understanding and appropriate use of touch, silence, eye contact, greetings, and body language are vital to the nurse-client interaction. The nurse's capacity to assist the individual, family, and community to reach the desired health outcomes may be impaired by his or her inability to understand and accurately interpret the nonverbal patterns of the ethnic and cultural groups that he or she serves (c.f. Munoz & Luckman, 2005; Purnell & Paulanka, 2003; Spector, 2004; Wilson-Stronks & Galvez, 2007).

Touch. Use of touch in the communication process is culturally dependent and varies significantly from culture to culture. Some cultures seek bodily contact; others carefully avoid contact. For example:

- Greetings among many Americans include traditional handshakes or hugging.
- Among Native American Navajos, touch is unacceptable except when one knows the person well or when it is part of therapeutic treatments (Still & Hodgins, 1998).
- For Nigerian Americans, touching or casual hand holding between members of the same or opposite sex usually signals friendship (Andrews & Boyle, 2008).
- In some Middle Eastern cultures, women do not shake hands with men, nor do men and women touch each other outside of marriage (Andrews & Boyle, 2008).
- Afghan and Afghan American extended family members and close friends often touch each other on the shoulder or leg during conversations and greet with a kiss on each cheek or a hug (Lipson et al., 2004).

Understanding the relevance of touch is important for the community/public health nurse, because touch is part of the process of providing health care. Nurses should be sensitive to and accommodate, whenever possible, cultural and ethnic differences in patterns of touch. For example:

- Examining the genitalia (and discussing reproduction) may be embarrassing in some cultural groups, and Chinese Americans, Hispanics, Muslims, and individuals from other racial, ethnic, and/or religious groups may prefer same-sex health care providers.
- In some Arab and Hispanic cultures, male health care providers are prohibited from examining all or parts of the female body (Purnell & Paulanka, 2003; Spector, 2004).

Touching children is of particular concern. For example, in Asian cultures touching a child on the head may be interpreted as a sign of disrespect, because the head is thought to be the source of a person's strength. Examining the fontanels of a Southeast Asian infant should be avoided if possible or done only with the permission of the parent. An alternative method would be to make other observations to assess for increased intracranial pressure or premature fontanel closure while the parent holds the child on his or her lap. The nurse might place his or her hand over the mother's hand on the fontanels while asking for a description for what the mother feels (Andrews, 2008).

Silence. Use of silence as a communication element varies across cultures. Silence may indicate approval, disapproval, a lack of understanding, respect, or disrespect. In Asian cultures, silence may indicate respect for elders. Silence and nodding during the nurse-client interaction must be carefully evaluated, because understanding or agreement of the message may or may not necessarily be conveyed. Silence and nodding may mean, "Yes, I hear you," "Yes, we are interacting," or some other message. For example, some American Navajos are comfortable with long periods of silence, because active listening demonstrates an interest in what an individual is saying. Responding with quick answers may suggest immaturity on the part of the client. Nurses need to provide ample time for elderly Navajos to respond to questions and allow more silent time than the nurse might ordinarily use in conversation (Still & Hodgins, 1998). Silence may indicate agreement or disagreement. For example, in French, Spanish, and Russian cultures silence may be interpreted as a sign of agreement; in Vietnamese cultures, in which direct expressions of emotion are considered bad taste, silence may mean "No" (c.f. Andrews & Boyle, 2008; Galanti, 2004; Munoz & Luckman, 2005).

An African American woman was being interviewed to determine suitable home health services. As the nurse questioned the client regarding support from her spouse, the client remained silent. The nurse interpreted this silence as indicating a possible situation of domestic disharmony. She continued the interview while assuring the client that she could feel comfortable sharing any information relative to domestic problems. The client finally responded sharply, "That's none of your business," indicating that she thought the discussion was inappropriate.

The preceding clinical example provides several points to ponder. Questions about interpersonal relationships are often considered an intrusion into an individual's privacy. Spousal support (financial) may prevent families from accessing various community and federal programs. If the nurse understands these points, he or she can attempt to put the client at ease by opening the discussion with an explanation of the types of questions to be asked and the reason for asking them.

For example, "To better help you and your family, I will need to ask you a list of questions to best determine which types of resources and supports are available to you."

Eye Contact. Eye contact is one of the most important non-verbal communication tools and can easily be misinterpreted. Nurses use direct eye contact during interpersonal contact with clients. Clients from different countries and different cultural backgrounds may be less comfortable with direct eye contact, depending on the degree of acculturation, length of time in America, age, and education. For example:

- Many Asian Americans, Mexican Americans, Appalachians, and American Indians consider eye contact rude and impolite (c.f. Giger & Davidhizar, 2004; Leininger & McFarland, 2006).
- Some Egyptian Americans think people who fail to maintain eye contact or have shifty eye contact should not be trusted (Meleis & Meleis, 1998).
- Among the Irish, the absence of direct eye contact may be interpreted as a sign of disrespect, guilt, or mistrust (Wilson, 2003).
- Avoiding direct eye contact with elders, superiors, or persons in authority is a sign of respect among many American Indians, Hispanics, and Filipino Americans (c.f. Cantos & Rivera, 1996; Munoz & Luckman, 2005).

PREFERRED GREETINGS AND BODY LANGUAGE

Greetings are important to all groups. A handshake is expected in first-time greetings for Americans. For Vietnamese clients, shaking a woman's hand is considered inappropriate for the nurse unless the woman offers her hand first. Ethiopians and Eritreans engage in handshakes only with persons who are unfamiliar. The standard greeting for familiar people in this culture is to kiss on the cheek three to four rounds, and hugging between men is common. Koreans greet with a bow of the head. Russians may shake hands or kiss on the cheek, depending on the relationship (Evanikoff, 1996).

Names are also an important part of the greeting and convey a sense of respect for the individual. In America, friends and relatives use first names. In the nurse-client interaction, the formal use of a title (Mr., Mrs., and Ms.) is appropriate. First names should be used only if the client permits it. In Cambodia, Korea, and the Philippines, name sequencing is reversed. A woman named Pak Yon is formally called Mrs. Pak, because the sequence of the names denotes that Pak is the last name and Yon is the first name. Addressing the person as Mrs. Yon is inappropriate. In both Appalachian and African American cultures, a common practice of respect for older adults is to address the person by the first name preceded by the title Miss or Mr., for example, Miss Alice or Mr. Jeremy, despite the fact that Miss Alice may or may not be married. Names in most Spanish-speaking populations are more complex, and for women include the name of the father, the mother's surname, and the husband's surname, for example, Rachel Sanchez-Ramirez Aldes (Rachel's father-mother and husband). Among American Navajos, elders are addressed as grandmother or grandfather, or mother or father, by members of their clan. As a sign of respect, the nurse may call an older Navajo client *grandmother* or *grandfather;* however, all clients should always be addressed in a formal manner and never by first names except on request (c.f. Andrews & Boyle, 2008; Galanti, 2004).

Correct interpretation of body language and gestures is important. The nurse may signal for someone to come by crooking the index finger, a common American gesture. Among the Vietnamese, however, this same signaling practice is a provocation, usually done to a dog. The *OK gesture* given as a response may have a different connotation for other cultural groups. In Latin American countries, the OK gesture may mean that you are referring to the individual in a derogatory manner. In the south of France, the sign may mean *worthless,* and in the German culture, the practice is rude. An important part of establishing rapport with clients is knowledge of the different meanings of gestures and body language in different cultures. Misinterpretation of traditional U.S. gestures can often be devastating to clients, especially to recent immigrants (c.f. Giger & Davidhizar, 2004; Leininger & McFarland, 2006).

RITES AND RITUALS

Rites and rituals are markers of important events within a culture. A **rite** is a ceremony or act that often marks an important event or life transition. A rite of passage is an event that marks a change in status from a lower to a higher level (Van Gennep, 1960). A **ritual** is a prescribed series of actions or process closely related to a culture's ideology (Herberg, 1995). Each cultural group has defined rituals that may be related to both critical and calendrical life events. Critical events include marriage, birth, death, and graduation. Examples of calendrical events include Thanksgiving, Christmas, and Halloween. Rites and rituals can indicate health and life in a community. For example, towns may have a carnival for a patron saint or an Independence Day parade every year. Residents are celebrating a calendrical rite of identification. They are saying: "This is who we are; we rejoice in it." Families that have ritual celebrations of Christmas or Hanukkah are celebrating both their identity and the holiday. Youths who are confirmed or bar/bat mitzvahed mark passage to a state of greater maturity.

The community/public health nurse must have an understanding and appreciation of the various rites and rituals that may influence the individual, family, and community health behaviors. One of the most significant types of rituals relates to birth and care of the newborn and mother. Cultural practices surround pregnancy and labor care, parental roles during the birth process, breast-feeding, and recuperation after childbirth. For example, American Indians' labor practices vary somewhat among tribes, but many include having the mother of the pregnant woman or other female kin in attendance during the birth. Stoicism and self-control are encouraged, and pain control may include meditation or use of indigenous plants (Kramer, 1996).

During pregnancy, labor, and the postpartum period, there are many prescriptive and restrictive taboo practices. For example, among American Navajos, wearing two hats at one time is considered taboo because one will then have twins (traditionally undesirable and believed to be the work of a witch). American Navajos do not purchase clothing for an infant before birth and bury the placenta following birth as a symbol of the child's being tied to the land (Still & Hodgins, 1998). Chinese Americans may express the belief that going to the zoo during pregnancy will cause the baby to take on the appearance of one of the animals (Chin, 1996). Postpartum practices may include avoiding any housework or strenuous activity from 7 to 40 days after delivery among Puerto Ricans, Mexican Americans, and Colombians;

avoiding a full shower for 2 to 4 weeks after delivery among the Vietnamese; and ritual baths among West Indians (Hill, 1996).

A community/public health nurse visits Mrs. Wong, a Chinese American, after delivery of a healthy infant boy. The nurse advises Mrs. Wong to be attentive to diet, suggesting that a healthy breakfast might include items such as orange juice, cold cereal, and milk. Startled, the client responds, "I can't eat that." For Mrs. Wong, postpartum practices are related to the belief that imbalance occurs as a result of disharmony caused by the pregnancy and birth. In this situation, beliefs about pregnancy are based on the hot-cold theory of disease causation. Because heat is lost during the birth process, the postpartum period should be marked by a return to balance and avoidance of cold food or cold air.

Death rituals also vary. A great deal of symbolism and ritual can be found surrounding the death or impending death of a family member. These symbols and rituals include, for example, reciting special prayers; using spiritual amulets, religious medallions, or rosary beads; sitting by the window of a dying family member to keep out night spirits and chase them away; or having all family members touch the body of the deceased. The deceased's body may require special care, such as ritual washing of the body by family members. These practices are of special significance to the family and should be respected and facilitated by the health care provider whenever possible.

RELIGION

Religion and spirituality are linked strongly to our identity as humans. Whenever possible, health care must fit into a client's belief system. If clients do not believe that treatments are religiously justified or morally acceptable, then the likelihood that they will comply with prescribed regimens is diminished.

One question of critical importance for community/public health nurses is: How does religion influence health behaviors? Some religious groups fast or feast or have specific food or drink regulations. Some religious ceremonies use alcohol or drugs as an integral part of the ceremony; other religions forbid their use. Religious beliefs may allow the use of faith healers. Some religions discourage participation in the modern medical system. For example, Christian Scientists are more likely to rely on a Christian Scientist practitioner than they are to seek medical care from a physician or nurse practitioner. Religion may also influence a person's willingness to participate in immunization, screening, and medical or nursing treatment. For example, Jehovah's Witnesses are opposed to blood transfusions and may be at greater risk during surgery if hemorrhage occurs. They are also likely to refuse a surgery in which blood transfusion is essential, such as some types of organ transplantation. Electronic or printed religious calendars may also be useful to alert community/public health nurses to upcoming religious events or ceremonies during which time individuals, families, groups, and communities might prefer to defer health-related appointments and might have significant changes in diet, such as fasting or feasting (Andrews & Hanson, 2008).

ROLE OF FOOD

Food habits are inextricably linked with culture. The perceptions and practices surrounding food provide important information about a cultural group and are so deeply rooted that they may be difficult to change. The health care provider should carefully investigate and evaluate food preferences and eating habits for nutritional adequacy. Cultural food practices should not be labeled *wrong* simply because they do not conform to established nutritional practices.

Food taboos are often linked to religious belief systems that are rooted in the history and culture of a people. Food customs can be so rooted in the past that people do not always know their origins. For example, prohibitions against pork are thought by many to have originated because of health reasons, such as fear of trichinosis. Farb and Armelagos (1980) disagree; they see the prohibition in Genesis 9:3 as a reaction of the Israelites to their Egyptian captors' worship of swine rather than as a safeguard against illness. This explanation, of course, does not account for the Muslim and Seventh-Day Adventist beliefs and practices that call for the avoidance of pork and pork derivatives. Although it is sometimes difficult for community/public health nurses to be familiar with the religious beliefs and practices related to diet for all religions, they are encouraged to discuss this matter with clients, especially those following special diets (low cholesterol, low carbohydrate, etc.) and to search for reference sources pertaining to the major religious groups (Andrews & Hanson, 2008).

In assessing dietary patterns in clients from diverse cultures, community/public health nurses should not only ask for a 24- or 48-hour diet recall but also be sure to ask about heavy weekend or holiday eating patterns, which are customary among most cultures and subcultures. Food customs are so deeply rooted in members of any cultural group that a kind of cultural revulsion can occur when they are presented with foods of other cultures. For example, what would a native-born American think of eating rats, cats, worms, or dogs? In France and Germany, corn is considered animal feed, whereas in the United States, it is a popular vegetable for human consumption.

The sharing of food often involves meaning and symbolism (the use of something to point to something beyond itself). Wine, grape juice, bread, and cake are used in some Christian services and can stand for blood and body, life supported by food and drink, the work involved in transforming grapes and grain, or the unity of sharing. An understanding of the meanings of food for various peoples and the context and manner in which food is shared (or not shared) is important for community/public health nurses who work with clients who belong to different cultural groups.

FAMILY AND KINSHIP

Community/public health nurses look to the individual's family members as important caregivers. Families provide, coordinate, and influence much of the care in the home. To work with families, nurses need to identify family members and the hierarchical structure of the family unit. Nurses often define the family as the next of kin or as the people living in the same household. This definition, however, may not match the perception of an individual or family.

A family has many different forms and structures, depending on individual and family selection and culture. The family may be nuclear or extended. Family members may be family by blood, marriage, consensual union, or friendship (see Chapter 12). Members may include children who were *given* to an individual or couple to be reared and other individuals who, although not related by blood, are considered family members. For example, in many African American and Mexican American families, extended families and kin residence sharing is characteristic; and in Amish circles, the entire community is viewed as part of the extended family.

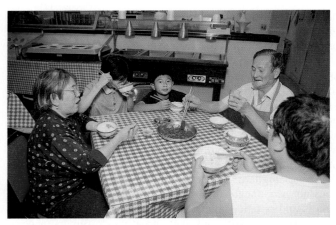

Asian family enjoying a traditional cultural meal eaten with chopsticks. (From Hockenberry, M. J., Wilson, D., Winkelstein, M. L., et al. [2003]. *Wong's nursing care of infants and children* [ed. 7]. St. Louis: Mosby.)

How a family defines itself and its members may be different from the definition of their family unit imposed by outsiders. People who are given children to rear may have no legal right to sign for hospitalization or surgical procedures. Gay partners may not have the legal right to hospital visits or to consent to medical treatment for their partners. Complications in providing nursing care can and do occur when the family defines itself one way and the nurse and health care system another. Efforts must be made by both sides to achieve a workable definition of the family that will best serve the family and take into account the family's view, however culturally different from the nurse's view (Boyle, 2008).

SEXUALITY

Gender is more than a biologic fact of life; it is also a cultural construct with expectations about behaviors associated with being a boy or a girl, a man or a woman. Sexual orientation involves beliefs and practices about sexual behavior, as well as the social roles a person assumes as a straight, gay, lesbian, bisexual, or transsexual. Culture also determines how people define a sex-related health problem.

Sexual beliefs and practices are emotionally charged issues in many cultures and serve as an arena for the airing of political, religious, and scientific differences. Some areas for exploration by community/public health nurses include how people learn about sexuality and how they are socialized into their sex roles. In some cultures, little information regarding sexuality is provided to children and adolescents. When this situation exists, the nurse needs to be sensitive to the problems associated with providing sexual education to children and teens. A clash may develop between the parents' wishes and the delivery of sound health education at school or the treatment of sexually related health problems in children and adolescents. Issues surrounding circumcision, menstruation, mate selection, sexual intercourse, conception and birth, contraception, menopause or climacteric, sexual taboos, and sexual deviations from the norm are all areas for nonjudgmental assessment, literature review, and verification.

BIOLOGIC VARIATIONS

Nurses may encounter important biocultural (racial and ethnic) variations during physical examinations. Individuals may differ in body structure, vital signs, general appearance, skin, enzyme levels, electrocardiographic patterns, nutritional deficiencies, psychologic characteristics, laboratory test values, response to drug therapy, and disease incidence. The biologic models that use normative data based on white populations may not hold true for members of other racial and ethnic populations.

Community/public health nurses have a responsibility to understand normative differences among racial and ethnic groups in order to perform an accurate physical assessment and separate normal from abnormal differences and reactions. Without knowledge of differences, the nurse runs the risk of alarming people unnecessarily (in the event of a normal variation) or, more importantly, missing a cue to a serious health hazard.

Normal variations in skin can be found between different racial and ethnic groups. For example, children of African, Asian, or Latin descent may have Mongolian spots. These irregular areas of deep-blue pigmentation are usually located in the sacral and gluteal areas. Mongolian spots may resemble bruising and be mistakenly interpreted as signs of child abuse.

Another issue encountered with skin assessments of clients from various cultures is correctly recognizing and interpreting jaundice, cyanosis, and pallor; erythema; petechiae; and ecchymosis. Persons with highly pigmented skin should be assessed initially for baseline skin color. The surfaces with the least amount of pigmentation (volar surfaces of the forearms, soles of the feet, palms of the hand, abdomen, and buttocks) should be checked. All skin, even in highly pigmented persons, has an underlying red tone, and its absence may indicate pallor. In highly pigmented persons, jaundice may be observed in the sclera or the hard palate, and cyanosis, pallor, or petechiae may be assessed in the conjunctiva or mouth. Pallor or cyanosis may also be detected by applying pressure to the nail and observing how rapidly the color returns to the nail beds.

An increased incidence of certain diseases may be found in select populations or ethnic groups. Some examples include glucose-6-phosphate dehydrogenase deficiency among Mediterranean people, African Americans, and Chinese; sickle cell disease in African Americans; cystic fibrosis in English populations; and cleft lip or palate in Japanese people (c.f. Andrews & Boyle, 2008; Giger & Davidhizar, 2004; Overfield, 1995).

Biocultural variations may occur in some laboratory test results. One of the most significant is serum transferrin levels: the mean level is higher for blacks than it is for whites. Because transferrin level increases in the presence of anemia, it is a valuable marker for use in diagnosing and treating children with anemia (Andrews & Boyle, 2008).

Significant differences exist among racial and ethnic groups in the metabolism, clinical effectiveness, and side effects of different drugs. Racial and ethnic groups metabolize drugs for diabetes, depression, and hypertension differently, and some persons of African, Asian, and Hispanic descent metabolize drugs more slowly than does the majority population. Few data are available on the differences in drug metabolism and effectiveness in subpopulations, because few drug trials have sufficient minority representation. Burroughs and colleagues (2002) have identified some of the environmental, genetic, and cultural factors underlying variations in responses among different population groups. Box 10-3 provides a few examples.

Box 10-3   Examples of Variations in Drug Metabolism in Selected Racial and Ethnic Groups

- African American and white clients have been shown to differ significantly in their responses to beta-blockers, angiotensin-converting enzyme inhibitors, and diuretics used either alone or in combination for the treatment of hypertension.
- Some populations of Chinese are considerably more sensitive than whites to the effects of the beta-blocker propranolol on heart rate and blood pressure.
- African Americans and Chinese Americans metabolize nicotine more slowly than do whites, and genetic variations associated with slower metabolism are more common in some Asian populations.
- Compared with some whites, certain Asian groups are more likely to require lower dosages of a variety of different drugs used to treat mental illness, including lithium, antidepressants, and antipsychotics.
- Hispanic clients have been reported to require lower dosages of antidepressants and to experience more side effects than whites.

Data from Burroughs, V. J., Maxey, R. W., Crawley, L. M., et al. (2002). *Cultural and genetic diversity in America: The need for individualized treatment.* Washington, DC: National Pharmaceutical Council and National Medical Association.

CULTURE-BOUND SYNDROMES

Culture-bound syndromes are often referred to as disorders restricted to a particular culture or group of cultures because of certain psychosocial characteristics of those cultures. Community/public health nurses and other health care providers may encounter people with symptoms that are difficult to interpret or explain and must be understood within the context of the clients' cultural beliefs. These very real symptoms may have emotional or spiritual causes. For example, an individual who presents with vomiting, diarrhea, and hallucinations may believe that he or she has been *conjured* or had a spell placed on him or her by persons who are skilled in witchcraft. The individual who firmly believes that the underlying cause of the illness is witchcraft is not likely to be receptive to treatments that do not involve casting out the spell (c.f. Andrews & Boyle, 2008; Giger & Davidhizar, 2004; Purnell & Paulanka, 2003; Spector, 2004).

Some African Americans use the expression *high blood,* which means that the blood is too rich because of consumption of too much red meat or other rich foods. Conversely, *low blood* is related to an insufficiency in the quantity of blood, and treatment would be dietary supplements. Hispanics may attribute a sudden onset of crying, fitful sleep, and diarrhea in children to *mal ojo,* or the *evil eye.* Anxiety—trembling from sudden fright—may be diagnosed as *susto.* In Western cultures, anorexia nervosa is a syndrome that is linked to sociocultural emphasis on body type and is an excessive preoccupation with thinness, a self-imposed starvation. This syndrome is seen in the United States, Europe, Japan, and Hong Kong, and among certain Asian populations and immigrants under Westernizing influence but not in other cultures. Table 10-2 lists select culture-bound syndromes found in various regions or cultures.

CULTURAL PATTERNS OF CARE

Leininger (1993) notes that one of the most significant challenges for the health professions is to study transcultural health-illness patterns of caring and curing systematically and critically. Individuals, families, and communities have various beliefs that influence their health seeking and acceptance of care. Decisions are based on personal experiences, nationality, ethnicity, culture, and family background. To ensure culturally competent care, nurses must understand and appreciate these differences.

CULTURE'S RELATIONSHIP TO HEALTH AND HEALTH BELIEFS

Culture is related to health in that culture teaches us the meaning of health and illness and the appropriate practices related to our beliefs. Wide variations exist in cultural belief systems and practices. In many cultures, concepts such as cause and effect may not be relevant. Cultural groups that adhere to the great traditions of Buddhism, Confucianism, and Taoism accept the fate of an illness and may not necessarily seek to discover the cause or cure. In fact, many cultural groups do not believe in natural causation (e.g., germs, stress, organic deterioration) but instead hold theories of supernatural causation, allowing fate to guide their lives and trying to live in simplicity and harmony with nature. Many cultures also do not accept the germ theory. Murdock (1980) describes 186 different cultural groups, only 31 of which have expressed theories concerning infection.

Andrews and Boyle (2008) describe three major health belief systems that people embrace: magico-religious, scientific, and holistic systems (Table 10-3). Community/public health nurses are likely to encounter individuals for whom the belief in health and illness is tied to the religious belief that illness is a result of God's will. Individuals may also wear amulets (objects such as charms worn on a string or chain) around the neck, waist, or wrist to ward off *evil spirits.* A special amulet called a *manu negro* is placed on babies of Puerto Rican descent to prevent the evil eye (Spector, 2004).

Some cultural groups may rely on the *hot and cold theories of disease*: four body humors—yellow bile, black bile, phlegm, and blood—must be balanced within the body for health. If imbalance occurs, the individual becomes ill. Imbalance is treated by consumption of prescribed foods or elements that are hot, cold, wet, or dry. Disease states, foods, beverages, and drugs are thus classified as hot or cold. Treating disease is accomplished by correcting the imbalance of hot or cold by adding or subtracting the substances that affect the humors. For example, an illness attributed to a problem with blood (e.g., hot and wet) would require a cold and dry treatment to reestablish and maintain equilibrium. The definitions of what are hot and cold entities vary with the cultural group. A community/public health nurse may encounter people who refuse certain foods and drugs because of the belief that they will not restore the body's imbalance.

SEEKING HEALTH CARE

An individual's decision to seek health care is influenced by family, community, and culture. Typical patterns of behavior, such as when, where, why, and how to seek care, are learned from parents, neighbors, religion, and the health care system.

The availability and acceptability of care and the ability to reciprocate or pay in some way for the care received also influence care-seeking decisions. In some countries, including the United States, goods or services are exchanged in lieu of

TABLE 10-2 **Select Culture-Bound Syndromes**

Syndrome	Group or Region	Description of Syndrome
Amok or mata elap	Malaysia	A dissociative episode characterized by a period of brooding followed by outburst of violent, aggressive, or homicidal behavior directed at people and objects
Anorexia nervosa	North America, Western Europe	An excessive preoccupation with thinness; self-imposed starvation; severe restriction of food intake associated with morbid fear of obesity
Dhat	India	Semen-loss syndrome, characterized by severe anxiety and hypochondriacal concerns with the discharge of semen, whitish coloration of urine, and feelings of weakness and exhaustion
Falling out, blacking out, or low blood	Southern United States, Caribbean (blacks, Haitians)	Episodes characterized by sudden collapse, dizziness, not enough blood or weakness of the blood that is often treated with diet; Individual's eyes are usually open, but person claims inability to see; person usually hears and understands what is occuring around him or her but feels powerless to move and is unable to move
Ghost sickness	Native Americans	Preoccupation with death and the deceased, sometimes associated with witchcraft; symptoms may include bad dreams, weakness, feelings of danger, loss of appetite, fainting, dizziness, confusion, feelings of futility, and a sense of suffocation
Hwa-byung or Wool-hwa-bung	Korea	Multiple somatic and psychologic symptoms; *pushing up* sensation of chest; palpitations, flushing, headache, *epigastric mass*, anxiety, irritability, and difficulty concentrating
Koro	Chinese, Southeast Asia, Malaysia	An episode of sudden and intense anxiety that the penis (or in the rare female cases, the vulva and nipples) will recede into the body and possibly cause death
Locura	Latin America	A severe form of chronic psychosis, attributed to an inherited vulnerability, the effect of multiple life difficulties, or a combination of the two; symptoms include incoherence, agitation, auditory and visual hallucinations, inability to follow rules of social interaction, unpredictability, and possible violence
Pibloktoq or Arctic hysteria	Greenland Eskimos	An abrupt dissociative episode accompanied by extreme excitement of up to 30-minutes' duration and frequently followed by convulsive seizures and coma lasting up to 12 hours; individual may be withdrawn or mildly irritable for hours or days before the attack and will typically report complete amnesia for the attack
Shenkui	Chinese	Marked anxiety or panic symptoms with accompanying somatic complaints for which no physical cause can be demonstrated; symptoms include dizziness, backache, fatigue, general weakness, insomnia, frequent dreams, and complaints of sexual dysfunction; symptoms are associated with excessive semen loss from frequent intercourse, masturbation, nocturnal emissions, or passing of *white turbid urine* believed to contain semen
Shin-byung	Korea	A syndrome characterized by anxiety and somatic complaints (general weakness, dizziness, fear, loss of appetite, insomnia, and gastrointestinal problems) followed by dissociation and possession of ancestral spirits
Spell	Southern United States	A trance state in which individuals *communicate* with deceased relatives or with spirits; at times is associated with brief periods of personality changes; spells may be misconstrued as psychotic episodes in a clinical setting
Mal de ojo	Spain and Latin America	The Spanish term for the *evil eye*; occurs as a common idiom of disease, misfortune, and social disruption throughout the Mediterranean, Latin American, and Muslim worlds
Rootwork	Southern United States and Caribbean	Idiom is described as a set of cultural interpretations that explain illness as the result of hexing, witchcraft, voodoo, or the influence of an evil person
Susto	Latinos in the United States and Latin America	Described as an illness that is attributed to a frightening event that causes the soul to leave the body, leading to symptoms of unhappiness and sickness; symptoms are extremely variable and may occur months or years after the supposedly precipitating event

Adapted from: Andrews, M. M., & Boyle, J. S. (2008). *Transcultural concepts in nursing care* (5th ed.). Philadelphia: Lippincott, Williams & Wilkins; First, M. B., & Frances, A. (2002). *DSM-IV-TR, Handbook of differential diagnoses.* Washington, DC: American Psychiatric Association.

TABLE 10-3   Health Belief Paradigms

Paradigm	Beliefs	Cultural Groups that Practice	Intervention
Magico-religious	Supernatural forces dominant. Fate of the individual depends on the actions of God, or the gods, or other supernatural forces for good or evil. Gods also punish humans for their transgressions. Illness is caused by sorcery, breach of taboo, intrusion of disease object or disease—causing spirit, loss of soul, and punishment form of God, and may be initiated by a supernatural agent or another person.	Many African American, Latino, and Middle Eastern cultures are grounded in this belief. Christian Scientists believe that physical healing can be effected through prayer alone. Some West Indians, Africans, and African Americans believe that sorcerers are the cause of many conditions. *Mal ojo*, or the evil eye, common in Latino and other cultures can be viewed as a disease-causing spirit.	Healing is through magic or religion, such as laying on of hands or anointing the sick with oil.
Scientific	Life (health and disease) is controlled by a series of physical and biologic processes that can be manipulated by humans (e.g., infection, communicability of a disease). Every disease has a specific cause and a specific effect.	Most western cultures, including the dominant cultural groups in the United States and Canada	Healing is through physical or chemical interventions specific to the identified cause (e.g., antibiotics for bacterial infection, chemotherapy or surgery for cancer, depending on type of cancer and body site).
Holistic	Health is the natural balance of the forces of nature (the laws of nature). Everything in the universe is a part of nature, including human life. Disturbing the laws of nature creates imbalance, chaos, and disease. Holistic theory incorporates the scientific or biologic aspects of disease, but maintains that it is not the only cause for the disease or illness.	North American Indian cultures and Asian cultures	Healing is through identifying disharmonies (imbalance), restoring body functioning, and seeking to reduce or eliminate the cause or causes. Great emphasis is on preventive health and maintenance measures.

Adapted from Andrews, M. M., & Boyle, J. S. (2008). *Transcultural concepts in nursing care* (5th ed.). Philadelphia: Lippincott, Williams & Wilkins.

money or health insurers' reimbursement. Lack of health insurance poses the most significant barrier to seeking care among racial and ethnic minorities.

Other barriers to seeking health care for racial and ethnic minorities include attitudes of fear, fatalism, and pessimism; mistrust of the system; poor availability of and access to services; inconvenience, such as office hours at difficult times; prejudice and discrimination; linguistic barriers; lack of cultural competence by providers; and low level of general health knowledge. African American, Asian American, and Hispanic American adults are reported to be less likely than are white adults to have a regular doctor, and fewer than one half of Hispanic and Asian Americans, when asked, feel confident in their ability to get needed care (Collins et al., 2002).

FOLK MEDICINE AND FOLK HEALERS

Folk healers are practitioners of lay medicine who work face to face with families and communities. Folk healers and their remedies are indigenous to many cultures. Because folk healers are present in both rural and urban communities, migrants to a different or new locale can often find a healer from their own cultural group. The healer helps them link their new life to their former life and ties.

The folk healer's scope of practice and treatment vary and may include diagnosis, prevention, and treatment of illness; interpretation of signs and omens; prayer; use of amulets; witchcraft; assistance with personal, financial, spiritual, or physical problems; blessings; and exorcisms. The types of healers seen in various communities include the following (c.f. Andrews & Boyle, 2008; Giger & Davidhizar, 2004; Leininger & McFarland, 2006; Purnell & Paulanka, 2003; Spector, 2004):

- *Curandero, espiritualista* (spiritualist), *yebero*, and *sanador* (Hispanic)
- Old Lady, spiritualist, and voodoo priest or priestess (African American)
- Herbalist and acupuncturist (Chinese)
- *Braucher* or *baruch-doktor* and lay midwife (Amish)
- *Magissa* or magician, bonesetter, and orthodox priest (Greek)
- Shaman (Native American)

COMPLEMENTARY AND ALTERNATIVE THERAPIES

Complementary and alternative medicine (CAM) is a growing concept in health care. CAM is a collective of diverse medical and health care systems, practices, and products that are beyond the realm of conventional Western medicine. Holistic health care practitioners incorporate CAM, recognizing that empirical science and technology do not necessarily have the answers to every health concern.

Complementary medicines are therapies that are used *together* with conventional medicine (e.g., aromatherapy to lessen postsurgical discomfort). *Alternative* medicines are used *in place of* conventional medicine (e.g., a special diet to treat cancer instead of conventional treatments such as surgery, radiation, or chemotherapy). Some clients combine both mainstream medical therapies and CAM therapies to enhance wellness and quality of life. An increasing number of major medical centers have large integrative health centers (IHCs). Integrative health centers focus on the science and practice of combining conventional and alternative therapies. The range of CAM therapies is expansive and changes as therapies are adopted into conventional treatments. This book's website provides a detailed list of CAM therapies in **Website Resource 10C.**

WEB

MEANING OF PAIN AND SUFFERING

Both pain and suffering have cultural as well as physical aspects. Pain—whether physical, mental, or spiritual—is experienced, influenced, and handled by individuals and groups in the context of their cultures. How pain is interpreted and expressed varies across cultures. Some cultural groups minimize or emphasize pain and the expression of pain. For example, some people see the suffering associated with pain as redemptive, whereas others view suffering as punishment (just or unjust), as fate, or as plain bad luck. An early anthropologic study by Wissler (1921) reported on the use of skewers inserted into chest incisions as part of the ritual *sun dance* performed by Plains Native Americans. Young men who were able to complete the dance gained esteem and warrior status. Studies show that complaining, demanding behavior is expected *sick role behavior* in American Jews and Italians; on the other hand, ill Asians and Native Americans are quiet and compliant (Ludwig-Beymer, 2007).

When clients and families minimize or emphasize pain, unknowledgeable health care providers can misinterpret what is taking place. Clients who minimize pain can be viewed as resting quietly and without pain, whereas those who emphasize pain can be viewed as nuisances, hypochondriacs, or malingerers. Nurses also tend to expect clients to *handle* pain in the same way the nurse has learned to handle pain. If nurses are stoic, they tend to expect clients to be stoic; if nurses are very verbal in expressing pain, they usually expect clients in pain to be verbal rather than silent. Any of these inaccurate assessments can impede appropriate diagnosis, referral, and treatment (Ludwig-Beymer, 2007).

COMMUNITY/PUBLIC HEALTH NURSE'S ROLE IN A CULTURALLY DIVERSE POPULATION

Culture and the values learned within a cultural group are critical to how people perceive health, health care, and nursing care providers. Whether community/public health nurses focus on an individual, group, or community as the unit of care, these concepts must be understood to provide the best possible nursing care. If community/public health nurses do not know what people believe about health and how they value health, then how can they change anything for the better with regard to groups or individual members of society? Cultural competence should be a goal for every community/public health nurse (American Nurses Association [ANA], 2007).

CULTURALLY COMPETENT NURSING CARE

When the author recently conducted an Internet search on **cultural competence** using the popular search engine Google, more than 27,700,000 results appeared. These fell into two major categories: (1) *organizational cultural competence*; and (2) *individual cultural competence,* usually in reference to nurses, physicians, social workers, or those in other health care, education, or social services professions.

According to the National Center for Cultural Competence *(www.gucchd.georgetown.edu/nccc)*, cultural competence requires that *organizations* do the following:

- Have a defined set of values and principles, and demonstrate behaviors, attitudes, policies, and structures that enable them to work effectively cross-culturally
- Have the capacity to (1) value diversity, (2) conduct self-assessment, (3) manage the dynamics of difference, (4) acquire and institutionalize cultural knowledge, and (5) adapt to diversity and the cultural contexts of the communities they serve
- Incorporate the previously mentioned actions into all aspects of policy making, administration, practice, and service delivery, and systematically involve consumers, key stake holders, and communities

Individual cultural competence refers to a complex integration of knowledge, attitudes, beliefs, skills, and encounters with those from cultures different from one's own that enhances cross-cultural communication and the appropriateness and effectiveness of interactions with others (American Academy of Nursing, 1992; Campinha-Bacote, 1998, 2007; USDHHS, 2001c). Cultural competence has been defined as a process, as opposed to an end point, in which the nurse continuously strives to work effectively within the cultural context of an individual, family, or community from a different cultural background (Andrews & Boyle, 2007; Campinha-Bacote, 1998, 2007; Campinha-Bacote & Munoz, 2001). Campinha-Bacote (2007) defines *cultural competence* as an ongoing process in which the health care professional continuously strives to achieve the ability and availability to work effectively within the cultural context of the client (individual, family, community). This process involves the integration of cultural desire, cultural awareness, cultural knowledge, cultural skill, and cultural encounters (Campinha-Bacote, 1998, 2002, 2007).

Given that community/public health nurses are likely to encounter clients from literally hundreds of different cultures and subcultures, as well as clients of mixed cultural heritage, it is virtually impossible for them to know about the culturally based health-related beliefs and practices of them all. It is possible, however, to master the knowledge and skills associated with cultural assessment and learn about some of the cultural dimensions of care for clients representing the groups most frequently encountered.

Cultural Self-Assessment

Before nurses provide culturally competent care to people from backgrounds different from their own, it is important for nurses to engage in **cultural self-assessment.** This includes developing an awareness of one's own cultural values, attitudes, beliefs, and practices. These insights also enable nurses to overcome ethnocentric tendencies and cultural stereotypes, which can lead to cultural imposition, prejudice, and discrimination against members of certain groups.

After engaging in a cultural self-assessment, community/public health nurses should conduct a cultural assessment of others—individuals, families, groups, and communities.

Cultural Assessment of Individuals, Families, and Groups

Cultural assessment is the foundation for culturally competent and culturally congruent nursing care; however, many nurses report that they lack cultural knowledge and skill. This problem is compounded by the fact that the nursing profession fails to reflect the diversity of the society at large (Sullivan Alliance, 2007; USDHHS, 2005).

Although the number of registered nurses has almost doubled during the past 24 years, nurses from racial and ethnic minorities are still underrepresented in the United States (Figure 10-5). Of the 2.4 million registered nurses, 82% are white compared with 67% of the total U.S. population. Eighteen percent of registered nurses are from racial and ethnic minority backgrounds. Hispanics or Latinos still remain the most underrepresented group among registered nurses compared with their representation in the overall population. Although Hispanics or Latinos account for 14.1% of the population, only 2.2% of nurses are from this ethnic group. Such homogeneity reduces the chances for nurses to learn about other cultures from members of their own profession. Cultural competency in nursing care can be improved by actively recruiting members of minority racial and ethnic groups to the profession and

improving the cultural knowledge of current nurses (Sullivan Alliance, 2007; USDHHS, 2005).

Cultural Frameworks and Assessment Tools

The existing body of information on cultural competency, as well as several models and frameworks, can assist nurses in delivering culturally competent care. Leininger (1978, 1988; Leininger & McFarland, 2006) was an early pioneer in the field. Other authors in this field include Murdock (1971), Tripp-Reimer and colleagues (1984), Fong (1985), Kim-Godwin and colleagues (2001), Campinha-Bacote (2002), Giger and Davidhizar (2004), Purnell and Paulanka (2003), Spector (2004), and Andrews and Boyle (2008).

The model proposed by Campinha-Bacote (2002) recognizes that achieving cultural competence is a continuous process in which the health care provider constantly strives to work effectively within the cultural context of the client (individual, family, and community) (Figure 10-6). This model has widespread applicability and outlines the integration or intersection of five processes:

- Cultural awareness—sensitivity to the values, beliefs, and customs of others and examination of a person's own cultural values and beliefs, biases, and prejudices toward other cultures
- Cultural knowledge—understanding of the beliefs and value systems of others developed through a scientific base of information about their similarities and differences
- Cultural skill—learning to collect cultural information by way of cultural assessments and culturally based physical assessments
- Cultural encounters—engagement in cross-cultural interactions with clients, including individuals and groups, so

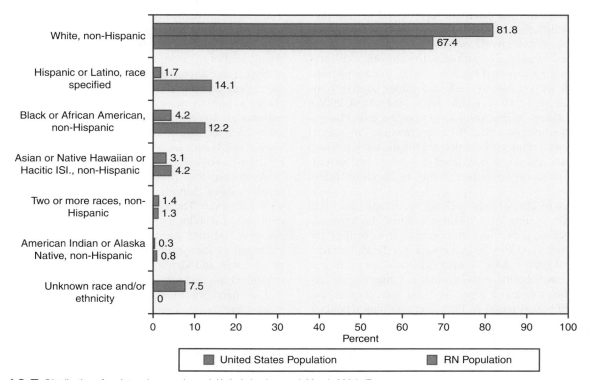

FIGURE 10-5 Distribution of registered nurses by racial/ethnic background, March 2004. (From U.S. Department of Health and Human Services, Health Resources and Services Administration, Bureau of Health Professions. [2005]. *The registered nurse population: Findings from the 2004 National Sample Survey of Registered Nurses. II: The registered nurse population 1980-2004.* Retrieved July 28, 2007, from *http://bhpr.hrsa.gov/healthworkforce/rnsurvey04/2.htm.*)

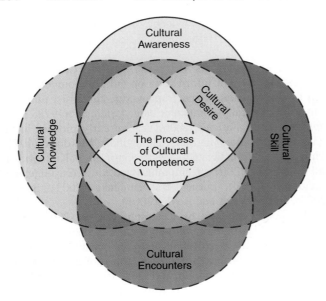

The Process of Cultural Competence in the
Delivery of Healthcare Services
(Campinha-Bacote, 1998)

FIGURE 10-6 Campinha-Bacote model of cultural competence. (From Campinha-Bacote, J. [2007]. The process of cultural competence in the delivery of healthcare services: The journey continues. Cincinnati: Transcultural C.A.R.E. Associates.)

as to explore the nurse's perceptions and knowledge about specific cultures and ethnic groups

• Cultural desire—motivation on the part of the health care provider, who wants to engage in the process of becoming culturally competent rather than having to do so

The Campinha-Bacote tool defines a continuum from simple awareness to in-depth discovery of and competence in one or more different cultures. The critical first step is cultural awareness. A caregiver's lack of awareness about his or her own values, beliefs, and attitudes toward other cultures may lead to nursing care that is *ethnocentric,* or care planned for individuals with cultural beliefs and values similar to his or her own (Leininger, 1978; Leininger & McFarland, 2006). For example, a nurse might value the importance of a baby's sleeping in his or her own bed. If the nurse comes in contact with a family who thinks it is important for the baby to sleep with the parents, the nurse may label that act as bad parenting, rather than simply a different way of handling infant care.

The process of deliberately seeking out interactions with individuals and groups from diverse cultural backgrounds is valuable because it provides an opportunity to explore the nurse's perceptions and knowledge about a specific culture with members of that group. These exchanges help nurses validate or negate their knowledge base and correct any misconceptions. This process helps to avoid generalizations, stereotyping, and development of beliefs based on limited cross-cultural contact. **Stereotyping** is an exaggerated, usually negative, belief or image applied to both an entire category of people of a racial or ethnic group and to each individual within it that is false or greatly distorts the real characteristics of the group. Recognizing that *even within a specific culture, individual differences in values and beliefs can be found* is important.

Two models are specifically proposed for delivering culturally competent community care: the Bernal model (1993) and the culturally competent community care model (Kim-Godwin, et al., 2001). Another model for use with families and communities is introduced later in this chapter. Other nursing scholars have developed cultural assessment tools (Andrews & Boyle, 2008; Giger & Davidhizar, 2004; Leininger & McFarland, 2006; Purnell & Paulanka, 2003; Spector, 2004).

CULTURAL ASSESSMENT FOR THE COMMUNITY/PUBLIC HEALTH NURSE

The cornerstone of community/public health nursing is the concept of *community as client* (Association of Community Health Nursing Educators, 2000). Community/public health nursing practice must operate within a framework and structure that focus on strategies for decreasing racial and ethnic disparities. Because individuals comprise a community, the community is a reflection of the characteristics of the community residents.

The **cultural assessment** is "a systematic appraisal or examination of individuals, groups, and communities as to their cultural beliefs, values, and practices to determine specific needs and interventions within the cultural context of the people being evaluated" (Leininger, 1978, pp. 85-86). Cultural assessment helps the nurse understand from where clients derive their ideas about disease and illness and helps determine beliefs, values, and practices that may influence client care and health behaviors.

The first step of a cultural assessment, before collection of any data, is to establish a rapport or beginning trust relationship. Building the trusting relationship acknowledges respect for the individual and the community and demonstrates the principle of caring. Trust allows the client to become relaxed. The nurse must master the skill of careful listening, recognizing that all information has subjective and objective components and should be validated. An equally important component of the assessment process is providing clear information to the client regarding the purpose of the assessment, the expected process, the anticipated use of the data, and the choice to participate or not participate in the process. In some cultural groups note taking is considered disrespectful, and terms such as *okay* or *you guys* may be unclear to the client. Use of words such as *dear, honey, baby, mama,* and *papa* is to be strictly avoided.

Assessing the cultural dimensions of the community involves more than eliciting facts and data during one interview encounter. The systematic *process* suggests the need for continuity involving numerous data points and numerous data sources. The data gathering process is enhanced by holding community focus group discussions, interviewing key community leaders, and identifying and listing community resources, organizations, and social outlets.

Leininger (1978) identified nine key areas in a cultural assessment:
1. Lifestyle patterns
2. Cultural values and norms
3. Cultural taboos and myths
4. The culture's world view and ethnocentric tendencies
5. The culture's perception of its similarities with and differences from other cultures

6. Health care rites and rituals
7. Degree of culture change
8. Caring behaviors
9. Folk and professional health-illness systems being used

The framework presented in Table 10-4 is designed to structure the assessment of families and communities within a cultural perspective and incorporates most of Leininger's original suggestions. Answers are *discovered* from observing and participating with people in a caring context, as well as interviewing people about their culture, family history, and beliefs and practices related to the health of individuals and groups. Some general community assessment tools address culture. However, when health care providers recognize that they are working with a cultural group that contrasts sharply with their own, a more extensive cultural assessment needs to be conducted using a tool such as the one presented here.

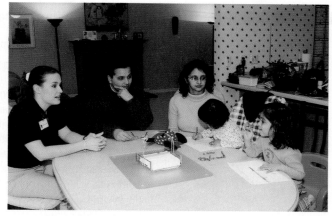

A nurse visiting a family at home. The nurse and family are of different racial/ethnic origins. (Copyright CLG Photographics.)

TABLE 10-4   Community and Family Cultural Assessment Guide

Cultural Category	Questions for Community Assessment	Questions for Family Assessment
Definition of self	How does the community view itself? What are its cultural groups? What are its calendrical events, and how are they ritualized? What is the history of the community? What is the community's view of its future?	How does the family view itself? Are there fictive kin? Does the family have more or fewer members than the household? How do family members define the role and status of each member? How does sex and gender influence family roles? Do family members live close by? How do they communicate? What are the family calendrical events, and how are they ritualized? What critical events have occurred in the family, and how are they marked? What is the history of the family? What stories are told about the family? What does the family see as its future? What does the family tree (genogram) look like?
Definition of others	Who are the helping agencies? Who are the key informal helpers?	Who are the helping people? Who would help in a time of need? What kind of help might be requested?
Definitions of health and illness	What groups does the community identify as well, worried and well, early ill, or ill? How are well and ill groups identified? What are the potential health problems of specific age and cultural groups? Who are the health and illness care providers in the community?	How does the family describe its health as a unit and the health of individuals within it? How and who within the family determines when a member is sick and how? Who within the family decides when to seek help for illness, and what type of help will be sought?
Beliefs about health and illness	How do cultural groups perceive health and illness in terms of accepting, adapting, and controlling? What are the prevailing illnesses? Do biocultural variations exist that are important to the health of the community? How does the community view the cause, diagnosis, and treatment?	Does the family accept fate or use health-promotion and illness-prevention strategies? How do they view cause, diagnosis, and treatment? What illnesses or biologic variation is the family susceptible to? Who do they view as health practitioners? Do family members practice folk medicine, traditional healers or alternative and complimentary therapies? What are usual home treatments and nutritional remedies?
Life ways and meaning	What are the major cultural values about life, nature, and relationships? What are the cultural standards of behavior? What is the prevailing meaning of life? How is life lived? What do people do each day?	What is the meaning of life to the family? How does the family live? What do the family members do each day?

Developed by Judith Strasser. Copyright Elsevier.

Continued

TABLE 10-4   Community and Family Cultural Assessment Guide—cont'd

Cultural Category	Questions for Community Assessment	Questions for Family Assessment
Communication	What is the major language and dialect spoken among community members? What are common patterns related to verbal and nonverbal communication? What is the relationship of personal space to the communication process? Are interpreters available in the community and health care settings?	What is the language and dialect spoken in the home and at social gatherings? How well do the family members speak and write English? Is the use of an interpreter necessary? What physical gestures do family members use during conversation? How much distance do family members place between each other when speaking?
Time	How is time structured? Is time viewed as a gift to be appreciated, as a commodity to be used, or in some other way? Are people present, past, or future oriented?	How is time structured? Is time viewed as a gift, a commodity, or in some other way? Are schedules used? Are schedules valued? Is the family past, present, or future oriented?
Space	How is space structured in the community? Is open space available? Are public buildings welcoming? Where are churches, shops, restaurants, bars, food stores, malls, public buildings, and health providers located?	How does the family structure space? Is the yard fenced? Who makes most use of what space? Where do family members eat and sleep? How close do family members get? How is observable touch used?
Physical objects	What visible objects represent the community? How are buildings characterized in terms of condition, cleanliness, and access? How are public facilities equipped and used?	What possessions are displayed? Does misplaced matter exist? Is the house cared for? Is clothing clean, stylish, and in good condition? Does evidence exist of conspicuous consumption ("keeping up with the Joneses")?
Food customs	What kinds of eateries are present in the community? How are eating places patronized and by whom? Is some ethnic style of eating noted? How do people communicate during meals?	Does the family eat together? Does the family eat at a set time? What kinds of food are eaten? Who prepares the food? What and when do family members drink? What foods are adult foods? What foods are children's foods? Are any foods or drinks taboo? Do family members talk during meals? To whom is food given and in what order?
Religion	How many churches, mosques, or synagogues are located in the community? What denominations are represented? Do the organized religious groups provide any health care services? Are designated healers or *nurses* available in the churches? Do the churches sponsor health fairs or screenings?	Do family members participate actively in one religion or more than one religion? Does church, mosque, or synagogue membership provide social support for the family now or if needed? Do, or might, religious beliefs or practices affect health? What are the rituals and taboos related to birth, death, and illness?
Clubs	What kinds of clubs are active in the community? What political parties are active in the community? What resources do the clubs have available? What kinds of people participate in clubs? Do separate groups for men, women, and children exist?	To what clubs do family members belong? Are clubs available to which the entire family belongs? How active are family members at the present time in the club? What actual or potential resources can the club provide?
Work	What occupations exist in the community? How many people in the community work outside the home? How many work inside the home? What work hazards exist in the major occupations? How many people cannot find work? What employment support resources exist? Do people know about them? Are they accessible? What is the value and meaning of work?	What family members work outside and inside the home? What potential or actual work hazards are encountered by family members? What kind of health insurance plans do family members have from their jobs? How do members prepare for and cope with retirement, layoffs, or a company closing? What are the work duties in the household? What is the value and meaning of work?
Education	What kinds of schools are located in the community? Who attends these schools? What are the absence rates in the schools? Is health care provided in the schools? What kind of health care is provided? What is the role of nursing with regard to school health? Does the school play an active part in the community?	Do the children in the family attend school regularly? Is the family generally satisfied with the schools the children are attending? Do the parents or grandparents attend school? Are family members active in school activities? Is school seen as a way to a good or better life? Does the family identify specific problems with the school?

TABLE 10-4   Community and Family Cultural Assessment Guide—cont'd

Cultural Category	Questions for Community Assessment	Questions for Family Assessment
Play	What leisure activities are available in the community for various age groups? Are recreation facilities being used? What groups use what kinds of resources? What is the value and meaning of play?	How many hours do family members spend in leisure activities? What kinds of activities do they enjoy as individuals and as a family? What is the value and meaning of play?
Power	How is official (formal) power structured in the community? Can informal power groups be identified?	How is power structured in the family? Who makes health decisions for family members?
Environment	Does the community environment (physical and social) foster health in the community? How?	Does the family environment (physical and social) foster its own health and the health of other community members? How?
In- and out-migrants and in- and out-migration	Who are the groups coming and going? How are in-migrant groups socialized to the community? How is out-migration justified?	How does the family accept newcomers and the loss of family members? Is the family open or closed to new groups in the community?
Deviance	How is deviance handled in the community? Who are the individual deviants and the deviant groups?	Who are the deviants in the family? How does the family cope with deviance? Is the family itself a deviant group within the community?
Change	What major changes have occurred in the community? How did the changes occur? Were the changes planned, unplanned, valued, or disvalued? How did the community accept or attempt to control the changes?	What major changes (anticipated and unanticipated) have occurred in the family? How did the family accept or attempt to control the changes? How does the family view change?
Sick role	Do ways of identifying sick, frail, chronically disabled, and mentally ill individuals and populations exist in the community? How are these groups described? What are the expectations for sick role behavior among various cultural groups?	How is a family member identified as being *sick*? What are the behavioral expectations for members in the sick role? What are the behavioral expectations for chronically ill family members? Who assumes the role of caregiver? Who makes decisions for entry into a health care system?
Death ways and meaning	How are deaths marked by the community? Do variations concerning the meaning of death among different groups exist in the community?	How are deaths marked by the family? What is the meaning of death? What are the rituals enacted at the time of a death? What are the expectations for individual family members?
Sexuality and sex roles	How do schools and religious groups socialize children with regard to male and female roles? How, where, and when is formal sex education taught? What are the prevailing ideas in the community about sexual behavior? Who are the sexual deviants? How is sexual deviance handled?	What are the sex role expectations across the life span? How, when, and by whom is sexuality discussed in the family? Who is responsible for monitoring the sexual conduct of family members? What are the rules for sexual conduct? How are boys and men supposed to act? How are girls and women supposed to act? When and how does a boy become a man? When and how does a girl become a woman? What are the sexual taboos?
Childbearing	What are the shared practices of the community with regard to pregnancy and childbirth? Who attends the mother during delivery? Is early nurturing and mother-child bonding encouraged? Do purification rituals exist for the mother? Is male (or female) circumcision practiced? What are the prevalent childbearing myths?	How are family members involved in the birth prenatally and at delivery? What are the expected roles of family members surrounding the birth experience? Who cares for the infant immediately after delivery? How is a newborn assimilated into the family?
Child rearing	What are community expectations with regard to child rearing? Does the community play a part in disciplining children?	Who are the main child rearers and caretakers? What is the expected role of siblings, other relatives, and fictive kin with regard to child rearing? Who are the sex role models? What are the privileges and responsibilities of children? What are the rules for child behavior? What are the patterns of discipline?

Continued

TABLE 10-4 Community and Family Cultural Assessment Guide—cont'd

Cultural Category	Questions for Community Assessment	Questions for Family Assessment
Growth and development across the life span	How does the community provide resources for all age groups? What health, education, and recreational resources are available for the needs of each age group?	How does the family provide for the very old and the very young? What are the expectations for behavior of each age group? How are life milestones marked?
Reciprocity and exchange	What is the means of exchange in the community (e.g., money, goods, services)? How is debt perceived?	When are gifts shared? Who purchases gifts, pays bills or taxes, and so forth? What is the meaning of money, debt, wealth, and poverty? When and how does one give and receive?
Customs and laws	What laws and customs are followed in the community? Who are the law and customs enforcers? Who are the cultural heroes?	What are the implicit and explicit family rules? Who makes the rules? Who breaks the rules? What are the consequences of rule breaking?
Health care providers	Who are the health providers (traditional and folk) in the community? What is the perception concerning the various kinds of health providers? How do cultural groups differ in their perceptions of health care providers?	What health care providers does the family use? How does the family perceive health care providers? When (under what circumstances) does the family use a health care provider? What does the family know about the traditional health care delivery system, including health insurance?

CULTURALLY APPROPRIATE STRATEGIES FOR THE COMMUNITY/PUBLIC HEALTH NURSE WORKING WITH DIVERSE COMMUNITIES

The diversity among communities is enormous, and local community consultation is important to understand what is culturally appropriate and acceptable within each community.

To promote health in diverse cultural groups, providers must do the following:

- Learn about the history of the culture, the traditional ways of life, and the communication patterns
- Spend time in the community attending community events
- Incorporate the community's input in planning
- Incorporate many of the traditional values, beliefs, and ways of life into program design and use of educational materials

WEB

Website Resource 10D provides a more detailed list of strategies to use in culturally diverse settings. Important resources for a thorough cultural assessment are library materials and good cultural informants. Although most nurses know how to conduct a literature search, the criteria for selecting an informant may be new knowledge. Spradley (1979) has delineated the following four characteristics of a good informant:

- Thoroughly acculturated—part of the group for a long time
- Currently involved in the culture—an active participant in the culture
- Capable of nonanalytic reporting—describes things in local terms rather than the way the informant thinks the nurse wants to hear it
- Willing to participate—willing to share his or her time and knowledge about the culture

Informants should be historically and actively a part of the culture. A good informant should be able to talk about what is a typical belief or behavior of the cultural group in the language of the people.

CONTEMPORARY ISSUES AND TRENDS

A considerable number of important issues are of interest to community/public health nurses who wish to become culturally competent. The following discussion identifies some of the most current issues.

REFUGEE AND IMMIGRANT POPULATIONS

People migrate both across national borders and within them, doing so in official (legal) and unofficial ways and for a wide variety of reasons. Migration involves *hellos* and *good-byes*. If a person migrates alone to a sharply contrasting culture, severe *culture shock* may occur. Culture shock is associated with feelings of panic, anger, denial, and depression and a sense of separation from others and even from a one's own self-identity. This experience can have serious health consequences. Culture shock can lead to acts of aggression toward self or others, a loss of appetite and sleep, and general malaise that can result in death.

People who come to a country to take up permanent residence are called **immigrants.** Illegal or undocumented immigrants are in a country without the appropriate documentation and permission. **Refugees** are persons who migrate to escape persecution based on race, religion, nationality, or political persuasion and come to this country under special legal procedures, usually requiring congressional action. **Asylees** are individuals seeking political asylum from persecution in their own countries. These classifications are of importance to the community/public health nurse, because they often determine the rights of individuals to health and social services.

All immigrants are at considerable risk for health and social problems because of language and employment difficulties, limited economic resources, and, often, past traumatic life events. Existing studies suggest that youth and adults suffer a disproportionate burden of mental health problems and disorders, and the suicide rate is 50% higher among immigrants than in the population as a whole (USDHHS, 2006). Immigrants disproportionately lack health insurance coverage, receive fewer health services than do native-born citizens, and experience other barriers, including linguistic issues and eligibility changes that have limited their ability to qualify for Medicaid (Kaiser Family Foundation, 2007; see also Chapters 4 and 21).

Newer immigrants are most in need of special care. These families must cope with a bewildering array of new experiences, including the health care system. Many of these individuals have come from countries with different methods of health care delivery and different ways of interacting with health care providers. Over time, many immigrant families adapt their health practices and lifestyles to accommodate their new country's patterns and practices, a process called *acculturation*.

Foreign-born individuals account for 11.7% of the total U.S. population. Nearly one half of all legal immigrants came from just 10 countries: Mexico, India, China, the Philippines, Cuba, Vietnam, the Dominican Republic, Korea, Colombia, and the Ukraine (Office of Immigration Statistics, 2006). Host countries have various ways of controlling both in- and out-migration. In the United States, although in-migration is limited by a quota system and by visa requirements, many people enter illegally without following the prescribed procedures. The terrorist attacks of September 11, 2001, significantly affected the number of refugee approvals and admissions. Nonetheless, in 2005, a total of 1,122,373 immigrants were admitted for lawful permanent residence in the United States, an increase of 17.2% over the previous year (Office of Immigration Statistics, 2006). Figure 10-7 shows the proportion of legal immigrants to this country from various regions of the world.

Data on undocumented residents (also called *unauthorized* or *illegal aliens*) in the United States vary widely, ranging from 4.6 to 5.3 million (National Conference of State Legislatures, 2007) to 7 million (Office of Immigration Statistics, 2006) to 10.3 million (Passel, 2005). Data from a study conducted by the Pew Hispanic Center reveal that undocumented migrants represent about 29% of the nearly 36 million foreign-born residents. Mexicans comprise the largest group of undocumented migrants at 5.9 million or 57% of the total estimates. Another 2.5 million (24%) come from Latin America, 9% from Asia, 6% from Europe or Canada, and 4% from other parts of the world (Passel, 2005).

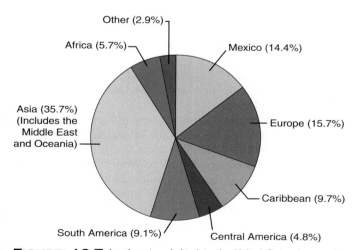

FIGURE 10-7 Immigrants admitted to the United States by country of birth, 2005. (Data from Office of Immigration Statistics. [2006]. *2005 Yearbook of immigration statistics.* Washington, DC: U.S. Department of Homeland Security, Office of Immigration Statistics.)

SOCIOECONOMIC STATUS OF MINORITIES AND HEALTH

An increasing body of evidence suggests that risk factors for health outcomes are related to socioeconomic status and race. Rabin (1993) and Williams and Collins (2002) suggest that the root cause of observed racial and ethnic differences in health status actually is social factors such as lifestyle, behavior, attitudes, and socioeconomic status, not racial or ethnic influences. Evidence indicates that socioeconomic inequalities in health are often larger than racial and ethnic inequalities in health and may be the single most important influence on health and health disparities among racial and ethnic groups (Rabin, 1993; Williams & Collins, 2002).

In the United States, minorities are at greater risk of poverty and its associated problems: higher unemployment, lower educational levels, and shorter life expectancy. The nation's official poverty rate rose from 11.7% in 2001 to 12.6% in 2004 and 2005 (DeNavas-Walt, Proctor, & Lee, 2006). People of limited economic means have fewer resources to pay for food, clothing, and shelter and are frequently unable to access or pay for health services and treatment (see Chapters 4 and 21). Many individuals forgo medical care to purchase other necessities. Preventive care is a luxury that few low-income people can afford. Poverty is related to other stressors that also affect health: occupational and educational opportunities are limited, housing is often substandard and hazardous, and neighborhoods are not safe. These and other social conditions create a highly stressful environment that affects the health of individuals. Nonetheless, racial differences often persist even when socioeconomic levels are *equivalent*. For example, at each socioeconomic level, African Americans generally have worse health status than do whites.

SEXUAL ORIENTATION

Other subpopulations with special needs experience disparities and barriers to care that result in unmet needs or lack of appropriate care or both. The health and quality of life of lesbian, gay, bisexual, transgendered, and intersexed (having a physically ambiguous gender with components of both male and female anatomy) (LGBTI) individuals are too often overlooked. LGBTI populations experience significant disparities in health status and health care. Barriers are related to sexual identity, sexual behavior, and gender identity, and most of the unique health care needs of this group have gone unmet within the nation's mainstream health care system (Gay and Lesbian Medical Association, 2001). As a result, many LGBTI individuals avoid or delay care or receive inappropriate or inferior care because of perceived or real homophobia and discrimination by health care providers and institutions.

Negative attitudes of nurses, as well as fear, ignorance, and homophobia, have served as obstacles to providing culturally competent care for LGBTI persons. As recently as 1998, a survey of nursing students showed that 8% to 12% 'despised' lesbian, gay, and bisexual people; 5% to 12% found them "disgusting"; and 40% to 43% thought that LGB people should keep their sexuality private (Eliason, 1998). The health of the LGBTI population involves a wide range of health care issues, not unlike that of their non-LGBTI counterparts; but they also have some LGBTI-specific health needs related to HIV infection and AIDS, mental health problems (such as suicide), exposure to violence, and other serious public health challenges. What may perhaps be of most importance are the clinical encounter and the health care experience.

The Gay and Lesbian Medical Association provides a wealth of resources and guidance on providing culturally competent care to this population. Box 10-4 provides a summary of community standards for quality health care services for the LGBTI population. The complete list of standards and suggestions for creating a safe clinical environment for this population are provided on the book's website as **Website Resources 10E and 10F.** This information is a useful resource to assist the nurse in developing culturally appropriate approaches and providing quality nursing care.

RACISM AND DISCRIMINATION

Racism and discrimination are important variables in the health of individuals and communities. Both of these practices are added stressors for minority populations. **Racism** commonly refers to institutional and individual practices that create and reinforce oppressive systems of race relations that adversely restrict the lives of individuals of certain races (Krieger, 2000). **Discrimination** is the "differential and negative treatment of individuals based on their race, ethnicity, gender, or other group membership" (Smedley et al., 2003, p. 95). Discrimination occurs in the broader context of American life and is evidenced in disparate practices in education, mortgage lending, housing, employment, and criminal justice. In health care, discrimination is reflected in documented differences in care that result from biases, prejudices, stereotyping, and uncertainty in clinical communication and decision making.

The experiences of minority clients with the health care system are very different from those of white Americans. Many minority clients perceive higher levels of racial discrimination in health care than do whites (LaVeist et al., 2000; Lillie-Blanton et al., 2000). Studies suggest that discrimination and stereotyping are present in health care. In one experiment, physicians treating black and white actors were less likely to recommend cardiac catheterization for the black actors than for white actors who were exhibiting the same symptoms (Schulman et al., 1999). In a review of actual clinical encounters, doctors rated black clients as less intelligent, less educated, more likely to abuse drugs and alcohol, less apt to comply with medical advice, more likely to lack social support, and less likely to participate in cardiac rehabilitation than were white clients, even when income, education, and personality characteristics were controlled for (van Ryn & Burke, 2000).

Some studies suggest that racial bias, restricted socioeconomic opportunities and mobility, residence in poor neighborhoods, the stress of experiences of discrimination, and the acceptance of the societal stigma of inferiority all have deleterious consequences for health (Williams, 1999). Personal negative emotional and stress responses associated with discrimination are linked to hypertension, cardiovascular disease, and mental illness (Finch et al., 2001; Karlsen & Nazroo, 2002; Williams & Williams-Morris, 2000).

Community/public health nurses must be aware of differences in health care perceptions among health care providers and the impact this may have on minority clients and community attitudes toward health care services. Watts (2003) suggests a four-step process to focus nurses in this area:
- Conduct a comprehensive self-appraisal of racial and ethnic heritage
- Launch a *culture interest group,* with a focus on the health concerns of a specific racial and ethnic group
- Participate in continuing education or professional development programs to increase knowledge regarding minority groups
- Develop a philosophy of lifelong learning

The ANA position statement on discrimination affirms the professional nurse's role in eradicating discrimination and racism in the profession of nursing, in the education of nurses, and in the practice of nursing, as well as in the organizations in which nurses work (ANA, 1992). All nurses must work to ensure a level of cultural and linguistic competence in addressing the needs of our increasingly culturally diverse population.

> **BOX 10-4** **Sample Community Standards of Practice for Provision of Quality Health Care Services for Gay, Lesbian, Bisexual, and Transgendered Clients**
>
> - **Personnel**—Agency provides a nondiscriminatory workplace for gay, lesbian, bisexual, and transgendered (GLBT) employees, including equal benefits, compensation, and terms of employment.
> - **Client's rights**—Agency assures nondiscriminatory delivery of services to GLBT clients, staff use culturally appropriate language, and agency has a policy to file and resolve grievances, and broadly interprets the term *family* to include domestic partners.
> - **Service planning and delivery**—Staff are familiar with GLBT issues as they pertain to health care services, and direct care staff are competent to deliver appropriate care.
> - **Confidentiality of documents**—Agency ensures the confidentiality of documents, including information about sexual orientation and gender identity.
>
> Data from *Community standards of practice for the provision of quality health care services for lesbian, gay, bisexual, and transgender clients.* Retrieved February 16, 2008, from *http://www.glbthealth.org/CommunityStandardsofPractice.htm.*

> **KEY IDEAS**
>
> 1. The changing demographics of the nation and the enduring health disparities among racial and ethnic groups present challenges and opportunities for community/public health nurses to improve the health of communities.
> 2. Cultural and linguistic competence is essential for providing appropriate health care for diverse racial, ethnic, and cultural groups.
> 3. Concepts of health, illness, and wellness and treatments evolve from a cultural perspective and are a part of the total cultural belief system.
> 4. Cultural competence is an ongoing process that involves cultural awareness, cultural knowledge, cultural skill, cultural encounters, and cultural desire.
> 5. Nurses need to explore the use of Western formal medical practices and other formal and informal health practices to ensure that clients receive optimal health care and care that is sensitive to clients' cultural values and beliefs.
> 6. Community/public health nurses need to be sensitive to the diversity that exists in communities and populations with regard to culture, ethnicity, race, age, health status, religious affiliation, language, physical size, disability, geographic location, political orientation, economic status, occupational and educational orientation, gender, sexual orientation, and life experiences.

7. Nurses should seek to avoid labeling or stereotyping and assuming that all members of a culture are alike. Different individuals within a specific culture will demonstrate variations in their beliefs and behaviors.

LEARNING BY EXPERIENCE AND REFLECTION

1. Caring for Miss Geraldine: an individual or group exercise in culturally competent care

   Miss Geraldine, an elderly African American woman, comes to the clinic complaining of shortness of breath. On initial cursory examination, you find that she is obese, is in moderate respiratory distress, has moderately elevated blood pressure, and complains of tiredness. She tells you that she "has been big, like my family, all my life"; was born with a veil over her face; and has had "high blood" all her life. She says her blood is very "thin." She has frequent blackout spells as a result of her "high blood." She has obvious large irregular patchy unpigmented areas of skin over her face and neck. Her skin appears to have a yellowish hue.

   a. From your knowledge of cultural variations, answer these questions:
      - What additional important questions will you ask Miss Geraldine?
      - What is the relevance of her sharing with you that she was born with 'a veil over her face'?
      - What are the probable unpigmented areas over her face and neck?
      - How will you assess whether the yellowish tint is jaundice?

   b. After conducting an extensive physical examination and interview, the nurse practitioner prescribes a single hypertensive drug for Miss Geraldine and orders a clinical nutrition assessment and intervention that is to include weight reduction and client education (the usual treatment for hypertension is a course of diuretics and a beta-blocker for most clients).

      Given your cultural and clinical knowledge:
      - Is it likely that the nurse practitioner is demonstrating incompetence in the treatment protocol by ordering a different course of therapy?
      - What information do you have regarding African American cultural practices that would be relevant to this assessment?

2. Group exercise

   Divide into two groups. Assume the following individuals, Sue Toms and John Adams. Each group selects one of these individuals and specifies a cultural or ethnic group of their choice for the individual. The other group selects a cultural or ethnic group for their individual that is different from the first group's selection. (For example, Sue may be an American Piscataway and John may be a Hispanic from El Salvador.)

Designating Sue as a member of cultural or ethnic group No. 1 and John as a member of cultural or ethnic group No. 2, answer the following questions based on your cultural knowledge and research. The two groups should come back together to share what they learned from their discussion, questions, and concerns.

   a. Describe characteristic cultural phenomena that may be associated with each individual (e.g., what is the time orientation, space relations). Discuss the health care beliefs, practices, and behaviors commonly associated with the cultural group for each individual.
   b. List two reasons for learning cultural health care practices for each individual.
   c. Describe one cognitive, one affective, and one behavioral strategy in overcoming communication barriers with each individual.
   d. Discuss the correlation between race, culture or ethnicity, and class, and health and illness as related to Sue Toms.
   e. Discuss the initiative to eliminate racial and ethnic disparities in health care as it may relate to John Adams.
   f. Identify any biocultural variations that may be of significance in the cultural assessment of both Sue and John.

COMMUNITY RESOURCES FOR PRACTICE

Information about each of the following organizations is found on its website, which can be accessed through the **WebLinks** section of this book's website at *http://evolve.elsevier.com/Maurer/community/*.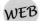

The Access Project
American Medical Student Association
Center for Cross-Cultural Health
Cross Cultural Health Care Program
EthnoMed
Diversity in Medicine
Gay and Lesbian Medical Association
Multicultural Mental Health Australia
National Center for Cultural Competence
National Council of La Raza's Institute for Hispanic Health
National Multicultural Institute
Transcultural C.A.R.E. Associates
Transcultural Nursing Society

The following sites provide cultural tools and other resources related to cultural care:
Compendium of Cultural Competence Initiatives in Health Care
Cultural Medicine
Multilingual Glossary of Medical Terms
Multicultural Pavilion
Provider's Guide to Quality and Culture
Resources for Cross-Cultural Health Care

STUDY AIDS   http://evolve.elsevier.com/Maurer/community/

Visit the Evolve website for this book to find the following study and assessment materials:

- Quiz
- Web Scenario
- Critical Thinking Questions and Answers for Case Studies
- Care Plans
- *Healthy People* Updates
- Glossary

WEBSITE RESOURCES

The following items supplement the chapter's topics and are also found on the Evolve site:

- 10A: Summary of Recommendations for Elimination of Health Disparities
- 10B: Recommended Standards for Culturally and Linguistically Appropriate Services in Health Care
- 10C: Alternative and Complementary Medicine Categories
- 10D: Working with Culturally Diverse Communities: Strategies for the Community Health Nurse

- 10E: Community Standards of Practice for Provision of Quality Health Care Services for Gay, Lesbian, Bisexual, and Transgendered Clients
- 10F: Guidelines for Creating a Safe Clinical Environment for Gay, Lesbian, Bisexual, Transgendered, and Intersex Patients

REFERENCES

Agency for Healthcare Research and Quality. (2005). *National healthcare disparities report, 2005.* Rockville, MD: Author. Retrieved July 28, 2007 from *http://www.ahrq.gov/qual/nhdr05/nhdr05.htm.*

American Academy of Nursing. (1992). Culturally competent nursing care. *Nursing Outlook, 40*(6), 277-283.

American Nurses Association. (1992). *Position statement of cultural diversity in nursing practice.* Washington, DC: Author.

American Nurses Association. (2007). *Public health nursing: Scope and standards of practice.* Silver Spring, MD: Author.

Andrews, M. M. (2008). Transcultural perspectives on the nursing care of children. In M. M. Andrews & J. S. Boyle (Eds.), *Transcultural concepts in nursing care* (5th ed.). Philadelphia: Lippincott Williams & Wilkins.

Andrews, M. M, & Boyle, J. S. (2003). *Transcultural concepts in nursing* (4th ed.). Philadelphia: Lippincott Williams & Wilkins.

Andrews, M. M., & Boyle, J. S. (2008). *Transcultural concepts in nursing* (5th ed.). Philadelphia: Lippincott Williams & Wilkins.

Andrews, M. M., & Hanson, P.A. (2008). Religion, culture and nursing. In M. M. Andrews & J. S. Boyle (Eds.), *Transcultural concepts in nursing* (5th ed.). Philadelphia: Lippincott Williams & Wilkins.

Association of Community Health Nursing Educators. (2000). *Graduate education for advanced practice in community/public health nursing.* Pensacola, FL: Author.

Bernal, H. (1993). A model for delivering culture-relevant care in the community. *Public Health Nursing, 10*(4), 228-232.

Bloche, M. G. (2001). Race and discretion in American medicine. *Yale Journal of Health Policy, Law, and Ethics, 1,* 95-131.

Boyle, J. S. (2008). Culture, family and community. In M. M. Andrews & J. S. Boyle (Eds.), *Transcultural concepts in nursing care* (5th ed.). Philadelphia: Lippincott Williams & Wilkins.

Burroughs, V. J., Maxey, R. W., Crawley, L.M., et al. (2002). *Cultural and genetic diversity in America: The need for individualized treatment.* Washington DC: National Pharmaceutical Council and National Medical Association.

Campinha-Bacote, J. (1998). African Americans. In L. Purnell & B. Paulanka (Eds.), *Transcultural health care: A cultural competent approach* (pp. 53-74). Philadelphia: F. A. Davis.

Campinha-Bacote, J. (2002). The process of cultural competence in the delivery of healthcare services: A model of care. *Journal of Transcultural Nursing, 13*(3), 181-184.

Campinha-Bacote, J. (2007). *The process of cultural competence in the delivery of healthcare services: The journey continues.* Cincinnati: Transcultural C.A.R.E. Associates.

Campinha-Bacote, J., & Munoz, C. (2001). A guiding framework for delivering culturally competent services in care management. *Case Manager, 12*(2), 48-52.

Cantos, A., & Rivera, E. (1996). Filipinos. In J. G. Lipson, S. L. Dibble, & P. A. Minarik (Eds.), *Culture and nursing care: A pocket guide* (pp. 115-125). San Francisco: UCSF Nursing Press.

Centers for Disease Control and Prevention. (2006). *Health, United States, 2006, with chartbook on trends in the health of Americans.* Hyattsville, MD: U.S. Department of Health and Human Services, Centers for Disease Control and Prevention, National Center for Health Statistics.

Chin, P. (1996). Chinese Americans. In J. G. Lipson, S. L. Dibble, & P. A. Minarik (Eds.), *Culture and nursing care: A pocket guide* (pp. 74-81). San Francisco: UCSF Nursing Press.

Collins, K., Hughes, D., Doty, M., et al. (2002). *Diverse communities, common concerns: Assessing health care quality for minority Americans.* New York: Commonwealth Fund.

DeNavas-Walt, C., Proctor, B., & Lee, C. (2006). *Income, poverty, and health insurance coverage in the United States, 2005* (Current Population Reports, P60-231). Washington, DC: U.S. Government Printing Office.

Eliason, M. J. (1998). Correlates of prejudice in nursing students. *Journal of Nursing Education, 37*(1), 27-29.

Evanikoff, L. J. (1996). Russians. In J. G. Lipson, S. L. Dibble, & P. A. Minarik (Eds.), *Culture and nursing care: A pocket guide* (pp. 239-249). San Francisco: UCSF Nursing Press.

Farb, P., & Armelagos, G. (1980). *The anthropology of eating.* Boston: Houghton Mifflin.

Federal Register, 65(247), 80865-80879.

Finch, B. K., Hummer, R. A., Kolody, B., et al. (2001). The role of discrimination and acculturative stress in the physical health of Mexican-origin adults. *Hispanic Journal of Behavioral Science, 4,* 399-429.

First, M. B., & Frances, A. (2002). *DSM-IV-TR: Handbook of differential diagnoses.* Washington, DC: American Psychiatric Association.

Fong, C. M. (1985). Ethnicity and nursing practice. *Topics in Clinical Nursing, 7*(3), 1-10.

Fullilove, M. T. (1998). Abandoning "race" as a variable in public health research—An idea whose time has come. *American Journal of Public Health, 88*(9), 1297-1298.

Galanti, J. (2004). *Caring for patients in diverse cultures.* Philadelphia: University of Pennsylvania Press.

Gay and Lesbian Medical Association. (2001). *Healthy People 2010 companion document for lesbian, gay, bisexual, and transgender (LGBT) health.* San Francisco: Author.

George, T. (2000). Defining care in the culture of the chronically mentally ill living in the community. *Journal of Transcultural Nursing, 11*(2), 102-110.

Giger, J. N., & Davidhizar, R. (2004). *Transcultural nursing* (4th ed.). St. Louis: Mosby Year Book.

Government Accountability Office. (2005). *Health care services are not always available to Native Americans.* Report to the Committee on Indian Affairs, U.S. Senate. Indian Health Service. Government Accountability Office No. 05-789. Washington, DC: U.S. Government Printing Office.

Hall, E. (1963). Proxemics: The study of man's spacial relations. In I. Gladson (Ed.), *Man's image in medicine and anthropology* (pp. 109-120). New York: International Universities Press.

Herberg, P. (1995). Theoretical foundations of transcultural nursing. In M. Andrews & J. Boyle (Eds.), *Transcultural concepts in nursing care* (2nd ed.; pp. 30-47). Philadelphia: J. B. Lippincott.

Hill, P. (1996). West Indians. In J. G. Lipson, S. L. Dibble, & P. A. Minarik (Eds.), *Culture and* nursing care: A pocket guide (pp. 291-303). San Francisco: UCSF Nursing Press.

Hockenberry, M. J., Wilson, D., Winkelstein, M. L., et al. (2003). Wong's nursing care of infants and children (ed. 7). St. Louis: Mosby.

Indian Health Service, Division of Diabetes Treatment and Prevention. (2007). Fact sheets: Diabetes in American Indians and Alaska Natives. Retrieved July 28, 2007 from http://www.ihs.gov/medicalprograms/diabetes/.

Kaiser Family Foundation. (2007). The Kaiser Commission on Medicaid and the uninsured: Fact sheet (Publication No. 7235-02). Menlo Park, CA: Kaiser Family Foundation. Retrieved July 21, 2007, from http://www.kff.org/medicaid/7235.cfm.

Karlsen, S., & Nazroo, J. Y. (2002). Relation between racial discrimination, social class, and health among ethnic minority groups. American Journal of Public Health, 92(4), 624-631.

Kim-Godwin, Y. S., Clarke, P. N., & Barton, L. (2001). A model for the delivery of culturally competent community care. Journal of Advanced Nursing, 35(6), 918-925.

Kramer, J. (1996). American Indians. In J.G. Lipson, S. L. Dibble, & P. A. Minarik (Eds.), Culture and nursing care: A pocket guide (pp. 11-22). San Francisco: UCSF Nursing Press.

Krieger, N. (2000). Discrimination and health. In L. Berkman & I. Kawachi (Eds.), Social epidemiology (pp. 36-75). Oxford, England: Oxford University Press.

LaVeist, T. A., Nickerson, K. J., & Bowie, J. V. (2000). Attitudes about racism, medical mistrust, and satisfaction with care among African-American and white cardiac patients. Medical Care Research and Review, 57(1), 146-161.

Leininger, M. (1978). Transcultural nursing: Concepts, theories, and practices. New York: John Wiley & Sons.

Leininger, M. (1988). Leininger's theory of nursing: Culture care diversity and universality. Nursing Science Quarterly, 1(4), 152-160.

Leininger, M. (1993, Winter). Towards conceptualization of transcultural health care systems: Concepts and a model (classic article for 1976). Journal of Transcultural Nursing, 4(2), 32-40.

Leininger, M. M., & McFarland, M. R. (2006). Transcultural nursing: Concepts, theories, research and practices (4th ed.). New York: McGraw-Hill Medical.

Lillie-Blanton, M., Brodie, M., Rowland, D., et al. (2000). Race, ethnicity, and the health care system: Public perceptions and experiences. Medical Care Research and Review, 57(1), 218-235.

Lipson, J. G., Askatyar, R., & Omidian, P. A. (2004). Afghans and Afghan Americans. In J. N. Giger, & R. E. Davidhizar (Eds.), Transcultural nursing (4th ed.; pp. 363-378). St. Louis: Mosby.

Ludwig-Beymer, P. (2007). Transcultural concepts of pain. In M. M. Andrews & J. S. Boyle (Eds.), Transcultural concepts in nursing care (5th ed.). Philadelphia: Lippincott Williams & Wilkins.

Meleis, A. I., & Meleis, M. (1998). Egyptian Americans. In L. Purnell & B. Paulanka (Eds.), Transcultural health care: A cultural competent approach (pp. 217-244). Philadelphia: F. A. Davis.

Munoz, C., & Luckman, J. (2005). Transcultural communication in nursing. Clifton Park, NY: Thomson/Delmar Learning.

Murdock, G. (1971). Outline of cultural materials (4th ed.). New Haven, CT: Human Relations Area Files.

Murdock, G. (1980). Theories of illness—A world survey. Pittsburgh: Pittsburgh University Press.

National Conference of State Legislatures. (2007). The Immigrant Policy Project. Retrieved July 28, 2007 from http://www.ncsl.org/programs/immig/immigpolicyoverview.htm.

Office of Immigration Statistics. (2006). 2005 Yearbook of immigration statistics. Washington, DC: U.S. Department of Homeland Security, Office of Immigration Statistics. Retrieved July 28, 2007, from http://www.dhs.gov/ximgtn/statistics/publications/yearbook.shtm.

Office of Minority Health. (2007a, July 28). Fact sheet: Eliminating health disparities among minority populations. Closing the Health Gap campaign. Retrieved July 28, 2007 from http://www.omhrc.gov/healthgap/2006factsheet.aspx.

Office of Minority Health. (2007b, May 11). Eliminating racial and ethnic disparities. Retrieved February 16, 2008, from http://www.cdc.gov/omhd/About/disparities.htm.

Osborne, N. G., & Feit, M. D. (1992). Using race in medical research. Journal of the American Medical Association, 267(2), 275-279.

Overfield, T. (1995). Biologic variation in health and illness: Race, age and sex differences. New York: CRC Press.

Passel, J. S. (2005). Estimates of the size and characteristics of the undocumented population. Washington, DC: Pew Hispanic Center. Retrieved July 28, 2007, from http://pewhispanic.org/reports/report.php?ReportID=44.

Polyakova, S., & Pacquiao, D. (2006). Psychological and mental illness among elder immigrants from the former Soviet Union. Journal of Transcultural Nursing, 17(1), 40-49.

Purnell, L., & Paulanka, B. (2003). Transcultural healthcare: A culturally competent approach (2nd ed.). Philadelphia: F. A. Davis.

Rabin, S. A. (1993). A private sector view of health surveillance and communities of color. Morbidity and Mortality Weekly Report, Recommendations and Reports, 42(RR-10), 1-17.

Rowland, D., & Hoffman, C. (2005). The impact of health insurance coverage on health disparities in the United States. Human Development Report 2005, Human Development Office, Occasional Report. Retrieved July 28, 2007, from http://hdr.undp.org/en/reports/global/hdr2005/papers/hdr2005_rowland_diane_and_catherine_hoffman_34.pdf.

Schulman, K. A., Berlin, J. A., Jarless, W., et al. (1999). The effect of race and sex on physician's recommendations for cardiac catheterization. New England Journal of Medicine, 340(8), 618-626.

Smedley, B. D., Stith, A. Y., & Nelson, A. R. (2003). Unequal treatment: Confronting racial and ethnic disparities in healthcare. Washington, DC: National Academy Press.

Spector, R. E. (2004). Cultural diversity in health and illness (6th ed.). Stamford, CT: Appleton & Lange.

Spradley, J. (1979). The ethnographic interview. New York: Holt, Rinehart and Winston.

Still, O., & Hodgins, D. (1998). Navajo Indians. In L. Purnell, & B. Paulanka (Eds.), Transcultural health care: A cultural competent approach (pp. 423-448). Philadelphia: F. A. Davis.

Sullivan Alliance. (2007). Summary proceedings of the National Leadership Symposium on Increasing Diversity in the Health Professions, March 12, 2007. Washington, DC: Kaiser Family Foundation.

Transcultural nursing: Basic concepts and case studies, Asian community. (2005). Retrieved July 28, 2007, from http://www.culturediversity.org.

Tripp-Reimer, T., Brink, P., & Sauners, J. (1984). Cultural assessment: Content and process. Nursing Outlook, 32(2), 78-82.

U.S. Bureau of the Census. (2000). Detailed list of languages spoken at home for the population 5 years and over by state: 2000. Retrieved June 8, 2007, from http://www.census.gov/prod/cen2000/doc/sf3.pdf.

U.S. Bureau of the Census. (2003). Health insurance coverage in the United States: 2002. Washington DC: U.S. Government Printing Office.

U.S. Bureau of the Census. (2005). S1601: Language spoken at home (2005 American Community Survey). Retrieved June 8, 2007 from http://factfinder.census.gov/servlet/STTable?_bm=y&geo_id=01000US&-qr_name=ACS_2005_EST_G00_S1601&-ds_name=ACS_2005_EST_G00_.

U.S. Bureau of the Cenusus. (2006). Current population survey: 2004 to 2006. Annual social and economic supplements. Washington, DC: U.S. Government Printing Office.

U.S. Bureau of the Census. (2007, May 17). Minority population tops 100 million. Retrieved July 28, 2007, from http://www.census.gov/Press-Release/www/releases/archives/population/010048.html.

U.S. Department of Health and Human Services. (2000). Healthy People 2010: Understanding and improving health. Washington, DC: U.S. Government Printing Office.

U.S. Department of Health and Human Services, Health Resources and Services Administration, Bureau of Health Professions. (2005). The registered nurse population: Findings from the 2004 National Sample Survey of Registered Nurses. II: The registered nurse population 1980-2004. Washington, DC: U.S. Government Printing Office. Retrieved July 28, 2007, from http://www.bhpr.hrsa.gov/healthworkforce/rnsurvey04/2.htm.

U.S. Department of Health and Human Services, Office of Civil Rights. (2006). *Guidance to federal financial assistance recipients regarding title VI prohibition against national origin discrimination affecting limited English proficient persons.* Retrieved July 28, 2007, from *http://www.hhs.gov/ocr/lep/revisedlep.html.*

U.S. Department of Health and Human Services, Office of Minority Health. (2001b). *National standards for culturally and linguistically appropriate services in health care: Final report* (Contract No. 282-99-0039). Washington, DC: U.S. Government Printing Office.

U.S. Department of Health and Human Services, Office of Minority Health, Center for Linguistic and Cultural Competence. (2001c). *Cultural competence resources.* Retrieved July 28, 2007, from *http://www.omhrc.gov.*

U.S. Department of Health and Human Services, Office of the Surgeon General, Substance Abuse and Mental Health Services Administration. (2001a). Chapter 5: Mental health care for Asian Americans and Pacific Islanders. In *Mental health: Culture, race, ethnicity supplement.* Retrieved July 28, 2007, from *http://www.mentalhealth.org/cre/ch5.asp.*

Van Gennep, A. (1960). *The rites of passage* (M. B. Vixedom & G. L. Coffee, Trans.). Chicago: University of Chicago Press.

van Ryn, M., & Burke, J. (2000). The effect of patient race and socio-economic status on physician's perception of patients. *Social Science and Medicine, 50*(6), 813-828.

Watts, R. J. (2003). Race consciousness and the health of African Americans. *Online Journal of Issues in Nursing,* 8(1), manuscript 3. Retrieved February 18, 2008, from *http://nursingworld. org/MainMenuCategories/ANAMarketplace/ ANAPeriodicals/ojin.aspx.*

Williams, D. R. (1999). Race, socioeconomic status, and health: The added effects of racism and discrimination. *Annals of the New York Academy of Sciences, 896,* 173-188.

Williams, D. R., & Collins, C. (2002). U.S. socioeconomic and racial differences in health: Patterns and explanations. In T. A. LaVeist (Ed.), *Race, ethnicity and health* (pp. 391-432). San Francisco: John Wiley & Sons.

Williams, D. R., & Williams-Morris, R. (2000). Racism and mental health: The African American experience. *Ethnicity and Disease, 5*(3-4), 243-268.

Wilson, S. A. (2003). People of Irish heritage. In L. Purnell & B. Paulanka (Eds.), *Transcultural health care: A cultural competent approach* (pp. 194-204). Philadelphia: F. A. Davis.

Wilson-Stronks, A., & Galvez, E. (2007). *Hospital, language, and culture: A snapshot of the nation. Exploring cultural and linguistic services in the nation's hospitals.* Report by the California Endowment and the Joint Commission on the Accreditation of Healthcare Organizations. Los Angeles: California Endowment. Retrieved July 21, 2007, from *http://www.calendow.org/ references/publications/pdf/cultural/hospitallanguageculture.pdf.*

Wissler, T. (1921). The sun dance of the Blackfoot Indians. *American Museum of Natural History Anthology Papers, 12,* 223-270.

Youdelman, M., & Perkins, J. (2002). *Providing language interpretation services in health care settings: Examples from the field.* New York: Commonwealth Fund.

SUGGESTED READINGS

Boyle, J. S. (2008). Chapter 2: Culturally competent nursing care; Chapter 11: Culture, family and community; Chapter 14: Religion, culture and nursing. In M. M. Andrews & J. S. Boyle (Eds.), *Transcultural concepts in nursing care* (5th ed.). Philadelphia: Lippincott Williams & Wilkins.

Campinha-Bacote, J. (2007). *The process of cultural competence in the delivery of healthcare services: A culturally competent model* (5th ed.). Wyoming, OH: Transcultural

C.A.R.E. Associates Press. Retrieved June 7, 2007 from *http://Transculturalcare.net/ Cultural_Competence_Model.htm.*

Loeb, S. J. (2006). African American older adults coping with chronic health conditions. *Journal of Transcultural Nursing, 17*(2), 139-147.

Nailon, R. E. (2006). Nurses' concerns and practices with using interpreters in the care of Latino patients in the emergency department. *Journal of Transcultural Nursing, 17*(2), 119-128.

Schim, S. M., Doorebnos, A., Benkert, R., et al. (2007). Culturally congruent care: Putting the puzzle together. *Journal of Transcultural Nursing, 18*(3), 103-110.

Yehieli, M. (2005). *Health matters: A pocket guide to working with diverse cultures and underserved populations.* Yarmouth, ME: Intercultural Press.

Family as Client

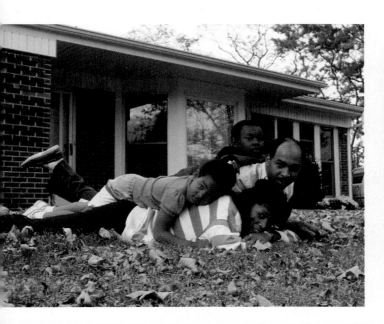
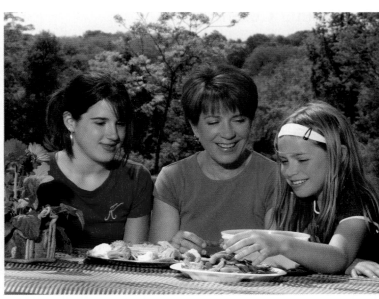

11 Home Visit: Opening the Doors for Family Health

Claudia M. Smith

FOCUS QUESTIONS

Why are home visits conducted?

What are advantages and disadvantages of home visits?

How is the nurse-client relationship in a home similar to and different from nurse-client relationships in inpatient settings?

How can a nurse's family focus be maximized during a typical home visit?

What promotes safety for community/public health nurses?

What happens during a typical home visit?

How can client participation be promoted?

CHAPTER OUTLINE

KEY TERMS

Agreement	Family focus	Presence
Collaboration	Genuineness	Referral
Consultation	Home visit	
Empathy	Positive regard	

Nurses who work in all specialties and with all age groups can practice with a **family focus,** that is, thinking of the health of each family member and of the entire family per se and considering the effects of the interrelatedness of the family members on health. Because being family focused is a philosophy, it can be practiced in any setting. However, a family's residence provides a special place for family-focused care.

Community/public health nurses have historically sought to promote the well-being of families in the home setting (Zerwekh, 1990). Community/public health nurses seek to promote health; prevent specific illnesses, injuries, and premature death; and reduce human suffering. Through home visits, community/public health nurses provide opportunities for families to become aware of potential health problems, to receive anticipatory education, and to learn to mobilize resources for health promotion and primary prevention (Kristjanson & Chalmers, 1991; Raatikainen, 1991). In clients' homes, care can be personalized to a family's coping strategies, problem-solving skills, and environmental resources (see Chapter 13).

During home visits, community/public health nurses can uncover threats to health that are not evident when family members visit a physician's office, health clinic, or emergency department (Olds et al., 1995; Zerwekh, 1991). For example, during a visit in the home of a young mother, a nursing student observed a toddler playing with a paper cup full of tacks and putting them in his mouth. The student used the opportunity to discuss safety with the mother and persuaded her to keep the tacks on a high shelf. The quality of the home environment predicts the cognitive and social development of an infant (Engelke & Engelke, 1992). Community/public health nurses successfully assist parents in improving relations with their children and in providing safe, stimulating physical environments.

All levels of prevention can be addressed during home visits. Research has demonstrated that home visits by nurses during the prenatal and infancy periods prevent developmental and health problems (Kitzman et al., 2000; Norr et al., 2003; Olds et al., 1986). Olds and colleagues demonstrated that families who received visits had fewer instances of child abuse and neglect, emergency department visits, accidents, and poisonings during the child's first 2 years of life. These results were true for families of all socioeconomic levels but greater for low-income families. The health outcomes for families who received home visits were better than those of families who received care only in clinics or from private physicians. Furthermore, the favorable results were still apparent 15 years after the birth of the first child (Olds et al., 1997), and the home visits reduced subsequent pregnancies (Kitzman et al., 1997; Olds et al., 1997). The U.S. Advisory Board on Abuse and Neglect advocates such home-visiting programs as a means to prevent child abuse and neglect (U.S. Department of Health and Human Services, 1990). Other research shows that home visits by nurses can reduce the incidence of drug-resistant tuberculosis and decrease preventable deaths among infected individuals (Lewis & Chaisson, 1993). This goal is achieved through directly observing medication therapy in the individual's home, workplace, or school on a daily basis or several times a week (see Chapter 8).

Several factors have converged to expand opportunities for nursing care to ill and disabled adults and children in their homes. The American population has aged, chronic diseases are now the major illnesses among elderly persons, and attempts are being made to limit the rising hospital costs. As the average length of stay in hospitals has decreased since the early 1980s, families have had to care for more acutely ill adults and children in their homes. This increased demand for home health care has resulted in more agencies and nurses providing home care to ill persons and teaching family members to perform the care (see Chapter 31).

The degree to which families cope with a chronically ill or disabled member significantly affects both the individual's health status and the quality of life for the entire family (Burns & Gianutsos, 1987; Harris, 1995; Whyte, 1992). Family members may be called on to support an individual family member's adjustment to a chronic illness, as well as take on tasks and roles that the ill member previously performed. This adjustment occurs over time and often takes place in the home.

Community/public health nurses can assist families in making these adjustments.

Since the late 1960s, deinstitutionalization of mentally ill clients has shifted them from inpatient psychiatric settings to their own homes, group homes, and the streets (see Chapter 33). Nurses in the fields of community mental health and psychiatry began to include the relatives and surrogate family members in providing critical support to enable the person with a psychiatric diagnosis to live at home (Mohit, 1996; Stolee et al., 1996).

The hospice movement also recognizes the importance of a family focus during the process of a family member's dying (American Nurses Association [ANA], 2007a). Care at home or in a homelike setting is cost-effective under many circumstances. As the prevalence of acquired immunodeficiency syndrome (AIDS) increases and the number of older adults continues to increase, providing care in a cost-effective manner is both an ethical and an economic necessity.

Nurses in any specialty can practice with a family focus. However, the specific goals and time constraints in each health care service setting affect the degree to which a family focus can be used. A home visit is one type of nurse-client encounter that facilitates a family focus. Home visiting does not guarantee a family focus. Rather, the setting itself and the structure of the encounter provide an opportunity for the nurse to practice with a family focus.

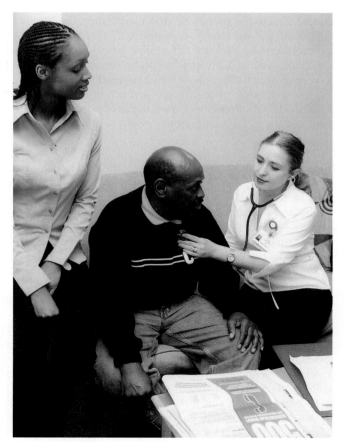

A nurse visiting a client in his home listens to the man's heart while his daughter looks on.

Nurses who graduate from a baccalaureate nursing program are expected to have educational experiences that prepare them for beginning practice in community/public health nursing. Family-focused care is an essential element of community/public health nursing. One of the ways to improve the health of populations and communities is to improve the health of families (ANA, 2007b).

Home visits may be made to any residence: apartments for older adults, group homes, boarding homes, dormitories, domiciliary care facilities, and shelters for the homeless, among others. In these residences, the family may not be related by blood, but rather they may be *significant others:* neighbors, friends, acquaintances, or paid caregivers.

Nurses who are educated at the baccalaureate level are one of a few professional and service workers who are formally taught about making home visits. Some social work students, especially those interested in the fields of home health and protective services, also receive similar education. The American Red Cross and the National Home Caring Council have developed training programs for homemakers and home health aides; not all aides have received such extensive training, however. Agricultural and home economic extension workers in the United States and abroad also may make home visits (Murray, 1968; World Health Organization, 1987).

HOME VISIT

DEFINITION

A **home visit** is a purposeful interaction in a home (or residence) directed at promoting and maintaining the health of individuals and the family (or significant others). The service may include supporting a family during a member's death. Just as a client's visit to a clinic or outpatient service can be viewed as an encounter between health care professionals and the client, so can a home visit. A major distinction of a home visit is that the health professional goes to the client rather than the client coming to the health professional.

PURPOSE

Almost any health service can be accomplished on a home visit. An assumption is that—except in an emergency—the client or family is sufficiently healthy to remain in the community and to manage health care after the nurse leaves the home.

The foci of community/public health nursing practice in the home can be categorized under five basic goals:

1. Promoting support systems that are adequate and effective and encouraging use of health-related resources
2. Promoting adequate, effective care of a family member who has a specific problem related to illness or disability
3. Encouraging normal growth and development of family members and the family and educating the family about health promotion and illness prevention
4. Strengthening family functioning and relatedness
5. Promoting a healthful environment

The five basic goals of community/public health nursing practice with families can be linked to categories of family problems (Table 11-1). A pilot study to identify problems common in community/public health nursing practice settings revealed that problems clustered into four categories: (1) lifestyle and living resources, (2) current health status and deviations,

(3) patterns and knowledge of health maintenance, and (4) family dynamics and structure (Simmons, 1980). Home visits are one means by which community/public health nurses can address these problems and achieve goals for family health.

ADVANTAGES AND DISADVANTAGES

Advantages of home visits by nurses are numerous. Most of the disadvantages relate to expense and concerns about unpredictable environments (Box 11-1).

TABLE 11-1 Family Health-Related Problems and Goals

Problem*	Goal
Lifestyle and resources	Promote support systems and use of health-related resources
Health status deviations	Promote adequate, effective family care of an ill or disabled member
Patterns and knowledge of health maintenance	Encourage growth and development of family members, health promotion, and illness prevention
	Promote healthful environment
Family dynamics and structure	Strengthen family functioning and relatedness

* Problems from Simmons, D. (1980). *A classification scheme for client problems in community health nursing* (DHHS Pub No. HRA 8016). Hyattsville, MD: U.S. Department of Health and Human Services.

BOX 11-1 Advantages and Disadvantages of Home Visiting

Advantages

Home setting provides more opportunities for individualized care.

Most people prefer to receive care at home.

Environmental factors impinging on health, such as housing condition and finances, may be observed and considered more readily.

Collecting information and understanding lifestyle values are easier in family's own environment.

Participation of family members is facilitated.

Individuals and family members may be more receptive to learning because they are less anxious in their own environment and because the immediacy of needing to know a particular fact or skill becomes more apparent.

Care to ill family members in the home can reduce overall costs by preventing hospitalizations and shortening the length of time spent in hospitals or other institutions.

A family focus is facilitated.

Disadvantages

Travel time is costly.

Home visiting is less efficient for the nurse than working with groups or seeing many clients in an ambulatory site.

Distractions such as television and noisy children may be more difficult to control.

Clients may be resistant or fearful of the intimacy of home visits.

Nurse safety can be an issue.

NURSE-FAMILY RELATIONSHIPS

How nurses are assigned to make home visits is both a philosophic and a management issue. Some community/public health nurses are assigned by geographic area or *district*. The size of the geographic area for home visits varies with the population density. In a densely populated urban area, a nurse might visit in one neighborhood; in a less densely populated area, the nurse might be assigned to visit in an entire county. With geographic assignments, the nurse has the potential to work with the entire population in a district and to handle a broad range of health concerns; the nurse can also become well acquainted with the community's health and social resources. The potential for a family-focused approach is strengthened because the nurse's concerns consist of all health issues identified with a specific family or group of families. The nurse remains a clinical generalist, working with people of all ages.

Other community/public health nurses are assigned to work with a population aggregate in one or more geopolitical communities. For example, a nurse may work for a *categorical* program that addresses family planning or adolescent pregnancy, in which case the nurse would visit only families to which the category applies. This type of assignment allows a nurse to work predominantly with a specific interest area (e.g., family planning and pregnancy) or with a specific aggregate (e.g., families with fertile women).

PRINCIPLES OF NURSE-CLIENT RELATIONSHIP WITH FAMILY

Regardless of whether the community/public health nurse is assigned to work with an aggregate or the entire population, several principles strengthen the clarity of purpose:
- By definition, the nurse focuses on the family.
- The health focus can be on the entire spectrum of health needs and all three levels of prevention.
- The family retains autonomy in health-related decisions.
- The nurse is a guest in the family's home.

Family Focus

To relate to the family, the community/public health nurse does not have to meet all members of the household personally, although varying the times of visits might allow the nurse to meet family members usually at work or school. Relating to the family requires that the nurse be concerned about the health of each member and about each person's contribution to the functioning of the family. One family member may be the primary informant; in such instances, the nurse should realize that the information received is being *filtered* by the person's perceptions.

The community/public health nurse should take the time to introduce herself or himself to each person present and address each person by name. Building trust is an essential foundation for a continued relationship (Heaman et al., 2007; Zerwekh, 1992). The nurse should use the clients' surnames unless they introduce themselves in another way or give permission for the nurse to be less formal. Interacting with as many family members as possible, identifying the family member most responsible for health issues, and acknowledging the family member with the most authority are important. The nurse should ask for an introduction to pets and ask for permission before picking up infants and children unless it is granted nonverbally.

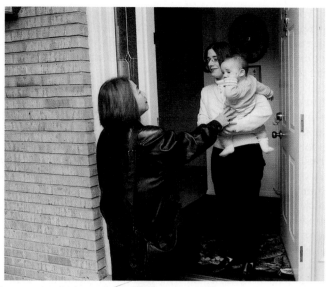

A nurse enters the home of a client with a young child.

All Levels of Prevention

Through assessment, the community/public health nurse attempts to identify what actual and potential problems or concerns exist with each individual and, thematically, within the family (see Chapter 13). Issues of health promotion (diet) and specific protection (immunization) may exist, as may undiagnosed medical problems for which referral is necessary for further diagnosis and treatment. Home visits also can be effective in stimulating family members to seek appropriate services, such as prenatal care (Bradley & Martin, 1994) and immunizations (Norr et al., 2003). Actual family problems in coping with illness or disability may require direct intervention. Preventing sequelae and maximizing potential may be appropriate for families with a chronically ill member. Health-related problems may appear predominantly in one family member or among several members. A thematic family problem might be related to nutrition. For example, a mother may be anemic, a preschooler may be obese, and a father may not follow a low-fat diet for hypertension.

Family Autonomy

A few circumstances exist in our society in which the health of the community, or *public,* is considered to have priority over the right of individual persons or families to do as they wish. In most states, statutes (laws) provide that health care workers, including community/public health nurses, have a right and an obligation to intervene in cases of family abuse and neglect, potential suicide or homicide, and existence of communicable diseases that pose a threat of infection to others. *Except for these three basic categories, the family retains the ultimate authority for health-related decisions and actions.*

In the home setting, family members participate more in their own care. Nursing care in the home is intermittent, not 24 hours a day. When the visit ends, the family takes responsibility for their own health, albeit with varying degrees of interest, commitment, knowledge, and skill. This role is often difficult for beginning community/public health nurses to accept; learning to distinguish the family's responsibilities from the nurse's responsibilities involves experience and consideration of laws and ethics. Except in crises, taking over for the family in areas in which they have demonstrated capability is usually inappropriate.

For example, if family members typically call the pharmacy to renew medications and make their own medical appointments, beginning to do these things for them is inappropriate for the nurse. Taking over undermines self-esteem, confidence, and success.

Nurse as Guest

Being a guest as a community/public health nurse in a family's home does not mean that the relationship is social. The social graces for the community and culture of the family must be considered so that the family is at ease and is not offended. However, the relationship is intended to be therapeutic. For example, many elderly persons believe that offering something to eat or drink is important as a sign that they are being courteous and hospitable. Because your refusal to share in a glass of iced tea may be taken as an affront, you may desire to accept the tea. However, you certainly have the right to refuse, especially if infectious disease is a concern.

Validate with the client that the time of the visit is convenient. If the client fails to offer you a seat, you may ask if there is a place for you and the family to sit and talk. This place may be any room of the house or even outside in good weather.

PHASES OF RELATIONSHIPS

Relatedness and communication between the nurse and the client are fundamental to all nursing care. A nurse-client relationship with a family (rather than an individual) is critical to community/public health nursing. The phases of the nurse-client relationship with a family are the same as are those with an individual. Different schemes have been developed for naming phases of relationships. All schemes have (1) a preinitiation or preplanning phase, (2) an initiation or introductory phase, (3) a working phase, and (4) an ending phase (Arnold & Boggs, 2007). Some schemes distinguish a power and control or contractual phase that occurs before the working phase.

The initiation phase may take several visits. During this phase, the nurse and the family get to know one another and determine how the family health problems are mutually defined. The more experience the nurse has, the more efficient she or he will become; initially, many community/public health nursing students may require four to six visits to feel comfortable and to clarify their role (Barton & Brown, 1995).

The nursing student should keep in mind that the relationship with the family usually involves many encounters over time—home visits, telephone calls, or visits at other ambulatory sites, such as clinics. Several encounters may occur during each phase of the relationship (Figure 11-1). Each encounter also has its own phases (Figure 11-2).

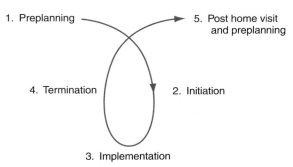

FIGURE 11-2 Phases of a home visit. (Redrawn from Smith, C. [1980]. *Phases of a home visit* [unpublished manuscript]. Baltimore, MD: University of Maryland School of Nursing.)

Preplanning each telephone call and home visit is helpful. Box 11-2 lists activities in which community/public health nurses usually engage before a home visit. The list can be used as a guide in helping novice community/public health nurses organize previsit activities efficiently.

The visit begins with a reintroduction and a review of the plan for the day; the nurse must assess what has happened with the family since the last encounter. At this point, the nurse may renegotiate the plan for the visit and implement it. The end of the visit consists of summarizing, preparing for the next encounter, and leave-taking. Box 11-3 describes the community/public health nurse's typical activities during a home visit.

CHARACTERISTICS OF RELATIONSHIPS WITH FAMILIES

Some differences are worth discussing in nurses' relationships with families compared with those with individual clients in hospitals. The difference that usually seems most significant to the nurse who is learning to make home visits is the fact that

---

Box 11-2	**Planning before a Home Visit**

1. Have name, address, and telephone number of family with directions and a map.
2. Have telephone number of agency by which supervisor or faculty can be reached.
3. Have emergency telephone numbers for police, fire, and rescue personnel.
4. Clarify who has referred family to you and why.
5. Consider what is usually expected of a nurse in working with a family who has been referred for these health concerns (e.g., postpartum visit) and clarify the purposes of this home visit.
6. Consider whether any special safety precautions are required.
7. Have a plan of activities for the home visit time (see Box 11-3).
8. Have equipment needed for hand-washing, physical assessment, and direct care interventions, or verify that client has the equipment in the home.
9. Take any data assessment or permission forms that are needed.
10. Have information and teaching aids for health teaching as appropriate.
11. Have information about community resources as appropriate.
12. Have gasoline in your automobile or money for public transportation.
13. Leave an itinerary with the agency personnel or faculty.
14. Approach the visit with self-confidence and caring.

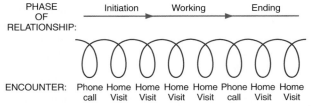

FIGURE 11-1 A series of encounters during a relationship. (Redrawn from Smith, C. [1980]. *A series of encounters during a relationship* [unpublished manuscript]. Baltimore, MD: University of Maryland School of Nursing.)

Box 11-3　Nursing Activities during Three Phases of a Home Visit

Initiation Phase of Home Visit

1. Knock on door and stand where you can be observed if peephole or window exists.
2. Identify self as [name], the nurse from [name of agency].
3. Ask for the person to whom you were referred or the person with whom the appointment was made.
4. Observe environment as regards your own safety.
5. Introduce yourself to persons who are present and acknowledge them.
6. Sit where family directs you to sit.
7. Discuss purpose of visit. On initial visits, discuss services to be provided by agency.
8. Have permission forms signed to initiate services. This activity may be done later in the home visit if more explanation of services is needed for the family to understand what is being offered.

Implementation Phase of Home Visit

9. Complete health assessment database for the individual client.
10. On return visits, assess for changes since the last encounter. Explore the degree that family was able to follow-up on plans from previous visit. Explore barriers if follow-up did not occur.
11. Wash hands before and after conducting any physical assessment and direct physical care.
12. Conduct physical assessment as appropriate and perform direct physical care.
13. Identify household members and their health needs, use of community resources, and environmental hazards.
14. Explore values, preferences, and clients' perceptions of needs and concerns.
15. Conduct health teaching as appropriate, and provide written instructions. Include any safety recommendations.
16. Discuss any referral, collaboration, or consultation that you recommend.
17. Provide comfort and counseling as needed.

Termination Phase of Home Visit

18. Summarize accomplishments of visit.
19. Clarify family's plan of care related to potential health emergency appropriate to health problems.
20. Discuss plan for next home visit and activities to be accomplished in the interim by the community/public health nurse, individual client, and family members.
21. Leave written identification of yourself and agency, with telephone numbers.

---

the nurse has less control over the family's environment and health-related behavior (McNaughton, 2000). The relationship usually extends for a longer period. A more interdependent relationship develops between the community/public health nurse and the family throughout all steps of the nursing process.

Families Retain Much Control

The family can control the nurse's entry into the home by explicitly refusing assistance, establishing the time of the visit, or deciding whether to answer the door. Unlike hospitalized clients, family members can just walk away and not be home for the visit. One study of home visits to high-risk pregnant women revealed that younger and more financially distressed women tended to miss more appointments for home visits (Josten et al., 1995). Being rejected by the family is often a concern of nurses who are learning to conduct home visits. As with any relationship, anxiety can exist in relation to meeting new, unknown families. Families may actually have similar feelings about meeting the nurse and may wonder what the nurse will think of them, their lifestyle, and their health care behavior.

A helpful practice is to keep your perspective; *if the clients are home for your visit, they are at least ambivalent about the meeting!* If they are at home to answer the door, they are willing to consider what you have to offer.

Most families involved with home care of the ill have requested assistance. Because only a few circumstances exist (as previously discussed) in which nursing care can be forced on families, the nurse can view the home visit as an opportunity to explore voluntarily the possibility of engaging in relationships (Byrd, 1995). The nurse is there to offer services and engage the family in a dialogue about health concerns, barriers, and goals. As with all nurse-client relationships, the nurse's commitment, authenticity, and caring constitute the art of nursing practice that can make a difference in the lives of families. Just as not all individuals in the hospital are ready or able to use all of the suggestions made to them, families have varying degrees of openness to change. If after discussing the possibilities the family declines either overtly or through its actions, the nurse has provided an opportunity for informed decision making and has no further obligation.

Goals of Nursing Care Are Long Term

A second major difference in nurse relationships with families is that the goals are usually more long term than are those with individual clients in hospitals. Clients may be in hospice programs for 6 months. A family with a member who has a recent diagnosis of hypertension may take 6 weeks to adjust to medications, diet, and other lifestyle changes. A school-age child with a diagnosis of attention deficit disorder may take as long as half the school year to show improvement in behavior and learning; sometimes, a year may be required for appropriate classroom placement.

For some nurses, this time frame is judged to be slow and tedious. For others, the time frame is seen as an opportunity to know a family in more depth, share life experiences over time, and see results of modifications in nursing care. For nurses who like to know about a broad range of health and nursing issues, relationships with families stimulate this interest. Having had some experience in home visiting is helpful for nurses who work in inpatient settings; it allows them to appreciate the scope and depth of practice of community/public health nurses who make home visits as a part of their regular practice. These experiences can sensitize hospital nurses to the home environments of their clients and can result in better hospital discharge plans and referrals.

Because ultimate goals may take a long time to achieve, short-term objectives must be developed to achieve long-term goals. For example, a family needs to be able to plan lower calorie menus with sufficient nutrients before weight loss is possible; a parent may need to spend time with a child daily before unruly behavior improves.

Nursing interventions in a hospital setting become short-term objectives for client learning and mastery in the home setting. In an inpatient setting, *giving medications as prescribed* is a nursing action. In the home, *the spouse giving medications as prescribed* becomes a behavioral objective for the family; the related nursing action is teaching.

Human progress toward any goal does not usually occur at a steady pace. For example, you may start out bicycling faithfully three times a week and give up abruptly. Similarly, clients may skip an insulin dose or an oral contraceptive. A family may assertively call appropriate community agencies, keep appointments, and stop abruptly. Families can be committed to their own health and well-being and yet not act on their commitment consistently. Recognizing that setbacks and discouragement are a part of life allows the community/public health nurse to be more accepting of reality and have the objectivity to renegotiate goals and plans with families. Box 11-4 includes evidence-based ways to foster goal accomplishment.

Changes are sometimes subtle or small. Success breeds success, at least motivationally. The short-term goals on which everyone has agreed are important to make clear so that the nurse and the family members have a common basis for evaluation. Goals can be set in a logical sequence, in small steps, to increase the chance of success. In an inpatient setting, the skilled nurse notices the subtle changes in client behavior and health status that can warn of further disequilibrium or can signal improvement. Similarly, during a series of home visits, the skilled nurse is aware of slight variations in home management, personal care, and memory that may presage a deteriorating biologic or social condition.

Nursing Care Is More Interdependent with Families

Because families have more control over their health in their own homes, and because change is usually gradual, greater emphasis must be placed on mutual goals if the nurse and family are to achieve long-term success.

Except in emergency situations, the client determines the priority of issues. A parent may be adamant that obtaining food is more important than obtaining their child's immunization. A child's school performance may be of greater concern to a mother than is her own abnormal Papanicolaou (Pap) smear results. Failure of the nurse to address the family's primary

priority may result in the family perceiving that the nurse does not genuinely care. At times, the priority problem is not directly health related, or the solution to a health problem can be handled better by another agency or discipline. In these instances, the empathic nurse can address the family's stress level, problem-solving ability, and support systems and make appropriate referrals. When the nurse takes time to validate and discuss the primary concern, the relationship is enhanced.

Families are sometimes unaware of what they do not know. The nurse must suggest health-related topics that are appropriate for the family situation. For example, a young mother with a healthy newborn may not have thought about how to determine when her baby is ill. A spouse caring for his wife with Alzheimer's disease may not know what safety precautions are necessary. Community/public health nurses seek to enhance family competence by sharing their professional knowledge with families and building on the family's experience (Reutter & Ford, 1997).

Flexibility is a key. Because visits occur over several days to months, other events (e.g., episodic illnesses, a neighbor's death, community unemployment) can impinge on the original plan. Family members may be rehospitalized and receive totally new medical orders once they are discharged to home. The nurse's clarity of purpose is essential in identifying and negotiating other health-related priorities after the first concerns have been addressed.

INCREASING NURSE-FAMILY RELATEDNESS

What promotes a successful home visit? What aspects of the nurse's presence promote relatedness? What structures provide direction and flexibility? The nursing process provides a general structure, and communication is a primary vehicle through which the nursing process is manifested. The foundation for both the nursing process and communication is relatedness and caring (ANA, 2003; Roach, 1997; Watson, 2002; Watson, 2005).

FOSTERING A CARING PRESENCE

Nursing efforts are *not* always successful. However, by being concerned about the impact of home visits on the family and by asking questions regarding her or his own motivations, the nurse automatically increases the likelihood that home visits will be of benefit to the family. The nurse is acknowledging that the intention is for the relationship to be meaningful to both the nurse *and* the family.

Building and preserving relationships is a central focus of home visiting and requires significant effort (Heaman et al., 2007; McNaughton, 2000). The relatedness of nurses in community health *with* clients is important (Goldsborough, 1969; Zerwekh, 1992).

Involvement, essentially, is caring deeply about what is happening and what might happen to a person, then doing something with and for that person. It is reaching out and touching and hearing the inner being of another....For a nurse-client relationship to become a moving force toward action, the nurse must go beyond obvious nursing needs and try to know the client as a person and include him in planning his nursing care. This means sharing feelings, ideas, beliefs and values with the client....Without responsibility

---

| Box 11-4 | **Best Practices in Fostering Goal Accomplishment with Families** |

1. Share goals explicitly with family.
2. Divide goals into manageable steps.
3. Teach family to do for themselves.
4. Do not expect family to do something all of the time or perfectly.
5. Be satisfied with small, subtle changes.
6. Be flexible.

and commitment to oneself and others...[a person] only exists. It is through interaction and meaningful involvement with others that we move into being human (Goldsborough, 1969, pp. 66-68).

Mayers (1973, p. 331) observed 16 randomly selected nurses during home visits to 37 families and reported that "regardless of the specific interaction style [of each nurse], the clients of nurses who were client-focused consistently tended to respond with interest, involvement and mutuality." A client-focused nurse was observed as one who followed client cues, attempted to understand the client's view of the situation, and included the client in generating solutions. Being related is a contribution that the nurse can make to the family, independent of specific information and technical skills, a contribution that students often underestimate.

Although being related is necessary, it is inadequate in itself for high-quality nursing. A community/public health nurse must also be competent. Community/public health nursing also depends on assessment skills, judgment, teaching skills, safe technical skills, and the ability to provide accurate information. As a community/public health nurse's practice evolves, tension always exists between being related and doing the tasks. In each situation, an opportunity exists to ask, "How can I express my caring *and* do (perform direct care, teach, refer) what is needed?"

Barrett (1982) and Katzman and colleagues (1987) report on the differences that students actually make in the lives of families. Barrett (1982) demonstrated that postpartum home visits by nursing students reduced costly postpartum emergency department and hospital visits. Katzman and co-workers (1987) considered hundreds of visits per semester made by 80 students in a southwestern state to families with newborns, well children, pregnant women, and members with chronic illnesses. Case examples describe how student enthusiasm and involvement contributed to specific health results.

Everything a nurse has learned about relationships is important to recall and transfer to the experience of home visiting. Carl Rogers (1969) has identified three characteristics of a helping relationship: positive regard, empathy, and genuineness. These characteristics are relevant in all nurse-client relationships, and they are especially important when relationships are initiated and developed in the less-structured home setting. **Presence** means being related interpersonally in ways that reveal positive regard, empathy, genuineness, and caring concern.

How is it possible to accept a client who keeps a disheveled house or who keeps such a clean house that you feel as if you are contaminating it? How is it possible to have positive feelings about an unmarried mother of three when you and your spouse have successfully abstained from pregnancy? Having positive regard for a family does not mean giving up your own values and behavior (see Chapter 10). Having positive regard for a family who lives different from you does not mean you need to ignore your past experiences. The latter is impossible. Rather, having positive regard means having the ability to distinguish between the person and her or his behavior. Saying to yourself, "This is a person who keeps a messy house" is different from saying, "This person is a mess!" Positive regard involves recognizing the value of persons because they are human beings. Accept the family, not necessarily the family's behavior. All behavior is purposeful; and without further information, you cannot determine the meaning of a particular family behavior. **Positive regard** involves looking for the common human experiences. For example, it is likely that both you and the family members experience awe in the behavior of a newborn and sadness in the face of loss.

Empathy is the ability to put yourself in someone else's shoes and to be able to walk in her or his footsteps so as to understand her or his journey. "Empathy requires sensitivity to another's experience...including sensing, understanding, and sharing the feelings and needs of the other person, seeing things from the other's perspective" according to Rogers (cited in Gary & Kavanagh, 1991, p. 89). Empathy goes beyond self and identity to acknowledge the essence of all persons. It links a characteristic of a helping relationship with spirituality or "a sense of connection to life itself" (Haber et al., 1987, p. 78). Empathy is a necessary pathway for our relatedness.

However, what does understanding another person's experience mean? More than emotions are involved. A person's experience includes the sense that she or he makes of aspects of human existence (van Manen, 1990). Being understood means that a person is no longer alone (Arnold, 1996). Being understood provides support in the face of stress, illness, disability, pain, grief, and suffering. When a client feels understood in a nurse-client partnership (side-by-side relationship), the client's experience of *being cared for* is enhanced (Beck, 1992).

To understand another person's experience, you must be able to imagine being in her or his place, recognize commonalities among persons, and have a secure sense of yourself (Davis, 1990). Being aware of your own values and boundaries is helpful in retaining your identity in interaction with others. To understand another individual's experience, you must also be willing to engage in conversation to negotiate mutual definitions of the situation. For example, if you are excited that an elderly person is recovering function after a stroke, but the person's spouse sees only the loss of an active travel companion, a mutual definition of the situation does not exist. Empathy will not occur unless you can also understand the spouse's perspective.

We like to perceive that we have some control in our environment, that we have some choice. We avoid being dominated and conned. The nurse's genuineness facilitates honesty and disclosure, reduces the likelihood that the family will feel betrayed or coerced, and enhances the relationship. Genuineness does not mean that you speak everything that you think. **Genuineness** means that what you say and do is consistent with your understanding of the situation.

The nurse can promote genuine self-expression in others by creating an atmosphere of trust, accepting that each person has a right to self-expression, "actively seeking to understand" others, and assisting them to become aware of and understand themselves (Goldsborough, 1969, p. 66). When family members do not believe that being genuine with the nurse is safe, they may tell the nurse what they think she or he would like to hear. This action makes developing a mutual plan of care much more difficult.

The reciprocal side of genuineness is being willing to undertake a journey of self-expression, self-understanding, and growth. Tamara, a recent nursing graduate, wrote about her growing self-responsibility:

"Although I felt out of control, I felt very responsible. I took pride in knowing that these families were my families, and I was responsible for their care. I was responsible for their health teaching. This was the first semester where there was not a faculty member around all day long. I feel that this will help me so much as I begin my nursing career. I have truly felt independent and completely responsible for my actions in this clinical experience."

This student, who preferred predictable environments, was able to confront her anxiety and anger in environments in which much was beyond her control. A mother was not interested in the student's priorities. A family abruptly moved out of the state in the middle of the semester. Nonetheless, the student was able to respond in such circumstances. She became more responsible, and she was able to temper her judgment and work with the mother's concern. When the family moved, the student experienced frustration and anger that she would not see the "fruits of her labor" and that she would "have to start over" with another family. However, her ability to respond increased because of her commitment to her own growth, relatedness with families, and desire to contribute to the health and well-being of others.

In a context of relating with and advocating for the family, the relationship becomes an opportunity for growth in both the nurse's and the family's lives (Glugover, 1987). Imagine standing side-by-side with the family, being concerned for their well-being and growth. Now imagine talking to a family face-to-face, attempting to have them do things your way. The first image is a more caring and empathic one.

CREATING AGREEMENTS FOR RELATEDNESS

How can communications be structured to increase the participation of family members? Without the family's engagement, the community/public health nurse will have few positive effects on the health behavior and health status of the family and its members.

Nurses are expert in caring for the ill; in knowing about ways to cope with illness, to promote health, and to protect against specific diseases; and in teaching and supporting family members. **Family members are experts in their own health.** They know the family health history, they experience their health states, and they are aware of their health-related concerns.

Through the nurse-family relationship, a fluid process takes place of matching the family's perceived needs with the nurse's perceptions and professional judgments about the family's needs. Paradoxically, the more skilled the nurse is in forgetting her or his own anxiety about being the *good nurse,* the more likely the nurse is to listen to the family members, validate *their reality,* and negotiate an adequate, effective plan of care.

One study of home visits revealed that more than half of the goals stated by public health nurses to the researcher could not be detected, even implicitly, during observations of the home visits. Therefore half of the goals were known only to the nurse and were therefore not mutual. The more specifically and concretely the goals were stated by the nurse to the researcher, the greater the likelihood that the clients understood the nurse's purposes (Mayers, 1973). To negotiate mutual goals, the client needs to understand the nurse's purposes.

The initial letter, telephone call, or home visit is the time to share your ideas with the family about why you are contacting them. During the first interpersonal encounter by telephone or home visit, explore the family members' ideas about

the purpose of your visits. This phase is essential in establishing a mutually agreed on basis for a series of encounters. As a result of her qualitative research study of maternal-child home visiting, Byrd (2006, p. 271) states that "people enter…relationships with the expectation of receiving a benefit" that may be information, status, service, or goods. Byrd asserts that it is important for nurses to create client expectations through previsit publicity about (marketing) home-visiting programs. Also it is essential to understand the expectations of the specific persons being visited.

Family members may have had previous relationships with community/public health nurses and students. Family members may be able to share such information as what they found to be most helpful, why they are willing to work with a nurse or student again, and what goals they have in mind. Other families who have had no prior experience with community/public health nurses may not have specific expectations. Asking is important.

A contract is a specific, structured **agreement** regarding the process and conditions by which a health-related goal will be sought. In the beginning of most student learning experiences, the agreement usually entails one or more family members continuing to meet with the nursing student for a specific number of visits or weeks. Initially, specific goals and the nurse's role regarding health promotion and illness prevention may be unclear. (If this role was already clear, undergoing a period of study and orientation would be unnecessary.)

Initially, the agreement may be as simple as, "We will meet here at your house next Tuesday at 11:00 until around noon to continue to discuss what I can offer related to your family's health and what you'd like. We can get to know each other better. We can talk more about how the week has gone for you and your family with your new baby." These statements are the nurse's oral offer to meet under specific conditions of time and place. The process of mutual discussion is mentioned. The goals remain general and implicit: fostering the family's developmental task of incorporating an infant and fostering family-nurse relatedness. For the next week's contract to be complete, the family member or members would have to agree. The most important element initially is whether agreement about being present at a specific time and place can be reached. If 11:00 AM is not workable for the family, would another time during the day when you both are available be mutually agreeable? For families who do not focus as much on the future, a community/public health nurse needs to be more flexible in scheduling the time of each visit.

The word *contract* often implies legally binding agreements. This is not true of nurse-client contracts. Nurses are legally and ethically bound to keep their word in relation to nursing care; clients are not legally bound to keep their agreements. However, establishing a mutual agreement for relating increases the clarity of who will do what, when, where, for what purposes, and under what conditions. Because of some people's negative response to the word contract, agreement or discussion of responsibilities may be better.

An agreement may be oral or written. For some families, written agreements, especially early in the relationship, may be a threat. For example, a family who has been conned by a household repair scheme may be very suspicious of written agreements. Families who are not legal citizens may not want to sign an agreement for fear that if it is not kept they will be punished. Do not push for a written agreement if the family is uncomfortable. If you do notice such discomfort, this may be a good opportunity to explore their fears. Written agreements are required when insurance is paying for the care provided by nurses working with home health agencies and to comply with the Health Insurance Portability and Accountability Act (HIPAA).

Helgeson and Berg (1985) describe factors affecting the contracting process by studying a small convenience sample of 15 community/public health nursing students and 12 client responses. Of the 11 students who introduced the idea of a contract to clients, all did so between the second and the fourth visits of a 16-week series of visits; 9 students did so orally rather than in writing. There was not one specific time that was best. Eight clients were very receptive to the idea because they liked the idea of establishing goals to work toward and felt the contract would serve as a reminder of their responsibility. The very process of developing a draft agreement to present to families provides the novice practitioner with an increased focus of care, clarity of nurse and family responsibilities and activities, and a basis from which to negotiate modifications in client behaviors (Helgeson & Berg, 1985; Sheridan & Smith, 1975).

The Home Visiting Evaluation Tool in Figure 11-3 lists nurse behaviors that are appropriate for home visits, especially initial home visits and those early in a series of home visits. Nurses can use this list as a preplanning tool to identify their readiness to conduct a specific home visit. Additionally, students and community/public health nurses have used the tool to evaluate initial home visits and identify their behaviors that were omitted and needed to be included on the second home visits. The tool also has been used jointly as an evaluation tool by nurses and supervisors and students and faculty.

INCREASING UNDERSTANDING THROUGH COMMUNICATION SKILLS

The nurse's ability to *be* with family members determines the success of the nurse-family relationship. A nurse can employ techniques of speaking and listening appropriately and still not have a working relationship because of the absence of caring. Mayers (1973) reports that each of the community/public health nurses studied had her or his own interactional style: some were nondirective listeners, calm, and relatively quiet; others were more verbally active and directive. Most nurses did not demonstrate a balanced use of communication techniques, yet those who were unable to *be* with the families had a successful relationship in spite of their imperfect technique.

Communication techniques do have their place as skills for community/public health nurses. Through communication, the

HOME VISITING EVALUATION TOOL

This Home Visiting Evaluation Tool is built upon behaviors of initiation, implementation, and termination within each visit.

Directions: Place a check in the appropriate box below:

Family name	Date and time of home visit					
Nursing Activities	Present	Absent	N/A	Present	Absent	N/A
1. Determines name, etc., of client						
2. Has planned the visit						
3. Introduces self						
4. Links self with others						
5. Accepts client non-judgmentally						
6. Identifies household members						
7. Assesses client's capacity to comprehend						
8. States with whom you will communicate						
9. Initiates contract						
a. Time						
b. Day						
c. Beginning week						
d. Ending week						
e. Attendance						

FIGURE 11-3 Home Visiting Evaluation Tool. (From Chichester, M., & Smith, C. [1980]. *Home visiting evaluation tool* [unpublished manuscript]. Baltimore, MD: University of Maryland School of Nursing.)

Continued

Family name	Date and time of home visit					
f. Cancellations						
g. Purpose						
h. What you will offer						
i. Your constraints						
j. Exploration of expectations						
k. What client may offer						
10. Negotiates mutually acceptable contract						
11. Reduces distraction						
12. Listens actively						
13. Allows and supports distance						
14. Explores client's ideas						
15. Relates own understanding of what has been said						
16. Seeks shared meanings of words						
17. Explores ambivalence						
18. Tolerates silence						
19. Has verbal/nonverbal communications that are congruent						
20. Focuses discussion appropriately						
21. Completes a relevant tangible intervention						
22. Reinforces positive behaviors						
23. Avoids giving disapproval						
24. Avoids defending others						
25. Avoids "talking down" to client						
26. Avoids cliches/stereotyping						
27. Avoids prolonging the contact						
28. Gives client in writing						
a. Your name						
b. Agency phone number						
c. Other significant information						
29. Summarizes agreed upon points						
30. Leaves promptly						

FIGURE 11-3, CONT'D

nurse discovers the meanings of particular things to families and validates these meanings. Through communication, the nurse comes to understand the family and their circumstances, goals, and preferences.

Leitch and Tinker (1978) discuss clusters of communication skills and their purposes and guidelines for use. Listening, leading, reflecting, and summarizing are important communication skills. Listening skills assist nurses in clarifying and validating messages. Leading skills assist nurses in focusing and questioning for the purposes of expanding the scope and depth of factual and emotional messages and reducing confusion. These skills are basic to all nursing relationships, and they are especially important to community/public health nurses because the nurse is probably the sole collector of information. Time passes between home visits, during which events occur in the family's life. Unlike in a hospital setting, in which records or reports are given from nurses on previous shifts, on home visits the nurse must update the assessment based mainly on what the family says. Reflecting skills allow community/public health nurses to understand the family's frame of reference and the meaning of its concerns. Reflecting also allows the family members to know that they have been understood.

In working with families and individuals over time, the opportunity to identify themes of communication emerges. Analytic skills can be of assistance. When themes become clearer, the family and nurse can work on more basic issues rather than on piecemeal episodes. For example, during week 2 of a series of home visits, a young mother had missed a well-child appointment; during week 4, she missed her own appointments to a general practitioner to monitor the blood levels of her antiseizure medications and to the dentist to treat her related gum problems. By week 6, she had not made any new appointments. The student, Juanita, was able to recognize a theme of unkept appointments and summarize the past weeks with the mother.

When Juanita confronted her own feelings, she realized that she was frustrated and angry that the mother had not kept her word and had not made progress toward what Juanita believed had been mutual goals. Juanita expressed the intensity of her own feelings to faculty and peers rather than directly with the client. She wanted neither to blame nor to attack the mother with her own anger. Rather, she expressed herself calmly to the mother by describing the pattern of making, missing, and not remaking appointments.

When Juanita asked the mother to explain, the mother agreed that the infant's shots were important, that she had been "worried about her living arrangements and felt tired," and that she would make and keep the infant's future appointments. She explained that because she had suffered from seizures for so long, she knew to go to the physician when she was seriously ill but would not go routinely. Although Juanita did not like the mother's response about her own health, she accepted it as the mother's own frame of reference. Juanita pointed out that more frequent medical appointments might help to prevent seizures. The mother still said she would not go to the physician.

Juanita returned from the home visit no longer angry. She expected that the mother would have her son immunized before the end of the semester (twelfth visit) and that she would not obtain medical care for herself at this time. Her expectations were fulfilled.

The efficiency of identifying themes usually increases with the nurse's experience. Discussing families with your peer group and faculty or supervisor allows you to identify others' perceptions of family themes, while maintaining confidentiality. Expanding possible meanings provides you more flexibility and depth of interpretations. You have an opportunity to return to the family with renewed ability to validate the meaning of behavior with the family. This process may result in the family having a clearer understanding or interpretation of their own behavior.

REDUCING POTENTIAL CONFLICTS

Acknowledging that the nurse can feel uneasy because of reduced control during home visits, how is mutuality facilitated?

Because coercion has little place in public health and nursing, how can a nurse exert influence over the health of family members?

The truth is that the one person you can change is yourself. Changing yourself is under your direct control. Through changes in *yourself*, you *may* be able to affect your relationship with a client so that a shift in her or his being and behavior may take place. A paradox of relationships is that the more you focus on changing, fixing up, or making another person "better," the more likely that person is to feel dominated and to resist change. Through managing your own anxiety and your degree of self-attention, you may shift your being and behavior sufficiently to provide the family members with openness and self-expression. By attuning to their perception of reality, you have a basis for dialogue, therapeutic relationship, and practical problem solving.

How does a nurse manage her or his own anxiety or self-absorption in a home that is likely very different from the nurse's own home? Expectations, role insecurity, value interference, and the client's reaction to the nurse are potential sources of conflict (Friedman, 1983).

MATCHING THE NURSE'S EXPECTATIONS WITH REALITY

Surprises often shock or unnerve and reduce a person's ability to feel in control. Have you ever attempted to use a piece of medical equipment that you have never seen before? Did you wonder how to make it work? Did you feel anxious that you might do something foolish? Were you thinking that other people were watching you and thinking that you were an incompetent nurse? If someone had described the machine to you ahead of time, talked you through the procedure, and warned you of the machine's idiosyncrasies, might you have felt more prepared, more in control, and less anxious? For many of you, the answer is yes.

Similarly, learning about a neighborhood and a family before your home visit can allow you to anticipate what you will find, reduce surprises, and promote your feelings of calmness and self-control. In such a state, you are much more likely to be attentive in your relationship with family members.

Learning about the family before the home visit can be accomplished by gathering as much information as possible. These data may be obtained by calling the person who initiated the referral to you, by having the liaison nurse or discharge planner obtain the information from the hospitalized family member, by calling the family, and by looking at the family identification information if you are working in a health maintenance organization or health department.

1. Who is in the family? How old are they? Who is likely to be there during your home visit? If you know that three preschoolers are at home, you can be mentally prepared for relating with children and for the possible exuberance of their presence.

2. What are the related developmental tasks of the family members? Anticipating these tasks can suggest possible situations in the family that are timely topics for discussion. For example, if it is autumn, is a child adjusting to kindergarten or first grade?

3. How receptive might this family be to your visit? Has the family initiated the request for service? If not, what have

they been told about the referral to you? Has the family been visited previously by community/public health nurses or nursing students? What is the family's past or current relationship with the agency with which you are affiliated? Does the family usually keep outpatient office and clinical appointments? Nurses previously involved with the family may be able to describe the family's usual way of presenting themselves.

4. With what other health and social service agencies and providers are the family involved? Are all of the relationships voluntary, or are some of them court ordered? This information assists you in clarifying part of the family's support system, as well as to initiate discussion about persons already known to the family.

5. What will the environment be like? In some neighborhoods, predicting what the inside of a home looks like based on the exterior of the building is misleading.

A disadvantage of collecting information about the family before your initial home visit is that the information may bias your point of view about the family. Some nurses prefer to visit first and then validate their perceptions with data from other sources.

CLARIFYING NURSING RESPONSIBILITIES

The purpose of the visit constitutes another category of data to be collected in the preinitiation phase of the relationship before the home visit.

- What has the family been told about the purpose of your visit, and what are the family's expectations?
- If the family initiated the request for services, what specifically do they want?
- What is the goal of the agency or program for whom you are working?
- What is the job description for you and your peers?

Uncertainty and ambivalence are common responses of nurses who have little experience in home visiting. Talk about your anxieties with faculty, supervisors, or more experienced nurses.

For registered nurses who are skilled at providing nursing practice in inpatient settings, home visiting adds complexity. The reduced control, increased focus on family, expanded teaching, adaptation of care to the home, and increased primary prevention add complexity to the already-established role (see Chapter 1).

Once you have contacted the family by telephone or at their home, listen actively to the specifics and themes of what is communicated. What is not talked about may be as important as what is mentioned. Following up on cues can provide important information for you. For example, when reviewing the health of household members with the nurse during a home visit, a mother spoke positively about all of her children except Patti. When the mother did not even mention Patti, the nurse specifically commented, "We haven't talked about Patti yet." The mother hesitantly said they did not get along and changed the subject. The nurse now knew more about the meaning of the mother's omission.

The desire to have families be appreciative and cooperative can backfire. Families may test what the nurse is willing to do, or they may be so overwhelmed and looking for help that they make inappropriate or unrealistic demands. Families sometimes ask for time, money, rides, or assistance with tasks that they can accomplish themselves. Other families are so emotionally distraught that they seek relief from their uncomfortable feelings by placing unrealistic hopes on the nurse. The nurse tries to develop a relationship with a family that inspires their trust. Limit setting on the part of the nurse helps establish trust. For example, if a client asks for a loan to pay the rent, you might reply, "I will not loan you money, but I will help you think about other plans for paying your bills." Agreeing to demands that are unrealistic or uncomfortable for the nurse will eventually erode the relationship. The nurse needs to learn to be comfortable identifying and stating limits to the family starting at the very first visit.

You would not have come this far in your nursing education and practice were you not committed to being a successful nurse and contributing to the well-being of other persons. Rather than worry about your success in a new environment, attempt to experience your home visits as the next step in your nursing journey.

MANAGING THE NURSE'S EMOTIONS

As with all relationships in nursing, our emotions can get in the way of our providing client-centered care. Anxiety has already been mentioned; sadness, disgust, anger, joy, and fear can also be evoked. Our emotions are linked through associations to events and situations in our lives. Although our emotional responses are often automatic and certainly color our perceptions, they are usually not rational. What seems to be *the* only feeling possible at the moment is really one of many. Another person may associate the environmental cue with an entirely different meaning and thereby have an entirely different emotional response.

Although community/public health nurses are confronted with a variety of home settings, lifestyles, family types, and cultures, possibly triggering strong emotions, family members may end the relationship if nurses are judgmental. One goal in therapeutic nursing relationships is to be open to possible interpretations of the situation other than your initial, automatic one. For example, if on an initial home visit a mother does not maintain eye contact with the nurse and the preschoolers shelter themselves behind her, the nurse might automatically conclude that she or he is not wanted and act accordingly, by leaving the visit prematurely. Perhaps the mother has low self-esteem or is relatively shy with strangers. Not making eye contact may also be a respectful gesture, especially to authority figures. Considering these possible meanings of the family's reaction to the home visit will at least remind the nurse that the meaning of the mother's behavior is not known. *Not knowing* provides an opportunity for further discussion of the purpose of the visit and of the mother's perception of that purpose, as well as of the mother's concerns and possible ambivalence.

MAINTAINING FLEXIBILITY IN RESPONSE TO CLIENT REACTIONS

The nurse should not assume that a client's behavior is a reaction rationally linked to the nurse's behavior. Her or his culture, family values, and personal experience influence the way a particular individual behaves at a given moment. In the example given previously, the mother may rarely maintain eye contact with anyone except a close friend or sister. Because the nurse-family relationship is in the initiation stage, some testing behavior may automatically occur regardless of the nurse's behavior. The client may unconsciously ask, "Is the nurse sufficiently interested to continue caring for *me*?"

Conversely, do not assume that your behavior has no effect on the client's responses and behavior during the home visit. By definition, communication is interactive. How you present yourself with family members makes a difference with them.

CLARIFYING CONFIDENTIALITY OF DATA

If both the nurse and the family members are clear about who is working with the family and what information is being shared, the potential for conflict will be far less. The nurse and family expectations about shared information will be aligned.

Furthermore, nurses must follow the privacy regulations of the 1996 federal Health Insurance Portability and Accountability Act (HIPAA) that became effective in April 2003 (Frank-Stromber & Ganschow, 2002). These regulations cover any health care information that can be used to identify an individual. The regulations address privacy rights, confidentiality, and who should and should not have access to client information.

Clients have a right to know what information is being entered in the legal health record and with whom the nurse is sharing that information. Remember that individual clients have the right to read their own health records and the records of their children and of those under their guardianship. Keep the following in mind when recording: objective data, not inferences or generalizations, should be recorded. Describe client behaviors, but do not attribute motivation. For example, note that the "client spoke rapidly," and the client stated, "they can't make me give my child medicine." Do not record that the "client doesn't like health providers," which is an invalidated, overgeneralized conclusion.

Other health care providers employed by your health care agency may have access to the legal record if they are involved in providing direct care, consulting with you, or supervising your care. Identifying with the client the specific health care providers with whom you will share information routinely is honest and fair. For example, "I will share this information about your child with my supervisor, the nurses who work in the clinic, and the physician(s) there. Sometimes I may speak with Dr. X, your pediatrician."

Written permission of the client or of the parent or guardian of a minor is required to obtain or release written information from other agencies or disciplines in private practice (see Chapter 6). With the client's knowledge, you may share and seek information orally to collaborate in providing care. As discussed earlier, some situations are such that the nurse is required by law to share information without client consent. Even when you are initiating a referral for suspected abuse or neglect, discussing your problem solving with the available family members would be appropriate. Though these family members may be unhappy or angry, you have acknowledged them by providing information. Remember that the right of minors to sign for permission for their own treatment varies from state to state.

Before the home visit, clarify your state's laws that govern consent of minors and mandatory reporting of selected circumstances (such as child abuse) by health providers. With your supervisor or faculty, identify the usual and customary people within the agency with whom you will be sharing information.

PROMOTING NURSE SAFETY

The safety of community/public health nurses is critical. The purpose of the home visit is to offer or provide nursing services that make a contribution to the family's health *and* to do so while maintaining the nurse's safety. The purpose of a home visit is not to provide care *at all costs*. Assertiveness, not abandonment of one's own needs, is required, which is especially true when you are learning to be a community/public health nurse and testing yourself and the boundaries of your professional role.

CLARIFYING THE NURSE'S SELF-RESPONSIBILITY

Nurses will encounter some clients who are hostile, angry, volatile, or potentially violent. This type of encounter is true of individuals in an acute inpatient setting and in their homes (e.g., a person with dementia who is combative). Therefore why do many nurses who are beginning home visits (as well as their families) express anxiety and fear? The reason is largely because the nurse has less control over the environment on a home visit.

The experience of home visiting is new and unknown. There are no hospital or agency walls within which to practice, no backup personnel immediately available, no receptionist, and, often, no security guards. The community/public health nurse often visits alone.

Community/public health nurses visit in every type of household and neighborhood. Each nurse has grown up in a specific family constellation and neighborhoods, with particular socioeconomic, ethnic, religious, and racial compositions. We are more comfortable with people who are similar to ourselves and with environments similar to those to which we are most accustomed. Practicing as a community/public health nurse will probably expand these boundaries.

As the incidence of violence in our society has increased, concerns about safety in general have grown. This increase has become especially true in neighborhoods in which drug trafficking, gang activity, and violent crimes occur. Having acknowledged all these potentially dangerous circumstances, putting the potential threats in perspective is necessary. Community/public health nurses are generally known in communities and acknowledged as having special skills and relationships that contribute to the residents' well-being. Community/public health nurses collectively have been seen as caring, helpful, constructive persons throughout their history. As a visitor who represents nursing, you have the protection of this general community attitude.

Community/public health nurses are also usually perceived differently in a community than are police and social workers because nurses' roles are perceived to have less *threat of law*. As discussed elsewhere, community/public health nurses are usually invited in, or families at least have the opportunity to decline nursing services. Consequently, nurses are seen as being helpful rather than threatening.

What is done to promote the safety of community/public health nurses? In very high-risk neighborhoods, some nurses are accompanied by police, neighborhood volunteers, or paid security escorts (Nadwairski, 1992) (Box 11-5). Almost universally, nurses may request that another nurse or their supervisor accompany them on visits to neighborhoods and homes

Box 11-5   Safety and Home Visiting

1. If possible, obtain the family's permission to work with them by telephone before home visiting.
2. Ask for directions to their road, driveway, building, or apartment.
3. Always leave an itinerary with the agency for each clinical day that includes the name of the family to be visited, their address and telephone number, and the license plate number and make of the automobile you are driving.
4. Consider whether certain times of day are safer for visits in certain areas.
5. Do not carry purses or wear jewelry other than engagement or wedding rings. Do not wear rings with large gems.
6. Wear the appropriate dress (uniform or street clothes) determined by the agency.
7. Carry coins for telephone calls or a cell phone and a small amount of money for emergencies.
8. Carry an identification badge and wear a name pin.
9. Avoid secluded areas such as stairwells, alleys, basements, and empty buildings or obtain an escort.
10. Avoid areas where persons are loitering or obtain an escort.
11. Use discretion about visiting a family. If you feel unsafe—do not visit.
12. In the residence, sit between the client and the exit.
13. Consider asking for pets to be removed from the room.
14. If approached on the street by someone requesting a home visit, refer them to the office of the public health or home health agency.
15. Consider whether an escort is needed to avoid visiting a lone man if you are a woman or visiting a lone woman if you are a man.
16. Request a nurse partner or escort to a home visit if needed.
17. Avoid entering a home in which fights, drug use, or drug sales are in progress.
18. Always report back to the agency in person or by telephone at the end of the clinical day.
19. Visit only during your scheduled work hours. If you must make an exception to this time, permission from your supervisor must be obtained.

in which they are uncomfortable. In some agencies, the ethical decision has been made to forbid nursing visits to selected neighborhoods, apartment developments, or families for the nurse's protection. Family members can be invited to more neutral territory, such as a school, clinic, or library, for an interaction. Telephone visits may at times be substituted for some home visits.

PROMOTING SAFE TRAVEL

All community/public health nurses can benefit from basic crime prevention courses that local or state police provide regarding safety on the street and in automobiles. Knowing that she or he is incorporating basic self-protection behaviors is especially helpful for a community/public health nurse. For nurses driving in remote areas, having cellular telephones or citizen-band radios and knowing what to carry for weather emergencies are especially important. Some community health agencies supply nurses with telephones or radios.

HANDLING THREATS DURING HOME VISITS

Actual and potential threats can occur during home visits. What should a community/public health nurse do if the family is engaged in an altercation or fight when the nurse arrives? What if family members appear to be intoxicated or under the influence of drugs? What if someone in the family displays a weapon? Although no single, absolutely correct response exists, some guiding principles may be helpful. The first rule is to protect your own safety because you are of no assistance if you become entangled in an altercation or are harmed. If you are feeling sufficiently fearful or anxious that your functioning is compromised, or if you perceive that your presence is further aggravating the circumstances, then either do not enter the home or leave the home if you have already entered.

You can ask the family whether another time to visit would be better; or you can announce that you will not stay and that you will call or come at another time. By sometimes having their focus shifted by the presence of an outsider, the situation is temporarily defused. Always notify your supervisor or faculty as soon as possible. Remember, though, as a beginning community/public health nurse, you may feel less confident than someone with more experience. Erring on the side of being *too cautious* as regards your own safety is acceptable. If, however, you are finding that most home visits seem threatening, you must speak with your faculty, preceptor, or supervisor to help identify the source of perceived threats and ways to relieve them.

PROTECTING THE SAFETY OF FAMILY MEMBERS

The second principle is to protect the safety of each family member. How can you accomplish this task if you are no longer in their house? If you believe that someone is in imminent physical danger or is being injured, you need to call the policing authority that responds to domestic violence. If someone has been injured, you should call for both police and rescue workers. If you believe that dependent children or adults are being neglected or abused, you need to contact your faculty or supervisor and follow your school's or agency's policies and procedures. Short of these priorities, the community/public health nurse is not legally bound to respond.

After you have gained experience with a specific family or are more experienced in dealing with family anger in general, you can use communication and crisis intervention to alter the family's self-expression. All of your knowledge and experience in psychiatric and mental health nursing is of value in such circumstances. In some agencies, psychiatric nursing consultants are available to coach you in responding to family members who exhibit anger. Psychiatric emergency teams are available for home visits in some communities.

Families generally present a more reserved, social self to nurses, especially at first. Consequently, illegal behavior is often hidden from the nurse. As a beginner, do not probe your speculations about illegal behavior. For example, if several different people are coming in and out of a house during each of your visits, you might suspect that drug sales are taking place. However, you usually would not ask, "Is someone here dealing drugs?" Seek consultation from your faculty or supervisor instead. In some households, members may be intoxicated from consuming alcohol or may be using illicit drugs during the visit. Such individuals are likely to be cognitively impaired and will not benefit from your visit. You should indicate that you will return at another time and leave the home. If other family members who are at risk of harm, such as an infant who is not being supervised, are being cared for by the intoxicated person, you should follow the policies and procedures for notifying the appropriate authorities.

If clients have weapons that are unsafely displayed in the home, requesting that weapons be put away during or before your visits is your right. For example, an elderly man kept a loaded pistol with him for protection in his efficiency apartment. The nurse requested that, because he knew when she was coming, he put his gun away before he answered the door for her. When he refused, he was given a choice between keeping his gun out and having nursing visits. After some discussion, the man chose to store his gun when the nurse visited.

Ethically, you need to encourage family safety related to proper storage of weapons, especially when children or adults with compromised cognition or proneness to violence are present. Some states or local jurisdictions have legislation governing safe gun storage in homes.

MANAGING TIME AND EQUIPMENT

The community/public health nurse's effectiveness depends on planning the day for the efficient use of time and other resources. Physical resources are often limited to equipment carried by the nurse, or provided by the family at the home, or both. Consequently, *making do* with what is at hand and doing this consistent with basic principles of safety and infection control are the hallmarks of a skilled community/public health nurse, although more specialized equipment is being used in the home to care for sicker individuals (see Chapter 31). Box 11-2 discusses activities for planning a home visit that will increase efficiency.

STRUCTURING TIME

The time devoted to a home visit may vary; an hour is often used as a basis for planning. As many as seven visits per day may be expected of nurses in some home health agencies. Geographic location, travel time, and client priorities help establish the order of visits. Visits to persons with infected wounds should be scheduled after home visits to healthy or immunosuppressed individuals.

Some visits may last only the few minutes required to determine that a family either is absent from the home or is engaged in other activities that make home visiting inappropriate at that time. Other visits may approach 2 hours in length, especially an initial visit to a family with a member who is being admitted to the services of a home health agency. In such a case, consent forms must be signed, assessments must be performed, environmental evaluations must be done to determine equipment needs, and direct care techniques must be demonstrated to family members. An hour for novices usually proves sufficient time to accommodate some inefficiencies in interviewing, relating, and performing nursing care. If family members are especially anxious or upset, visits may take longer. If equipment must be improvised or modified, or if a health-related emergency exists, more time will probably be needed.

Conversely, visits may need to be shortened when the stamina of the family members is compromised. An interview with a person with shortness of breath, for example, needs to be paced so that the person does not become tired. Some family members think concretely rather than abstractly; thus short, frequent visits allow the nurse to focus on one or two items at a time. Shorter visits result in greater clarity and timely correction or reinforcement, or both, of the family's health-related behaviors.

HANDLING EMERGENCIES

Emergencies in the family may extend the length of the home visit and are *always* to be handled before the nurse leaves unless the safety of the nurse is threatened. If the nurse were *not* making the home visit, the family would probably handle the emergency without the nurse, unless the nurse was one of the resources that the family contacted. More likely, the family would contact other family members, their private physician, the emergency department of a hospital, an ambulatory emergency center, or the rescue system. However, once the nurse is made aware that an emergency exists, the nurse's professional and legal responsibility is to address the emergency within the scope of nursing and to support the family to obtain appropriate resources.

Medical Emergencies

Responding to a medical emergency in the home is similar to responding to a client's emergency in the hospital in that in both circumstances the nurse has knowledge of basic assessment skills, cardiopulmonary resuscitation (CPR), asepsis, and nursing interventions to reduce client anxiety, conserve client energy, promote comfort, and prevent further dysfunction. However, the nurse in the home does not have the equipment and team members that are available to the hospital nurse. Equipment in the home is probably limited to what the nurse brings—soap, clean gloves, a sphygmomanometer, a stethoscope, thermometers, and clean dressings. The only medication available is that of the respective family members. The medical orders are those of the family member's physician or nurse practitioner, which may be known to the nurse from written medical orders to the nurse or from written and oral instructions to family members. Many agencies also have written policies and procedures for handling a variety of emergencies. Knowledge of basic and advanced first aid is appropriate for any nurse making home visits (American Red Cross, 2000). In addition to knowing what family members are taught to do in emergencies, a nurse who starts with first-aid skills and incorporates basic nursing practice and agency policy will be functioning on a firm foundation.

As presented in CPR classes, the priorities in physiologic emergencies are the ABCs—airway, breathing, and circulation. In these three emergencies, appropriate use of CPR is required, which includes activating the emergency rescue system.

Poisoning is usually considered the fourth life-threatening priority. Nurses should always carry their state's poison control telephone number; nurses are to call this number to verify the importance of any suspected poisoning and to ascertain the need for any immediate treatment before medical treatment.

Other physical emergencies include acute deficits in hydration or nutrition and environmental safety hazards that may be life-threatening. Of similar magnitude are the psychologic emergencies of potential suicide, homicide, and abuse, which have been discussed previously.

Community/public health nurses often encounter family members who exhibit signs or symptoms that have not yet been diagnosed by a physician or nurse practitioner. Are these signals of normal variations that bother the family member? Is a referral for medical diagnosis appropriate? Are these signals of an unstable condition or an impending emergency that requires immediate referral? These are distinctions that community/public health nurses assist families to make.

Other Family Emergencies

Families, in addition to individual family members, also have emergencies. Unexpected situations requiring immediate action do constitute emergencies for families. Emergencies often relate to an unhealthy environment, such as loss of heat, potable water, or refrigeration for food. Families may have insufficient funds to pay heating bills or repair a refrigerator, or community disasters, such as storms or fires, may have interrupted utilities. A family may be experiencing an impending or actual eviction. Food, water, clothing, shelter, and safety are basic for survival, and their loss usually constitutes an emergency.

Families may also experience crises in which the stressors exceed their coping skills. A birth, death, unemployment, or chronic illness may tax their coping. Stress may manifest as acute physical or psychiatric illness in one or more family members.

How does a community/public health nurse relate to such emergencies? What does the nurse do? Referrals are appropriate for emergency food, clothing, and shelter. The local or state department of social services has some resources for emergency food stamps and shelter. Agencies such as the Salvation Army and Red Cross, as well as religious and civic organizations, supply emergency provisions. Members of the extended family, neighbors, or volunteers may be mobilized to stay with the family for support during the crisis.

PROMOTING ASEPSIS IN THE HOME

The goals of infection control in the home are to prevent the spread of communicable organisms from one family member to another and from one household to another, to protect individual family members who are especially susceptible to infection, and to protect the nurse from infection. The Centers for Disease Control and Prevention (CDC, 1998; Siegel et al., 2007) publishes infection-control standards for the hospital and other settings. The community health nurse adapts these standards to the circumstances of each household and to the specific needs of the family. See Box 11-6 for some ways to promote asepsis during home visits.

Some visits will be entirely *talking* visits and involve no direct physical care. For example, you might be making a home visit to a mother of school-age children when they are in school. If your initial purposes are to introduce yourself, obtain the mother's agreement to work together, and collect identifying information and health history for the record, no direct physical contact may occur. Unless the mother herself is ill and requires some physical assessment or she exhibits risk factors that indicate the need for screening (e.g., high blood pressure), you need not wash your hands and use equipment from the nursing bag. Your hands are clean from having washed them before leaving the agency or the previous home visit.

Hand-Washing

Hand-washing is as an essential component of infection control in homes as it is in all other settings of practice. In the hospital, nursing home, or clinic, the sink with water, soap, and paper towels is an expected part of the environment. Running water will not always be available in homes. The water may be temporarily shut off while the pipes or hot water heater is being fixed. In one instance, a family owned its own condominium and had faucets that leaked excessively. Rather than pay for a plumbing bill, the family turned the water off under each sink until it was needed. Some homes have well or cistern water that must be carried in from outside, sometimes over a great distance.

All sinks in homes are considered to be dirty. This determination is not meant as a judgment of the family's house-cleaning skills; rather, it is a basic principle of medical asepsis. The community/public health nurse does not know what else has touched the sink or how the sink has been used.

Some homes will have sinks, running water, liquid soap, and separate hand towels for guests. Unless a known infection exists in the home, the nurse may use these family supplies for hand-washing. Other homes will have sinks and running water but will have a bar of soap and towel that everyone in the household uses. In this case, neither the soap nor the towel is

---

| Box 11-6 | **Asepsis during a Home Visit** |

1. Airborne organisms can be transmitted to and from you and among family members, even without direct contact. Noticing respiratory symptoms among family members offers an opportunity to *teach family members about managing coughs and sneezes and performing hand-washing and other infection-control measures.*

2. If you have a respiratory illness yourself, you need to identify the likely degree of communicability; as in the hospital, nurses need to distinguish their allergies from colds, manage their symptoms, and avoid clients with compromised immunity. In community/public health nursing, the nurse may wear a mask and be fastidious about hand-washing, postpone the visit until another day, or have another nurse act as a substitute.

3. Lice and scabies can be transmitted from clothing, bedding, and upholstered furniture. In some households, the furniture is multipurpose—for sleeping and for sitting. When this situation occurs, *sitting in un-upholstered furniture, if available, such as a wood or plastic chair is best.* Routinely avoid sitting on beds, both as a protection to

yourself and so as not to transmit any organisms from your clothing to the bedding.

4. When you remove your coat, either continue to sit on it, or remove it completely and fold it with the outside out; the outside is considered less clean to you. Washing uniforms in hot water (55° C or 131° F for 20 minutes) or dry cleaning or driers set on the "hot cycle" promotes infection control (Heymann, 2004).

5. Direct physical contact and using equipment introduce the necessity for medical asepsis or clean technique by the community/public health nurse. *Take as little equipment into the home as you anticipate you will need;* do not carry purses, knapsacks, extra records, or books. If you travel by car, you can stock extra supplies and resources there. Usually sufficient is to take a pen, paper, permission forms to be signed, health records to be completed, emergency telephone numbers, educational materials, and a nursing bag (with hand-washing equipment and basic physical assessment equipment) into the home. Some agencies also provide small policy and procedure handbooks.

clean enough for the nurse to use. Sometimes, no waste receptacle will be available. Consequently, the nurse must always include soap, paper towels, and bags for waste as a part of the standard equipment for home visiting (Box 11-7).

Handling Equipment

Proper handling of equipment prevents the spread of communicable organisms. Each agency usually specifies the standard equipment each nurse is to have on a home visit; minimally,

equipment for physical assessments is included. When sterile equipment is needed, the family usually obtains it from a supply company. Cleansing equipment in the home is sometimes needed to prevent contamination of the nursing bag and subsequent transmittal of organisms to other households and individuals (Box 11-8).

The Centers for Disease Control and Prevention has recommended that *all* individuals receive care as though they are potentially positive for human immunodeficiency virus and

---

Box 11-7   Hand-Washing Procedures

Hand-Washing Procedure with Running Water
Equipment
1. Liquid soap in squeeze bottle (Antimicrobial soap is needed only when contact precautions are required, a client is severely immunosuppressed, or invasive procedures will be done [Rhinehart & Friedman, 1999].)
2. Paper towels
3. Trash receptacle (paper or plastic bags)

Procedure
1. Remove soap and paper towels from nursing bag.
2. Place one paper towel down as a clean field.
3. Squeeze soap into the palm of one hand, and place the soap container on the clean field.
4. Carry the remaining paper towels to the sink area. Place paper towels under one arm and hold them against your side. This action prevents them from getting wet or being placed on the dirty sink.
5. Turn on the water, adjust temperature to warm, and wash and rinse hands.
6. Dry hands with paper towels.
7. Turn off water with paper towels.
8. Dispose of paper towels in household receptacle or return to nursing bag and use the receptacles provided.

    A major advantage of this procedure is that the equipment does not have to be taken to the dirty sink where it can get wet and contaminated. The disadvantage is that the soap may be left out of sight of the nurse, which may present a poisoning hazard to a confused family member or a child. If you have any doubts, take the soap with you,

replace it in the bag before going to the sink, or assign a responsible person to guard the equipment. Other procedures involve taking the soap to the bathroom.

Hand-Washing Procedure with Poured Water
Substitute the previous step 5 with the following:
5. Have another person pour a small amount of water from a clean pitcher, glass, jar, or other utensil over your hands. (To warm the water, water may be heated in a small saucepan on a stove, burner, or fire, and then cooled with additional water as needed.)

Hand-Washing Procedure without Water
Germicide liquids and aerosols are commercially available for hand-washing without water and can be carried in the nursing bag. Avoid scented products, which may act as asthma triggers.

Equipment
1. Bottle or can of waterless, antimicrobial hand-washing product

Procedure
1. Squeeze or spray small amount onto hand.
2. Rub germicide onto all surfaces of hands, fingers, and fingernails for 30 seconds. The germicide evaporates, and no towel is needed (Trotter, 1996).
3. Hand-washing with a germicide is only effective for four cleansings. Water must be used for the fifth washing.

Box 11-8   Cleaning Equipment in the Home

Remember: The rule of thumb is to bring as little equipment in and out of the home as possible to decrease the possibility of cross-contamination.

Equipment
1. Article to be washed
2. Soap
3. Running water
4. Paper towels
5. Plastic bags
6. Disposable gloves

Procedure
1. Don disposable gloves when working with equipment contaminated with any body fluids or blood.
2. Rinse article with cold running water. (Rationale: Cold water releases organic material from the equipment, whereas warm or hot water will make the material adhere.)

3. Wash with hot, soapy water using friction.
4. Rinse well with clean water.
5. Dry thoroughly.
6. Disinfect equipment or article as indicated: one part household chlorine bleach to nine parts water or phenolic germicidal detergent solutions, such as Lysol, diluted according to product label.
7. Dry thoroughly.
8. Remove disposable gloves.
9. Dispose of gloves (inside out) into plastic trash bag using blood and body fluid precautions.
10. Wash hands.

Data from Rhinehart, E., & Friedman, M. (1999). *Infection control in home care.* Gaithersburg, MD: Aspen (an official publication of the Association for Professionals in Infection Control and Epidemiology, Inc.).

other blood-borne infections. All health agencies adopt universal precautions when handling blood and body fluids, needles, and other materials (see Chapter 8). Infection-control guidelines for people living with infections (including AIDS) in the community also are included. Waste material contaminated with blood or body fluids should be double-bagged in plastic before disposal (Trotter, 1996).

MODIFYING EQUIPMENT AND PROCEDURES IN THE HOME

From its inception, district nursing involved teaching families in the home about the care of the ill and preventive hygiene practices. The nurse assisted the family in using available equipment, in modifying household items for health-related purposes, and in making equipment. How can a family make bed tables and bed rails? How can a drawer become an infant bed?

The need to modify home equipment has been reduced by the availability of durable medical equipment for purchase and rent (such as hospital beds and commodes) and disposable equipment (such as dressing trays). Medicare and some other health insurance and assistance plans often pay for such equipment. However, many people are not eligible for reimbursement because they are not eligible for skilled home health care (see Chapter 31). Therefore improvised equipment is a cost-effective means of assisting families to care for such individuals. Some home health books for nurses discuss equipment modifications (Humphrey, 1998).

While en route to homes, the nursing bag is to be kept clean and safe from theft. Always keep the bag in your sight, or have it locked in the vehicle's trunk or covered hatch or in a covered box. For example, do not drive to a restaurant for lunch, open the trunk, and place the bag in the trunk. Rather, immediately before leaving a home, put the bag in the trunk, and then drive away. The bag is safe and out of sight until it is needed at another home visit.

Just as the floor in a hospital is considered dirty, so too are streets, sidewalks, the ground, vehicle floors, and floors in homes. Do not place a nursing bag on any of these surfaces. Newspapers are considered clean and provide a field on which to place your nursing bag.

Modifications in using assessment equipment may also be needed. For example, infant scales are not always available. An alternative procedure is to weigh a parent on the bathroom scale, weigh the parent again with the infant, and subtract the first value from the second value. Although the parent should be dressed similarly at each visit to reduce variation, this procedure provides a gross estimate of infant weight.

Teaching family members to assess their own health status is often a responsibility of community/public health nurses. By using the family's equipment, the procedures can be tailored to specific circumstances. For example, using the thermometer that is available in the home and assisting the family members in effective, safe, clean use may be more appropriate. Cool water can be used as a lubricant for taking rectal temperature if clean petroleum jelly is not available. Family members can be taught that inserting thermometers into a jar of petroleum jelly that is also used for chapped hands and lips is unhygienic.

When families give medications, especially liquids, validating the type and size of spoons and droppers used is important to ensure that the doses given match the doses prescribed.

Alarm clocks and prefilled medication boxes can be used to assist families in remembering medication schedules.

POSTVISIT ACTIVITIES

You have prepared yourself for a home visit, considered your own safety, and conducted a home visit. You have considered your relatedness with the family and management of time and equipment. You have a right to feel successful and pleased with yourself. What comes next?

Postvisit activities provide a time for your evaluation and work on behalf of the family: **collaboration,** referral, and documenting. This conclusion of one visit becomes the beginning or preinitiation for the next encounter. A plan of care is derived from the information you have assessed. The initial home visit, the first of few or many visits in your nurse-family relationship, is complete.

EVALUATING AND PLANNING THE NEXT HOME VISIT

How does a community/public health nurse determine whether the home visit has been successful? What criteria are used to determine the success of any nurse-client encounter? The nurse usually looks at the scope and specificity of the nursing process, the degree of client satisfaction, the quality of the nurse-client relationship, and the health behavior and status of the client.

How can these criteria be applied to evaluating a specific home visit? Box 11-9 lists questions that were derived from the criteria; you may wish to develop more.

CONSULTING AND COLLABORATING WITH THE TEAM

Consultation is seeking the advice or opinion of an expert. Community/public health nurses may consult with a wide array of practitioners in other disciplines, such as medicine, physical therapy, and environmental hygiene. Nurses with specialties are also available. For example, psychiatric nurses can assist in formulating a plan of care for an interpersonally intense family situation; pediatric nurses in regional neonatal intensive care units can demonstrate the use of monitoring equipment to you and the parents before an infant who is at risk for sudden infant death syndrome is discharged to home. Your supervisor and peers are also available to share opinions about family care in formal and informal conferences.

Even if you are just beginning community/public health nursing practice, you are the individual who has made the home visit and experienced meeting the family in their environment. You are therefore in a position to collaborate with nursing and multidisciplinary teams. You are in a position to share assessment information, determine what it means to the family, and discuss nursing inferences you have derived. You are also able to contribute ideas for realistic goals and time frames. Developing a plan on which the entire team has agreed helps prevent duplication and gaps in care. For example, will home visits be made jointly by disciplines to prevent family confusion, or will home visits be made separately to promote intermittent reinforcement?

Consultation and collaboration may occur via the telephone (or other telecommunications, such as fax), by mail, or in person, depending on the complexity and urgency of the situation.

Box 11-9   Determining the Success of Your Home Visit

Preinitiation

- Was your preplanning adequate in scope to assist you in anticipating the needs of the family?
- How did a review of nursing literature before the home visit strengthen your knowledge base, promote evidence-based practice, and foster your role security?

Home Visit

- To what degree were you able to express your purpose for the home visit and to elicit the perception of family members?
- How were you able to address the purpose?
- Did any major issues arise for which you were not prepared? If so, how did you handle them?
- What data do you have to support your inferences about the family's satisfaction with the home visit? To what degree did you validate the accuracy of your inferences with the family members?
- How satisfied were you with your visit? What contributed to your satisfaction?
- What cues indicate that you and the family are engaged in the relationship?

- What cues indicate that the interactions were appropriate to the phase of the relationships?
- What health care behaviors did one or more family members agree to initiate or modify? What information did they indicate they better understood?
- Can you identify any changes in the health status of one or more family members?

Postvisit Activities

- How complete was your documentation? Were gaps in your database revealed? If so, what plans are necessary for collecting the missing data?
- What activities are necessary to complete any referrals?
- What consultation with your faculty, supervisor, or other members of the health care team would be helpful?
- What plans are evolving for your next home visit in the areas of data collection, teaching, other direct care, and referral?
- What changes, if any, in equipment, asepsis, or safety require planning before the next home visit?

Adapted from Smith, C. (1987). *Determining the success of your home visit* (unpublished manuscript). Baltimore, MD: University of Maryland School of Nursing. Used with permission.

Emergencies are best handled with telephone calls or citizens-band radio followed by written communications. Complex situations are best handled by face-to-face conferences (including teleconferencing), in which all disciplines can hear the same information simultaneously. One participant can be designated to write and circulate a meeting summary.

As a beginner, reporting to your supervisor about changes in family health status and functioning, emergencies, threats to your safety, and situations that you do not understand clearly is always the safest course of action. This process is considered necessary for sound legal practice.

MAKING REFERRALS

Referral is the act or instance of sending or directing someone for treatment, aid, information, or a decision. If the family members have needs that cannot be satisfied with available resources and the problem is not within the scope of your responsibility and capability (or that of your team), making a referral may be necessary.

Referrals may be indicated for the following reasons: screening procedures; medical diagnostic consultations, laboratory tests, or procedures; emergency services; nursing home placement; educational, vocational, and social services; or consultations with medical, nursing, and other disciplines regarding the treatment and care regimen (Smith, 1972).

Referral always consists of communication among three individuals: the client, the person making the referral, and the person or persons to whom the client has been referred. The most short-term goal is that the family member or members and the person to whom they are referred make contact. The intermediate goal is for the family to receive the desired treatment, aid, or information. The ultimate goal is that the family's needs will be met because of the relationship with the third person. Staying involved with the family until connections have been made between the family and the third person

is ideal for the nurse. The nurse can evaluate the degree to which the family and agency are satisfied with the referral. At times, the original referral proves to be inappropriate for family needs, and additional referrals are necessary.

The nurse initiating the referral must have prior knowledge of both the family and the agency or specialist to whom the family is being referred. The nurse must then decide what information about the family needs to be shared with the agency and what information the family needs to be given about the agency. In many cases, it may take up to 6 months for a community/public health nurse to learn the details about health and social agencies and private practitioners in the specific geographic area of practice. Because personnel and policies frequently change, keeping up to date is a continual process (see Chapter 19).

LEGAL DOCUMENTATION

All home visits are to be documented on the legal record. Telephone calls from and to the family and with other disciplines involved are also to be recorded. Ineffective telephone calls and home visits are recorded to show effort and timeliness of nursing attempts to provide care.

Most community/public health agencies use some version of the problem-oriented recording (POR) system, which consists of forms for databases, including identifying information; problem lists; selected flow sheets; progress notes; and discharge summaries. In agencies that do not use POR, narrative progress notes and flow sheets are used. Computerized record systems are becoming more prevalent.

THE FUTURE OF EVIDENCE-BASED HOME-VISITING PROGRAMS

At the beginning of this chapter, we discussed populations for whom home-visiting programs exist. Given the trend of increased numbers of frail elderly and those with chronic diseases and disabilities, the demand for home visiting is expected to increase for these populations. Home visiting for care of the frail elderly, ill, and disabled has proved to be cost-effective when compared with providing care in hospitals and nursing homes.

Other home-visiting programs seek to empower families with children, especially those that live in poor communities with health disparities (Donovan et al., 2007; Wisconsin Department of Health and Family Services, 2007). Evaluations of some prenatal and postnatal home-visiting programs that target low-income, unmarried women demonstrate improved pregnancy outcomes, reductions in child abuse and neglect, and improved maternal life course (Olds, 2004). The David Olds' Nurse-Family Partnership program has produced consistent effects in three different trials, including white, African American, and Hispanic populations; it has been partially replicated in the United Kingdom (Barlow et al., 2006). Similar programs show promise of improving infant attachment and behaviors (Olds, 2004), as well as reduced criminal and antisocial behavior in adolescents (Olds et al., 1998). Compared with paraprofessionals, nurses have been shown to produce larger effects (Olds et al., 2002).

Community/public health nurses need to continue to demonstrate the cost-effectiveness of programs of home visiting for health promotion and primary prevention to reduce disparities among various aggregates/populations. Community/public health nurses are exploring creative models of nursing care that reintegrate care of the sick with health promotion and primary prevention within families.

KEY IDEAS

1. Home visiting is a traditional and evidence-based activity of community/public health nurses for providing health promotion and all levels of illness prevention to individuals and families.
2. Home visits provide opportunities for family-focused care, for persona lizing care within the environment in which the care will actually be implemented, and for modifying care to family preferences. Home visits also provide an opportunity for detecting health threats of which the family may be unaware.
3. Practice and research indicate that positive preventive health outcomes result from home visits by community/public health nurses. Although the health results obtained from home visits can exceed those obtained by visits to clinics and private physicians, political debate continues regarding the cost-effectiveness of home visiting for health promotion and primary prevention.
4. Home visiting involves a process of initiating relationships with family members, negotiating and implementing a family-focused plan of care, and evaluating health outcomes and family satisfaction.
5. Each home visit involves several phases or steps: preplanning the visit, traveling to the home and initiating the visit, accomplishing the interventions, evaluating and summarizing the visit with the family, ending the visit and leaving the home, and conducting postvisit activities. Efficiency is increased when community/public health nurses wisely manage their time and equipment.
6. Relationships with families within their homes are different from nurse-client relationships in inpatient settings. Families retain more control over the environment; the relationship may extend over weeks, months, or years; and goal achievement depends more on an interdependent partnership between the nurse and the family.
7. Nurses can reduce potential conflicts in their relationships with families by clarifying the purpose of the visits, carefully negotiating contracts/agreements with family members, being aware of their own feelings and values, and honoring confidentiality.
8. Maintaining nurse and family safety and appropriately handling emergencies are important responsibilities when making home visits. Promoting personal hygiene and a clean home environment reduces the likelihood of the transmission of communicable diseases among family members and between households.
9. Postvisit activities include evaluating the visit and the plan of care, collaborating with other team members, conducting referrals, documenting in the legal health record, and planning for future contacts with the family.
10. Community/public health nurses need to continue to demonstrate the cost-effectiveness of home visits for health promotion and primary prevention to reduce disparities among various populations. Home visiting for care of the ill and disabled has proved to be cost-effective when compared with providing care in hospitals and nursing homes. Community/public health nurses are exploring creative models of nursing care that reintegrate care of the sick with health promotion and primary prevention within families.

CASE STUDY Home Visiting

A community/public health nurse employed by a suburban county health department in a maternal-child health program received a referral from the local hospital for a young mother and her newborn daughter. The nurse who initiated the referral was employed by the health department and the hospital for the express purpose of interviewing and identifying families at risk for child health problems.

Planning for the Home Visit

The community/public health nurse reviewed the referral for identifying information, information about the family, and the purpose of the referral. The referral included the parents' and infant's names, address, and telephone number; a brief delivery history (normal, 5-lb, 7-oz female infant born of vaginal delivery); the results of screening tests for illicit drugs and sexually transmitted diseases (negative); the method of infant feeding (breast-feeding); and a description of mother-infant interactions (anxiety regarding breast-feeding and living arrangements) observed by the hospital nurse. The mother had agreed to be contacted by a community/public health nurse for home visits.

The referral further stated that the mother had moved to the county 2 months ago, interrupting her prenatal care. She was staying with her cousin while her husband traveled to a neighboring state in search of employment. Therefore the nurse inferred that further

CASE STUDY   Home Visiting—cont'd

assessment of the mother's support systems, knowledge of health care resources, and finances would be especially important.

When the community/public health nurse telephoned the home to make an appointment for a home visit, she heard the voices of children in the background; their volume made hearing the mother difficult. The nurse introduced herself by name, stated that she worked for the health department, and indicated that she had been notified by the hospital that the mother had delivered a baby girl. The nurse asked how the mother and infant were doing. The mother replied that she was very tired and was not sure that her infant was getting enough to eat; she was giving her infant formula from a bottle and trying to breast-feed at alternate feedings. Yes, she was eager to have the nurse visit in her cousin's home. The nurse arranged a visit for the next day at a time when the infant was usually being fed.

The nurse determined that the family lived in a mobile home behind an old farmhouse near a new housing subdivision. The nurse found the address on her county map and decided that she believed that the area was adequately safe to visit alone.

After completing the telephone call, she reflected that the purpose of the maternal-child health program was to promote the well-being of families with infants, to prevent problems such as infant failure to thrive and injuries, to ensure that family members received appropriate immunizations and health care, and to promote positive parent-child relationships and child development. Her focus would be on the infant, the mother, and other household members.

In preparation for the visit, the nurse obtained the appropriate agency forms for recording postpartum and newborn care in the home and obtaining the mother's written permission for services. She restocked her nurse's bag with soap, towels, disposable tape (used to measure infant head circumference), thermometers, sphygmomanometer, and stethoscope. She obtained an infant scale. To be prepared for teaching the mother, the nurse collected pamphlets on postpartum care, care of a newborn, breast-feeding, infant safety, and community resources. Before leaving the office, the nurse left an itinerary of her visits for the next day; she would go directly from her home to her first visit.

Initiating the Home Visit

As the nurse drove to the home, she noticed a "for sale" sign on the farm property and that tall grass and weeds grew in the field. A relatively new mobile home sat next to a farmhouse, which was in disrepair. The yard around the mobile home was mowed and contained a plastic swimming pool and several children's bikes. No animals appeared.

As she parked her car and approached the mobile home, a woman appeared at the door and called, "Are you the nurse?" The nurse replied that she was and introduced herself by name. The woman introduced herself, stated that her cousin and the cousin's infant were inside, and motioned for the nurse to come in.

On entering the mobile home, the nurse noticed three preschoolers playing on the floor and a young woman sitting with an infant on a sheet-covered sofa. The nurse introduced herself and so did the mother. The nurse said hello to the children as well. The chairs were piled with clothes and there was nowhere in the room to sit. The nurse noticed the dinette chairs and asked if she might move one to the living room to sit down; the cousin agreed.

The nurse repeated that she was from the health department and was there to be of assistance to the mother and her newborn. The nurse sat quietly, looking at the mother and newborn, waiting for the mother to speak. The mother smiled faintly and asked if the nurse would like to hold her infant. The mother was dressed in nightclothes, her hair was uncombed, and she had dark circles under her eyes. The nurse stated that she would be delighted to hold the infant but that she would like to wash her hands first.

Implementing the Home Visit

After washing her hands, the nurse held the infant, looked into her face, and spoke softly about how alert she was. She asked the infant's name. The nurse noticed that the infant's respirations were regular and her color was good; her fontanels were not depressed or bulging, and her mucous membranes were moist; her umbilical cord was drying without exudate; she did not appear to be in any distress. Therefore the nurse focused on the mother.

The mother stated that she was tired because the infant did not yet sleep through the night. She was sleeping on the couch, and the infant slept in an infant car seat that belonged to her cousin. She was disappointed that her husband had not yet come to see his daughter. He had telephoned about his job interviews and had wired her some money from his unemployment check. Yes, she was able to purchase some diapers and had a few bottles. Her cousin had loaned her some infant clothes.

When asked specific questions about her postpartum status, the mother replied that her vaginal bleeding was getting lighter and did not contain any clots. She did not have any bothersome pains in her abdomen or her legs. Her blood pressure was 130/76 mmHg. She was eating two meals a day but wondered what to eat to "help make my milk." Her breasts were engorged, and she reported difficulty getting the infant to latch onto her nipples.

The infant began to fret and root as if she were hungry. The mother noticed the infant's behavior and stated it was time for her to eat. The nurse stated she would like to observe the breast-feeding so she might make suggestions; the mother eagerly agreed. The nurse used the opportunity to demonstrate several positions for holding the infant during breast-feeding and how to use the rooting reflex and position her nipples to assist her daughter. The nurse explained that the more the infant sucked and emptied the breasts, the more milk would be produced. The nurse suggested that the mother empty one breast before going to the second. The nurse affirmed what the mother was doing correctly and worked with the mother to improve her technique. The nurse discussed how to check for wet diapers to ensure that the infant was receiving enough breast milk.

As the infant fell asleep, the nurse had the mother sign the permission form for home-visiting services. Most of the visit was devoted to teaching related to breast-feeding because this was the immediate concern of the mother and was also essential for the hydration and nutrition of the infant. The nurse assessed that the mother had completed high school and had worked in an office for a while. The nurse reviewed the written pamphlets on breast-feeding, postpartum changes in mothers, safety for newborns, and medical emergencies. She gave the mother the telephone numbers of a local church, which supplies infant clothes and equipment, and the local La Leche League group, which provides information and support for breast-feeding women.

The nurse further assessed the mother's living arrangements, financial circumstances, and plans for obtaining a postpartum examination for herself and well-child care for the infant. The mother had no health insurance but had initiated application for medical assistance while in the hospital. She had applied for Women, Infants, and Children (WIC)

Continued

CASE STUDY Home Visiting—cont'd

vouchers to help obtain nutrition for herself while she breast-fed. She would return to the hospital for a postpartum visit, but she did not know where to obtain care for her infant. The nurse provided a list of pediatricians who participated in medical assistance managed care, as well as the health department's immunization clinics.

The cousin and the mother both confirmed that the mother planned to stay for a "couple of months," until her husband returned for her. Yes, it was crowded in their mobile home, but "families need to help each other out and I know a lot about caring for babies," the cousin asserted.

Ending the Home Visit

The nurse stated that it was almost time for her to leave. The mother volunteered that she felt much more confident with her breast-feeding and that she understood that she did not have to feed both formula and breast milk. She would call the church for more infant clothes and call the La Leche League. The nurse reinforced that she was doing well caring for her infant and had a plan for obtaining medical care when she needed it.

The nurse left her name, agency address, and telephone number in writing. The nurse stated that she would telephone the next day to see how the breast-feeding was working and whether the mother's breast engorgement had decreased. A second home visit was planned for the next week.

Postvisit Activities

During the evaluation of her home visit, the community/public health nurse was pleased that she had been able to establish a relationship with the mother and to offer information related to breast-feeding that was immediately helpful. No additional referrals or consultations were needed.

The community/public health nurse completed her legal documentation on the client identification form, postpartum assessment form, newborn infant assessment form, and progress note. She identified the problems as altered breast-feeding, potential for growth related to care of firstborn, knowledge deficit related to community resources, and income deficit related to unemployment.

The family strengths included the father's motivation to seek employment, the mother's education and readiness to learn, the mother's attentiveness to her newborn, and the support from her extended family. The nurse concluded that she needed more information about the social situation before she was able to predict how long she would need to continue the home visits. Her assessment priorities for the next home visit included information about the spousal relationship and the mother's coping skills, more information about the cousin's family and their health needs, a home safety assessment, and a developmental assessment of the infant.

The community/public health nurse would start her next home visit by inquiring about how the week had gone, how the mother was feeling, and whether breast-feeding had improved. She would also evaluate whether the mother had contacted the church and La Leche League and the degree to which these resources had been helpful.

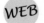 See **Critical Thinking Questions** for this Case Study on the book's website.

LEARNING BY EXPERIENCE AND REFLECTION

1. Describe experiences you have had with visits to homes in which you did not know anyone (e.g., selling newspapers, collecting money for charities). Recall your feelings. What did you do that was usually effective? Share your ideas with others.
2. Describe your own home and compare it with another home that is much different. Notice what categories you use for comparison: (a) What are the themes in your comparison (e.g., did you compare the level of activity in the home, or did you compare the amount and type of furniture)? (b) Which of your senses are represented in your comparison, in addition to sight?
3. After an initial home visit to a family, describe the physical features of the home without including value judgments or generalized conclusions, such as, "The furniture was in good shape."
4. Have another person critique how successful you were in answering question 3. Notice which of your values or biases were revealed.
5. After a home visit to a family, describe several behaviors of a family member or members that you believe to have been in response to your interactions. Speculate on at least three possible meanings of the behaviors. Create a plan to validate which of the meanings is most accurate.
6. Write an agreement that you desire to negotiate with a family on the first home visit. Role-play how this might be expressed verbally to the family members; be certain to validate with the *clients* to what they actually agree.
7. Discuss how a family focus can be fostered during a home visit when only one household member is present.
8. After an initial home visit, use the Determining the Success of Your Home Visit guide (see Box 11-9) or the Home Visiting Evaluation Tool (see Figure 11-3) to help preplan for your second visit.
9. Create an artistic expression of what *relating with a family and being concerned for their well-being and growth* means to you. (You might work with drawing, painting, music, prose, dance, or poetry, for example.)

COMMUNITY RESOURCES FOR PRACTICE

Information about each organization listed below is found on its website, which can be accessed through the **WebLinks** section of the book's website at *http://evolve.elsevier.com/Maurer/community/*.

Association for Professionals in Infection Control and Epidemiology, Inc.
Center for Home Visiting
Centers for Disease Control and Prevention
National Association for Home Care and Hospice
Nurse-Family Partnership
Visiting Nurse Association of America

STUDY AIDS   http://evolve.elsevier.com/Maurer/community/

Visit the Evolve website for this book to find the following study and assessment materials:

- Quiz
- Web Scenario
- Critical Thinking Questions and Answers for Case Studies
- Care Plans
- *Healthy People* Updates
- Glossary

REFERENCES

American Nurses Association. (2003). *Nursing's social policy statement*. Washington, DC: American Nurses Publishing.

American Nurses Association. (2007a). *Hospice and palliative nursing: Scope and standards of practice*. Silver Spring, MD: NursesBooks.org.

American Nurses Association. (2007b). *Public health nursing: Scope and standards of practice*. Silver Spring, MD: NursesBooks.org.

American Red Cross. (2000). *Responding to emergencies* (3rd ed.). Yardley, PA: Staywell.

Arnold, E. (1996). Points of intersection: Therapeutic communication. In Carson V. & Arnold E. (Eds.), *Mental health nursing: The nurse-patient journey* (pp. 191-229). Philadelphia: W. B. Saunders.

Arnold, E., & Boggs, K. (2007). *Interpersonal relationships: Professional communication skills for nurses* (5th ed.). St. Louis: Saunders.

Barlow, J., Davis, H., McIntosh, E., et al. (2006). Role of home visiting in improving parenting and health in families at risk of abuse and neglect: Results of multicentre randomized controlled trial and economic evaluation. *Archives of Disease in Childhood, 92*, 229-233.

Barrett, J. (1982). Postpartum home visits by maternity nursing students. *Journal of Obstetric, Gynecologic, and Neonatal Nursing, 11*(4), 238-240.

Barton, J., & Brown, N. (1995). Home visitation to migrant farm workers: An application of Zerwekh's family caregiving model for public health nursing. *Holistic Nursing Practice, 9*(4), 34-40.

Beck, C. (1992). Caring among nursing students. *Nurse Educator, 17*(6), 22-27.

Bradley, P., & Martin, J. (1994). The impact of home visits on enrollment patterns in pregnancy-related services among low-income women. *Public Health Nursing, 11*(6), 392-398.

Burns, P., & Gianutsos, R. (1987). Reentry of the head-injured survivor into the educational system: First steps. *Journal of Community Health Nursing, 4*(3), 145-152.

Byrd, M. (1995). The home visiting process in the contexts of the voluntary vs. required visit: Examples from fieldwork. *Public Health Nursing, 12*(3), 196-202.

Byrd, M. (2006). Social exchange as a framework for client-nursing interaction during public health nursing maternal-child home visits. *Public Health Nursing, 23*(3), 271-276.

Centers for Disease Control and Prevention. (1998). *Guidelines for prevention and control of nosocomial infections* (PHS-CDC 83-8314). Springfield, VA: National Technical Information Service. Also available at *http://www.cdc.gov/niosh/hcwapp8.html*.

Chichester, M., & Smith, C. (1980). *Home visiting evaluation tool* (unpublished manuscript). Baltimore, MD: University of Maryland School of Nursing.

Davis, C. (1990). What is empathy, and can empathy be taught? *Physical Therapy, 70*, 707-711.

Donovan, E., Ammerman, R., Besl, J., et al. (2007). Intensive home visiting is associated with decreased risk of infant death. *Pediatrics, 119*(6), 1145-1151.

Engelke, M., & Engelke, S. (1992). Predictors of the home environment of high-risk infants. *Journal of Community Health Nursing, 9*(3), 171-181.

Frank-Stromberg, M., & Ganschow, J. R. (2002). How HIPAA will change your practice. *Nursing, 32*(9), 54-57.

Friedman, M. (1983). *Manual for effective community health nursing practice*. Monterey, CA: Wadsworth.

Gary, F., & Kavanagh, C. (1991). *Psychiatric mental health nursing*. Philadelphia: J. B. Lippincott.

Glugover, D. (1987). Community health nurses: Role models for change in our lives and in our client's lives. *Caring, 84*, 14-15.

Goldsborough, J. (1969). Involvement. *American Journal of Nursing, 69*(1), 66-68.

Haber, J., Hoskins, P., Leach, A., et al. (1987). Self-awareness. In Haber J., Leach A., & Sideleau B. (Eds.), *Comprehensive psychiatric nursing* (pp. 77-86). New York: McGraw-Hill.

Harris, M. (1995). Caring for individuals in the community who are mentally retarded/developmentally disabled. *Home Healthcare Nurse, 13*(6), 27-36.

Heaman, M., Chalmers, K., Woodgate, R., et al. (2007). Relationship work in an early childhood home visiting program. *Journal of Pediatric Nursing, 22*(4), 319-330.

Helgeson, D., & Berg, C. (1985). Contracting: A method of health promotion. *Journal of Community Health Nursing, 2*(4), 199-207.

Heymann, D. (Ed.). (2004). *Control of communicable diseases manual* (18th ed.). Washington, DC: American Public Health Association.

Humphrey, C. (1998). *Home care nursing handbook* (3rd ed.). Gaithersburg, MD: Aspen.

Josten, L., Mullett, S., Savik, K., et al. (1995). Client characteristics associated with not keeping appointments for public health nursing home visits. *Public Health Nursing, 12*(5), 305-311.

Katzman, E., Cohen, C., & Lukes, E. (1987). Students *do* make a difference. *Journal of Community Health Nursing, 4*(1), 49-56.

Kitzman, H., Olds, D., Henderson, C., et al. (1997). Effect of prenatal and infancy home visitation by nurses on pregnancy outcomes, childhood injuries, and repeated childbearing: A randomized controlled trial. *Journal of the American Medical Association, 278*(8), 644-652.

Kitzman, H., Olds, D., Sidora, K., et al. (2000). Enduring effects of nurse home visitation on maternal life course: A 3-year follow-up of a randomized trial. *Journal of the American Medical Association, 283*(15), 1983-1989.

Kristjanson, L., & Chalmers, K. (1991). Preventive work with families: Issues facing public health nurses. *Journal of Advanced Nursing, 16*, 147-153.

Leitch, C., & Tinker, R. (1978). *Primary care*. Philadelphia: F. A. Davis.

Lewis, J., & Chaisson, R. (Sept 1993). *Tuberculosis: The reemergence of an old foe*. Paper presented at the Baltimore City Health Department 200th Anniversary Celebration Conference, Baltimore, MD.

Mayers, M. (1973). Home visit—ritual or therapy? *Nursing Outlook, 21*(5), 328-331.

McNaughton, D. (2000). A synthesis of qualitative home visiting research. *Public Health Nursing, 17*(6), 405-414.

Mohit, D. (1996). Management and care of mentally ill mothers of young children: An innovative program. *Archives of Psychiatric Nursing, 10*(1), 49-54.

Murray, S. (1968). *Farm and home visits: A guide for extension workers in many countries*. Washington, DC: U.S. Department of Agriculture.

Nadwairski, J. (1992). Inner-city safety for home care providers. *Journal of Nursing Administration, 22*(9), 42-47.

Norr, K., Crittenden, K., Lehrer, E., et al. (2003). Maternal and infant outcomes at one year for a nurse-health advocate home visiting program serving African Americans and Mexican Americans. *Public Health Nursing, 20*(3), 190-203.

Olds, D. (2004). Prenatal/postnatal home visiting programs and their impact on the social and emotional development of young children (0-5). In R. Tremblay, R. Barr, & R. Peters (Eds.), *Encyclopedia on early childhood development* (online) (pp. 1-7). Montreal, Quebec: Centre of Excellence for Early Childhood Development. Accessed January 16, 2008, at *http://www.child-encyclopedia.com/documents/OldsANGxp.pdf*.

Olds, D., Eckenrode, J., Henderson, C., et al. (1997). Long-term effects of home visitation on maternal life course and child abuse and neglect: Fifteen-year follow-up of a randomized trial. *Journal of the American Medical Association, 278*(8), 637-643.

Olds, D., Henderson, C., Chamberlin, R., et al. (1986). Preventing child abuse and neglect: A randomized trial of nurse home visitation. *Pediatrics, 7*(1), 65-78.

Olds, D., Henderson, C., Cole, R., et al. (1998). Long-term effects of nurse home visitation on children's criminal and antisocial behavior: 15-year follow-up of a randomized controlled trial. *Journal of the American Medical Association, 280*(14), 1238-1244.

Olds, D., Henderson, C., Kitzman, H., et al. (1995). Effects of prenatal and infancy nurse home visitation on surveillance of child maltreatment. *Pediatrics, 95*(3), 365-372.

Olds, D., Robinson, J., O'Brien, R., et al. (2002). Home visiting by paraprofessionals and by nurses: A ramdomized, controlled trial. *Pediatrics, 110*(3), 486-496.

Raatikainen, R. (1991). Self-activeness and the need for help in domiciliary care. *Journal of Advanced Nursing, 16*, 1150-1157.

Reutter, L., & Ford, J. (1997). Enhancing client competence: Melding professional and client knowledge in public health nursing. *Public Health Nursing, 14*(3), 143-150.

Rhinehart, E., & Friedman, M. (1999). *Infection control in home care*. Gaithersburg, MD: Aspen (an official publication of the Association for Professionals in Infection Control and Epidemiology, Inc.).

Roach, M.S. (1997). *Caring from the heart: The convergence of caring and spirituality*. New York: Paulist Press.

Rogers, C. (1969). *Freedom to learn*. Columbus, OH: Charles E. Merrill.

Sheridan, A., & Smith, R. (1975). Family-student contracts. *Nursing Outlook, 23*(2), 114-117.

Siegel, J., Rhinehart, E., Jackson, M., et al. (2007). *Guidelines for isolation precautions: Preventing transmission of infectious agents in healthcare settings 2007*. Atlanta: Centers for Disease Control and Prevention. Retrieved February 29, 2008, from *http://www.cdc.gov/ncidod/dhqp/pdf/guidelines/Isolation2007.pdf*.

Simmons, D. (1980). *A classification scheme for client problems in community health nursing* (DHHS Pub No. HRA 8016). Hyattsville, MD: U.S. Department of Health and Human Services.

Smith, C. (1972). *Referral as triadic communication*. Unpublished manuscript.

Smith, C. (1980a). *Phases of a home visit* (unpublished manuscript). Baltimore, MD: University of Maryland School of Nursing.

Smith, C. (1980b). *A series of encounters during a relationship* (unpublished manuscript). Baltimore, MD: University of Maryland School of Nursing.

Smith, C.. (1987). *Determining the success of your home visit* (unpublished manuscript). Baltimore, MD: University of Maryland School of Nursing. Used with permission.

Stolee, P., Kessler, L., & LeClair, J. K. (1996). A community development and outreach program in geriatric mental health: Four years' experience.

Journal of the American Geriatrics Society, 44(3), 314-320.

Trotter, J. (1996). Home care management. In Smith S. & Duell D. (Eds.), *Clinical nursing skills* (4th ed.). Stamford, CT: Appleton & Lange.

U.S. Department of Health and Human Services, Office of Human Development Services, U.S. Advisory Board on Child Abuse and Neglect. (1990). *Child abuse and neglect: Critical first steps in response to a national emergency*. Washington, DC: Author.

van Manen, M. (1990). *Researching lived experience: Human science for an action sensitive pedagogy*. London, Ontario: State University of New York.

Watson, J. (2002). *Assessing and measuring caring in nursing and health science*. Springer: New York.

Watson, J. (2005). *Caring science as sacred science*. Philadelphia: F. A. Davis.

Whyte, D. (1992). A family nursing approach to the care of a child with a chronic illness. *Journal of Advanced Nursing, 17*, 317-327.

Wisconsin Department of Health and Family Services. (2007). *Initial report on the Empowering Families of Milwaukee Home Visiting Program: July 2005-December 2006*. Retrieved January 16, 2008, from *http://www.dhfs.wisconsin.gov/aboutDHFS/OPIB/policyresearch*.

World Health Organization. (1987). *The community health worker*. Geneva: Author.

Zerwekh, J. (1990). Public health nursing legacy: Historical practical wisdom. *Nursing and Health Care, 13*(2), 84-91.

Zerwekh, J. (1991, October). Tales from public health nursing: True detectives. *American Journal of Nursing, 91*(10), 30-36.

Zerwekh, J. (1992). Laying the groundwork for family self-help: Locating families, building trust, and building strength. *Public Health Nursing, 9*(1), 15-21.

SUGGESTED READINGS

American Red Cross. (2000). *Responding to emergencies* (3rd ed.). Yardley, PA: Staywell.

Aston, M., Meagher-Stewart, D., Sheppard-Lemoine, D., et al. (2006). Family helath nursing and empowering relationships. *Pediatric Nursing, 32*(1), 61-67.

Brofman, J. (Oct 1979). An evening home visiting program. *Nursing Outlook, 27*(10), 657-661.

Centers for Disease Control and Prevention. (1989). Guidelines for prevention of transmission of human immunodeficiency virus and hepatitis B virus to health-care and public-safety workers (No. S6). *Morbidity and Mortality Weekly Report, 38*, 1-37.

Helvie, C., Hill, A., & Bambino, C. (Aug 1968). The setting and nursing practice: Part I. *Nursing Outlook, 16*(8), 27-29.

Keeling, B. (March 1978). Making the most of the first home visit. *Nursing, 78*, 24-28.

Lentz, J., & Meyer, E. (Sept 1979). The dirty house. *Nursing Outlook, 27*(9), 290-293.

Nadwairski, J. (1992). Inner-city safety for home care providers. *Journal of Nursing Administration, 22*(9), 42-47.

Olds, D., Hill, P., Robinson, J., et al. (2000). Update on home visiting for pregnant women and parents of young children. *Current Problems in Pediatrics, 30*(4), 107-141.

Price, J., & Broden, C. (Sept 1978). The reality in home visits. *American Journal of Nursing, 78*(9), 1536-1538.

Pruitt, R., Keller, L., & Hale, S. (1987). Mastering distractions that mar home visits. *Nursing and Health Care, 8*(6), 345-347.

Rhinehart, E., & McGoldrick, M. (2006). *Infection control in home care and hospice* (2nd ed.). Sudbury, MA: Jones & Bartlett (an official publication of the Association for Professionals in Infection Control and Epidemiology, Inc.).

Sargis, N., Jennrich, J., & Murray, K. (1987). Housing and health: A crucial link. *Nursing and Health Care, 8*(6), 335-338.

Stulginsky, M. (1993a). Nurses' home health experience—part I: The practice setting. *Nursing and Health Care, 14*(8), 402-407.

Stulginsky, M. (1993b). Nurses' home health experience—part II: The unique demands of home visits. *Nursing and Health Care, 14*(9), 476-485.

U.S. General Accounting Office. (1990). *Home visiting: A promising early intervention strategy for at-risk families*. Washington, DC: U.S. Government Printing Office.

12 A Family Perspective in Community/ Public Health Nursing

Marcia L. Cooley

FOCUS QUESTIONS

Why use a family perspective in community/public health nursing?

How do families differ? How are they the same?

What different family approaches have been proposed in the past?

How can these approaches be integrated?

What is family nursing?

How is the family perspective used in the practice of community/ public health nursing?

CHAPTER OUTLINE

A Family Perspective
Family as Client
Why Choose a Family Perspective?
What Is a Family?
Definition of Family
How Are Families Alike and Different?

Historical Frameworks
Family Development
Family as a System
Bowen's Family Systems Theory
Family Structure and Function
Family Interaction and Communication

Distinctive Characteristics of Families
Family Coping with Stress
How Can These Approaches Be Integrated?
Family Perspectives in Nursing
What Is Family Nursing?
How Is Family Nursing Practiced?

KEY TERMS

Anxiety	Hierarchy	Stages
Appraisal	Interactional style	Strengths
Boundary	Level of differentiation	Structure
Coping	Metacommunication	Style
Developmental tasks	Needs	Subsystems
Double-bind communication	Process	Transition
Dysfunctional	Resilience	Triangle
Family	Resources	Values
Function	Roles	

A FAMILY PERSPECTIVE

All nurses can and should practice family nursing. People are born into and grow, live, and die within their families. Everyone has a family. Families have different structures and sizes, have different levels of connection and ways of operating with each other, and may be geographically close or distant. Families can offer support and love and can also bring their members disappointment and grief. People grow older, may move away, or may sometimes try to pretend that they do not have a family; but ultimately, the person that one becomes is a reflection of the family from which one came.

FAMILY AS CLIENT

The family as a unit of care has been a focus in community/public health nursing since its beginning (Whall, 1993).

Nurses and other workers in the community recognized that the family was a major source of support and influence in many situations. Whether the issue was an ill family member, a change in the family (e.g., birth, death), or disease prevention, the community/public health nurse learned to include the family in nursing care. People's lifestyles and, consequently, their health are intimately tied to the culture, values, beliefs, practices, and socioeconomic status they share with their families.

Appreciation of the family as a unit of care evolved naturally as community/public health nurses worked within the community. With this work came a recognition that not all families are able to provide all their members with what they need to reach optimal levels of health. Community/public health nurses have a unique position because they are broadly educated and able to integrate different perspectives that

327

contribute to an understanding of family functioning. Nurses also have a unique role within the community that offers them access to family situations. Focusing on the family is a helpful step to take in working toward a broader perspective of caring for the individual, the family, and the entire community.

Can a difference be found in using a family rather than an individual perspective? Consider the following example.

> Michelle is a 13-year-old girl who was referred to the community/public health nurse by administrators at her middle school. Her attendance has been very poor, she is irritable and rebellious in class, her previously good grades are dropping, and she has recently gained so much weight that the school nurse wonders if Michelle is pregnant. Depending on the professional's point of view, many different ideas may be formulated about her *problem*. The school system views her behavior as truant, the school psychologist wonders about depression, and her teacher views her as a behavior problem. Repeated attempts to involve her mother have had little success.
>
> Suppose the community/public health nurse has been alerted to the need to visit and assess the family. During the visit, she realizes that Michelle is staying home from school to watch her younger brother and sister on days her grandmother goes to work and has no other baby-sitter. Michelle is unhappy about having to miss school but does not want anyone to know the situation at home. Her mother, who had been taking care of the children, is abusing drugs and is not a reliable person to care for them. The younger children, aged 6 and 8, have had repeated throat infections during the winter. No one has been able to take them to the clinic. Michelle is not pregnant, but she has been so unhappy that she is overeating and gaining weight.

The opportunity to look at a bigger picture gives a very different perspective than the one presented when an individual view of Michelle is taken. Viewing the situation solely as *Michelle's problem* is difficult. The community/public health nurse may still choose to focus only on Michelle's difficulties but realizes that these difficulties are connected to other issues and to the health of other people. Not only is Michelle's health a concern, but the health of the family is also at risk. The family can either be supportive of Michelle or block attempted interventions. Community/public health nursing recognizes the importance of the family and defines the entire family as the unit of treatment. Michelle will be involved, but the whole family will become the focus for nursing care.

A problem can be viewed in many ways. In the past, science has often used a cause-and-effect way of thinking: *Germ A causes sickness B. Applying medicine C cures the sickness.* This example is a type of cause-and-effect thinking that became popular in the medical field after medications and inoculations proved to be successful in combating specific infectious illnesses.

Real life, however, is more complex than simple cause-and-effect thinking implies. Not every person exposed to a certain pathogen becomes ill. Becoming infected depends on variables such as general level of health, stress level at the time, previous antibody development, and genetic susceptibility. Many different events occur at the same time. When the organism confronts these events while various factors are

in balance, health is usually maintained. When imbalance exists, illness or dysfunction may occur—not because of any one event, but because of a combination of factors. This recognition of the complexity and interconnectedness of a living organism is a systemic, rather than a cause-and-effect, way of thinking.

Individuals in a family can be thought of as a *living* system. Each person is one of the elements that are interrelated with one another. A **boundary** or imaginary wall exists around the family, similar to the thin membrane of a cell wall. This boundary can vary; it can be rigid and impenetrable, or it can be a permeable membrane that allows exchange in and out of the system. Each member, although only a part of the system, has the potential to change the patterns and organization of the entire system. Together, the individuals within the family make up something new that is different from and greater than the simple sum of its members.

Living systems have parts that undergo growth and change. At any given point in time, the individuals in the family will be undergoing change themselves. The members are growing, developing, learning, and changing, usually on trajectories or paths that are recognizable as part of the life cycle. Thus the family as a living system is constantly changing.

The boundaries of the system permit some exchange of information between the inside and the outside. The family is one system; the community outside the family is another. Bronfenbrenner (1979), while studying children in families, proposed the idea of different levels of systems: a mesosystem, a macrosystem, and an endosystem. The three levels constitute broader and broader environmental contexts in which the child will grow. Scheflen (1981) takes a similar approach in explaining different perspectives on schizophrenia. The author describes how this one phenomenon can be viewed from genetic, biochemical, individual, family, community, and societal perspectives. Figure 12-1 depicts some different levels of analysis that can be used when thinking about family nursing care. Notice that family is not the only perspective but is one piece in an ever-broader context of conceptualizing the appropriate target of intervention.

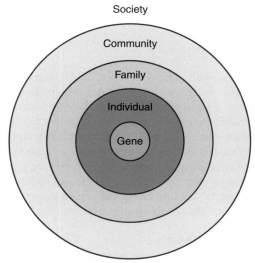

FIGURE 12-1 Levels of systems.

WHY CHOOSE A FAMILY PERSPECTIVE?

- *Family thinking gives a broader picture.* Viewing an individual in a smaller framework may narrow the information and understanding of the problem. This view assumes that individuals act independently and in an isolated way when they are actually intimately connected with larger systems. When a family member is being assessed, that person may be able to be completely understood only if he or she is viewed within the context of the gestalt—the whole situation. Assessment using an individual perspective may miss important interrelated aspects of the problem or resources that can be used to promote health and alleviate distress.
- *The family is a unit of care.* People often live in households as families. Families are organized in a structure with identified roles and leadership, and society expects families to assume some responsibility for each of their members. The family divides its economic resources. Family members also have emotional ties to each other. Even though society is assuming more and more of the family's functions, the family remains a workable unit.
- *The family assumes a crucial role in maintaining health.* Such a strong relationship exists between the family and health care that the role of the family becomes paramount in maintaining health. Health beliefs, values, and behaviors are learned and supported in the family. Health promotion activities are taught and implemented. Denham (2003) developed the Family Health Model after finding that the mother plays a key role in transmitting health beliefs about issues such as food choice and preparation, exercise, rest, and sleep patterns to children. The family is also a critical resource in the delivery of health care. How decisions are made about when to seek care, how health care is paid for, and how the recommended treatment regimens are carried out are all enacted within the family. The family is sometimes the primary care provider for its ill and dependent members. Changes in lifestyle are often required of the whole family if the level of wellness of one of the members is affected. Research evaluating the effectiveness of service delivery validates a family-centered approach. Families that form a partnership with care providers who recognize the parents as experts on their children's needs have more positive outcomes for their children (Law et al., 2003). This approach is considered as the *best practice* for families with children with disabilities (King et al., 2002).
- *Dysfunction in one member may be related to disturbance in the whole family.* Because a family operates as a system, a symptom in one member may be a signal that something is happening in the family as a whole. The family will sometimes work hard on one health problem, with some good results, only to have another health problem present in a second family member. A familiar example of this concept is an alcoholic family in which one spouse stops drinking, only to have the marriage break up or the *healthy* spouse become ill. Physical, emotional, and social problems are considered to be related to the degree of anxiety and emotional immaturity present and shared among family members in the entire system.
- *Dysfunction in one member may lead to added stress and depletion of resources for a family.* Some believe that any family member who is dysfunctional will ultimately affect the health of the entire system. Caring for an ill or dependent member can deplete financial resources, physical energy, and other sources of family support. The health of other members is sometimes disturbed. In many instances, the ability of the family to fulfill its maintenance functions for its members, such as giving time and attention to young children or sharing recreational activities, is affected by the illness of a member. The following clinical example demonstrates how illness in one member affects the health of other members and the entire family.

> The Johnson family is a family that had a very successful early life, but this changed when the father, Mike, became ill. Jennifer and Mike Johnson worked hard to put themselves through college and later graduate school. Mike worked as an accountant, and Jennifer was a teacher. Their two children, Stephanie and Chad, had typical ups and downs during the teenage years. Stephanie is now married and expecting a child. Chad is working hard at starting a computer business.
>
> Jennifer and Mike had been planning a happy retirement until 6 months ago. Then a second mortgage was taken out on the house to help Chad start his business. Mike found out 2 months ago that he needs bypass surgery, at about the same time that his company laid off workers, including him. He now has health coverage that will pay for only approximately 50% of the cost of the surgery. He cannot work for at least 3 months. Jennifer cannot cover the mortgage with her salary. She had planned to baby-sit for Stephanie, but now she must keep her teaching job. The worry about finances and Mike's health has led to migraines for Jennifer and is adding to Mike's stress and his high blood pressure. Both Chad and Stephanie are very concerned about asking their parents for the help that was previously planned.

- *Family and intimate relationships are important for tracking the occurrence and incidence of disease.* To community/public health nurses who are attempting to prevent, track, and record disease processes, the relationships within families and with other intimate partners are clearly significant. Family information is used in assessing needs, determining health care priorities, finding cases, tracking and preventing the spread of communicable diseases, educating for preventive purposes, and organizing the delivery of care to special and large populations. The family is an essential piece of these epidemiologic health care functions.
- *The unique goals of family nursing—individual health, supportive interpersonal relationships, and an effective family unit—can be achieved only by using a family perspective.* Hanson (2005) suggests that family is the umbrella under which all other nursing should be practiced. Family nursing is a movement in nursing that is coming into its own identity. By definition, all nursing practice is oriented toward achieving goals that are beneficial to the health and well-being of individuals within society. The goals that are put forth in family nursing—goals for individuals, relationships, and the family unit—can be addressed only by using a family perspective.

WHAT IS A FAMILY?

DEFINITION OF FAMILY

Thus far, this text has talked about families as if all families are alike and as if everyone understands what is meant when the word *family* is used. In the United States, however, many different kinds of families can actually be found. Community/public health nurses need a definition broad enough to encompass the many ways they will be interacting with families. Box 12-1 presents various definitions that have been proposed by family theorists and experts. The definition of family must not ignore the atypical or nontraditional family forms that are often encountered in current communities. The definition should also provide some structure to the way nurses think about families to establish a framework for intervention. The definition adopted by this text is as follows: a **family** is an open and developing system of interacting personalities with a structure and process enacted in relationships among the individual members, regulated by resources and stressors, and existing within the larger community.

HOW ARE FAMILIES ALIKE AND DIFFERENT?

All living systems need some sort of organization and pattern to function. Families also have this organization. Many people use a framework of structure, process, and function to describe the complex nature of families.

Structure

Structure refers to the elements of the family and the organization of these elements within the family. Over the life of a family, structure does not remain exactly the same, but a certain continuity of structure is maintained. Structure is defined in several ways. Some people define structure anthropologically, using family types defined in terms of lineage and power. For example, families may be matriarchal or patriarchal. Other people look at the arrangement of members within the system in terms of subsystems, coalitions, and other structures that have hierarchies and boundaries; this is explored in more depth in the structural-functional approach discussed later in this chapter. Still other persons believe that structure means the diversity of family forms.

Family Forms

Some type of family exists in all societies, although there is a wide diversity of forms. Variations may even exist among classes within the same society. In Greece and America, for example, slaves were prevented by law from forming legal families. Even so, the family in some form (although not necessarily the traditional nuclear family) is an ideal that most people try to attain.

Family structures have changed across societies and over time. Our idea of the traditional American family living in a household with extended family members such as grandparents is actually a myth that has been popularized through the years (Hareven, 1982). Current family types are varied and changing. Of all the households in the United States, only 67.8% were families, defined by the census as two or more persons related by birth or marriage and living together under one roof (U.S. Bureau of the Census, 2006). Nonfamily households, including single people living alone, nonrelatives living together, and cohabiting couples, now comprise 32.2% of the population (Figure 12-2). Some trends affecting families include higher age at first marriage, increased divorce, declines in childbearing rates resulting in smaller families, and increased numbers of Americans who are 55 years or older (Urban Institute, 2006). The total percentage of single-parent families has actually dropped since the 1990s but remains high (53.4%) for African American families. Ten percent of African American children in the United States are now in living situations with no parents (Wherry & Finegold, 2004). Households also have changed since the 1990s due to the large migration of Hispanics to the United States. One out of every five children in the United States in living in an immigrant family (Annie E. Casey Foundation, 2007). Migration is also affecting families by increasing stress during transitions and adding numbers of people with varying legal and economic status. In 2006, 5% of all children lived in the home of a grandparent (Child Trends Data Bank, 2007). Box 12-2 presents some different family forms.

BOX 12-1   Definitions of Family

- A family cooperates economically, may share a common dwelling place, and may rear children (Strong & DeVault, 1992).
- The family is a haven in a heartless world (Lasch, 1995).
- A family is a unity of interacting personalities (Burgess, 1926).
- The family is the basic unit of society and the social institution that has the most marked effect on its members (Friedman, 1986).
- The family is an open system that functions in relation to its broader sociocultural context and that evolves over the life cycle (Walsh, 1993).
- A family is two or more persons who are joined together by bonds of sharing and emotional closeness and who identify themselves as being part of a family (Friedman, 1998).
- Definition adopted in this text: a family is an open and developing system of interacting personalities with a structure and process enacted in relationships among the individual members, regulated by resources and stressors, and existing within the larger community.

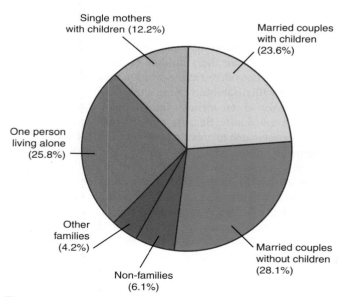

FIGURE 12-2 Household composition in the United States in 2000. *N* = 105.5 million households. (Data from U.S. Bureau of the Census. [2002]. *Statistical abstract of the United States, 2002* [122nd ed.]. Washington, DC: U.S. Government Printing Office.)

Box 12-2 Family Forms

- **Nuclear:** a father, mother, and child living together but apart from both sets of the father's and mother's parents.
- **Extended:** members of three generations, including married brothers and sisters and their families.
- **Three-generational:** any combination of first-, second-, and third-generation members living within a household.
- **Dyad:** husband and wife or other couple living alone without children.
- **Single-parent:** divorced, never married, separated, or widowed man or woman and at least one child. Most single-parent families are headed by women.
- **Step-parent:** a household in which one or both spouses have been divorced or widowed and have remarried into a family with at least one child.
- **Blended or reconstituted:** a combination of two families with children from one or both families and sometimes children of the newly married couple.
- **Single adult living alone:** a never married, divorced, or widowed individual maintaining a separate household, an increasingly common occurrence.
- **Cohabitating:** an unmarried couple living together.
- **No-kin:** a group of at least two people sharing a relationship and exchanging support who have no legalized or blood tie to each other.
- **Compound:** one man (or woman) with several spouses.
- **Gay:** a homosexual couple living together with or without children. Children may be adopted, from previous relationships, or artificially conceived.
- **Commune:** more than one monogamous couple sharing resources.
- **Group marriage:** group of individuals who all are married to each other and are considered parents of all the children.

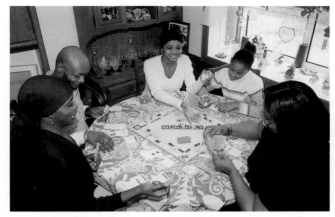

Sharing leisure time and humor through playing games is a family strength.

forefront. Focusing on family strengths not only helps bring sometimes forgotten qualities to light, but also reminds us of the incredible power and support families continue to offer. Family strengths are present in many areas of family functioning. All families, especially families at risk, have some **strengths** that are working or have worked in the past to maintain some health for their members.

Otto (1973) is one of the earliest authors to identify family strengths. The author's framework for assessing family strengths is presented in Box 12-3. Curran (1983) also identifies family strengths such as teaching respect for others, displaying a sense of play and humor, teaching children a sense of right and wrong, having a shared religious core, sharing leisure time, respecting privacy, and developing shared rituals and traditions. Many researchers studying family stress and coping have started to focus on family strengths—as well as strains and stressors—that affect families (Bomar, 2004; Feeley & Gottlieb, 2000). Some of the tools and assessment strategies for these ideas are presented in Chapter 13.

Process

A process is a phenomenon that occurs over time. Families, individuals, and society go through processes of growth, development, and change. The term implies change, but within every change, some pattern and connectedness with previous and future patterns is often found.

Family **process** can be defined as predictable and repetitive interaction patterns within families. For example, mom always watches Johnnie's behavior very closely. Johnnie gets upset with her attention and complains to dad. Dad goes to mom and complains that she is too harsh with Johnnie. Mom backs off for a while but soon resumes her attention. Such interaction can be observed in dyads, or two-person groups, or in interconnecting triangles (three-person groups) within the family.

Families also seem to have a characteristic way of interacting as a unit in relation to the outside world. This process can be open or closed, separate or connected. Families may allow information from the environment to help them problem solve or close themselves off from outside influence. Families may act together in a cohesive manner, withdraw from each other, or even split apart. The behavior of the family may be random and chaotic or rigid and predictable.

Strengths

When one is discussing families or focusing on health needs, weaknesses or deficits of families frequently jump to the

Box 12-3 Family Strengths

Ability to provide for physical needs
Ability to provide for emotional needs
Ability to provide for spiritual needs
Respect for parental views and decisions on child rearing
Ability to communicate openly and in depth
Consensual decision making
Provision of security, support, and encouragement
Ability to relate to each other and to foster growth-producing relationships
Responsible community relationships
Ability to grow with and through children
Ability to help itself and accept help when needed
Flexibility of family functions and roles
Mutual respect for individuality
Ability to see crisis as a means of growth
Family unity and loyalty and intrafamily cooperation
Flexibility of family strengths

Adapted from Otto, H. (1973). A framework for assessing family strengths. In A. Reinhardt & M. Quinn (Eds.), *Family-centered community nursing* (pp. 87-93). St. Louis: Mosby.

Function

In the past, some who wrote about the family used the term *functioning* to describe the activities the family provided for the well-being of its members. In this text, the term family **function** is used to describe results or the effectiveness of families. Does the family operate in a way that successfully provides for the needs of its members? Successful functioning is a measure of normality or health. Examining how well individual family members care for self and others is a way of assessing that family's level of health. Unhealthy families are called **dysfunctional.**

Family functioning is best viewed as a continuum. When the words *functional* and *dysfunctional* are used, family functioning can be considered as *good* or *bad*. There is no such thing as a good or bad family. All families fall somewhere along a continuum from minimal functioning to optimal functioning in which all members benefit. Many different means can be used to assess families according to different views of optimal family functioning. Bowen (1978) describes families as more or less healthy according to (1) their ability to separate thinking from feeling and (2) the amount of anxiety that is present in the family. Tapia (1997) defines levels of family functioning from chaotic to adult according to the family's degree of emotional maturity. Olson and McCubbin (1982) suggest that families should have moderate degrees of cohesion, coordination, and adaptability for healthy family functioning.

For optimal family functioning, the structure and process must combine in a way that allows the family to be effective. Understanding the particular stresses and history that have shaped a specific family's current way of operating helps the nurse understand that family. Conversely, the typical level of functioning of a family may determine its developing processes and structure (e.g., divorce, single parenthood, the arrangement of subsystems). Structure, process, and function are interrelated, and all of these aspects must be considered when assessing a family. However, no one structure, process, or type of function is proposed here as the *right* one. Many variations exist within these dimensions that can lead to healthy families. See Chapter 10 for a further discussion of diversity and cultural differences.

HISTORICAL FRAMEWORKS

The study of family does not fit neatly into any one field, be it genetics, physiology, anthropology, sociology, or psychology; many disciplines have contributed to the understanding of family functioning. The study of family is interdisciplinary, and theories of family have been broadly adapted and used. However, most frameworks used to study family have been drawn from family sociology or family therapy.

Sociologists have studied families since the nineteenth and early twentieth centuries because of the need to solve emerging social problems. The 1950s saw the development of conceptual frameworks in family theory. At approximately that time, interest in the family as a unit of treatment emerged in the psychiatric field. Family therapists began focusing on pathologic factors within families. Relatively recent trends have included the formulation of family theories attempting to describe the characteristics of healthy families, the development of theories of family coping with stressful situations, and the emergence of frameworks for family nursing.

Family approaches can be separated into several areas that provide different viewpoints that describe the complexity of the family. Families develop, interact, communicate, have structures, cope with stress, develop identity, and operate as systems. The following sections describe these approaches in more detail.

FAMILY DEVELOPMENT

Sharon, a new community/public health nurse, is visiting the Mitchell family. Myra Mitchell has three children aged 18, 14, and 9. Brenda, the 14-year-old, recently had a baby boy who is now living with the family. Marcia, the 18-year-old, is in her first year of college but is living at home. Her mother was helping pay Marcia's tuition by working a second job. This work schedule has stopped so she can help with care of the new baby. Marcia finds that studying with the baby in the house is difficult. Brenda planned to continue high school but is thinking of dropping out. Both girls are failing to accomplish their developmental tasks. For Marcia, her progress in completing her education, finding a career and a mate, and establishing her independence is threatened. Brenda is now out of the dating and high school scene with her peers and cannot even think of her dream to join the Air Force right now. Myra, who was hoping for some time for herself, is now busier than ever. Sharon knows that the family is having difficulty completing expected developmental tasks because of these events.

The family development approach attempts to track change over time in a family. Families and individuals are engaged in a developmental process of growth, aging, and change over the life span. In this approach, a longitudinal view of the family classifies and predicts differences in families as they develop. The assumption is that both individuals in the family and the family as a whole need to accomplish certain tasks at specific times in their life cycles. As the family confronts various **stages** of the life cycle, **developmental tasks** must be achieved if the stage is to be negotiated successfully. These tasks carry certain role expectations. If the tasks are not achieved at specific times as a result of stress, crises, lack of resources, or unhealthy family structure and process, they may never be completely achieved. The better equipped a family is to help each member complete his or her developmental tasks and help the family meet its group tasks, the more successful the development of the family will be. The theory assumes that commonalities exist for all families.

Duvall (1977) adapted this approach from the theory of individual developmental tasks proposed by Havighurst. Duvall defined nine ever-changing family developmental tasks that span the family life cycle and outlined eight stages of the family life cycle and specific tasks for each stage (Table 12-1). Family stages are defined by the age of the oldest child. For example, a family that has two children aged 7 and 2 would be considered a school-aged family rather than a preschool family.

In the cycle of family development, the **transition** from one stage to the next is the critical period. The ease with which a family progresses through these critical phases is determined, to some extent, by the completion of earlier tasks. For example, a family in the launching stage typically has a young adult who is preparing to leave home. The family in this stage must successfully release the young adult, maintain a supportive home base, and reestablish the relationships and structure

TABLE 12-1   **Family Developmental Tasks**

Stage		Tasks
Establishing	Marital couple	Establishing a marriage
		Establishing a functional household
		Family planning
		Relating to extended family
		Promoting achievement of developmental tasks for all members
Early childbearing	Adding an infant	Managing time and energy
		Stabilizing the family unit
		Developing parenting skills
Preschool	Children (3-5 years old)	Maintaining a stable marriage
		Making employment decisions
		Nurturing young children
School age	Children (6-12 years old)	Promoting school and skill achievement
		Socializing children
		Balancing work and family
Adolescent	Teenage children	Balancing adolescent independence with responsibility
		Building an economic and emotional base for the future
		Maintaining open communication
Launching	Child leaves home	Disengaging
		Readjusting the marriage and family roles
		Caring for aging parents
Middle age	Parents in midlife	Preparing for retirement
		Rediscovering couplehood
		Maintaining intergenerational relationships
		Developing recreational activities
Aging	Late adulthood	Adapting to retirement
		Dealing with loss of function
		Managing health issues
		Preparing for death of self and spouse

Adapted from Duvall, E. M. (1977). *Family development* (5th ed.). Chicago: J. B. Lippincott; Friedman, M. M. (1992). *Family nursing: Theory and assessment* (3rd ed.). Norwalk, CT: Appleton & Lange.

within the family to adjust to the lack of the missing member. The transition is easier if the family has completed earlier transitions successfully. For example, what if a family is trying to launch a young adult but has never worked out a way to share the responsibilities involved in day-to-day life? The member who is about to be launched might be unprepared to accept adult responsibilities.

Duvall's ideas provide a structured and logical way of looking at family life. However, the early framework tended to view all families as nuclear (i.e., mother-father-children). The organization of the developmental stages is based on the assumption that every family will experience the birth and eventual release of children. This portrait of family life does not represent modern families.

Others have expanded Duvall's ideas to include varied family forms and transitions such as presence of younger siblings (McGoldrick et al., 1993), divorced families (Melnyk & Alpert-Gillis, 1997), adoptive families (Peterson, 1997), single-parent families, and families in poverty (Hines, 1986). McGoldrick and colleagues (1993) recognized that families take different forms and are often three generational. In their model, the family life cycle spans more than one generation, and families react to both the past and the future. For many families, for example, when the youngest child leaves home,

increased responsibilities for elderly parents often arise. The examination by Carter and McGoldrick (1989) of stages and tasks for the divorcing family is outlined in Table 12-2.

A community/public health nurse who is aware of developmental family theory will attempt to determine the family's stage in the life cycle and to assess the family's knowledge of current developmental demands, the strategies they are using to meet these demands, and their success at accomplishing these tasks. Some families need information about the *usual* course that can be expected. Other families may benefit from interventions that help them arrange some balance between the developmental demands and other demands such as illness, job loss, or scarce family resources. In families with an ill member, the needs of a healthy child will occasionally get lost in the shuffle. The goal is to enable the family to accomplish its function for all its members, not just the ones who are ill or otherwise in the forefront.

FAMILY AS A SYSTEM

Thinking about the family as a system is so common that many other approaches actually combine their ways of thinking about families with a systems perspective. The systems perspective views the family as a unit and was first proposed by von Bertalanffy (1968) as the general systems

TABLE 12-2   Stages of Divorce and Remarriage

Stage	Developmental Tasks
Divorce	
Deciding to divorce	Acceptance of one's own part in failure of marriage
Planning the breakup	Working cooperatively with problems of custody and finances
	Dealing with extended family
Separation	Mourning the loss of the family
	Restructuring marital and parent-child relationships
	Realignment of relationships with spouse's family
Divorce	Overcoming hurt, anger, guilt, and fantasies of reconciliation
	Staying connected with extended families
Postdivorce	
Custodial single parent	Maintaining flexible arrangements with ex-spouse
	Rebuilding own social network
	Managing finances
	Supporting emotional adaptation of children
Noncustodial parent	Finding ways to continue effective parenting
	Maintaining financial responsibilities for children
	Rebuilding own social network
Planning Remarriage	
Entering relationship	Recovery of loss of first marriage
	Recommitment to formation of a marriage and family
	Willingness to deal with complexity and ambiguity
Planning new family	Planning for cooperative financial and parenting arrangements with ex-spouses
	Allowing time and patience for adjustment of all
	Adjusting to multiple new roles, boundaries, space, time, membership, and discipline practices
	Dealing with own and children's fears, guilt, and loyalty conflicts
Remarriage	Acceptance of a different model of family
	Restructuring parental boundaries and adjusting to permeable boundaries of new family
	Maintaining relationships of children with all family members
	Enhancing new family integration and identity
	Sharing memories of history of family and creating new traditions and memories

Adapted from Carter, B., & McGoldrick, M. (1989). *The changing family life cycle* (2nd ed.). Boston: Allyn and Bacon.

theory (see Chapter 1). Certain principles are applicable to all systems:

- A system is a unit in which the whole is greater than the sum of its parts.
- Predictable rules govern the operation of these systems.
- Every system has a boundary that is somewhat open or closed.
- Boundaries allow exchange of information and resources into (external influences) and out of (outcomes) the system.
- Communication and feedback mechanisms between parts of the system are important in the functioning of the system.
- Circular causality helps explain what is happening better than linear causality. A change in one part of the system leads to change in the whole system.
- Systems operate on the principle of equifinality. The same end point can be reached from a number of starting points or in different ways.
- Systems appear to have a purpose. This purpose is often the avoidance of entropy or complete randomness and disorganization.
- Systems are made up of subsystems and are themselves part of suprasystems.

Family therapists were the first to apply systems theory to families. Approaches such as those of Minuchin and Fishman (1981) and Satir (1972), described later in this chapter, are based on the idea of the family as a system in which the whole is different and greater than the individual members. A family system perspective recognizes that change in one part of the system will affect the entire family. Because the system has a tendency to want to stay the same (morphostasis), the family will usually attempt to resist the change even if the change is helpful. Nurses who are planning interventions with families must take into account this resistance and the implications for the entire system.

Suppose a family with a child with disabilities is not adhering to daily treatments. Planning an intervention that encourages the mother to spend more time on these treatments may help the disabled child, but doing so may take the mother away from tasks that need to be accomplished for her other children. Viewing families as an interconnected system makes nursing care more difficult to plan and perform but is a more accurate way to think about families.

Families have boundaries differing in openness to the environment. Some boundaries will allow information and resources to pass back and forth freely, and others shut off this exchange. Families are exposed to stress over time. When stress is present in an open system, it can result in adaptation and growth in the individuals. When stress is present in a more closed family system, it can result in maladaptation; distorted perceptions, thoughts, and feelings; and less capable individuals. Community/public health nurses who interact with families need to be aware of the character of a particular family's boundaries. Helping a family become aware of its tendencies to use resources from the environment often promotes family health.

Family systems tend to want to reach relatively steady states, but change can occur. Change occurs most often when at least one member of the system, often the one who is the most flexible or free of constraints and has some power in the family, makes a change in his or her way of functioning within the family. From this perspective, interventions for families are not directed at the member who is ill, injured, or at risk, but at the members who are strongest and most able to change. This means that the nurse will plan and target interventions with the members of the system who have some freedom and strength to carry out the interventions. A community/public health nurse who is working with a family that is caring for an aging mother may choose to spend more time with a daughter-in-law who has indicated a willingness to help than with the aging mother or her ill spouse, who is having difficulty himself. Family interventions include the entire family, building on its strengths, rather than focusing on its weaknesses.

BOWEN'S FAMILY SYSTEMS THEORY

Murray Bowen is the founder of a school of family therapy that developed the family systems approach in more specific ways (Bowen, 1978). Several concepts from this theory help nurses work more effectively with families.

A key concept is the **level of differentiation,** or a person's ability to separate his or her emotions and thoughts. People exist along a continuum that ranges from being able to separate decisions and emotional reactions to being totally driven by automatic emotional responses. When an individual is operating in a high feeling state, the need to be approved of or close to other people is paramount; operating in an autonomous or self-directed way is difficult. A person's level of differentiation will affect his or her ability to operate successfully in the many spheres of life, including employment, parenting, money management, and health habits. A person's physical, emotional, and social functioning is related to his or her level of differentiation and to the amount of anxiety present in the family system.

The **triangle** is another concept that is helpful in understanding family operations (Figure 12-3). Any two-person system is unstable. Within a short period, tension develops between the two people and results in the automatic *triangling in* of a third person. Each triangle has three sides: a close one in which two people are allied, a conflictual one in which two people are in disagreement, and a distant one in which two people are emotionally separated (Triangle A). In periods of calm, the distant position is uncomfortable. The distant person (person 2) will usually try to move into a closer position (Triangle B). In periods of anxiety, the distant position is preferred. People try to maneuver this position to escape the tension. Triangles are usually dynamic (i.e., constantly changing), although, in families, they often have predictable and rigid forms.

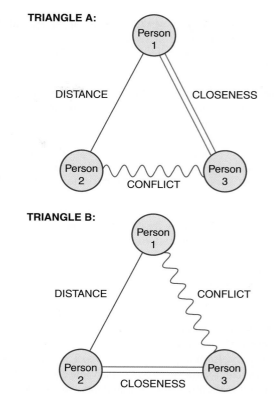

FIGURE 12-3 Triangles are dynamic. (See text for explanation.)

Community/public health nurses who interact with a family can use this knowledge of triangles. Remembering that nurses will automatically become a member of one or several triangles when interacting with a family, nurses can monitor their behavior and be aware of the pull toward automatic behaviors. For instance, a nurse interacting with two brothers trying to make plans about moving their mother into a nursing home may find himself or herself taking sides with the brother who first contacted him or her. Being able to operate in somewhat neutral ways and to maintain contact with all participants is likely to be more helpful than taking sides with one of the family members. Nurses cannot avoid triangles, but they can be aware of the behaviors within them.

Anxiety is another concept that is important in this theory. The more anxiety that is present, the more likely that people will react with automatic rather than thoughtful actions. These automatic reactions tend to escalate triangles and patterns of interactions within the system that have developed over time in attempts to manage tension.

The Levine family is a family that has had conflictual family relationships for some time. Carl Levine is a quiet man who works at a retail store. His wife, Jackie, is an optometrist. The family has always operated with a high level of anxiety in their daily life that is noticeable in their everyday relationships. Jackie jumps at anything Carl says that is slightly critical. She is very quick to start a conflictual conversation. Carl reacts by becoming very quiet. The couple's son, Sam, is frequently caught up in this conflict and is asked to moderate the arguments. When the family is experiencing additional stress, Sam will react with migraine headaches that keep him out of school. The level of differentiation of this family is demonstrated by reactivity under minimal stress. Adding more anxiety is likely to increase family patterns of blame and decrease the family's ability to function effectively.

A community/public health nurse applying family systems ideas with families realizes that monitoring self-functioning is the prerequisite to any intervention. A person who is anxious and not thinking clearly will take this anxiety into the family. Being in contact with a family without being anxious, being overresponsible, or taking sides is sometimes difficult. The nurse who can remain in contact and continue to relate to the family in a way that enables the nurse to see the *problem* calmly and in a broad and thoughtful way is believed to be more helpful to a family system than is a nurse who is determined to find a way to *fix* the family. If a nurse can enter an anxious system and retain a somewhat calm presence in the midst of great tension, others in the system may be able to do so as well. Nurses cannot change the functioning of the system, but they can change the ways they operate within it.

FAMILY STRUCTURE AND FUNCTION

In a structural-functional approach, the family is viewed as an organization arranged in a structure with a hierarchy that enables it to perform necessary functions. The family is organized into smaller parts, or subsystems. Some concepts relevant to this framework are values, boundaries, roles, hierarchies, and interactional style.

Structural-functional theory has an outcome orientation: what does the family do in relation to society at large? Sociologists emphasize three major areas of function: the functions of the family for society, the functions of subsystems within the family for the family, and the functions of the family for individual members (Nye & Berardo, 1981). Examples of functions of family that are frequently mentioned include socialization of new members into society, reproduction, maintenance (of the family as an organization), affective functions (stabilization of adult personalities), and economic functions (provision of food, clothing, and shelter for members). To carry out these functions, family members assume certain **roles** or expected ways of behaving and make contributions. **Values** or beliefs about priorities are often learned or shared with similar societal groups.

Structural-functional concepts also emerged in family therapy. According to Salvatore Minuchin, a structural family therapist, symptoms of family members can be resolved through appropriate family organization (Minuchin & Fishman, 1981). The concept of boundaries between subsystems is emphasized in his approach. Boundaries represent rules that define participants in a subsystem and regulate their behavior. Families with clear and age-appropriate boundaries are believed to function better than families with rigid or ill-defined boundaries. **Subsystems** enable the family to perform its functions. Each subsystem has different territories and makes certain demands on its members. Commonly discussed family subsystems include spousal, parental, and sibling subsystems. Each of these subsystems has a different place in the **hierarchy** of family life and has different power in relation to others.

Interactional style describes the way family members relate to each other. Families sometimes develop repetitive patterns of interaction that prescribe their behavior. A family therapist observing a family would ask: Do certain patterns reappear that seem to be regulated by the structure and past behaviors within the family? Are these patterns functional in that they help the family achieve its goals? Do they function to keep things the same, or do they seek change?

How is the family organized in general? Is it enmeshed, with boundaries blurred and a strong feeling of overinvolvement? Are family members disengaged, with members barely connecting with each other? Are they somewhere in between? Are boundaries so rigid that no growth or adaptation is possible? Structural family therapists often use a tool called a *family map* to diagram the spatial and relationship qualities within a family system. This subject is discussed in more detail in Chapter 13.

FAMILY INTERACTION AND COMMUNICATION

Burgess (1926) described the family as "a unit of interacting personalities." Family sociologists began using the term *symbolic interaction* to describe the way family members interact with each other. Interaction is defined as a set of processes taking place among individuals that cannot be separated into isolated parts. Behaviors of one person are both the cause and the effect of behaviors in another. A representation of self is also learned through values and symbols communicated to the actor by other people.

Symbolic interaction is perhaps most clearly demonstrated when we think about the process of child development—how a child learns about himself or herself and his or her position and status within the environment. This concept is appropriate for all family interactions. For example, in every marriage, many actions become regulated through symbols and shared meanings that define the situation and each spouse's relationship to the other. Playing a part (e.g., the *competent husband,* the *comforting wife*) may typify many of the interactions in a marriage.

Communications theory, which is based on systems theory, was developed by family therapists. This theory, in which communication is the primary tool for looking at and working with families, grew out of the work of Watzlawick and colleagues (1967) and of Satir (1972). For example, double-bind communication may be seen in schizophrenic families. A **double-bind communication** sends two conflicting messages. For example, a mother may say, "Come here, I love you" to a child, yet remain rigid and cold when the child approaches. Not only is the child in a double bind by being unable to respond to both messages, but also the communication usually includes the unspoken message, "Don't comment on how incongruent this communication is."

Early observations of communication and interaction among people gave rise to several basic concepts of communications theory:

1. Not communicating is impossible, because every verbal or nonverbal behavior includes a message. Even silence is communication.

2. Communication has several levels. On one level, the content or literal meaning of the message is communicated: "I want you to go to the store." On another level, information about intimacy, power, or conflict is transmitted. This level is known as **metacommunication.** "I want you to go to the store" can be said in many different ways intending to communicate power, helplessness, intimacy, conflict, or many other messages about the relationship between the communicators.

3. Communication implies an exchange of information. Within a family, these interactions become patterns that are predictable and repeated. For example, in one family, the only way to complain about something may be for the mother to talk to the son, who will then talk to the father. This communication may always occur in a derogatory way so that the father is blamed for what is happening. Because families have a long history of repeated contacts with each other, these patterns tend to repeat themselves in somewhat predictable ways.

4. In functional families, communication is usually one of the following:
    a. A tool to help children learn about the environment
    b. A way to communicate rules about how people in the family should think and act
    c. A tool for conflict resolution
    d. A nurturing method that leads to the development of self-esteem

5. Healthy communication is open, honest, direct, and congruent with internal feelings.

6. Family members assume certain roles relating to family communication.

Virginia Satir (1972) emphasized the messages about self-esteem communicated within families. Her book *Peoplemaking* provides interesting exercises and reading for those who want to learn more about family communication.

The community/public health nurse using communication theory principles with families would first assess the family's style of communication. Families will have certain rules that govern the way they communicate. The family's patterns of interaction will repeat themselves and can be used as a source of information about its communication and members' relationships with each other. These patterns determine how a family will solve conflict, communicate respect or worth, assert power and authority, and develop closeness or distance. The nurse will want to observe what kinds of messages family members receive about themselves as people and about the problem at hand. Ideally, communication will be open (members discuss events with each other rather than engage in circuitous ways of transmitting the information), honest (members feel free to say what they think and feel), direct (members go directly to the person involved rather than communicate through another), and congruent (verbal messages match internal feelings); however, the family may not be able to communicate in these ways. On some occasions, helping family members alter their communication may be appropriate; in other circumstances, the nurse may choose to alter interventions to match the family communication. For example, if a family has a rule that all communication goes through the father, the nurse may choose to communicate with the family in the preferred way.

Even if the situation is not conducive to changing family communication, the community/public health nurse can influence the family situation by being careful of his or her own communication. Taking steps to ensure that communication is open, honest, direct, and congruent accurately sends information to the family and increases the chance that the family will perceive the information accurately. The nurse may sometimes intervene most effectively simply by being a role model of an effective communicator. The nurse's *meta* position—having the ability to be outside the family and observe more accurately what goes on—sometimes enables him or her

to communicate information about family communication patterns that the family cannot observe. All members in the family deserve communication from the health care system that recognizes their importance and worth as individuals in the family. How the nurse communicates to each member may be as important as what is said.

DISTINCTIVE CHARACTERISTICS OF FAMILIES

Other family scholars have attempted to describe families by identifying their distinctive characteristics. How do families differ from each other? Do *types* of families exist? Many of these models focus on healthy or *normal* families in contrast to earlier theories, which focused on family problems.

Beavers and Hampson (1993) studied healthy families and developed a model that describes levels of family functioning that range from *healthy* to *midrange* to *severely dysfunctional*. The authors used two dimensions—family competence and family **style**—to describe families. Style is centripetal or centrifugal; that is, families tend to look for gratification within the family or outside of it, respectively. Family styles tend to vary along developmental lines. For example, a family that is newly formed will often be centripetal, whereas a middle-aged family is often centrifugal.

Olson, Sprenkle, and Russell (1982) advanced the Circumplex Model of families based on the family dimensions of cohesion and adaptability. Cohesion is the tendency of the family to interact as a unit and can vary from open to closed. Adaptability or flexibility refers to the family's ability to adopt new ways of operating. Families vary from rigid to extremely flexible; 16 different types are possible. The model suggests that a balanced level of cohesion and adaptability is most functional, but no one family type is believed to be the *best* (Figure 12-4).

These different models suggest that many variations exist in the ways families can operate and still be *healthy*. When working with families, the community/public health nurse should assess for different family styles. Knowing a family's style will help the nurse plan the best way to proceed in order to fit into the family's usual way of dealing with the world. For example, a family that is operating in a disconnected way may not be able to present all its members together at a prearranged conference. However, the nurse may be able to see different family members at different times and discuss issues with individuals. Families that prove to be at either extreme of the continuum may find themselves in trouble if their conventional way of operating is not working for the current situation. Some families may be receptive to suggestions about alternative ways to do things, but others may not. The goal for the nurse is to maximize what can be done within the family style.

FAMILY COPING WITH STRESS

Interest in how families cope with stress has been growing, and the emphasis in family theories has changed from concentrating on the pathology within families to focusing on family strengths, resources, and adaptability. This focus has resulted in attempts to maximize families' abilities to cope with expected and unexpected stressors in their lives.

As early as 1949, Hill proposed a model that describes family reaction to stress as a process in which the family experiences several phases or changes (Figure 12-5). In the ABCX Model (crisis model) of family coping, A (the event) interacts with

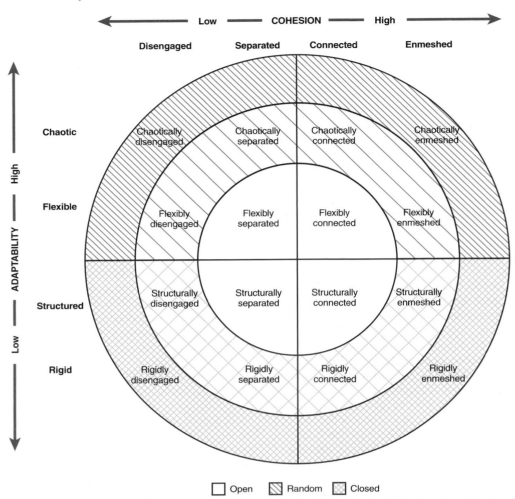

FIGURE 12-4 The Circumplex Model of family systems. (Redrawn from Olson, D. H., & McCubbin, H. I. [1982]. Circumplex Model of marital and family systems: V. Application to family stress and crisis intervention. In H. I. McCubbin, A. E. Cauble, & J. M. Patterson [Eds.], *Family stress, coping, and social support* [p. 54]. Springfield, IL: Charles C. Thomas.)

B (resources), which interacts with C (the definition the family makes of the event) to produce X (the crisis). The family is thought to experience a roller-coaster course of adjustment, a process involving disorganization, recovery, and a subsequent level of reorganization. Burr (1973) added the concepts

of vulnerability and regenerative power to Hill's framework, stressing that families vary in their internal resources or abilities to respond to crisis.

The following clinical example is of a family coping with stress.

> The Bower family has recently been told that the 7-year-old son, Anthony, has a learning disability. This news is coming right on top of learning that the mother, Eve, has diabetes. Eve has been occupied with learning how to take care of her new health problem and is committed to some rigid rules in the family about mealtimes, exercise, bedtime, homework, and chores. In addition, she is recovering from the recent death of her father in an automobile accident. Her husband, Tom, and her daughter, Lisa, will be helping her learn how to manage Anthony's new requirements, which include frequent medication and behavior management strategies. In the past, Eve managed these types of problems mostly by herself. She is feeling quite overwhelmed. The community/public health nurse, Dawn, knows that the way the family appraises the situation, its resources, and their problem-solving abilities will play a big part in its ability to adjust and eventually adapt to these new demands. The present situation is the first time the family will really be presented with problems that test its resilience.

FIGURE 12-5 Hill's ABCX Model of family coping. (Redrawn from McCubbin, H. I., & Patterson, J. M. [1982]. Family adaptation to crisis. In H. I. McCubbin, A. E. Cauble, & J. M. Patterson [Eds.], *Family stress, coping, and social support* [p. 46]. Springfield, IL: Charles C. Thomas.)

In 1982, McCubbin, Cauble, and Patterson proposed the Double ABCX Model of family stress and adaptation. This model adds the concepts of pileup of demands, family system resources, and postcrisis behavior. How a family responds to crisis will depend, in part, on its response to previous crises. When crises pile up, the family is more at risk for being unable to maintain sufficient resources and healthy coping behaviors. The Double ABCX Model is a clear model to use when trying to understand and explain family reactions to stress. Refinements have been made to this model as presented in Figure 12-6.

In 1987 the concept of family type was added. Families can be regenerative, resilient, and rhythmic. Boss (1987) emphasized the meaning the family gives to an event as the most crucial factor determining a family's experience of stress. In 1993, McCubbin, McCubbin, and Thompson defined the concept of family schema, which includes shared family values, goals, expectations, and world views.

The Resiliency Model of Family Stress, Adjustments, and Adaptation is a refinement of the original Double ABCX Model (McCubbin & McCubbin, 1993). According to this model, families respond to life events and life transitions in two phases: adjustment and adaptation. The adjustment phase involves the transitory changes families make in response to an event. The adaptation phase is a longer phase that occurs when a family's attempts to make minor adjustments are not effective and result in crisis.

For example, consider the case of a family that experiences the birth of a child with a severe disability. When the community/public health nurse encounters this family, the degree of family vulnerability should be appraised. The family vulnerability will be related to the current pileup of demands, such as financial obligations, developmental changes being experienced with other siblings, or job pressures. The more events being experienced by the family, the more vulnerable the family will be. However, the community/public health nurse knows that different families will respond to a birth in different ways. The family type or amount of **resilience**—plus **resources,** problem-solving and **coping** behaviors, and **appraisal** of the stress—leads to its adjustment to the event. If this family is

resilient, has already developed effective problem-solving and coping behaviors, and appraises the birth as a challenge that can be dealt with, then members will probably manage the period of adjustment fairly well. The community/public health nurse would find on the initial visits that the family experienced a period of disorganization at first but was able to make changes that will help the family care for the child. Family members sought resources of time and physical help from extended family and friends. The wife adjusted her work schedule so that she would be home during the day and gone in the evening. The husband took over child care when he came home from work. Family meals and routines were simplified.

This family is faced with caring for a son who will require respiratory care, physical therapy, and fairly frequent monitoring for many years. After the initial adjustment, the family will continue to make changes in its way of operating to deal with the longer-term demands. As the family enters the adaptation phase, the amount of stressors, strains, and transitions occurring adds to the pileup of events. However, newly instituted patterns of functioning, family resources, and social support can moderate the impact. The family will assign a meaning to the disability and its impact on the family. The community/public health nurse can work with the family members to help them assign a meaning that includes a view of themselves as succeeding and living with some joy in the face of the demands. This view will interact with their problem-solving and coping mechanisms to determine a new level of adaptation. Eventually, the family will stabilize in ways that are different from the way the family was before the birth.

Suppose, however, that family resilience was limited. Perhaps shortly before the birth of the child the father had taken a new job, the family had moved to a new community, and the grandmother, who had helped when the older children were young, had fallen and needed some help herself. The pileup of demands for this family might exhaust their resources and drive them into less effective coping behaviors. Or suppose that the family appraisal of the birth left its members with feelings of incompetence and failure. Perhaps the family problem-solving ability was rigid, and they were unable to trust themselves in trying new coping behaviors. Family

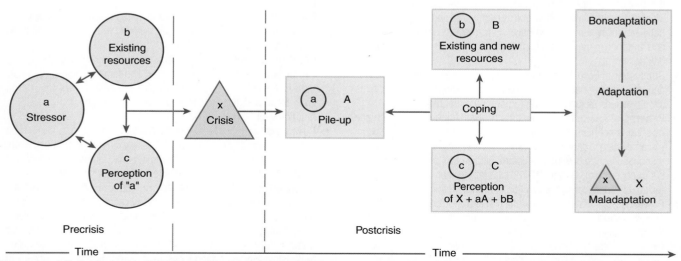

FIGURE 12-6 The Double ABCX Model of family stress and adaptation. (Redrawn from McCubbin, H. I., & Patterson, J. M. [1982]. Family adaptation to crisis. In H. I. McCubbin, A. E. Cauble, & J. M. Patterson [Eds.]. *Family stress, coping, and social support* [p. 46]. Springfield, IL: Charles C. Thomas.)

members' lessened capability to pull new patterns of functioning into the situation would drive them into a less healthy adaptation. Multiple factors enter into the effectiveness of the family adaptation.

The outcome for this family must be considered in terms of the effect on the individual members and the family as a whole. Possibly, resources might be effectively mobilized to provide safe care for the child, but the marriage of the parents might end in divorce. Anyone who works with families should understand this requirement of simultaneous balancing of individuals' needs and family needs.

HOW CAN THESE APPROACHES BE INTEGRATED?

Understanding the family is not a simple task. The models and theories presented here provide a wide array of ideas about how families work. Some characteristics of families that are functional, however, seem to be universal and are brought up over and over in these theories. A summary of these characteristics is presented in Box 12-4.

FAMILY PERSPECTIVES IN NURSING

Concepts and principles from family theories must be used within a framework that considers the role of the nurse and the relationship between the nurse and the client. Some early nursing theorists have included the idea of family in their theories. One of the major concepts of King (1981) was that the family is a social system. Other theorists did not include family in their early work but added the component later (Newman, 1979; Orem, 1971; Rogers, 1970). All theorists discuss the family as a unit that can be the focus of care (Newman, 1983; Orem, 1980; Rogers, 1983). However, none of these nursing theories describes the family or interventions for the family in enough detail to direct family nurse interactions.

WHAT IS FAMILY NURSING?

Family nursing is a relatively new approach to nursing science. Although those in nursing can learn from other disciplines such as sociology and family therapy, nursing theory must direct nursing practice. Nursing theorists began to formulate frameworks specifically for family nursing in the 1980s. Family nursing has now evolved to include multiple approaches to family care.

Some nurses began to suggest more strongly that the focus of family nursing should be on health. Gillis and colleagues (1989) began with an interest in family health and illness. Bomar (2004) emphasizes family health promotion. Denham (2003) provides a framework for studying and improving family health. Denham defines family health as the "ways families communicate, cooperate, and provide care for each other and maintain and sustain health routines." Denham further

---

BOX 12-4   Characteristics of Functional Families

- **Developmental stages and tasks:** A family goes through predictable stages according to the age and development of its members. If tasks are not achieved at the stage-appropriate time, they may never be achieved. Maturational crises are predictable. Some crises are unpredictable and interfere with achievement of tasks.
- **Roles:** Define certain patterns of expected behavior. Are often male or female linked. Need to be appropriate for age and sex. Also need to be flexible, not rigid, and able to support family functioning.
- **Boundaries:** Exist around the system to handle exchange between the family and the environment. Also exist between subsystems to differentiate members belonging to each subsystem. Need to be permeable to allow information and resources in and out. Boundaries between subsystems should have clear generational lines and support a strong parental coalition. Should be neither too rigid nor too diffuse.
- **Subsystems:** Each member of the family belongs to several simultaneously: spouse, parent-child, sibling, and grandparent. Subsystems should include all (and only) age-appropriate members.
- **Patterns of interaction:** Repeat themselves. Are healthier when one member is not blamed, left out, or put down in the interaction. Should be somewhere in between enmeshed and disengaged. Communication theorists describe how people communicate (e.g., placatory, blaming, superresponsible). Bowen (1978) talks about four ways of handling fusion: distance, conflict, projection, and dysfunction.
- **Power:** Results from clear role definition and appropriate rules. Should be somewhat shared, appropriate to age, and within the parental subsystem until the children are independent.
- **External stressors:** Usually present at some point. If they vary, are not very intense, and are spread out over time, the family has a chance to adapt. Illness brings its own set of demands to the family.

- **Open or closed system:** As the system closes, all variables and patterns become fixed and less adaptable. Energy is used in dysfunctional ways. Open systems can adapt and change as feedback is received from within and outside the system. This aspect is related to permeability of boundaries.
- **Communication:** Healthier when it is clear, honest, direct, congruent, and specific and when the family is able to use it as a mechanism to resolve conflict.
- **Values:** Related to cultural, socioeconomic groups. Provide some stability, rules, and guidelines. Need to be able to change with changing times.
- **Encouragement of autonomy and acceptance of difference:** A balance needs to exist between autonomy of members and the need to be a cohesive group.
- **Level of anxiety:** When the family is calm, people in the family can think and solve problems better. The family tends to do better than in times of stress. Anxiety can be transitional or long-term. Long-term anxiety tends to wear down the ability of the family to function well.
- **Resources and social support:** Available to most families from within and outside the family, but the family must be able to use them. Extended family is often used. Socioeconomic status and geographic location tend to influence these. All families have some strengths.
- **Meaning, perception, and paradigm:** The way a family perceives a situation, the meaning it attaches to the events, and its typical way of relating to the outside environment influence the ways families react.
- **Adaptability:** Flexibility, adaptability, and resilience are necessary for a family to be able to cope with changing demands. A family needs to maintain a certain degree of flexibility and yet a certain degree of cohesiveness and predictability.

identifies common family health routines, including dietary habits, sleep and rest, activity patterns, care of dependent members, avoidance behaviors, medical consultation, and health recovery activities.

Three approaches are strong examples of integrated family nursing theory. Hanson (2005) and colleagues developed the Family Assessment and Intervention Model using the Family System Stressor-Strengths Inventory to measure family stress and guide interventions built on family strengths. The Friedman Family Assessment Model (Friedman, Bowden, & Jones, 2003) looks at families within the larger community. It draws on developmental, structural-functional, stress and coping, and environmental approaches. The Calgary Family Assessment and Intervention Model is a systems model that uses communication and change theory to address family affect, behaviors, and function (Wright & Leahey, 2005).

Interest has also increased in shifting the focus of family nursing practice from a deficit-based to a strength-based perspective. The concept of individual and family strengths is central to the McGill Model of Nursing (Allen, 1999). Feeley and Gottlieb (2000) identify different types of strengths that reside in individuals and families. Bomar (2004) suggests that the role of nursing is to identify and call forth strengths and to mobilize and regulate resources.

Who Is the Client?

In the frameworks described earlier, family is viewed in two ways in nursing: family as client and family as context for the individual (Whall, 1993; Wright & Leahey, 2005). Viewing the family as the unit of care means that the entire family is the recipient of the nursing intervention. This viewpoint recognizes the standard put forth in the American Nurses Association (ANA) public health nursing standards of practice (ANA, 2007), which identifies clients as individuals, families, communities, and populations. In contrast, viewing the family as context recognizes the impact the family has on an individual. This viewpoint underscores the need to understand the family environment in which the individual exists.

At what level do family health nurses intervene? If the family is the client, do nurses intervene with individuals, some members, the family as a unit, or even larger systems? Friedemann's framework (1995) outlines system-based family nursing practiced on three levels. The individual level is directed at the family as a composite of individuals. The interpersonal level is directed at dyads and other small groups of people within the family. The family system level is directed at the total system as it interacts with the environment. This text adds a fourth level: the environmental level. Sometimes, the environment itself may need to be addressed. Novice community/public health nurses can reduce environmental hazards, link families with community resources, and develop resources that are external to families. Community/public health nurses are often involved at a level at which they are addressing legislation, policies, and practices at a local, state, national, or even international level. The community or even the larger system of society is also an appropriate level of intervention. Thus the four levels of intervention for the community health nurse are the individual, the interpersonal, the family system, and the environmental levels (Figure 12-7), all of which are discussed more in Chapter 13.

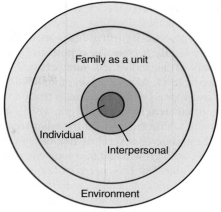

FIGURE 12-7 Levels of intervention in family nursing.

What Is the Appropriate Area of Concern for Intervention?

Which aspects of the family's experience need intervention? Is directing practice to physical dimensions of health and illness enough, or are other areas of family functioning appropriate to address in the role of the family health nurse? As discussed in Chapter 11, health promotion and primary, secondary, and tertiary prevention are all appropriate with families. Bomar and McNeely (1996, p. 5) integrate these ideas and then describe a global view of family health nursing as the "assessment and enhancement of family health status, family health assets, and family potentials."

Definition of Family Nursing

Some people believe that a nurse who practices with families as clients should be a specialist with advanced preparation in family nursing; others suggest that all nurses practice family-centered care (Hanson, 2005). Different nurses bring different amounts of knowledge and experience to the family situation. All nurses practice family nursing at the individual level, but only a nurse who guides family communication can practice interpersonal family nursing. Community/public health nurses practice at the interpersonal level when they assist parents in communicating with their preschool children or assist family members in sharing their thoughts with a terminally ill member. Nurses who provide family therapy or family systems nursing need to have advanced education (Friedman et al., 2003). However, all baccalaureate-level nursing graduates can conduct basic family assessments and interventions such as those discussed in Chapter 13.

The definition of family nursing proposed in this text is as follows: family nursing is the practice of nursing directed toward maximizing the health and well-being of all individuals within a family system. Two views of family are incorporated into this definition: family as the unit of care and family as context. Family nursing views the family as a system existing within a larger system. As noted earlier, levels of intervention are the individual, the interpersonal, the family system, and the environmental level. The goals of family nursing include optimal functioning for the individual and for the family as a unit. For community/public health nurses, improving the health of families is one way to improve the health of communities.

How Is Family Nursing Practiced?

Family nursing practice, like any nursing practice, begins with the nursing process. By using this process, the nurse who practices with a family perspective is potentially able to intervene effectively at the individual, interpersonal, family unit, or environmental level. After assessing the individuals, dyads, family unit, and suprasystem, the nurse is ready to begin identifying areas of concern or **needs.** Smith (1985) suggests that nurses who work within the community will discover that family needs fall into one or several of five categories: needs of families dealing with growth and development, needs of families coping with illness or loss, needs of families dealing with external stressors, needs of families with inadequate resources or support, and needs of families with disturbances in organization. In addition to needs, family strengths are identified that will help the family move toward optimal functioning and health. The family style, or process, must be considered as the nurse works with the family. This consideration helps the nurse choose appropriate ways of interacting. Finally, family function—an evaluation of the effectiveness of the family—must be assessed to determine if the goals are realistic. This *family needs* framework for family nursing is based on four assumptions:

1. Improvement in the functioning of an individual will elicit improvement in the functioning of the whole family.
2. Because of the systemic nature of family, interventions can be directed at any of several levels with a resultant change in family operation.
3. Nurse-client interaction is a crucial part of family nursing intervention.
4. Family nursing interventions need to be modified to match different family needs, family strengths, family styles, and levels of family functioning.

To begin this transition to using a family perspective, theorists have suggested that the nurse guide his or her family practice by considering some questions about the nature of the contact:

- What have I learned during my assessment of family structure, process, and function that best explains the phenomena happening in this family?
- What does the family want from me? What are they expecting me to do?
- What does the larger system expect or require of me? What is a community/public health nurse's responsibility in this situation?
- What level of expertise and skill am I bringing to the situation? What do I have the skills to do? What are my relationship skills?
- What have I learned from evidence-based science and theory that seems to apply to this situation?
- What might I know or be able to offer to help the individuals and the family achieve a more optimal level of health? How do I present this as a choice to the system?
- At what level of the system will I intervene (individual, interpersonal, family system, or environment)?

The decisions and actions of a nurse with regard to families are performed within the nursing process. How family nursing is actualized within each step of the process—assessment, planning, implementation, and evaluation—is discussed in more detail in the next chapter. Working toward family health is a goal that will support people today and strengthen our society for the future. Family nursing is an essential basis of community/public health nursing practice. Healthier families contribute to healthier communities.

KEY IDEAS

1. Using a family perspective is necessary for the community/public health nurse.
2. The nature of the American family is changing, which has led to the emergence of many different family forms.
3. No one type of healthy family exists. Families organize themselves in different ways that work for them.
4. Historic frameworks from social sciences and family therapy provide information about the nature of families.
5. Recent efforts in the development of nursing frameworks identify the family as the context in which an individual lives or as the unit of care.
6. Community/public health nurses can intervene with families at any of several levels: individual, interpersonal, family system, and environmental.
7. Family nurses need to identify family needs, family strengths, family styles, and family level of functioning.
8. Helping individuals maintain or restore their functioning will ultimately help strengthen the family.
9. Nurse-client interaction is a crucial part of family nursing and is adjusted for differing family situations.

LEARNING BY EXPERIENCE AND REFLECTION

1. Write a description of an ideal family. Take a moment to reflect on where these ideas originated. In what ways is your family similar to and different from your ideal?
2. Compare the characteristics of a functional family with those of a clinical family with which you are providing care (see Box 12-4). In what ways does the latter family exhibit the ideal and in what ways is it weak? Can you see at which point some of the concepts begin to relate to each other? For example, are boundaries between subsystems related to communication patterns?
3. Observe a family in a public place, such as a restaurant or shopping center. What does the members' interaction tell you about the family? Do you get a sense of the emotional tone and what it would be like to live in this family?
4. Mentally review the families living in your neighborhood. How many of these families are a traditional family? What other family forms do you recognize? From your knowledge of any of these families, do you think family form determines family health?
5. Watch a television show depicting family life. What form does this family represent? In your opinion, is it a healthy or not-so-healthy family? From where is the drama or comedy in the show originating? Is the show making fun of the family, using it to explain the drama, or presenting it as the answer to the heroic dilemma in the plot?
6. Think about intervening at the individual, interpersonal, family, or environmental level. At what levels have your past interventions been? At what levels do you feel comfortable intervening now? What additional experience or skills would you eventually like to have to intervene at all these levels?
7. Write a plan for improving your family's health.

COMMUNITY RESOURCES FOR PRACTICE

Information about each of the following organizations is found on its website, which can be accessed through the **WebLinks** section of this book's website at *http://evolve.elsevier.com/Maurer/community/*.

Caring for Every Child's Mental Health
Center for Mental Health Services

Grandparents Raising Grandchildren
Helping Us KIDS
National Mental Health Association
National Council on Family Relationships
Stepfamily Association of America
Strengthening America's Families
U.S. Department of Health and Human Services

STUDY AIDS   http://evolve.elsevier.com/Maurer/community/

Visit the Evolve website for this book to find the following study and assessment materials:

- Quiz
- Web Scenario
- Critical Thinking Questions and Answers for Case Studies

- Care Plans
- *Healthy People* Updates
- Glossary

REFERENCES

Allen, F. M. (1999). Comparative theories of the expanded role in nursing and implications for nursing practice. *Canadian Journal of Nursing Research, 30,* 83-90.

American Nurses Association. (2007). *Public health nursing: Scope and standards of practice.* Silver Spring, MD: Author.

Annie E. Casey Foundation. (2007). *KIDS COUNT.* Retrieved September 7, 2007 from *http://www.aecf.org/MajorInitiatives/KIDSCOUNT.aspx.*

Beavers, W. R., & Hampson, R. (1993). Measuring family competence: The Beavers systems model. In F. Walsh (Ed.), *Normal family processes* (2nd ed.; pp. 73-103). New York: Guilford Press.

Bomar, P. (2004). *Promoting health in families: Applying family research and theory to nursing practice* (3rd ed.). Philadelphia: Saunders.

Bomar, P., & McNeely, G. (1996). Family health nursing: Past, present, and future. In P. Bomar (Ed.), *Nurses and family health promotion: Concepts, assessments, and interventions* (2nd ed.; pp. 3-21). Philadelphia: Saunders.

Boss, P. G. (1987). Family stress. In M. Sussman & S. Steinmetz (Eds.), *Handbook on marriage and the family* (pp. 695-723). New York: Plenum.

Bowen, M. (1978). *Family therapy in clinical practice.* New York: Jason Aronson.

Bronfenbrenner, U. (1979). *The ecology of human development.* Cambridge, MA: Harvard University Press.

Burgess, E. W. (1926). The family as a unit of interacting personalities. *Family, 7,* 3-9.

Burr, W. (1973). *Theory construction in the sociology of the family.* New York: John Wiley & Sons.

Carter, B., & McGoldrick, M. (1989). *The changing family life cycle* (2nd ed.). Boston: Allyn & Bacon.

Child Trends Data Bank. (2007). Retrieved September 6, 2007 from *http://www.childtrendsdatabank.org/.*

Curran, D. (1983). *Traits of the healthy family.* Minneapolis: Winston.

Denham, S. (2003). *Family health: A framework for nursing.* Philadelphia: F. A. Davis.

Duvall, E. M. (1977). *Family development* (5th ed.). Chicago: J. B. Lippincott.

Feeley, N., & Gottlieb, L. N. (2000). Nursing approaches for working with family strengths and resources. *Journal of Family Nursing, 6*(1), 9-24.

Friedman, M. (1986). *Family nursing: Theory and assessment* (2nd ed.). Norwalk, CT: Appleton-Century-Crofts.

Friedman, M. (1998). *Family nursing: Research, theory, and practice* (4th ed.). Stamford, CT: Appleton & Lange.

Friedman, M. M. (1992). *Family nursing: Theory and assessment* (3rd ed.). Norwalk, CT: Appleton & Lange.

Friedman, M. M., Bowden, V. R., & Jones, E. G. (2003). *Family nursing: Research, theory, and practice* (5th ed.). Saddle River, NJ: Prentice Hall.

Friedemann, M. L. (1995). *The framework of systemic organization: A conceptual approach to families and nursing.* Thousand Oaks, CA: Sage.

Gillis, C. L., Roberts, B. M., Highley, B. L., et al. (1989). What is family nursing? In G. L. Gillis, B. Highley, B. M. Roberts, et al. (Eds.), *Toward a science of family nursing* (pp. 63-74). Menlo Park, CA: Addison-Wesley.

Hanson, S. M. H. (2005). Family nursing assessment and intervention. In S. Hanson, V. Gedaly-Duff, & J. Kaakinen. *Family health care nursing: Theory, practice, and research* (3rd ed.). Philadelphia: F. A. Davis.

Hareven, T. K. (1982). American families in transition: Historical perspectives in change. In A. Skolnick & J. Skolnick (Eds.), *Family in transition.* Boston: Little, Brown.

Hill, R. (1949). *Families under stress.* New York: Harper & Row.

Hines, P. M. (1986). The family life cycle of poor black families. In B. Carter & M. McGoldrick

(Eds.), *The changing family life cycle* (2nd ed.: pp. 513-542). Boston: Allyn & Bacon.

King, G., King, S., Law, M., et al. (2002). *Family-centered service in Ontario: A "best practice" approach for children with disabilities and their families.* Hamilton, Ontario: CanChild Centre for Childhood Disability Research, McMaster University.

King, I. (1981). *A theory of nursing: Systems, concepts, process.* New York: John Wiley & Sons.

Lasch, C. (1995). The family as a haven in a heartless world. In A. Skolnick & J. Skolnick (Eds.), *Family in transition* (8th ed.). Boston: Little, Brown.

Law, M., Hanna, S., King, G., et al. (2003). Factors affecting family-centered service delivery for children with disabilities. *Child Care, Health and Development, 29*(5), 357-366.

McCubbin, H. I., Cauble, A. E., & Patterson, J. M. (1982). *Family stress, coping, and social support.* Springfield, IL: Charles C. Thomas.

McCubbin, H. I., & McCubbin, M. A. (1993). Families coping with illness: The Resiliency Model of Family Stress, Adjustment, and Adaptation. In C.B. Danielson, B. Hamel-Bissel, & P. Winsted-Fry (Eds.), *Families, health and illness: Perspectives on coping and intervention* (pp. 21-63). St. Louis: Mosby.

McCubbin, H. I., McCubbin, M. A., & Thompson, A. I. (1993). Resiliency in families. In T. H. Brubaker (Ed.), *Family relations: Challenges for the future.* Newbury Park, CA: Sage.

McCubbin, H. I., & Patterson, J. M. (1982). Family adaptation to crisis. In H. I. McCubbin, A. E. Cauble, & J. M. Patterson (Eds.), *Family stress, coping, and social support* (pp. 26-47). Springfield, IL: Charles C. Thomas.

McGoldrick, M., Heiman, M., & Carter, E. A. (1993). The changing family life cycle. In F. Walsh (Ed.), *Normal family processes* (pp. 405-443). New York: Guilford Press.

Melnyk, B. M., & Alpert-Gillis, L. (1997). Building healthier families: Helping parents and children cope with divorce. *Advanced Practice Nursing*, *2*(4), 35-43.

Minuchin, S., & Fishman, H. C. (1981). *Family therapy techniques*. Cambridge, MA: Harvard University Press.

Newman, M. (1979). *Theory development in nursing*. Philadelphia: F. A. Davis.

Newman, M. (1983). Newman's health theory. In I. Clements & F. Roberts (Eds.), *Family health: A theoretical approach to nursing care* (pp. 161-175). New York: John Wiley & Sons.

Nye, F. I., & Berardo, F. E. (1981). *Emerging conceptual frameworks in family analysis*. New York: Praeger.

Olson, D., Sprenkle, D., & Russell, C. (1982). Circumplex model of marital and family systems. *Family Process*, *18*(3), 3-27.

Olson, D. H., & McCubbin, H. I. (1982). Circumplex model of marital and family systems: V. Family stress and crisis intervention. In H. I. McCubbin, A. E. Cauble, & J. M. Patterson (Eds.), *Family stress, coping, and social support* (pp. 48-68). Springfield, IL: Charles C. Thomas.

Orem, D. (1971). *Nursing: Concepts of practice*. New York: McGraw-Hill.

Orem, D. (1980). *Nursing: Concepts of practice* (2nd ed.). New York: McGraw-Hill.

Otto, H. (1973). A framework for assessing family strengths. In A. Reinhardt & M. Quinn (Eds.), *Family-centered community nursing* (pp. 87-93). St. Louis: Mosby.

Peterson, E. A. (1997). Supporting the adoptive family. *MCN: American Journal of Maternal/Child Nursing*, *4*(2), 147-152.

Rogers, M. (1970). *An introduction to the theoretical basis of nursing*. Philadelphia: F. A. Davis.

Rogers, M. (1983). Science of unitary beings: A paradigm for nursing. In I. Clements & F. Roberts (Eds.), *Family health: A theoretical approach to nursing care* (pp. 219-228). New York: John Wiley & Sons.

Satir, V. (1972). *Peoplemaking*. Palo Alto, CA: Science and Behavior Books.

Scheflen, A. E. (1981). *Levels of schizophrenia*. New York: Brunner/Mazel.

Smith, C. (1985). *Goals for community health nursing* [Unpublished manuscript]. Baltimore, MD.

Strong, B., & DeVault, C. (1992). *The marriage and family experience*. CA: West Group.

Tapia, J. A. (1997). The nursing process in community health. In B. W. Spradley & J. Allender (Eds.), *Readings in community health nursing* (5th ed.; pp. 343-350). Philadelphia: Lippincott–Raven.

Urban Institute. (2006). *Current population survey*. Washington, DC: National Center for Health Statistics.

U.S. Bureau of the Census. (2006). *Statistical abstract of the United States, 2007* (126th ed.; pp. 39-67). Retrieved September 7, 2007 from *http://www.census.gov/prod/www/statistical-abstract.html*.

von Bertalanffy, L. (1968). *General systems theory*. New York: George Braziller.

Walsh, F. (1993). *Normal family processes* (2nd ed.). New York: Guilford Press.

Watzlawick, P., Beavin, J., & Jackson, D. (1967). *Pragmatics of human communication*. New York: W. W. Norton.

Whall, A. L. (1993). The family as the unit of care in nursing: A historical review. In G. Wegner & R. Alexander (Eds.), *Readings in family nursing* (pp. 3-12). Philadelphia: J. B. Lippincott.

Wherry, L., & Finegold, L. (2004, September). *Marriage promotion and the living arrangements of black, Hispanic, and white children*. New Federalism: National Survey of America's Families series, Series B, No. B-67. Washington, DC: Urban Institute.

Wright, L., & Leahey, M. (2005). *Nurses and families: A guide to family assessment and intervention* (4th ed.). Philadelphia: F. A. Davis.

SUGGESTED READINGS

Betz, C. L. (1996). A systems approach to adolescent transitions: An opportunity for nurses. *Journal of Pediatric Nursing: Nursing Care of Children and Families*, *11*(5), 271-272.

Black, K., & Lobo, M. (2008). A conceptual review of family resilience factors. *Journal of Family Nursing*, *14*(1), 33-55.

Bomar, P. J. (2004). *Promoting health in families: Applying family research and theory to nursing practice* (3rd ed.). St. Louis: Saunders.

Cody, W. K. (2000). Nursing frameworks to guide practice and research with families: Introductory remarks. *Nursing Science Quarterly*, *13*(4), 277-284.

Denham, S. (2003). *Family health: A framework for nursing*. Philadelphia: F. A. Davis.

Faux, S. A., & Knafl, K. A. (1996). Family–health care provider relationships: The new paradigm [Guest editorial]. *Journal of Family Nursing*, *2*(2), 107-110.

Ford-Gilhoe, M. (1997). Family strengths, motivations, and resources as predictors of health promotion behavior in single-parent and two parent families. *Research in Nursing and Health*, *20*(3), 205-217.

Gilbert, R. M. (2006). *The eight concepts of Bowen theory*. Falls Church, VA: Leading Systems Press.

Hanson, S., Gedaly-Duff, V., & Kaakinen, J. R. (2005). *Family health care nursing: Theory, practice, and research* (3rd ed.). Philadelphia: F. A. Davis.

Ingoldsby, B., Smith, S., & Miller, J. E. (2004). *Exploring family theories*. Oxford, England: Oxford University Press.

Kerr, M. (2003). *One family's story: A primer on Bowen theory*. Washington, DC: Bowen Center for the Study of Family.

McCubbin, H., Joy, C., Cauble, A., et al. (1980). Family stress and coping: A decade review. *Journal of Marriage and the Family*, *10*, 855-871.

Rolland, J. (1987). Chronic illness and the life cycle: A conceptual framework. *Family Process*, *11*(4), 203-221.

Scanzoni, J. (2001). From the normal family to alternate families to the quest for diversity with interdependence. *Journal of Family Issues*, *22*, 688-710.

Skolnick, A. S., & Skolnick, J. H. (1993). *Family in transition* (8th ed.). Boston: Little, Brown.

Steinglass, P. (2006). The future of family systems medicine: Challenges and opportunities. *Families, Systems and Health*, *24*(4), 396-411.

Sussman, M., & Steinmetz, S. (1987). *Handbook of marriage and the family*. New York: Plenum.

Wright, L. M., & Leahey, M. (2005). *Nurses and families: A guide to family assessment and intervention* (4th ed.). Philadelphia: F. A. Davis.

Zinn, M. B., & Eitzen, D. S. (1987). *Diversity in American families*. New York: Harper & Row.

CHAPTER

13

Family Case Management

*Claudia M. Smith**

FOCUS QUESTIONS

What is family case management?

What is the purpose of family assessment?

What methods and tools are used for assessing individuals? Subsystems? The family unit? The family within the environment?

How does the nurse analyze family data?

What are family nursing diagnoses?

How are priorities determined in family nursing?

What principles will help the nurse and family develop an effective plan of care?

How do family style, family strengths, and family functioning influence care planning?

How do family-nurse interventions vary with different family needs?

What are the possible outcomes of the evaluation phase of the nursing process?

How does the nurse coordinate termination with a family in a way that will benefit the nurse and the family?

CHAPTER OUTLINE

Family Case Management

Family Assessment

Assessing Individual Needs

Assessing Family Subsystems

Assessing the Family as a Unit

Assessing the Family within the Environment

Analyzing Family Data

Determining Family Needs

Determining Family Style

Determining Family Strengths

Determining Family Functioning

Determining Targets of Care

Determining the Nurse's Contribution

Determining Priorities of Identified Needs

Developing a Plan

Principles of Family Care Planning

Implementing the Plan

Helping the Family Cope with Illness or Loss

Teaching the Family Experiencing Developmental Changes

Connecting the Family to Needed Resources and Support

Coaching the Family to Change Its Internal Dynamics

Helping the Family Remain Healthy within the Environment

Evaluation

Methods

Factors Influencing Evaluation

What to Evaluate

Outcome of Evaluation

Terminating the Nurse-Family Relationship

KEY TERMS

Eco-map

Family case management

Family functioning

Family map

Family needs

Family strengths

Family style

Formative evaluation

Genogram

Priorities

Social support

Summative evaluation

Targets of care

---

*This chapter incorporates material written for previous editions by Marcia L. Cooley.

The betterment of human communities is the goal of community/public health nursing. To achieve this, community/public health nursing interventions may be directed to the community and its populations, community systems, and individuals/families within populations at risk (Minnesota Department of Health, 2001). Improving the health of families can improve the health of the community (American Nurses Association [ANA], 2007). As part of their scope of practice, baccalaureate-prepared community/public health nurses are expected to be able to implement programs of care targeted toward families.

Family health nursing is the practice of nursing directed toward maximizing the health and well-being of all individuals within a family system. Two views of a family are incorporated: family as the unit of care and family as context for individuals and family subsystems. When working with families, the community/public health nurse's goal is to promote optimal health for each member of the family and for the family as a unit. Bringing a family perspective to the arena in which the nurse will meet with the family will change the way the nurse practices. The nurse begins to consider more complex needs and more complex interactions as care is offered. The Family Needs Model of family health nursing introduced in Chapter 12 will be used as the guide in this text (Figure 13-1). Using the Family Needs Model, the community/public health nurse assesses and analyzes family needs, family style, family strengths, and family functioning. Identifying family needs allows the nurse to determine the areas in which the family needs help. Assessing family style allows the nurse to adjust interpersonal interactions to match the family's preferred style of communicating and relating. Describing family strengths enables the nurse to suggest ways to build on the family competencies. Determining family functioning allows the nurse to set realistic goals with the family. As with all nursing practice, the practice of family health nursing builds on the foundation of the nursing process. Community/public health nurses assess, diagnose, plan, implement, and evaluate their nursing care for and with families.

For nurses who work with families, extra challenges are posed in the complexity and skill that are sometimes required to deal with these larger and more intensely connected groups of people. The nurse's ability to establish a relationship that respects the family's rights and strengths becomes more important than any other task. Trust, open communication, and acceptance of diverse family values are essential. Although the community/public health nurse has responsibilities to the community and wishes to affect the health of each family member and the family as a whole, she or he must always remember that the family is ultimately responsible for its actions. The nurse's role is limited to that of a facilitator, educator, or advocate, except in the most extreme cases of personal safety or abuse. Success depends primarily not on what the nurse does, but on her or his talent at empowering the family to act for itself.

FAMILY CASE MANAGEMENT

Case management of families seeks to "optimize the self-care capabilities" of families regarding their health and well-being (Minnesota Department of Health, 2001, p. 93). A public health nursing perspective for **family case management** includes outreach to find families in need, focus on prevention, and reliance on health teaching, counseling, and referral and follow-up with families (Minnesota Department of Health, 2001). Nurses consult with family members in problem solving, as well as coordinate services and resources on behalf of families. Public health nursing case management is "client-centered and relationship-based" (Minnesota Department of Health, 2001, p. 100). Additionally, advocacy and collaboration within the community or community systems may emerge from the relationship(s) with families. Family case management in public health nursing is *neither* disease management nor benefits' management for managed care or an insurance company. The above aspects of case management in community/public health nursing are considered

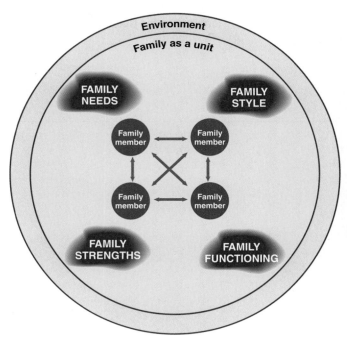

FIGURE 13-1 The Family Needs Model of family health nursing, created by Marcia Cooley and Claudia Smith. (See text for explanation.) (Copyright [1995]. Used with permission.)

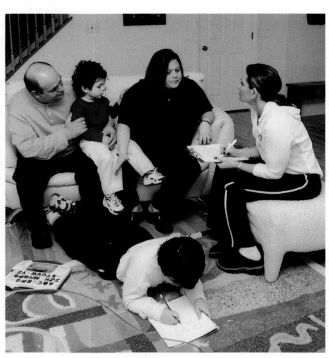

A nurse taking a health history during a family home visit. (Copyright CLG Photographics.)

best practices (Minnesota Department of Health, 2001) and are integrated with the nursing process (ANA, 2007).

FAMILY ASSESSMENT

As with all assessment, the nurse uses as many possible sources of data as is practical to help complete a comprehensive picture of the family and each member. Of course, before discussing a family or reviewing the family's records with a member of the health care team from another agency, the family's permission must be obtained. Sources of data can include, but should not be limited to, charts and written health records, biologic data such as blood pressures or specimens, telephone calls and conversations with other health care team members, information from social service agencies involved with the family, and environmental and community information. However, the most accurate and complete information can be obtained only by observing and interviewing the family itself.

Interviewing families can be more difficult than interviewing an individual client and, for a nurse who is not familiar with this situation, a little frightening. After all, the family has been together for a long time and has a history together that gives even the most dysfunctional family strength and a collective power. Interviewing families can also be a rich source of information and a path to establishing relationships that are fulfilling and meaningful for both the nurse and the family members.

Families may first be seen in the hospital, clinic, community setting, or in their own home. Meeting families in their own environment is preferable because the nurse can observe firsthand the physical and environmental conditions, as well as the way family members interact with each other on their own turf. Preparing for a home visit is discussed in Chapter 11. Ideally, the nurse will keep these principles in mind when planning the first meeting with the family.

The nurse should try to include as many family members as is possible in the interview. Each family will have a communicator (someone who tends to speak for the other members of the family) and usually a leader (someone who takes charge of family operations). Often, but not always, the communicator and the leader are the same person. Although the nurse can work through this strength, be aware that, to be accurate, perceptions of the problem or concern and other data must be gathered from all persons. Being able to see the family together often gives the observer information about family interaction that is useful.

The goal of family assessment is to gather information that allows the nurse and family to identify family needs together and to plan care that will allow the family to work toward more optimal health for individual family members and for the family as a whole. Families can then be assessed on several levels: assessing individuals within the family, assessing interactions among subsystems, assessing the family as a unit, and assessing the family within the environment. A comprehensive family assessment should include information gathered about and from all of these levels. Data that are essential to collect include household composition, health status and behaviors of all members, interaction among the family members, and the relationship of the family with its community.

ASSESSING INDIVIDUAL NEEDS

Typically, one member of the family is identified as the client who is to be the recipient of nursing care. This client may have an identified health problem (e.g., a recent discharge from a hospital after a stroke, a communicable disease), a chronic illness that needs continued monitoring (e.g., diabetes), or a potential problem (e.g., a new mother who needs education about her infant). Adequate identification and collection of information about the client's response to these actual or potential health problems is the first priority in family assessment.

However, many families will have more than one member with actual or potential health problems. Because family members are interconnected, the health of all members is a concern to the nurse. Depending on the mission and guidelines of the agency and the nurse's role, all family members are potential targets of individual assessment. For example, suppose the identified client is a 55-year-old man who has developed a foot ulcer. He may eventually need assistance with moving and transferring. What if the only other member of the family, his wife, has chronic obstructive pulmonary disease and is unable to help? Family health is interconnected because members share their environment and depend on each other.

Individual assessment will vary with the age and particular health status of each person. Included in the assessment may be comprehensive health or physical assessment, assessment of developmental level, mental status assessment, focused information about specific health problems such as incontinence or decubiti, or assessment of coping and adaptation. Some specific individual assessments are outlined in Box 13-1.

All family members can benefit from health promotion and disease or injury prevention. Community/public health nurses need to assess the history of immunizations and screening tests for each family member. By comparing this information with recommended schedules for immunizations (see Chapter 8) and screening tests (see Chapter 19), nurses can identify the immunizations and screening tests that each family member needs.

ASSESSING FAMILY SUBSYSTEMS

Families interact in small interpersonal groups. Understanding the interactions and functioning of these dyads and triangles is important to understanding the functioning of the family and ascertaining available support. Subsystems such as the parent-child subsystem, the marital pair, and the sibling subsystem should always be assessed. Other, less obvious, subsystems might be grandparent-grandchild, foster parent–child, or parents–young married couple. Tools that can be used include maps of social interaction, tools that assess the health of developmental bonds such as mother-child interaction, and tools that target problems in dyads, such as elder abuse screening tools. Examples of these assessments are presented in Box 13-1.

ASSESSING THE FAMILY AS A UNIT

Although assessing families in smaller segments is helpful, these assessments do not capture the nature of the family as a whole. Families have unique identities that cannot be understood when thinking about only the segments. Parameters that are often assessed include family processes, roles, communication, division of labor, decision making, boundaries, styles of problem solving, coping abilities, and health-promotional practices. Some specific tools are outlined in Box 13-1, and some of the more widely used family assessments are discussed in the following sections.

Box 13-1   Examples of Assessments

Individual Assessments
Physical assessment of the newborn
Adult physical examination
Diet history
Discharge Planning Risk Screen (Blaylock & Cason, 1992)
Mental status examination (Jernigan, 1986)
Incontinence assessment (Kane et al., 1993)
Mortality Risk Appraisal (Pender, 1987)
  Spiritual assessment (Zerwekh, 1989)
Levels of Cognitive Functioning Assessment Scale (Flannery & Korchek, 1993)
Denver Eye Screening Test (Wong & Whaley, 1995)

Interpersonal Assessments
Brief Screening Inventory for Postpartum Adaptation (Affonso, 1987)
Elder Abuse Assessment Tool (Fulmer, 1984)
Neonatal Perception Inventory (Broussard & Hartner, 1995)
Social Assessment of the Elderly (Kane et al., 1993)

Family Assessments
Calgary Family Assessment Model (CFAM) (Wright & Leahey, 2005)
Family Inventory of Life Events and Changes (FILE) (McCubbin & Thompson, 1987b)
Family Nutritional Assessment Tool (James & Flores, 2004)
Family Social Support (Roth, 1996)
Family Systems Stressor-Strength Inventory (FS3I) (Berkey & Hanson, 1991)
Family Nursing Scale (Astedt-Kurki et al., 2002)
Family Coping Oriented Personal Scales (F-COPES) (McCubbin & Thompson, 1987a)

Environmental Assessments
Assessment of Immediate Living Environment (Skelley, 1990)
Building Accessibility Checklist (Mumma, 1987)
Eco-map (Hartman, 1978)
Home Observation for Measurement Environment (HOME) (Caldwell, 1976)
Occupation/Environment Health History (Wiley, 1996)

Family Maps

A **family map** is used to diagram spatial and relationship qualities of a family system. The tool originated with structural-functional family therapists (Minuchin & Fishman, 1981). These researchers began observing the structure and interaction of families in therapeutic situations and mapping families to understand their hierarchies, roles, and power. After an interview in which the family is observed in an interactive situation, a map is drawn that details the subsystems, the boundaries between subsystems, and interactive patterns, such as coalitions, conflict, and avoidance.

A healthy family will demonstrate age-appropriate subsystems. Power will reside with parents, and children will have the nurturant guidance they need to grow. Spousal subsystems will have a clear identity. Boundaries between subsystems will be clear and permeable. Diffuse boundaries allow too much confusion because members move back and forth without clear definition of roles. Rigid boundaries serve to shut off necessary interaction and discourage flexibility and adaptiveness. Interactive patterns tend to repeat themselves and provide information about who will communicate and in what way the communication may occur. Symbols for the maps are shown in Figure 13-2.

Genograms

A **genogram** is a format for drawing a family tree that records information about family members and their relationships for at least three generations (Cain, 1981; McGoldrick & Gerson, 1985). Genograms help community/public health nurses remember the family members, patterns, and significant events that are important in the family's care. The picture of the family that is presented in the genogram helps the observer think about the family systemically and over time. Occasionally, when a larger picture is presented, connections between events and relationships become clearer and are viewed in a more objective way.

Genograms serve several other functions. The process of collecting and recording information for constructing a genogram serves as a way for the interviewer and family to connect in a personal but emotionally safe way. The genogram also provides the interviewer with information about how the members of the family think about family problems and interact with other members. Recording information on a genogram can serve to detoxify issues or reduce anxiety about the family problem. During the process, family members are required to think, organize, and present facts. The nurse helps the family normalize and reframe problems so that they are viewed in a larger context. This type of interaction can help family members step back and think about an issue in a calm way.

Typically, the genogram is constructed in the first or an early session and revised as new information becomes available. Genogram construction may be divided into three parts:

1. Mapping the family structure
2. Recording family information
3. Delineating family relationship

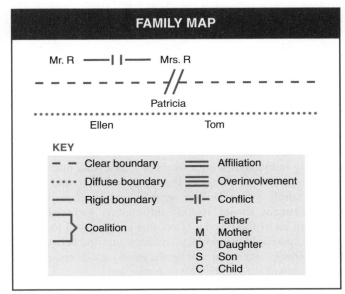

FIGURE 13-2 Family map using family example from the Nursing Practice in Process at the end of the chapter. (Adapted from Minuchin, S. [1974]. *Families and family therapy.* Cambridge, MA: Harvard University Press.)

To map the family structure, a diagram of family members in each generation is drawn using horizontal and vertical lines. Symbols used to represent pregnancies, miscarriages, marriages, and deaths are presented in Figure 13-3. Male family members are placed on the left of the horizontal line; female members on the right. Birth order is represented by placing the oldest sibling on the far left and progressing toward the right. In the case of multiple marriages, the earliest is placed on the left and the most recent on the right.

Family information that is usually helpful includes ages, dates of birth and death, geographic location, occupation, and educational level. Critical family events and transitions such as moves, marriages, divorces, losses, and successes are recorded. Family members' physical, emotional, or social problems or illnesses are identified. A chronology, or time line, of family events is often useful to help people see relationships between events and behavior changes.

Observing and describing family relationships is the stage that is the most crucial and often the most helpful to the family but is often ignored. Relationship patterns can be quite complex and are inferred from observations and from family members' comments and analyses. The nurse should identify patterns of closeness, conflict, and distance. When relationships are too close, this intensity is also noted. Some symbols

that are used to represent relationships are presented in Figure 13-3. Triangles are present in every family (see Chapter 12). Attempting to map the primary or most influential triangles in the family is a part of describing the family relationships.

The genogram is an assessment tool that can be useful throughout the contact with the family. At some point, the genogram may also be used as a therapeutic tool whereby information is interpreted and used to help individuals define the way they would like to operate within the group. Although the nurse may yield to thinking that she or he knows what the family should do, interpretations that come from family members themselves are usually more accurate and useful for change.

Family Cultural Assessment

At this point, competence in family cultural assessment is also required. When working with diversity in families, the nurse needs to develop an awareness of her or his own existence, thoughts, and environment without letting it have undue influence on others. The nurse should be able to demonstrate knowledge and understanding of the family's culture and also respect for cultural differences. If language is a barrier, interpreters can be used, but be sure to provide time for translation, and avoid using children as interpreters. Cultural norms about personal space, touch, and eye contact vary; thus the nurse needs

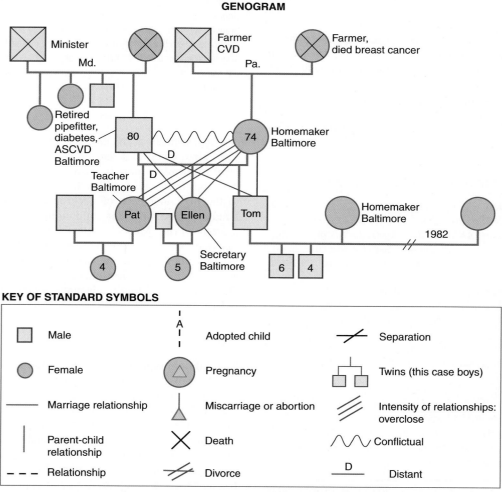

FIGURE 13-3 Genogram using family example from the Nursing Process in Practice at the end of the chapter. (Adapted from Cain, A. [1981]. Assessment of family structure. In J. Miller & E. Janosik [Eds.], *Family-focused care* [p. 117]. New York: McGraw-Hill.)

to be aware of nonverbal behavior and adjust it as necessary. Box 13-2 presents Purnell and Paulanka's model (1998) of cultural competence with hints for areas of family life to assess. See Table 10-4 for a more detailed guide to family cultural assessment.

ASSESSING THE FAMILY WITHIN THE ENVIRONMENT

The family is a group of interacting people who also live within an external physical and interpersonal environment. Data about the family's physical environment, such as the presence of accident hazards, window screens, plumbing, and cooking facilities, help the nurse (1) plan care that matches or supplements family resources and (2) identify potential health problems. Some physical conditions that should be assessed are presented in Box 13-1. Home Observation for Measurement Environment (HOME), an observation tool developed to assess the potential of the environment for development of children from birth to 6 years of age, is an example of a tool that can be used to collect data about the physical environment (Caldwell, 1976) (see also Chapter 9).

Community resources and facilities that are available to the family should also be noted. However, some families can live within a fairly resource-rich environment and be unable to maintain the connections that are needed to tap these resources. An **eco-map** (Hartman, 1978) is a tool that can be used to help the nurse and family discover the patterns of energy flow into and outside of the family. The family's relationships with significant community resources, activities, and agencies are diagrammed. Are these connections strong, tenuous, or stressful? The diagram illustrates the amount of energy that a family uses to maintain its system and what support is available. After the nurse helps the family prepare the diagram, the eco-map helps family members visualize how relationships with external systems are affecting their state of well-being. An eco-map is presented in Figure 13-4.

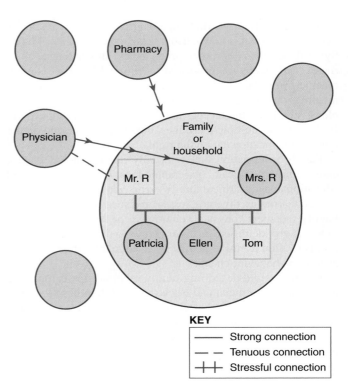

KEY

——	Strong connection
– –	Tenuous connection
┼┼	Stressful connection

FIGURE 13-4 An eco-map using family example from the Nursing Practice in Process at the end of the chapter. **Directions:** Fill in connections where they exist. Indicate their nature by descriptive words or different lines. Draw arrows along lines to signify flow of energy and resources. Identify significant people. Fill in empty circles as needed. (Adapted from Hartman, S. [1978]. Diagrammatic assessment of family relationships. *Social Casework, 59,* 470. Reprinted with permission from Families in Society [http://www.familiesinsociety.org], published by the Alliance for Children and Families.)

BOX 13-2   Family Cultural Assessment

1. Who is the head of the household? Who has the final say? For example, some families are patriarchal; some are matriarchal.
2. Does the family operate with specific assigned roles, or are the roles less defined? Who is responsible for maintaining health? For example, some families have clear separations for what men and women should do.
3. Do family members exhibit essential or taboo behaviors? For example, some families have prescriptive behaviors such as purging their children with laxatives; others have restrictive behaviors such as not allowing unchaperoned dating.
4. What are the family's goals for members?
5. What is the cultural significance of children, elderly members, and extended family?
6. What is the family's acceptance of different lifestyles?
7. How does the family respond to living with a partner without marriage? Homosexuality? Divorce?
8. What are the family's health-related behaviors?
9. What do they do to promote and maintain health? To prevent illness? What home remedies are used?

Adapted from Purnell, L. D., & Paulanka, B. (1998). *Transcultural health care: A culturally competent approach.* Philadelphia: F.A. Davis; and Spector, R. E. (2000). *Cultural diversity in health and illness.* Upper Saddle River, NJ: Prentice Hall.

Other aspects of the environment, such as chemical exposure, air quality, and danger in neighborhoods with a high level of criminal activity, also affect families. Kuster (1997) describes inner-city families that are at risk for asthma related to the high incidence of cockroaches in their environment. Lead exposure for young children in older buildings is another example of risk. Musculoskeletal injuries, accidents, exposures to radiation and carcinogens, and sound damage to hearing are examples of danger in the workplace. An example of a tool to assess a family's occupational and environmental history is the Occupational and Environmental Health History (Wiley, 1996) in Box 13-3.

ANALYZING FAMILY DATA

The different types of assessments discussed in the preceding section provide not only a comprehensive assessment but also a massive amount of data. Family assessments can be complex and confusing if these data are not sorted and analyzed in some way. What does this information mean, and in what way can it be used to help the nurse and family plan their work together? The information must be integrated and analyzed before decisions about the plan of care can be made. Once the information is summarized and targets of care are identified, the process of intervention is clearer for the nurse and the family. Neglecting to accomplish this task carefully can lead to

Box 13-3   Occupational and Environmental Health History

Identifying Data

Name: _____

Address: _____

Telephone number: _____

Social security number: _____

Gender: _____

Age: _____ Date of birth: _____

Chief Complaint and Stressors Perceived by the Client: _____

_____

Key Questions

1. Describe the health problem or injury you are currently experiencing. _____

   _____

2. Are any other members of your family experiencing this problem? Any co-worker? Any acquaintance? _____

3. Do you smoke? _____ Use chewing tobacco? _____ Consume alcohol? _____ Use any other drugs? _____
   (Packs of cigarettes per day, quantity, frequency, number of years in which ciagarettes used)_____

   _____

4. Do you smoke while on the job? _____ At home? _____ Do your co-workers smoke on the job? _____ Do family members smoke while you are in the room? _____

5. Have you missed work within the last 6 weeks? _____ When did these symptoms begin? _____ Have you stayed in bed since this condition started? _____ Are you distressed by your disability now? _____

6. Have you ever worked at a job or other activity that has caused you to have this problem before? _____ If so, describe the pattern of illness or difficulty. _____

7. Have you ever found yourself short of breath, light-headed, dizzy, with a cough, or wheezing at work? _____ After work? _____
   At the beginning of the workweek? _____ At the end of the workweek? _____ During the weekend?_____

8. Have you ever changed jobs, homes, or hobbies because of a health problem?

9. Have you ever experienced muscle or moving difficulties (back pain, fractures, sore muscles, decreased ability to move around, joint pain) related to work, home, or play?

10. Name the chemicals and compounds with which you work and the frequency of your contact with each substance. _____

    _____

11. Name the chemicals and compounds with which your spouse or other family member works. _____

    _____

12. Does your skin ever come in contact with any chemicals or substances at work or play?_____

13. Describe your neighborhood. _____
    Map out the location of industrial areas, waste disposal sites, water sources, and waste disposal processes. _____

    _____

14. Have any community environmental problems evolved recently?_____

15. Have there been any toxic spills, sewage breakage, smog changes, or Occupational Safety and Health Administration investigations pertinent to your condition?_____

16. What types of pesticides, cleaning solutions, glues, solvents, metals, or poisons are used in your home?_____

    _____

17. What type of heating and cooling system is used in the home? _____

    _____

18. What is its impact on the illness pattern?_____

Adapted from Wiley, D. (1996). Family environmental health. In P. Bomar (Ed.), *Nurses and family health promotion: Concepts, assessment, and interventions* (2nd ed.; p. 351). Philadelphia: W.B. Saunders.

feelings of being overwhelmed or to nonfocused, constantly changing interventions. The following steps can be used to help organize these data:

- Determining *family needs* or areas of concern
- Determining *family style*
- Determining *family strengths*
- Determining *family functioning*
- Determining *targets of care*
- Determining *nursing's contribution*
- Determining *priorities* of identified health needs

DETERMINING FAMILY NEEDS

When looking at **family needs,** the nurse is asking the following questions: *"What?" "In what areas does the family need help?" "What concerns do the nurse and family want to explore?"* These needs are identified on multiple levels: needs of individual members, needs of family subgroups, needs of the family as a whole, and needs related to the family interacting with the environment. Nursing diagnoses can be developed that represent each of these areas. The North American Nursing Diagnosis Association (NANDA International) has been identifying and listing diagnostic nomenclature since the early 1970s (NANDA International, 2007). These diagnoses are formulated to help nurses choose and focus nursing interventions by concentrating on client responses to health promotion and actual or potential health problems rather than on the disease process. Each diagnosis consists of two parts: the unhealthy response and an indication of the factors contributing to the response. Problems may be those that exist currently *(actual)* or may possibly exist in the future *(potential),* or the problems may relate to *health promotion.*

Nursing diagnoses for individual family members are identified just as they are when an individual is the sole target of care. Diagnoses that represent responses to health problems are organized according to patterns or clusters of behaviors such as sleep and rest, elimination, and activity and exercise (Cox et al., 1997).

Interpersonal nursing diagnoses may include needs that represent the interaction of more than one person, such as "Breast-feeding: Ineffective," or diagnoses that affect more than one person, such as "Social Interaction: Impaired." Examples of individual and interpersonal nursing diagnoses are presented in Box 13-4.

Family nursing diagnoses have also been identified by NANDA International. The nomenclature used includes Family Processes: Interrupted; Family Processes: Readiness for Enhanced; Family Coping: Compromised or Disabled; and Family Coping: Readiness for Enhanced. The major defining characteristics that correspond to these diagnoses include most of the concepts discussed within the family chapters in this book and are presented in Box 13-5.

However, some authors find that the NANDA International family nursing diagnoses are not sufficiently specific. Smith (1985) suggests that five major areas exist in community health nursing in which families and nursing intersect (Box 13-6). This delineation may help the nurse identify more specific family needs. Families meeting normal growth and developmental challenges often benefit from health-promotion and illness-prevention education or supportive contact as family members master behaviors appropriate for their new stage of life. Families coping with illness or loss not only need emotional support but also need concrete help, such as direct care, education, and connection to services. Families dealing with external stressors, such as natural disasters, unemployment, or societal violence, benefit from emotional and physical support. During this time of crisis, the family may be strained and not as functional. However, a crisis period may also be a time for the family to grow and discover strength under stress.

Inadequate resources or support can be temporary or long term. For example, a family with several events happening at once (e.g., children in college, an illness, an aging parent) may find its usually sufficient resources inadequate. Other families deal with the chronic problem of poverty, lack of access to resources, and inadequate energy to maintain self-esteem and meet other persons' emotional needs (see Chapter 14).

Families with disturbances in internal dynamics create stress from within. The unhealthy way in which they operate tends to provoke rather than mediate their stress. Of course, families can have combinations of these problems, or some of the problems may potentiate others. However, this framework covers most of the needs families will present in the community/ public health setting.

Environmental problems for families are described in the Omaha System problem classification scheme (Martin, 2005). Problems with material resources and physical surroundings include income, sanitation, residence, and neighborhood and workplace safety (Table 13-1).

Family problems related to the social environment may occur in the areas of communication with community resources and social contacts (Table 13-2). Each problem may have actual or potential impairments or opportunities for health promotion.

Different family needs require different intervention strategies from the nurse. Specific interventions for each of the five categories of family needs are discussed later in this chapter.

DETERMINING FAMILY STYLE

Most families have characteristic processes they use to meet challenges and deal with others. Identifying this style will help the nurse choose appropriate actions and ways of working with the families. Determining the **family style** helps the nurse answer the following questions: *"How?" "How should I adjust my interpersonal interactions to match the family style?"*

| BOX 13-4 | **Individual and Interpersonal Nursing Diagnoses** |

- Adjustment: Impaired
- Breast-Feeding Pattern: Ineffective
- Caregiver Role Strain
- Home Maintenance Management: Impaired
- Individual Coping: Ineffective
- Parenting: Impaired
- Role Performance: Ineffective
- Self-Care Deficit
- Sexual Dysfunction
- Social Interaction: Impaired
- Social Isolation
- Verbal Communication: Impaired
- Violence, Risk for: Self-Directed or Directed at Others

From North American Nursing Diagnosis Association. (2007). *Nursing diagnoses: Definitions and classification, 2007-2008.* Philadelphia: Author.

Box 13-5   Major Defining Characteristics of Family Diagnoses

Family Processes: Altered*

The state in which a family that normally functions effectively experiences a dysfunction

In families with this diagnosis, the family system or family members have the following characteristics:

1. Family is unable to meet physical needs of members.
2. Family is unable to meet emotional needs of members.
3. Family is unable to meet spiritual needs of members.
4. Parents do not demonstrate respect for each other's views on childrearing practices.
5. Family members are unable to express or accept a wide range of feelings.
6. Family members are unable to express or accept feelings of other members.
7. Family is unable to meet security needs of its members.
8. Family is unable to relate to each other for mutual growth and maturation.
9. Family is uninvolved in community activities.
10. Family is unable to accept or receive help appropriately.
11. Family is rigid in function and roles.
12. Family members do not demonstrate respect for individuality and autonomy of its members.
13. Family is unable to adapt to change or deal with traumatic experiences constructively.
14. Family members fail to accomplish current or past developmental tasks.
15. Family exhibits unhealthy decision-making process.
16. Family members fail to send and receive clear messages.
17. Boundary maintenance is inappropriate.
18. Family exhibits inappropriate or poorly communicated family rules, rituals, or symbols.
19. Unexamined family myths are exhibited.
20. Family has inappropriate level and direction of energy.

Family Processes: Interrupted†

Change in family relationships and/or functioning; often related to development transitions, family role shifts, interaction with community, changes in family finances or social status, shift in health status of family member, or situational transitions or crises

In families with this diagnosis, the family system or family members have the following characteristics:

1. Changes in assigned tasks
2. Changes in affective responsiveness or availability of emotional support
3. Changes in communication patterns
4. Changes in effectiveness in completing assigned tasks
5. Changes in expressions of conflict with community resources
6. Changes in expressions of conflict within family
7. Changes in intimacy
8. Changes in mutual support
9. Changes in participation in decision making or power alliances
10. Changes in rituals
11. Changes in satisfaction with family
12. Changes in somatic complaints
13. Changes in stress-reduction behaviors

Family Coping: Ineffective—Compromised and Disabled

Compromised: insufficient, ineffective, or compromised support, comfort, assistance, or encouragement, usually by a supportive primary person

(e.g., family member or close friend). [Individual] client may need support to manage or master adaptive tasks related to his or her health challenge

1. Compromised†
   a. Subjective
      (1) Client expresses or confirms a concern or complaint about significant other's responses to his or her health problem.
      (2) Significant person describes preoccupation with personal reactions (e.g., fear, guilt, anticipatory grief, anxiety) to client's illness, disability, or situational or developmental crisis.
      (3) Significant person describes or confirms inadequate understanding or knowledge base that interferes with effective assistive or supportive behavior.
   b. Objective
      (1) Significant person attempts assistive or supportive behavior with less than satisfactory results.
      (2) Significant person withdraws or enters into limited or temporary personal communication with the client at the time of need.
      (3) Significant person displays protective behavior disproportionate to the client's abilities or need for autonomy.

Disabled: behavior of a significant person (e.g., family member or other primary person) that disables his or her own capacities and the client's capacities to effectively address tasks essential to either person's adaptation to the health challenge

2. Disabled†
   a. Neglectful care of the client in regard to basic human needs or illness treatment
   b. Distortion of reality regarding the client's health problem, including extreme denial
   c. Intolerance
   d. Rejection
   e. Abandonment or desertion
   f. Carrying out usual routines, disregarding client's needs
   g. Psychosomaticism
   h. Taking on illness signs of client
   i. Decisions and actions by family that are detrimental to economic or social well-being
   j. Agitation, depression, aggression, hostility
   k. Impaired restructuring of meaningful life for self, impaired individualization, prolonged overconcern for client
   l. Neglectful relationship with other family members
   m. Client development of helpless, inactive dependence

Family Coping: Readiness for Enhanced‡

Effective management of adaptive tasks by family member involved with the client's health challenge who now is exhibiting desire and readiness for enhanced health and growth in regard to self and in relation to the client

1. Family member attempting to describe growth impact of crisis on her or his own values, priorities, goals, or relationships
2. Family member moving in direction of health-promoting and health-enriching lifestyle
3. Individual expressing interest in making contact with another person who has experienced a similar situation

*North American Nursing Diagnosis Association. (1995). *Taxonomy I with complete diagnosis.* St. Louis: Author.
†North American Nursing Diagnosis Association. (2007). *Nursing diagnoses: Definitions and classifications, 2007-2008.* Philadelphia: Author.
‡North American Nursing Diagnosis Association. (2003). *Nursing diagnoses: Definitions and classifications, 2003-2004.* Philadelphia: Author.

Box 13-6 Determining Family Needs

1. **The family dealing with normal growth and development**
   - Transitions such as births, divorces, and a child going to college are stressful for all families.
   - As family members grow older, the family must adjust and learn new roles and ways of operating as a group.
   - Normal age-related behaviors may be unexpected or unfamiliar to the family.
   - All families must adjust health-promotion and illness-prevention behaviors for their life stages.
2. **The family coping with illness or loss**
   - Illness may be acute or chronic but is almost always accompanied by stressors such as financial demands or inability to perform family roles.
   - The family often needs to accomplish health care tasks such as special diets, exercises, or tracheostomy care.
   - Myth: All people should be encouraged to talk about their feelings. Individuals cope in different ways—humor, action, denial, intellectualizing, seeking support of others.
   - Myth: Family coping requires simple, open communication. Families cope in different ways—pulling together, depending on one member, distancing, seeking help from the community.
3. **The family dealing with external stressors**
   - Stress from the environment is usually unexpected and is therefore more difficult to manage.

- An event may be positive or negative but is still stressful because the family is required to rearrange itself or to adjust emotionally.
- The environment may be hazardous.

4. **The family with inadequate resources and support**
   - The family may lack equipment, money, tools, space, or other materials.
   - The family may lack emotional or social support.
   - The family may have never had resources, may have depleted them, or may not know how to connect with available supports.
5. **The family with disturbances in internal dynamics**
   - Internal dynamics lead to relationships that are problematic and ineffective.
   - Power and authority are not appropriately placed.
   - Organization may be chaotic and unpredictable or too rigid and inflexible.
   - Family members are not responsible for self: they either push things onto others or assume extra responsibility that should belong to another.
   - Unhealthy patterns are used, such as blaming, conflict, scapegoating, withdrawal, or sacrifice of one member.

Categories adapted from Smith, C. (1985). *Goals for community health nursing* (unpublished manuscript).

"How will the way the family typically acts affect planning and implementation of care with this family?" "How will I even get in the door or get the family to accept my presence?" "In what ways does the family usually act to process information, solve problems, and open or close itself to the environment?"

Family style usually has two components: internal family interactions and relationship to the outside world. These patterns remain fairly consistent over time. The styles describe family patterns of meeting challenges and dealing with others. Some families are organized within themselves and are receptive to interactions with a helper. Other families have more trouble with organization, are resistive, or are distant. Identifying this style will help the nurse choose appropriate actions and ways of working with the family. Information gained from tools that assess the family's coping ability, patterns of interaction, and use of support from others can be integrated to complete this analysis. Table 13-3 presents a format for thinking about family style.

Different family styles require different interactions from the nurse. The competent family health nurse will be able to adjust her or his own personal way of relating to others to

TABLE 13-1 Nursing Diagnoses for Environmental Problems

Problem	Signs and Symptoms
Income	Low/no income, uninsured medical expenses, difficulty with money management, able to buy only necessities, difficulty buying necessities, other
Sanitation	Soiled living area, inadequate food storage/disposal, insects/rodents, foul odor, inadequate laundry facilities, allergens, infectious/contaminating agents, mold, excessive pets, other
Residence	Structurally unsound, inadequate heating/cooling, steep stairs, inadequate/obstructed exits/entries, cluttered living space, unsafe storage of dangerous objects/substances, unsafe mats/throw rugs, inadequate safety devices, presence of lead-based paint, unsafe gas/electric appliances, inadequate/crowded living space, homeless, other
Neighborhood and workplace safety	High crime rate, high pollution level, uncontrolled animals, physical hazards, unsafe play areas, other

Adapted from Martin, K. (2005). *The Omaha System: A key to practice, documentation and information management* (2nd ed.). St. Louis: Elsevier/Saunders.

TABLE 13-2 Nursing Diagnoses Related to the Use of Social Resources

Problem	Signs and Symptoms
Communication with community resources	Unfamiliarity with options/procedures for obtaining services, difficulty understanding roles/regulations of service providers, unable to communicate concerns to service provider, dissatisfaction with services, cultural or language barrier, inadequate/unavailable services, transportation barrier, other
Social contract	Limited social contract, uses health care provider for social contact, minimal outside stimulation/leisure time activities, other

Adapted from Martin, K. (2005). *The Omaha System: A key to practice, documentation and information management* (2nd ed.). St. Louis: Elsevier/Saunders.

TABLE 13-3   **Determining Family Style**

Family Style	Defining Characteristics
Receptive	• Is open to suggestions. • Is eager to work with the system. • Will accept part of the responsibility for the problem and solution.
Distancing	• Understands the problem but has difficulty making connections with resources. • Is embarrassed or tries to deny the problem's existence. • Has difficulty dealing with the emotions surrounding the contact.
Resistive	• Denies or disagrees with institutional interpretation of the problem or the solutions. • Feels powerless in the face of the larger system. • May play along without really cooperating or following through on suggestions.
Disorganized	• Is flexible and experiences frequent and quick changes. • May be extremely adaptive or so disorganized or pressured that this problem is only one of many. • May have difficulty cooperating with planning or solutions because family life is unpredictable and unstructured.
Rigid	• Has a fixed way of dealing with things that cannot easily be changed to accommodate new demands or behaviors. • May see itself as incapable of carrying out new routines, even if the family accepts the solutions.
Lopsided	• Power or responsibility lies mostly with one adult member. • Member may be too burdened to accomplish all that needs to be done. • The "doer" may have to struggle with another adult to accomplish the changes.
Ordered	• Hierarchy, roles, and lines of communication are clearly spelled out. • The way the family usually works together results in success and accomplishments.
Tight	• Family members depend on each other for physical assistance and emotional support. • Talking to one member usually means the rest of the family will receive the information quickly. • The family prefers to look to its own rather than to persons outside the family unit.
Teeter-totter	• Family members trade the roles of caregiver and care receiver; often occurs when a strong family member becomes sick or disabled. • Or more than one family member may trade the role of caregiver; often happens when different family members provide care at different times for the receiver. • Family members need to adjust to new roles as others around them adjust also.
Dependent	• The family as a unit prefers to look to others to provide direction and supply their needs; often happens when no member is available to take a leadership role. • The family may have learned this behavior from previous generations. • Dependency may be accompanied by anger when external systems cannot supply what is needed.

Developed by Marcia Cooley.

match the family style. If a family is distant in the face of emotional and private events, moving in too quickly makes them retreat even more. Each nurse should examine personal ways of behaving and practice a flexible repertoire of interactions to be used when the family situation requires it. Principles for interacting with different family styles are presented in Table 13-4.

In this example, the nurse modifies her communication pattern to match the family's style.

Vonda, a community/public health nurse, was having difficulty connecting with the Baker family, which had a mother-in-law who was recovering from a major stroke. Whenever Vonda called to make an appointment, Mr. Baker would answer the phone and indicate that she should talk to his wife. Vonda left a message, but Mrs. Baker would never call back. Vonda talked to her supervisor, who knew the family, and she suggested that the Baker family would benefit from the contact but were using a distant style. Vonda decided to send the family a list of common problems of stroke victims with a suggestion that she had some equipment that might help. Vonda was feeling anxious at this point because she knew the family had five authorized home visits that were about to expire, and she had no accurate assessment of the grandmother's status. Mrs. Baker called back the next day and asked for some help with the catheter. Vonda offered to come out that day, but Mrs. Baker wanted to wait until next week. Vonda carefully explained the date that the authorization would end. Mrs. Baker decided to make an appointment for the next day and Vonda visited. At that time, she made arrangements for four more visits, once a week at the same time each week. She was not pushy or anxious. At the end of the visits, Mrs. Baker indicated how grateful she was for the help.

DETERMINING FAMILY STRENGTHS

Clients and families in the community are often categorized according to their weaknesses. In spite of problems, families have many helpful and healthy behaviors that carry them through. **Family strengths** are positive behaviors or qualities that help maintain family health. Family strengths are really the key to a successful intervention. After all, the family will be doing the work, not the nurse. A list of some possible family strengths is presented in Box 12-3 (Otto, 1973). Feeley and Gottlieb (2000) suggest three aspects to using strengths in nursing: (1) identifying strengths, (2) developing strengths, and (3) calling forth strengths.

TABLE 13-4　Principles for Adjusting Interactions to Family Style

Family Style	Principles for Interaction
Receptive	• Be clear about boundaries and keep to professional role. • Be realistic about time and skill. • Take the opportunity to use family strengths to focus on growth for the family. • Education and linkage with resources will be helpful here.
Distancing	• Move carefully. Watch timing and do not pursue too much • Be aware of your own anxiety. Be aware of increased emotionality and try to be calm and patient. • Expect to have repeated contacts.
Resistive	• Make stronger attempts to connect. • Follow the family interpretation of the situation and focus on their priority. • Be concrete; provide information, but do not argue. • Watch your own frustration.
Disorganized	• Be creative and loose about connecting. • Have very simple plans. • Go after only a few changes. • Do not try to structure the family or the family operations. • Use flexibility.
Rigid	• Assess the family's expectations, and make every attempt to meet them if reasonable; work hard to match the plan of care to the family's routine. • Role model or gently suggest new ways. • Support their original way; stroke it.
Lopsided	• Work through strength; work to get the "doer" to pull back; coach others to do more. • Get additional resources. • Stress that taking care of self is helpful and in the long run benefits others in the family.
Ordered	• If it is not broken, do not try to fix it; find out the family's way of operation and follow it. • Help them determine what they need or want and offer resources.
Tight	• Find the family communicator; give concrete assistance first; feed information and resources to that family member. • Do not try to take a family member's place, especially the communicator's.
Teeter-totter	• Be aware that the active member and the expenditure of energy change; work through the member in action at the present time. • Keep a connection to all members though, especially the previous active member. • Help members see the cycle of overdoing, getting tired, underdoing. Reframe blame, disappointment, guilt, and so forth as reactions to changes in energy patterns.
Dependent	• Decide on your own limits and goals at the beginning of the contact; keep this in mind through the relationship. • Be aware of a family tendency to wait or expect you to do for them; clearly communicate what you can or will do with warmth, not anger. • Translate requests into simple plans of action that family members can perform for themselves. • Step in immediately when the safety of any member is in danger.

Copyright Marcia L. Cooley. (1994). Used with permission.

Identifying the family's good points and competencies is the secret to helping a family be effective in their ability to change and grow. Simply asking the questions to identify strengths often starts the change process. This action helps the nurse develop a caring relationship with the family and emphasizes the power the family will have in making decisions and carrying out the implementation. When determining family strengths, the nurse is asking the following questions: *"Who and where?" "Who in the family is most able to respond to this crisis, and where does the family show talents or areas of pride?"*

Developing strengths includes discussion in concrete terms that both validates the presence of a strength and also links the strength specifically to its effects. This action may change the family perspective on the behavior and present a forum for change. Discussing strengths also helps the family see the value of using more of their strengths for the desired effects. The nurse can also help the family transfer the use of a strength from one context to another and to develop new skills.

Nurses need to be creative, though, in assessing family strengths. Frequently, many family strengths are not evident. When the nurse is viewing a family this way, *reframing* can be a tool to help identify some strengths. For example, a family that is messy and chaotic can be reframed as permissive and creative. Calling forth new strengths may involve focusing on a minor one that can become more evident or teaching new ones. The following clinical example provides a description of this concept.

Ed, a community/public health nurse, was working with a family he did not like very much. The Peters family includes Susan, age 51, her daughter, Carol, and her son, Mark. Mark was using drugs and asked his mother for money and transportation frequently. He was not able to keep a job. Carol was working at a department store, but was having a hard time managing her diabetes and her weight. Ed had been called in to help with dressing changes and intravenous therapy for an ulcer on Carol's leg. Susan was depressed about both situations and her finances. No matter what Ed suggested, the family seemed unable to follow through with any suggestions for improvements in their health.

Ed tried a different tact and began focusing on what the family did well. Together, he and Susan began talking about Carol's laissez-faire style and Susan's ability to organize. By identifying these strengths, Ed demonstrated that Susan was able to set up a plan for meals and wound care that Carol might more easily complete given that she was able to follow directions well. Ed knew that Susan needed to be more firm with Mark about finances and began focusing on those times she was able to set limits. Finding strengths related to Mark was more of a challenge, but Ed realized that Mark's interest in social activities extended to Carol. Ed reframed his own behavior by emphasizing Mark's concern for other people. The family began asking Mark to extend this concern to Carol and his mom. By focusing on strengths rather than deficits, the family made more movement toward health.

DETERMINING FAMILY FUNCTIONING

The final component of the Family Needs Model is the area of family functioning. Remember that, in this context, **family functioning** means family effectiveness in achieving and maintaining physical, emotional, interpersonal, and occupational health. Looking at family functioning helps the nurse answer the following questions: *"To what extent can goals be accomplished?" "What is the potential for change?" "How much energy is available for growth and change?"* To determine the level of family functioning, the nurse may want to integrate information about family resources and coping. Families with stable internal patterns, plenty of support, and the widest ranges of coping behaviors are more able to manage multiple stresses and strains. A family with limited health may appear functional in times of calm but fall apart with relatively

little stress. Conversely, a healthy family may be able to function well in the presence of crushing adversity. A family with greater functional and adaptive ability will be able to progress more quickly and with less dependence on the nurse than will a family with less ability.

Many schema to measure functioning can be used. For example, the McMaster Family Assessment Tool examines the level of family functioning across a range of behaviors, such as communication, problem solving, and emotional support to members (Epstein et al., 1978). This text suggests that beginning nurses use Tapia's criteria (1972). Families are classified according to their level of maturity and potential to function independently (Table 13-5). Even though family functioning can be measured in other ways, Tapia (1972) provides suggestions to guide nurses' decisions about setting goals.

DETERMINING TARGETS OF CARE

Targets of care are different levels of the system, including individuals, dyads, the whole family unit, or the community, that may be recipients of nurse and family actions. Determining targets of care asks the following questions: *"Who will be involved in the care?" "Who is the most likely person in the family to be able to change her or his own behavior?" "Who is likely to communicate with or assert power over other members?" "What members are so burdened by problems that they need support rather than new challenges?"*

The family assessment may reveal many actual needs or potential problems. Too many needs and problems may be present to manage at once, and some people may not wish to be involved in the care. Because families act as systems, an action applied to one member will influence the other members. The nurse may need to make predictions about how certain actions may affect individual members and the family as a whole. For instance, if a child who is afraid of school is successfully encouraged to return to school, another child in the

---

TABLE 13-5 Criteria for Selection of Family Functioning

Characteristics	Nursing Goal
Level I: The Chaotic Family	To establish a trusting relationship; to help family obtain basic necessities and safety
1. Disorganization in all areas of family life	
a. Barely meets needs for security and physical survival	
b. Unable to secure adequate wages or housing	
c. Unable to budget money	
d. Unable to maintain adequate nutrition, clothing, heat, and cleanliness	
e. No future orientation	
2. Inability to provide for healthy emotional and social functioning of its members (apparent alienation from community)	
a. Distrusts outsiders	
b. Unable to use community services and resources	
c. Becomes hostile and resistant to offers of help	
3. Poor role identification	
a. Immature parents unable to assume responsible adult roles (child neglect or abuse often seen)	
b. Parents unable to act as mature role models for children	
4. Family fails to provide support and growth for its individual members	
a. Exhibits depression and feelings of failure	
b. Insecurity of family members prevents change	
5. Family sees the nurse as a *good parent* and will test her or him for consistency and try to be dependent	

TABLE 13-5   Criteria for Selection of Family Functioning—cont'd

Characteristics	Nursing Goal

Level II: The Intermediate Family
1. Lesser degree of disorganization of family life than Level I family
  a. Slightly more able to meet the needs for security and physical survival
  b. Economic level may fall within a wide range
  c. More hope for better way of life
2. Family unable to support and promote growth of members
  a. Members appear unable to change
  b. Defensive and fearful
  c. Lacks resources to gain a sense of accomplishment
  d. Does not seek help actively
  e. Requires much assistance to acknowledge problems realistically
3. Role identification
  a. Parents are immature; socially deviant behavior may occur
  b. Distortion and confusion of roles exists, but parents are more willing to work together for benefit of whole family
  c. Children not neglected to the extent that they must be removed from the home
4. Family will see the nurse as a sibling; that is, they will vacillate between dependence and independence and compete for attention and control
	To increase the ability of family members to understand themselves in their interaction as a group and to grow to the point at which they can work on solutions to some of their problems

Level III: The Adolescent Family
1. Essentially normal but has more than the usual amount of conflicts and problems
  a. More capable of physical survival and providing security for its members (abilities may vary greatly)
  b. Economic level may fall within a wide range
  c. Future oriented, even though present may be painful
2. Increased ability to provide healthy emotional and social functioning of its members
  a. Greater trust in people
  b. Have knowledge and ability to use some community resources
  c. Less openly hostile to outsiders
  d. Increased ability to face some of its problems and look for solutions
3. Role identification
  a. Usually one parent appears more mature than the other
  b. Children have less overall difficulty adjusting to changes in family, school, environment
  c. Difficulty in providing sexual differentiation and training of children
  d. Because one parent may appear quite immature, adult role model for one or more of the children may be lacking (physical care usually adequate, but emotional conflicts usually present)
4. Family members experience achievements and successes outside the family to replace missing satisfaction within family life
5. The nurse will be seen by the family as an adult helper with expertise in the solution of problems
	To help family members improve the ability to manage their roles and tasks as they proceed from one problem to another

Level IV: The Adult Family
1. Normal organization in most areas of family life
  a. Capably provides for physical security and survival
  b. Steady adequate wage earner
  c. Enjoys present and plans for future
2. Capably provides for emotional and social functioning
  a. Has ability to adapt and change in crisis situations
  b. Is able to handle most problems as they arise; however, may show anxiety over these problems
  c. Often refers to outside services for help
  d. Individual and group needs and goals are usually brought into harmony
3. Family confident in roles
4. Main problems center on stages of growth and developmental tasks
5. Family sees the nurse as an expert teacher and partner and is able to use this partnership
	To provide preventive health teaching to enable the family to maintain and promote its health and to increase the members' self-understanding and effectiveness in group functioning

Adapted from Tapia, J. (1972). The nursing process in family health. *Nursing Outlook, 20*(4), 267-270.

family may begin to act out. Of course, the most useful care plan will develop from the wishes of the family members who will be responsible for implementing it. Targeting some individuals as recipients of care without their cooperation will be less helpful than if the idea to participate comes from within. Every assessment should include identifying the most functional and most willing members. These people will usually be the ones to follow through with the intervention plan.

DETERMINING THE NURSE'S CONTRIBUTION

Determining the nurse's contribution asks the following question: *"What can the nurse do for and with this family?"* The nurse needs to define a focus not only for the family but also for self. The needs of the family may be beyond the scope of the nurse's competence or energy, and time and resources become a factor in making decisions about what a nurse can do. The agency and reimbursement mechanisms also dictate the nurse's role. A successful community/public health nurse will be aware of her or his strengths and preferences and try to use them whenever possible. Being able to say *no* or to give up responsibilities is helpful in the long run when potential nursing actions are not realistic. Friedemann's description (1989) of nursing roles is helpful here. The nurse, depending on the analysis of the family and the nurse's experience, chooses to focus on individuals, interpersonal interactions, the family as a whole, or the family's interface with its community.

DETERMINING PRIORITIES OF IDENTIFIED NEEDS

When determining priorities of needs, the nurse asks the following questions: *"What is most crucial?" "What is the most essential or necessary?" "What is possible given current constraints?" "What is most likely to empower the family to act in healthy ways on behalf of itself in the future?"* Some people will use a framework such as that developed by Maslow (1972) to help them determine priorities. **Priorities** are areas of concern or tasks to be accomplished that require immediate action of additional energy from the family and the nurse. In most instances, anything that is life-threatening or a threat to physical safety will be the top priority. Beyond this, certain decisions need to be made to help ensure that the care of the family will be effective. Dunst and colleagues (1989) suggest that the key to working with families is recognizing their need for empowerment. Helping the family discover or regain its sense of power and hope is the basis for the members to be able to continue to build adaptive behaviors and strengths. **When working with families, the need that assumes top priority (after life-threatening emergencies) is the need that the family itself identifies as most important.** This concept may sometimes conflict with the nurse's ordering of priorities. Dunst and colleagues (1989) urge the nurse to choose the family's identified need first, achieve some success and trust when a realistic and achievable goal is accomplished, and then continue with priorities that the nurse suggests.

Once the family and the nurse have identified the family needs and strengths and established priorities, plans for action can be made. Interventions with the family system are the most exciting and challenging part of the nurse's role in family nursing. However, the nurse who enters into this role without an appropriate understanding of some principles risks frustration

and disappointment. Inexperienced nurses sometimes believe that they must change the internal dynamics of the family system if their nursing care is to be successful. However, a change to the family system can come only from within the family. Other goals (e.g., strengthening support systems, engaging in health-promotion behaviors, learning to cope with an illness, promoting a healthful environment) are helpful and more appropriate when working with families.

DEVELOPING A PLAN

Planning family nursing care occurs after the family system is assessed and data are analyzed in a systematic way. Priorities are determined with the family. Remember that nursing interventions are primarily directed toward the five areas of needs that are identified through most family-nurse interactions: growth and development, coping with losses and illness, adapting to the demands of or modifying the environment, strengthening inadequate resources and support, and dealing with disturbances in internal dynamics. The target of the interventions may be an individual, a subsystem, the family unit, or the interaction with the environment. The level of family functioning will affect the type and extent to which goals can be achieved. For example, families with lower levels of functioning benefit from goals that are short term, realistic, concrete, and compatible with their definitions of what is needed. Additionally, family style will determine the way the nurse applies interventions.

PRINCIPLES OF FAMILY CARE PLANNING
Mutuality

The biggest mistake a nurse can make is to forget that the care plan is supposed to benefit the family. If the family has identified the problem and some solutions toward which they are willing to work, their energy and attention will be directed toward a goal that both the nurse and the family support. Dunst and colleagues (1989, p. 13) remind us, "a need is an individual's judgment of the discrepancy between actual states or conditions and what is considered normative, desired or valued *from a help seeker's and not a help giver's perspective.*" Unless an indicated need exists on the part of the help seeker, a need may not exist, regardless of what the professional believes to be the case. Mutuality in family-nurse interactions must occur during identification of the family's needs, definition of goals, choices for nurse and family actions, and evaluation of effectiveness.

Personalization

Even though many families experience similar issues and have common health problems, each family care plan must be unique for that family. The family structure, style of operation, values, strengths, perception of the problem, resources, preferred goals, and level of functioning will all influence the way nursing care should be planned. Two families may have the same health problem and yet require a different nursing intervention.

Realistic Goals

When a nurse first connects with a family, the tendency is to do everything at once. An outsider looking in on a family can often see many things that hinder the growth and happiness of some of the members. Problems that are identified as potential problems by the nurse, however, do not mean that these problems concern the family or that the family wants to change. Time and resources are also limited, and goals must be adjusted to the limitations determined by the nurse's employer or by funding. To some extent, family functional level will also determine the level of goals that can be achieved. According to Tapia (1972), a family that is operating on an adult level will be able to achieve goals that involve health prevention and minimization of potential problems. In contrast, a realistic goal for a chaotic family would be connecting the family to a resource that will perform some of the family maintenance functions and then coaching them to use the resource appropriately.

Values and Health Care Beliefs

Behavior begins with thoughts and feelings about the present situation. The family's beliefs and values will direct their responses to any situation. A care plan that takes the family's values into account will have a greater chance of success than a plan that works against family values (see Chapter 10).

Coordination with the Health Care Team

Neither the nurse nor the family operates in isolation from other professionals and institutions within the community. The plan must be coordinated with all parties involved for it to be successful, avoid duplication, and maximize the use of resources. Nothing is more frustrating to a family than to be pulled or advised in two different directions by two agencies that are supposed to be helping them.

Defining Self

For the nurse who works within the community, the demands and needs that she or he sees will be great and sometimes overwhelming. In a community in which many people are operating with scarce resources, many people must do as much as they can. The nurse who wants to work in a community setting for any extended period will soon realize that choices must be made about how time and resources are spent. Being aware of her or his own beliefs and purpose within the setting will help the nurse to make these choices in ways that continue to be satisfying and do not overextend the capabilities of any one person. The nurse will sometimes encounter a situation that is at odds with her or his personal beliefs. Being clear about a person's operating principles helps her or him respond in a thoughtful and ethical way rather than an automatic, emotional way.

A traditional care plan format is presented in Table 13-6 and completed in The Nursing Process in Practice feature later in this chapter.

IMPLEMENTING THE PLAN

When the nurse is implementing the plan, she or he asks the following questions: *"What?" "How?" "Who?" "Where?" "To*

what extent can goals be achieved?" Most nurses are well prepared to address family needs by borrowing previous skills and knowledge from prior practice settings. For example, the nurse might teach a family how to feed an infant, to clean a tracheostomy, or to role model communication with an adolescent. Each one of the need categories requires knowledge and competencies. While the needs are being addressed, the nurse is also managing self to fit the family style. Summaries of principles used in these actions are presented in Tables 13-4 and 13-7.

HELPING THE FAMILY COPE WITH ILLNESS OR LOSS

Nurses often view their role as one that supports a family's coping. Most nurses think this role means that the nurse is expected to provide emotional support for a family that is experiencing stress. This task is often accomplished in conversations in which the nurse is available and empathetic to family concerns. However, many families actually need other, different types of interventions to support their coping.

Coping is a set of behaviors that emerge whenever a person or family is confronted with a stressor that requires some mobilization of energy. The stressor can be a positive or negative event, but some adaptation or change in behavior is often demanded from a member or the family as a whole. Effective coping will result in an outcome that is positive not only for one family member, but also for the whole family. Coping requires both instrumental and affective actions. *Instrumental actions* are coping behaviors that accomplish a task, such as changing a dressing, locating a source of oxygen supply, or making a clinic appointment. *Affective actions* are coping behaviors that help modify negative emotions that might arise during the stressful situation. Examples of affective coping include talking to others, putting the illness out of one's awareness, or using humor to diffuse tension.

Families and individuals within families already have a repertoire of coping behaviors that they use when stress arises. These coping behaviors are sometimes effective, and sometimes they are not. Table 13-8 lists possible family coping strategies.

When a stressful situation first arises, the nurse can be most helpful in assisting a family to think about its meaning. How a family perceives the events may greatly affect how it is able to deal with them. The same situation may be perceived by one family as a crisis from which no recovery is available and by another family as an opportunity to forge new bonds. After the crisis is identified and an accurate perception of what is happening is shared, some family members may benefit from discussing their emotional reactions to the crisis, and some may be uncomfortable with this strategy. In this early stage of the crisis, the nurse can help the family identify its typical coping behaviors and support or encourage their use. A family in crisis should not try to change unless what it is doing is dysfunctional or not working.

TABLE 13-6	Components of a Care Plan				
Nursing Diagnosis	**Goals and Objectives**	**Nurse-Family Actions**	**Rationale**	**Evaluation**
Individual, interpersonal, family, and environmental diagnoses	Long- and short-term	Interventions to be performed	Evidence-based: derived from research or theory; individualized	Criteria are observable; outcomes are measurable

TABLE 13-7	**Principles Guiding Interventions with Family Needs**
Family Need	**Principles Guiding Interventions**
Growth and development	• Provide anticipatory guidance/education regarding tasks of normal life transitions; give feedback to affirm. • Plan for difficulties of unusual transitions or of multiple transitions occurring at the same time. • Advocate for policies that support family development and self-determination. • Provide guidance for health promotion.
Coping with illness or loss	• Provide information and instrumental and emotional support. • Teach individual and caregiver details of medical regimen and nursing care. • Be case manager to coordinate care. • Collaborate with multiple disciplines, including physicians. • Monitor individual health status and adjust interventions as necessary. • Help family define coping styles and their effectiveness; suggest new behaviors if needed.
Strengthening resources and support	• Facilitate mobilization of resources internal to the family. • Facilitate mobilization of friends and other informal support. • Strengthen support systems by referring family to external resources. • Help family identify barriers to their use of resources, including family style. • Collaborate with others in the community to create community support groups or services.
Changing family dynamics	• Manage participation in family triangles to decrease triangling behavior; stay in contact with all family members without taking sides. • Do not pursue a distancer; offer services and stay in touch. • Assist family members to make decisions consistent with their values and based on thinking rather than automatic emotional reactions. • Explore alternatives and choices that encourage responsibility of individual members.
Remain healthy within the environment	• Remove hazards from family or vice versa. Teach family about environmental factors that may interfere with health or well being. • Teach family to modify the environment to meet needs. • Report unhealthy environmental factors to appropriate agencies. • Advocate for healthful environmental policies.

Copyright Claudia M. Smith. (1995). Used with permission.

No single right or wrong way to cope exists. For example, denying a problem or distancing oneself from it may, in some cases, be protective and necessary until the situation changes. In some instances, the coping that the family chooses does not work or does not work in a healthy way for the entire family. At this point, the nurse can help the family identify alternative coping behaviors. Developing a list of alternatives can be accomplished jointly with the nurse, who may have more ideas or information than the family.

The nurse then helps the family select alternative coping behaviors that seem workable to the family members. As the family tries these new ways of coping, the nurse is available to offer feedback, reinforce new behaviors, and act as a sounding board as the family makes decisions about the next course of action.

When families are dealing with illness, the community/public health nurse can gather nursing knowledge from other health care settings to help the family manage the illness. The nurse needs to help the family deal with three areas of knowledge and adjustment to illness: *knowledge of the specific illness, adjustment to the changes common with all illness,* and *adjustment to different stages of illness* (Cooley, 1989).

Each illness requires that the family have information and skills necessary to manage the demands of that particular illness. For example, a client with chronic obstructive pulmonary disease may need to monitor the weather, prevent exposure to infections, learn how to set up oxygen equipment, and learn to use inhalers appropriately. However, a client with chronic pain may need to learn to use an infusion device, practice daily exercises, and monitor stress. Each illness has specific information and skills to be learned for proper management. The nurse's responsibility is to anticipate the need for and teach this information until the family has mastered the process.

Additionally, many common family reactions and changes exist to illness. Most illnesses bring changes in family roles and responsibilities, occupational and financial changes, alterations in social opportunities, feelings of loss and grief, and a need to adjust expectations of future functioning. Health behaviors and routines need to change to accommodate the illness and to prevent future problems. Changes in daily living such as sleep and rest, exercise and activity, diet, recreation, and sexual activity are commonly required. The community/public health nurse can help the family by providing information and support about these normal and common changes.

Illnesses also have different phases. The earliest phase of diagnosis often involves preparation and cooperation with diagnostic testing, dealing with anxiety and uncertainty, and mobilizing support while awaiting the diagnosis. After the illness is identified, the client and family then enter a working phase during which people are learning illness-management techniques and making adjustments in daily living to manage the care. A period of rehabilitation may precede the return to functioning for some illnesses. Chronic illnesses often have periods of remission and exacerbation that need to be predicted, identified, and managed. Finally, some clients enter a terminal stage, and families and clients are helped toward the end of life.

TABLE 13-8   Family Coping Strategies: Family Crisis Oriented Personal Scales (F-COPES)

When We Face Problems or Difficulties in our Family, We Respond by:	Strongly Disagree	Moderately Disagree	Neither Agree Nor Disagree	Moderately Agree	Strongly Agree
1. Sharing our difficulties with relatives	1	2	3	4	5
2. Seeking encouragement and support from friends	1	2	3	4	5
3. Knowing that we have the power to solve major problems	1	2	3	4	5
4. Seeking information and advice from persons in other families who have faced the same or similar problems	1	2	3	4	5
5. Seeking advice from relatives (grandparents, etc.)	1	2	3	4	5
6. Seeking assistance from community agencies and programs designed to help families in our situation	1	2	3	4	5
7. Knowing that we have the strength within our own family to solve our problems	1	2	3	4	5
8. Receiving gifts and favors from neighbors (e.g., food, taking in mail)	1	2	3	4	5
9. Seeking information and advice from the family physician	1	2	3	4	5
10. Asking neighbors for favors and assistance	1	2	3	4	5
11. Facing the problems *head-on* and trying to get a solution right away	1	2	3	4	5
12. Watching television	1	2	3	4	5
13. Showing that we are strong	1	2	3	4	5
14. Attending religious services	1	2	3	4	5
15. Accepting stressful events as a fact of life	1	2	3	4	5
16. Sharing concerns with close friends	1	2	3	4	5
17. Knowing that luck plays a big part in how well we are able to solve family problems	1	2	3	4	5
18. Exercising with friends to stay fit and reduce tension	1	2	3	4	5
19. Accepting that difficulties occur unexpectedly	1	2	3	4	5
20. Doing things with relatives (get-togethers, dinners, etc.)	1	2	3	4	5
21. Seeking professional counseling and help for family difficulties	1	2	3	4	5
22. Believing that we can handle our own problems	1	2	3	4	5
23. Participating in church activities	1	2	3	4	5
24. Defining the family problem in a more positive way so that we do not become too discouraged	1	2	3	4	5
25. Asking relatives how they feel about problems we face	1	2	3	4	5
26. Feeling that no matter what we do to prepare, we will have difficulty handling problems	1	2	3	4	5
27. Seeking advice from a minister or other religious leader	1	2	3	4	5
28. Believing that the problem will go away if we wait long enough	1	2	3	4	5
29. Sharing problems with neighbors	1	2	3	4	5
30. Having faith in God	1	2	3	4	5

From McCubbin, H. I., & Thompson, A. I. (1987). *Family assessment inventories*. Madison: University of Wisconsin–Madison.

Families are the primary social environment for children with chronic illnesses. Chronically ill children have higher social-emotional coping and become more adaptive adults if their fathers participate in their care (Hovey, 2005). Furthermore, when the father supports the mother in her role as primary caregiver, the mother deals with stress better. Family emotional closeness is associated with less depression in teenagers with diabetes (Cole & Chesla, 2006). Conversely, when children must care for a parent with a chronic disease such as multiple sclerosis, it is important to consider child adjustment (Pakenham & Bursnall, 2006). Adolescents are often at greater risk of psychological distress than young children (Pedersen & Revenson, 2005). When illness of a family member is more severe and the family has low cohesion, the risk of conflict is higher.

Families who are dealing with illness and loss may encounter experiences in which nothing that they do will make the situation better. When tragedy strikes, a loved one dies, or a family must confront an irreversible loss, no actions will make the situation right again. In these situations, both the nurse and the family often resolve the situation by searching for some meaning within what has happened. Dass and Gorman (1986) ask, "How can I help?" The nurse who can find meaning in what she or he does when she or he cannot help is valuable to a family in this situation. Having a compassionate and thoughtful contact within the health care system is useful for almost any family dealing with a crisis.

TEACHING THE FAMILY EXPERIENCING DEVELOPMENTAL CHANGES

Every family deals with the experience of members who grow older and confront day-to-day life in new ways. Many families add or lose members as the family reproduces, the children grow to adulthood, and the family ages. The developmental stage of a family will indicate typical tasks that need to be completed (see Chapter 12). Even the most functional families are novices during the experience of growing into a new stage. Other families confronted with *situational,* as well as *maturational* tasks, may be more overwhelmed by dealing with many new things simultaneously. Families at lower functional levels may be poorly prepared to deal with any additional demands and may view new behaviors of developing members with anger or misunderstanding (see Chapter 14).

The nurse's role when dealing with families who are confronting developmental demands is primarily educational. Providing information about normal growth and development and the adaptations that parents, children, and extended family members require can prevent potential problems and help families manage current ones. The information that is provided may be new to the family, or it may be a reinforcement of what the family already knows but has not recognized as important. For example, Bantz and Siktberg (1993) urge nurses to teach families to evaluate age-appropriate toys that will not frustrate or overstimulate the child. This action enables all parents, regardless of income or education, to promote their child's growth and skill development. Smith (1989) found that a group of postnatal mothers had major concerns related to care of selves and their new babies that were not addressed during their hospital stay with their new baby. All the mothers viewed teaching sessions in the home after discharge as very valuable.

Families will differ in their ability to hear information that the nurse presents, especially if the timing competes with other demands that seem more pressing (Hausman & Hammen,

1993). To teach families with developmental needs effectively, the nurse must assess each member's current knowledge of the developmental issue and then gain agreement from family members that this is something they would like to learn more about. Teaching-learning interactions should be planned for maximal effectiveness, considering timing, the learner's ability, and the method of presentation. After each session, the nurse validates the family's understanding of the content. Finally, the nurse helps the family formulate problem-solving solutions that will satisfy the current or potential developmental demands.

Through this entire process, the nurse is concerned with normalizing the situation for the family. In other words, the more family members can perceive this situation as something through which all families face, the more objective they may be about it. Even though a situation is normal, families may feel pressured or uncomfortable. Not all families will or should adapt to the situation in the same way. Helping the family use its knowledge of its strengths and values to choose operating principles that are compatible must be done on an individual basis for each family. Table 13-9 presents some family research related to parenting

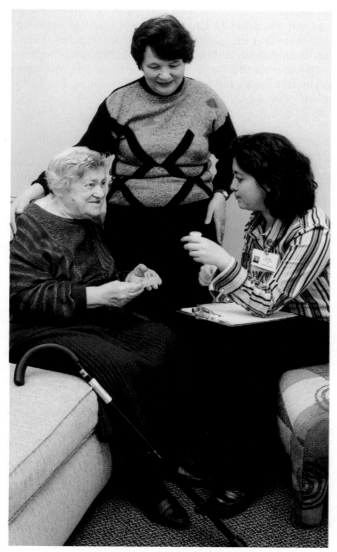

A nurse reviewing medication dosage and frequency with a client and her daughter.

and parenting programs; nurses either conducted the research or were involved in implementing the programs.

Some families will have special needs for education. For example, adoptive families have had a different developmental experience than a biologic family. Asking the right questions at the right time can have a great impact on the well-being of a family who may be faced with situations that they did not anticipate (Peterson, 1997). Other families may have normative development, but they may be limited in their knowledge of normal developmental sequences. For example, Wayland and Rawlins (1997) studied a group of unmarried teenage mothers and found that their perceptions of parenting were based on their own limited experiences. These mothers lacked information about breast-feeding, common childhood illnesses, basic growth and development, safety, and discipline; they also had problems dealing with crying and conflicts with family members. These adolescents often depended on grandmothers to care for the children.

Based on the age of family members and the stage of family development, each family can benefit from knowledge of health-promotion and illness-prevention activities. Health-promotion strategies across the life span are discussed in Chapter 18, and screening tests appropriate for various ages are discussed in Chapter 19. All families experience developmental changes and need to learn to adapt their health-promotion and health-screening behaviors appropriately for their life stages. An important focus of community/public health nursing practice is educating families for health promotion.

CONNECTING THE FAMILY TO NEEDED RESOURCES AND SUPPORT

Resources, including social support, contribute to family well-being. Families who access resources and experience social support are better able both to prevent and to cope with life stressors. For example, one qualitative research study conducted by nurses explored how families managed mental illness (Walton-Moss et al., 2005). Families who were stable or doing well reported adequate support. Families who reported living with uncertainty and frustration had limited finances and limited social support. Community/public health nurses assist families to mobilize resources and strengthen social support.

Mobilizing Resources

Resources are supplies or support that enable the family to meet and handle its situations. Some families do not have necessary resources; other families have difficulty accessing them. Resources are both internal and external—that is, within both the family and the community. Resources can be tangible (e.g., money, clothing, transportation, shelter) or intangible (e.g., strong values, emotional support, religious beliefs, a sense of family solidarity). Resources for health promotion, illness prevention, and early detection of health problems are especially important (see Chapters 18 and 19). One of the most obvious responsibilities of the community/public health nurse is helping families identify and access resources. Families may not know their way around the community or the health care system as well as does an effective community/public health nurse. The ability to act as a provider of information, referral agent, liaison,

TABLE 13-9	**Selected Family Research Related to Parenting and Social Support**			
Researcher	**Target Population**	**Intervention**	**Type of Study**	**Outcomes**
Fergusson et al. (2006)	443 families in an Early Start Program in New Zealand	Community health nurses conducted home visits to promote well-being. Social learning model: Assessment Partnership Collaborative problem-solving Support	Evaluation of Early Start Program Randomized, controlled trial of home visitation on parent and family outcomes; assessed at 6, 12, 24, and 36 months	• Positive parenting and child-related outcomes related to child health, education, and parenting • Absence of family level changes related to stress exposure, economics, and family functioning
Haggman-Laitila & Pietila (2007)	Families with Children Project: 123 parents and 58 children in Finland	Small goal-oriented groups of 14 members meeting 7 times over 10 months; led by multiple professional disciplines, including public health nurse	Qualitative evaluation of parental perceptions of small group benefits. Videotaped interviews after group meetings	• Information • Motivation to seek info • Rest and "company" • Stronger social support networks • Stronger awareness of own personal resources • Reliance on own coping, confidence, future orientation
Black & Ford-Gilboe (2004)	Convenience sample of 41 single, white, adolescent mothers in Ontario, Canada	Not applicable	Assessment of resilience, family health promotion, and own health-promoting lifestyle. Verbal responses to questionnaires	• Mothers' employment, professional support, and resilience predicted mothers' health-promotion behaviors

or coordinator of resources is essential for community/public health nurse case managers.

The nurse who desires to help families access resources will thoroughly assess tangible and intangible resources that have the potential for being useful in the situation. Many families have a need for multiple resources; identifying the one or two that are most helpful to the need will target the nurse's and family's energies.

In some instances, resources that are not typically seen as helpful may be used creatively in certain situations. For example, the family may think that no one is available to care for an ill member but may be ignoring a family member who is able to do so, but typically does not perform this role. Encouraging the family to open itself up to new ways of using internal resources is useful.

Families that are relatively closed—that is, families with boundaries that are not very permeable—often attempt to deal with problems themselves. These families may have strong beliefs that they should manage troubles themselves. Helping them accept aid from extended family members, the community, or professionals may involve exploring their beliefs and offering help while acknowledging their preferred tight style. Other families may have had experiences with resources that have turned out to be ineffectual or inadequate. Making sure that resources are reliable and that the family has realistic expectations of what the resource can provide are ways to prevent repeats of earlier negative experiences.

Strengthening Social Support

Social support is the perceived positive value of the interpersonal relationships or contacts of the family. Social support is a resource that affects health and well-being by (1) directly providing a sense of belonging, approval, and social contact, (2) helping prevent life stresses by providing information about how to avoid hazards and prevent stressors, and (3) buffering the effect of life stresses by helping to reduce threats or increase coping, or both (Uphold, 1991). Therefore social support is relevant to health promotion and all three levels of illness prevention.

Deficits in social support may be episodic or chronic. For most families, the primary sources of social support are family members, extended family, close friends, and neighbors. When these relationships are disrupted through death, divorce, or relocation, family members may experience deficits in social support. Deficiencies in social support also may occur when health or other problems exceed the family's usual capacity for problem solving (Bullock, 2004). Community/public health nurses can assist family members to strengthen social support. The nurse assists the family to identify what help they need and possible sources of that support. The first priority is to mobilize social support from inside the family or from informal support networks such as friends, neighbors, and religious communities. These relationships are more likely to be long lasting and to be the most culturally appropriate. When specialized assistance is needed or families are in crisis, the nurse refers families to appropriate professional sources such as home health agencies, grief counseling, vocational rehabilitation services, or legal services. The goal is for families to access meaningful and supportive relationships.

Community/public health nurses can collaborate with others to create community support groups and services where none exist. Drury-Zemke (1997) describes her experience in starting an amputee support group in her city of 300,000 peo-ple. Support groups such as these provide opportunities for persons to network with others who understand each other's problems and experiences.

Some families experience chronic deficiencies in social support. For example, one study in the United Kingdom explored the perceptions of family caregivers of persons with developmental disabilities and challenging behavior. Almost half of the caregivers reported that they did not receive professional support, or that the input was not helpful (Papachristoforou & Cooper, 2006). The community/public health nurse needs to assess the barriers to social support and work with the family to remove these barriers. For example, if a caregiver spends most of her or his time caring for a bed-bound spouse, rarely leaves the home, and is experiencing loneliness, the caregiver may regain social support through telephone calls and by having others visit her or his home.

When internal family relationships are unhealthy and stressful, family members may have difficulty establishing and maintaining a social network outside the family because they have not learned to trust others or have not been taught necessary interpersonal skills. Community/public health nurses can work with the family members most ready for change and assist them to seek positive relationships outside their family. For example, children of alcoholics might be referred to self-help groups such as Adult Children of Alcoholics.

COACHING THE FAMILY TO CHANGE ITS INTERNAL DYNAMICS

The process of change within a family will occur naturally as the family grows and adapts to new and ever-changing environmental circumstances. Most families do not need help to change their way of operating in general; instead, they need help to adapt and cope with new developmental, situational, and environmental challenges. The nurse assists the family to change not because something is wrong with the family, but rather because the family style and organization are not effectively meeting the current demands.

Sometimes, however, families do not effectively meet the needs of their members even in times that are relatively calm. These families with disturbances in internal dynamics are candidates for change in the family system.

The community/public health nurse who is informed about the dynamics of families and has some training in family coaching is in the perfect position to serve as a catalyst for change. Most baccalaureate-prepared nurses do not receive this education; family coaching is taught most frequently at the graduate level, especially among psychiatric/mental health/behavioral nurses.

The following principles of change must be kept in mind when working with a family toward change:

1. *Many families are resistant to change.* Even when the change would probably be beneficial to the family, families may prefer to remain as they are. Remaining in what is known is easier than exerting energy to move into the unknown.
2. *Sequencing or timing will affect the outcome.* Families have difficulty changing during times of crisis or stress. However, this period is often the best time to change because the family sees the need for it then. Change is most likely to happen after perceptions of the situation begin to change. Working on the family's cognition or thinking about the problem is the first step in an intervention. Helping the family modify affect and behavior comes next.

3. *Past patterns must be interrupted.* Families tend to operate in patterns of interaction that repeat themselves. Triggers set up behaviors to which all family members respond automatically. Breaking these patterns and starting healthier behavioral sequences is difficult, but it can be done.

4. *A change in one part of the system will affect the whole system.* No person can change another, but any person can change herself or himself. What we do and the way we react have an impact on others. When any one person in a system changes, the system will automatically change.

5. *The more important a family member is to the family's functioning, the more impact a change in that family member will have.* Not all family members will change equally or have equal capacity to change. Identifying the family member who is most likely to be able to change is a good strategy for the nurse who desires to help the family modify its functioning.

6. *Family strengths are as important as family problems.* The perception of the family problem is often unhealthier than is the problem. When one family member is blamed or held responsible for others, the shared nature of the family problem cannot be recognized. For example, at times Harry is lazy and irresponsible. Is it also possible that Harry adds humor and genuineness to a restricted family environment? Can the problem be reframed and seen as an asset?

7. *A family's capacity to change is related to its level of functioning.* The family has probably operated at a certain level of health for some time before the nurse appears on the scene. Having realistic ideas about what can be accomplished for each family is necessary. The nurse who can help the family think about issues in ways that lead to a small improvement in or maintenance of functioning will mean that the family is in better shape than having no intervention at all.

Techniques that advanced practice nurses use to help families change include contracting, tracking family process, increasing cognitive awareness, reframing, aligning or maintaining neutral connections to family members, exploring affect, restructuring, suggesting direct interventions, and offering paradoxical interventions (Minuchin & Fishman, 1981). Contracting, tracking family process, reframing, and maintaining neutral connections with family members are appropriate for baccalaureate-educated nurses.

Formulating a contract with the family at the beginning of the interaction, having a definite goal, and limiting the number of sessions help keep the interaction focused. At different times during the sessions, the professional carefully chooses a position in relation to family members, such as aligning with a weak member or maintaining neutral but meaningful connections to all.

Reframing is a way to label negative as positive. Something that is perceived as negative can be explored and renamed in a positive way. This action breaks up the family's typical way of thinking about the problem and helps family members begin to think of alternatives. Cognitive perceptions and knowledge about family dynamics can be broadened. When this expansion happens, objectivity about the family problem is increased, and family members are able to act in less reactive ways.

During early sessions, the family process or patterns of interaction are tracked by the professional and brought into the awareness of the family. Seeing the repetitive nature of the behavior sequences and recognizing the behavioral triggers are the first step to being able to modify behavior. Affect or feelings that accompany behavioral sequences can be named and examined. Many times, if the behavioral sequence is changed, the emotion that accompanies it will also change.

Helping a family change its internal dynamics is not a goal that every nurse should attempt. However, with practice and training, many nurses become effective family coaches.

HELPING THE FAMILY REMAIN HEALTHY WITHIN THE ENVIRONMENT

The world in which families live is resource rich, and our society performs many functions that used to be the responsibility of the family. Families and family members are healthier and have access to many more living aids than did families in the past. However, today's world is also a potential threat to health in many ways. Pollutants in the air, water, soil, food, homes, schools, and occupational settings are threats to family health. The social environment also exposes us to unsafe situations of crime, violence, drug abuse, and deteriorating interpersonal behavior. Many families make plans for their lives only to have them affected by situations beyond their control, such as buy-outs and mergers of employers, changes in health and retirement benefits, and a changing economy.

The community/public health nurse who is interested in family health will consider family-environment interactions (see Chapter 9). Actual health problems may be related to or aggravated by environmental issues, and potential health problems related to environmental issues may be diverted. For example, Kuster (1997) urges community/public health nurses to help families reduce the risks of house dust mite and cockroach exposure. Recent evidence has linked these environmental exposures to asthma in inner-city children. Surveillance, detection, and correction of environmental threats become a way to help families maintain their health. For example, Arvidson and Colledge (1996) urge school nurses to develop lead screening programs for their populations. Lead poisoning is one of the most preventable conditions of childhood with devastating effects on a young child. For lead and other environmental issues, educating families and communities is crucial to help the public become aware of potential health threats and strategies for dealing with them. Nurses also have the opportunity to intervene by providing data that influence health care decisions and by participating in legislative and executive processes that formulate health policy.

EVALUATION

Even though evaluation is the final step of the nursing process, it is also a step that starts at the beginning of the contact and occurs continually as the contact progresses. The word *evaluate* means to determine the worth of something. Many methods can be used to evaluate nursing care, but the key to evaluation is to determine the correct criteria that demonstrate the value of the nursing contact. Criteria for evaluating client outcomes are derived from the objectives developed with the family. Because the outcomes of nursing interventions occurring during one visit may not be apparent until later, both long-term and short-term evaluative criteria should be developed.

METHODS

Two methods of evaluation are formative and summative evaluation. **Formative evaluation** occurs during the course of nurse-family interactions. This form of evaluation can be used to guide decisions about modification of goals, objectives, nursing actions, and priorities as the nursing encounters unfold. Data are collected once or multiple times during the home visiting process, clinic visits, telephone conversations, and health-education classes and events. Examples of formative evaluation methods include keeping daily records of blood glucose levels, holding monthly health care team meetings to discuss family progress, or asking the family for feedback at the end of each nurse-family encounter. Formative evaluation helps the nurse and family modify nursing care in a more effective way.

Summative evaluation occurs at the end of the family-nurse relationship and is used to summarize the value of the interaction to the family. A description of the extent of goal accomplishment and remaining family needs helps the family make choices about termination or referral. The family can review with the nurse the actions that it used to achieve its goals and can leave the relationship with a sense of accomplishment. Summative evaluation can also help inform the nurse about her or his effectiveness and provide feedback about specific nursing actions and suggestions for working with other families in the future. Examples of summative evaluation include an oral quiz about a client's knowledge of her or his medication, a discharge planning meeting with the health care team, or a conversation with a family about the series of visits.

FACTORS INFLUENCING EVALUATION

Many factors influence evaluation; an example is the availability of data. If data are easy to obtain and have been carefully collected, the evaluation is likely to be accurate and complete. The resources available to the nurse and health care team also influence the outcomes being judged during evaluation. In a community health situation that is resource rich, the expectation is that many of the family's needs will be met. In a situation with fewer resources, outcomes are likely to be judged more leniently. Family expectations also influence evaluation. If the family begins the encounter(s) with a realistic expectation of what can be accomplished and under what circumstances the nurse would leave, then the family is more likely to be satisfied with what has happened. Families who expect something the professionals are unlikely to deliver will naturally leave the interaction disappointed. Additionally, the nature of the family-nurse–health care team interaction often influences the way people view the encounter. Relationships that have been pleasant and mutually satisfying are more likely to lead to perceptions that the nursing care has been effective than are relationships in which some or all of the parties have been dissatisfied or uncomfortable.

Finally, the nurse's attitudes will influence her or his judgment of success. Many new nurses enter community/public health situations with unrealistic expectations of their own power. Although nurses cannot fix families, they can help families maintain or improve their level of wellness within realistic limits.

WHAT TO EVALUATE
Examination of Goals

At the beginning of the planning process, the nurse and family state the criteria for goal achievement. If these criteria are clearly stated and data are available, then it is a simple matter to determine goal achievement. Goals should be written in the form of outcomes so that the true impact of the nursing intervention can be determined. For example, knowing that a family member read a pamphlet about parent-child communication is not the same as seeing the parent interact with the child.

Remember that both short-term and long-term objectives exist. During the evaluation process, examining short-term objectives may make evident that the long-term goal is not going to be achieved. Revision of either the long-term goal or the actions performed to accomplish the goal may be necessary.

Examining the Effect on the Ill Member

Many family nursing encounters are initiated because someone in the family has been identified as sick. The person who is the focus of care, especially one who has been identified by an agency or reimbursement mechanism, is the primary person to be evaluated. What effect did nursing actions have on the ill family member? Is her or his health status improved? Has her or his position and role within the family changed in any way? To what extent is this person satisfied with the nursing contact?

Examining the Effect on Individuals

In many cases, other individuals within the family have health needs of their own. Other members will be involved in offering care to the ill person, coping with necessary changes, or promoting health. Family nursing interventions often upset the balance within a family. What is the impact on each member of the family? To what extent have individual health needs been met? To what extent is each person satisfied with the nursing contact?

Examining the Effect on Subsystems

A subsystem of the family may have been the target of care or may be particularly affected by the activities of the family. For example, the nurse may have been working with a single mother with regard to her parenting of a toddler. The sibling subsystem—two older children in the family—may feel left out or may have benefited by the mother's new skills. As families learn new behaviors, other groups of people within the family may be affected. Have the changes been beneficial and satisfying for all the members of the system? Do interventions need to be planned for another portion of the family to balance recent activity?

Examining the Effect on the Family Unit

A family is more than a collection of individuals; it is a unit that can stand on its own. How has the family as a whole benefited or responded to the nursing interventions? Is the family able to function more effectively? Does the family operate more smoothly as a unit? What is the affective response to the interactions? Is the family more able to master situations and solve problems for itself?

Examining the Interaction with the Environment

The family is not isolated; it lives within an environmental context. How has the family-environment interaction changed? Is this change beneficial to the family? Is the change beneficial to the community? Is there reason to plan more or different actions directed toward the family's interaction with their context?

Examining the Nursing Performance

The nurse also will benefit from evaluating herself or himself. Was the nurse prepared for each nursing visit? What knowledge did the nurse bring to the visit? What new knowledge would have been helpful? How skillful was the nurse while performing her or his tasks? Does the nurse need to acquire other skills? How did the nurse's own values and attitudes influence the interactions? Did the nurse use feedback to modify performance? How much effort was put into communicating and coordinating care with other members of the health care team? To what extent is the nurse satisfied with the family interactions? These insights can be used to maintain the quality of the current family care and for the nurse's future family contacts.

OUTCOME OF EVALUATION

People sometimes think of evaluation as the end of the nursing process. In many situations, however, evaluation is just the beginning. If evaluation is used properly at several predetermined times during the nurse-family relationship, it should help the nurse refine the nursing care plan and improve its quality. Three outcomes are possible: modification, continuation, and resolution.

Modification

Modification, or change, may be necessary in any part of the nursing care plan, including identifying needs, establishing priorities, selecting short-term or long-term goals, or choosing nursing or family actions. The nurse and family may change their ideas about timing or which family member will perform certain tasks. Modification is a necessary step in a nursing care plan if it is to be a plan that the family really needs.

Continuation

The evaluation may show that the plans that have been made are working or are likely to work. Continuing the plan is evidence of successful planning but does not imply that termination is imminent.

Resolution

Hopefully, some or all of the original needs will be resolved or no longer require nurse and family actions. A need is resolved when outcome criteria have been achieved or when the family no longer perceives intervention as a need. Resolution of some needs may allow the family to proceed to needs perceived as having less priority or to decide that terminating the nurse-family relationship is appropriate.

TERMINATING THE NURSE-FAMILY RELATIONSHIP

Ending a meaningful relationship always elicits feelings for the family and for the nurse. In any relationship that has been defined as potentially therapeutic for the family, attention should be paid to the termination process. During termination, everyone involved must deal with her or his personal feelings about separation. Many people have a preferred form of separation: they may distance themselves; attempt to prolong the contact; become angry, sad, or *act out;* or deny that the relationship has been important. The type of reaction depends to some extent on the way separations have happened in the past.

In the community health setting, the nurse frequently experiences termination. Clients may experience terminations all too often when community/public health nurses are transferred or families move to another jurisdiction without much notice. Careful planning, providing advance notice, and talking about the emotions and issues that arise are helpful for everyone involved. The nurse will often bring up the issue of termination before the client is ready. Allowing clients to express reactions and helping families perceive themselves as being able to master upcoming situations independently will help the family make the transition to independence and termination.

During the final encounters, the nurse begins to prepare the family by reminding them that the time together is limited. A date or goal should be set that is understood as the marking point for termination. Goal accomplishment, satisfaction with the process, and plans for continuing health maintenance should be discussed. If referrals or transfers are needed, they are arranged at this time. Criteria should be established for the family to know when to seek health care again; for example, reappearance of the signs and symptoms of a chronic mental illness would be a signal for the family to contact the clinic. Hopefully, the nurse will find a way to frame the outcomes of the visits in a way that indicates success for the family even if the original goals were not met. In almost every contact, the nurse and family have learned something, or they grew in some way that can be presented as a success.

KEY IDEAS

1. Family nursing takes place within the framework of the nursing process.
2. Family needs, style, strengths, and functioning are assessed with the Family Needs Model of family nursing. Families are assessed on several levels: individual, subsystem, family unit, and family-environment interaction.
3. The goal of family assessment is mutual identification of needs and care planning that includes both the nurse and the family. The success of family health care depends on setting realistic goals related to the level of family functioning.
4. Several diagrams help assess families. A family map diagrams the structure and organization of the family and its subsystems. A genogram identifies family facts and process, including illnesses and multigenerational patterns of relationships. An eco-map describes the energy exchanges between the family and the environment.
5. Analysis of family data helps the nurse determine family needs, family style, family strengths, and family functioning. Analysis of family data includes determination of the targets of care, nursing contribution, and the priorities of family needs.
6. NANDA International has specified several nursing diagnoses related to families, focusing on family processes and family coping. The Omaha System identifies family problems related to the use of social resources and the environment.
7. Different nursing intervention strategies are used for each family need: developmental and health-promotion needs, coping with illness or loss, inadequate resources and support, disturbances in internal dynamics, and coping with the environment. Nursing interactions are adjusted to the family style. Family strengths are as important as family problems.
8. Families are resistant to change, but a time of crisis is often the best opportunity for change. As the importance of the family member increases, the impact of a change in that member on the family increases. Helping a family change its internal dynamics is not a goal for every community/public health nurse or every family.
9. Evaluation should include examination of goals and the effect of intervention on an ill family member, other individuals, family subsystems, the entire family, and the environment. Evaluation should also include evaluation of the quality of nursing performance. The outcome of evaluation may be modification of the plan, continuation of the plan, or resolution of the problem.

Formulating a Family Care Plan

Mr. R. is an 80-year-old retired pipe fitter who lives with his wife; he has had diabetes for 15 years. Although his diabetes has been moderately controlled with diet and daily insulin, some complications have occurred. He experiences arteriosclerotic cardiovascular disease and peripheral neuropathy, and he recently spent 2 months in the hospital with circulatory problems in his left leg. The progressive deterioration of circulation resulted in an amputation below the knee. Although fitting him with a prosthesis would be possible, he has refused this and is wheelchair bound. Mr. R. currently depends on someone else to help with transfers. He is cranky, irritable, and demanding to almost everyone. He recently has stopped following his diabetic regimen because he claims, "It just doesn't matter anymore."

Mr. R.'s wife, Doris, is a 74-year-old woman who has been a homemaker most of her life. She has always been the "watchdog" for Mr. R.'s health. Mostly through her changes in food preparation and her lifestyle adjustments, Mr. R.'s diabetes has been managed. She schedules his physician appointments, buys his medical supplies, and administers his insulin. He is now refusing to accept her help, and she is anxious and angry about his behavior. They frequently argue, after which Mrs. R. retreats to her room.

Mr. and Mrs. R. have three children and four grandchildren who live in the same city. The eldest daughter, Patricia, calls or stops by about once a week. The other children, Tom and Ellen, are busy with their families and see their parents mostly on holidays; they have very little communication with Patricia or their parents. When the children do come to visit, Doris tries to put on a happy expression and pretend that everything is going well so she will not worry them. She is also embarrassed about Mr. R.'s behavior and does not want anyone from outside the family to see what is happening.

On her initial home visit to this family, the community health nurse noted that Mr. R. appeared somewhat drowsy and unkempt. Mrs. R. looked anxious and tired, her skin color was slightly ashen, and she had circles under her eyes. When the nurse asked them what they hoped to get out of the nursing visits, Mrs. R. said, "Actually, you don't need to keep visiting. In a few weeks we'll be back to normal and doing fine."

Based on a thorough assessment of the family, the community health nurse may begin to develop a mutually acceptable plan of care with the family.

ASSESSMENT

In the initial interview, the community health nurse completed a genogram and an eco-map with the family (see Figures 13-3 and 13-4). After the second family interview, the nurse also completed a family map that described the members' interactions with each other (see Figure 13-2). A family guide to help structure a family assessment is presented in Box 13-7.

Completing the genogram helped break the ice to get the family to talk about their situation. The genogram provided a safe and thought-provoking way for Mrs. R. to supply appropriate information about the situation. During this process, the nurse obtained information about other family members, their general levels of functioning, and the possibility of acting as resources. She identified family members' patterns of closeness and distance.

The eco-map presented a picture to both the nurse and Mr. and Mrs. R. of a family that was not well connected to outside resources. Little energy was coming in or going out of the immediate family system, with the exception of intervention by the health care system, which the family wanted to discontinue. When the community health nurse later completed a family map, she became aware of Mrs. R.'s tendency to act as a parent and

---

BOX 13-7   Family Assessment Guide

I. Identifying Data

Name: _____

Address: _____

Phone number(s): _____

Household members (relationship, gender, age, occupation, education): _____

_____

_____

Financial data (sources of income, financial assistance, medical care; expenditures): _____

_____

_____

_____

Ethnicity: _____

Religion: _____

Identified client(s): _____

Source of referral and reason: _____

_____

_____

_____

II. Genogram

Include household members, extended family, and significant others

Age or date of birth, occupation, geographic location, illnesses, health problems, major events

Triangles and characteristics of relationships

Continued

BOX 13-7   **Family Assessment Guide—cont'd**

III. Individual Health Needs (for each household family member)
Identified health problems or concerns: _____

_____

Medical diagnoses: _____

_____

Recent surgery or hospitalizations: _____

_____

Medications and immunizations: _____

_____

Physical assessment data: _____

_____

Emotional and cognitive functioning: _____

_____

Coping: _____
Sources of medical and dental care: _____
Health screening practices: _____

IV. Interpersonal Needs
Identified subsystems and dyads: _____
Prenatal care needed: _____
Parent-child interactions: _____
Spousal relationships: _____
Sibling relationships: _____
Concerns about elders: _____
Caring for other dependent members: _____
Significant others: _____

_____

_____

V. Family Needs
A. Developmental
Children and ages: _____

_____

Responsibilities for other members: _____

_____

Recent additions or loss of members: _____
Other major normative transitions occurring now: _____

_____

Transitions that are out of sequence or delayed: _____

_____

Tasks that need to be accomplished: _____

_____

Daily health-promotional practices for nutrition, sleep, leisure, childcare, hygiene, socialization, transmission of norms and values: _____

_____

_____

Family planning used: _____

_____

B. Loss or Illness
Nonnormative events or illnesses: _____

_____

Reactions and perceptions of ability to cope: _____

_____

Coping behaviors used by individuals and family unit: _____

_____

Meaning to the family: _____
Adjustments family has made: _____
Roles and tasks being assumed by members: _____

_____

Any one individual bearing most of responsibility: _____
Family idea of alternative coping behaviors available: _____

_____

Box 13-7   Family Assessment Guide—cont'd

Level of anxiety now and usually: _____
_____

C. Resources and Support
General level of resources and economic exchange with community: _____
External sources of instrumental support (money, home aides, transportation, medicines, etc.): _____
Internal sources of instrumental support (available from family members): _____
External sources of affective support (emotional and social support, help with problem solving): _____
_____
Internal sources of affective support (who in family is most helpful to whom?): _____
_____
Family more open or closed to outside? _____
Family willing to use external sources of support? _____

D. Environment
Type of dwelling: _____
Number of rooms, bathrooms, stairs; refrigeration, cooking: _____
_____
_____
Water and sewage: _____
Sleeping arrangements: _____
Types of jobs held by members: _____
_____
Exposure to hazardous conditions at job: _____
Level of safety in the neighborhood: _____
Level of safety in household: _____
Attitudes toward involvement in community: _____
Compliance with rules and laws of society: _____
How are values similar to and different from those of the immediate social environment? _____
_____

E. Internal Dynamics
Roles of family members clearly defined? _____
Where do authority and decision-making rest? _____
Subsystems and members: _____
Hierarchies, coalitions, and boundaries: _____
Typical patterns of interaction: _____
Communication, including verbal and nonverbal: _____
Expression of affection, anger, anxiety, support, etc.: _____
_____
Problem-solving style: _____
Degree of cohesiveness and loyalty to family members: _____
_____
Conflict management: _____
_____

VI. Analysis
Identification of family style: _____
Identification of family strengths: _____
Identification of family functioning: _____
What are needs identified by family? _____
_____
What are needs identified by community health nurse? _____
_____

Mr. R.'s tendency to act as a child. This blurring of boundaries had set up a behavior pattern in which Mr. R. gave away responsibility for his own health. At the same time, however, the rigidity of these boundaries kept the children out of these interactions. After assessing the family, the nurse tried to guide her practice with some questions. She asked herself about the family's needs, strengths, functioning, and style. She examined the family's priorities and the resources they were using or potentially able to use. She looked at her own skills and abilities and attempted to define her responsibility to the family system. These questions helped her begin to analyze the family data. This analysis led to several determinations.

FAMILY HEALTH NEEDS

The family needs help coping with this illness and connecting with resources and sources of support. Some minor disturbances in internal dynamics are influencing the way the family is dealing with the problem. The nurse assigns the family the nursing diagnosis of "Family Coping: Ineffective, Compromised."

FAMILY STYLE

This family is a distancing family that prefers to keep its problem-solving activities to itself. However, this isolation limits family members' ability to support each other. The community health nurse must adjust her nursing interactions to accommodate this family's style of operating. The nurse should respect the family's need for distance, approach them cautiously, and observe for cues that indicate that they are becoming anxious.

FAMILY STRENGTHS

This family has some ability to organize activities that need to be accomplished to maintain Mr. R.'s health. Family members are concerned about each other and may be able to adjust schedules or routines. Mrs. R. is committed to Mr. R.'s health care and will try to do what is required. The family has a long history together and in the past has developed a sense of identity and common purpose.

FAMILY FUNCTIONING

Even though the family is currently stressed, long-term functioning is fairly healthy. No one member has consistently been a problem or has failed to fulfill her or his role. The adult children are not acting in their age-appropriate roles of support to parents. This status seems to reflect the family style but can possibly be modified.

TARGETS OF CARE

The community health nurse believes several levels of this family— the individuals with health problems (both Mr. and Mrs. R.), the couple, and the family as a unit—are potential targets for care. When she reviews who the most likely person in the family is to be able to change behavior, she looks for someone who seems willing to change. She decides this person is Mrs. R. and potentially the children.

NURSE'S CONTRIBUTION

The community health nurse reviews her own caseload and her available time and attempts to make an accurate assessment of her skills. She is fairly comfortable in dealing with families and decides she will intervene on three levels: individual, subsystem, and family unit. Her contribution will be to offer information, counseling, and connection with other resources. She can visit one time per week and will try to schedule these visits when some of the children can be present.

PRIORITIES

The family has several needs. What is most crucial? Any life-threatening situation must be top priority, but nothing will be accomplished without the family's agreement that this is their concern. After discussing these ideas with the family, the nurse and the family decide to first address individual health concerns. Mr. R.'s hyperglycemia is noted, and he admits it is making him feel bad. Mrs. R.'s cardiac status is to be assessed next week at an appointment with the family physician. Although Mr. R. seems agreeable to resuming his insulin injections, he has no desire to change his diet or learn how to walk with a prosthesis. The community health nurse puts aside these problems for the time being and addresses Mrs. R. She wonders if Mrs. R. would be interested in exploring her current care for herself. Mrs. R. tentatively agrees. Using additional resources to help Mr. R. transfer in and out of his wheelchair is something that can be accomplished, but the family is still reluctant about this course of action. This problem, too, is put off to a later time.

PLANNING

The community health nurse and the family together develop both long-term and short-term goals.

Mr. R.:
- Will monitor and record blood glucose levels every morning
- Will accept administration of insulin by Mrs. R.
- Will begin range-of-motion and strengthening exercises to promote mobility for eventual transfer of self to chair
- Will communicate to Mrs. R. his ability to take care of any of his own needs as each opportunity arises
- Will demonstrate improved blood glucose levels within 1 month

Mrs. R.:
- Will have her cardiac status evaluated within 2 weeks
- Will self-monitor her health and record her health status for 1 week
- Will decide on one goal to take care of herself within 2 weeks
- Will practice this behavior for 1 month
- Will allow Mr. R. to care for himself when he desires

Mr. and Mrs. R. together:
- Will experience decreased frequency of arguments within 1 month
- Will spend some relaxed time together every evening

The family:
- Will discuss new ways of coping with this situation as a group
- Will try out two behaviors that use different family members within 2 weeks
- Will accept one resource to help within 1 month

IMPLEMENTATION

The community health nurse is aware that the disturbances in the family's coping ability are fairly recent. The behaviors they have used in the past—self-reliance, appropriate action, distancing, and some denial of the problem—are not working in this situation. The first goal for nursing implementation addresses individual health needs. The second goal involves helping Mr. and Mrs. R. think about the crisis and identify their present coping strategies. Because the nurse knows that the family style is distant, she will proceed slowly with this step, adjusting to suit the family's pace. She will initially keep the discussion focused on thoughts and facts rather than feelings. Mr. R. perceives the situation as hopeless. It is important to help the family reframe this perception so that the current crisis is seen as being able to be modified. Subsequent plans with regard to family coping would include identifying alternative coping behaviors and practicing them. Because significant strengths are present and the family level of functioning is fairly high, the community health nurse would expect the family to use information to appropriately problem solve in this crisis. The family may also use the situation as a way of growing into new behaviors that foster family health.

Connecting the family with resources must be done in a way that allows this family to make the choice about outside care. Providing information about the extent to which other modern families use these resources may help them accept this intrusion into their world. Internal resources that are available to the family include the adult children, who may be able to offer instrumental or emotional support simply by being made aware of the extent of the need.

The internal dynamics of the family, in which the couple's roles are unbalanced, given that the wife has assumed more and more responsibility for the husband, are likely to be long-term patterns. Expecting a family at this stage of life to change a formerly effective pattern of relating to each other is unrealistic and ill advised. Instead, helping Mrs. R. focus on herself more so that she can care for her own needs and helping Mr. R. increase his awareness about his responsibility for his health and to his wife are more appropriate interventions.

EVALUATION

The community health nurse reviewed the care plan periodically with the family and at the end of the contact. This evaluation included examination of goals. As the family crisis subsided, goals were quickly accomplished and revised weekly.

Continued

The family also examined the effect of the interaction on the ill member (Mr. R.). His hyperglycemia was modified the first week, and his blood glucose levels dropped to a normal range within several weeks of contact. He accepted his insulin and even expressed interest in administering it himself. His stance about eating whatever he wanted also changed, and he began to follow his diet recommendations more closely. He continued to resist attempts to be fitted for a prosthesis but eventually learned to assist with his transfers. When the community health nurse left this family, a goal still to be accomplished was Mr. R.'s learning to use a walker.

Examination of the intervention's effect on individuals included looking at Mrs. R.'s health status and that of the adult children. Mrs. R.'s cardiovascular status had deteriorated. She began some cardiotonic medication and was urged to moderate her activity and stress level. All three of the adult children began sharing in the care of their father. Although the children were busier than before, the impact on them was manageable.

Examination of the effects on the subsystem included effects on the interactions of the marital couple. Mr. and Mrs. R. both began to assume more appropriate responsibility for themselves. The arguments and anger lessened, although their long-term way of relating to each other did not change a great deal.

The effect on the whole family was also examined. Incorporating additional resources led to a decreased perception of crisis and an increased calm in the family. As the members began to renew connections with each other, they discovered new sources of emotional support. Several months later, Mr. R. died after experiencing a pulmonary embolus. The children were able to support their mother during this time of loss.

In examining the family's interaction with the environment, it became apparent that the family members had become more aware of the community resources available to them. Members were still very private but began to use available resources appropriately. Members' home environment was relatively safe.

As she was working with this family, the community health nurse continually sought feedback to evaluate her own performance. She carefully monitored the family's reactions to her interventions and her reactions to the family. She was frustrated at the need to proceed slowly with the family but was satisfied with her choice when she saw that the strategy had worked. Her contact with the family led her to enroll in a course about client nonadherence. She learned to be patient during this experience and took these behaviors with her in her future contacts with families.

LEARNING BY EXPERIENCE AND REFLECTION

1. Choose one of the family assessment tools and apply it to a family you know. In what ways does the tool help you identify information to collect? Would you have considered this information important without the guidance of the tool? In what ways does the tool restrict your thinking about the family? What important information was not included?

2. Trace the origins of one of the assessment tools back to the original theoretical concepts from which it evolved. Is the theory appropriate for thinking about this family? Would different concepts seem to fit better?

3. Draw a structural-functional map of an ideal family. Then draw a structural-functional map of a family you know from television programs such as "The Simpsons," "The Hughleys," or "Everybody Loves Raymond." In what ways does the television family match your ideal?

4. Complete a genogram of your own family for at least three generations. What was it like to ask family members questions about your family? Did you find out information that was not known to you before you began? How did family members respond to thinking about past generations? Can you figure out the relationships, as well as the facts, of the family? Where would you go to find the missing information?

5. What categories of needs exist within your family of origin? What data support your analysis? What developmental and health-promotion issues are relevant in your family? In what ways does your family experience needs related to illness or loss, inadequate resources and support, family dynamics, and environmental threats?

6. What style would you assign to your family of origin? What data support your analysis? What suggestions would you give to a community health nurse about how to interact with your family?

7. What are the strengths within your family of origin? How are these strengths valuable to your family, especially in stressful times?

8. What functional level would you assign to your family of origin? What data support your analysis?

9. Think about a patient you have known in an inpatient capacity. Can you apply some of the family concepts to her or his situation? How might knowing more about the family have helped you with her or his care?

10. Think about the family you have in your community/public health clinical practicum. What categories of needs does this family have? Do the family needs fit into more than one category? Which category of needs do you believe you are most prepared to deal with as a nurse? In which category are you the least informed? What do you need to learn to prepare yourself to deal with these types of needs?

11. Assess your clinical family's environment. How does the environment affect your thinking about your care planning?

12. How many different dyads (two-person groups [e.g., mother-infant]) can you conceive that might occur in a family? Where do health priorities and problems fit into these dyads?

13. In a student group, role-play an initial encounter with a family. Introduce yourself, engage the family, make some initial assessment, and set up a contract for your repeated visits.

14. In a student group, role-play a visit in which you and the family are planning mutual goals. Have an observer set up the situation so that the goals of the family and the goals of the nurse are slightly different. Can you negotiate and come to an agreement?

15. Think of three examples of summative evaluation and three examples of formative evaluation in your clinical area. What formative and summative evaluation methods would be appropriate for your clinical family?

16. Identify the family style of one family that you know. Try different interpersonal approaches with this family. Which ones seem to work best? Does the family give you any clues about how they would like you to interact with them?

17. Watch a movie that demonstrates family interaction (e.g., *My Family*, *One True Thing*, *Smoke Signals*, *Arranged*,

The Debaters, or *Into the Wild*). Try to apply family assessment tools to the family in the film. Can you make a care plan that addresses that family's needs, style, strengths, and level of functioning?

COMMUNITY RESOURCES FOR PRACTICE

Information about each organization listed here is found on its website, which can be accessed through the **WebLinks** section of this book's website at *http://evolve.elsevier.com/Maurer/community/.*

Association for Conflict Resolution
Council for Exceptional Children

Educational Resources Information Center (ERIC)
Grandparents Raising Grandchildren
National Mentoring Partnership
Nurse-Family Partnership
Parent Help USA

STUDY AIDS   http://evolve.elsevier.com/Maurer/community/

Visit the Evolve website for this book to find the following study and assessment materials:

- Quiz
- Web Scenario
- Critical Thinking Questions and Answers for Case Studies

- Care Plans
- *Healthy People* Updates
- Glossary

REFERENCES

Affonso, D. (1987). Assessment of maternal postpartum adaptation. *Public Health Nursing, 4*(1), 9-16.

American Nurses Association. (2007). *Public health nursing: Scope and standards of practice.* Silver Spring, MD: Author.

Arvidson, C. R., & Colledge, P. (1996). Lead screening in children: The role model of the school nurse. *Journal of School Nursing, 12*(3), 8-13.

Astedt-Kurki, P., Tarkka, M., Paavilainen, E., et al. (2002). Development and testing of a Family Nursing Scale. *Western Journal of Nursing Research, 24*(5), 567-579.

Bantz, D. L., & Siktberg, L. (1993). Teaching families to evaluate age-appropriate toys. *Journal of Pediatric Health Care, 7*(3), 111-114.

Berkey, K. M., & Hanson, S. M. (1991). *Pocket guide to family assessment and intervention.* St. Louis: Mosby.

Black, C., & Ford-Gilboe, M. (2004). Adolescent mothers: Resilience, family health work and health promoting practices. *Journal of Advanced Nursing, 48*(4), 351-360.

Blaylock, A., & Cason, C. (1992). Discharge planning: Predicting patients' needs. *Journal of Gerontological Nursing, 18*(7), 5-10.

Broussard, E., & Hartner, S. (1995). Neonatal perception inventory. In M. Stanhope & J. Lancaster (Eds.), *Community health nursing: Process and practice for promoting health* (pp. 953-954). St. Louis: Mosby.

Bullock, K. (2004). Family social support. In P. Bomar (Ed.), *Nurses and family health promotion: Concepts, assessment, and interventions* (3rd ed.; pp. 142-161). Philadelphia: W.B. Saunders.

Cain, A. (1981). Assessment of family structure. In J. Miller & E. Janosik (Eds.), *Family-focused care* (pp. 115-131). New York: McGraw-Hill.

Caldwell, B. (1976). *Home observation measure of the environment.* Little Rock: University of Arkansas Center for Child Development and Education.

Cole, I., & Chesla, C. (2006). Interventions for the family with diabetes. *Nursing Clinics of North America, 41*, 625-639.

Cooley, M. (1989). *A family process model of coping with illness.* Paper presented at the National Council for Family Relations Theory and Methodology Workshop. Nov 1989, New Orleans, LA.

Cox, H., Hinz, N., Lubno, M. A., et al. (1997). *Clinical applications of nursing diagnosis.* Baltimore: Williams & Wilkins.

Dass, R., & Gorman, P. (1986). *How can I help?* New York: Knopf.

Drury-Zemke, L. (1997). Mutual support groups. In B. Spradley & J. Allender (Eds.), *Readings in community health nursing* (pp. 422-431). Philadelphia: Lippincott-Raven.

Dunst, C., Trivette, C., & Deal, A. (1989). *Enabling and empowering families: Principles and guidelines for practice.* Cambridge, MA: Brookline Books.

Epstein, N., Bishop, D., & Levin, S. (1978). The McMaster Model of Family Functioning. *Journal of Marriage and Family Counseling, 4*, 19-31.

Feeley, N., & Gottlieb, L. N. (2000). Nursing approaches for working with family strengths and resources. *Journal of Family Nursing, 6*(1), 9-24.

Fergusson, D., Grant, H., Horwood, J., et al. (2006). Randomized trial of the Early Start Program of Home Visitation: Parent and family outcomes. *Pediatrics, 117*, 781-786.

Flannery, J., & Korchek, S. (1993). Use of the levels of cognitive functioning assessment tool (LOCFAS) by acute care nurses. *Applied Nursing Research, 6*(4), 167-169.

Friedemann, M. L. (1989). The concept of family nursing. *Journal of Advanced Nursing, 14*, 211-216.

Fulmer, T. (1984). Elder abuse assessment tool. *Dimensions of Critical Care Nursing, 3*(4), 216-220.

Haggman-Laitila, A., & Pietila, A. (2007). Perceived benefits on family health of small groups for families with children. *Public Health Nursing, 24*(3), 205-216.

Hartman, S. (1978). Diagrammatic assessment of family relationships. *Social Casework, 59*(8), 465-476.

Hausman, B., & Hammen, C. (1993). Parenting in homeless families: The double crisis. *American Journal of Orthopsychiatry, 63*(3), 358-369.

Hovey, J. (2005). Fathers parenting chronically ill children: Concerns and coping strategies. *Issues in Comprehensive Pediatric Nursing, 28*, 83-95.

James, K., & Flores, E. (2004). Family nutrition. In P. Bomar (Ed.), *Nurses and family health promotion: Concepts, assessments and interventions* (3rd ed.; pp. 371-389). St. Louis: Saunders.

Jernigan, D. (1986). Mental health assessment and intervention: An integral part of nursing service. *Caring, 5*(7), 4-10.

Kane, R., Ouslander, J., & Abrass, I. (1993). Social assessment of the elderly. In R. Kane (Ed.), *Essentials of clinical geriatrics.* New York: McGraw-Hill.

Kuster, P. A. (1997). Reducing risk of house dust mite and cockroach allergen exposure in inner-city children with asthma. *Pediatric Nursing, 22*(4), 297-305.

Martin, K. (2005). *The Omaha System: A key to practice, documentation and information management* (2nd ed.). St. Louis: Elsevier/Saunders.

Maslow, A. (1972). *Toward a psychology of being.* New York: Van Nostrand Reinhold.

McCubbin, H., & Thompson, A. (1987a). Family coping-oriented personal scales (F-COPES). In H. McCubbin & A. Thompson (Eds.), *Family assessment inventories for research and practice.* Madison: University of Wisconsin—Madison.

McCubbin, H., & Thompson, A. (1987b). Family inventory of life events and changes (FILE). In H. McCubbin & A. Thompson (Eds.), *Family assessment inventories for research and practice.* Madison: University of Wisconsin—Madison.

McGoldrick, M., & Gerson, R. (1985). *Genograms in family assessment.* New York: W.W. Norton.

Minnesota Department of Health, Division of Community Health Services, Public Health Nursing Section. (2001). *Public health interventions: Applications for public health nursing practice.* St. Paul: Author.

Minuchin, S. (1974). *Families and family therapy.* Cambridge, MA: Harvard University Press.

Minuchin, S., & Fishman, H. C. (1981). *Family therapy techniques.* Cambridge, MA: Harvard University Press.

Mumma, C. M. (1987). Building accessibility checklist. In C. Mumma (Ed.), *Rehabilitation nursing, concepts and practice: A core curriculum.* Evanston, IL: Rehabilitation Nursing Foundation.

North American Nursing Diagnosis Association. (1995). *Taxonomy I with complete diagnosis.* St. Louis: Author.

North American Nursing Diagnosis Association. (2003). *Nursing diagnoses: Definitions and classifications, 2003-2004.* Philadelphia: Author.

North American Nursing Diagnosis Association. (2007). *Nursing diagnoses: Definitions and classification, 2007-2008.* Philadelphia: Author.

Otto, H. (1973). A framework for assessing family strengths. In A. Reinhardt & M. Quinn (Eds.), *Family-centered community nursing* (pp. 87-93). St. Louis: Mosby.

Pakenham, K., & Bursnall, S. (2006). Relations between social support, appraisal and coping and both positive and negative outcomes for children of a parent with multiple sclerosis and comparisons with children of healthy parents. *Clinical Rehabilitation, 20,* 709-723.

Papachristoforou, P., & Cooper, V. (2006). Support for family carers of children and young people with developmental disabilities and challenging behaviour. *Child: Care, Health & Development, 32*(2), 159-165.

Pederson, S., & Revenson, T. (2005). Parental illness, family functioning, and adolescent well-being: A family ecology framework to guide research. *Journal of Family Psychology, 19*(3), 404-409.

Pender, N. J. (1987). *Health promotion in nursing practice* (2nd ed.). Norwalk, CT: Appleton & Lange.

Peterson, E. A. (1997). Supporting the adoptive family: A developmental approach. *MCN: American Journal of Maternal/Child Health Nursing, 22*(3), 147-152.

Purnell, L. D., & Paulanka, B. (1998). *Transcultural health care: A culturally competent approach.* Philadelphia: F.A. Davis.

Roth, P. (1996). Family social support. In P. Bomar (Ed.), *Nurses and family health promotion: Concepts, assessment and Intervention* (2nd ed.; pp. 107-120). Philadelphia: W.B. Saunders.

Skelley, A. (1990). Assessment of immediate living environment. In B. Bullough & V. Bullough (Eds.), *Nursing in the community.* St. Louis: Mosby.

Smith, C. (1985). *Goals for community health nursing* (unpublished manuscript).

Smith, M. P. (1989). Postnatal concerns of mothers: An update. *Midwifery, 5*(4), 182-188.

Spector, R. E. (2000). *Cultural diversity in health and illness.* Upper Saddle River, NJ: Prentice Hall.

Tapia, J. (1972). The nursing process in family health. *Nursing Outlook, 20*(4), 267-270.

Uphold, C. (1991). Social support. In J. Creasia & B. Parker (Eds.), *Conceptual foundations of professional nursing practice* (pp. 445-470). St. Louis: Mosby.

Walton-Moss, B., Gerson, L., & Rose, L. (2005). Effects of mental illness on family quality of life. *Issues in Mental Health Nursing, 26,* 627-642.

Wayland, J., & Rawlins, R. (1997). African American mothers' perceptions of parenting. *Journal of Pediatric Nursing: Nursing Care of Children and Families, 12*(1), 13-20.

Wiley, D. (1996). Family environmental health. In P. Bomar (Ed.), *Nurses and family health promotion: Concepts, assessment, and interventions* (2nd ed.; pp. 339-364). Philadelphia: W.B. Saunders.

Wong, D., & Whaley, L. (1995). *Clinical manual of pediatric nursing* (4th ed.). St. Louis: Mosby.

Wright, L. M., & Leahey, M. (2005). *Nurses and families: A guide to family assessment and intervention* (4th ed.). Philadelphia: F.A. Davis.

Zerwekh, J. (1989). Homecare of the dying. In I. Martinson & J. Widmer (Eds.), *Home health nursing care* (pp. 217-236). Philadelphia: W.B. Saunders.

SUGGESTED READINGS

Barnfather, J. S. & Lyon, B. L. (Eds.). (1994). *Stress and coping: State of the science and implications for nursing theory, research, and practice.* Indianapolis: Sigma Theta Tau International.

Black, K., & Lobo, M. (2008). A conceptual review of family resilience factors. *Journal of Family Nursing, 14*(1), 33-55.

Bomar, P. J. (2004). *Promoting health in families: Applying family research and theory to nursing practice* (3rd ed.). St. Louis: Saunders.

Bullock, K. (2004). Family social support. In Bomar, P. (Ed.), *Nurses and family health promotion: Concepts, assessment, and interventions* (3rd ed., pp. 142-161). Philadelphia: Saunders.

Danielson, C. B., Hamel-Bissell, B., & Winstead-Fry, P. (1993). *Families, health, and illness: Perspectives on coping.* St. Louis: Mosby.

Hanson, S., Gedaly-Duff, V., & Kaakinen, J. (2005). *Family health care nursing: Theory, practice and research* (3rd ed.). Philadelphia: F.A. Davis.

Hardy, K. (1993). Implications for practice with ethnic minority families. In P. G. Boss, W. J. Doherty, R. LaRossa et al. (Eds.), *Source book of family theories and methods.* New York: Plenum.

Hupcey, J. (1998). Social support: Assessing conceptual coherence. *Qualitative Health Research, 8*(3), 304-318.

McCubbin, H., Joy, C., Cauble, A., et al. (1980). Family stress and coping: A decade review. *Journal of Marriage and the Family, 10,* 855-871.

McFarland, J. (1988). A nursing reformulation on Bowen's family systems theory. *Archives of Psychiatric Nursing, 2*(5), 319-324.

McGoldrick, M., & Shellenberger, S. (1999). *Genograms in family assessment.* New York: W.W. Norton.

McKenry, P., & Price, S. (Eds.). (2005). *Families & change: Coping with stressful events and transitions* (3rd ed.). Thousand Oaks, CA: Sage.

Miller, S. R., & Winstead-Fry, P. (1982). *Family systems theory in nursing practice.* Reston, VA: Reston.

Pendagast, E., & Sherman, C. (1979). A guide to the genogram. In E. Pendagast (Ed.), *The best of the family: 1973-1978* (pp. 101-112). New Rochelle, NY: Center for Family Learning.

Pesnecker, B., & Zerwekh, J. (1989). The mutual-participation relationship: Key to facilitating self-care practices in clients and families. *Public Health Nursing, 6*(4), 197-203.

Walsh, F. (1998). *Strengthening family resilience.* New York: Guilford.

Wright, L., & Leahey, M. (2005). *Nurses and families: A guide to family assessment and intervention* (4th ed.). Philadelphia: F. A. Davis.

Zerwekh, J. (1991). A family caregiving model for public health nursing. *Nursing Outlook, 39*(5), 213-217.

Multiproblem Families

Marcia L. Cooley

FOCUS QUESTIONS

What characterizes a family in which members are unable to meet basic needs or maintain optimal levels of health?

What constitutes a resilient family or resilient individual? How do they deal with problems and challenges?

What feelings are experienced by nurses who work with multiproblem families?

How do nurse and family values interact in these nurse-client relationships?

How does the nurse work toward mutual goal setting with multiproblem families?

What guidelines can the nurse use in searching for strategies that are effective with multiproblem families?

How does a nurse transcend labeling, blame, and cutoff when a multiproblem family is encountered?

To what extent does clear definition of the nursing role play a part in moderating a nurse's frustration?

What are appropriate and achievable goals for multiproblem families?

CHAPTER OUTLINE

Families Experiencing Crisis
Families with Chronic Problems
  Multiproblem Families
  Vulnerable Families
  Families with Negative Choices
  Families in Poverty

Families with Disturbances in Internal
  Dynamics
Resilience
Responsibilities of the Community/
  Public Health Nurse
  Assessment

Planning
Issues in Intervention
Realistic Goals and Outcomes

KEY TERMS

Appraisal
Coherence
Crisis
Family of promise

Family resilience
Hardiness
Multiproblem family
Resources

Stressor
Vulnerable families

Working with families is challenging, but the true challenge for a community/public health nurse is working with families that have problems in several areas simultaneously. These families can be called *multiproblem families* to indicate that they face several concurrent difficulties. The problems may be serious, such as abuse, neglect, substance abuse, illegal activities, homelessness, chronic mental illness, and major deficits in ability to care for members (Berne et al., 1990; Black et al., 2001; Jaffe et al., 2007). Families that experience this level of stress or disorganization often have little capacity to organize health promotion behaviors as they try to deal with immediate and serious problems.

Many health professionals base their appraisal of family behavior on their own comfort zone, which defines what they consider normal. Biased definitions of appropriate family functioning or the importance of self-sufficiency can create barriers to working with multiproblem families. Terms such as *vulnerable families* and *families at risk* help us recognize that certain families have an increased probability of experiencing acute or chronic problems. The term **family of promise** might better be used to describe these families to decrease our tendency to blame these families and to convey an attitude of hopefulness (Swadener & Lubeck, 1995). Any family, no matter how distressed, may be viewed as a family of promise, because all families have the potential to stabilize and grow from difficult experiences. Most vulnerable families can be divided into two general types: families that are experiencing crisis and families with chronic problems.

FAMILIES EXPERIENCING CRISIS

The families of today's world are exposed to multiple intense events such as natural disasters and acts of terrorism like 9/11. More of our families face catastrophic fears, loss, and disruptive transitions (Walsh, 2006). Even the healthiest family, when it encounters multiple stressors and stress of long duration, can be pushed beyond its resources to crisis. Most families can be supported through the crisis and can regain some measure of their previous level of health. In crisis, some families even develop emergent behaviors to help them face the future. But families pushed to the limit are more vulnerable to future problems. What leads a family to crisis?

Family **crisis** is a continuous disruption, disorganization, or incapacitation of the family social system (Burr, 1973). Families in crisis may have serious disturbances in family organization and require basic changes in family patterns of functioning to restore stability. Crises come in many forms. The Resiliency Model of Family Stress, Adjustments, and Adaptation (McCubbin & McCubbin, 1993) reminds us that the **stressor** along with the family's resources and appraisal of the stressful event interact to drive the family to a state of crisis or to adaptation (see Figure 12-6 in Chapter 12). The family's response is influenced in part by the characteristics of the stressor, including the predictability, extent, onset, intensity, perceived solvability, and content of the stressor (McKenry & Price, 2005). Each dimension differs in its ability to affect the family. For example, an intense, unpredictable event such as a sudden death is more stressful than is the expected loss of an elderly family member.

The family's perception of the event may be the most important mediating factor (Boss, 2002). When presented with a stressor, the family makes an appraisal of the situation. An **appraisal** is the perception of or assignment of meaning to a stressful event. The family schema or shared family view of the world shapes this appraisal. If family members judge themselves as inadequate to meet the demands, the tension increases.

Another factor is the family's **resources,** including inherent family strengths and specific coping abilities. Resources can include personal assets, such as innate intelligence or a sense of humor; family system resources, such as communication and problem-solving ability; and social support.

During the initial process of situational appraisal, including evaluation of the stressor, assessment of the family's capabilities and strengths, and consideration of alternative courses of action and coping strategies, the family ultimately comes together as a unit to manage the stress. The process of coping begins. The successful family has several coping strategies that include internal and external mechanisms. Such a family knows how to use the coping mechanism that is most appropriate to the problem presented. The family manages stress, often adjusting behaviors as time goes on to adapt to new demands and changing environments (Boss, 2002). Adaptation is not an outcome but an ongoing process. This process occurs within the context of the community in which the family lives, which

will greatly affect a family's decisions and also suggests pathways for intervention (Patterson, 1988).

Sometimes, however, the coping measures themselves become stressors. For example, taking time off work to attend a health appointment may endanger a job. In many lower-income families, dependence on an older daughter for help with the household becomes burdensome, endangering the young female's growth and development (Crouter et al., 2001).

Families that have experienced a pileup of demands—that is, long-term accumulation of and exposure to multiple stressors—will sometimes exhaust their ability to be resilient. These families are more vulnerable to stress when it is presented again. Such families may then find themselves in crisis.

In the family described in the following clinical example, pregnancy, illness, and unemployment pile up as demands that reduce the adaptability of the family. When the parents' son is born prematurely with developmental delays, the family is overwhelmed.

> Martha and John Galt married and had two children by the time Martha was 19 years old. John worked as a plumber's apprentice while Martha went to school to get her GED and took care of the kids. Things were actually going pretty well. Both of the couple's families were supportive, and the two bought a small house near Martha's mother. Then, Martha got pregnant again and found out that she was diabetic. At about that time, John lost his job and was unable to find another. A son was born prematurely, and he spent several weeks in the neonatal intensive care unit, which resulted in a large bill. After he came home, the child's developmental problems became clear. The family was now in crisis.

Helping families cope with crisis is within the scope of the community/public health nurse's role. Interventions useful to this process are presented in Box 14-1.

FAMILIES WITH CHRONIC PROBLEMS

Ever since nurses began visiting in the community, they have encountered families that have had chronic problems and many

---

BOX 14-1   Helping Families Cope with Crisis: Best Practices

1. Start by recognizing sources of family resilience and strength.
2. Offer hope.
3. Help the family identify and describe the nature of the stressors.
4. Explore the family's appraisal of the situation, including its meaning to members and their judgment of their ability to respond.
5. Provide information about the nature and demands of the stressor that may not be known to the family.
6. Help the family divide the tasks required by the stressor into manageable pieces.
7. Help the family explore current and alternative coping mechanisms.
8. Validate and emphasize the use of internal family resources, including personal and family strengths.
9. Pull in external sources of social support.
10. Arrange for tangible sources of external support such as financial assistance, health care, home visitors, support groups, food assistance, and transportation.
11. Encourage a positive reappraisal of the situation as the family moves from adjustment to adaptation to their new state.

barriers to gaining optimal health. Some of the families have experienced generations of poverty, as well as problems in many areas of functioning, such as physical, psychologic, and social. Many of these families have disturbances in their internal dynamics. The personal and family resources available to them, their range of coping behaviors, and their willingness and ability to use external sources of support combine to keep them in a perpetual state of stress.

Some families experience multiple situational stressors simultaneously (multiproblem families). Some families are vulnerable, some are presented with only negative choices, some struggle with poverty, and some have disturbances in internal dynamics. Many families with chronic problems have combinations of these situations at the same time. Experienced community/public health nurses recognize this situation and become aware of their own frustrations in dealing with families that seem unable or unwilling to change. The interface between multiproblem families and community/public health nurses is the focus of the remainder of this chapter.

MULTIPROBLEM FAMILIES

A **multiproblem family** has needs in several areas simultaneously: difficulty in achieving developmental tasks, illness or loss, inadequate resources and support, disturbances in internal dynamics, or environmental stressors (see Box 13-6). Multiproblem families are families in which combinations of low functional level, multiple stresses, multiple symptoms, and lack of support interact to threaten or destroy the family's ability to meet the physical, social, and emotional needs of its members. A family need not have disturbances in family dynamics to have multiple problems. Circumstances beyond the family's control and a pileup of demands can result in a family's having multiple problems. However, disturbances in internal dynamics predispose a family to having multiple problems.

The multiproblem family in the following example has needs in at least four categories: developmental tasks, illness or loss, inadequate support, and internal dynamics.

> Keith, 9 years old, has muscular dystrophy and attends a school in your district. His mother has been married twice. Her new husband, Keith's stepfather, is abusive to Keith. A great deal of conflict is present, so Keith recently moved to his grandmother's house. She is also caring for his two cousins; they lost their mother to a drug overdose, and their father is in jail. Keith visits his mother on the weekends, but often an argument breaks out and he is returned to his grandmother's house early. None of the family members seems to be able to work out the problems. You suspect that Keith's mother lies to you and that she and her mother barely speak to each other. Keith is not only losing some muscular function but is also having difficulty in school. He is aggressive and manipulative in his classroom. His grandmother is not following through with needed care for his braces, exercise, and skin care at home.

Developmental needs exist for the school-aged child, Keith, and adult family members. Illness needs are related to Keith's muscular dystrophy and to his aunt's substance abuse, and inadequate family resources exist for Keith's physical care. Underlying all the other needs are disturbances in family dynamics manifested as child abuse, substance abuse, illegal behavior, and emotional cutoffs.

VULNERABLE FAMILIES

Vulnerable families are families at increased risk because of the intensity and clustering of stressors associated with life events (Gillis, 1991; Janko, 1994). Examples of families at high risk for future health problems are families with members who are chronically ill or have Down syndrome or alcoholism. Special events such as assaults, teenage pregnancy, and sexual abuse can also predispose a family to subsequent physical, emotional, and social problems. Many vulnerable families live in social situations in which loss of members through death, institutionalization, abandonment, or incarceration is common. The combination of intense stressors and depletion of resources can push the family beyond its capacity to cope.

FAMILIES WITH NEGATIVE CHOICES

Community/public health nurses assist families in coping with stress by helping them identify their previous coping style, their resources, and their alternatives for action. For some families, however, coping with stress remains a problem even after nursing intervention, because the choices for action are all negative (Wilson, 1989). In some instances, none of the available choices will modify the problem, and sometimes the consequences of the choices are all negative and create more problems. For example, suppose a family is dealing with a husband and father who has Alzheimer's disease. The wife, having assumed the caregiver role, is exhausted and needs to spend some time out of the house. However, her husband becomes anxious and more confused whenever any other person takes over his care. None of the choices available to this family solves or completely alleviates the problem. The wife must choose among solutions with negative implications. Families that must cope when all the choices are undesirable are also a special risk group.

FAMILIES IN POVERTY

The impact of poverty or living in a resource-depleted or hostile environment is also a factor in family coping. The poor, as both individuals and a group, are continually faced with multiple and chronic stressors, including frustration over employment options, inadequate and unsafe housing conditions, repeated exposure to violence and crime, inadequate child care assistance, and insensitive attitudes and responses of health and

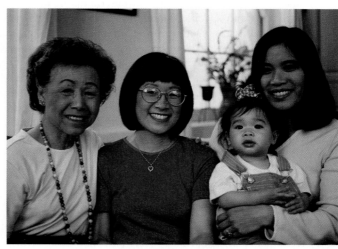

Four generations of one family.

social service agencies (Berne et al., 1990). As family coping abilities are strained by unpredictable and unrelenting stressors, mastery of the situation decreases. Relationships are strained, feelings of helplessness and hopelessness increase, and self-esteem suffers (Cutrona et al., 2003; Mistry et al., 2002). The spiral continues as people become anxious and depressed, feel powerless, and thus are less able to marshal energy to meet the next day's problems.

Poverty also brings its own set of health problems. Correlates of poverty include increased incidence of communicable diseases, especially tuberculosis and human immunodeficiency virus infection; more episodes of illness; less use of preventive care; and higher rates of chronic disease, premature death, occupational hazards, and unsafe housing. Unfortunate correlates for children include delayed development, childhood depression and anxiety, and increased separation from families into foster care. Poor neighborhoods may also have greater environmental risks such as industrial sites, landfills, and toxic waste sites. Living within a poverty area may contribute to excess mortality, independent of an individual's own health behaviors (Waitzman & Smith, 1998). Poor individuals are also more likely to be homeless and to lack access to health care (Berne et al., 1990). The recent large increase in the number of working poor in the United States is notable. Although the Work Opportunity Reconciliation Act of 1996 moved many families off the welfare rolls, these families may have even less access to adequate health care, housing, and child care than do others who are not working (Meyers & Lee, 2003).

Differences in family structures in poor families are often mentioned as the cause or source of multiple family problems. In actuality, family structures can serve to strengthen resilience rather than undermine it. Many multiproblem poor families have strong ongoing family connectedness even though single parenthood or teenage birth is the norm. The three-generational nature of these families adds support and buffers some of the stress (Chatman, 1996; Cooley & Unger, 1991). At times, however, the burden a grandmother feels when caring for younger family members is stressful for her and leads to poor outcomes for others in the family (Unger & Cooley, 1992). Poor families often have developmental phases or attitudes that are different from those of other families. For example, Sachs and colleagues (1997) found that many low-income single mothers with young children held unrealistic expectations for child behavior, viewed their own parenting responsibilities as overwhelming, and perceived their children as unappreciative of the family unit. Discipline was often punitive.

Fulmer (1989) describes the family life cycle of poor families enmeshed in chronic unemployment and discrimination, vulnerable to problems, and intruded on by various agencies that affect their lives. Constantly reminded of their lack of power in the current system, some families turn to illegal activities to meet their basic needs. Hines (1989) cautions that many variations can be found in poor families and suggests a shorter life cycle with three predominant phases (outlined in Table 14-1). Four characteristics of the life cycle are: (1) it is more truncated (less time is available to allow unfolding of developmental stages), and life transitions are not clearly delineated; (2) households are frequently headed by women and include extended family members; (3) the life cycle is punctuated by numerous unpredictable life events; and (4) families have few resources available and must rely on governmental assistance to meet basic needs.

FAMILIES WITH DISTURBANCES IN INTERNAL DYNAMICS

Multiproblem families are often unable to provide for security, physical survival, emotional and social functioning, sexual

TABLE 14-1 Family Life Cycle of the Poor

Stage	Characteristics
Unattached young adult	• May start as early as age 11 or 12 • Young adult on his or her own not accountable to adults • May need to distance self from burdens of family • Attaches self to peers • Blurring of boundaries between adolescence and young adulthood minimizes availability of role models • Difficult to establish self in work • Difficult to establish intimate relationships with partner • Early transition to parenthood • Missing accomplishment of early tasks weakens ability to accomplish later ones
Families with children	• Occupies most of the life span • Common to involve three- or four-generation households • Often begins without marriage • Combines tasks of two stages—the marital couple stage and family with young children stage • Negotiation with extended family related to interconnectedness and role demands is difficult
Family in later life	• Phase of the nonevolved grandmother (no growth for self) • Grandmother involved in central childrearing role in old age • Not likely to be empty nest • Death may occur before or shortly after retirement

Data from Carter, B., & McGoldrick, M. (1989). Overview of the changing family life cycle: A framework for family therapy. In Carter, B. & McGoldrick, M. (Eds.), *The changing family life cycle: A framework for family therapy* (2nd ed., pp. 3-28). New York: Gardner Press; Fulmer, R. (1989). Lower-income and professional families: A comparison of structure and life cycle process. In Carter, B. & McGoldrick, M. (Eds.), *The changing family life cycle: A framework for family therapy* (2nd ed., pp. 545-578). New York: Gardner Press; Hines, P. (1989). The family life cycle of poor black families. In Carter, B. & McGoldrick, M. (Eds.), *The changing family life cycle: A framework for family therapy* (2nd ed., pp. 513-544). New York: Gardner Press.

differentiation, training of children, and promotion of growth of individual members (Tapia, 1997). These families are characterized by insufficient internal support, frequent or intense emotional conflict, inability to conform to societal expectations, and acting out of family members. It is unclear if disturbances in dynamics lead to more family problems or if response to problems leads to unhealthy family dynamics.

Family systems theory provides some thoughts about how the level of health of a family might develop. Multigenerational patterns that are passed down from one generation to another can be adaptive or maladaptive. The tendency to repeat these patterns is great, especially considering that the family members have known no other family experience. Doing what an individual knows, even if it brings unhappiness and failure, is often easier than is changing behavior to something unfamiliar and unknown.

The level of differentiation of a family is a crucial variable in the appearance of symptoms (Kerr & Bowen, 1989). Families have varying levels of differentiation or ability to separate emotion from thought. Families on the low end of the continuum have greater difficulty living their lives in a thoughtful way. Instead, these families respond to situations automatically in attempts to manage their high levels of anxiety. At the opposite end of the continuum are families with the ability to distinguish thought from feeling. These families have members who are able to think of themselves as separate persons, as well as group members, and who can define life goals and pursue them in a thoughtful way. Families on the thoughtful end of this continuum have fewer life problems than do families that are caught in automatic emotional reactivity. Most multiproblem families tend to fall on the more emotional side of differentiation

of self. Family theory suggests that these levels of differentiation are transmitted from generation to generation through the process of projection, which is the degree of the child's relationship dependence or the extent to which each child is involved in maintaining the emotional lives of the parents. Some researchers suggest that stressors and events that occur during the formation of early attachments predispose the parent-child relationship to problems. Separation of premature infants from their parents, prolonged hospitalizations or illness, unexpected crises such as homelessness or imprisonment, deaths, and emotional illnesses are examples of disruptions in family life that can interfere with parenting and early development. Tension or lack of nurturing during the child's earliest interactions influences the growth and development of the child and the child's subsequent ability to nurture his or her own children. Not only multigenerational patterns but also perhaps even basic emotional health is passed from generation to generation.

Box 12-4 contains a list of healthy family characteristics. A comparison list of characteristics of families with disturbed internal dynamics is presented in Box 14-2. The multiproblem family may have disturbances in many of these areas, such as inadequate support, multiple stressors, high levels of anxiety, dysfunctional family boundaries, unhealthy communication patterns, dysfunctional expression of emotion, inadequate problem-solving skills, underorganization or rigid organization, unclear roles, and repetitive patterns of interaction that blame or shift responsibility.

Scapegoating, or identifying one family member as the *problem,* is one pattern that may be used. *Distancing* and cutting off of family members can occur when the anxiety rises to the point that family members can no longer tolerate contact

---

BOX 14-2 Characteristics of Families with Disturbances in Internal Dynamics

Developmental stages and tasks: The family has difficulty achieving tasks at the stage-appropriate time. Situational and maturational crises occur simultaneously. Tasks for the next stage are delayed or not accomplished.

Roles: Patterns of expected behavior are not appropriate to age and ability, roles are rigidly assigned and are unable to support family functioning.

Boundaries: Closed and impermeable or completely diffuse. Members fail to allow appropriate exchange with the environment or fail to define the family unit. Boundaries between subsystems have no clear generational lines and do not support a strong parental coalition. Subsystem boundaries may be unclear, rigid, or diffuse.

Subsystems: As in most families, each member of the family belongs to several subsystems simultaneously: spouse, parent-child, sibling, grandparent. However, subsystems may include inappropriate members.

Patterns of interaction: Repetitive and fixed. The focus is on one member who is blamed, left out, or put down in the interaction. Family cohesion is extremely enmeshed or disengaged. Communication patterns of placater, blamer, superresponsible one, and distractor are often used. Distance, conflict, projection, and overresponsibility or underresponsibility are common.

Power: No clarity of role definition and appropriate rules. Power is not shared, appropriate to age, or within the parental subsystem until the children are independent.

External stressors: Very intense, numerous, and occur simultaneously. The family has little chance to adapt. Chronic illness adds to family stress.

Open or closed system: As the system closes, all variables and patterns become fixed and less able to adapt. Energy is used in dysfunctional ways.

Communication: Unclear, not honest, and indirect; contains incongruent feelings and words; and is nonspecific. The family is not able to use communication as a mechanism to resolve conflict.

Values: Do not provide guidelines for behavior acceptable to society and culture. Values are unable to be modified to adapt to changing times.

Encouragement of autonomy and acceptance of difference: A balance does not exist between autonomy of members and the need to be a cohesive group. Strong pressures to conform and to sacrifice individual needs for the purpose of the group are present.

Level of anxiety: Extremely high. People in the family have difficulty thinking and solving problems. Long-term anxiety tends to wear down the ability of the family to function well.

Resources and social support: Family has few internal and external sources of support. Members who are available are not used to their capacity or are overused. All families have some strengths, but the strengths may be different from those expected by society.

Meaning, perception, and paradigm: The family agrees to allow myths and secrets to structure the meaning of many situations. Life problems are viewed as unsolvable problems rather than challenges. The family views itself as powerless.

Adaptability: Resilience is necessary for a family to be able to cope with changing demands. The family is not able to be flexible or is so chaotic that cohesiveness and predictability are missing.

with each other. In some areas, having members of a family who live on the same street but who have not spoken to each other in years is not unusual. Repetitive patterns of emotional conflict occur in which the conflict seems to be resolved and then erupts again. These families often contain many active and interlocking triangles and may use this pattern with outsiders when tension rises. *Triangling in* the social worker, police officer, or nurse helps relieve anxiety.

RESILIENCE

What makes a family resilient or adaptive? What are the characteristics of families that are able to bounce back from stress?

Garbarino (1992, p. 101) defined resilience as "the capacity to develop a high degree of competence in spite of stressful environments and experiences." The term *resilience* has been used to describe an individual's response to adversity. Many researchers propose that some trauma or major stressor must first be present for resilience to develop. This view suggests that an individual develops resilience while experiencing trauma within a dysfunctional family. The concept of family resilience proposes instead that family resilience parallels individual resilience. Family resilience may develop in response to a specific adversity, but it may also be a response in any family facing risks in life (Patterson, 2002). **Family resilience** can be defined as "the ability of the family to respond positively to a situation and emerge feeling strengthened and more resourceful than before" (Simon et al., 2005, p. 427).

Each family has risk factors and protective factors that work to promote competence to handle stress. McCubbin (1998) suggested that the protective factors are the family's coherence and hardiness. **Coherence** is a fundamental coping strategy in which the family emphasizes acceptance, loyalty, and shared respect and pride to manage the stressor. **Hardiness** is an "internal sense of control of life events and its meaningfulness and a commitment to learn and explore new experiences" (McCubbin, 1998, p. 5). Lietz (2007) studied family resilience and uncovered several protective factors that increase resilience. They are internal and external social support, boundary setting, the ability to take action or take charge, and communication.

The resilient family will proceed through several stages after the presentation of a stressor: struggling to survive, adapting, accepting, growing stronger, and sometimes helping others (Lietz, 2007). This type of family creates an emotional atmosphere that fosters trust, cooperation, and acceptance; but more importantly, a sense of hopefulness is maintained. The family has several coping strategies, including using insight, humor, spirituality, creativity, and boundary setting. Most important, the family will be able to take charge, communicate with each other and the outside, and use the support of each other and external sources. Finally, the resilient family engages in productive and adaptive activities to meet the family's own needs and to meet society's expectations.

RESPONSIBILITIES OF THE COMMUNITY/ PUBLIC HEALTH NURSE

Families that are defined as multiproblem families are often the most challenging, most time-consuming, and least rewarding families in a community/public health nurse's caseload (Fox, 1989). Nurses often need support to continue working in situations in which their efforts are frustrated. As experienced and educated health care workers, we expect that we will have the answers and that our expertise will be accepted and acted on. This assumption is in direct conflict with the family's perception of a health care worker as someone whom they are unable to trust and whose advice does not seem to affect their quality of life. If the assumption is made that families have the right to self-determination and know what is best for them, then a conflict exists between these two ways of viewing family care. Only after examining his or her own values and resolving this conflict can the community/public health nurse be effective in caring for multiproblem families.

ASSESSMENT

Most of the time, but not always, multiproblem families operate at a low level of functioning, according to Tapia (1997) (see Table 13-5). Families at level I (chaotic families) are characterized by disorganization in all areas of life. In these extremely immature families, adults may be unable to fulfill their roles and responsibilities. Children or others may be expected to assume these roles, which is inappropriate and interferes with normal growth and fulfillment of nurturing needs. Physical and emotional resources may be inadequate. Family members are often depressed, with a sense of hopelessness and powerlessness. These individuals may have little self-esteem, a high sense of failure, and little reason to trust another health care worker who comes with promises that are most often unfulfilled.

Families at Tapia's level II (intermediate families) are able to meet their basic survival needs but are immature and unable to meet many needs of family members. These individuals are often defensive, unable to trust, and alienated from the community. However, these families retain some hope and have some capacity to change and improve their functioning.

Assessment of multiproblem families includes a three-generational time frame, because many families are cooperating across generations to meet basic needs. Assessment should especially evaluate the interactions among the family's many needs, strengths, styles, functional level, coping patterns, resources and supports, and past experiences with health care workers (see Chapter 13). Special areas of focus should include the number and duration of stressors the family has experienced over time, the family's perception of the events, an estimation of the severity of any symptoms the family may be experiencing (e.g., depression, alcohol use, physical abuse), and contacts with other health care resources. Tools such as the Family Inventory of Life Events (FILE) by McCubbin and Thompson (1987) or the Family Systems Stressors–Strength Inventory (Mischke & Hanson, 1991) may be especially helpful. The Family Coping Index (Lowe & Freeman, 1981) helps determine coping patterns, and the ecomap (Hartman, 1978) helps describe the family's connection with resources.

PLANNING

After analyzing the data, the nurse will have a better understanding of realistic goals and expectations of what will happen in the family encounters. Perfection should not be sought. Goals should be concrete and realistic and mutually defined by family and nurse. In the presence of what seem to be overwhelming problems, identifying family strengths is sometimes difficult for a nurse. The nurse's values set up expectations that block his or her identification of strengths. As the community health nurse truly listens and asks the family to identify its strengths, they become more apparent. As discussed in Box 12-3, Otto (1973) was one of the first to emphasize family strengths. Karpel (1986) suggests that some personal strengths are often hidden, such as self-respect, protectiveness, caring in action, hope, tolerance, affection, humor, and playfulness. Relational strengths include respect, reciprocity, reliability, the ability to repair, flexibility, and family pride. Karpel also suggests that loops of family interactions repeat themselves to amplify resources and that symptoms can be reframed to allow people to see the situation in a positive way. For example, suppose one of the daughters loses her job. When her sisters and brothers become aware of this, the situation is redefined as one that allows her to spend more time with her young children. The sisters and brothers engage in a series of telephone calls and conversations in which all agree to offer a little financial help and a lot of emotional support until the situation changes. This family has maximized its resources.

Alterations in the Nurse-Family Relationship

Sometimes the multiproblem family's past experiences with health care workers have led the family to distrust other encounters. After hoping to have some of its needs met and then being left with problems that are unresolved, the family may pull away or be reluctant to engage with another health care worker. Especially when values are different, the family may *play along* with the nurse, feeding the nurse inaccurate information that the family believes he or she wants to hear. Members may agree to make appointments and then not keep them, preferring to break the contact rather than be disappointed. The family may test the nurse while trying to determine his or her reliability and consistency. The nurse may even interpret this action as manipulation. However, this action is frequently a pattern that the family has found helpful in the past to maintain some control. Zerwekh (1992) describes three responsibilities of the community/public health nurse in response to this pattern: locating (tracking down) families, building trust, and building strength.

Burton, a home health nurse, was about to visit the Carter family when he realized that the assignment would be difficult because of the family's past relationships with nurses. The Carter family had a history of bad experiences with home nurses, including one nurse who was overbearing and critical. Mr. Carter, who had lung cancer, actually had had an unnecessary hospital admission because a nurse did not believe Mrs. Carter when she called to ask the nurse for an immediate assessment of Mr. Carter's labored breathing. The Carters had lost their medical assistance eligibility for not following through with the agency's suggestions several times. The family blamed their loss of medical assistance on the agency.

How would Burton deal with this understandable reluctance on the part of the family to accept a new nurse? He called the Carters before he visited and introduced the idea that he wanted to start fresh with a family plan of care. He told them his priorities, which were keeping Mr. Carter safe and comfortable and making sure that the medical assistance coverage was monitored carefully; he then asked what their priorities were. Mrs. Carter admitted tearfully that her husband seemed worse, and she feared his illness was near its end. She was not sure that she wanted Burton's help but allowed him to visit. He spent the visit working on the family priorities of helping Mr. Carter with his comfort.

When the time comes for problems to be identified, the nurse may find that the family cannot agree on or clearly identify problems. The family's ability to sort through multiple priorities and clearly see the problem and what can be done may be weakened by its anxiety and its sense of being overwhelmed. The family members may have no previous experience with this style of thinking and so may resort to impulsive and automatic patterns as explanations for their distress.

For the family to continue to engage in care, some commitment and resources are necessary. Other needs may compete for priority. For instance, the usual time a nurse might meet with a family member is during the day. A mother who has a 9-to-5 job may be unable to take time off to keep up with nurse contacts, and a mother caring for a toddler with an earache may find herself at the pediatric clinic waiting to be seen and then spend several hours getting home on the bus. Families with fewer resources seem to have to work harder and deal with more obstacles to get done things that others take for granted.

Mutual Goal Setting

A mutual goal is one that is shared by both the family and the community/public health nurse, meaning that the family and the nurse agree on the need for the goal and agree to work together toward meeting it. Carey (1989) identifies the process of mutual goal setting as the single most important skill to bring to multiproblem families. Individuals have a right to knowledge about themselves and to participate in decisions that influence their lives and health. Health professionals have a responsibility to share information that helps individuals make informed decisions about their care. Nurses' education and knowledge sometimes get in the way of family interactions. People tend to resist being told what to do and are therefore more likely to work toward goals they choose and support. Instead of investing himself or herself in the outcome, the nurse should let go of the outcome and invest in respect and support of the client.

Determination of Level of Intervention

Potential levels of intervention include the individual, small interpersonal groups, the family as a unit, and the family within the environment. How does the community/public health nurse determine the appropriate level of intervention with multiproblem families? For some families, working with the family as a unit may not be possible because of access, time constraints, or disconnected relationships. For example, the community/public health nurse may be referred to work with a mother who has lost permission to see her children because of abuse. In multiproblem families, the nurse takes every opportunity to work with any part of the family, recognizing that more optimal ways may be unavailable.

Working at the individual level will include interventions directed at individual health problems and at strengthening individual functioning and resilience. For example, the nurse who works to prepare the previously mentioned mother for the return of her children may be educating her about parenting skills, helping her find and maintain employment, and connecting her to resources in her community. Developing personal strengths is always beneficial to someone in the family.

Working at the interpersonal level is often a choice the community/public health nurse will make. Multiproblem families will frequently exhibit problems in areas related to interpersonal relationships, such as inadequate prenatal care, unsafe parent-child interactions, marital conflict, or elder abuse. Neglected children can be at great risk for other problems, including serious damage to emotional, physical, and cognitive development. Chronic neglect is more a way of life than it is a series of individual events (Turner & Tanner, 2001). Helping subsystems within the family learn new ways of interacting and coping ultimately helps the whole family (Niemeyer & Proctor, 1995; Scannapieco, 1994).

Some thoughts about working with the family as a unit are outlined later. For many family health nurses, this strategy is preferred. Knowing that the family functions as a unit makes the experienced nurse wary of addressing it in segments.

One argument asserts that the most appropriate role for a nurse is at the macro, or environmental, level. In fact, the realities of life for many multiproblem families are related to factors that are beyond their internal control. Coping with exposure to environmental hazards, health risks in air and water, violence in the street, deterioration of the neighborhood, inadequate education, limited access to health care, and unavailability of adequate employment would tax the resilience of any person or family. Nurses who assume the role of advocate for families within a larger social context may ultimately have the most impact on family health.

ISSUES IN INTERVENTION
Family Participation and Family Choice

Nurses who offer care to families in the community use two basic approaches. In the first, nurses approach families with the expectation that the members will participate equally with the nurse in the process of planning and implementing care. Families are asked on what problems they want or need to work. Clients identify their own problems and monitor their own progress. Nurses assist the family by clarifying ideas, breaking problems down into more manageable units, helping families set priorities, and giving feedback and positive support. When a goal is reached, the family may start working toward a new goal.

With less functional families, this nursing approach may not work. We have already discussed families that may not have the ability to identify their needs or ask for specific kinds of help. These families may have difficulty engaging and continuing in the relationship. Impulsivity and competing demands may alter the ability to adhere to the care plan. With these families, the nurse must alter the approach. From the beginning, the nurse must be consistent and reliable in his or her contact. A regular and continued physical presence on which the family can count is necessary to reassure the family that the relationship can be trusted.

If the family cannot identify its own goals, the nurse acts as an information giver, sharing the assessments and diagnoses. Visual or concrete portrayals of the assessment, such as a pie chart, a score on a test, or a photograph may help engage the family's interest. The nurse can suggest possible goals but must carefully validate whether the family shares the same concerns and wants to work toward the goals that the nurse suggests. If the family is uninterested, then the nurse presents the assessment again to gain feedback about the client's perception of the situation. The feedback process continues until a concern and goal that are shared by the family are identified (Zander, 1996).

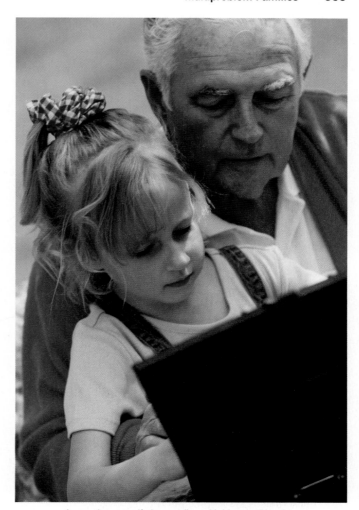

A caregiver grandfather reading with his granddaughter.

Incorporation of Evidence-Based Practice

Using *evidence-based practice* helps the nurse and family achieve desired goals and outcomes. Reviews of evidence-based practice with multiproblem and vulnerable families have identified several principles that should be incorporated into the choice of practices, including providing early intervention, offering concrete support such as transportation and food during interventions, and arranging longer and more frequent sessions (Kumpfer & Alvarado, 2003). Nursing roles will vary and may include educator, facilitator of family decisions, liaison to community resources, provider of emotional support and direct care, and advocate for the client within the community systems, if necessary.

Nurses who wish to promote the development of resilience in individuals and families should pay particular attention to some interventions tested in the literature. Interventions demonstrated effective in supporting resilience in African American youth include formation of strong ethnic and racial identity, contact with supportive social networks, and involvement in meaningful activities in safe community environments (Barrow et al., 2007). Development of strong belief systems, optimism, and healthy communication patterns has also proved effective in fostering resilience (Tusale et al., 2007). Van Riper

(2007) found that enhanced family problem solving was significantly associated with positive outcomes for families with children with Down syndrome. All approaches emphasize the importance of developing and using strong relational networks (Black & Lobo, 2008; Walsh, 2007).

The fact that some individuals and families respond to hardships with resilience cannot always protect them from negative outcomes, however. And again, the individuals and families that cannot respond should not be blamed. Jaffee and colleagues (2007) found that children residing in multiproblem families with substance abuse, low social cohesion, and informal social control are not likely to be resilient to maltreatment. This provides evidence that the social context sometimes overrides individual and family efforts.

Families That Do not Respond

The goals of the nursing contacts are not to *fix* the family or to address all the problems of family members. Helping family members gain awareness of the distinctions between feelings and behaviors may curb some of the impulsivity and encourage members to think before they act. Unhealthy family behavior patterns are recognized by describing and tracking them with family members (Reimel & Schindler, 1994). The patterns can then be reframed and sometimes modified to be more functional for the family.

Using circular communication is often helpful for families with multiple problems (Bell, 2003; Wright & Leahey, 2005). The affect, cognition, and behavior of the individuals are observed, and the nurse gives feedback that illustrates the mutual influence each person has on another's feelings, thoughts, and actions. As family members begin to understand this reciprocity or the effects one member has on another, breakthroughs can sometimes be achieved.

Helping the family feel a sense of power can break through the hopelessness. Working with the family toward a small but achievable success helps empower it to take similar actions in the future (Dunst et al., 1989). The possibility of additional problems is great, however, and continued support and recognition of the family's attempts and strengths are necessary. This assistance must be balanced against the family's possible tendency to depend on the nurse when it needs to learn to develop itself (Box 14-3). The nurse becomes a compassionate and informed companion as the family struggles with its daily tasks of living.

Nurse Self-Management

Triangling is a fact of life with all families but especially with families that are anxious (see Chapter 12). Nurses cannot avoid triangles, but they can learn to manage themselves within them. When tension rises in the family, the tendency will be for a family member to try to escape uncomfortable feelings by pulling in a third or fourth or fifth person. This additional person serves to distract the family from its original tension. The distraction does not always help the family move toward a problem solution. When a community/public health nurse or anyone else is pulled into a triangle through the family's wish for that person to be closer and to take over, providing a calm and thoughtful presence can help diffuse the emotion. Instead of participating in the emotionality, the nurse should resist the temptation to jump in to help and instead be a thoughtful observer in the situation. Asking questions, maintaining neutrality, and demonstrating thoughtfulness will be most helpful.

During the contact, nurses should be aware of their tendency to feel hopeless, to discount the value of the time and effort spent with the family, or to feel angry and want to withdraw when family problems continue. Many nurses build in regular support by talking with colleagues or making a plan to take care of themselves in the midst of a heavy workload. Carefully defining a nursing role that includes realistic expectations of self is one way the nurse can help manage these feelings.

REALISTIC GOALS AND OUTCOMES

Although the successful community/public health nurse will *not* be able to move all families toward health, helping multiproblem families feel a sense of competency and power may assist them in developing more effective ways of managing family life. To believe that a family that may have had troubles for generations will be without concerns after limited nursing contact is unrealistic. However, all families should be recognized as *families of promise* that have the potential for growth (Swadener & Lubeck, 1995). Some examples of goals that can be achieved with multiproblem families are given in the sections that follow. Specification of clear family outcomes helps the nurse and family direct efforts in a focused and prioritized way. Table 14-2 gives examples of some family outcomes.

Selected Stressors Are Prevented or Reduced

The family may have many members with health or social problems. Not all of these problems can be corrected. However, solid action aimed at one or two specific needs may improve the quality of the family's life.

In the following clinical example, the community/public health nurse successfully addressed the problems of (1) inadequate nutrition and (2) fear about safe child rearing.

Box 14-3   Strategies for Working with Multiproblem Families

1. Foster continuity of care.
2. Be patient—do not expect instant solutions.
3. Help the family identify its strengths.
4. Work on small pieces of problems.
5. Help the family recognize opportunities for moving forward or doing things differently.
6. When all choices are undesirable, help the family cope more positively with the choice that is made.
7. Ensure that all contacts are characterized by caring and respect.
8. Organize possible sources of tangible support.
9. Encourage use of sources of intangible support.
10. Remember that the ultimate goal is empowerment and resilience of the family and development of individual self-esteem.

Martin, an elderly man who had been cut off from his family in the community, had multiple health problems, including emphysema, severe hypertension, fatigue, decubiti, depression, and nutritional deficits. His disorganized family had difficulty maintaining contact with him because of their own legal and parenting concerns and anger about past conflicts. Shari,

| TABLE 14-2 | **Family Outcomes** |

Goal	Examples of Family Outcomes
Selected stressors are prevented or reduced	• The family will identify a number of stressors currently impacting the family. • At least one family member can identify a preventable or reducible stressor. • At least one family member implements a strategy to prevent or reduce a stressor. • The family verbalizes an awareness of the impact of decreasing the stressors.
Support system is strengthened	• The family will identify at least one human service resource available to them. • The family will identify an advocate or person who can help them get information about available human services. • The family verbalizes a list of informal sources of social support. • At least one family member tries using a social support not previously used. • The family verbalizes blocks internally or externally to use of social support. • The family verbalizes reactions to services offered.
Family organization is improved	• The family accepts a behavior of a member that respects individual difference. • One overworked member sets limits on availability. • The family negotiates a cooperative decision. • The family rearranges roles necessary to maintain family functioning. • The family develops a sense of tradition and identity. • The family practices an activity dedicated to caring and continuity.
Coping processes are more adaptive	• The family can state some past ways of coping and effectiveness. • At least one family member appraises the current challenge and degree of family effectiveness in coping. • The family agrees to try a new coping behavior. • The family discusses the impact of the new coping behavior. • The family increases their sense of competence and shares affirmation of the behavior with other members.

the community/public health nurse, worked on getting Martin a continuing supply of food that he would eat (he rejected Meals on Wheels). His nutritional status improved, which led to decreased fatigue, lower blood pressure, and healing decubiti. He was extremely worried about the physical safety of one of the preschool children of his daughter, who was abusing substances and neglecting her child. His sister agreed to care for the child in her home with the permission of his daughter, who knew she was not able to function as a parent.

The family continued to have multiple problems, but two specific stressors were reduced, which helped the family members to maintain health and safety that year.

Support System Is Strengthened

Multiproblem families report more feelings of loneliness and social isolation, and less social support than other families (Ortega, 2002; Wilkins, 2003). The feelings of isolation persist even when the actual social network includes a large number of members. Some families do not know about the resources available to them or lack skills to access them. This may be especially true for families new to the community. The nurse has more than one responsibility in helping families use resources. These tasks can include identifying resources, helping the family mobilize and use them, and sometimes limiting and regulating their input (Feeley & Gottlieb, 2000). The nurse works at providing information or guiding the family through actions to access these resources, but some sources of support may be overlooked. Family members who appear dysfunctional may be able to do more than expected.

Once support is started, feedback loops are set up that serve to continue the supportive behaviors. Being supported feels good, as does being acknowledged for the support.

Consider the following clinical example in which resources were mobilized and support strengthened from within the family itself.

In one family, an elderly grandmother had cancer and was being cared for in the home. Zelda, the middle-aged mother, was coping with caring for several preschoolers, maintaining a job, and monitoring her 20-year-old daughter, who had cognitive developmental delays. The daughter's help was enlisted to bathe her grandmother and keep her company. Although the daughter had not been counted on as a resource in this family before, once her potential was tapped, she was delighted to be able to help. Zelda got some respite for a time before the grandmother entered a hospice program.

Family Organization Is Improved

The chaotic family may have little experience with a more ordered existence and may not recognize the benefits of simple structuring and rules. The very rigid family may never have experimented with a different way of doing things. Assisting the family in making minor changes in organization may help it move in the needed direction.

How a family's organization is improved depends on the unique circumstances. Creative thinking and personalized interventions were displayed by the community/public health nurse who worked with the following family.

Marylee, 7 years old, was not attending school. She stayed home to take care of her mother, who was often "ill." Her mother, who had dropped out of school herself at age 16, would turn off the alarm clock in the morning and sleep late, and, as a result, Marylee missed the school bus. Repeated attempts by the school system to address the problem failed. With the community/public health nurse's help, Marylee's mother asked an older neighbor who rose early to call her every morning at 7:30. With the older neighbor's support, the mother began to see herself as able to parent Marylee, and, as a result, Marylee's school attendance improved.

In this family, the external support system was first strengthened to help Marylee's mother improve her organization. The nurse might have had the neighbor call Marylee directly to awaken her, but that would have bypassed the responsibility of the mother to parent her own child.

Coping Processes Are More Adaptive

Many multiproblem families have learned dysfunctional coping behaviors as part of their lifestyle. For a family that tends to blame others or depend on others to help it out of any situation, the concept of planning and acting may be quite foreign. Drinking alcohol, acting out emotions, and procrastinating are examples of unhealthy coping behaviors.

In the following clinical example, the community/public health nurse assisted the mother to become more assertive in her problem solving.

One family had a son, Andy, with spina bifida, who was extremely dependent on various health care systems and social service agencies. The family became angry every time a problem occurred with Andy at school, with his catheter, with his wheelchair, or with his braces. They blamed the agencies or others for not managing his care correctly. When a new set of braces caused a pressure sore on his skin, the community/public health nurse coached the mother to be active in contacting the supply company, which made needed adjustments. This success moved the mother to a more self-confident stance in dealing with her son's care.

KEY IDEAS

1. Multiproblem families include families in crisis and families with chronic problems.
2. Some families can be supported through a crisis and will regain their previous level of health. Strategies for working with families in crisis include identifying stressors, reframing appraisals, locating resources, and considering alternative ways to cope.
3. Families at risk for multiple chronic problems include vulnerable families, families with negative choices, families in poverty, and families with disturbances in internal dynamics.
4. All families have some strengths, which must be tapped for intervention to be successful.
5. Resilience is a quality of individuals and families that helps them rebound and deal with intense stress and everyday life. Some protective factors associated with resilience include internal and external social support, boundary setting, taking charge, and communication (Lietz, 2007).
6. Nurse-family interventions may be influenced by the family's previous negative contacts with the health care

---

BOX 14-4   Competencies for Community/Public Health Nurses Working with Multiproblem Families

The community/public health nurse working with multiproblem families must demonstrate competence in the following areas:
- Engaging families that are distant, resistive, or disorganized or that have had previous negative experiences with the health care system
- Assessing individual member's safety within the family context and taking immediate action to protect a threatened member
- Applying knowledge of the relationship of family diversity to family strengths, family style, and family functioning
- Identifying the interrelationships of multiple family problems while helping the family choose a priority for intervention
- Intervening with a family group with frequently changing membership or attendance
- Communicating hopefulness
- Brokering contacts with multiple agencies and services available to the family
- Maintaining an awareness of one's own feelings of helplessness and frustration
- Helping the family perform activities that add to a sense of power and competence

---

Community/public health nurses interface with families in serious trouble within communities. Avoiding multiproblem clients is increasingly impossible; in fact, the clients who need nurses the most have multiple problems. Experienced community/public health nurses develop competencies in helping multiproblem families find solutions (Box 14-4). To gain access to these families, nurses need to examine their own values and approach families with respect and a willingness to allow them to define their care. Nurses who learn to expect less than perfection from themselves and the families they care for can be extremely influential as mutual progress is made in little steps. Restoring a family's sense of power and hope greatly enriches a nurse's satisfaction.

system. Strategies to counteract this failure include locating (tracking down) the family, creating trust, and building strength (Zerwekh, 1992).
7. A community/public health nurse makes choices about the level of intervention (individual, family subsystem, family as a unit, or family within the environment) based on the family assessment and on practical limitations to practice.
8. A community/public health nurse considers the level of family functioning when making choices about realistic goals and specific interventions.
9. Realistic goals in families with multiple, chronic problems include reducing stressors, strengthening the support system, improving family organization, introducing more adaptive coping behaviors, and altering the environment. The goals of nursing contact do not include trying to "fix" the family.
10. Maintaining and communicating hope are especially important for community/public health nurses working with multiproblem families.

The Walker family consists of Edna, age 29; William, age 31; and their children, Mary, 13; Sean, 9; and Mark, 3½. The Walkers are a struggling urban family living in their third apartment within the last 2 years. William has a high school education but no formal job training. He has supported the family off and on with his job as a house painter. He has a back injury and works sporadically because of his physical problems and the limited availability of work. Their average annual income is $31,000. The Walker's financial situation adds to the constant stress within the family. Although the Walkers care for each other, their interactions are usually disorganized and tense.

Mr. and Mrs. Walker were married when he was 18 and she was 16. Edna has an eighth-grade education, having dropped out of school after experiencing learning problems. She is a very concrete learner, has never worked, and has no job skills. Edna is currently 70 lb overweight and smokes approximately 1 pack of cigarettes a day. She spends most of her day caring for the children or talking on the telephone to her mother, who lives about 15 miles away. Edna's mother tries to be supportive of the family but is getting older. She used to baby-sit and help the family out financially but has not been able to do so recently because of her own health problems and her lack of transportation.

Mary, in the seventh grade, is a help to her mother. She has few outside interests other than watching television and occasionally cooking. Her younger brother, Sean, has been diagnosed with a learning disability and is failing in school. Mark, a preschooler, has asthma in addition to elevated blood lead levels.

The family's health problems require frequent clinic appointments, but the Walkers' automobile is often nonfunctional. Relations with the health care clinic are strained because of the clinic's perception that the Walkers are noncompliant. The stress of making it to these appointments leads to frequent cancellations and sporadic contact with the clinic.

This family has survived an earlier bout with illness. When Mark was born, he was premature and spent 2 months in the neonatal intensive care unit. He had problems with his lungs and has subsequently been small for his age and has frequent colds and illnesses. The family managed at that time with the help of Edna's mother and father and her neighbors. Edna's father drove her to the hospital and Edna's mother watched her children. William was working at the time, and the family had a health insurance plan. They pulled through that illness with a sense of pride about their ability to manage it and a commitment to each other.

ASSESSMENT

After receiving the referral, the community/public health nurse makes an appointment to meet the Walkers; but when she arrives, no one is home. She later learns that the Walkers had gone earlier to the clinic for Mark's asthma appointment but that their automobile would not start on the way home. At a second scheduled appointment, the Walkers again are not there. Later, by telephone, she finds out that Edna's mother fell and had to be taken to the hospital. The appointment is rescheduled. Edna is careful to be there on this occasion and has obviously attempted to clean up the house and make herself presentable. She has on lipstick and has carefully combed her hair and set out cookies and coffee for the nurse.

Mary, who is home from school that day with a cold, pops in and out of the room during the visit. The nurse meets with Edna, William, and Mark; Sean is at school. William has just returned from trying to get temporary work, but he has been unsuccessful.

During the initial visit, the community/public health nurse asks questions, completes a family assessment form (Box 14-5), and has the family begin to help her construct a genogram (Figure 14-1). She is also observing the family's interactions and the environment. She inquires about connections with community resources through use of an ecomap (Figure 14-2, A).

When the community health nurse first entered the house, William was in the bedroom. Edna yelled for him to come out several times and finally went back to the bedroom to get him, complaining about his behavior to the nurse. They sit on opposite sides of the room, with Edna doing most of the talking. Mark runs back and forth between them, carrying a piece of paper torn from the telephone book on which he is coloring.

The apartment, which is in a poorer section of the city, is on the third floor of an older building, with trash in the yard. The stairs up to the apartment are dirty and unlit, and the paint is peeling. The Walkers' apartment is cheery, with some curtains and knickknacks. Space appears to be a problem, because some of the pots and pans are stored in a corner in the front room, the kitchen table is covered with bills and schoolbooks, and the family shares two bedrooms.

ANALYSIS

On discussing the situation with the family, the community/public health nurse identifies the following family health needs: the family is experiencing demands from normal growth and development, is coping with illness and the external stress of the job market and the family's environment, and has inadequate resources. The nurse does not believe that severe disturbances in family dynamics exist but is concerned about parenting style and communication in the family. Family strengths include the ability to share and a commitment to make things work out for all members. The family has demonstrated some resilience since Mark's birth but has lost some resources and has more stressors to deal with since then. The nurse identifies the family style as disorganized but somewhat receptive and the family level of functioning as Tapia level II (see Chapter 13).

She compiles the following list of problems specific to individuals, subsystems, the family, and the environment:

William:
- Impaired physical mobility related to previous back injury as evidenced by (AEB) decreased range of motion (ROM)
- Chronic pain related to previous back injury AEB complaints of physical pain and decreased physical activity

Edna:
- Imbalanced nutrition: more than body requirements related to excessive food intake AEB obesity
- Altered health maintenance related to denial of effects of smoking AEB continuation of smoking and "I don't feel any effects from smoking now" statement
- Deficient knowledge of health maintenance and effects of smoking related to cognitive limitation/learning disorder

BOX 14-5 **Family Assessment Guide with Data of the Walker Family**

I. Identifying Data

Name: Walker

Address:

Phone:

Household members (relationship, sex, age, occupation, education):

William	Father	M	31	Part-time house painter	High school
Edna	Mother	F	29	Homemaker	Eighth grade
Mary	Daughter	F	13	Student, seventh grade	
Sean	Son	M	9	Student	
Mark	Son	M	3½		

Financial data (sources of income, financial assistance, medical care, expenditures): $31,000 per year income; no health insurance; applied for medical funds for children with special needs for Mark's medicines

Ethnicity: English/Irish descent

Religion: None practiced

Identified client(s): Mark

Source of referral and reason: Asthma clinic for repeated failure to keep appointments

II. Genogram (see Figure 14-1)

Include household members, extended family, and significant others

Ages or date of birth, occupation, geographic location, illnesses, health problems, major events

Triangles and characteristics of relationships

III. Individual Health Needs (for each household family member)

Identified health problems or concerns: William: back injury with pain; Edna: concrete learner, obese, smokes; Mary: little socialization; Sean: school failure

Medical diagnoses: Sean: learning disability; Mark: asthma, elevated lead level

Medications and immunizations: Mark up to date on immunizations; no asthma medications in house; and prescriptions not refillable

Physical assessment data: Mark: temperature: 98.4° F; pulse: 86 beats/min; respirations: 18 breaths/min; breath sounds clear; no wheezing; good hydration

Emotional and cognitive functioning: Mark: age-appropriate play

Coping: Strained relations with asthma clinic caused by unkept appointments; Edna frightened by Mark's asthma

Sources of medical care and dental care: None, except well-child clinic and asthma clinic for Mark

Health screening practices: Not explored

IV. Interpersonal Needs

Identified subsystems and dyads: Spousal, parent-child, sibling

Prenatal care needed: Not applicable

Parent-child interaction: Little concern re: Sean's school failure

Spousal relationships: Married 13 years; traditional spousal roles clear

Sibling relationships: "Get along OK"

Concerns about elders: Maternal grandmother (gm) recently ill and hospitalized with a fall

Caring for other dependent members: Not applicable

Significant others: Not applicable

Box 14-5   **Family Assessment Guide with Data of the Walker Family—cont'd**

V. Family Needs

A. Developmental

Children and ages: 13, 9, 3½

Responsibilities for other members: Mary helps mother; has few outside interests

Recent additions or loss of members: None

Other major normative transitions occurring or delayed: None

Transitions that are out of sequence or delayed: Development of personal interests and peer relationships for Mary

Family proceeding at expected sequence: Might use anticipatory guidance

Tasks that need to be accomplished: Learning successes for Sean; socialization for Mary; school readiness for Mark

Daily practices for nutrition, sleep, leisure, child care, hygiene, socialization, transmission of norms and values: Adequate hygiene; maternal gm was only baby-sitter; nutrition not explored

Family planning used: Tubal ligation

B. Loss or Illness

Nonnormative events or illnesses: Maternal gm in hospital

Reactions and perceptions of ability to cope: Edna worried about care of her mother following hospital discharge

Coping behaviors used by individuals and family unit: Cannot visit because of lack of transportation

Meaning to the family: Threat

Adjustments family has made: None yet, seems paralyzed

Roles and tasks being assumed by members: Edna assuming most responsibility, Mary's responsibility increased

Any one individual bearing most of responsibility: Edna

Family idea of alternative coping behaviors available: No ideas right now

Level of anxiety now and usually: High

C. Resources and Support (see Figure 14-2, *A*)

General level of resources and economic exchange with community: Low

External sources of instrumental support (money, home aides, transportation, medicines, etc.):   Unreliable care; chronic financial stress; able to buy only necessities

Internal sources of instrumental support (available from family members):   Maternal gm baby-sat before her illness

External sources of affective support (emotional and social support, help with problem solving):   None

Internal sources of affective support (who in family is most helpful to whom?):   Maternal gm

Family more open or closed to outside?   Does not actively seek resources

Family willing to use external sources of support?   Yes

D. Environment

Type of dwelling: Third-floor apartment; walk-up; dirty yard and stairs

Number of rooms, bathrooms, stairs; refrigeration, cooking: Two bedrooms, one bath; working stove, refrigeration, heating; decorated; cluttered because of inadequate storage

Water and sewage: Public

Sleeping arrangements: Parents together; boys together; Mary on folding bed in living room

Types of jobs held by members: Painter

Exposure to hazardous conditions at job: Yes—paint and height

Level of safety in the neighborhood: Moderate crime and air pollution

Continued

BOX 14-5   Family Assessment Guide with Data of the Walker Family—cont'd

Level of safety in household: Peeling paint in hallway of 40-year-old building; unlit stairs; working smoke detector; no pets; dust could be allergen for Mark

Attitudes toward involvement in community: Only recently moved to apartment; "keep to themselves"

Compliance with rules and laws of society: Very compliant

How are values similar to and different from those of the immediate social environment?   This family has higher expectations for self than neighbors; expects members to follow rules and contribute to each other

E. Internal Dynamics

Roles of family members clearly defined?   Yes

Authority and decision-making rest where?   Health care with Edna

Subsystems and members: See Interpersonal Needs section

Hierarchies, coalitions, and boundaries: Mary helpful to Edna; spouses' activities are goal directed, and roles complement each other

Typical patterns of interaction: Expression of feelings by children; Edna blames William

Communication, including verbal and nonverbal: Spouses: some intense verbal interactions; Edna: more vocal, complains

Expression of affection, anger, anxiety, support, etc.:   Anxiety, hope

Problem-solving style: Deal with immediate needs

Degree of cohesiveness and loyalty to family members: Cohesive, caring, loyal, "stick together"

VI. Analysis

Identification of family style: Disorganized (see Chapter 13)

Identification of family strengths: Ability to share; commitment to each other

Identification of family functioning: Tapia level II

What are needs identified by family?   Edna: care for her mother, Mark's asthma, better housing; William: work, car repair

What are needs identified by community/public health nurse?   See problem list in Analysis section of Nursing Process in Practice box

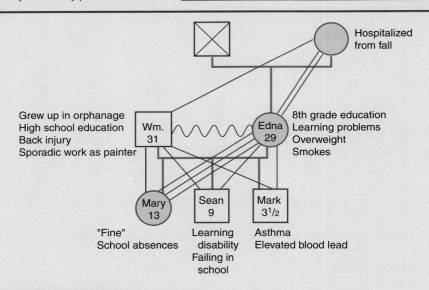

FIGURE 14-1   The Walker family genogram. (Adapted from Cain, A. [1981]. Assessment of family structure. In J. Miller & E. Janosik [Eds.], *Family-focused care* [p. 117]. New York: McGraw-Hill.)

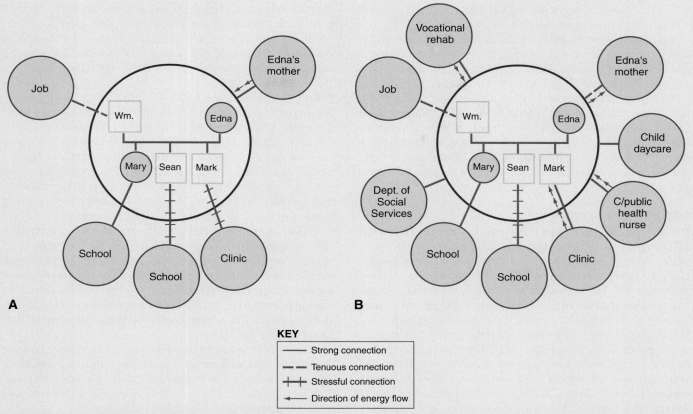

KEY

——	Strong connection
– –	Tenuous connection
—|—|—	Stressful connection
←——	Direction of energy flow

FIGURE 14-2 A, Ecomap of Walker family on first home visit. **B,** Ecomap of Walker family after 6 months of nursing care. (Adapted from Hartman, S. [1978]. Diagrammatic assessment of family relationships. *Social Casework, 59,* 470. Reprinted with permission from *Families in Society [http://www.familiesinsociety.org],* published by the Alliance for Children and Families.)

and lack of teaching AEB continuance of smoking around asthmatic son

Mary:
- Impaired social interaction related to lack of transportation and nearby friends AEB self-reported lack of friendships
- Disruption in completion of developmental tasks

Sean:
- Deficient knowledge of educational subjects related to cognitive impairment/learning disorder AEB failing grades in school
- Situational low self-esteem in response to learning disorder diagnosis related to failing grades AEB statements such as "It's now worth trying to learn. I can't learn anyways"

Mark:
- Ineffective airway clearance related to tracheobronchial narrowing AEB wheezing
- Poisoning related to flaking, peeling paint in the presence of young children AEB increased blood lead levels
- Risk for delayed development related to lead poisoning

Subsystems:
- Concern about Edna's mother's health and well-being
- Expenditure of resources for Edna's mother post-hospitalization

Family unit:
- Compromised family coping
- Potential for resilience
- Limited social contact

Environment:
- Residence: presence of environmental hazards (lead)

- Income: difficulty buying necessities and no health insurance
- Neighborhood: moderate crime and pollution

Edna and William are asked their perceptions of what is happening and what they would like to work on. William is most concerned with finding work and keeping the automobile running. Edna is worried about her mother and how she will cope by herself when she is released from the hospital and about Mark's asthma, which frightens her. She is less concerned with Sean's school problems or Mark's lead poisoning and thinks Mary is doing fine. Her wish for the family is for them to get their own house with a yard in which the kids can play. When asked how she and William get along, she just shrugs her shoulders.

PLANNING

Before formulating a plan of care, the nurse analyzes the data and tries to determine priorities. She is concerned about what the family identifies as its needs and what she and the health care system can realistically help with, and about setting some realistic goals. Together, she and the family come up with the following short-term goals:
- To contact the health care system about Edna's mother within the next 3 days and determine what plans are being made for her care after discharge
- To arrange for alternative transportation for Mark and Edna to get to the clinic for next week's appointment
- To call the state vocational rehabilitation department to get information for William about job retraining

- To apply for the State Children's Health Insurance Program (SCHIP) for the three children

Long-term goals include (1) safe care for Edna's mother, (2) stabilization of the family income, (3) appropriate treatment and family response for Mark's asthma, and (4) a move to a dwelling that has no chipping paint.

Goals that the community/public health nurse would like to achieve but that are not yet seen as needs by the family include further assessment and improved family response to Sean's learning disability, support for Mark's developmental functioning, and increased socialization for Mary. Edna's smoking and weight are also targets of concern, as is the family's repertoire of coping strategies.

IMPLEMENTATION

Because the family is functioning at Tapia level II and the family style is considered disorganized, the community/public health nurse alters her approach to the family. She takes special care to set realistic short-term goals that can be achieved within a week. She is aware that the family style may necessitate frequent changes in goals and plans and is careful to keep her contract with the family clear and reasonable on both sides. Her goal is to take small steps so that the family can begin to see some successes and to pay special attention to pointing out these successes and what the family did to achieve them. She will shape and role-model behaviors toward more successful coping. However, crises must be managed first. The family developed a sense of coherence and feeling of competence

after Mark's birth. Helping the family restore these feelings is important. Finding more connections with sources of relational support within the community is also essential. With this family, the unpredictable should be expected and must be considered as the family moves toward maintaining itself.

EVALUATION AND OUTCOMES

After 6 months, the nurse and the family are able to see some successes. William has been evaluated by the vocational rehabilitation department and is waiting to hear about retraining as a security guard. Edna has heard about a program as a daycare mother and is considering a job herself. Her mother fell again and has been placed in a rehabilitation nursing home that is on the opposite side of the city. The family cannot get to the nursing home very often but did visit her near Christmas.

Mark has been reevaluated at the asthma clinic, and medications have been prescribed. Edna gives the medicine more regularly now that the nurse has taught her how it helps prevent asthma attacks. Edna says that she is more comfortable now because she can recognize these attacks earlier. She usually goes outside to smoke but has not cut down on her use of cigarettes. Overall, the family is now connected with more community resources (see Figure 14-2, *B*).

Although little has changed with Mary or Sean, the state department of social services is finding funds to help move the family into new housing because of Mark's lead poisoning. This housing does not have a yard, so a home with a yard will remain Edna's dream for a while longer.

LEARNING BY EXPERIENCE AND REFLECTION

1. In what ways do family environment, family dynamics, and family stress influence how an individual will cope and behave? What has been the greatest influence for you?
2. Pick a major social problem in which you already have some interest (e.g., pollution, global warming, poverty, teenage pregnancy, drug abuse, violence). In what ways might a community/public health nurse intervene with regard to this environmental issue to advocate a change for family health?
3. Read your local newspaper, paying particular attention to the events and crimes occurring that day. How many of these news items are related to symptoms in families—that is, families in which the family unit is unable to support its members? Do you agree that dysfunction or inadequacy in the family should be considered when someone is being judged for a crime? Why or why not?
4. In a small group, discuss the ways in which your family has coped with problems in the past. How much pileup of stress was occurring at the time? What resources did you use? What were your coping strategies? Would you use these strategies again? What would have helped your family at that time? Can you envision help from a community/public health nurse? Why or why not?
5. Role-play a visit of a community/public health nurse to a family that has multiple problems. Have someone set up the situation so that no matter what the nurse does, the situation seems unresolvable. Break and discuss your feelings and reactions to this situation.

6. Role-play the same visit with the same family, but this time, have the director set up the situation so that the family members are confidentially instructed to feel some hope and will attempt to work on a little piece of the issues. Break and discuss your feelings and reactions to this situation. What was different?
7. Identify which family you would be more comfortable working with—a family in crisis or a family that has chronic problems. Why?
8. Spend some time with magazines, scissors, and glue. Compose a collage that depicts the life of a family with which you are interacting in the community. What does the collage evoke in you and in others in your group?
9. Locate a family that has experienced a particular hardship. Observe how that family copes with life now.

COMMUNITY RESOURCES FOR PRACTICE

Information about each of the following organizations is found on its website, which can be accessed through the **WebLinks** section of this book's website at *http://evolve.elsevier.com/Maurer/community/*.

Asian American Legal Defense and Education Fund
Child Welfare League of America
Consumer Credit Counseling Services
The Finance Project
Head Start Bureau
The Incredible Years: Parents, Teachers, and Children Training Series
Mixed Folks

National Association for the Advancement of Colored People
National Council on Child Abuse and Family Violence
Office of Civil Rights
U.S. Department of Health and Human Services

The following are national toll-free hotlines:
Child Abuse Hotline: (800) 422-4433
Domestic Violence Hotline: (800) 799-7233
Elder Abuse Hotline: (800) 879-6682

STUDY AIDS   http://evolve.elsevier.com/Maurer/community/

Visit the Evolve website for this book to find the following study and assessment materials:

- Quiz
- Web Scenario
- Critical Thinking Questions and Answers for Case Studies

- Care Plans
- *Healthy People* Updates
- Glossary

REFERENCES

Barrow, F. H., Vargo, A., & Boothroyd, R. A. (2007). Understanding the findings of resilience-related research for fostering the development of African American adolescents. *Child and Adolescent Psychiatric Clinics of North America, 16*(2), 393-413.

Bell, J. (2003). Encouraging nurses and families to think interactionally. *Journal of Family Nursing, 6*(3), 203-209.

Berne, A. S., Dato, C., Mason, D. J., et al. (1990). A nursing model for addressing the health needs of homeless families. *Image: Journal of Nursing Scholarship, 22*(1), 8-13.

Black, D. A., Heyman, R. E., & Slep, A. M. S. (2001). Risk factors for child physical abuse. *Aggression and Violent Behavior, 6*, 121-188.

Black, K., & Lobo, M. (2008). A conceptual review of family resilience factors. *Journal of Family Nursing, 14*(1), 33-55.

Boss, P. G. (2002). *Family stress management: A contextual approach* (2nd ed.). Thousand Oaks, CA: Sage.

Burr, W. (1973). *Theory construction and the sociology of the family.* New York: John Wiley & Sons.

Cain, A. (1981). Assessment of family structure. In J. Miller & E. Janosik (Eds.), *Family-focused care* (p. 117). New York: McGraw-Hill.

Carey, R. (1989). How values affect the mutual goal setting process with multiproblem families. *Journal of Community Health Nursing, 6*(1), 7-14.

Carter, B., & McGoldrick, M. (1989). Overview of the changing family life cycle: A framework for family therapy. In Carter, B. & McGoldrick, M. (Eds.), *The changing family life cycle: A framework for family therapy* (2nd ed., pp. 3-28). New York: Gardner Press.

Chatman, D. M. (1996). *Social support in African American adolescent mothers: An exploratory study.* Doctoral dissertation. Ohio State University, Columbus, Ohio.

Cooley, M., & Unger, D. (1991). The role of family support in determining developmental outcomes in children of teen mothers. *Child Psychiatry and Human Development, 21*(4), 39-42.

Crouter, A. C., Head, M. R., Bumpas, M. F., et al. (2001). Household chores: Under what conditions do mothers lean on daughters? In A. J. Fuligini (Ed.), *Family obligation and assistance*

during adolescence (pp. 23-41). New York: John Wiley & Sons.

Cutrona, C. E., Russell, D. W., Abrahm, W. T., et al. (2003). Neighborhood context and financial strain as predictors for marital interaction and marital quality and instability. *Journal of Marriage and the Family, 52*, 643-656.

Dunst, E., Trivette, C., & Deal, A. (1989). *Enabling and empowering families: Principles and guidelines for practice.* Cambridge, MA: Brookline Books.

Feeley, N., & Gottlieb, L. (2000). Nursing approaches for working with family strengths and resources. *Journal of Family Nursing, 6*(1), 9-24.

Fox, M. (1989). The community health nurse and multiproblem families. *Journal of Community Health Nursing, 6*(1), 3-5.

Fulmer, R. (1989). Lower-income and professional families: A comparison of structure and life cycle process. In B. Carter & M. McGoldrick (Eds.), *The changing family life cycle: A framework for family therapy* (2nd ed.; pp. 545-578). Boston: Allyn & Bacon.

Garbarino, J. (1992). *Children and families in the social environment.* New York: Aldine de Grayter.

Gillis, C. L. (1991). Family nursing research: Theory and practice. *Image: Journal of Nursing Scholarship, 23*(1), 19-22.

Hartman, S. (1978). Diagrammatic assessment of family relationships. *Social Casework, 59*, 470.

Hines, P. M. (1989). The family life cycle of poor black families. In B. Carter & M. McGoldrick (Eds.), *The changing family life cycle: A framework for family therapy* (2nd ed.; pp. 513-544). Boston: Allyn & Bacon.

Jaffee, S. R., Caspi, A., Moffitt, T. E., et al. (2007). Individual, family and neighborhood factor distinguish resilient from non-resilient maltreated children. *Child Abuse and Neglect, 31*(3), 231-253.

Janko, S. (1994). *Vulnerable children, vulnerable families: The social construction of child abuse.* New York: Teachers College Press.

Karpel, M. (1986). Testing and promoting family resources. In M. Karpel (Ed.), *Family resources: The hidden partner in family therapy.* New York: Guilford Press.

Kerr, M., & Bowen, M. (1989). *Family evaluation.* New York: W. W. Norton.

Kumpfer, K., & Alvarado, R. (2003). Family-strengthening approaches for the prevention of youth problem behaviors. *American Psychologist, 58*(6-7), 457-465.

Lietz, C. (2007). Uncovering stories of family resilience: A mixed methods study of resilient families. *Families in Society: The Journal of Contemporary Social Services, 88*(1), 147-155.

Lowe, M., & Freeman, R. (1981). Family coping index. In R. Freeman & J. Heinrich (Eds.), *Community health nursing practice* (pp. 555-566). Philadelphia: W. B. Saunders.

McCubbin, H. (1998). *Stress, coping, and health in families: Sense of coherence and resiliency.* Thousand Oaks, CA: Sage.

McCubbin, H., & Thompson, A. (Eds.). (1987). *Family assessment inventories for research and practice.* Madison, WI: University of Wisconsin.

McCubbin, H. I., & McCubbin, M. A. (1993). Families coping with illness: The Resiliency Model of family Stress, Adjustment, and Adaptation. In C. B. Danielson, B. Hamel-Bissel, & P. Winsted-Fry (Eds.), *Families, health, and illness: Perspectives on coping and intervention* (pp. 21-63). St. Louis: Mosby.

McKenry, P. C., & Price, S. J. (2005). Families coping with change: A conceptual overview. In P. C. McKenry & S. J. Price (Eds.), *Families and change: Coping with stressful events and transitions* (pp. 1-24). Thousand Oaks, CA: Sage.

Meyers, M. K., & Lee, J. M. (2003). Working but poor: How are families faring? *Children and Youth Services Review, 25*(3), 177-201.

Mischke, K., & Hanson, S. (1991). *Pocket guide to family assessment and intervention.* St. Louis: Mosby.

Mistry, R. S., Bandewater, E. A., Huston, A. C., et al. (2002). Economic well-being and children's social adjustment. *Child Development, 73*, 935-951.

Niemeyer, J. A., & Proctor, R. (1995). Facilitating family-centered competencies in early intervention. *Infant Toddler Intervention: The Transdisciplinary Journal, 5*(4), 315-324.

Ortega, D. (2002). How much support is too much? Parenting efficacy and social support. *Children and Youth Services Review, 24*(11), 853-876.

Otto, H. (1973). A framework for assessing family strengths. In A. Reinhardt & M. Quinn (Eds.), *Family-centered community nursing* (pp. 87-93). St. Louis: Mosby.

Patterson, J. M. (1988). Families experiencing stress: The family adjustment and adaptation response model. *Family Systems Medicine, 6*, 202-237.

Patterson, J. M. (2002). Understanding family resilience. *Journal of Clinical Psychology, 58*(3), 233-246.

Reimel, B., & Schindler, R. (1994). Family-of-origin work with multi-problem families. *Journal of Family Psychotherapy, 5*(1), 61-75.

Sachs, B., Pietrukowicz, M., & Hall, L. A. (1997). Parenting attitudes and behaviors of low-income single mothers with young children. *Journal of Pediatric Nursing: Nursing Care of Children and Families, 12*(2), 67-73.

Scannapieco, M. (1994). Home-based services program: Effectiveness with at risk families. *Children and Youth Services Review, 16*(5), 363-377.

Simon, J. B., Murphy, J. J., & Smith, S. (2005). Understanding and fostering family resilience. *Family Journal, 13*(4), 427-436.

Swadener, B., & Lubeck, S. (Eds.). (1995). *Children and families "at promise": Deconstructing the discourse of risk*. Albany: State University of New York Press.

Tapia, J. (1997). The nursing process in family health. In B. Spradley & J. Allender (Eds.), *Readings in community health nursing* (5th ed.; pp. 343-350). Philadelphia: J. B. Lippincott.

Turner, D., & Tanner, K. (2001). Working with neglected children and their families. *Journal of Social Work Practice, 15*(2), 193-204.

Tusale, K., Puskar, K., & Sereika, S. M. (2007). A predictive and moderating model of psychosocial resilience in adolescents. *Journal of Nursing Scholarship, 39*(1), 54-60.

Unger, D., & Cooley, M. (1992). Partner and grandmother contact in black and white teen parent families. *Journal of Adolescent Health, 13*, 546-552.

Van Riper, M. (2007). Families of children with Down syndrome: Responding to a change in plans with resilience. *Journal of Pediatric Nursing, 22*(2), 116-128.

Waitzman, N., & Smith, K. (1998). Phantom of the area: Poverty-area residence and mortality in the United States. *American Journal of Public Health, 88*(6), 973-976.

Walsh, F. (2006). *Strengthening family resilience* (2nd ed.). New York: Guilford Press.

Walsh, F. (2007). Traumatic loss and major disasters: Strengthening family and community resilience. *Family Process, 46*(2), 207-227.

Wilkins, W. P. (2003). Support networks and well-being. *Children and Schools, 25*(2), 67-68.

Wilson, H. S. (1989). Family caregiving for a relative with Alzheimer's dementia: Coping with negative choices. *Nursing Research, 38*(2), 94-98.

Wright, L., & Leahey, M. (2005). *Nurses and families: A guide to family assessment and intervention* (4th ed.). Philadelphia: F.A. Davis.

Zander, K. S. (1996). Negotiating outcomes with patients and families. *Seminars for Nurse Managers, 4*(3), 172-177.

Zerwekh, J. V. (1992). Laying the groundwork for family self-help: Locating families, building trust, and building strength. *Public Health Nursing, 9*(1), 15-21.

SUGGESTED READINGS

Allison, S., Stacey, K., Dodds, V., et al. (2003). What the family brings: Gathering evidence for strengths-based work. *Journal of Family Therapy, 25*(3), 263-284.

Anderson, K. H. (2000). The family health system approach to family systems nursing. *Journal of Family Nursing, 6*(2), 103-119.

Carten, A. J. (1996). Mothers in recovery: Rebuilding families in the aftermath of addiction. *Social Work: Journal of the National Association of Social Workers, 41*(2), 214-223.

Ehreneich, B. (2001). *Nickel and dimed: On (not) getting by in America*. New York: Henry Holt and Company.

Garbarino, J. (1999). *Raising children in a socially toxic environment*. Hoboken, NJ: John Wiley & Sons.

Guiao, I. Z., & Esparza, D. (1997). Family interventions with "troubled" Mexican American teens: An exploration from a review of the literature. *Issues in Mental Health Nursing, 18*(3), 191-207.

McCubbin, H., McCubbin, M. A., Thompson, A. I., et al. (1998). *Resiliency in families: A conceptual model for predicting family adjustment and adaptation*. Thousand Oaks, CA: Sage.

Murata, J. M. (1995). Family stress, mother's social support, depression, and son's behavior problems: Modeling interventions for low-income inner city families. *Journal of Family Nursing, 1*(1), 41-62.

Pokorni, J. L., & Stagna, J. (1996). Community and home care. Caregiving strategies for young infants born to women with a history of substance abuse and other risk factors. *Pediatric Nursing, 22*(6), 540-544.

Provan, K. (1997). Services integration for vulnerable populations: Lessons from community mental health. *Family and Community Health, 19*(4), 19-30.

Sachs, B., Hall, L. A., & Pietrukowicz, M. A. (1995). Moving beyond survival: Coping behaviors of low-income, single mothers. *Journal of Psychiatric and Mental Health Nursing, 2*, 207-216.

Schorr, L. (1998). *Common purpose: Strengthening families and neighborhoods to rebuild America*. New York: Doubleday.

Scrandis, D. (2006). Home health clinicians can find and help women with postpartum depression. *Home Healthcare Nurse, 24*(9), 564-571.

Shami, M., & Sharlin, S. (1996). Who writes the "therapeutic story" of families in extreme distress? Overcoming the coalition of despair. *Journal of Family Social Work, 1*(4), 65-82.

Webster-Stratton, C. (June 2000). The Incredible Years Training Series. *Juvenile Justice Bulletin*. Retrieved February 29, 2008 from *http://www.ncjrs.gov/html/ojjdp/2000_6_3/contents.html*.

Whittaker, J., Kinney, J., Tracy, E., et al. (1990). *Reaching high-risk families: Intensive family preservation in human services*. New York: Aldine de Gruyter.

Zerwekh, J. (1992). Laying the groundwork for family self-help: Locating families, building trust, and building strength. *Public Health Nursing, 9*(1), 15-21.

Zerwekh, J. (1992). The practice of empowerment and coercion by expert public health nurses. *Image: Journal of Nursing Scholarship, 24*(2), 101-105.

Zerwekh, J., Primomo, J., & Deal, L. (1992). *Opening doors: Stories of public health nursing*. Portland, OR: Celebration of the Public Health Nurse Committee for the Oregon and Washington State Public Health Associations Joint Conference.

Community as Client

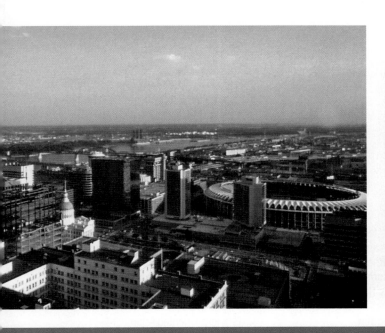
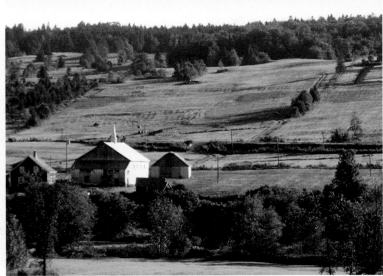

Community Assessment

Frances A. Maurer and Claudia M. Smith

FOCUS QUESTIONS

What is community-focused nursing?

How are communities defined?

What are the critical components of a community?

How are groups and aggregates considered as different types of populations?

What are different types of community boundaries?

What are goals of communities?

What are frameworks for assessing communities?

What is a general systems framework for assessing communities?

What are factors to consider in assessing the health of communities?

What are sources of data regarding communities?

What are approaches to community assessment?

How do community/public health nurses analyze community data?

CHAPTER OUTLINE

Community Assessment: Application to Community/Public Health Nursing Practice

Community Defined

Literature Review

Critical Components of a Community

Basic Community Frameworks

Nursing Theories Applicable to Community Assessment

Nursing Frameworks for Community Assessment and Practice

Systems-Based Framework for Community Assessment

Overview of Systems Theory

Components to Assess

Tools for Data Collection

Personal Observation

Existing Data Sources: Secondary Data

Surveys

Interviews with Key Informants

Meetings with Community Groups

Geographic Information Systems

Approaches to Community Assessment

Comprehensive Needs Assessment Approach

Problem-Oriented Approach

Single Population Approach

Familiarization Approach

Analysis

KEY TERMS

Aggregate	Geopolitical	Population
Asset	Group	Population "at risk"
Census tract	Healthy community	Target population
Community	Phenomenological	

The community/public health nurse is concerned with the health of the individual, the family, populations, and the community (American Nurses Association, 2007). This unit focuses on applying the nursing process with the community as client. What is the role of the nurse in population-focused nursing? What does it mean to be a nurse who is responsible for the health of a community? Where does the nurse start in considering community? What is a healthy, competent community?

Take a moment to reflect on this scene:

You are driving down a city street on a warm, sunny day. The row houses you see are in various physical states; some are painted and appear to be cared for, and others are in

disrepair and dilapidated; no grass is growing in the yards, and the street is littered with trash. People are sitting on the steps and front porches, talking and watching the traffic pass by. Several young female adolescents are sitting on the steps holding infants. Children of different ages are playing on the sidewalk and in the streets. The neighborhood is alive with noise and activity. As you continue your drive, you enter an area in which the houses are detached. The houses have small yards with green grass that are carefully maintained, and the streets are lined with lovely flowering trees. A few adults are working in their yards; a few children are playing in a nearby park. The scene is very quiet.

What is it like for residents who live here? Would you like to live here? What kinds of things would lead you or others to want to live here?

Healthy communities have "environmental, social, and economic conditions in which people can thrive" (Quad Council of Public Health Nursing Organizations, 1999, p. 3). A **healthy community** is one in which residents are happy with their choice of location and which exhibits characteristics that would draw others to the location. The majority of community residents are relatively functional for their age and health status. What are other characteristics of a healthy community? Kotchian (1995) suggests that a healthy community would be a safe community with little crime, supportive interaction between families and neighborhoods, a healthy environment (e.g., clean air, clean water, safe food), good schools, available and good quality health care services, and a sense of community cohesion. Green and Kreuter (1999) identify affordable housing and the availability of employment as prerequisites for healthy communities.

Besides these factors that immediately and obviously affect health, many social circumstances and other less tangible issues affect community living. For example, high crime rates and high levels of poverty in a neighborhood can seriously affect the health and welfare of residents. Ervin (2002) suggests that a healthy economy is key to a functional, healthy population. Although difficult to quantify, most people can identify characteristics of a healthy community that would influence their decision to reside there (Box 15-1).

COMMUNITY ASSESSMENT: APPLICATION TO COMMUNITY/PUBLIC HEALTH NURSING PRACTICE

Assessment, the *first step* of the nursing process, forms the foundation for determining the client's health, regardless of whether the client is an individual, a family, or a community. Nurses gather information by using their senses, as well as cognition, past experiences, and specific tools. These data are analyzed to make diagnoses about the community's health status and allow

---

BOX 15-1   Components of Healthy Communities

- Low crime rates
- Good schools
- Strong family life
- Robust economy, good jobs
- High environmental quality (clean air, water)
- Accessible and quality health services
- Adequate housing
- Civic involvement
- Nice weather
- Good transportation (roads, public transportation)
- Wide variety of leisure activities
- Exposure to the arts
- Reasonable taxes

Data from Asner, M., Polyak, I., & Weigel, D. (2003). The best places to retire. *Money, 32*(7), 83-90; Perdue, W. C., Stone, L. A., & Gostin, L. O. (2003). The built environment and its relationship to the public's health: The legal framework. *American Journal of Public Health, 93*(9), 1390-1394; Garb, M. (2003). Health, mortality and housing: The "Tenement Problem" in Chicago. *American Journal of Public Health, 93*(9), 1420-1430.

---

the nurse to answer the question, "Is this a healthy community or one with many problems and concerns?"

The assessment process affords nurses the opportunity to experience what it is like to be in the community, to get to know its people and their strengths and problems, and to work with them in planning and implementing programs to meet their unique needs. Just as all individuals and families are different, communities, too, are different. What makes one community different from another? To understand, nurses must get to know the community, its people, its purpose, and how it functions. Assessment tools provide a framework, a method of systematically gathering important information to help the nurse and other health professionals know the community.

How does the nurse become acquainted and familiar with a community? One way is to read about a community through newspapers, community histories, and objective statistical reports. Another way is to visit the community, talk to the people, and attend meetings—that is, *be with* the people. A visit to or a walk or a drive through the community provides *a feel* for the community that cannot be obtained from just reading about it. The walk or drive-through is frequently referred to as a *windshield survey*. Being in the community allows the nurse to subjectively experience a community and to learn how community members experience their community.

In the preceding example of community, two neighborhoods are presented, geographically close but different. Who lives in the two neighborhoods? What would it be like to live in these communities? What would it be like to be a community health nurse responsible for the health of these communities? What type of nursing care do you think this community needs?

Before we go any further, we need to define community. What is the meaning of a community? Is the community only the neighborhood in which one lives, or does it have other meanings?

COMMUNITY DEFINED

If you were to ask five people to define the word *community,* you would probably get five different answers: "a place where people dwell," "a group of people with common interests," "a place with specific boundaries." Some people may speak about an academic community, a religious community, or a nursing community, and others may define community as the neighborhood or city in which they live. Depending on the circumstances, each definition is correct.

In this text, **community** is defined as an open social system that is characterized by people in a place who have common goals over time. The term is applicable to a variety of situations. A community includes a place, and groups or aggregates. An **aggregate** is any number of individuals with at least one common characteristic (Williams, 1977). The terms population group and aggregate are synonyms for population (Williams, 1977). A **population** is a collection of individuals who share one or more personal or environmental characteristics, the most common of which is geographic location (Schultz, 1987). How a person defines community depends on the situation and that person's purpose. To community health nurses working for a county health department, community might mean a geographic area and its residents (population), such as the county or health district to which they are assigned. This description

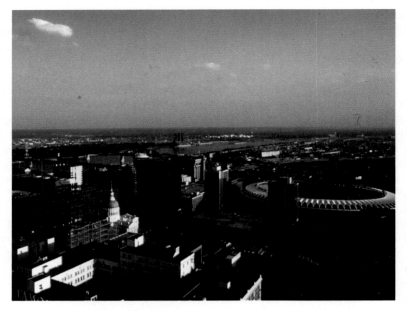

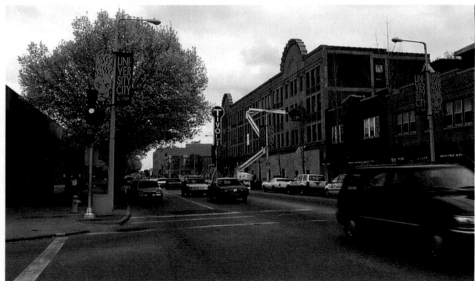

FIGURE 15-1 Geopolitical communities. In geopolitical communities, place is designated by a geographic or political boundary. The people who live, work, learn, and play in the community constitute the population. In most suburban and urban geopolitical communities, the individuals know only some of the residents on a face-to-face, personal basis. In less densely populated rural areas, most people may know each other on a personal basis.

is the classic definition of community. Nurses working with the homeless, the elderly, or a special interest group (e.g., smokers) may define community as people with common characteristics (aggregate) within a specific place.

LITERATURE REVIEW

Community health literature offers a variety of definitions. Behringer and Richards (1996) describe community as a web of people shaped by relationship, interdependence, mutual interests, and patterns of interaction. Shamansky and Pesznecker (1981) provide an operational definition of community considering the following three factors: (1) *who* (people factors), (2) *where* and *when* (space and time factors), and (3) *why* and *how* (for what purpose?). Ervin (2002) stresses that community assessments always occur at a particular time, for example, July 2008, or during the year 2009.

Anderson and McFarlane (2008) define community in terms of a core dimension (people) and eight subsystems: physical environment, education, safety and transportation, politics and government, health and social services, communication, economics, and recreation.

Other authors define community by describing types or categories. Communities may be geographically or socially bound (Hawe, 1994); categorized as emotional, structural, or functional (Archer, 1985); or defined in terms of relational and territorial bonds (Turner & Chavigny, 1988).

One of the most comprehensive definitions of community found in community health literature is formulated by Higgs and Gustafson (1985): "A community is a group of people with a common identity or perspective, occupying space during a given period of time, and functioning through a social system to meet its needs within a larger social environment." This definition is most closely related to the concept of community discussed in this text.

CRITICAL COMPONENTS OF A COMMUNITY

For the purpose of this text, a community may be defined as a community if three critical components or defining characteristics are included: *people, place,* and *social interaction or common characteristics, interests, or goals.* All communities contain all three of these components.

People

Population is the most obvious of the necessary community components. The number of people included in the community depends on the other two critical components. A population can be a relatively small number (a group of 20 pregnant adolescents enrolled in a clinic) or a large number of people (a city of 1,000,000). The ages, gender, race/ethnicity, religion, occupations, and socioeconomic status may be similar or diverse.

Place

Traditionally, communities were described in relation to geographic area. However, population aggregates such as older adults, the poor, people with acquired immunodeficiency syndrome (AIDS), or any population in which the members share one or more common characteristics, goals, or interests are sometimes used to identify a community for assessment purposes. Therefore communities may be defined by one of two designations: geopolitical (spatial) or phenomenological (relational). Figures 15-1 and 15-2 illustrate some geopolitical and phenomenological communities.

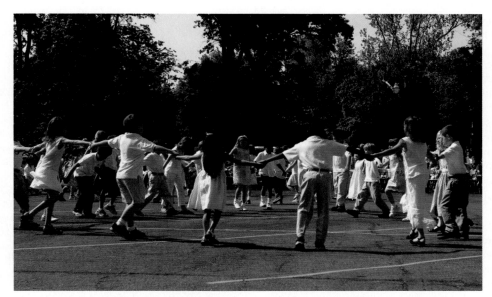

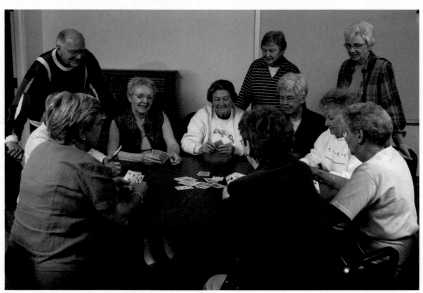

FIGURE 15-2 Phenomenological communities. In phenomenological communities, place is designated by a sense of belonging among its members. Although all human communities exist in a physical place, the members of a phenomenological community are bound together by their interpersonal connectedness rather than by geography. For example, individuals may belong to the U.S. military community even though they live throughout the entire world. A sense of belonging occurs in phenomenologic communities such as clubs, schools, gangs, senior centers, businesses, and churches and other religious organizations.

Geopolitical. The **geopolitical** community is a spatial designation—a geographic or geopolitical *area* or *place*. This view is the most traditional in the study of community.

Geopolitical communities are formed by either natural or human-made boundaries. A river, a mountain range, or a valley may create a natural boundary; for example, the Chesapeake Bay separates Maryland into the eastern and western shores. Human-made boundaries may be structural, political, or legal. Streets, bridges, or railroad tracks may create structural boundaries. City, county, or state lines create legal boundaries. Political boundaries may be exemplified by congressional districts or school districts.

Why does a community/public health nurse need to be concerned about geopolitical boundaries? A geopolitical view of community focuses the nurse's attention on the environment, housing, transportation, education, and political process subsystems. All of these elements are related to geographic locations, as well as the population composition and distribution, health services, and resources and facilities. Statistical and epidemiologic studies are frequently based on data from specific geopolitical areas.

Phenomenological. Most people initially think of community in terms of geographic location. Another way of thinking about community is in terms of the members' *feeling of belonging* or *sense of membership*, rather than geographic or political boundaries. Such a community is a **phenomenological** community, a *relational* rather than a spatial designation. A sense of *place* emerges through the members' awareness of their experiences together. This *place* is more abstract than a geopolitical place but is just as real to its members. People in a phenomenological community have a group perspective that differentiates them from other groups. A **group** consists of two or more people engaged in an interdependent relationship that includes repeated face-to-face communication. A group's identity may be based on culture, beliefs, values, history, common interests, characteristics, or goals. Examples of phenomenological communities include populations of people with common interests, such as a common religious conviction or professional or academic interest; with common beliefs, such as beliefs about human rights including women's rights or racial equality; or with a common goal, such as Students Against Drunk Driving (SADD), whose common goal is to decrease alcohol-related accidents among student drivers.

Another example of a phenomenological community is a *community of solution*. This type of phenomenological community has special significance for health planning. The National Commission on Community Health Services (1966) suggests that, when health services are considered, the boundaries of each community are established by the boundaries within which a problem can be identified, dealt with, and solved. A community of solution includes (1) a *health problem shed* (i.e., an area that has similar health problems) and (2) a *health marketing area* (i.e., an area that has similar solutions to the problem or an adequate supply of health resources to meet the problem).

For example, an oil spill in the Chesapeake Bay would affect more than one county. Parts of several counties in Maryland and Virginia may be affected. All of the communities affected become the health problem shed. All of the communities that join together and pool their resources to meet the need create a health marketing area. Figure 15-3 illustrates one city's communities of solution. The concept of

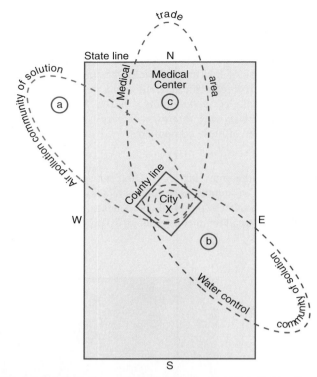

FIGURE 15-3 Communities of solution for city X. Note that health solution boundaries extend beyond city, county, and state lines. *A,* Because of air currents, air pollution may be displaced to the northwest. *B,* Because of the topography of the land, the water and sewage drain toward the southeastern portion of the state, which constitutes another "health problem shed." If the state and neighboring states joined together to solve the problem, this would constitute a health marketing area. *C,* A similar principle holds true for the medical trade area: the state emergency medical services system territory includes part of the adjoining state to the north. (Adapted from National Commission on Community Health Services. [1966]. Health is a community affair. Cambridge, MA: Harvard Press.)

a community of solution is especially important in coordinating health care and decreasing duplication and fragmentation of services.

Social Interaction or Common Interests, Goals, and Characteristics

Communities, similar to families, have their own patterned interaction among individuals, families, groups, and organizations; this interaction varies from community to community depending on needs and values. In a geopolitical community, this interaction may go beyond talking to one's neighbor and may include interactions with agencies and institutions within the community. In a phenomenological community, this attribute is inherent. A phenomenological community exists because of a common interest or feeling of belonging.

Each of us lives in a *geopolitical* community, but we may be members of several *phenomenological* communities. Figure 15-4 illustrates one individual's community membership.

BASIC COMMUNITY FRAMEWORKS

Now that we have defined the concept of community, how do you approach or study the community as a client? There are many theoretical approaches to communities. Perspectives on community come from diverse fields of study, including anthropology, sociology, epidemiology, social psychology, social planning, and nursing. Community/public health nurses have adapted and used theories from other disciplines. Several frameworks that are especially helpful in community/public health nursing include developmental, epidemiologic, structural-functional, and systems frameworks. Box 15-2 provides examples of frameworks used to study communities.

Box 15-2 Basic Frameworks Used to Assess Communities

Developmental Framework

Information about the community is collected from several points in time because communities change (McCool & Susman, 1990). Exploring the history of the community allows the community health nurse to consider the past. For example, even if a community has inadequate resources for treatment of substance abuse, it may currently have many more resources than it did 5 years ago.

Changes in a community are related to the needs of the population, changes in the societal context, changes in the physical environment, and the history of the community itself. For example, the U.S. population is currently aging; as the population ages, more health services are needed for older adults. Loss of population within a community may result in decay of existing buildings. An incorporated area may change its form of governance from a city manager and council to a city mayor and council.

Single events and trends should be considered. Events may be linked with the age of the community (e.g., the opening of the first local health department office), with changes in the environment (e.g., the closing of a business because of shifts in the national economy), and with unexpected situations (e.g., a flood) (McCool & Susman, 1990). Patterns of change may form trends. For example, trends in the health status of the community members are identified by analyzing epidemiologic data from several points in time.

Epidemiologic Framework

An epidemiologic perspective focuses on the health of the population. In this approach to community assessment, the nurse identifies persons who are at greater risk of illness, injury, disability, and premature death so that targeted interventions aim at reducing the risk or preventing the problem (Timmreck, 1998).

A recipe does not exist for identifying which epidemiologic data should be collected about a community. As discussed in Chapter 7, more data exist regarding mortality and the use of hospital services in the United States than exist about morbidity and the use of primary care services. However, we do know that health problems are not distributed evenly among all persons but instead vary with human characteristics such as age, gender, and socioeconomic status. Additionally, human behavior, quality of social support, and degree of environmental hazards are important factors that contribute to the distribution of health and the well-being among populations. Because of this fact, nurses who work with communities must consider the different health needs among various aggregates (e.g., elderly persons, pregnant women, workers in a specific occupation, poor individuals). The concept of aggregate/population is essential when using an epidemiologic approach to community assessment.

At-Risk and Vulnerable Populations

Epidemiologic data can identify which populations in a community are at higher statistical risk for experiencing illness, injury, or premature death. All populations have some risk, but risks for multiple illness conditions and premature death are much higher for specific populations (Feder et al., 2001; Sultz & Young, 2001). Community health nurses need to explore the multiple factors that contribute to the vulnerability of the population. Vulnerability is the predisposition or susceptibility to injury, illness, or premature death. To improve health status and reduce risk in high-risk populations, nurses must work with communities to identify and change, where possible, the factors that contribute to the populations' vulnerability (ANA, 2007).

Health programs and health policies aimed at reducing vulnerability to poor health must address a broad range of factors. Refer to other chapters for more in-depth discussions of risk factors: demographic factors in Chapter 7, socioeconomic and cultural factors in Chapter 10, human behavior in Chapter 18, high-risk populations in Chapter 21, and environmental factors in Chapter 9. Unit VII addresses the subject of community support for three vulnerable populations: persons with disabilities, children, and older adults.

Structural-Functional Framework

Structural-functional approaches to community emerged from anthropology and sociology. As social systems, communities have structures, processes, and functions. Structures are the parts of the community, and their organization and processes are the interactional patterns that change with time. Functions are the purposes and actual outcomes that result from community structures and processes. This approach asks: What structures and patterns of human interaction foster community goal achievement?

The following functions of the community can be identified:
- Creating and distributing goods and services
- Providing socialization
- Controlling social behavior
- Providing a sense of identity and mutual support
- Coordinating, controlling, and directing activities to attain other community goals (Katz & Kahn, 1966; Warren, 1987)

These social functions of the community may be achieved through a variety of social structures and processes. In other words, the same or similar results can be achieved in different ways. Communities differ by degree of autonomy, presence of service areas, psychological identification, and pattern of relationships (Warren, 1987).

A large urban area would generally be more autonomous and provide employment, a varied production of basic goods and services, its own police authority, and a network of formal groups that socialize and support the people. A suburban community might supply a strong social network and support of its members, but be less autonomous with fewer opportunities for employment and no formal production of goods. A rural community might have a strong social network and also provide some employment. Both suburban and rural communities may be dependent on a larger urban area for the functions of production and distribution. A community may have multiple service areas. For example, the suburban community may consist of two school districts, one election district, and the market area of two hospitals. The degree to which members identify with the locale may be strong or weak.

A community's relationship with other communities and the larger society affects the community. For example, many of the structures within a community, such as a hospital, nursing home, or home health agency, may be owned by corporations outside the community. Communities must be concerned with their internal functioning and their relationships to their social environments.

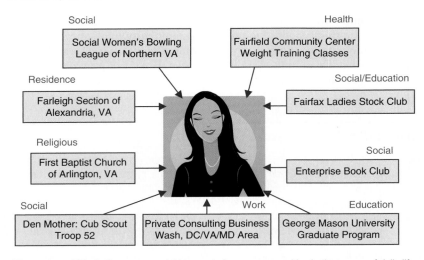

FIGURE 15-4 One person might be part of many communities in the course of daily life.

NURSING THEORIES APPLICABLE TO COMMUNITY ASSESSMENT

Most nursing theories were developed for individual clients, not communities (Hanchett, 1988; Marriner-Tomey & Alligood, 2006). Many nursing theories view the community as the environmental system influencing individuals and families.

Only a few nursing theories view the community as client (Hamilton & Bush, 1988). Goeppinger and colleagues (1982) proposed the development of a community assessment tool using Cottrell's characteristics (1976) of a competent community as a framework. Community competence is based on eight variables: commitment, self and other awareness and clarity of situation definitions, articulateness, communication, conflict containment and accommodation, participation, management of relations with the larger society, and machinery for facilitating participant interaction and decision making (Cottrell, 1976; Moorhead et al., 2004). Most of these characteristics of a competent community are community processes that can contribute to the inclusion and participation of community members.

The theories of Johnson (1980), Roy (1984), King (1971), Neuman (1982), and Watson (Rafael, 2000) may be used to view the community as client. All theories are based, in part, on general systems theory. As discussed in Chapter 1, general systems theory can be applied to any social system, including a community. Table 15-1 presents views of the health of a community from the perspectives of these nursing theories.

NURSING FRAMEWORKS FOR COMMUNITY ASSESSMENT AND PRACTICE

Several frameworks have emerged that are either nurse developed or used in public health practice. Two such frameworks view the community as partner. Anderson and McFarlane's (2008) Community as Partner model and Helvie's (1998) Energy Theory are nurse-developed frameworks. Both views consider *community* as a network of interrelating relationships, characteristics, and supports. Using these models, community/public health nurses act in partnership with others (health professionals *and* community members)

to address the community's health concerns (ANA, 2007). Several models are based on the epidemiologic framework. Two of these models have particular value to community health nurses: the GENESIS and MAPP models. All four models are influenced, to some degree, by systems theory and are briefly summarized in Box 15-3.

SYSTEMS-BASED FRAMEWORK FOR COMMUNITY ASSESSMENT

Although many useful strategies and frameworks are available for community assessment, the assessment tool used in this text is based on systems theory. A systems framework ensures that the dynamics within and external to each system, or community, are identified and explored. In addition, the tool incorporates aspects of the structural-functional framework (which identifies community goals and analyzes internal community functioning) and the epidemiologic framework (which analyzes the health status of the people/populations within the community).

The advantage of this systems-based community assessment tool is that it incorporates multiple frameworks simultaneously. If considered useful, a developmental framework can be incorporated to explore the history of the community.

OVERVIEW OF SYSTEMS THEORY

A systems framework views the community as a dynamic model in which the community is constantly in the process of responding and adapting to internal and external stimuli. The responses are aimed at developing and maintaining a sense of balance or equilibrium. The systems model (Figure 15-5) serves as a tool to help the nurse identify, collect, and organize appropriate data, including the critical components and their relationship to each other.

The components of the systems model for both geopolitical and phenomenological communities are the same and consist of the following:

- *Boundaries:* factors that separate a community from its environment and maintain the integrity of the community
- *Goals:* purpose or reason for which the community exists

- *Characteristics:* physical and psychosocial characteristics of the community that affect behavior
- *External influences:* resources or stressors from the suprasystem

TABLE 15-1 Perspective on the Health of Communities in Selected Nursing Theories

Theorist	Health of a Community
Dorothy Johnson	Successful community functioning and adjustment to environmental factors
Sister Callista Roy	Effectiveness of the community in accomplishing its functions and adapting to external stimuli
Imogene King	Quality interactions between individuals, groups, and the entire community that contribute to community functioning and development
Betty Newman	Competence of the community to function and maintain balance and harmony in the presence of stressors
Jean Watson	A healthy community is a holistic community, one which is able to integrate social and personal resources and capacities to attain or maintain health for its members

Data from Anderson, E., McFarlane, J., & Helton, A. (1986). Community-as-client: A model for practice. *Nursing Outlook, 34*(5), 220-224. Hanchett, E. (1988). *Nursing frameworks and community as client—Bridging the gap.* Norwalk, CT: Appleton & Lange; Marriner-Tomey, A., & Alligood, M. (2006). *Nursing theorists and their work* (6th ed.). St Louis: Mosby/Elsevier. Dixon, E. (1999). Community health nursing practice and the Roy Adaptation Model. *Public Health Nursing, 16*(4), 290-300; Rafael, A. R. F. (2000). Watson's philosophy, science, and the theory of human caring as a conceptual framework for guiding community health practice. *Advances in Nursing Science, 23*(2), 34-49.

- *Internal functioning:* structures and processes of the community, divided into four functional subsystems: economy, polity, communication, and values (University of Maryland School of Nursing, 1975)
- *Outcomes:* products, energy, and information created within the community, including health behavior and health status of the population(s) and degree of community competence
- *Feedback:* information that is returned to the system regarding its functioning

Although the components of geopolitical and phenomenological communities are the same, the types of data collected and the resources for those data vary. The environment external to the community in Helvie's model (1998) is referred to as the suprasystem in our model (von Bertalanffy, 1968). For the holistic assumptions and review of general systems theory refer to Chapter 1.

COMPONENTS TO ASSESS
Box 15-4 presents the basic systems model for community assessment, identifies important data to collect, and suggests possible data sources. **Website Resource 15A** expands the information on the tool in Box 15-4. The tool differentiates how the model would be used for both a *geopolitical* and a *phenomenological* community assessment, and suggests some of the questions nurses would need to ask. The following discussion examines the important features in each component in the assessment process.

Boundaries
The essential first step in community assessment is identifying the boundaries or parameters of the community. Remember that a community is defined in terms of the three critical components: *people, place,* and *social interaction or*

BOX 15-3 Sample Nursing Frameworks for Community Assessment and Practices

Community-as-Partner Model
The community-as-partner model evolved at the University of Texas School of Nursing at Galveston. Based on Betty Neuman's system model of a total-person, the community-as-partner model focuses on two central factors: the community as partner and the nursing process (Anderson & McFarlane, 2008). The community is composed of a core population and eight subsystems. These are depicted visually as a wheel with the population at the hub surrounded by the subsystems. The subsystems are physical environment, education, safety and transportation, politics and government, health and social services, communication, economics, and recreation. The core population and each subsystem may be influenced by other segments, as well as by stressors, beyond the community (external factors). The community/public health nurse works in partnership with the community to plan, implement, and evaluate strategies to reduce stressors, reestablish equilibrium, and prevent future problems. Interventions address primary, secondary, and tertiary prevention.

Helvie Energy Framework
The community (population) is an energy field that is ever changing (Helvie, 1998). The community influences and is influenced by other energy fields or subsystems in the environment such as health, educa-

tion, and economics. Changes in the community environment may come from internal (between community components) or external (outside the community) influences. The nurse works to identify stressors and to plan strategies to bring stressors into balance and improve health.

Epidemiologic Framework Models
GENESIS: General Ethnographic and Nursing Evaluation Studies in the State was developed by the University of Colorado School of Nursing. This model integrates epidemiologic and ethnographic data to develop a comprehensive view of a community's health status and health needs (Stoner et al., 1992). Areas of assessment include history, politics, services, economies, employment, education, environment, and a community's sense of belonging. Community members' feelings about health, health needs, and values are incorporated in the assessment process.

MAPP: Mobilization for Action through Planning and Partnerships. This tool is designed for use by local health departments in planning with geopolitical communities to improve health status and public health system capabilities (National Association of County and City Health Officials [NACCHO], 2000). The tool emphasizes community ownership of the process. It also helps instruct nurses and other public health personnel in the most effective ways to use collected data to develop effective intervention plans.

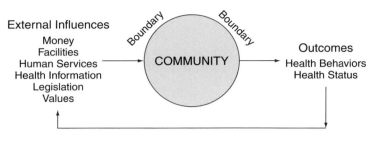

ENVIRONMENT
(Includes Suprasystem)

External Influences

Money
Facilities
Human Services
Health Information
Legislation
Values

Boundary   Boundary

COMMUNITY

Outcomes

Health Behaviors
Health Status

EXTERNAL FEEDBACK

FIGURE 15-5 Community as system.

BOX 15-4   Community Assessment Tool: A System-Based Approach

1. Identify the boundaries of this community.
   a. People
   b. Place
   c. Social interaction—common goals, interests, or characteristics
      Sources of data: **Geopolitical:** maps, census tract maps, libraries, city clerks, health departments, printed material describing the community. **Phenomenological:** interviews, printed material describing the community (e.g., pamphlets), philosophic and membership statements.
2. Identify the goals of this community.
   Sources of data: **Geopolitical:** charter of incorporation, printed material about the community, interviews of key informants (e.g., community leaders). **Phenomenological:** printed material about the community, statement of philosophy and goals, interviews of key informants (e.g., community leaders, community members).
3. Describe the community's physical and psychosocial characteristics.
   a. Physical characteristics
      (1) How long has the community existed?
      (2) Obtain demographic data about the community's members (age, race, gender, ethnicity, housing, density of population).
      (3) Identify physical features of the community that influence behavior.
   b. Psychosocial characteristics
      (1) Religion
      (2) Socioeconomic class
      Sources of data: **Geopolitical:** census tract data, GIS databases, health planning agencies, libraries, city/county clerks, Chamber of Commerce, printed matter about the community, telephone books listing places of worship and schools, a visit to the neighborhood (for information on set factors of the community), written surveys, local realtors (for information on housing). **Phenomenological:** a visit to the community, health and membership records, surveys, interviews with key informants.
4. Identify the suprasystem and explain the importance of looking at the suprasystem during a community assessment.
5. Which external influences from the environment (suprasystem) are resources? Which are demands?

	Resources	Demands
Money:		
Facilities:		
Human services:		
Formal:		
Informal:		
Health information:		
Legislation:		
Values of suprasystem (i.e., what external values affect this community?):		

Sources of data: **Geopolitical:** windshield survey, census tract data, GIS databases, health planning agencies, libraries, city/county clerks, Chamber of Commerce, printed matter about the community, telephone books listing places of worship and schools, a visit to the neighborhood (for information on set factors of the suprasystem), written surveys, local realtors (for information on housing). **Phenomenological:** a visit to the suprasystem, health and membership records, surveys, interviews with key informants.

6. Internal functions: identify resources and demands within the community that influence its level of health. (See pages 412-414 and **Website Resource 15A** for additional details.)
   a. Economy
      Areas of assessment include formal and informal human services; money; facilities, equipment, and goods; education; analysis of economy subsystem functioning; and are the services, facilities, finances, and education in this community accessible, adequate, and appropriate?
      Sources of data: **Geopolitical:** budget, interviews, drive or walk through the community, telephone book, and service directories. **Phenomenological:** budget, interview, surveys.
   b. Polity: describe the political system within the community used to attain community goals.
      Areas of assessment include basic organizational structure, formal and informal leaders, pattern of decision making, methods of

WE1

Box 15-4   Community Assessment Tool: A System-Based Approach—cont'd

social control, and analysis of polity subsystem: What is the ratio of demands to resources?

Sources of data: **Geopolitical:** organizational chart and charter, interviews and meetings with the community, laws. **Phenomenological:** by-laws, procedure and policy books, attending meetings, being with the group.

c. Communication: describe the communication within the community that fosters a sense of belonging and provides identity and support to its members.

Areas of assessment include nonverbal communications, verbal communications, and analysis of communication subsystem: How well does the community communicate a sense of identity or belonging to its members? How adequate is the communication?

Sources of data: **Geopolitical:** interviews, newspapers, kiosks, meetings, visit to the community. **Phenomenological:** interviews, newsletters, meetings, classes, committees, being with the community.

d. Values: identify the ideas, attitudes, and beliefs of community members that serve as general guides to behavior.

Areas of assessment include tradition, subgroups, environment, health attitudes and values, homogeneity versus heterogeneity of values and beliefs, and analysis of values subsystem: How well does the community provide guidelines for the behaviors of its members?

Sources of data: **Geopolitical:** surveys of agencies to determine utilization, surveys of community members, newspapers, and community announcements. **Phenomenological:** observation and interaction with members, charts or records, surveys of members.

7. Health behavior and health status (outcomes).

(Be sure to refer to the community assessment tool in **Website Resource 15A** for this portion of the assessment, because some differences exist between the geopolitical community and the phenomenological community.)

a. People factors:

(1) Describe the general trends regarding size of community.

(2) What are the trends in mortality and morbidity?

(a) What is the mortality rate?

(b) What are the major causes of death?

(c) What major diseases and illnesses are present?

(d) Who are the vulnerable groups? What are the risky behaviors?

(e) What presymptomatic illness or problems might be expected?

(f) What is the level of social functioning in this community?

(g) What types of disabilities or impairments, or both, are present or might be found in this community?

Sources of data: **Geopolitical:** local and state vital statistics (available through local and state health departments); *Morbidity and Mortality Weekly Report (MMWR),* published by the Centers for Disease Control and Prevention (available at libraries and health departments); reports of screening programs; interviews with key informants. **Phenomenological:** agency or community records, interviews with key informants, review of the literature pertaining to aggregates (e.g., literature about elderly individuals will provide information about most morbidity and mortality).

b. Environmental factors

(1) Physical environmental factors: What is the quality of the physical environment (air, water, housing, work or home environment)?

(2) Social environmental factors: What is the emotional tone and stability of the population?

Sources of data: **Geopolitical:** visit to community; reports such as Air Quality Index (AQI). **Phenomenological:** visit to community.

8. Describe feedback from the environment about the community's functioning.

9. Make inferences about the level of health of this community.

a. What are some actual health problems or needs?

b. What are some potential health problems or needs?

c. How well is the community working to meet its health needs? What is its proposed action to meet its health needs?

d. How has the community solved similar problems in the past?

e. What are the strengths of the community?

10. Identify one actual or potential health need for which you, as a nurse, could plan an intervention.

Adapted from Community Health Faculty, Undergraduate Program, University of Maryland School of Nursing. (1975). *Community assessment tool.* Baltimore: University of Maryland School of Nursing.

common interests. The definition of a community determines its boundaries. Consider the boundary as the *skin* or outside limit of the community. Establishing the boundary helps the nurse determine what data will be collected and considered internal to the community, in other words community information. Defining the boundary also identifies the suprasystem, the environment outside the community. Data collected from the suprasystem are considered external influences, or inputs, and may impact or influence the community.

Boundaries, similar to the skin of an individual, maintain the integrity of the system and regulate the exchange between a community and its external environment, the suprasystem. Boundaries of a geopolitical community are *spatial* and

concrete; they can be natural or human-made, as discussed earlier. Because the boundaries of geopolitical communities are real and concrete, they are often visible on maps. For example, the Potomac River and the Maryland state line can be visualized on a map as indicators of the boundaries of Washington, DC. The Rocky Mountains divide the western part of the United States from the Great Plains. The river and mountains are natural boundaries and the state line a human-made boundary.

Another type of human-made boundary is a **census tract.** The U.S. Bureau of the Census divides the United States into census tracts for the purpose of reporting demographic data about the U.S. population every 10 years. Census tract data are valuable for health planning. Census tract maps are

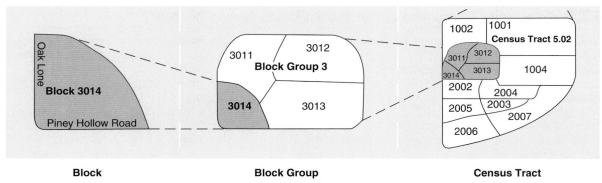

Block	Block Group	Census Tract

FIGURE 15-6 Census small-area geography map illustrates the relationship between block 3014 (the smallest geographic area of the census), its block group (several adjacent blocks 3011, 3012, 3013, and 3014), and census tract 5.02, which contains other block groups. (From U.S. Bureau of the Census. [2001]. Introduction to Census 2000 data products [Publication No. MSO/01-ICDP, June 2001]. Washington, DC: U.S. Department of Commerce.)

 available in libraries and health departments. Figure 15-6 illustrates how an area is incorporated into a census tract. **Website Resource 15B** provides additional information on census tracts.

The boundaries of *phenomenological* communities are more *relational* or *conceptual* than they are geopolitical boundaries and usually relate to the reason the community exists or to the criteria for membership. To determine the boundary of a phenomenological community, the following questions would be asked: Why does the community exist? Who can belong? What criteria are necessary for membership? What brings the members together? For example, the boundary of the nursing community would be its criterion for membership—that is, the person must be a nurse to belong. The boundary of a Cub Scout pack would be the criteria of age (7 to 10 years old) and gender (boys).

> The Morgan Center is a nutrition center for frail elderly persons. The center consists of 25 senior participants, a site manager, and 3 staff members. To attend Morgan Center, the participants must be 65 years of age or older, live in Allen County, be classified as frail (having difficulty with at least one activity of daily living), and be continent. The goals of the Morgan Center are to provide socialization, encourage activities of daily living, and ensure adequate nutrition for its clients.

A nurse assessing the community might determine some characteristics from the data provided. This community is a *phenomenological* community; it is an *aggregate* of the elderly (the frail elderly) attending Morgan Center. The *criteria for membership* (65 years of age and older, residents of Allen County, frail, and continent) determine the *boundaries*. Another way to define the community would be to view the Morgan Center in its entirety, including the frail elderly, the site manager, and the staff. In this case, the criteria for membership change to persons who work at or attend the center. Either definition is correct, depending on the reason or purpose for the assessment.

As you can see, the parameters of the community must be defined because they determine what data will be collected. In the first situation, the nurse will collect data about the frail elderly persons only, and the site manager and the staff will be external influences to the community; in the second example, the nurse will collect data about frail elderly persons, the site manager, and the staff as part of the community. Boundary definition is especially important when examining the external influences and the internal functioning of a community.

Permeability of Boundaries. The boundaries of any system may be relatively permeable (open) or impermeable (closed). For example, entrance or membership into a religious community may be contingent on certain beliefs and rituals, making the boundary impermeable to someone who does not hold these beliefs. In a phenomenological community, the criteria for membership often define the boundary's permeability or openness. A geographic community that has a gated entrance and homes that cost $250,000 or more is impermeable to people with an annual income of $25,000 to $30,000. Communities with greater variety of housing prices and rental units would be open to more people; thus the boundaries would be permeable.

The openness or closeness of a community has implications for health planning. A closed, rigid system is resistant to change, whereas an open, flexible system is more receptive to change and to help from the health care delivery system.

Suprasystem. Once you have determined the boundary of the community, anything *outside the boundary* becomes the *suprasystem*. No system (individual, family, or community) can exist in isolation. Therefore every client system operates within a larger system. The larger system, the suprasystem, is defined as the environment external to, or outside, the community that affects the community system. The suprasystem of a geopolitical community is concrete. For example, the immediate suprasystem of Ridgely's Delight, a neighborhood in Baltimore, is Baltimore itself. The suprasystem of Baltimore is the state of Maryland. Identifying a specific suprasystem for a geopolitical community is usually easier than it is in a phenomenological community.

In a phenomenological community, the suprasystem becomes anything outside of the community that affects or is affected by the community. Identifying a single suprasystem for a phenomenological community is sometimes difficult; many suprasystems may be found. For example, what is the suprasystem for an aggregate such as the elderly individuals in Orange County? It might be the Orange County Office on Aging, the entire Orange County government, the American Association of Retired Persons, or the Orange

County Social Security Office, all four of these entities, or these four entities and still others. The sources of external influences from the larger society must be examined, such as legislation, services, and money that influence (positively or negatively) the elderly community. For some phenomenological communities, however, identifying a specific suprasystem may be possible. For example, Girl Scout Troop No. 201 is a phenomenological community; its suprasystem is the Girl Scouts of Central Ohio.

Goals

Goals of communities vary with the type of community, but in general they are focused on maximizing the well-being of members, promoting survival, and meeting the needs of the community members. What are the goals of the community in which you live? Are they to provide safe housing for residents? One goal of the Morgan Senior Center is to provide socialization for its members. The community health nurse can assess the goals of the community by asking questions such as, "What is the purpose of the community?" A written statement of the community's philosophy and goals, if available, is another source.

Characteristics

Characteristics are the physical, biologic, and psychosocial factors of the community. These characteristics are often referred to as *demographics*. Characteristics are usually not easily changed or change slowly.

Physical Characteristics. Physical characteristics include (1) the length of time the community has been in existence, (2) pertinent demographic data about the community's members (e.g., age, race, gender, ethnicity, education, income, housing, density of population), and (3) physical features of the community that influence behavior.

The length of time the community has been in existence (the age of the community) has implications regarding stability, health services, and needs. A very new community may have few services simply because the supply has not caught up with the demand. On the other hand, communities that have been in existence for a long time may have many resources, or they may have resources that reflect past population needs but not the current needs (if population shifts have occurred).

Pertinent demographic data such as age, race, gender, ethnicity, and density of the population have significant meaning in the planning of health care and services. By looking at the age, race, and gender of members of the community, the community/public health nurse can make some inferences about possible health needs. A community with a large population of elderly individuals will have very different needs from persons of a community with a predominantly young population. Generally, elderly individuals need more services than do younger persons. Race is a factor in certain diseases (e.g., sickle cell anemia in the black population; Tay-Sachs disease in Jewish populations). A population with an unusually high number of women will need more women's health care services, and a community with a high number of adults may need blood pressure screening programs to detect early hypertension.

Ethnicity is reflected in customs, beliefs, and values and may affect how the community addresses certain health practices (refer to Chapter 10). The community/public health nurse must understand these customs and beliefs when assessing needs and planning interventions. In some areas, the cultural and ethnic backgrounds of the population have become the basis for the community. Some cities have sections that reflect the ethnic and cultural heritage of certain groups (e.g., Little Italy and Chinatown in San Francisco). Groups such as the Sons of Norway, the Sons of Italy, and the Polish Home Club have formed phenomenological communities on the basis of their ethnic and cultural heritage.

The type, condition, and amount of housing and density of the population are environmental factors that have implications for health. Crowded living conditions have long been associated with the increased transmission of some communicable diseases (e.g., tuberculosis, pediculosis). Also important to note is the condition of the housing and whether the housing is available and financially accessible to people in the community. The type and condition of housing may say a lot about the resources and values of the people living in the community.

In a phenomenological community, the environment or the place in which the group meets might be examined. This review takes into consideration the environmental factors and the aesthetics that contribute to or interfere with members' ability to feel comfortable in the physical environment.

Physical features of the community can influence the community's behaviors. A community with fences around all houses demonstrates a value of privacy and may imply little social interaction or the presence of dogs or pools. A school with open classrooms influences the interaction among students. Other physical features such as living or working in a community with toxic substances may influence the level of health of the residents or workers.

Psychosocial Characteristics. Psychosocial characteristics that affect the emotional tones of the community include religion, socioeconomic class, education, occupation, and marital status. Some ways these characteristics may affect health behavior include the following:

- *Religion:* Beliefs may involve the use or nonuse of contraceptives, abortion, living will, circumcision, and organ donation.
- *Socioeconomic level:* Poverty reduces access to health care services and increases health risks (see Chapters 4 and 21).
- *Educational level:* Higher education levels are associated with higher rates of preventive health behaviors.
- *Occupation:* A person's livelihood may influence the risk of disease or injury. For example, coal miners are prone to silicosis and lung cancer, typists to carpal tunnel syndrome, and white-collar technology professionals to stress-related conditions such as coronary artery disease.

Collecting demographic information can provide the nurse with some idea of the possible health needs of the community. Looking at a number of people with common characteristics and planning programs to meet their unique health needs are the basis for aggregate/population health planning. Sources of demographic information are identified later in Tools for Data Collection.

External Influences

All communities have external influences that affect their functioning. External influences are matter, energy, and information that come from outside the community—that is, from the suprasystem. External influences may be either resources (assets or strengths) or demands (liabilities or weaknesses) on the community and may be mandated (required) or voluntary. Some of the most important external influences are money, facilities, human services, health information, legislation, and values of the suprasystem. Some of the areas to explore for each of these influences are summarized here:

- *Money.* Outside sources would include taxes, state or federal funds, contributions, grants, or endowments. Finding money that may be used to fund health services is important.
- *Facilities.* Look for the following potential outside facilities: health care facilities such as hospitals, health maintenance organizations, nursing homes, home care agencies, and facilities and clinics that promote safety and transportation. Consider accessibility of facilities regarding location and cost, as well as transportation and attitude of staff. Ease of access and low cost are resources; excessive distance and poor staff attitudes are demands.
- *Human services.* These resources may be formal or informal. Examples of formal human services include professional resources, nurses, physicians, the local health department, and health insurance companies. Examples of informal services are often voluntary services, individuals, and organizations such as religious groups and other volunteer support groups for a variety of health conditions (e.g., Alcoholics Anonymous). Physicians and nurses outside the community who will see community members are a resource; physicians or clients who will not accept community members are a demand.
- *Health information.* Health information is communicated through printed matter, radio, television, or person-to-person. If the suprasystem has helpful information but does not have an effective way to communicate this information, this represents a demand.
- *Legislation.* This type of influence takes the form of laws, policies, and procedures that may affect a community in either a positive (resource) or a negative (demand) manner. The geopolitical community has laws that affect the community's health, including environmental pollution and zoning laws; the phenomenological community can be affected by external legislation, policies, and procedures. For example, legislation affects the health and health care of older adults (the Older Americans Act and Medicare legislation).
- *Values of the suprasystem.* Consider if the suprasystem's values are consistent or inconsistent with the values of the community. When the two sets of values are consistent, little conflict takes place, and there is increased likelihood that the suprasystem will be supportive of community requests. When the two sets of values differ, conflict is more likely, and the suprasystem will be less supportive of community needs and requests.

Data Sources for Suprasystem Information. Because the external influences come from the suprasystem, obtaining data about the suprasystem is important. Where can these data be found? A wealth of information is provided by review of the suprasystem budget, local telephone book and newspapers, health or human service directories, and information and referral services; systematic tours of services and agencies; interviews with members of the community; and review of legal and policy and procedure books.

Internal Functions of the Community

Internal functioning of the community occurs through its internal structures and processes. For the purpose of data collection and analysis, the tool examines four functional areas: economy, polity, communication, and values (University of Maryland School of Nursing, 1975). Resources and demands may be found within each of these subsystems.

When assessing individual human functioning, it is essential to determine areas of strength as well as areas of need. Nurses work with individuals to build on their strengths in order to overcome and adapt to health deficits. The same is true when assessing a community. **Asset** models of community assessment stress the positive abilities and capacities of communities to identify their own health problems and plan solutions (World Health Organization Regional Office for Europe, 2005). Such a model encourages community participation and has the potential to empower communities.

Economy. *The goal of the economy subsystem is production and distribution of goods and services.* Economy includes categories such as human services; money; facilities, equipment, and goods; and education. These factors are the same as those discussed in the assessment of external influences. However, the factors to examine here are those *within* the community itself.

1. *Human services.* Services available within the community may be either formal (e.g., nurses and physicians) or informal (e.g., volunteers). Questions to ask include the following:
   - What human services are available within the community to meet the community's health needs?
   - Are services adequate and sufficiently accessible to meet the community's needs, or are services available only to a certain segment of the population, such as persons who can afford to pay or who have transportation?
   - Are the human services responsive to the needs of the community?
2. *Money.* What is the budget? How does the community get its money? How is revenue generated from within the community? What are the fund-raising activities? For what is the money spent?
3. *Facilities, equipment, and goods.* What health care facilities (e.g., hospitals, clinics, home health agencies, nursing homes, daycare centers) are available within the community? How are they used? Are they accessible, appropriate, and adequate for the population in the community? Does the facility have the equipment and supplies it needs to produce its goods? What does it produce? What is its contribution to the larger society? For example, is this a high-technology geopolitical community that supplies research and development, or is it a phenomenological community, such as Mothers Against Drunk Driving (MADD), that provides support to its members and information to the larger suprasystem? These are examples of positive production (resources). Producing a negative effect on the larger society is possible for a community. For example, a community with many drug abusers may produce a negative effect (demand) on the system and the suprasystem. A community with many illegal drug users will require more health services and put greater demand on health facilities than would a community with fewer drug users.

4. *Education.* Education assists people in learning how to function productively in society so it is included in this subsystem. How are the members educated? In a geopolitical community, we can examine the numbers and types of schools, as well as the level of education. In a phenomenological community, we examine the needs for education of the group and what types of education are taking place. For example, what education is being provided to pregnant adolescents about their pregnancy?

In addition to assessing these factors, we need to begin to analyze the findings. Are the resources and assets outweighing the demands? Are the finances, services, facilities, and education appropriate, accessible, and adequate to members of the community? What is the ratio of demands to resources and assets?

Polity. Polity is the politics of a community. *The goal of polity is coordination, control, and direction of activities to maintain the community and attain the system goals.* The formal government, as well as informal leadership, serves these functions. The polity subsystem of a community provides organizational structure, leadership, decision making, and social control to its members in return for members' compliance and support.

1. *Organizational structure.* The organizational structure represents the way in which a population group has organized to facilitate collective action and to exert some control over its collective behavior. An organizational chart of a community will provide information about how the community is organized, its formal leadership positions, and its decision-making process. How is the community organized? Is it an incorporated city with a mayor and city council? Is it a charter government? Is it a volunteer group with no elected leaders?
2. *Leadership.* Both formal and informal leadership are present in any group; identifying both types is important. Who are the formal leaders? Formal leaders may be elected or appointed; they have the authority in decision making, but informal leaders often have the power. To effect any kind of change, a thorough understanding is needed of both the formal and the informal leadership dynamics. For example, if a strong leader pattern prevails, attention should be placed on reaching and convincing the leaders before any attempt is made to contact the **target population** (i.e., the population in which change is desired).
3. *Decision making or problem solving.* Finding out how the community approaches its problems and its pattern of decision making is important. To effect any type of change, the individual must know not only whom to approach, but also how the community has acted in the past to solve its problems. What is the decision-making process? Who have been the key decision makers for health issues? How have problems been approached and solved in the past? What problem-solving approaches have not worked in the past? Answers to these questions will provide a basis for determining the action pattern of the community and how capable it will be at solving its problems (Freeman & Heinrich, 1981); they will also give the nurse a clue as to what role is necessary in planning health programs. A community that is relatively competent may be quite independent and function with a minimal amount of assistance from the nurse. A dependent community may need the nurse to take a more active and direct role in developing leadership skills of community members.

4. *Social control.* Social control refers to the rules and norms of a community that affect behavior. The rules in a geopolitical community usually refer to local laws or control measures, often enforced through police, sheriffs, law agencies, courts, and the government; examples include curfews, speed limits, and "blue laws" governing the sale of alcohol. In a phenomenological community, the rules are the control enforced by bylaws, policies, and procedures. The norms in a geopolitical community are social sanctions enforced by the members of the neighborhood and by institutions such as the schools and faith communities, whereas in a phenomenological community, the group (e.g., peer pressure among adolescents) enforces the norms.

Communication. The goal of the communication subsystem is to provide identity and support to its members—that is, to provide a sense of belonging. People in the community offer group participation in exchange for support and identity from the community.

The communication subsystem includes the many affective relationships that exist among community members. These relationships provide the emotional tone of the community. Emotional tone is communicated through nonverbal and verbal communication.

1. *Nonverbal communication.* What personality or emotional tone is communicated to you when you visit the community? Does it feel warm and inviting? Does it feel cold and hostile? How do members describe their community? What are the nonverbal messages that the community communicates to the external environment and among community members? How are strangers and newcomers treated?
2. *Verbal communication.* Who communicates with whom? Is communication horizontal (egalitarian) or vertical (hierarchical)? How is communication achieved (e.g., by newspaper, television, radio, newsletters, posters, fliers, person-to-person communication, informal gatherings, formal meetings)? What is the focus of the communication? Is it "business" or goal directed, social, or a combination? When does the communication occur?

Values. *The goal of the values subsystem is to provide guidelines for behavior.* This component addresses the general orienting principles that guide the socialization and behavior of members of the community. Community members accept and conform to the standards of the community in return for approval. Important to examine are patterns of behavior that reflect values, beliefs, standards, culture, and ethnic background (see Chapter 10) because these patterns help determine the health action pattern of the community. The patterns of behavior that are examined include traditions, presence of identifiable subgroups, aesthetics and environment, health, and homogeneity of the group.

1. *Traditions.* Some communities are steeped in tradition, and others have few traditions. Traditions often reflect the ethnic background of a community's members and can also vary with the age of the community. A new, young community may have no or only a few traditions, whereas an older community may have many long-standing traditions. The celebration of traditions often provides a sense of identity to a community's members and stability to the community. In considering the impact of traditions, a nurse may need to address the following questions: Are traditional ways followed, or is individuality stressed? Are kinship bonds

strong, or is each individual expected to cope with his or her own problems? What traditions are upheld? How are they celebrated?

2. *Subgroups.* Subgroups may be present within a community. For example, subgroups may exist based on ethnic or racial identity, social class, and age of community members. These identifiable subgroups have their own values, customs, problems, and strengths.

3. *Aesthetics and environment.* Observation of the environment can tell you a lot about what the people value. That is, do they value clean, tidy environments that are pleasing to the eye? Is the environment in decay or disrepair, showing little or no evidence of attention to aesthetics (because the focus is on survival and basic life support instead)?

4. *Health.* People vary with regard to the value and priority they place on health. To assess needs and plan health care, nurses must know what the community values in the way of health. Even though health care professionals value preventive health, a given community may not. The people in the community may have some very different ideas about what they want in a health program. If health care professionals do not consider the community's needs and values, then health care programs will not be effective. Therefore it is important to answer questions such as the following: What types of health facilities are used? How often are they used? What are the attitudes about health, health care, and health care professionals? What priority do members place on health? How do community members define health? (See Chapter 18.)

5. *Homogeneity.* Is the community homogeneous or heterogeneous in its beliefs and values? Communities may be very similar in their values or very diverse. The level of homo- or heterogeneity influences the community health nurse when planning care. In more heterogeneous communities, interventions need to be tailored to the various and different subgroups and populations.

Outcomes (Health Behavior, Health Status, Community Competence)

Outcomes include measurable, *health-related behaviors* and *health status* of the populations in the community. Outcomes also include *community competence.* Outcomes influence the community and its suprasystem(s). The health status of the community includes two interrelated factors: people and environment. Identifying trends in health behavior and health status over time, rather than simply looking at health behaviors at one point in time, gives a clearer picture of health outcomes. We will look first at people factors and then at environmental factors.

People Factors. The people factors that the community health nurse needs to investigate include general trends, trends in mortality (death) and morbidity (illness), the presence of vulnerable groups or aggregates with at-risk behaviors, the prevalence of presymptomatic illness, and the level of social functioning. All of these factors impact or reflect the health status of a community.

1. *Growth trends.* The stability and growth of the community have implications for health and health planning. Therefore the nurse must examine the current size of the community and compare it with its original size or size at a particular point in time. Is the community growing or decreasing in size? What is the relationship between the birth and death rates (geopolitical community)? What is the relationship between immigration and emigration? What are the changes in demographic characteristics? Is the community becoming a younger or an older population, or staying the same? How mobile is the population?

2. *Trends in mortality and morbidity.* Trends in mortality and morbidity are indicators of a community's health status (see Chapter 7). The medical cause of death is a valuable indicator. For example, a high infant mortality rate may reflect evidence of inattention to or lack of value for preventive health care and identifies a need to provide preventive prenatal health services. However, medical cause of death alone may be inadequate because the cause of disease may be related to personal or social phenomena. For example, extreme poverty is a social condition that contributes to the cause of death. In the example just given, the high infant mortality rate may be caused by a combination of inadequate preventive health services and malnutrition related to poverty. Epidemiologic questions the community health nurse will want to address are the following: What are the trends related to death and illness? What is the mortality rate? What are the major causes of death? What major diseases are present in the population? What is the prevalence or incidence of diseases?

3. *Mortality.* Consider the number of deaths, age-specific rates of death, and the major causes of death in the community. If working with a geopolitical community, this information can be obtained from local and state vital statistics and health departments. Additionally, the *Morbidity and Mortality Weekly Report,* published by the Centers for Disease Control and Prevention, is available at libraries, by subscription, and on-line.

4. *Morbidity.* The nurse must know what diseases and conditions are present in a community and their incidence and prevalence. For a geopolitical community, these data can be obtained by reviewing statistics collected officially. In a phenomenological community, the nurse would need to collect data by surveying records, preparing questionnaires, or arranging interviews. In the United States, morbidity data are not systematically collected and are therefore sketchy and inadequate in scope.

5. *Vulnerable aggregates and risky behavior.* Is the **population "at risk"** of developing certain health conditions or problems? What risky or vulnerable types of behavior are present in this community? Groups may exist within a geopolitical community who do not have a disease or condition that requires medical care but do have a personal or social condition that makes them unusually susceptible or lowers their ability to deal with disease or disability (see Chapter 21). Examples include the homeless, people living below the poverty level, multiproblem families, and malnourished and pregnant adolescents. Risky behaviors include those that place people at risk for disease. For example, intravenous drug use is a risky behavior associated with the human immunodeficiency virus (HIV); cigarette smoking increases the risk of lung cancer; and driving without a seat belt is associated with vehicular trauma.

6. *Prevalence of presymptomatic illness.* What is the prevalence of presymptomatic illness in a community? Although precise data on the prevalence of a presymptomatic illness

are difficult to obtain, estimates based on special surveys or screening programs can be made (see Chapter 19). Some examples of presymptomatic illness are increased blood pressure, increased blood cholesterol level, and seropositive HIV individuals.

7. *Level of social functioning.* What is the level of social functioning in a community? The level of social functioning refers to the quality of life and the relationship of dependency to independency in a community. If a large number of people are dependent on a small number for support or help, the demand on the community for resources is much greater than if the proportion is balanced. People may be dependent for a variety of reasons, such as age, lack of finances, illness, or disability. For example, a community that has a high preponderance of elderly individuals will need more health facilities and services because of the increased medical needs of that age group. As you learned in Chapter 7, ratios are used to show relationships. A dependency ratio shows the proportion of dependents to independents. An example of a dependency ratio is shown as follows:

Dependency ratio =

$$\frac{\text{Population under} <18 \text{ years} + \text{population} >65 \text{ years}}{\text{Population of persons between 18 and 65 years}}$$

For example, Elmhurst has a population of 6784 people. According to the census information, 1604 people under the age of 18 and 2422 people over the age of 65 live in the area. To calculate the dependency ratio:

$$\frac{1604 \text{ (under 18)} + 2422 \text{ (over 65)}}{2758} = 1.45$$

This ratio means that there are almost 1.5 dependent persons for each person considered to be able to care for others.

8. *Disabilities and impairments.* Are disabilities or impairments present? These disabilities or impairments can be physical or emotional. People with impairments or disabilities require special care from the community (see Chapter 26). Therefore the nurse must identify numbers of people and types of impairments or disabilities so as to identify whether their needs are being met by the community or further services are necessary.

Environmental Factors. Environmental factors include the physical and the social environment. Indicators of the health status of the physical environment include the air, food, and water quality; the adequacy of housing; and the quality of home, school, and work sites (see Chapter 9). Solid waste disposal and hazardous waste disposal are also relevant.

Indicators of the health status of the social environment include the emotional tone of the community, the stability of the population (an extremely mobile population or rapid turnover of members in either a geopolitical or a phenomenological community can be a measure of dissatisfaction and instability within the community), levels of violence, and the reported quality of life in the community. The quality of life may include personal satisfaction with the community, as well as the measures of community competence previously discussed in this chapter.

Feedback

Feedback may be internal or external. Internal feedback is information from within the community that helps the community monitor its functioning. For example, if the city council or township receives information that tax revenues are lower than projected, the community may need to modify its budget and reduce spending.

External feedback is information from the suprasystem and larger environment about a community's functioning. This type of information provides an opportunity for the community to modify itself, adapt to changing environmental conditions, and negotiate interchanges with its environment. For example, community health nurses within a local health department may receive information about new state regulations that require directly observed medication therapy for persons with newly diagnosed tuberculosis. This information would necessitate that the nurses institute these services. Dialogue between nurses in the local and state health departments and with community members would help determine realistic ways to initiate such services. In this case, feedback from the suprasystem mandates that the community institute new services in response to changing regulations.

TOOLS FOR DATA COLLECTION

Community health nurses can use a systems-analysis framework to guide data collection for a community assessment. Where does the nurse go to collect all of these data? What tools are needed? Figure 15-7 identifies many of the data sources used to assess a community. An important tool is the use of self, particularly your senses. Of course, an automobile or other means of travel, a map, and a few resource materials are also helpful.

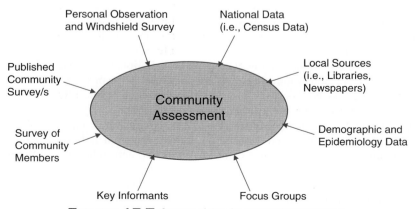

FIGURE 15-7 Sources of data for community assessment.

PERSONAL OBSERVATION

Use your eyes, ears, nose, hands, and body to *inspect, auscultate, palpate,* and *percuss* the community. You can tell a lot about a community just by using your own senses.

- *Eyes.* What do you see? Describe the people, what they are doing, and the environment.
- *Nose.* Smell the environment. Is it pleasant, polluted, fresh, or stale?
- *Ears.* Is the community noisy or quiet? Are the people talking to one another?
- *Palpate and percuss.* What is the feeling of the community? Is it warm, open, and friendly, or is it cold, hostile, and suspicious?

Be alert and collect data at every opportunity. A simple drive through the community, called a windshield survey, provides an opportunity to observe, listen, and collect information provided in the guide. **Website Resource 15C** provides a guide for collecting data in a *windshield survey.* During your visit to the community, talk to the people—the community members and leaders, health care professionals, clergy, real estate agents, and business people. These individuals can tell you a lot about the community. Read about the community in newspapers, literature, or printed materials distributed by the community or by other organizations. Look for bulletin boards, kiosks, information centers, or cable television programs in which community activities and information are posted.

EXISTING DATA SOURCES: SECONDARY DATA
National Sources

Many sources of demographic and epidemiologic data already collected can be used and are often available on the Internet. The National Center for Health Statistics, a federal agency established to collect and disseminate data about the health of U.S. residents, conducts the National Health Interview Survey. Many other agencies and organizations collect data on specific diseases, conditions, or aggregates. Box 15-5 lists some of these data sources. *The United States Government Manual,* available from the U.S. Government Printing Office in Washington, DC, is a good reference for information about federal programs and agencies that have health data. Most states have at least one library designated as a depository for federal publications. Your local librarian can refer you to the nearest depository.

The U.S. Bureau of the Census collects information on the demographic characteristics (age, gender, race, ethnicity, socioeconomic level, marital status, educational level, and housing) of the U.S. population every 10 years. Although these data are valuable, if you are using 2000 data in the year 2009, the data may need to be supplemented with other, more current data. State and local planning offices use a variety of statistical methods to estimate the size of populations between censuses. The census data are helpful for viewing patterns over time to identify trends. Census tract information is available in the reference section in some libraries, in local and state health departments, and on-line.

Many special interest groups collect and publish data about their particular group. For example, the American Heart Association, the American Lung Association, and MADD have publications that provide useful information about their respective topic and the aggregate characteristics.

Longitudinal research is being done with large populations in several areas of the United States. Although these populations are not national samples, they are large community samples that allow conclusions to be made about demographic risk factors and the long-term effects of various health-related behaviors on morbidity and mortality. Schools of public health are conducting longitudinal epidemiologic studies in several communities, including Alameda, California; Evans County, Georgia; Framingham, Massachusetts; and Ypsilanti, Michigan. Findings appear in health research and professional journals.

State and Local Sources

Chapter 7 defines vital and demographic data. Local and state health departments collect and disseminate information about the vital statistics in their localities. County and city planning and zoning boards often have current demographic data and a list of many resources. Health departments, agency records, libraries, business people, clergy, telephone books, and service directories are additional sources of information.

Many local areas publish a community resource guide that includes resources within a given geographic area. These books are often written in an annotated bibliographic format and are valuable resources to a community health nurse. Check with the health department or the health and welfare council in your area to see if one is available.

SURVEYS

If you cannot locate sources of data for the community under study, you may need to develop a survey to obtain needed information. This alternative is especially true when working with segments of a geopolitical community in which the only data available may be for a larger area that includes the community segment under study. Surveys are also needed in a geopolitical community when different, more specific information is desired. In a phenomenological community, developing data collection tools may be necessary because data may not be available.

Surveys include a series of questions that the investigator asks to obtain information from individuals within a population. Questions help describe the prevalence, distribution, and interrelationships of health and illness conditions, beliefs, attitudes, knowledge, or health-related behaviors within a population (Polit & Hungler, 2005). Ideally, surveys should be written in the primary language of the persons being surveyed.

The purpose of a survey might be to collect demographic data, obtain information on assets and problems, conduct a needs assessment, identify utilization patterns of services and facilities, or determine health interests of community members. The survey may be written or verbal. Written surveys can be mailed or conducted on a person-to-person basis. Low return rates and the cost of mailing are the major disadvantages of mailed surveys. Interviews or questionnaires often yield additional valuable information because direct contact can be made with community members. However, surveys, whether done by mail, face-to-face, or on the telephone, are time consuming.

If communities have small populations, surveying the entire population is best. When surveying the entire population is impractical because of time, cost, or difficulty reaching the community members, random sampling of the community is recommended (Polit & Hungler, 2005). Random sampling allows the results from the sample to be generalized to the entire population.

Box 15-5   Sample Sources of Health and Population Data*

Public Health Service, Centers for Disease Control and Prevention

Website: *www.cdc.gov*
Morbidity and Mortality Weekly Report (MMWR)

Publishes provisional and summary data on reportable infectious diseases and other health concerns by state. Reports include special topics of health concerns related to trends, control, or treatment recommendations and other health-related discussions. *MMWR* is available by subscription and can also be found at local or state health departments and in some libraries.

National Center for Health Statistics, Hyattsville, MD

Website: *www.cdc.gov/nchswww/index.htm*
Vital and Health Statistics Series

For community/public health nursing practice (series are periodically updated with new volume numbers):

Series 5, Comparative International Vital and Health Statistics. Compares U.S. vital and health statistics with other countries.

Series 10, Data from the National Health Interview Survey. A continuing national household interview survey that reports on illness; accidental injuries; disability; mental health and substance use; the use of hospital, medical, dental, and other services; as well as other health-related topics. Examples:

No. 233, Current estimates from the National Health Interview Survey, 2005 (January 2007). Includes incidence of acute conditions and episodes of persons injured, disability days, physician contacts, prevalence of chronic conditions, limitation of activity, and self-assessed health status. Data estimates are reported by subgroups of population, including by age, gender, race, income, and geographic region. This publication is updated yearly.

No. 230, Health Behaviors of Adults: United States, 2002-2004 (September 2006).

No. 321, Summary of health statistics for U.S. children (December 2006).

No. 232, Summary of health statistics for U.S. adults (December 2006).

Series 11, Data from the National Health Examination Survey and the National Health and Nutrition Examination Survey. Data collected by direct examination, testing, and measurement of national samples of population are the basis for estimates of prevalence of specific diseases and their distribution in the U.S. population with respect to physical, physiologic, and psychologic characteristics. This series has infrequent publications. Examples:

No. 248, Trends in oral health status: United States, 1988-1994 and 1999-2004. Published April 2007.

No. 245, Dietary intake of macronutrients, mircronutrients, and other dietary constituents: United States, 1988-1994. Published July 2002.

Series 13, Data on utilization of health manpower and facilities providing long-term care, hospital care, and family planning services. Examples:

No. 164, Characteristics of office-based physicians and their practices: United States, 2003-2004. Published January 2007.

No. 162, National hospital discharge survey: 2004 annual summary with detailed diagnosis and procedure data. Published October 2006.

For advanced practice and nursing researchers:

Series 1, reports describe general programs of the National Center for Health Statistics, its offices and divisions, and the data collection methods used. Reports include questionnaires, surveys, sampling, and other data collection techniques. Example:

No. 44, An introduction to the national nursing assistance survey. Published March 2007.

Series 2, studies new statistical methodology, reports on data evaluation and methods research. Example:

No. 143, Assessing the potential of national strategies for electronic health records for population health monitoring and research. Published January 2006.

Series 4, documents and committee reports, presents the final reports of major committees concerned with vital and health statisitics and documents such as the *Report on Recommended Model Vital Registration Law.*

Series 15, statistics on health and health-related topics not part of the continuing data system for the National Center for Health Statistics. Example:

No. 3, Summary statistics from the National Survey of Early Childhood Health, 2000. Published June 2002.

Series 20, data on mortality.

Series 21, data on natality, marriage, and divorce.

Advance Data from Vital and Health Statistics

Special reports concentrating on a specific health issue or topic. Examples:

No. 389, National Hospital Ambulatory Medical Care Survey: 2005 Outpatient Department Summary. Published June 29, 2007.

No. 343, Complementary and alternative medicine use among adults: United States, 2002. Published May 27, 2004.

Health, United States

Annual report presented to the President and Congress. In 2006 the report entitled *Health, United States, 2006* highlighted the current status of national health.

Bureau of the Census, Department of Commerce, Washington, DC

Website: *www.census.gov*
Statistical Abstract of the United States

Compiles detailed statistics at the city, county, state, and national levels on births, marriages, divorces, and deaths. Available on-line or selected statistics published in book form approximately 2 years after the reporting year ends.

National Vital Statistics Report

Provides provisional up-to-date tallies on births, marriages, divorces, and deaths on a monthly basis. Data are usually published 3 to 5 months after data are gathered.

Current Population Reports

Series are periodically updated with new volume numbers.

Current Population Reports, Series P-25

Reports on population estimates and projections with local, state, and national summaries. Example:

P25-1135, *Domestic net migration in the United States: 2000 to 2004.* Published April 2006.

Current Population Reports Series P-23, Special Studies

Provides a wide range of sample survey and census data on demographic, social, and economic trends in the foreign-born population of the United States. Examples:

P23-209, *65+ in the United States: 2005.* Published December 2005.

P23-208, *Computers and Internet use in the United States: 2003.* Published October 2005.

P23-211, *The older foreign born population in the United States: 2000.* Published September 2002.

Current Population Reports, Series P20

---

*Most states have at least one library designated as a depository for government publications. Your local librarian can refer you to the nearest depository.

Continued

BOX 15-5 Sample Sources of Health and Population Data—cont'd

Reports of population characteristics for subgroups of the population. Examples:

P20-555, *Fertility of American women: June 2004.* Published December 2005.

P20-553, *America's families and living arrangements: 2003.* Published November 2004.

P20-545, *The Hispanic population in the United States: March 2002.* Published June 2003.

Current Population Reports, Series P-60

Reports on consumer income issues. Examples:

P-60-232, *Income, poverty, and health insurance coverage in the United States: 2006.* Published August 2007.

P60-232, *The effects of taxes and transfers on income and poverty in the United States: 2006.* Published March 2006.

Governmental Accounting Office

Website: *www.gao.gov*

Develops and publishes reports requested by all branches of the federal government, including health-related issues. Usually reports are done in response to policy issue. Example: Problems remain in planning for and providing health screening and monitory services for responders (GAO-07-1253T). Published September 20, 2007.

Congressional Budget Office

Website: *www.cbo.gov*

Develops and publishes studies requested by members of Congress on policy issues including health issues. Example: CBO Testimony before the Committee of the Budget, U.S. Senate: Health care and the budget: Issues and challenges for reform. Testimony given June 21, 2007.

Centers for Mental Health Services, Substance Abuse, and Mental Health Services Administration

Performs targeted sample surveys on mental health and addictions. Surveys are also done on specialty mental health organizations every 2 years.

U.S. Department of Justice, Bureau of Justice Statistics

Performs national crime victimization survey that samples households for crime incidents, victims, and trends in violence and crime.

Occupational Safety and Health Administration

Concerned with workplace safety. Conducts workplace safety inspections and issues regulations regarding workplace safety procedures.

U.S. Environmental Protection Agency

Collects data on airborne and water pollution via 4000 stations nationwide. Has reporting systems that track water and waste discharge and toxic chemical releases.

In one urban city, nurses who were interested in determining the dietary habits of middle-school children used a survey approach. A food habits questionnaire was distributed to 223 sixth-, seventh-, and eighth-grade students (Frenn & Molin, 2003). Surveys were distributed during science class after parental approval was obtained. Of the 223 targeted students, only 2 did not complete the survey.

Whenever you develop a tool or survey, be sure to first perform a pilot study with a small sample of a similar population. That is, if you are planning to survey elementary school children, have five or six children of the same age complete the survey. The pilot study helps determine whether the survey was tailored to the characteristics of the study population with respect to reading level and the time needed to complete it. In addition, the pilot study can help illuminate any ambiguous or confusing directions or whether any questions are asked that allow different interpretations.

Either the survey format or specific questions might need to be altered based on the results of the pilot study. Directions may need to be clarified, the time allowed may need to be lengthened, or the survey itself may need to be shortened. Questions may need to be modified to reduce confusion or to obtain more detailed information.

When conducting a knowledge survey, knowing if the pilot group can answer all or most of the questions without a health intervention would be helpful. For example, if you were planning a health-education program on safety and found that the pilot group was able to correctly answer most of the questions, the value of proceeding with your intervention as initially designed would be in question. You might conclude that no knowledge deficit really exists or that you need to increase the sophistication of the material to be taught.

INTERVIEWS WITH KEY INFORMANTS

Interviews with *key informants*—people in the community and leaders of the community—are valuable sources of data. These interviews and conversations can provide focus, as well as a great deal of information. The community health nurse should use every opportunity to interact with the people in the community. These individuals are the richest sources of information about their health status, interests, community problems and strengths, and possible solutions.

Interviews may be open ended in which the interviewer starts by asking a few broad questions. Interviews also may be highly structured, using formal surveys. To prevent misunderstandings, interviews should be conducted in the primary language of the persons who are being interviewed. When using the primary language is not possible, bilingual interviewers or translators will be needed.

Vulnerable populations can be targeted for interviews. For example, in preparation for developing an intervention program to target the prevention of sexually transmitted diseases, Van Devanter and colleagues (2002) interviewed an aggregate of adolescents and young adults. The goal was to assess the youths' use and access to health care services. Interviews revealed that the youths had limited use and access to preventive health care. The authors designed their intervention program with this information in mind. Similar assessments can be conducted with the chronically mentally ill, elderly, disabled, or formerly homeless living in other communities.

MEETINGS WITH COMMUNITY GROUPS

Community forums are regular or special public meetings that provide an opportunity to obtain input from members of the community regarding their opinions about needs, services, or specific health-related topics. Forums can be open to the entire community, or they can focus on a small segment or subgroup of the community. Town meetings are one example of a community forum. The advantage of the forum approach is that it is a relatively cost-efficient and cost-effective way of obtaining opinion data from the community.

Focus groups are conversations held in a group with a small number of people (usually 6 to 12) to identify different perceptions and viewpoints about a subject (Gillis & Jackson, 2002). Focus groups are usually held with more than one group to identify patterns in perception. For example, focus groups might be held in a community early in the assessment process to identify patterns or themes regarding perceived community strengths and health problems.

Focus groups can be used to include vulnerable and previously underserved members of a community to understand their health problems and strengths and to identify possible culturally competent interventions. A health educator describes the process of using a community network strategy in a Midwestern state to identify needed and culturally appropriate health services for underserved Korean immigrants (Kim et al., 2002). Four different resource groups participated, including representatives of the Korean community, Korean health professionals, and representatives for the targeted population of low-income Korean immigrants. To succeed, the authors used group participants to (1) identify an appropriate service site accessible to the target population, (2) identify appropriate communication strategies to inform the target group of available services, and (3) identify the mental health needs of the target population, as well as barriers to seeking mental health services. In another example, in focus group conversations with women in abusive relationships, nurses were able to identify facts that inhibit, support, or sustain a woman's ability to leave and stay out of an abusive relationship (Lutenbacher et al., 2003).

As you can see, many types of data collection can be used. Only a few examples have been described here. Table 15-2 summarizes the pros and cons of various methods of data collection.

GEOGRAPHIC INFORMATION SYSTEMS

Geographic information systems are computer-based programs used to store and statistically manipulate geographic and location-based data to provide visual maps. Traditionally, public health professionals plotted communicable disease outbreaks on wall maps; these could be overlaid with transparent sheets to show changes in cases over time. Computers allow multiple data to be overlaid. Data can include demographics, morbidity and mortality, cases of communicable diseases, reported health behaviors, housing types, distribution of health facilities and services, and sources of environmental exposures, among others. This assists public health practitioners to analyze health disparities, disease outbreaks, availability and use of resources, and the relationship of environmental exposures with health problems (Choi et al., 2006; Riner et al., 2004). This expanded analysis fosters improved health planning and evaluation.

One *Healthy People 2010* objective advocates for expanded development and use of GIS in the public health infrastructure. Several metropolitan areas, such as Indianapolis, have publicly accessible GIS data as do several cities coordinated by the Urban Institute (Riner et al., 2004) (see **Website Resources 15D** and **15E** for additional information about GIS).

TABLE 15-2	Pros and Cons of Data Collection Methods	
Data Collection Method	**Pros**	**Cons**
Surveys written	Reliable	Low return rate; costly (i.e., mailing and printing costs)
Verbal (person to person or by telephone)	Good return rate; participants may provide additional information that is valuable.	Time consuming
Interview of key informants	Inexpensive: valuable subjective data that may be difficult to obtain on written survey.	Biased view
Community forums	Provide opportunity for wide variety of community members to supply input on wide range of topics regarding community; may find an otherwise unidentified need.	May be difficult to keep the forum from becoming a grievance or gripe session
Census tract data	Readily available; show trends over time	Collected only every 10 years
Preexisting reports and publications	Readily available; show trends over time	May not include data for specific community being assessed by nurse

APPROACHES TO COMMUNITY ASSESSMENT

Just as assessment of the individual or family can be approached in a variety of ways, so also can assessment of the community be approached in several ways. The approach taken depends on the type of community and the reason for the assessment.

COMPREHENSIVE NEEDS ASSESSMENT APPROACH

As the name implies, the comprehensive needs assessment is the most thorough assessment of the community; it is also the most traditional and the most time consuming. In the comprehensive approach, the nurse begins with the total community (geopolitical or phenomenological) and uses a systematic process to assess all aspects of the community to identify or validate actual and potential health problems.

In a previous cited example, Kim and colleagues (2002) describe the comprehensive process nurses used in conducting an assessment among Chicago area Korean immigrants to determine what culturally appropriate health education and services were needed. First, interviews with selected Korean community leaders were conducted and then interviews with selected health and social services providers. Next, focus groups of the targeted Korean immigrant were conducted. Periodic assessments and reevaluations were conducted over the 4-year development phase for this bilingual, interdisciplinary project.

PROBLEM-ORIENTED APPROACH

In the problem-oriented approach, the community/public health nurse assesses a community in relation to a specific topic or health problem. The nurse begins the process with the problem or topic area and then assesses a specific community in relation to that subject.

A group of nursing students was interested in AIDS. The group's community/public health clinical course expected the students to plan and implement a community-oriented health project. Because the students were interested in AIDS, they decided to do an AIDS-related project (the problem). The literature review identified potential communities in which AIDS was a serious problem.

Potential aggregates for intervention included intravenous drug abusers or sexually active homosexuals. The literature also identified the need for health-promotion and illness-prevention programs for sexually active adolescents and female sexual partners of intravenous drug users. The students chose an adolescent population of eleventh graders and assessed the population in relation to the topic. As a result of a survey, the students determined that a knowledge deficit regarding HIV transmission existed, and a primary prevention program was developed.

In another community, in response to local concerns about the health needs of older adults, a community assessment of Escalante, Arizona, was completed. The assessment led to the development of a multifaceted intervention model designed to improve and maintain the functional health of community seniors (Nunez et al., 2003). The Escalante Health Partnership has a two-pronged intervention approach. First, community resources such as city officials, hospitals, community leaders, and health professionals were targeted to expand the coalition so as to increase participation and expand services to seniors. Second, community seniors were targeted with the intent of reducing disease and disability in this vulnerable population.

SINGLE POPULATION APPROACH

Some community/public health nurses may be employed by a health department or a nonprofit organization to work with a single population. In the single population approach, the community/public health nurse assesses one population in a community (e.g., women of reproductive age, teenagers, homeless, migrants). The nurse begins the process with defining the population and then assesses the population in a specific community. Often the population has already been determined to be an especially vulnerable one. The process of assessment is the same, but more narrow in scope because it focuses on one population. Data and literature are collected related to the health behaviors and health status of the specific population.

The Farm Worker Family Health Program (FWFHP) is a 13-year-old partnership that serves migrant farm workers (a single population). The partnership is comprised of five colleges and universities, a federally funded farm worker health clinic, the local school system, and area health education centers (AHEC) (Connor et al., 2007). The purpose of the partnership is to increase the delivery of health care services to migrant farm workers and their family members. An urban school of nursing coordinates the partnership in the southeast United States. Undergraduate nursing students and nurse practitioner students work with students from other professional schools to supplement services of the clinic and the summer school for children of migrant families.

FAMILIARIZATION APPROACH

Familiarization involves studying data already available about a community (e.g., census tract data, surveys, and other official data from the health departments). This approach helps the community/public health nurse focus on special populations (aggregates or groups) that have similar characteristics and may have health needs. Table 15-3 provides examples of census tract data to be used in the geopolitical case study at the end of the chapter. Information from these data indicated that many children and adolescents lived in this census tract. Having identified the youth as a target population, the community health nurse would focus the assessment on this aggregate.

Peterson and colleagues (2002) describe using secondary data sources to document the health-promotion needs of church attendees. Demographic data from the *National Vital and Morbidity Statistics,* the task force of the *National Institutes of Health Women's Health Research Agenda,* and the *Healthy People 2010 National Health Objectives* were used to support the need for a midlife women's health-promotion program designed to increase physical activity and reduce risk of cardiovascular disease.

ANALYSIS

The areas of consideration for data analysis include community assets, major problems, major health-related problems, current and proposed community action for problem resolution, and the community's pattern of action involving past problems.

When applying a systems analysis to the data, three parameters are used to make inferences about the level of health:

- Congruency must exist among the physical, psychological, and social data and imperatives.
- The community requires a minimum amount of energy to function (efficiency).
- The health status behaviors must be satisfying to the population and the community (University of Maryland School of Nursing, 1975).

Physical imperatives include safe air, food, and water. Nonabusive interpersonal relationships are an example of a psychosocial imperative. For an example of efficiency, consider communities X and Y. Both have similar health behavior trends regarding the incidence of heart disease in their communities. However, the average length of hospital stay in community X and the cost of treatment are 20% higher than those in community Y. From these data, the nurse can infer that community X is not operating as efficiently as community Y. Similarly, a community may appear to have an acceptable level of health, but community members may express dissatisfaction about the way they are treated at health care facilities. From these data, the nurse can infer that the community is not functioning up to its capacity because it is not meeting one of the parameters.

Through analysis of the relationships between the component parts of a community system and its external environment

TABLE 15-3   2000 Census Tract Data for Census Tract 1 in City X (to Use with The Nursing Process in Practice: A Geopolitical Community)

	Number	Percentage*		Number	Percentage*
I. Population statistics	7924		Native of foreign country or mixed	82	1.0
A. Total population			Foreign born	4	0.1
B. General characteristics			2. School enrollment	3785	
1. Race			Elementary	2544	67.2
White	8	0.1	High school	834	22.0
Black	7899	99.7	College	108	2.9
2. Age (years) by sex			3. Years of school completed		
Male			Persons 25 and over	2217	
Total	3408	43.0	No school completed	50	2.3
Under 5	548	6.9	Elementary, 1-4	194	8.8
5-9	743	9.4	Elementary, 5-7	531	24.0
10-19	1280	16.2	Elementary, 8	333	15.0
20-34	401	5.1	High school, 1-3	615	27.7
35-54	293	3.7	High school, 4	427	19.3
55-64	89	1.1	College, 1-3	47	2.1
65-74	33	0.4	College, 4 or more	20	0.9
75 and above	21	0.3	Median school years completed	9	
Female			4. Mobility of residents, 1985-1990		
Total	4516	57.0	Same house	3791	50.1
Under 5	522	6.6	Different house		
5-9	782	9.9	Central city	1744	22.0
10-19	1323	16.7	Other part of SMSA	72	0.9
20-34	930	11.7	Outside SMSA	20	0.3
35-54	701	8.8	Abroad	11	0.1
55-64	140	1.8	Unknown	2116	26.7
65-74	80	1.0	5. Means of transportation and place of work		
75 and above	41	0.5	Total number of workers	1620	
3. Persons per household	Mean = 4.48		a. Transportation		
4. Type of family			Private auto (driver)	234	20.6
Total number of families	1586		Private auto (passenger)	245	15.1
Families with children under 18	1363	85.9	Bus	931	57.5
Husband-wife families	471	29.7	Subway, train	0	0
Families with other male head	42	2.6	Walk	102	6.3
Families with female head	1002	63.2	Work at home	0	0
5. Marital status			Other	8	0.5
Male			b. Place of work		
Total (over 14)	1502		Inside SMSA	1149	70.9
Single	878	58.4	City X central business district	118	7.3
Married	543	36.2	Remainder of City X	874	54.0
Separated	39	2.6	Surrounding counties	156	9.6
Widowed	31	2.1	Outside SMSA	14	0.9
Divorced	11	0.7	Not reported	457	28.2
Female			D. Labor force characteristics		
Total (over 14)	2577		1. Employment status		
Single	1036	40.2	Male		
Married	572	22.2	Age 16 and over	1285	
Separated	582	22.6	In labor force	832	64.7
Widowed	246	9.6	Female		
Divorced	141	5.5	Age 16 and over	2334	
C. Social characteristics			In labor force	938	40.2
1. Nativity, parentage, and country of origin					
All persons	7924				
Native of United States	7838	98.9			

*Numbers may not add up to 100% because of rounding or missing data.

SMSA, Standard Metropolitan Statistical Area.

Continued

TABLE 15-3   2000 Census Tract Data for Census Tract 1 in City X (to Use with The Nursing Process in Practice: A Geopolitical Community)—cont'd

	Number	Percentage		Number	Rate per 100,000
2. Occupation			III. Vital statistics		
Total employed	1596		A. Births		
(age 16 and over)			Total live births	140	18
Professional, technical, and	90	5.6	Neonatal deaths (before 28 days	3	21.4
kindred workers			of age)		
Managers and administrators	37	2.3	Infant deaths (before 1 year of	2	14.2
Sales workers	75	4.7	age)		
Clerical and kindred workers	260	16.3	Premature single live births	20	3
Craftsmen, foremen, and	136	8.5	Single live births	140	18
kindred workers			Live births to mothers		
Operatives	365	22.9	Below 17 years of age	32	4
Laborers	125	7.8	Below 20 years of age	67	17
Service workers	403	25.3	Live births to mothers		
Private household workers	105	6.6	With inadequate prenatal care	11	78.6
E. Income characteristics			With less than tenth grade	33	235.7
1. Mean income	$14,220		education		
2. Source of income			Live births to mothers with five or	23	164
Number of families	1525		more children		
Wage or salary	806	52.8	B. Mortality (SMSA)		
Self-employed	18	1.2	Total deaths	36	454
Farm self-employed	0	0	Maternal deaths	1	13
Social Security	200	13.1	Coronary heart disease	7	88
Welfare	501	32.9	Cancer	7	88
3. Income below the poverty level			Stroke	0	0
Number of families	742	48.7	Diabetic deaths	2	25
II. Housing characteristics			Liver cirrhosis	2	25
Total units	1770		Influenza and pneumonia	1	13
Vacancy status	6	0.3	Drug dependence	1	13
Owner occupied	138	7.8	All accident deaths	3	38
Renter occupied	1626	91.9	Motor vehicle deaths	0	0
Lacking plumbing	9	0.5	Homicides	7	88
Number of rooms			Suicides	1	13
1-2	21	1.2	Congenital anomalies	4	50
3-4	1013	57.2	IV. Morbidity: reportable diseases		
5-8	734	41.5	Total incidence	498	6285
9 or more	2	0.1	Tuberculosis (all forms)	2	25
Median	4.3		Syphilis	19	240
Persons per room			Gonorrhea	462	5830
1.00 or less	1035	58.7	Hepatitis B	3	38
1.01-1.50	534	30.3	Hepatitis A	1	13
1.51 or more	195	11.1	Chickenpox	11	139
Contract rent (per month)			Mumps	2	25
Less than $150	21	1.5	Rubella	1	13
$150-199	41	3.0	Salmonellosis	7	88
$200-249	48	3.5	Shigellosis	2	25
$250-299	471	34.6	Streptococcal infection	1	13
$300-349	489	36.0	Lead poisoning	1	13
$350-399	239	17.6	Bacterial meningitis	1	13
$400-449	49	3.6	HIV	7	88
$450 or more	1	0.7			
No cash rent	2	1.5			

(suprasystem), the health status of the community may be determined; its strengths, assets, and health needs identified; priorities established; and programs planned and implemented. The next chapter focuses on analysis of the data and planning and implementing appropriate interventions.

KEY IDEAS

1. Community/public health nurses assess communities to determine the assets and critical health needs as a basis for planning and implementing effective nursing care.
2. A community contains three essential elements: people, place, and social interaction or common characteristics.
3. An organized framework for gathering data will help the community/public health nurse comprehensively assess a community and identify missing information.
4. Developmental, epidemiologic, structural-functional, and systems frameworks may be used to assess communities. This text uses a systems framework for community assessment.
5. The first step in community assessment is determining the community's boundaries. The boundaries help the nurse

The Nursing Process in Practice box describes a geopolitical community and a phenomenological community. Use the community assessment tool in Box 15-4 to organize the data available for each community. Then, compare your assessments with the completed assessment tools included for each of the applications.

identify which processes and resources are internal to the community and which affect the community from the external environment, or suprasystem.
6. Influences from the suprasystem and the internal processes of the community may be positive (resources) or negative (demands).
7. For the community/public health nurse, the process of data collection in community assessment may include observing the community, interviewing community members, reviewing community records, reading local newspapers and periodicals, examining government documents, reviewing the professional literature, and conducting surveys of community members.
8. A community/public health nurse may approach community assessment comprehensively or focus on a preselected health problem or population.

THE NURSING PROCESS IN PRACTICE ▶ A Geopolitical Community and a Phenomenological Community

A GEOPOLITICAL COMMUNITY*

Census tract 1 (CT 1), located in city X, is bounded on the north by First Avenue, on the south by Tenth Avenue, on the west by A Street, and on the east by J Street. Although this CT is zoned for residential use, previously existing stores are allowed to remain but cannot expand. Most people within this CT do not know that CT boundaries exist. Therefore the residents do not form any real bonds based on location alone. Neighborhood schoolyards and recreation centers, a library, a multipurpose center, and churches contribute to a sense of community. Several clubs and organizations within the CT also contribute to a sense of community, including various church groups, Boy and Girl Scouts, the urban 4-H Club, the senior citizens center, the Young Men's Christian Association (YMCA), Big Brothers and Big Sisters, and a soup kitchen. Churches within the CT are primarily Baptist, Methodist, or storefront churches. This community recognizes several church leaders as community leaders.

CT 1 is located in an inner city. The streets look relatively clean, but some alleys and backyards have litter and broken glass. Stray dogs abound, and places for rats to breed are abundant. The crime rate is almost twice that of city X overall. Property crime rates are higher than are violent crime rates. A police station is located within the CT, and a fire station is nearby. The city coordinates emergency medical services. A neighborhood watch program has recently been implemented to attempt to reduce crime. This program resulted from combined efforts of the local police, church leaders, school officials, and

the city council. City X has a mayor and a city council, with one city council member basically representing CT 1.

CT 1 suffers from moderate air and noise pollution. The major source of pollutants is traffic, which contributes sulfur dioxide, carbon monoxide, and hydrocarbons. Several industries, an airport, and a train station are located within a 10-mile radius of this CT and also contribute pollutants. Residents benefit from both city water and a city sewage system. Drinking water is chlorinated and fluoridated.

In times of need, community members tend to turn to certain people within the community for advice and assistance. These individuals include church leaders, the director of the YMCA, a worker at the soup kitchen, the manager of Paul's Corner Store, and the owner of Gibby's Pawn Shop.

Within the CT are numerous small businesses, such as restaurants, barbershops, cleaners, fast-food carryouts, corner markets, pawnshops, and taverns. Numerous appliance, bakery, clothing, discount department, drug, florist, food, furniture, hardware, hobby, industrial supplies, jewelry, liquor, shoe, and wig stores are located within the CT. Most local stores extend credit but are also more expensive compared with larger stores outside of the CT. Local food stores accept food stamps. Several large shopping centers and malls are located outside the CT; some of these are accessible by bus, and others are accessible only by automobile. The CT is part of one school district composed of six elementary schools (grades K through 5), two junior high schools (grades 6 through 8), and one senior high school (grades 9 through 12).

*Adapted from Kidd, C. (1985). *Case study: Geopolitical community.* Baltimore, MD: University of Maryland School of Nursing Undergraduate Program.

Continued

Two community/public health nurses from the nearby district office of the city health department are assigned to provide nursing services to these schools. One nurse is assigned to the elementary schools, and the other is assigned to the junior and senior high schools. Each nurse spends 1 day (8 hours) per week divided among her assigned schools. According to state law, the nurses must follow up on designated communicable diseases and required immunizations as their top priorities. Health problems commonly referred to the nurses include communicable diseases and rashes, minor first-aid problems, pregnancy, chronic illnesses (e.g., diabetes, seizure disorders, asthma), head lice, personal hygiene, and dental problems; requests for birth control information and vision screening are also made.

Occasionally, the public health nurse teaches a class or large group on a health-related topic. Within four blocks of the CT is a Head Start Program offering daycare for children ages 2 to 5 years from 7:00 AM to 5:30 PM Monday through Friday. A waiting list is necessary, and families must be eligible on the basis of income.

Within the CT are one physician (general practice), one dentist, and one podiatrist. A Planned Parenthood office is located outside the CT but is accessible via the bus line. The district office of the city health department is located a few blocks from the CT and provides maternity, well-baby, well-child (through age 6 years), sexually transmitted disease, immunization, and chest radiography services. Home visiting services are provided to home health care clients and to some clients as follow-up to clinic services. Located next to the district health department is the inner city community mental health center, which provides five basic services: therapy, partial hospitalization, crisis intervention, referral to inpatient psychiatric settings, and consultation. The Inner City Nursing Home is a 314-bed long-term care facility that offers skilled nursing care for convalescent, chronically ill, and aged clients. Although the home is located near the CT, the occupants of the facility are drawn from a much larger geographic area.

The majority of CT residents use one or more of three public and nonprofit hospitals. Hospital emergency department services are used extensively for acute care; hospital outpatient department services are used less frequently. These three hospitals accept all third-party reimbursements and charity cases. Outside the CT but within a 20-mile radius are various other health care facilities, including two private home health agencies, six hospitals (some private and some public), and numerous physician and dentist offices (most requiring payment at the time of service). Health- and social-related associations and organizations outside the CT, but providing services to those who need it, include the Agricultural Extension Service, American Cancer Society, American Diabetic Association, American Heart Association, American Red Cross, Association for Retarded Citizens, Birthright, Child Development Center, Childbirth Education Association, Crisis Intervention, Services for Children with Special Needs, Drug Abuse Center, Family and Children's Society, Family Crisis Center, Goodwill Industries, Health and Welfare Council, La Leche League, League for the Handicapped, Legal Aid Bureau, American Lung Association, Meals on Wheels, National Association for the Advancement of Colored People, National Foundation, March of Dimes, Poison Control Center, Public Housing Authority, Rape and Family Abuse Center, Right to Life, Salvation Army, United Way, and Vocational Rehabilitation Center.

Table 15-3 presents 2000 census tract data for CT 1. Use these numeric data and the CT description to complete an assessment of this geopolitical community.

GEOPOLITICAL COMMUNITY ASSESSMENT OF CT 1
BOUNDARIES
- People: residents of CT 1 number 7924 people.
- Place: this is a geopolitical community with defined borders.

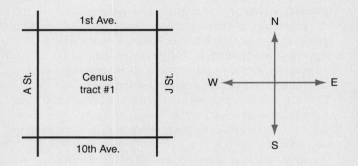

- Common interests or goals: the residents live in the same area.
- Suprasystem: city X. Look at the suprasystem to identify the resources and demands from outside the community (inputs) that affect the community.

GOALS
The goals of any geopolitical community are to promote the survival and maximize the well-being of the community. No specific goals are listed in the description.

CHARACTERISTICS
Physical Characteristics
1. *Length of existence* is not identified but might be determined by a review of city history.
2. *Demographic data* (see Table 15-3 for the source of the answers provided in this section):
   - Age: the largest age group is 10 to 19 years old (1280 boys + 1323 girls = 2603 of 7924 total population, or 33%).
   - Race: almost exclusively black (99%).
   - Gender: more girls and women (57%) than boys and men (43%) in the community.
   - Ethnicity: the community consists of mostly native-born citizens of the United States (98.9% native-born children of native-born parents).
   - Characteristics of housing: most individuals rent (1626 of 1770 households, or 92%) and live in small housing units. The median number of rooms is 4.3. Most residents pay between $250 and $349 per month (471 + 489 = 960 of 1626 renters, or 59%).
   - Density of population: the population is rather dense, with an average of 4.48 persons in each household.
3. *Physical features* of the community: the CT is urban, is relatively clean, and has residential and business areas.

Psychosocial Characteristics
1. *Religion:* the two denominations with the greatest number of churches are Baptist and Methodist.

2. *Socioeconomic class:* this community is poor, with a mean yearly income of $14,220. Forty-nine percent of families live below the poverty level (742 of 1525), and 33% are on welfare (501 of 1525).

3. *Education:* the median level of education is ninth grade; only 3% of individuals 25 years of age and older have some college education (67 of 2217).

4. *Occupation:* the three largest job categories for workers in this community are service jobs, operative jobs, and clerical positions.

5. *Marital status:* marital status data are collected on residents 14 years of age and older. Twenty-seven percent of persons report that they are married (1115 [543 men + 572 women] of the eligible population of 4079 [1502 men + 2577 women]). Forty-seven percent report their marital status as single (1914 [878 men + 1036 women] of 4079). Note the discrepancy between the number of men and women who list their marital status as either married or single. The community health nurse would want to explore the reasons for the discrepancy to reach a clearer understanding of the marital status of community residents.

6. Family composition: the community consists primarily of young families, the majority of which are headed by single females. Thirty percent of households are headed by a husband and wife; 63% are headed by single women. Eighty-six percent of all households have children under the age of 18 years.

EXTERNAL INFLUENCES FROM THE SUPRASYSTEM

	Resources	Demands
Money	No information is given about budget inputs or financial demands on the community from the suprasystem. The community health nurse should attempt to gather additional data on the question.	
Facilities	Inner-City Community Mental Health Center	
	Inner-City Nursing Home	Nursing home is not exclusive to community.
	Shopping centers and malls	Shopping access is limited.
	District office of city health department	
	Planned Parenthood Office	
	Six hospitals	
	Two private home health care agencies	
	Industry, airport, and train station (may provide employment)	These entities contribute pollutants to the community.
Formal human services	Numerous physicians and dentists	
	All social and health agencies listed at the end of the community description (e.g., Poison Control Center and American Cancer Society)	
	City water and sewer	
	Emergency medical services	
	Head Start Program	
	Bus transportation	
Health information	May be provided by the same social and health agencies listed at the end of the community description. The nurse would need to find out which of these do and which do not provide health information and education to the community.	
Legislation	No information is available at this time. However, the community health nurse should be aware of or attempt to discover what city legislation affects the community (e.g., city X Board of Education would determine school policies and plans and direct the activities of all schools in the city, including those in this community).	
Values		Crime rate of city X is less than that of the CT. City X's environmental pollutants affect the community.

INTERNAL FUNCTIONS OF THE COMMUNITY
Economy

	Resources	Demands
Formal human services	Public health nurses in schools	Services of school nurses are limited.
	Scouts	
	Urban 4-H Club	
	Big Brothers and Big Sisters clubs	
	Police	
	One physician, one dentist, one podiatrist	Services are not adequate to meet the needs of the community.
		No daycare facilities, community colleges, or technical schools are in the community.

Continued

Resources		Demands
Informal human services	Church groups Number of small businesses that extend credit and accept food stamps	There are higher prices in local stores compared with those outside the CT.
Facilities, equipment, goods	Schools Churches Recreational centers Library Senior Citizen Center YMCA	No parks or shopping malls Lack of cars for transportation High property crime rate Environmental hazards such as stray dogs and rats
Money	Little is known about this topic. One area to explore would include an appraisal of the money acquired and spent within the community. Because this community is part of a larger city, the budget for infrastructure support would come from the city. Information might be obtained about the taxes collected from residents of this community and that amount compared with the money spent by the city on providing services to the community. Is more money collected by the city than is spent on community needs, or is more money spent on community needs than is collected from residents?	
Education	Little is known about how members are socialized and educated to function productively. The educational level of this community is low, and many members live below the poverty level. Many of the persons who are employed are employed in occupations that require little advanced education.	

Analysis of Economy: The community has relatively few resources to meet the health-related needs of its members. The economy of the area is relatively weak in terms of goods and services, including many demands that are not being met. In planning health services for this community, funding should be considered. The nurse should explore getting funding sponsors or city funding or should pursue grants from philanthropic and government sources.

Polity
- Organizational structure: the community is part of city X; it does not have its own organizational structure.
- Leaders: the formal leaders include the local representative to the city council, church leaders, and local business owners. The informal leaders include the manager of the corner store, the pawnshop owner, the worker at the soup kitchen, and the director of the YMCA.
- Patterns of decision-making: because this community is only a portion of the larger city, many of the decisions that affect it are probably made from outside the community. For example, the City X Board of Education makes the decisions related to the local schools. Some of the questions a nurse might want to ask to get additional information in this category include the following: Does the council member meet with other leaders and community members to address concerns and problem solve, or does he or she make decisions without community input? How have past decisions been made? The Neighborhood Watch Program started with the combined efforts of local police, church leaders, school officials, and the city councilman.
- Methods of social control: in any geopolitical community, the police enforce the rules. Norms are established by schools, churches, neighborhood expectations, family standards of conduct, and peer group influences. The nurse would need to interview community members to get a sense of the norms set by the community; no information is available at this point.

Analysis of Polity: The community has a mix of formal and informal leaders, but little is known about the norms representative of the community. The nurse would need more data to complete an assessment of polity. In planning health care for the community, the nurse would be especially interested in discovering which community norms might be compatible with health care or health-seeking behavior.

Communication
- Nonverbal: residents feel a sense of community or belonging. Many clubs and organizations are available for residents.
- Verbal: informal communication occurs wherever people gather and talk (e.g., the corner store, in churches, in other group activities). A bulletin board is used to post notices, but it is not known if any community newspapers or periodicals are published.

Analysis of Communication: A variety of opportunities for social gathering and exchange of information are available. Little evidence exists to suggest that the community has the capacity to communicate easily with all its members (e.g., a newspaper). In planning health care, the nurse should be aware of the usual avenues of communication within the community so that he or she can use them to gather and disburse information to members.

In reference to communication on health-related matters, the nurse would want to know if community residents express their needs and concerns to health care providers and whether health care providers seek out or listen to community concerns. Do health care providers communicate among themselves? Are they involved in coordinating services? Do providers determine the care and service needs by themselves? More information is needed.

Values
- Traditions: no information is available in the description on community traditions.
- Subgroups: there are a number of subgroups and aggregates that can be identified by church attendance, age, and education.

With the number of churches within the community, a subgroup of individuals who are actively involved in religious practices is apparent. The age of the population would indicate a substantial number of young individuals (under 18 years old) as a subgroup. Single mothers as heads of household are another aggregate, and the median educational level reflects a large subgroup with minimal high school experience.

- Environment: the streets are clean; back alleys and backyards are littered with debris and glass, providing a haven for rats. Stray dogs are present. The crime rate is higher than that in the city, and residents are subject to both property and violent crime. The environment is relatively stark, and adherence to certain laws (e.g., littering, leash laws) is lax. The higher crime rate indicates a community that may contain a higher proportion of residents who are less concerned with adhering to laws related to private property and personal safety than is contained in the city as a whole.

- Health: community residents tend to rely on community hospitals for their health care needs. The emergency department is used more frequently than is the outpatient department, indicating that members place a greater priority on acquiring health care services when ill than on seeking preventive health care. Nothing is known from the data about residents' attitudes toward health professionals.

- Homogeneity versus heterogeneity: the community appears to be homogeneous with respect to race, socioeconomic status, education, and residential maintenance. With the existing high crime rate and the organization of a Neighborhood Watch Program, the community is apparently divided in its attitudes toward crime; however, many residents appear to be concerned about personal safety.

Analysis of Values: Because of the degree of homogeneity, community members appear to share similar values. Church groups and church attendance are valued, as is parenthood. Community members are moderately concerned about the physical appearance of their property. Education and preventive health care are not especially valued, based on the level of education and the type of health care services used. The nurse would need to consider community values in planning health programs or services to ensure community participation.

OUTCOMES (HEALTH BEHAVIORS AND HEALTH STATUS)
People Factors

- Size: information to identify trends related to the size of the community is inadequate. The nurse would need population statistics over several time periods to determine whether this community is growing, losing members, or remaining relatively stable. The total births during this time are greater than the total deaths. A majority of residents who were surveyed reported that they live in the same home or in a different home in the same general area. The two factors seem to indicate a growing population that is not very mobile and remains within the community limits.

- Mortality and morbidity: the mortality rate is 454 per 100,000 population. The three most common causes of death are heart disease, cancer, and congenital anomalies. The most common communicable diseases are gonorrhea, syphilis, and chickenpox. Several vulnerable or high-risk groups can

be identified: pregnant adolescents and their infants, sexually active teens, and poor individuals. The community has many young mothers. The nurse can use pregnant adolescents to illustrate some of the presymptomatic illnesses or problems that might be expected in this community: poor nutrition and anemia, inadequate prenatal care, poor self-efficacy, and inadequate family support systems. Why would these problems be expected? The nurse can use research to identify potential problems associated with specific situations. Chapter 24 documents research findings that identify the social and health-related impacts of pregnancy.

- Social functioning: the level of social functioning can be measured by calculating the dependency ratio:

$$\frac{\text{Number of persons} <20 \text{ years}^* + \text{number of persons} >65 \text{ years}}{\text{Number of persons ages 20 through 64}} \times 100$$

For this community the dependency ratio is:

$$\frac{5273}{2554}\left(\frac{548+743+1280+522+782+1323+33+21+80+4}{401+293+89+930+701+140}\right) = 2.1 \times 100 = 210$$

This community is very dependent on its adult members.

- Types of disabilities or impairments present or expected: congenital anomalies are known to be the third leading cause of death for this community. The nurse can expect that there may be a number of infants who survive with congenital health problems. In addition, the literature indicates that teenage mothers have a greater number of infants with learning disabilities; thus this community might be expected to experience this problem. To validate this expectation, the nurse might survey families, Head Start Program leaders, and school officials.

Environmental Factors

- Physical environment: housing is crowded and not well kept. The air contains a significant number of pollutants (i.e., sulfur dioxide, carbon monoxide, hydrocarbons). The city provides sewer and chlorinated and fluoridated water. No additional information about the quality of the water supply is available.

- Social environment: the community is relatively stable; many residents have remained in the area for some time, but they are subjected to a high rate of crime and the stress that accompanies concerns for personal and family safety.

Level of Health

- Actual needs: many health concerns can be identified from the existing data, including congenital anomalies; maternal, infant, and neonatal deaths; sexually transmitted diseases, particularly syphilis, gonorrhea, and HIV; poverty; heart disease; deaths from drugs and cirrhosis; cancer; chickenpox; and air pollution.

- Potential needs: a knowledge deficit may exist about community resources and the unacceptability or inaccessibility of community resources. The rates of deaths from drugs and cirrhosis suggest that drug and alcohol use is higher than are national

---

*The number of people under 18 years is not listed, so the calculations are based on the number of people 19 or younger (the information that was available).

Continued

rates. Congenital anomalies might be related to fetal alcohol syndrome, but more information is needed about the types of such anomalies before a correlation can be determined.

- Community action: some community action has been taken related to crime reduction, but community action related to health needs is not available. One way to ascertain the community's response to health needs would be to determine how the community has acted to solve other health-related problems or if it has not acted to solve past health problems. Either way, the nurse will have information that will help determine whether the community can effectively address health issues.

A PHENOMENOLOGICAL COMMUNITY*

Northview, a public high school (grades 9 through 12), is located in CT 1 in city X; it is 1 of 10 public high schools in that city. The Northview school district encompasses all of CT 1. Most of the students who attend Northview walk to school or take the city bus.

The school is a two-story red brick building built in 1962. The building and its grounds, which consist of a parking lot, an athletic field, and a small area of grass, cover one city block. The school is situated between B and C Streets and between Second and Third Avenues. The main entrance to the school is on B Street. When approaching the school, the observer is struck by the rather stark appearance of the complex—no trees, little grass, mostly concrete—and a moderate amount of litter (paper, broken glass, and beverage cans) around the schoolyard.

The interior of the building is traditional in appearance. The long halls, lined with lockers on either side, are painted a pale yellow; the floors are tiled, and the windows have grates over them for security. The entrance area next to the administrative offices has a display of trophies won in various sports events and a bulletin board that lists the football schedule and various notices for students, faculty, and visitors. The first floor consists of the administrative offices, health room, counselors' offices, auditorium, music room, gymnasium, cafeteria, kitchen, and faculty lounge area, a few small classrooms, and a common area. Students describe the common area as their place and is located just outside of the gymnasium; thus it is also convenient to use when ballgames are being played. The area resembles a small teen center. The second floor consists of classrooms and a large media center. Lockers and bathrooms are on both floors. The bathrooms have a lot of graffiti on the walls but are fairly clean. The classrooms have a traditional appearance, with green chalkboards, individual chairs with arm desks, a teacher's desk, and some visual materials such as posters and signs. In several rooms, hanging maps and screens appear to be in disrepair. The classrooms were designed to hold 30 to 35 students. The basement consists of the physical maintenance plant, the science laboratories, and the industrial arts classrooms. The stairways are at both ends of the halls.

The staff at Northview includes the principal, Mr. Johnson; 32 teachers; 3 full-time and 2 part-time counselors; a psychologist who visits weekly or when called; a community/public health nurse from the local health department who spends one-half day per week at the school; a truancy officer who covers 3 schools; secretaries; cooks; janitors; and volunteers who staff the health room. The teachers are members of the teachers' union and are active in its activities.

The mean age of the teachers is 28 years. Most of the teachers are women and have been teaching fewer than 10 years. The student to teacher ratio is 1:26, but this ratio includes special education and resource teachers. The average class size is 35. Each teacher is involved as a homeroom advisor in addition to having a regular teaching assignment. The homeroom is a 20-minute period at the beginning of each day. Each teacher is assigned approximately 25 students as advisees. The homeroom period serves as an attendance and announcement time, as well as a time for some small group activities.

The enrollment at Northview is 834: 275 ninth graders (140 female and 135 male students), 240 tenth graders (122 female and 118 male students), 200 eleventh graders (102 female and 98 male students), and 119 twelfth graders (61 female and 58 male students). The enrollment was 852 last year. The students range in age from 13 to 19; 817 of the students are black, and 17 are of Asian descent. The religion is predominantly Protestant.

Northview is an active school with many organizations, clubs, and activities. Joanne Riley, president of the Parent-Teacher Association (PTA), states, "It is very difficult getting a lot of the parents involved." The PTA meets once a month, and the average attendance is 30. The Student Government Association (SGA) is composed of representatives elected from each of the four classes. The group meets weekly to determine student policies and to plan and coordinate student activities. The president of the SGA, Pat Smith, says that the biggest problem he sees is that a lot of kids drop out of school as soon as they can. "It's hard to get some of these students involved in school activities. Take Harry over there [he points to a boy standing in the hall with about five other students around him]—whatever he says goes with many of the problem kids. Yeah, we definitely have two kinds of kids here—ones who want to better themselves and ones who are here because they have to be." Smith also says that students are proud of their football team, which has won the regional championship for the last 3 years. The school publishes a monthly newspaper, *The Viewer,* and an annual yearbook. The school is active in sports (football, basketball, track, and baseball) and has other activities such as drama club, dance club, chorus, band, and cheerleading. Many of the clubs and organizations have fundraisers to help support their activities. School dances are held at intervals during the school year, usually associated with special events such as the homecoming game or Valentine's Day. Schoolwide assemblies are held during the school day approximately three times per year.

Because Northview is part of the public school system, it must adhere to certain guidelines set forth by state and local authorities. The following policies are included:

1. All children must attend school until age 16.
2. Students must have at least 20 credits to graduate (1 physical education, 3 social studies, 2 mathematics, 2 science, 4 English, and 8 elective credits).
3. All students must pass mastery tests in reading and mathematics to graduate from high school.

*From Trotter, J. (1985). *Description of a phenomenological community: A case study.* Baltimore, MD: University of Maryland School of Nursing, Undergraduate Program.

4. Each school year must consist of a minimum of 180 instructional days.
5. All high schools in city X are in session from 8:00 AM to 3:00 PM, with 30 minutes for lunch.

The budget is determined by the city X Board of Education. Funds for the public schools are tax supported (city and state) and are allocated to schools based on a formula that considers full-time-equivalent students (FTEs). This year, the budget was cut in the areas of capital equipment and sports.

The school is organized by departments. Each department has a chairperson (who is a faculty member) and a team leader. Each team or department makes decisions about how to present the material, but the material must be within the overall curriculum guidelines. All faculty members report to the principal. Northview has 11 departments: art, business, English, foreign languages, home economics, industrial arts, mathematics, music, physical education, science, and social studies. The physical education teachers are responsible for teaching the health component of the curriculum. Occasionally, the community health nurse will teach a class on a health-related topic.

The community/public health nurse spends one-half day per week at the school. Because the meeting is not always held the same day each week, the school principal announces over the public address system when the nurse is in the building. The nurse then sees students in the health room based on self-referrals or referrals from teachers or other school personnel. The health problems most commonly referred to the nurse include communicable diseases and rashes, first-aid problems, pregnancy, chronic illnesses, personal hygiene, dental problems, and eating disorders (obesity and anorexia); requests for birth control information and vision screening are also made.

During a recent visit to the school, some of the following comments and concerns were overheard:

Students:
- "I can't wait until I get out of here. I'm quitting school as soon as I can."
- "I sure hope we win the trophy again this year."
- "My period is 3 weeks late; I think I might be pregnant. Do you know where I can get an abortion? My dad would kill me if he knew about it!"
- "I heard that if you take the pill too long, it does something to your blood."
- "Did you hear what happened to Angie? She got some kind of terrible infection from wearing a tampon. I sure hope that doesn't happen to me."
- "I never use a condom because it doesn't feel good."

Teachers:
- "If we don't get our raise this year, I'm quitting teaching."
- "We just can't handle all of these kids unless we get more help in the classroom."
- "I'm really concerned about the increasing number of pregnancies among our girls. Last year, there were 38, and there are already 45 this year. It's such a shame—they don't have any way to continue their schooling. They drop out of school before the baby is born; and even though they say they're planning to come back, there's no one to take care of the baby."
- "I really think we need to do something about the increasing number of substance abuse and sexually transmitted disease cases."

- "You know these students don't go for regular health and dental checkups; they only go when they're sick or have problems."

Principal:
- "I'm really pleased about how well our program is working to reduce absenteeism." (Last year the principal and the PTA worked together to identify components of the problem and then petitioned the school board for additional funds for a truancy officer, who works with volunteers to check on absent students.)

PHENOMENOLOGICAL COMMUNITY ASSESSMENT OF NORTHVIEW HIGH SCHOOL IN CT 1
BOUNDARIES
- People: students (834) and staff, consisting of 1 principal, 32 teachers, 5 counselors, janitors, and cooks
- Place: one city block in city X, census tract 1, between B and C Streets and Second and Third Avenues
- Common interests or goals: students' education; for staff, education, and employment
- Criteria for membership: students must have completed eighth grade; teachers, counselors, and staff must meet the employment criteria set by the school system for their occupation, unknown to us
- Suprasystem: city X school system and the board of education

GOALS
Education of students, grades 9 through 12. The nurse may find other goals described in the school's written philosophy.

CHARACTERISTICS
Physical Characteristics
1. In *existence* since 1962
2. Demographic data:
   - Ages: students, 13 to 19 years; faculty mean age, 28 years
   - Race: students: 817 black (98%); 17 Asian descent (2%); staff and faculty: unknown
   - Gender: students, 425 (51%) girls; 409 (49%) boys
   - Ethnicity: unknown; predominantly black student body
   - Housing: very little information is available about the housing situation of community members; this is a city environment. (However, the nurse might observe the housing and review census tract data.)
   - Density of population: teacher-to-student ratio is 1:35; classrooms are slightly crowded because they were built to hold 30 to 35 students
3. Physical features of the community: fairly young, fairly large student group; traditional school building

Psychosocial Characteristics
1. *Religion:* mostly Protestant
2. *Socioeconomic class:* no data (The nurse could ask the principal and review census tract data.)
3. *Education:* students, grades 9 through 12; faculty, presumably college education (the nurse should check this); staff, no information available
4. *Occupation:* faculty, teachers and counselors; staff includes secretaries, cooks, and janitors
5. *Marital status:* no information, but the nurse might expect that most of the students are single

Continued

EXTERNAL INFLUENCES FROM SUPRASYSTEM

	Resources	Demands
Money	Taxes fund budget	A smaller budget than previous year's budget
	Fund-raisers from PTA	
Facilities	Facilities are available in the surrounding census tract, but no information is available in this description.	No information
Formal human services	Community/public health nurse, ½ day per week	Not full-time
	Psychologist	
	Truancy officer	
Informal human services	Volunteers	Probably a lack of resources to assist pregnant adolescents to stay in school
	PTA	
Health information		City school district does not require sex education courses in the curriculum
		Lack of information is related to abstinence and birth control
Legislation	Laws related to attendance, mastery examinations, number of credits for graduation, curriculum, and number of instructional days	
	Immunization requirements for students not described	
	Union laws for teachers	
Values of suprasystem	Information related to budget	Budget adjustments indicate that school board values sports less than the community. With only ½ day per week of funding for the nurse, it appears health is not a high priority.

INTERNAL FUNCTIONS OF THE COMMUNITY
Economy

	Resources	Demands
Formal human services	Principal	Fewer teachers than needed based on teacher dissatisfaction and student to teacher ratio
	Teachers	
	Counselors	
	Staff	
Informal human services	Volunteers in health room (Some people would place this resource here, others in "External Influences from the Suprasystem.")	No resources for unwed mothers
		No formal health education program
Money	No information about amount of money generated within the community	
	Fund-raising within certain clubs	
	No information on how money is spent	
Facilities	Description indicates space, classrooms, common area for students, faculty lounge, health room	Lack of audiovisual equipment
		Some equipment in classroom in disrepair
Education	Mastery examinations are a criterion for productivity.	
	The curriculum appears to provide educational opportunities for students who wish to go on to college, as well as for students who are interested in jobs immediately out of high school (business, industrial arts); further assessment is necessary.	

Analysis of Economy: The school has a mix of resources and demands. The community is struggling with budget and personnel problems that affect the provision of services. Volunteers are available, and facilities are, for the most part, adequate. Any new health programs would have to be inexpensive or require additional fund-raising.

Polity
Organizational structure:

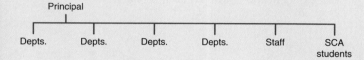

1. Leaders: the formal leaders are the principal, the department chairpersons, and the SGA president. Informal leaders include Harry, the leader of the problem students.
2. Patterns of decision making: decisions regarding the curriculum are made within the departments following school system guidelines. An example of a past decision is that made regarding absenteeism. In this decision, some efforts at democratic decision making were probable because the principal enlisted the PTA and school board. No other data are available.
3. Methods of social control: rules regarding attendance come from the suprasystem, with the SGA and PTA particularly mentioned in relation to absenteeism.

Analysis of Polity: Although the data are sparse, a variety of formal leaders and one informal leader are available. The formal leaders are resources, but the informal leader is not considered a positive leader by the formal leaders. Norms of conduct have been established, and no real information is available to suggest whether they are being largely ignored or violated, with the exception of absenteeism and dropping out. When planning for health care services, a variety of leaders and groups need to be involved.

Communication
- Nonverbal: teachers appear frustrated, and students cannot wait to leave. SGA activity indicates that some students are engaged in school. The school seems to support sports activities, and many clubs and student organizations (i.e., drama club, dance club, chorus, band, and cheerleading) are available. Several special events, such as homecoming, occur throughout the year.
- Verbal: no mention of schoolwide announcements, but a bulletin board is in use. The principal has established a task force with other personnel to study the dropout rate. Some evidence is suggestive of democratic or horizontal communication, but most communication appears to be vertical; this area needs further exploration. Announcements are made during the homeroom period, a school newspaper is published monthly, and a school yearbook is published annually. School assemblies are held three times a year.

Analysis of Communication: The school has a mix of resources and demands, but many more resources are identified, as well as a variety of verbal and nonverbal communication patterns and a variety of planned activities. Low morale would need to be considered when suggesting new health

activities. Time would need to be spent empowering faculty and students.

Values
- Traditions: school dances associated with special events (homecoming, Valentine's Day) and sports events.
- Subgroups: student activities' groups, sports groups, Harry's group, and the SGA.
- Environment: window grates for security; trophy displays; moderate litter on the school campus; common area for student use and relaxation; the description does not indicate that the complex is poorly maintained.
- Health: facilities consist of a health room, but no description of supplies or environment is provided. With regard to attitudes about health care, health priority, and health care professionals, students generally seek crisis-oriented care. Students appear to consider the nurse a valuable resource for health care and information. Some students do not appear to value preventive care (i.e., a need exists for sexual abstinence and birth control information; the pregnancy rate is high). Interviews or surveys are necessary to get additional information.
- Homogeneity versus heterogeneity: the description indicates that the students are racially homogeneous. Socioeconomic status is not known; the nurse would need additional information. Attitudes toward school and education appear to be polarized (i.e., some students are active in school organizations and pursue education; others drop out). No information is available to make an assessment about the staff.

Analysis of Values: The school values traditions, safety, and sports. Students are very homogeneous and are therefore more likely to have similar values than do those in another community with more widely variant characteristics. The school appears to be moderately concerned with cleanliness. The health care provider is valued, but preventive health care behavior is not a priority. If preventive health issues are linked with sports, some students may be interested.

OUTCOMES (HEALTH BEHAVIORS AND HEALTH STATUS)
People Factors
- Size: slightly fewer students than 2 years ago. No additional information is available.
- Mortality and morbidity: the number of students enrolled decreases with grade level. No information is available on how many students have died in recent years or about the reason for leaving the school or causes of death, if any have occurred. Major diseases and conditions are communicable diseases (specific diseases unknown) and rashes, accidents requiring first aid, pregnancy, and chronic illnesses (none specified), dental problems, and eating disorders. No information is available about the incidences and prevalences of these problems. Presymptomatic illness or problems that might be expected in students as per the literature include substance abuse, sex education needs, access to birth control, depression and suicide, pregnancy, sexually transmitted diseases and HIV infection, trauma and violence, and communicable diseases, such as mononucleosis, upper respiratory tract illnesses, and, if population is underimmunized, measles. Vulnerable or high-risk groups include pregnant adolescents (45 of 425 girls, or 11% [national rate in 2000 was 4.1% (U.S. Department of Health and Human Services,

Continued

2002)]), teenage parents, dropouts, substance abusers (including smokers), and sexually active adolescents.

- Social functioning: school attendance is problematic but may be improving, according to the principal.
- Types of disabilities or impairments present or expected: learning disabilities are likely to be present because the school has special education classes. No additional information is available, but a likely source would be health room records and children with individualized education plans related to disabilities.

Environmental Factors

- Physical environment: appears adequate from the description, except some classes may be crowded.

- Social environment: teachers appear dissatisfied, indicating a stressful environment.

Level of Health

- Actual needs: substance abuse; sexually transmitted diseases; pregnancy; health information needs related to hygiene, birth control, sexual abstinence; teenage parenting.
- Potential needs: depression, accident rate.
- Community action: no information is supplied, but remarks about health-related needs seem to indicate little action addressing health issues has been taken.

LEARNING BY EXPERIENCE AND REFLECTION

1. Write a definition of community. Does the definition include the three critical components? Does your definition relate more to a geopolitical or to a phenomenological community?
2. Draw a diagram depicting the communities to which you belong. Do you work or attend school in the same geopolitical community in which you live? How many phenomenological communities do you belong to? In which communities do you receive health care?
3. Interview at least two members from the same community regarding their perceptions of the health of their community members and the community's competence. Compare and contrast their responses. What questions emerge for further assessment?

4. Use the responses in guideline 3 to begin to develop a survey you might use with more community members.
5. Use the community assessment tool presented in this chapter to assess a community. Start by identifying whether the community is geopolitical or phenomenological.
6. Using the demographic characteristics of a community and epidemiologic and nursing literature, predict what health problems are likely to exist in the community.
7. Suppose that a state survey of public schools indicates increasing rates of alcohol and tobacco use among middle-school students. The parents and school administrators deny that a problem exists in the school in community A. As a school nurse, how might you begin to explore whether a problem exists in this community school?

STUDY AIDS   http://evolve.elsevier.com/Maurer/community/

Visit the Evolve website for this book to find the following study and assessment materials:

- Quiz
- Web Scenario
- Critical Thinking Questions and Answers for Case Studies

- Care Plans
- *Healthy People* Updates
- Glossary

WEBSITE RESOURCES

These items supplement the chapter's topics and are also found on the Evolve site:

15A: The Community Assessment Tool Applied to Geopolitical and Phenomenological Communities
15B: Census 2000: Geographic Areas
15C: Windshield Survey

15D: Geographic Information Systems (GIS)
15E: Using Geographic Information Systems (GIS) in Community Health Nursing

REFERENCES

American Nurses Association (ANA). (2007). *Public health nursing: Scope and standards of practice.* Silver Spring, MD: Author.

Anderson, E., & McFarlane, J. (2008). *Community as partner: Theory and practice in nursing.* Philadelphia: J.B. Lippincott.

Anderson, E., McFarlane, J., & Helton, A. (1986). Community-as-client: A model for practice. *Nursing Outlook, 34*(5), 220-224.

Archer, S. (1985). *Community health nursing* (3rd ed.). Monterey, CA: Wadsworth Health Services.

Asner, M., Polyak, I., & Weigel, D. (2003). The best places to retire. *Money, 32*(7), 83-90.

Behringer, B., & Richards, R. W. (1996). The nature of communities. In R. W. Richards (Ed.), *Building partnerships: Educating health professionals for the communities they serve* (pp. 82-101). San Francisco: Jossey-Boss.

Choi, M., Afzal, B., & Sattler, B. (2006). Georgraphic information systems: A new tool for environmental health assessment. *Public Health Nursing, 23*(5), 381-391.

Community Health Faculty, Undergraduate Program, University of Maryland School of Nursing. (1975). *Community assessment tool.* Baltimore: University of Maryland School of Nursing.

Connor, A., Rainer, L., Simcox, J., et al. (2007). Increasing the delivery of health services to migrant farm worker families through a community partnership model. *Public Health Nursing, 24*(4), 355-360.

Cottrell, L. (1976). The competent community. In B. Kaplan, R. Wilson, & A. Leighton (Eds.), *Further explorations in social psychiatry* (pp. 195-209). New York: Basic Books.

Dixon, E. (1999). Community health nursing practice and the Roy Adaptation Model. *Public Health Nursing, 16*(4), 290-300.

Ervin, N. E. (2002). *Advanced community health nursing practice.* Upper Saddle River, NJ: Prentice-Hall.

Feder, J., Uccello, C., & O'Brien, E. (2001). The differences different approaches make: Comparing proposals to expand health insurance. In C. Harrington & C. L. Estes (Eds.), *Health policy: Crisis and reform in the U.S. health care delivery system* (3rd ed.; pp. 298-313). Boston: Jones and Bartlett.

Freeman, R., & Heinrich, J. (1981). *Community health nursing practice.* Philadelphia: W. B. Saunders.

Frenn, M., & Molin, S. (2003). Diet and exercise in low-income culturally diverse middle school students. *Public Health Nursing, 20*(5), 361-368.

Garb, M. (2003). Health, mortality and housing: The "tenement problem" in Chicago. *American Journal of Public Health, 93*(9), 1420-1430.

Gillis, A., & Jackson, W. (2002). *Research for nurses: Methods and interpretation.* Philadelphia: F. A. Davis.

Goeppinger, J., Lassister, P., & Wilcox, B. (1982). Community health is community competence. *Nursing Outlook, 30*, 464-467.

Green, L. W., & Kreuter, M. W. (1999). *Health promotion planning: An educational and environmental approach* (3rd ed.). Blacklick, OH: McGraw-Hill Education.

Hamilton, P., & Bush, H. (1988). Theory development in community health nursing: Issues and recommendations. *Scholarly Inquiry for Nursing Practice: An International Journal, 2*(2), 145-160.

Hanchett, E. (1988). *Nursing frameworks and community as client: Bridging the gap.* Norwalk, CT: Appleton & Lange.

Hawe, P. (1994). Capturing the meaning of "community" in community intervention evaluation: Some contributions from community psychology. *Health Promotion International, 9*(3), 199-210.

Helvie, C. O. (1998). *Advanced practice nursing in the community.* Thousand Oaks, CA: Sage.

Higgs, Z., & Gustafson, D. (1985). *Community as a client: Assessment and diagnosis.* Philadelphia: F. A. Davis.

Johnson, D. (1980). The behavioral system model for nursing. In J. Riehl & C. Roy (Eds.), *Conceptual models for nursing practice* (2nd ed.). New York: Appleton-Century-Crofts.

Katz, D., & Kahn, R. (1966). *The social psychology of organizations.* New York: John Wiley and Sons.

Kidd, C. (1985). *Description of a geopolitical community: A case study.* Baltimore: University of Maryland School of Nursing.

Kim, M. J., Hyang-In, C., Cheon-Klessig, Y. S., et al (2002). Primary health care for Korean immigrants: Sustaining a culturally sensitive model. *Public Health Nursing, 19*(3), 191-200.

King, I. (1971). *Toward a theory for nursing: General concepts of human behavior.* New York: John Wiley and Sons.

Kotchian, S. (1995). Environmental health services are prerequisites to health care. *Family and Community Health, 18*(3), 45-53.

Lutenbacher, M., Cohen, A., & Mitzel, J. (2003). Do we really help? Perspectives of abused women. *Public Health Nursing, 20*(1), 56-64.

Marriner-Tomey, A., & Alligood, M. (2006). *Nursing theorists and their work* (6th ed.). St. Louis: Mosby/Elsevier.

McCool, W., & Susman, E. (1990). The life span perspective: A developmental approach to community health nursing. *Public Health Nursing, 7*(1), 13-21.

Moorhead, S., Johnson, M., & Maas, M. (2004). *Nursing outcomes classification (NOC)* (3rd ed.). St. Louis: Mosby/Elsevier.

National Association of County and City Health Officials. (2000). *Mobilizing for Action through Planning and Partnerships (MAPP).* Washington, DC: Author. Retrieved October 8, 2007 from *http://mapp.naccho.org/mapp_introduction.asp.*

National Commission on Community Health Services. (1966). *Health is a community affair.* Cambridge, MA: Harvard University Press.

Neuman, B. (1982). *The Neuman systems model: Application to nursing education and practice.* Norwalk, CT: Appleton-Century-Crofts.

Nunez, D. E., Armbruster, C., Phillips, W. T., et al. (2003). Community-based health promotion program using a collaborative practice model: The Escalante Health Partnership. *Public Health Nursing, 20*(1), 25-32.

Perdue, W. C., Stone, L. A., & Gostin, L. O. (2003). The built environment and its relationship to the public's health: The legal framework. *American Journal of Public Health, 93*(9), 1390-1394.

Peterson, J., Atwood, J. R., & Yates, B. (2002). Key elements for church-based health promotion programs: Outcome-based literature review. *Public Health Nursing, 19*(6), 401-411.

Polit, D., & Hungler, B. (2005). *Essentials of nursing research: Methods, appraisal, and utilization* (6th ed.). Philadelphia: J. B. Lippincott.

Quad Council of Public Health Nursing Organizations. (1999). *Scope and standards of public health nursing.* Washington, DC: American Nurses Association.

Rafael, A. R. F. (2000). Watson's philosophy, science, and theory of human caring as a conceptual framework for guiding community health nursing practice. *Advances in Nursing Science, 23*(2), 34-49.

Riner, M., Cunningham, C., & Johnson, A. (2004). Public health education and practice using geographic information system technology. *Public Health Nursing, 21*(1), 57-65.

Roy, C. (1984). *Introduction to nursing: An adaptation model* (2nd ed.). Englewood Cliffs, NJ: Prentice Hall.

Schultz, P. (1987). When the client means more than one. *Advances in Nursing Science, 10*(1), 71-86.

Shamansky, S., & Pesznecker, B. (1981). A community is... *Nursing Outlook, 29*(3), 182-185.

Stoner, M., Magilvy, J., & Schultz, P. (1992). Community analysis in community health nursing practice: The GENESIS Model. *Public Health Nursing, 9*(4), 223-227.

Sultz, H. A., & Young, K. M. (2001). *Health care USA: Understanding its organization and delivery* (3rd ed.). Gaithersburg, MD: Aspen Publishers.

Timmreck, T. C. (1998). *An introduction to epidemiology* (2nd ed.). Sudsbury, MA: Jones and Bartlett.

Trotter, J. (1985). *Description of a phenomenological community: A case study.* Baltimore: University of Maryland School of Nursing.

Turner, J., & Chavigny, K. (1988). *Community health nursing: An epidemiological perspective through the nursing process.* Philadelphia: J. B. Lippincott.

University of Maryland School of Nursing. (1975). *Conceptual framework.* Baltimore: Author.

U.S. Bureau of the Census. (2001). Introduction to Census 2000 data products (Publication No. MSO/01-ICDP, June 2001). Washington, DC: U.S. Department of Commerce.

U.S. Department of Health and Human Services. (2002). *Health, United States, 2002.* Washington, DC: U.S. Government Printing Office.

Van Devanter, N., Hennessy, M., Howard, J. M., et al. (2002). Developing a collaborative community academic, health department partnership for STD prevention: The Gonorrhea Community Action Project in Harlem. *Journal of Public Health Management and Practice, 8*(6), 62-68.

von Bertalanffy, L. (1968). *General systems theory*. New York: George Braziller.

Warren, R. (1987). *Perspectives on the American community*. Chicago: Rand-McNally.

Williams, C. (1977). Community health nursing—What is it? *Nursing Outlook*, *25*(4), 250-254.

World Health Organization Regional Office for Europe. (2005). *Socioeconomic deter-minants of health: Assets model—focusing on health rather than disease*. Retrieved September 21, 2007, from *http://www.euro.who.int/socialdeterminants/assets/20050628_1*.

SUGGESTED READINGS

American Nurses Association (ANA). (2007). *Public health nursing: Scope and standards of practice*. Silver Spring, MD: Author.

Anderson, E., & McFarlane, J. (2008). *Community as partner: Theory and practice in nursing*. Philadelphia: J.B. Lippincott.

Davis, J. (1986). Using participant observation in community based practice. *Journal of Community Health Nursing*, *3*(1), 43-49.

Dever, A. (1980). *Community health analysis: A holistic approach*. Rockville, MD: Aspen.

Finnegan, L., & Ervin, N. (1989). An epidemiological approach to community assessment. *Public Health Nursing*, *6*(3), 147-151.

Goeppinger, J., Lassister, P., & Wilcox, B. (1982). Community health is community competence. *Nursing Outlook*, *30*, 464-467.

McCool, W., & Susman, E. (1990). The life span perspective: A developmental approach to community health nursing. *Public Health Nursing*, *7*(1), 13-21.

Milio, N. (1971). *9226 Kercheval: The storefront that did not burn*. Ann Arbor, MI: The University of Michigan Press.

Phillips, L. (1995). Chattanooga Creek: Case study of the public health nursing role in environmental health. *Public Health Nursing*, *12*(5), 335-340.

U.S. Bureau of the Census. (2000). *2000 Census of population and housing*. Washington, DC: U.S. Department of Commerce.

U.S. Department of Health and Human Services. (2006). *Health, United States, 2006*. Washington, DC: U.S. Government Printing Office.

Zust, B., & Moline, K. (2003). Identifying underserved ethnic populations within a community: The first step in eliminating health care disparities among racial and ethnic minorities. *Journal of Transcultural Nursing, 14*(1), 66-74.

16 Community Diagnosis, Planning, and Intervention

Claudia M. Smith and Frances A. Maurer

FOCUS QUESTIONS

What is the history of contemporary health planning in the United States?

What are the responsibilities of community/public health nurses in planning health-related changes with communities?

How do models of community organization relate to health planning?

What principles and steps can assist the nurse and community in developing an effective plan?

What are examples of community diagnoses?

How are priorities determined in health planning with communities?

What is a target population?

What are common types of interventions typically planned by community/public health nurses?

What are strategies for implementing plans?

CHAPTER OUTLINE

Population-Focused Health Planning
Population Targets and Intervention Levels
History of U.S. Health Planning
Rationale for Nursing Involvement in the Health Planning Process
Nursing Role in Program Planning
Planning for Community Change
Community Organization Models
Structures for Health Planning

Steps of Program Planning
Assessment
Analysis of Data
Diagnosis
Validation
Prioritization of Needs
Identification of the Target Population
Identification of the Planning Group
Establishment of the Program Goal
Identification of Possible Solutions
Matching Solutions with At-Risk Aggregates

Identification of Resources
Selection of the Best Intervention Strategy
Delineation of Expected Outcomes
Delineation of the Intervention—Work Plan
Planning for Program Evaluation
Tools Used to Present and Monitor Program Progress
Implementation
Types of Interventions
Strategies for Implementing Programs

KEY TERMS

Community empowerment
Community organization models
Data gap
Gantt Chart
Management objectives
North American Nursing Diagnosis Association (NANDA) classification system

Nursing Outcomes Classification (NOC)
Omaha System
Outcome objectives
Planned Approach to Community Health (PATCH)
Planning, Programming, and Budgeting System (PPBS)

Population-focused health planning
Process objectives
Program Evaluation and Review Technique (PERT)
Social action
Social planning
Target population

Chapter 15 provides community/public health nurses with the basics of community assessment, the first step in the nursing process. The chapter illustrates the use of a systems-based community assessment tool to assist nurses in gathering information about a community. This chapter continues the nursing process with communities (Figure 16-1), introducing the process of planning and implementing population-focused health care in communities. The components of and steps used in program planning, the types of interventions appropriate for the community level, and the responsibilities of the com-munity/public nurse in planning and implementing care with populations are described. The nursing process is dynamic, not static, as the arrows in the figure illustrate. Health intervention plans may be modified as new information becomes available. It is important to include community members in as many steps in the process as is possible. Input from the population(s) should be elicited regarding analyzing the assessment data to determine population diagnoses and priorities, identifying desired outcomes, planning, and evaluation (American Nurses Association [ANA], 2007).

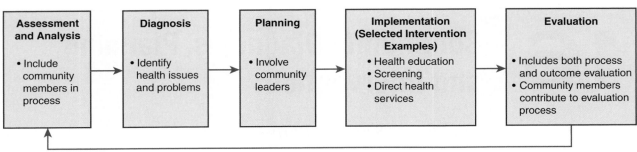

FIGURE 16-1 Illustration of the nursing process with communities.

POPULATION-FOCUSED HEALTH PLANNING

Health planning is a continuous social process by which data about clients are collected and analyzed for the purpose of developing a plan to generate new ideas, meet identified client needs, solve health problems, and guide changes in health care delivery. To date, you have been responsible primarily for developing a plan of care for the individual client. How do you go about developing a plan of action to meet the health needs of a community? How is the plan different from that for the health of an individual or a family? What types of nursing actions and interventions are appropriate for the community?

POPULATION TARGETS AND INTERVENTION LEVELS

Population-focused health planning is the application of a problem-solving process to a particular population. In population-focused health planning, communities are assessed, needs and problems are prioritized, desired outcomes are determined, and strategies to achieve the outcomes are delineated.

Persons for whom you desire change to occur are referred to as the *target population.* Planning care for groups or populations results in programs, and hence the term program planning is often used when planning care at the community level.

Programs may be aimed at the *primary, secondary,* or *tertiary* level of prevention. For example, a health-education program about safer sex is aimed at preventing sexually transmitted diseases through health-promotion measures (primary prevention); a program to screen preadolescent girls for scoliosis is geared toward early detection and treatment (secondary prevention); and an exercise program for stroke victims to limit or minimize their disability is an example of a tertiary level of prevention.

Population-focused health planning can range from planning health care for a small group of people to planning care for a large aggregate or an entire city, state, or nation. The planning process described in this chapter is applicable to all types of communities (phenomenological and geopolitical) and to all levels of planning (local, state, national, and international). Health planning can be proactive or reactive. The goal is to use a more proactive approach and for nurses to be an integral part of the planning process.

HISTORY OF U.S. HEALTH PLANNING

The history of health planning in the United States has alternated between the state and federal government. Before the 1960s, health planning occurred primarily at the state level.

In the 1960s, health planning became a federal effort. In 1966, the Comprehensive Health Planning and Public Health Service Amendment was passed to enable states and local communities to plan for better health resources. Inadequate funding allocation led to the The National Health Planning and Resources Development Act of 1974. This legislation created a national network of health system agencies and statewide coordinating councils responsible for health planning. The intent was to improve health status and care, while reducing cost. These goals were to be achieved by preventing unneeded or duplicate services, decreasing fragmentation of services, and coordinating resources. New services were encouraged based on regional needs assessments.

In the 1980s, President Reagan aimed to reduce both the size of the federal government and the influence the federal government had on states. His administration eliminated the federal budget and planning requirements while encouraging states to make their own planning decisions. The federal health objectives for the years 2000 and 2010 suggest targets for local communities and states to consider (U.S. Department of Health and Human Services [USDHHS], 1997, 2000).

Increasing costs have placed heavy demands on the health care system (see Chapters 3 and 4). As a result health planning has essentially become economically focused. The federal government has attempted to control its share of health care costs by changing reimbursement methods, and shifting some of the budget responsibilities to the states. Because the federal government mandates health care services in those specific programs, states are left with limited autonomy to plan and deliver health care services.

In 1980, the Omnibus Budget Reconciliation Act encouraged the use of noninstitutional services, such as home health care, to fight escalating costs. In 1983 the Prospective Payment System drastically changed hospital reimbursement, resulted in shorter hospital stays for patients, shifted care into the community, and placed greater responsibilities for care of relatives on family members (see Chapters 3, 4, and 28).

The Gramm-Rudman-Hollings Budget and Deficit Control Act of 1985 added additional budget controls and cutbacks to health care. Taken together, these and subsequent federal efforts have presented a challenge to all health care professionals to plan and implement cost-effective health care programs that meet the needs of the people they serve. It is imperative that nurses become more cognizant of the health care planning process and their role within it.

The 1990s and early 2000s offered new opportunities for nurses to be involved in efforts to reform the nation's health care system (ANA, 1991). Debate continues about the degree to which government should be involved in health planning and whether federal or state planning is preferred (see Chapter 3). Some states have passed their own health care legislation, ensuring access to health care, identifying standard health benefit packages, and budgeting or requiring finance mechanisms. A greater interest has developed in ensuring that planning efforts also address the quality of health care. Furthermore, *Healthy People 2010* includes a goal that federal, state, and local public health infrastructures should have the capacity to provide essential public health services (USDHHS, 1998).

Health care planning for specific geopolitical communities continues at the state and local levels. Community/public health nurses are involved with specific communities to assess community needs. Nurses explore how the *Healthy People 2010* objectives apply to these geopolitical or phenomenological communities. Based on the assessments, community/public health nurses participate with others to develop plans to meet the health care needs of the people.

RATIONALE FOR NURSING INVOLVEMENT IN THE HEALTH PLANNING PROCESS

Florence Nightingale and Lillian Wald pioneered health planning based on an assessment of the health needs of the communities they served (see Chapter 2). Additionally, nurses have long been involved in implementing programs planned by other disciplines. Both the ANA (2007) and the American Public Health Association (APHA, 1996) state that the primary responsibility of community/public health nurses is to the community or population as a whole and that nurses must acknowledge the need for comprehensive health planning to implement this responsibility. Both professional organizations identify program planning as a primary function of the community/public health nurse.

In addition to mandates from professional organizations, nurses should be involved in program planning for several reasons. Nurses make up more than one third of all health care workers in the United States and implement the majority of health care programs. Our involvement in numerous and diverse health programs has given us experience in seeing what works and what does not. This experience helps identify difficulties that can be avoided in the future.

Nurses spend a greater amount of time in direct contact with their clients than do any other health care professionals. We are with the clients in the community, gaining first-hand information about their health, their lifestyles, their needs, and what it is like to be a member of that community. This exposure to the community places us in the unique position of possessing valuable information that is useful to the planning and implementation of successful health programs.

Not only do nurses make up a large portion of health care providers, they also make up a large portion of health care consumers in the United States. With the emphasis on consumer participation in health planning, nurses are in a unique position to make an impact in the planning of population-focused health programs.

NURSING ROLE IN PROGRAM PLANNING

Planning for change at the community level is more complex than that at the individual level. Components to the

client system have been increased, and more people and more complex organizations are involved. Baccalaureate-prepared community/public nurses are expected to apply the nursing process with subpopulations or aggregates with limited supervision (American Association of Colleges of Nursing, 1986; ANA, 2007). If nurses practice in agencies with a broad public health mandate, they will find that the scope of their focus shifts to larger populations (APHA, 1996). Community/public health nurses prepared at the baccalaureate level are expected to collaborate with others to assess the entire population and multiple aggregates in a geopolitical community (ANA, 2007). Therefore community health planning often takes a multidisciplinary approach, which requires excellent teamwork and thorough communication. The roles of collaborator, coordinator, and facilitator are important when working with the community as client.

A necessary task is to collaborate with people from the community to validate nursing diagnoses made from the assessment; to plan with, not for, the community; and to enlist community members' support and assistance in implementing change. If the community is not involved from the beginning, the program may not be effective. Just as you will have better adherence and outcome from planning care with an individual client, so, too, you will have a more successful program if you involve the community in the assessment and planning phases.

The coordinator role emerges when working with a variety of community members and organizations within and outside of the community. The nurse is in a key position to coordinate the activities and facilitate the community's ability to achieve a higher level of health. However, to affect change at the community level, community organization must be understood.

PLANNING FOR COMMUNITY CHANGE

To plan and implement programs at a community level effectively, the community/public health nurse must understand how the community works, how it is organized, who are its key leaders, how the community has approached similar problems, and how other programs have been introduced in the past. The health care professional who is facilitating the community organization process with regard to a specific health need or problem must work with the community members. To be an effective change agent in applying the nursing process, the nurse must be aware not only of the community and how it works, but also of methods of community organization that facilitate change.

COMMUNITY ORGANIZATION MODELS

Rothman (1978, 2008) identifies three **community organization models** designed to facilitate change in a community: community development (now called empowerment), social planning, and social action. The three models can be used separately or in combination. Although the models are presented here in pure form, in reality, they are generally combined. Social planning was the model most used by community health nurses and other public health care practitioners between the 1970s and the early 1990s. However, community organization approaches used by Lillian Wald and others during the nineteenth century, as well as during the 1960s, are reemerging as models for community empowerment.

Each model contains four components: goals, strategy, practitioner role, and medium of change. Table 16-1 summarizes the salient points from each of the three models. A thorough understanding of the components is necessary in planning for change in a community. Each model involves community change.

Community Empowerment Models

The **community empowerment** model is an approach designed to create conditions of economic and social progress for the whole community and involves the community in active participation. The community empowerment approach is also referred to as the *locality development approach* because of its work within the community. The community-locality development model is a *grass roots approach* that uses a democratic decision-making process, encourages self-help, seeks voluntary cooperation from the members, and develops leadership within the group (Milio, 1971). In this approach, community members believe they have some control over their destiny and therefore become actively involved. The change strategy is characterized by, "We know we have a problem, let's get together and discuss it." The theory underlying this model is that if people are involved in determining their own needs and desires, they will become more active in solving their problems than if someone else comes in and solves the problems for them. If they are more active in working out solutions to their own problems, they will be more satisfied with the solution and will continue to expend energy to make it work. That is, if they are *vested* in the solution, they will have more of a commitment to it. This model seeks to build on community assets and strengthen community competence.

The community empowerment model is especially important for communities with vulnerable and underserved populations. This model is being used successfully in both urban and rural communities.

> *Urban example*. In the inner city of Chicago, Illinois, a team of nurses identified a community need to improve maternal and infant health outcomes because the community had higher rates of maternal and infant complications than the national norm. Assessment indicated that minority women (African American and Hispanic) in the community needed support to follow through with prenatal and postpartum care,

education to improve parenting skills, and encouragement to use health prevention behaviors, such as immunizations, to improve the health status of both the mothers and the infants. The nurses implemented the REACH-Futures program, which is a home visiting program designed to monitor the health status of participants, provide appropriate health services as needed, and improve the health and welfare of both young mothers and their infants. The project enrolled 588 minority African American and Hispanic pregnant women into an intervention program that used both health professionals (nurses) and community workers to deliver health services. Each team consisted of one nurse and two community workers. Home visits were initiated in the last trimester of pregnancy and continued at 1-month intervals, or more often as necessary, for a planned 36 months. The community workers, who did most of the home visits, were trained in child development milestones, appropriate parenting skills and techniques, the identification of home safety and health hazards, and strategies to improve compliance with immunization schedules and well-baby visits (Norr et al., 2003). Initial evaluation of the program, after 1 year, indicated that the community workers were effective in supporting young mothers and improving parenting skills and compliance with immunization schedules and well-baby visits.

> *Rural example*. Community health nurses enlisted the use of "community guides and community leaders" to identify health resources and solutions for elderly residents and their caregivers in a Mexican American community in Arizona (Crist & Dominguez, 2003). The health interventions were secondary and tertiary, aimed at increasing the knowledge and use of health care services by the older adults and their caregivers.
>
> The nurses recruited *nanas* (grandmothers) as actors in a short play or *telenovela* designed to reduce resistance to use of health services. Additional community collaborative efforts included development of an Elders Use of Services Community Advisory Council to assist and guide the nurses toward community-acceptable interventions.

This approach, then, has the potential of having the longest lasting effect of the three models to be discussed. However, the

---

TABLE 16-1   Three Models of Community Organization Practice According to Selected Practice Variables

Variables	Community Empowerment	Social Planning	Social Action
Goal categories of community action	Self-help; community capacity and integration (process goals)	Problem solving with regard to substantive community problems (task goals)	Shifting of power relationships and resources; basic institutional change (task or process goals)
Basic change strategy	Broad cross-section of people involved in determining and solving their own problems	Fact gathering about problems and decisions on the most logical course of action	Crystallization of issues and organization of people to take action against obstructive targets
Salient practitioner role	Enabler-catalyst; coordinator; teacher of problem-solving skills and ethical values	Fact gatherer and analyst; program and policy designer and implementer; facilitator	Activist or advocate; agitator; broker; negotiator; partisan
Medium of change	Guiding of small task-oriented groups	Guiding of formal organizations and of data	Guiding ongoing action groups and mobilizing of ad hoc mass action groups

Adapted from Rothman, J. (1978). Three models of community organization practice. In Cox, F., Erlich, J., Rothman, J., & Tropman, J. (Eds.), *Strategies of community organization: A book of readings* (pp. 25-45). Itasca, IL: Peacock Publications; Rothman, J. (2008). Approaches to community intervention. In Rothman, J., Erlich, J., & Tropman, J. (Eds.). *Strategies of community intervention* (7th ed., p. 163). Peosta, IA: Eddie Bowers Publishing Company.

task is also the most time consuming to initiate because time is required to discuss the problems, to make decisions democratically, and to develop leadership within the group that will be able to sustain the program. Therefore even though the community-locality development approach to community organization is successful, it may not always be used in pure form because of the amount of time required to accomplish the action.

Social Planning Model

The **social planning** approach emphasizes a process of rational, deliberate problem solving to bring about controlled change for social problems. This method is an *expert* approach in which knowledgeable people (experts) take responsibility for solving problems. The degree of community involvement may be very small or very great. (The greater the involvement is, the more successful the outcome will be.) The social planning approach is characterized by, "Let's get the facts and proceed logically in a systematic manner to solve the problem." Pertinent data are considered before decisions are made about a feasible course of action to meet the need.

Agencies and organizations frequently use this approach as they attempt to effect desired change. The legislative and regulatory process is one example of a social planning approach. Problems are identified, data are collected, and bills are introduced into local, state, or national legislative bodies to effect change. A social planning approach is also used when a local health department institutes a program of directly observed therapy for treating tuberculosis. Public health nurses use facts gathered about the prevalence of tuberculosis in the community, as well as public health and nursing literature about effective treatment programs, to plan a program to directly observe persons with active tuberculosis take their antituberculosis medications.

The social planning approach can be effective, but it has one major pitfall: the potential for lack of community involvement. Much money has been spent and many health programs have failed because experts have planned programs *for* the community instead of *with* the community. The health planners, the nurse experts, must develop a partnership with the community for effective health care planning (ANA, 2007).

Social Action Model

The **social action** approach is a process in which a direct, often confrontational action mode seeks redistribution of power, resources, or decision making in the community or a change in the basic policies of formal organizations, or both. In this approach, one group of people or segment of an organization or community is feeling *oppressed,* and the organization or community is viewed as needing basic changes in its institutions or practices. Aggressive actions or nonviolent civil-disobedience may be taken to facilitate these changes. This approach, which is direct and often confrontational and radical, may be characterized as follows: "Let's organize to rectify an imbalance of power." In the 1960s the social action approach was used a great deal. The civil rights movements and protests against the Vietnam War are examples of the social action approach. Current examples include welfare rights organizations and advocacy groups for the environment or for the homeless, as well as some antiabortion groups.

Citizens in the Chattanooga Creek area of Tennessee became concerned about the quality and safety of water in the Chattanooga Creek. A local environmental activist group, Stop Toxic Pollution (STOP), organized. STOP contacted local public health nurses, other health professionals, and the Agency for Toxic Substances and Disease Registry (ATSDR). ATSDR is a federal agency responsible for preventing and mitigating the health hazards of exposure to toxic wastes.

An assessment conducted by local health personnel, area residents, and a nurse researcher from ASTDR revealed several potential sources of pollution and 42 hazardous waste sites. A nursing diagnosis was developed:

Potential for injury—residents who were exposed to creek water or ate fish from the creek were at risk of short-term gastrointestinal and skin problems, and long-term skin or liver cancer.

The following three-pronged intervention strategy was devised:
1. Public education
2. Public protection
3. Clean up hazardous waste sites (Phillips, 1995)

STOP, community nurses, and other local health providers were actively involved in developing and implementing the public education program aimed at both adults and children. The group also cooperated in ensuring that the problems with the creek remained in the news. Publicity about the situation facilitated the public education aspect of the intervention and also spurred public officials to take remedial actions to isolate the hazards. Finally, the site was placed on the National Priorities list for pollution cleanup.

Change Theory

Each of the community organization models involves change. Change can be threatening and stressful or it can be exciting and rewarding. Understanding some theory about planned change will provide a guide to use in the planning process. Lewin (cited in Dever, 1991) describes change as being a three-stage process: unfreezing, moving, and refreezing. In the first stage, unfreezing, a need for change is identified. The stimulus for the perceived need may be within the client or come from an outside force. Disequilibrium exists or is created, making a disruption in the status quo (unfreezing), and change is initiated. Moving, the second stage of the change process, occurs when the proposed change is tried out by the people involved, old actions are questioned, and attitude changes occur, creating movement toward acceptance of the proposed change. This phase is a vulnerable time for the people involved, because change is threatening and anxiety producing. Individuals will need help and support while trying out the proposed change. Refreezing, the third stage of the change process, occurs when the change is established and accepted as a permanent part of the system. Stabilization of the situation occurs. Lewin also describes forces that facilitate (driving forces) or impede (restraining forces) change. Driving forces must exceed restraining forces for change to occur.

STRUCTURES FOR HEALTH PLANNING

Several structures or schemes have been developed by national organizations to help communities plan for improving their health. These structures encourage collaborative partnerships and comprehensive assessments as building blocks for community health planning.

Planned Approach to Community Health (PATCH) is a program initiated by the Centers for Disease Control and Prevention (Association for the Advancement of Health Education, 1992). PATCH attempts to engage entire geopolitical communities in a comprehensive assessment of their health needs rather than focusing solely on high-risk groups or those served by a specific health institution. PATCH depends on the participation of citizens, the cooperation of several organizations within the community, and vertical integration of local, state, and federal government resources.

The Institute of Action Research for Community Health at the University of Indiana School of Nursing is helping cities in the United States adopt the World Health Organization's Healthy Cities project (Flynn et al., 1992; World Health Organization, 1991). The Healthy Cities project seeks to promote the health of urban communities through developing local leadership, innovative health programs, and effective coordination of resources (World Health Organization, 1991).

The National Association of County and City Health Officials (NACCHO) developed a strategic planning tool, Mobilizing for Action through Planning and Partnerships (MAPP) (NACCHO, 2000). MAPP is intended for use by local health departments in planning with geopolitical communities to improve health status and public health system capacities (see Chapters 15 and 29). The tool emphasizes community ownership of the process. The action cycle of MAPP includes planning, implementation, and evaluation.

The *Healthy People 2010* objectives are introduced in Chapter 2 and used as examples throughout the text. Many state and local jurisdictions have developed health improvement plans that link the national perspective of *Healthy People 2010* with local needs.

STEPS OF PROGRAM PLANNING

The planning process consists of a series of specific steps. Although each of these steps is necessary, the steps do not have to occur in the exact sequence given here. Occasionally, several steps may be undertaken simultaneously, or they may occur in a slightly different order. Identification of the planning group may occur much earlier in the sequence. The steps are as follows:

1. Assessment
2. Diagnosis
3. Validation
4. Prioritization of needs
5. Identification of the target population
6. Identification of the planning group
7. Establishment of the program goal
8. Identification of possible solutions
9. Matching solutions with at-risk aggregates
10. Identification of resources
11. Selection of the best intervention strategy
12. Delineation of expected outcomes
13. Delineation of the intervention work plan
14. Planning for program evaluation

Some researchers call steps 8 through 14 operations planning (e.g., Hale et al., 1994).

ASSESSMENT

A thorough, accurate assessment of the community is the first essential step in program planning. Chapter 15 provides a framework for community assessment and assessments of a geopolitical and a phenomenological community.

ANALYSIS OF DATA

A systematic analysis of the data collected is necessary to identify the problems, needs, strengths, and trends in the community. Categorizing the data first is always helpful to identify the inferences that are descriptive of actual or potential health problems. The community assessment described in Chapter 15 provides a framework in which to categorize the data about community functioning. Within each subsystem, nurses identify resources (assets, strengths) and demands (deficits, weaknesses), looking not only at whether something is present, but also to what extent, how it is working, and how it relates to the past and future to provide an idea of trends over time. Nurses also consider the health status of the population. Typically, the nurse identifies high-risk aggregates among the population as well.

In addition to illustrating the community's strengths and weaknesses, an analysis will provide information about demographic and personal characteristics, which are important to consider when planning and implementing health programs. For example, if you are working with a group of senior citizens enrolled in a senior center and your assessment indicates a potential risk for injury by fire, what other factors should you consider in the assessment data before you plan a fire prevention program? One factor that comes to mind is the educational level of the senior citizens. Knowing the educational level provides information about the appropriate level at which to plan the teaching interventions. The level of disability and social functioning indicates the presence of visual or hearing impairments that might affect the type of teaching strategy you use. Additionally, if many seniors are in wheelchairs or need assistive devices, you would focus the program on fire safety involving limited mobility and would need to modify practice sessions to the participants' level of ability. In other words, analysis of community data provides information not only about what is needed, but also about what will be appropriate in the intervention.

Data Gaps

Assessment sometimes reveals areas in which all the information is not available. This lack of information is called a **data gap.** The nurse must identify areas of insufficient information and devise a strategy to collect additional data if possible. Data gaps themselves may sometimes be informative. For example, if you cannot find out the date of a town council meeting, it might imply that the council is not open to citizen input.

Ways to Display Data for Analysis

As shown in Chapter 7, displaying data that aid in the analysis process can be done in a variety of ways. Graphs, charts, histograms, and mapping techniques are some of the most common visual displays. Computer-based geographic information systems (GIS) that map data spatially are becoming more widely used (see Chapter 15).

Obtaining as much data as possible that are specific to the target population is important. Table 16-2 includes the age and sex of people living in census tract 1 and city X. Census tract 1

TABLE 16-2   Comparison of Age by Sex of Populations in Census Tract I and City X, 2000

Age (Year)	Census Tract 1		City X	
	Number	Percentage	Number	Percentage
Male				
Under 5	548	6.9	38,512	4.3
5-9	743	9.4	44,204	4.9
10-19	1280	16.2	84,037	9.3
20-34	401	5.1	85,373	9.4
35-54	293	3.7	95,793	10.6
55-64	89	1.1	41,788	4.6
65-74	33	0.4	25,938	2.9
75 and above	21	0.3	11,822	1.3
Total	3408	43.0	427,467	47.2
Female				
Under 5	522	6.6	37,567	4.1
5-9	782	9.9	43,502	4.8
10-19	1323	16.7	86,668	9.6
20-34	930	11.7	95,611	10.6
35-54	701	8.8	108,122	11.9
55-64	140	1.8	48,920	5.4
65-74	80	1.0	36,165	4.0
75 and above	41	0.5	21,737	2.4
Total	4516	57.0	478,292	52.8
Total population	7924	100	905,759	100

data are included in city X totals, but, as can be seen, census tract 1 is quite different from city X. The population of the census tract is younger than the total city population, and data from the city cannot be used to describe the residents of the census tract. Looking at city X data only and thinking that the data would apply specifically to census tract 1 would not be accurate.

DIAGNOSIS

After analyzing the data, the next step is to make a definitive statement (diagnosis) identifying what the problem is or the needs are. Nursing diagnoses for communities may be formulated regarding the following issues:
- Inaccessible and unavailable services
- Mortality and morbidity rates
- Communicable disease rates
- Specific populations at risk for physical or emotional problems
- Health-promotion needs for specific populations
- Community dysfunction
- Environmental hazards (ANA, 1986)

The format of the problem statement varies, depending on the philosophy of the agency conducting the assessment. For example, problems or needs may be stated simply in epidemiologic terms, such as a high rate of adolescent pregnancies, whereas in other instances you may be asked to state the problem or need as a nursing diagnostic statement.

Nursing diagnosis has evolved since 1973 as a result of the efforts of the North American Nursing Diagnosis Association (NANDA) (NANDA, 2007-2008). The initial **North American Nursing Diagnosis Association (NANDA) classification system** of nursing diagnoses focused on the physical needs of individual clients and was severely criticized because it was not applicable to the family and community situations faced by community health nurses (Hamilton, 1983; Muecke, 1984). Over the years, the NANDA classification system has expanded to include biologic, psychologic, and social needs of individuals and families but was still criticized for not adequately addressing the community as client. Starting in the 1980s, the National Group for the Classification of Nursing Diagnosis organized and refined a taxonomy of nursing diagnoses that, at present, has 12 functional health patterns. Tools have been developed to assess the community using the functional health pattern typology (Gikow & Kucharski, 1987; Wright, 1985). Newer NANDA diagnoses may also apply to communities; examples include the diagnoses *impaired home maintenance* and *impaired social interaction.*

Other classification systems have been developed in an attempt to address the community. One example is the **Omaha System,** written by community/public health nurses for community/public health nursing practice (Martin, 2005). The system was designed by the Omaha Visiting Nurse Association and has been used in home care, public health, and school health practice settings, among others. Client problems/needs/concerns are organized into four domains: physiologic, psychosocial, health-related behaviors, and environmental. Each domain may involve actual or potential problems or opportunities for health promotion. The system includes four categories of interventions: teaching, guidance, and counseling; treatments and procedures; case management; and surveillance. Although originally developed for application with individuals or families, users are now beginning to apply the problem domains and interventions with communities (Martin, 2005). The Omaha System includes more environmental and community factors than are considered in the NANDA system.

Because of the multiple nursing diagnostic and classification systems, the NNN Alliance has formed to develop a consistent classification system. The NNN Alliance is a collaboration of NANDA and the Center for Nursing Classification and Clinical Effectiveness (CNC). The taxonomy developed by the NNN Alliance has four domains (Dochterman & Jones, 2003). The one relevant to community health practice is the environmental domain, with three subsets: health care system, populations, and aggregates. All three subsets have diagnosis, outcome, and intervention arenas. Because the taxonomy is so new, information is scarce on how useful the system will be to community/public health nursing practice.

Because community/public health nursing is concerned with health promotion, other nurses have developed ways to add wellness diagnoses to the problem-focused diagnoses of NANDA. Neufield and Harrison (1990) recommend that wellness nursing diagnoses for populations and groups include three components: the name of the specific target population, the healthful response desired, and related host and environmental factors. For example, high school students with children (target population) have the potential for responsible parenting (desired response); this potential is related to a desire to learn about child development (host factor) and the presence of a family life education curriculum and an availability of teachers (environmental factor).

During the late 1990s and early 2000s, NANDA added three community-focused diagnoses: *readiness for enhanced community coping, therapeutic regimen management,* and *ineffective community coping* (NANDA, 2002). These diagnoses address a community's ability to adapt and solve problems.

How does the nurse formulate a community-focused nursing diagnosis? A diagnosis is a statement that synthesizes assessment data; it is a label that describes a situation (state) and implies an etiologic component (reason). A nursing diagnosis limits the diagnostic process to the diagnoses that represent human responses to actual or potential health problems that are within the legal scope of nursing practice.

A nursing diagnosis has three components: a descriptive statement of the problem, response, or state; identification of factors etiologically related to the problem; and signs and symptoms that are characteristic of the problem (Carpenito, 2000).

Using this information, let us take a moment to try to state nursing diagnoses for some problems on the community level.

Situation 1

Howard County is a suburban county with a rapidly increasing number of elderly people. The assessment data indicate the presence of only one taxicab company serving that area. No public bus system is available.

Obviously, the problem is lack of transportation; but how might this be worded in nursing diagnosis format?

Suggestion:

Altered health-seeking behaviors related to inadequate transportation services for senior citizens

However, inadequate transportation probably also affects other areas of seniors' lives, such as socialization and community participation. If this factor were validated through further assessment, an additional diagnosis might be as follows:

Impaired social interactions related to inadequate transportation for senior citizens

Situation 2

Students in Johnson High test very low on an acquired immunodeficiency syndrome (AIDS) awareness survey. Further investigation reveals that no information is provided to the students, and the parents do not want information taught in the school. Ninety-eight percent of the students stated that they do not believe they are in any danger of getting human immunodeficiency virus (HIV).

Suggestion:

Lack of knowledge about HIV/AIDS in high school students related to:

- *Inadequate information provided in school curriculum*
- *Parental attitudes about the disease*
- *Perceived perception that they are not at risk for the disease*

Situation 3

Assessment data indicate that a high number of children at Little Joy Day Care Center have low hematocrit levels and median household incomes less than $15,000 per year. Both parents and children scored very low on a nutrition game.

Suggestion:

Altered health maintenance among children at Little Joy Day Care Center related to lack of knowledge about foods high in iron and to low median household income.

VALIDATION

Validating data and nursing diagnoses with the community is important. Do community members really see this as a problem? If so, do they desire a solution? Have they adjusted to the problem and therefore may be resistant to change? For example, people living in a run-down housing area in a large city are offered better housing in a new project. However, many people choose to remain where they are rather than leave their friends and move to a strange environment. These people have adapted to the problem and are, for a variety of reasons, resistant to possible solutions. The restraining forces (friendships and fear of the unknown) are greater than the driving forces (desire for newer housing). Many programs have failed because the professionals planned care based on their own values and perceptions of the problem and did not validate clients' perceptions of the problem and their desire for change. Perhaps if the residents had been involved in the decisions to move together, the resistance would be lessened.

How is validation with the community carried out? Validation may be done in a variety of ways. You might use a questionnaire, conduct personal interviews, or make appointments with key community leaders or informants. Foremost, community members need to be included in planning groups.

PRIORITIZATION OF NEEDS

The community assessment identifies needs and problems. However, not all needs can be addressed simultaneously; priorities must be determined. Prioritization can be based on many factors, such as the seriousness of the problem, the desires and concerns of the community, time, cost, and availability of resources. Obviously, a life-threatening situation, such as a nuclear spill, will have priority over other less life-threatening situations. A health problem may also be identified as serious when the community rate is higher than the national rate for the same problem. The American Public Health Association (APHA) (1961) identified the first five of the following six factors to consider when determining priority of health needs at the community level:

1. Degree of community concern
2. Extent of existing resources for dealing with the problem (e.g., time, money, equipment, supplies, facilities, human resources)
3. Solubility of the problem
4. Need for special education or training measures
5. Extent of additional resources and policies needed
6. Degree to which community/public health nursing can contribute to the planning process

When attempting to prioritize the community's needs, assessment data and the nursing literature must be used to answer questions such as the following: How concerned is the community? How does the magnitude of the problem compare with national rates? Are enough resources available to deal with the problem? Can the problem be solved? What additional education and training measures, if any, will be needed to solve the problem? What additional resources will be needed? Are existing policies in place that need to be changed or modified for the problem to be solved? Are community/public health nurses likely to be effective? After answering these questions, priorities may change from those identified initially.

IDENTIFICATION OF THE TARGET POPULATION

The term **target population** is used to describe the identified group or aggregate in which change is desired as the result of a program or intervention. An assessment is sometimes conducted on an entire community, as was done with "city X" and "Northwood High" in Chapter 15. However, intervention can also target one segment of the population. For example, city X has a high rate of gonorrhea. If a community/public health nurse planned a program to decrease gonorrhea among high school students in census tract 1, the students enrolled in high school in census tract 1 would be the target population, that is, the group in which the nurse wishes to effect change. Can you identify the target populations in the following examples? What are the communities?

- *Example 1:* a program to decrease alcohol-related automobile accidents among students at Jackson High
- *Example 2:* an exercise program for the frail elderly at Hebron House Senior Center
- *Example 3:* a health-education program about first aid for 10- and 11-year-old girls enrolled in Girl Scout Troop No. 26

Students, the frail elderly, and 10- and 11-year-old Girl Scouts are the target populations in the three respective examples. Did you list Jackson High, Hebron House Senior Center, and Girl Scout Troop No. 26 as the phenomenological communities? If so, you are correct.

Can the target population and the community ever be one and the same? Even though they are listed separately in the previously mentioned examples, the community and the target population may be one and the same. Remember that Chapter 15 stressed the importance of defining the community, because the parameters delineated in the definition determine what data to collect. Therefore the community might be defined as the students enrolled at Jackson High. If this definition is accurate, the community and the target population would be one and the same. Similarly, the frail elderly at Hebron House and the 10- and 11-year-old girls of Girl Scout Troop No. 26 might be designated as the community; again, the community and target population would be the same.

IDENTIFICATION OF THE PLANNING GROUP

The nature and extent of the community's needs will determine who should be involved in developing the plan. Consideration should be given to (1) persons for whom the plan is designed, that is, the target population; (2) those who are concerned with the health problems; (3) those who appear best able to contribute resources to the plan; and (4) those who are most likely to follow through in carrying out the plan of action. The size of the planning group must also be considered. For logistical reasons, obviously, everyone concerned with the problem cannot be personally involved as a member of the planning group. However, the interests of persons who are concerned must be considered and handled in a representative manner throughout the planning process.

An important task is to identify the *opposition* early in the planning process and attempt to get these individuals involved. The opposition might help improve the plan by pointing out weaknesses. Participation also provides time to plan an appropriate rebuttal to opposition arguments. Involving opponents in the planning process is much better than waiting until the program is implemented and then facing resistance and program failure. Finally, the opposition may become involved and convert to supporters.

Keep in mind the following *general guidelines:* community members need to be included early in the assessment phase. However, an expanded or a different group may be formed before or after the target population is identified. Considerations about who should be involved in the planning group are summarized in Box 16-1.

ESTABLISHMENT OF THE PROGRAM GOAL

The program goal is a comprehensive statement of intent or purpose. A difference exists between the program goal and the desired outcomes (objectives). The goal is stated in general terms and gives no indication of possible means of achieving the desirable outcome (McKenzie & Smeltzer, 2000). Objectives, however, are stated in terms of a specific outcome that contributes in some way to the achievement of the goal. The following are two examples of program goals:

- To improve health knowledge regarding HIV/AIDS
- To decrease infant mortality rate

These positions are broad statements of purpose, not specific and measurable objectives.

BOX 16-1 Guidelines for Who Should Be Involved in the Planning Group

- Broad segments of the community, whenever possible, to provide widespread base of support for the program
- Leaders and others who control financial resources and have the legal authority to deal with the problem
- People in a position to promote acceptance of the program (e.g., media representatives, key community leaders, influential community members)
- People who will implement the program
- People who will be affected by the program
- People who are most likely to offer resistance, the opposition
- Specialists in the area who can contribute to the group's understanding of the problem and knowledge of possible alternative solutions

After the program goal is established, health planners will have to meet to discuss possible ways to achieve the goal and a feasible time frame within which to accomplish the goal.

IDENTIFICATION OF POSSIBLE SOLUTIONS

At this point in the process, the planning group has a *brainstorming* session to examine various strategies and to identify the pros and cons of each strategy for this particular community. What might work for one community may be inappropriate for another. Several factors influence the appropriateness of strategies. Physical, psychologic, social, cultural, economic, and political considerations affect the appropriateness of strategies to solve a problem in any given community.

Physical factors include demographic characteristics such as the age, race, gender, education, and income of the population. For example, a health-education program that uses a series of speakers might be appropriate for an adult population, whereas a group of children might need a more action-oriented, active participation program, such as a puppet show or a game.

The major area of concern in relation to psychologic factors is motivation. How will the strategies being proposed affect the community's motivation? Will members perceive this course of action as helping or hindering the solution of the problem? People's perceptions of a problem and individual motivational factors are important indicators of their health behavior. People will accept strategies or programs that are consistent with their value system and that they perceive as helping the problem. For example, many prevention-oriented programs have been aimed at people living in impoverished conditions. Many of these programs have failed because the people responsible for the programs did not consider motivational factors. Studies show that poverty contributes to an orientation to the present rather than to the future. Therefore people living in impoverished conditions tend to be more crisis or treatment oriented rather than prevention oriented.

What motivates people to accept or oppose a strategy? A variety of factors can influence acceptance or opposition. Opposition can be based on a rational decision-making process or an irrational emotional process. An important question to ask is the following: "Does the solution to the problem conflict with any basic religious or cultural beliefs held by this segment of the population?" For example, a program on birth control for adolescents may meet with much opposition from parents, or some faith communities, or both. As another example, opposition to HIV/AIDS education may exist within a school because many parents do not want sex education taught in the school.

Perceived vulnerability is another source of emotional opposition to programs. If people feel threatened, they may oppose the planned change. Although a small portion of the population will always oppose any change, identifying who might feel threatened by or vulnerable to the proposed action is important. Once these people are identified, the nurse can plan to work with them to explain the plan and solicit their help and cooperation rather than their opposition.

Social practices influence the acceptability of certain programs in a community. Understanding the community's social values and beliefs enables the nurse to plan a program that will be more consistent with these beliefs. For example, a rural community with a long history of self-sufficiency may prefer to raise money internally to fund a new program rather than apply for a grant from the state health department.

Cultural, ethnic, and religious values influence how people accept health care plans. People will not accept programs that are incongruent with their cultural, ethnic, and religious practices (see Chapter 10).

The level of education is crucial in knowing what type of interventions to plan. The level of education influences whether the nurse will plan a program that has a lot of reading or a visual, nonreading program. When printed materials of any kind are used in the intervention or to promote the program, the reading level must be considered (see Chapter 20).

Economic factors are also a consideration. We live in a cost-conscious era in which people ask, "Is the strategy cost effective?" If not, the nurse will probably have to plan a more cost-efficient alternative. Remember that cost-effectiveness refers to time and resources, as well as money. Generally, although the least costly alternative will be the most popular, an alternative that is more costly in money but saves time or resources will occasionally be favored.

What about political factors? You have heard people say, "It will probably go through this year because this is an election year," or "This would not be a very good proposal in this administration." These statements refer to the political climate and the importance of knowing when to propose certain programs. In election years, programs and strategies that appeal to the greatest number of voters for a politician in a given area would be more powerful strategies than ones that appeal to a small minority of the voting population. Knowing what community leaders and elected officials favor and approaching them for their support early are also extremely important. Knowing how to write letters to elected officials to elicit their support or to influence their vote is also important.

Power is closely associated with politics. Milio (1981) describes organizational effectiveness as the capacity of an organization to bargain for scarce resources. Whoever has the most power gets the resources.

MATCHING SOLUTIONS WITH AT-RISK AGGREGATES

Within the population assessed, you may determine that different subpopulations have different needs based on their risks, problems, and concerns. Consequently, you may want to identify specific solutions for different at-risk aggregates.

For example, in the clinical example provided in Chapter 15, when nurses assessed the members (population) of a Korean immigrant community, they identified numerous at-risk aggregates, each requiring a different health care service to address their needs (Kim et al., 2002). Hypertensive adults required prescription medication and exercise classes, and women needed breast cancer screening and education. An 8% case rate of hepatitis B (above the national average) dictated a two-pronged approach: health education for adults and young children and an immunization program for children.

IDENTIFICATION OF RESOURCES

Discussing the possible solutions in relation to the identified resources is an important part of planning. The nurse should identify the resources within the community, as well as outside the community, that can be used to help solve the problem.

These sources include both human and nonhuman resources. Human resources can provide expertise and people. Nonhuman resources include funding, facilities, supplies, and equipment. Knowing ahead of time that personnel, funding, or needed supplies are insufficient is better than aborting the mission for lack of resources after the intervention is begun.

> For example, in the Korean community identified in Chapter 15 and previously discussed, bilingual health professionals and social service personnel were identified as appropriate resources to assist with communication and values clarification, and to serve as educators to assist the non-Korean health professionals to deliver culturally competent care (Kim et al., 2002).

SELECTION OF THE BEST INTERVENTION STRATEGY

The nurse should select the best strategy for the population within the context of resources and time available. A problem can almost always be solved in more than one way. The key in this step of the planning process is selecting the best strategy for the population within the context of available resources.

The best intervention strategies are culturally appropriate and personalized to the preferences of the target population.

> *Example 1.* Smith Battle (2003) found that teen mothers accepted health-related assistance best when they felt they were in a reciprocal relationship, in which their views were considered important. Consequently, to be successful with teen mothers in this community and similar communities, Smith Battle (2003) recommends that community health nurses use a participatory rather than a nurse-focused strategy. Rather than be passive recipients of nursing care, the teens should be encouraged to contribute their knowledge to the community/public health nurse and community.
>
> *Example 2.* An assessment of health-education needs for Arab-American adolescent cigarette smokers in the Troy, Michigan, area revealed that they were eager to share their reasons for smoking and the efforts they had made to quit. The adolescents reviewed an existing smoking cessation program and offered suggestions to modify intervention strategies to customize it to their target group. These Arab-American teens also advised the nurses that including family and peer participation in the health-education project would be important (Kulwicki & Rice, 2003).

Having decided on a course of action, the next step is to plan the details of the intervention. First, however, specific, expected outcomes must be delineated.

DELINEATION OF EXPECTED OUTCOMES

Objectives for health programs include outcome objectives, process objectives, and management objectives (Hale et al., 1994). **Outcome objectives** address the health status or health behaviors desired in the target population or competencies desired in the community. **Process objectives** specify the implementation activities and health care delivery that are necessary to achieve the desired changes in the outcome objectives. **Management objectives** define the structures needed to carry out the process objectives. The *Healthy People 2010* objectives (USDHHS, 2000; USDHHS, 2006) are an important source of specific objectives.

For outcome objectives to be useful, they must meet a variety of criteria or indicators. Some criteria for the outcomes *community health status* and *community competence* are published in **Nursing Outcomes Classification (NOC)**, Appendix C (Moorhead et al., 2004). These criteria provide cues to measure the expected outcomes.

Outcome objectives (Ervin, 2002; Gronlund, 1970; Mager, 1962) should relate to the program goal or goals and the following:
- Identifying the program participants (who)
- Describing specific behaviors that program participants will exhibit to demonstrate accomplishment of the objectives (what)
- Describing the condition in which participants will demonstrate accomplishment (where and to what extent)
- Describing the standard performance expected to indicate accomplishment (how much)
- Describing the time frame (when)

How does writing objectives for the community differ from writing objectives for an individual client? Although the same criteria must be met, community-focused objectives are written for the group or population. When working with an individual client, the nurse may state the following objective: *After watching a film on diabetes, the client will state at least three signs of hyperglycemia.*

How would a similar objective be stated if the nurse was working with a group of diabetic clients? One example might be the following objective: *After watching a film on diabetes, 90% of the participants enrolled in the diabetic education program will state at least three signs of hyperglycemia.*

What is the difference? When working with the community, the nurse must consider the population and indicate whether all members of the population or a certain portion of the population needs to demonstrate the action. Examples of specific community-orientated behavioral objectives and differences between criterion and norm-referenced objectives are listed in Table 16-3.

In *criterion-referenced outcome objectives,* the objectives specify the behaviors desired in the target population or community. For example, the pregnancy rate of census tract 1 will be reduced to 40 pregnancies per 1000 female adolescents in 3 years. In *norm-referenced outcome objectives,* the desired outcome is compared with another population or an ideal. For example, the pregnancy rate of female adolescents in census tract 1 will be no higher than the national rate of pregnancies per 1000 female adolescents in 3 years. The population might also be compared with itself: the teenage pregnancy rate of census tract 1 will be reduced 50% in 3 years.

Process objectives specify incremental activities or service delivery that will lead to attainment of outcome objectives (Ervin, 2002). These objectives are monitored in short intervals to ensure that the program is on course to meet outcome objectives and program goals. The following is an example of a process objective: *75% of Northview High students will participate during the spring semester in an education session on reducing risky sexual behavior.* An objective such as this one would contribute to attainment of the program goal: to reduce risky sexual behavior among high school students.

Management objectives are concerned with funding; personnel; program support, such as equipment and record

TABLE 16-3 Behavioral Objectives/Outcomes

Sample Outcome Goal

At least 40% of the smokers among mothers enrolled in the central city Mom and Tots Center will have modified their smoking habits by June 2004.

Determine specific behavioral objectives: include who, behavior, condition, criteria, and when.

Sample Outcome Objective (Criterion-Referenced)

Given a smoking modification program, at least 80% of the interested mothers will devise and implement a contract to modify their smoking habits by the fifth week of the program.

1. Who—description of group participants	Interested mothers
2. Behavior—description of the behavior the participants will exhibit to demonstrate accomplishment of the objectives	Devise and implement a contract to modify smoking habit
3. Condition—description of condition in which participants will demonstrate accomplishment	Given a smoking modification program
4. Criteria—standard of performance expected to indicate accomplishment	At least 80% will actively participate
5. When—description of time frame	By the fifth week of the program

Sample Outcome Objective (Norm-Referenced)

After the presentation by the nursing students, the target population will demonstrate a statistically significant increase in knowledge as measured by a paper-and-pencil pretest and posttest.

1. Who—description of group participants	The target population
2. Behavior—description of the behavior the participants will exhibit to demonstrate accomplishment of the objectives	As measured by a paper-and-pencil pretest and posttest
3. Condition—description of condition in which participants will demonstrate accomplishment	After the presentation by the nursing students
4. Criteria—standard of performance expected to indicate accomplishment	Will demonstrate a statistically significant increase in knowledge

BOX 16-2 Steps in Establishing a Work Plan

1. Identify the specific target population to be served by the program.
2. Specify the number of people to be served during various time periods (called *utilization*).
3. Sequence the interventions logically, and specify when they are to be phased in and who is responsible to do so (perhaps using a Gantt Chart).
4. Determine the personnel needed. Anticipate learning needs of the personnel regarding implementing the program. (For example, if a program's purpose is to screen pregnant women for risk of abuse, nurses would need to know the factors indicating increased risk.)
5. Identify space, equipment, educational materials, and disposable supplies needed.
6. Develop a budget, including revenue sources and costs of personnel, equipment and supplies, publicity, use of buildings, and administrative services.
7. Develop mechanisms for managing the entire program, including supervising personnel, administering the budget, monitoring the planned sequence of activities (work plan), and conducting formative evaluation.
8. Develop mechanisms to communicate with interested parties and include the parties in program monitoring and decision making.

- WHEN will each action occur?
- HOW MUCH TIME will be required to accomplish the action?
- WHERE will the actions take place? This question includes obtaining the place and determining how much space is needed.

This work plan includes specific process and management objectives discussed earlier in the chapter.

Taking the time to make a detailed work plan in the beginning will save time and will make for a much smoother working phase. Nothing is more frustrating, or embarrassing, than coming to the intervention phase and realizing that a basic detail is missing.

PLANNING FOR PROGRAM EVALUATION

Although evaluation is the last step of the nursing process, evaluation planning should begin as soon as goals are established. All too often, evaluation is not even considered until the end. However, plans must also be made for evaluation. Evaluation is needed *throughout* the program to measure progress, as well as at the end to measure the overall value, adequacy, efficiency, outcomes, and effectiveness. Evaluation is a continuous feedback process that provides the stimulus for changes in the system.

Program evaluation is the process of determining whether the program is achieving its purpose, whether it should be continued or terminated, and how it can be improved or better managed (Glick & Kulbok, 2002). Process and management objectives are evaluated throughout the program to ensure that planned activities are being accomplished. Outcome objectives are measured primarily at the end of the program to determine whether the program goal was attained.

Many approaches can be used to program evaluation. Chapter 17 is devoted to exploring different methods of program evaluation in detail. Sufficient to mention in this chapter is that a plan for program evaluation must be seen

keeping; and publicity. The following is a management objective: *The health department will hire three community/public health nurses for school health within 4 months.*

DELINEATION OF THE INTERVENTION— WORK PLAN

In this step, the nurse plans the basics of the intervention and takes into consideration the specific what, how, who, when, and where (Box 16-2). A good plan will have the following questions answered *before* any intervention:

- WHAT actions are to be done?
- HOW are the actions to be accomplished?
- WHAT resources (equipment, space, money) are needed?
- WHO is responsible for the accomplishment of each action?

as an essential step in the planning process so that systematic program evaluation becomes a reality, not merely an afterthought. Box 16-3 summarizes some keys to success and pitfalls in planning and implementing health care for communities.

TOOLS USED TO PRESENT AND MONITOR PROGRAM PROGRESS

During implementation of the plan, evaluating progress is important. A visual guide to present and measure program progress is often helpful. Several tools are used to chart activity and anticipate management problems in the implementation phase. The three tools that are discussed here are the Gantt Chart, the Program Evaluation and Review Technique, and the Planning, Programming, and Budgeting System (Green & Kreuter, 1999; Rowland & Rowland, 1992).

Gantt Chart

Henry Gantt developed the Gantt Chart during World War I to identify the process needed to accomplish a result.

Starting with a final work result, major steps necessary to obtain the result are projected backward from results to actions; their timing and sequence are then considered (Drucker, 1974). The **Gantt Chart** considers the concepts of events and time (Figure 16-2). The events are listed down the left side of the chart. Time is represented across the chart for each event by lines showing when the event is to start and when it is to be completed.

Program Evaluation and Review Technique

The **Program Evaluation and Review Technique (PERT)** is a more complex tool. PERT is a network programming method developed during the 1950s through a joint effort between the U.S. Navy and private industry (Lockheed Aircraft Corporation and Booz Allen Hamilton, Inc.) for the Polaris Missile project. Similar to the Gantt Chart, PERT also looks at the concepts of events and time but is particularly useful for large-scale projects.

The intent of PERT is to accomplish the following:
- Focus attention on key developmental parts of the program
- Identify potential program problems
- Evaluate program progress toward goal attainment
- Provide a prompt, efficient reporting method
- Facilitate decision making

PERT involves the following three steps (Roman, 1969):
1. Identifying specific program activities
2. Identifying resources to accomplish these activities
3. Determining the sequence of activities for accomplishment

PERT uses a flowchart designed to estimate the time required to complete specific events necessary to complete the entire project. Events are shown on a chart by shapes (circles, ovals, squares, or triangles) with numbers. The number is not necessarily a sequential number; that is, number 3 does not have to occur after number 2. The numbers designate a task, not a sequential order. The activities to complete the events are the time-consuming element. Time is represented on the chart by lines and arrows. Unlike the Gantt Chart, each line has three different numbers representing three time estimates: optimistic, most likely, and pessimistic. *Optimistic* is the shortest amount of time possible to complete the activity if everything goes perfectly; *most likely* is the most likely amount of time needed to complete the activity; and *pessimistic* is the longest amount of time the activity might take (Ervin, 2002).

Planning, Programming, and Budgeting System

The **Planning, Programming, and Budgeting System (PPBS)** is an economical method of expressing a program plan. PPBS is an outcome-oriented accounting system designed to determine the most efficient method of resource allocation to attain measurable objectives (LaPatra, 1975).

The three components of the PPBS are as follows:
1. *Planning*: formulation of objectives and identification of alternatives and methods for accomplishing the objectives
2. *Programming*: delineation of resources for each identified alternative
3. *Budgeting:* assignment of dollar values to the resources required for the program implementation

Although designed by the U.S. Department of Defense to plan broad-scale programs, the PPBS can be used as a framework to plan programs for smaller organizations and population groups.

IMPLEMENTATION

Implementation is the action portion of the plan; in other words, the plan states what will occur in the implementation. Mobilizing people and resources to activate the plan of action is a challenging task for the community/public health nurse.

The role of the nurse during implementation varies based on the type of program, the community, and the community organization methods used. Baccalaureate-prepared community/public health nurses may directly implement the plan in partnership with others, coordinate programs and services, provide health education and health promotion, consult with others, and implement public health laws, regulations, and policies (ANA, 2007). In many health programs, community/public health nurses perform the interventions and manage the program.

BOX 16-3   Pitfalls and Keys to Success in Implementing Health Programs

Pitfalls to Success

Inaccurate assessment
Nonvalidation of data with community
No community involvement
Insufficient resources
Lack of coordinated planning
Lack of leadership
Poor communication

Keys to Success

Thorough, accurate assessment
Validation of assessment data with the community
Involvement of the community
Sufficient resources
Well-developed plan, with coordination among team members
Good leadership
Open communication

EXAMPLE OF GANTT CHART

This chart specifies time frame, tasks, and persons assigned to work on each task. Time frames listed below are suggested task allotment intervals; your group's progress may vary somewhat from these guidelines.

▲ Begin task ▲ Complete task ───────── Duration of task

Time (in weeks)

Tasks	1	2	3	4	5	6	7	8	9	10	11	12	13	14	15	16	Person assigned
1. Review task chart and delegate tasks	▲		▲														
2. a. Selection of health need/target population/ community and suprasystem	▲			▲													
b. Seek agency/ community approval to work with them			▲	▲													
3. Community assessment: a. Identify data needed			▲		▲												
b. Determine method(s) of data collection			▲			▲											
c. Collect data					▲		▲										
d. Analyze data						▲				▲							
e. Complete written community assessment and analysis																	
4. Health need of target population: a. Review literature of community health needs and risk areas for target population			▲			▲											
b. Identify additional data needed specific to selected population					▲			▲									
c. Determine method of data collection							▲	▲									
d. Identify or develop tool								▲	▲								
e. Pilot tool and revise										▲	▲						
f. Collect data										▲	▲						
g. Analyze data											▲		▲				
5. Propose nursing intervention(s) a. Select priorities											▲	▲					
b. Identify goals/objectives											▲		▲				
c. Identify possible interventions								▲				▲					
d. Select interventions													▲	▲			
6. Develop evaluation plan a. Review literature											▲		▲				
b. Selection of program evaluation method													▲	▲			

FIGURE 16-2 Example of a Gantt Chart, which specifies time frame, tasks, and persons assigned to work on each task. Time frames listed are suggested task allotment intervals; actual intervals may vary. (Adapted from Community Health Nursing Faculty, Undergraduate Program. [1985]. *Syllabus for nursing* [p. 325]. Baltimore: University of Maryland School of Nursing.)

Community/public health nurses often conduct health-education and screening programs and may provide primary health care. Community/public health nurses manage programs by supervising personnel, administering the budget, ordering equipment and supplies, maintaining program records, and ensuring that planned interventions are accomplished.

Throughout the implementation phase, the nurse continues to collaborate, coordinate, and consult with others. The role of facilitator increases because the nurse must facilitate the community's sense of ownership of the program. Active participation of the community is essential to the success of the program; the health program will be successful *only* if the community *owns it.* The nurse facilitates ownership by getting key people involved from the beginning and by facilitating increased involvement in the program. Therefore the nurse's role may change during implementation as the community begins to assume more responsibility.

Implementation results in change that can be stressful and threatening. Resistance to change is natural and inevitable, because every system attempts to maintain dynamic equilibrium. Change brings an initial state of disequilibrium. However, if the people in the community have been involved from the beginning in a plan that affects them, are informed about the benefits of the plan for them, and are convinced of the value of the plan, they are less apt to offer resistance.

TYPES OF INTERVENTIONS

Just as many different types of interventions can be made for the individual, so, too, a variety of interventions can be conducted for the community as client. All 17 public health nursing interventions discussed in Chapter 1 can be carried out with communities (Minnesota Department of Health, 2001). Several major types of community/public health intervention programs exist, including the following:

- Health-education programs
- Screening programs
- Establishing services
- Policy setting and implementation
- Increasing community self-help and competence
- Increasing power among disenfranchised individuals

Health-Education Programs

Much intervention at the community level is aimed at educating people about their health (see Chapter 20). Health-education programs can be geared toward one or more of the three levels of prevention. Programs provide information on how to promote health, prevent illness, manage care for those with illnesses, minimize the effects of illness or injury, and ensure a healthful environment.

Different health-education programs may be targeted to specific at-risk aggregates within the larger population or community that has been assessed.

> For example, in the Chattanooga Creek case study introduced earlier in this chapter, different health-education programs were planned for local health care providers, elementary school–age children, and adult residents to make them aware of environmental health hazards (Phillips, 1995).

Another example of targeting education occurred in 170 public and Catholic elementary schools in Ontario, Canada (Cicutto and colleagues, 2006).

> In Ontario, the schools had no school nurses and relied on public health nurses. A needs assessment conducted via questionnaire to teachers revealed that teachers did not know which students had asthma and 80% of teachers did not feel confident in handling asthma. To provide asthma-friendly schools, public health nursing interventions were targeted to children with asthma and to the broader school community. An asthma education program for children with asthma occurred once per week for 6 weeks. Multiple posters, newletter articles, teacher in-service education programs, and standardized asthma management forms targeted schools, teachers, staff, and parents.

The teaching methodology must be appropriate to the community. Using different methods of presentation that appeal to many senses (not just the lecture method, which is the least effective method) is important. U.S. society has been described as a media society. Use media that are well received by a given age group (e.g., for young children, use a puppet show or coloring books to teach content). Be creative! One example of a creative health-promotion program is a music video designed for adolescents in which the lyrics suggest birth control behaviors. This creative effort was designed by the Johns Hopkins Population Center for reaching populations in other countries. This approach has been popular in the Philippines and was released in Mexico.

Screening Programs

Screening programs are designed to provide early detection and diagnosis of health problems (see Chapter 19). An important point to remember is that screening does not prevent the disease but merely identifies risk factors or early signs so that appropriate treatment intervention may be obtained.

> To improve access to tuberculosis (TB) treatment among inner-city homeless, faculty and student nurses screened 327 residents of an addictions recovery program during an 18-month period (Lashley, 2007). Nursing students administered Mantoux tuberculin skin tests and provided assessments for TB symptoms. Those individuals with positive findings were referred to the city health department TB clinic for appropriate treatment. Nursing students educated the residents about TB infection, transmission, and control. The students also coached residents to keep clinical appointments and tracked those who missed appointments.

Important to note here is that when planning a screening program, referral and treatment resources must be included as part of the intervention. Saying, "You have a problem" is not enough. The nurse must also provide information about how and where to go for help. Community participation in screening activities and health fairs can be increased by using bilingual volunteers and paid community workers, as well as translators, when appropriate (Hecker, 2000).

Establishing Services

Many community health programs focus on establishing the services needed to meet the health needs of a given population. Some examples of services are school health clinics, home health care nursing services, grocery shopping services for home-bound elderly individuals, and adult daycare centers for elderly persons. Bremer (1987) has described the establishment of a community health nursing service to promote the health of elderly individuals in their homes and to prevent disability.

With the advent of nurse practitioners in the 1970s, contemporary community nursing centers began to emerge. Although the number of health centers is difficult to document, at least 250 of these centers have been established in the United States (Glick, 1999). In a study by the National League for Nursing, 170 community nursing centers were identified in 31 states (Barger & Rosenfeld, 1993). More than half of these centers were affiliated with another organization, often a school of nursing, and the rest were freestanding. The study found that community nursing centers provide direct access to nursing services, such as primary care, assessment and screening, education, case management, and counseling. The centers tend to provide care for traditionally underserved populations, such as children and poor, elderly, and homeless individuals. Approximately 30% of the care is financed directly by clients, almost 50% is paid for by insurance or gifts, and 20% is uncompensated. Planning for the establishment of community nursing centers is described further by several authors (Chalick & White, 1997; Hatcher et al., 1998; Shiber, 2002).

Innovation is basic to public health nursing practice.

> Sloand and Gebrian (2006) describe village-based fathers' clubs in Haiti, which has the poorest health indicators in the western hemisphere. Public health nurses supervise village health agents who are paraprofessionals. There are 40 active fathers' clubs with 700 members; fathers meet regularly for health education, support, and community building.

Policy Setting and Implementation

A community may have needs that must be met by policy changes (Williams, 1983). These changes might include legislation at the local or state level. Interventions that focus on policy setting may include lobbying, building coalitions, and participating in the political process. For example, a group of nurses initiated mandatory seat belt legislation as a result of the deaths and injuries they witnessed in emergency departments. In St. Louis, public health nurses were successful in getting the jurisdiction for a lead poisoning control program returned to the health department (Kuehnert, 1991). Previously, the responsibilities for lead screening and control had been transferred from the health department to the private sector, resulting in lower screening rates and a higher prevalence of lead poisoning.

Process evaluation of specific programs or interventions may result in recommendations for policy improvement.

> Personnel from a local health department responded to an outbreak of Norwalk-like virus at a church camp in Northwestern United States. Community/public health nurses who attended the camp were concerned about the perceived absence of partnership between the local health department personnel and the camp community (Sistrom & Hale, 2006). This led the nurses to recommend that community participation be identified as an essential part of outbreak investigation guidelines.

Increasing Community Self-Help and Empowerment

Locality development strategies focus on strengthening the processes that involve community members in solving their own problems (Rothman, 1978). These strategies do not result immediately in new educational programs on a specific health topic or in new services or policies. Instead, community competence is enhanced. Short-term results among community members include increased self-confidence, increased levels of problem-solving skills, and new or strengthened communication and problem-solving networks and coalitions. Milio's work (1971) with the Mom and Tots Center in Detroit is a classic example of this form of community development.

> Nurses who were concerned about the plight of elderly residents in rural Alabama found that older adults were often unable to perform chores or to pay to have chores and other activities done that would help maintain their independence and improve their quality of life. The nurses developed the Rural Elderly Enhancement Program to develop community volunteer coalitions; provide accessible and safe water, housing, and transportation; and conduct needs assessments of elderly persons (Farley, 1993). Community participation in the Alabama Rural Elderly Enhancement Program consisted of the following activities and services:
> Housing—Builds steps, ramps, porches; replaces roofs and windows
> Fund raising—Helps elders buy medications and obtain transportation and public water
> Education—After training by nurses, volunteers provide health education to elders
> Helping Hand—Trained volunteers provide friendly visits and homemaking, personal, and respite care

The REACH-Futures program discussed earlier in this chapter is an example of the empowerment of a community through the involvement of lay health workers (Norr et al., 2003).

Through locality development strategies, public health nurses can assist communities in strengthening their capabilities to engage in the core public health functions: assessment, policy development, and assurance (Kang, 1995). Community/public health nurses can facilitate partnerships among community groups and various subpopulations through which community members can become more active in identifying their health concerns, lobbying for changes in health policy, and ensuring culturally appropriate health promotion and disease or injury prevention. Thus self-help goes beyond empowerment of a specific population to strengthen the structures and competency of the entire community.

Changing Community Power Structures

Strategies that shift the power balance within or among communities can empower disenfranchised individuals. The power balance can be shifted if the ability of community members to help themselves is increased. However, the institutionalized structures of the community often must also be changed if the population is to have more equal access to community power. One example is the attempt to restructure employment opportunities so that a working adult is guaranteed a wage above the poverty level (Lewit et al., 1997).

STRATEGIES FOR IMPLEMENTING PROGRAMS

Several strategies can be used for implementing programs on the community level.

Single Action

In the single-action approach, programs are implemented one time for a specific purpose. In some instances, this approach is all that is necessary or all that resources will allow.

Phasing

Phasing in programs over a period is sometimes necessary or advantageous. Phasing in is often used in large programs and in programs in which a multitude of resources are needed. The problem is sometimes so multifaceted that several different stages of interventions are required to solve it.

Phasing has been used to implement the national injury prevention program. To reduce injuries and fatalities related to motor vehicle accidents, interventions have been added over time:

1. Mandatory seat belt laws passed by states
2. Mandatory helmets for motorcyclists by states
3. Improved safety standards for children's car seats
4. Federal funding eliminated or reduced if states did not pass mandatory seat belt laws
5. Laws tightened to allow police to stop a vehicle solely for nonuse of seat belts
6. Upgrading of manufacturing standards for car structures

Collaboration and Networks

Collaborative efforts between disciplines and agencies can be effective and efficient when planning care at the community level. A partnership between agencies and personnel results in better use of resources and often a much stronger program. A great deal more can be accomplished when resources are pooled.

A group of 10 nursing students enrolled in their senior community/public health course decided to do a community project in an elementary school. After consultation with the school principal, and because of time constraints (10 weeks), the students limited their community to a group, the third-grade students. The nursing students visited the school and classrooms to gather information. During their first visit, several students noticed two incidents of bullying during playground activities. This observation and subsequent collaborating data (interviews with teachers, the school nurse, the principal, and some third-grade students) identified a need to address bullying behavior as a health need.

In developing the intervention plan, the nursing students collaborated with the county police department, the university school of social work, and a high school student peer-counseling program. The ultimate intervention included an educational component, several play-acting sessions, and an ongoing peer-counseling program under the guidance of participants in the high school peer-counseling program. All the groups profited from the collaborative effort. The nursing students gained valuable experience working with multiple disciplines and agencies. The third-grade students gained an ongoing support program that continues to help them cope with bullying behavior. The school of social work and police department gained additional experience working with young children in violence prevention activities. The high school students learned how to modify their approach to peer counseling by making it age appropriate. The high school students also benefited because they acquired volunteer or credit hours needed to graduate from high school.

Coalitions

A coalition is a temporary union for a common purpose. Coalitions are effective strategies at the local, state, and national political levels and often are population oriented. For example, coalitions for women's health issues have been formed.

Ultimately, a program's success depends on many factors, including human resources, funding, political will, and community support. Community/public health nurses—with their unique knowledge of community resources and assets, community problems or lack of resources, and key players—are well situated to facilitate and empower community action.

KEY IDEAS

1. Health planning is a social process that many disciplines use to promote the health of populations and the competency of communities.
2. Health interventions planned for groups and populations are often called programs. Although programs may be single actions, they are more often ongoing interventions involving several different activities and phases.
3. Steps in health program planning are consistent with the nursing process and include assessment, analysis, planning, implementation, and evaluation.
4. Community/public health nurses work in partnership with other professionals, community leaders, and community members to plan and implement health care based on a community assessment.
5. Community health planning based on community assessment is a basic element of community/public health nursing.
6. Community nursing diagnoses address the community members' responses to actual and potential health problems. No single classification system exists for nursing diagnoses for communities.
7. Program goals are broad statements of desired health outcomes. Outcome, process, and management objectives contribute to goal attainment.
8. Community/public health nurses use *Healthy People 2010* objectives as guides to develop goals and objectives for health programs in specific communities.
9. Community/public health nurses often implement and manage community and public health programs.
10. Common health care interventions performed by community/public health nurses include health education, screening, policy formation, establishing new nursing services, and community empowerment.
11. Planning health programs for communities includes planning for evaluation.

In this case study, we use the community assessment of Northview High School given in Chapter 15 to plan and begin to implement health programs. Many of the steps of program planning discussed earlier in this chapter are evident.

A community/public health nurse, Marian Fields, is assigned full time to two high schools, Northview and South Central high schools. This assignment is new for her. She is expected to spend 5 days each 2-week period at each school. Previous to her appointment, the health department provided a nurse for one half day per week at each school. Her job description includes staffing a health room to address the complaints of ill students, maintaining the health and immunization records of all students, administering medications and providing treatments as ordered for chronically ill students (e.g., nebulizer treatments for asthmatic students), assisting with classroom instruction on health-related issues, and developing programs to address the major health-related concerns of the high school students.

Through the assessment of Northview High School in Chapter 15, the following health issues emerged:

- Substance abuse, including smoking
- Communicable diseases and rashes
- Injuries necessitating first aid
- Insufficient birth control information
- Unprotected sexual activity
- Teenage pregnancy
- Lack of daycare for infants of teenage parents
- High dropout rates for pregnant teens
- Sexually transmitted diseases
- Vision screening
- Chronic illnesses
- Personal hygiene
- Dental problems
- Obesity and anorexia

Ms. Fields decides to concentrate her initial program efforts on a single health issue rather than to address all the health problems of the high school at one time.

PRIORITIZATION

In selecting a health need for intervention, the community/public health nurse should consider how many students are affected by the problem, as well as the degree of risk associated with the problem. Risky sexual behavior is selected as the priority problem because it is of concern to both parents and faculty; community/public health nurses can contribute to the solution, and risky sexual behavior can be changed. Addressing risky sexual behavior also has the potential to contribute to other health status outcomes as well. The nurse's ultimate goal is to change the health status of her community by lowering the rates of teenage pregnancy and sexually transmitted disease through reducing the number of students engaging in unprotected sexual activity. When comparing the teenage pregnancy rate for this school with national statistics, the nurse finds the school's pregnancy rate (18%) is well above the national rate (4.1%) (USDHHS, 2002).

TARGET POPULATION

The target population is the students attending Northview High School.

PLANNING GROUP

Ideally, the planning group at Northview should include the following:

- The consumers (students in the high school)
- Individuals who are concerned with the problem (faculty, administrators, members of the parent-teacher association [PTA])
- Individuals with resources (health department, board of education)
- Individuals who will implement the plan (community/public health nurse, physical education teacher)

In this situation, Ms. Fields is charged by the principal to develop a plan and then bring it to him and the school board for consideration. Ms. Fields is able to arrange several meetings with a group consisting of some faculty (including the physical education teacher), health department personnel, and student representatives.

POSSIBLE SOLUTIONS

During the meetings, participants brainstorm the following possible solutions to the problem:

- Teen clinic on site
- Teen clinic near the school
- Educational program regarding sexually transmitted diseases and containing contraceptive information
- Educational program without contraceptive information
- Simulation experience: caring for a child (to increase motivation to avoid pregnancy)
- Peer counseling or partnership program
- Interviews with teenage parents to determine why they got pregnant
- Inviting adolescents with sexually transmitted diseases or HIV to speak (to increase perceived vulnerability to disease)
- Participatory programs to strengthen identity and self-efficacy and identify own goals or values

PROGRAM GOALS

After much discussion, the group incorporates a large number of solutions into a two-phase program design. The first phase is to develop a comprehensive sex education program aimed at changing risky health behaviors. The second phase is to improve access to health services for sexually active students. (*Planning for evaluation* is discussed in Chapter 17.)

PHASE 1: A SEX EDUCATION PROGRAM

Ms. Fields is responsible for designing the educational program. She reviews the literature on teenage pregnancy, birth control, sexual activity, attitudes, and knowledge level. Because of the various opinions about the inclusion of sexually transmitted disease and contraceptive information in a sexual education program for adolescents, Ms. Fields needs to identify the community's position on these topics. From conversations with parents, she knows that many people would support inclusion of this information in the educational program. She meets with the principal to determine his position, who informs Ms. Fields that he will support inclusion of the topics and that the school superintendent has informed him that five of seven school board members will support the position.

To validate that Northview High School students' needs are similar to those identified in the literature, the nurse designs a questionnaire to distribute to a sample of students. The aim of the questionnaire is to assess the level of student knowledge about the selected topics to tailor the educational program for the students at Northview High School. Her survey reveals that students are knowledgeable about the mechanics of sexual intercourse, and most acknowledge the importance of protection during sexual intercourse; nevertheless, they continue to engage in risky behavior and show knowledge deficits on a significant number of topic areas included in the following nursing diagnoses.

Nursing Diagnoses and Problems

1. *Population at risk for health problems as evidenced by a high rate of sexual activity (more than 50% of students sampled report engaging in sexual intercourse)*
2. *Knowledge deficit related to the risks of pregnancy during sexual activity*
3. *Inconsistent use of birth control*
4. *Knowledge deficit related to functioning of various birth control mechanisms*
5. *Knowledge deficit related to signs, symptoms, and potential consequences of untreated sexually transmitted diseases*

Nursing Goals and Actions

The *program goals* are as follows:

- Provide students with the skills needed to explore the benefits and risks of engaging in sexual activity during adolescence.
- Increase the knowledge level of students about sexually related information so that students can make informed choices about behavior.

Problem 1 Outcome Objective. Consistent with the *Healthy People 2010* objectives, reduce the number of students who begin sexual activity and increase the number of students who postpone beginning sexual activity until they are older.

The *nursing actions* are as follows:

1. Develop a seminar discussion program with student participation that explores the reasons students begin or continue to engage in sexual activity.
2. Identify the benefits and risks of beginning sexual activity.
3. Provide skill-developing exercises that help students practice the declining of sexual advances.
4. Develop a peer network that will support students who choose not to engage in sexual activity.

Problem 2 Outcome Objective. Increase student knowledge about the process of conception.

The *nursing actions* are as follows:

1. Explore the physiologic process of conception.
2. Examine the myths associated with preventing pregnancy during sexual intercourse and physical intimacy.

Problems 3 and 4 Outcome Objective. Increase student knowledge about birth control methods.

The *nursing actions* are as follows:

1. Review various birth control methods, including abstinence.
2. Discuss the benefits and risks of each method.
3. Identify the risk of pregnancy for each method.
4. Hold a discussion seminar that explores with students common reasons why some opt not to use birth control.
5. Link the myths associated with reduced risk of pregnancy, inconsistent contraceptive use, and actual pregnancy risks.

Problem 5 Outcome Objective. Increase student knowledge of sexually transmitted disease.

The *nursing actions* are as follows:

1. Review common sexually transmitted disease signs and symptoms.
2. Review treatment and potential complications of common sexually transmitted diseases.
3. Provide seminar discussion to explore with students the issues and concerns related to these health issues; correct misconceptions.
4. Relate the best ways to reduce the risk of sexually transmitted disease.

Implementation

Ms. Fields identifies a significant number of resources to assist with the program she has designed. The physical education teacher is willing to assist with the lecture portion of the program but does not want to conduct seminar discussions. The health department is willing to provide a social worker and a clinical psychologist to implement the first discussion groups and assist high school staff to become more comfortable with the discussion process. In addition, the health department is willing to provide posters, brochures, and other visual aids for classroom instruction.

Ms. Fields presents her plan to the principal, who agrees that the plan is appropriate and sends it to the school superintendent for review. The superintendent, with the principal and Ms. Fields in attendance, presents the plan to the school board, and it is approved by one vote. The principal assigns a volunteer biology teacher to help with classroom instruction. Ms. Fields intends to implement the program at the start of the second term, after the students return from winter vacation.

Process Objective. Seventy-five percent of students will participate in the instructional program during the spring semester.

PHASE 2: IMPROVE STUDENT ACCESS TO HEALTH SERVICES, INCLUDING SERVICES TO ADDRESS RISKY SEXUAL BEHAVIOR

To validate the need for additional adolescent health services, Ms. Fields surveys the resources for teenage health services in the surrounding geopolitical communities. She finds that a community health center is nearby. This site provides services to well children under the age of 6 years, prenatal care to pregnant women, and family planning services. No services are aimed specifically at adolescent health problems. Although teens can be served at the site for pregnancy and family planning, the clinic has not had the resources to actively target teens. From the assessment of the high school community (see Chapter 15), Ms. Fields knows that support services for teen parents are inadequate; many of the teens do not continue with school, and many drop out. The surrounding census

Continued

tract consists of families with moderately low income. Many are "gray area" families; that is, they have no health insurance but do not qualify for state medical assistance because their income exceeds the eligibility criteria. Two general practitioners are in the community, both with heavy client loads. These practitioners do treat adolescent members of families in their practice, but restrict the number of families who are unable to pay for services. Care is acutely focused rather than preventive in nature. Both practitioners report that they do not have the time or resources to target teens or emphasize preventive health practices. No other medical professionals are practicing within the community boundaries.

Nursing Diagnoses

1. *Inadequate services to provide adolescent health care*
2. *Inadequate services to address primary prevention with respect to pregnancy and sexually transmitted diseases*
3. *Inadequate support services for teenage mothers with respect to daycare, parenting skills, and continuation of their educational program*

Nursing Goals and Actions

The *program goals* are as follows:

• Improve health services for adolescents.
• Improve support services for teenage parents, especially teenage mothers.

Problems 1 and 2 Outcome Objective. Provide adequate health care services to students within 24 months.

The *nursing actions* are as follows:

1. Convene a committee of community and suprasystem representatives and health care providers to identify the types of health services needed.
2. Have the committee brainstorm ways to provide these services, including addressing the issues of cost and access.
3. Develop a proposal for providing health care services to the teenage population.
4. Present the proposal to the school board for approval.

Implementation

The proposal to improve health care services for adolescents resulted in a recommendation for a school-based clinic. This proposal was taken to the school board, which held hearings. A vocal minority of census tract residents opposed a school-based clinic because they were not in favor of providing contraceptives in a school-based setting. The committee then altered its plan to improve services to adolescents through the community health center. Funding for a pilot project was approved as a joint effort of the local school district and the health department, with each contributing $25,000. In addition, the health department will provide the space and the services of one community/public health nurse to staff the program. The program can use any existing equipment at the health center, but new equipment and other support personnel will have to come out of the program budget. The adolescent program is projected to start in approximately 3 months. Ms. Fields is in the process of developing a referral mechanism for students seen through the school health suite who require further medical attention or seek services not currently offered through student health services. Evaluation will be needed as the project unfolds.

Problem 3 Outcome Objective. Develop support services for teenage parents that will facilitate their educational progress and the well-being of their children within 18 months.

The *nursing actions* are as follows:

1. Meet with representatives of the teachers and administrative staff to identify problem areas for continued education.
2. Meet with a sampling of young mothers and fathers to help identify problem areas and the types of services they believe would be most beneficial to their educational advancement.
3. Convene a committee of professionals, students, and community representatives and leaders. Report your results with problems 1 and 2 as previously stated, assist the committee in developing a proposal for support services, and have committee members present the proposal to the school board.

Implementation

Ms. Fields met with both professionals and students in an effort to identify the problems associated with continued schooling during and after pregnancy. Some of the problems identified included the following:

• No in-school child daycare
• Limited daycare options in the community and the cost of these options
• Student families who are unable to provide daycare because of their employment responsibilities
• Poor preparation for parenting, including information related to managing infant illness, hygiene, infant growth and development, and discipline techniques
• Lack of emotional support for continued schooling, especially among peers

Ms. Fields is in the process of meeting with the committee to explore the information she has collected. Several parents of adolescent mothers, two teachers from the high school, a nurse practitioner from the community health center, and a minister active in adolescent counseling have agreed to serve on the committee, as well as two high school students who are mothers of infants. Ms. Fields would like to get representatives from the local school board or academic administrators (or both) to complete the committee. Her efforts to date have taken one half of the academic year. She hopes to have the committee intact and the work completed before the end of the school year.

Process Objectives. Several process objectives were developed for phase 2:

• Two years from inception of the adolescent health program, 75% of Northview High School students referred to the program will receive services at the health center or be referred to other community-based services to meet their needs.
• Within 2 years, all adolescent parents will have access to affordable, certified child care.
• Within 2 years, all adolescent parents who remain in school will be encouraged to attend a school-based parenting skills program.

LEARNING BY EXPERIENCE AND REFLECTION

1. Based on the assessment of census tract 1 in Chapter 15, apply the steps for program planning. Be sure to identify who needs to be involved in the planning process to ensure its success. Rewrite the health problems as nursing diagnoses. Develop at least one program goal and related outcome and process objectives. Discuss the rationale for your selection of the priority problem.

2. Attend a community meeting at which health concerns or health programs are discussed. Identify the key persons involved, and discuss with several of them why they are interested in health care. Identify differing points of view. Think about alternative solutions that might provide common ground, in other words, that would include as many points of view as possible.

3. Interview a community/public health nurse who has been involved in establishing a new health program. Discuss who was involved; how long the process took; and what the sources of money, equipment, and space were. Ask the community/public health nurse why the program was successful. Ask what aspects were unsuccessful and what might have been done differently.

4. Consider which model of community organization you are more inclined to use: community empowerment, social planning, or social action. What values and experiences contribute to your preference?

5. Read a major newspaper, watch the national news on television, or use other resources to identify examples of community empowerment, social planning, and social action. What are the advantages and disadvantages of each model for community change? How long range were the outcomes? What aspects of planning and implementing were especially difficult?

STUDY AIDS   http://evolve.elsevier.com/Maurer/community/

Visit the Evolve website for this book to find the following study and assessment materials:

- Quiz
- Web Scenario
- Critical Thinking Questions and Answers for Case Studies
- Care Plans
- *Healthy People* Updates
- Glossary

REFERENCES

American Association of Colleges of Nursing. (1986). *Essentials of college and university education for professional nursing: Final report.* Washington, DC: Author.

American Nurses Association. (1986). *Standards of community health nursing practice.* Washington, DC: Author.

American Nurses Association. (1991). *Nursing's agenda for health care reform.* Washington, DC: Author.

American Nurses Association. (2007). *Public health nursing: Scope and standards of practice.* Silver Spring, MD: Author.

American Public Health Association, Committee on Public Health Administration. (1961). *Guide to a community health study* (2nd ed.). Washington, DC: Author.

American Public Health Association, Public Health Nursing Section. (1996). *The definition and role of public health nursing: A statement of the APHA Public Health Nursing Section.* Washington, DC: Author.

Association for the Advancement of Health Education. (1992). PATCH: Planned approach to community health. *Journal of Health Education, 23*(3), 1-192.

Barger, S., & Rosenfeld, P. (1993). Models in community health care: Findings from a national study of community nursing centers. *Nursing and Health Care, 14*(8), 426-431.

Bremer, A. (1987). Revitalizing the district model for the delivery of prevention-focused community health nursing services. *Family and Community Health, 10*(2), 1-10.

Carpenito, L. (2000). *Nursing diagnosis: Application to clinical practice* (8th ed.). Philadelphia: J. B. Lippincott.

Chalick, T., & White, J. P. (1997). Providing primary care to poor urban women. *Nursing Forum, 32*(2), 23-28.

Cicutto, L., Conti, E., Evans, H., et al. (2006). Creating asthma-friendly schools: A public health approach. *Journal of School Health, 76*(6), 255-258.

Community Health Nursing Faculty, Undergraduate Program. (1985). *Syllabus for nursing* (p. 325). Baltimore: University of Maryland School of Nursing.

Crist, J. D., & Dominguez, S. E. (2003). Identifying and recruiting Mexican American partners and sustaining community partnerships. *Journal of Transcultural Nursing, 14*(3), 266-271.

Dever, G. E. (1991). *Community health analysis. Global awareness at the local level* (2nd ed.). Gaithersburg, MD: Aspen.

Dochterman, J. M., & Jones, D. A. (Eds.). (2003). *Unifying nursing language: The harmonization of NANDA, NIC, and NOC.* Washington, DC: American Nurses Association.

Drucker, P. (1974). *Management: Tasks, responsibilities, practices.* New York: Harper & Row.

Ervin, N. E. (2002). *Advanced community health nursing practice.* Upper Saddle River, NJ: Prentice Hall.

Farley, S. (1993). The community as partner in primary health care. *Nursing and Health Care, 14*(5), 244-249.

Flynn, B., Rider, M., & Bailey, W. (1992). Developing community leadership in healthy cities: The Indiana model. *Nursing Outlook, 40*(3), 121-126.

Gikow, F., & Kucharski, P. (1987). A new look at the community: Functional health pattern assessment. *Journal of Community Health Nursing, 4*(1), 21-27.

Glick, D. F. (1999). Advanced practice community health nursing in community nursing centers: A holistic approach. *Holistic Nursing Practice, 13*(4), 19-27.

Glick, D. F., & Kulbok, P. A. (2002). Revising programs. In N. E. Ervin (Ed.), *Advanced community health nursing practice* (pp. 451-462). Upper Saddle River, NJ: Prentice Hall.

Green, L. W., & Kreuter, M. W. (1999). *Health promotion planning: An educational and ecological approach* (3rd ed.). Mountain View, CA: Mayfield.

Gronlund, N. E. (1970). *Stating behavioral objectives for classroom instruction.* New York: Macmillan.

Hale, C., Arnold, F., & Travis, M. (1994). *Planning and evaluating health programs: A primer.* Albany, NY: Delmar Publishers.

Hamilton, P. (1983). Community nursing diagnosis. *Advances in Nursing Science, 5*(3), 21-35.

Hatcher, P. A., Scarinzi, G. D., & Kreider, M. S. (1998). A primary health care model for a community-based/nurse-managed health center. *Nursing and Health Care Perspectives, 19*(1), 12-19.

Hecker, E. J. (2000). Feria de Salud: Implementation and evaluation of a community wide health fair. *Public Health Nursing, 17*(4), 247-256.

Kang, R. (1995). Building community capacity for health promotion: A challenge for public health nurses. *Public Health Nursing, 12*(5), 312-318.

Kim, M. J., Hyang-In, C., Cheon-Klessig, Y. S., et al. (2002). Primary health care for Korean immigrants: Sustaining a culturally sensitive model. *Public Health Nursing, 19*(3), 191-200.

Kuehnert, P. (1991). The public health policy advocate: Fostering the health of communities. *Clinical Nurse Specialist, 5*(1), 5-10.

Kulwicki, A., & Rice, V. H. (2003). Arab American adolescents perceptions and experiences with smoking. *Public Health Nursing, 20*(3), 177-183.

LaPatra, J. W. (1975). *Health care delivery systems: Evaluation criteria.* Springfield, IL: Charles C. Thomas.

Lashley, M. (2007). A targeted testing program for tuberculosis control and prevention among Baltimore City's homeless population. *Public Health Nursing, 24*(1), 34-39.

Lewit, E. M., Terman, D. L., & Behrman, R. E. (1997). Children and poverty: Analysis and recommendations. *The Future of Children—The Journal, 7*(2), 222-229.

Mager, R. F. (1962). *Preparing objectives for programmed instruction.* San Francisco: Fearon Publishers.

Martin, K. (2005). *The Omaha system* (2nd ed.). St. Louis: Saunders.

McKenzie, J., & Smeltzer, J. L. (2000). *Planning, implementing, and evaluating health promotion programs: A primer* (3rd ed.). New York: Macmillan.

Milio, N. (1971). *9226 Kercheval: The storefront that did not burn.* Ann Arbor, MI: The University of Michigan Press.

Milio, N. (1981). *Promoting health through public policy.* Philadelphia: F. A. Davis.

Minnesota Department of Health, Divison of Community Health. (2001). *Public health interventions: Applications for public health nursing practice.* St. Paul: Author.

Moorhead, S., Johnson, M., & Maas, M. (2004). *Nursing outcomes classification (NOC)* (3rd ed.). St. Louis: Mosby/Elsevier.

Muecke, M. (1984). Community health diagnosis in nursing. *Public Health Nursing, 1*(1), 23-35.

National Association of County and City Health Officials. (2000). *Mobilizing for Action through Planning and Partnerships (MAPP).* Washington, DC: Author. Retrieved October 8, 2007, at *http:// mapp.naccho.org/mapp_introduction.asp.*

Neufield, A., & Harrison, M. (1990). The development of nursing diagnoses for aggregates and groups. *Public Health Nursing, 7*(4), 251-255.

Norr, K. F., Crittenden, K. S., Lehrer, E. L., et al. (2003). Maternal and infant outcomes at one year for a nurse-health advocate home visiting program serving African Americans and Mexican Americans. *Public Health Nursing, 20*(3), 190-203.

North American Nursing Diagnosis Association International. (2002). *Nursing diagnoses: Definition and classifications 2001-2002.* Philadelphia: Author.

North American Nursing Diagnosis Association International. (2007-2008). *Nursing diagnoses: Definition and classifications.* Philadelphia: Author.

Phillips, L. (1995). Chattanooga Creek: Case study of the public health nursing role in environmental health. *Public Health Nursing, 12*(5), 335-340.

Roman, D. (1969). The PERT system: An appraisal of program evaluation review technique. In H. Schulberg, A. Sheldon, & F. Baker (Eds.), *Program evaluation in the health fields.* New York: Behavioral Publications.

Rothman, J. (1978). Three models of community organization practice. In J. Cox, F. Erlich, F. Rothman et al. (Eds.), *Strategies in community organization: A book of readings.* Itasca, IL: F. E. Peacock Publishers.

Rothman, J. (2008). Approaches to community intervention. In Rothman J., Erlich, J., & Tropman, J. (Eds.). *Strategies in community intervention* (7th ed., p. 163). Peosta, IA: Eddie Bowers Publishing Company.

Rowland, H., & Rowland, B. (1992). *Nursing administration handbook* (3rd ed.). Gaithersburg, MD: Aspen.

Shiber, D. (2002). A win-win model for an academic nursing center: Community partnership faculty practice. *Public Health Nursing, 19*(2), 81-85.

Sistrom, M., & Hale, P. (2006). Outbreak investigations: Community participation and the role of community and public health nurses. *Public Health Nursing, 23*(3), 256-263.

Sloand, E., & Gebrian, B. (2006). Fathers' clubs to improve child health in rural Haiti. *Public Health Nursing, 23*(1), 40-51.

Smith Battle, L. (2003). Displacing the "rule book" in caring for teen mothers. *Public Health Nursing, 20*(5), 369-376.

U.S. Department of Health and Human Services. (1997). *Healthy People 2000, review 1997.* Washington, DC: U.S. Government Printing Office.

U.S. Department of Health and Human Services. (1998). *Healthy People 2010 objectives: Draft for public comment.* Washington, DC: U.S. Government Printing Office.

U.S. Department of Health and Human Services. (2000). *Healthy People 2010: National health promotion and disease prevention objectives* (2nd ed.). Washington, DC: U.S. Government Printing Office.

U.S. Department of Health and Human Services. (2002). *Health, United States, 2002.* Washington, DC: U.S. Government Printing Office.

U.S. Department of Health and Human Services. (2006). *Healthy People 2010: Midterm Review.* Washington, DC: U.S. Government Printing Office.

Williams, C. (1983). Making things happen: Community health nursing and the policy arena. *Nursing Outlook, 31,* 225-228.

World Health Organization. (1991). *City networks for health.* Geneva: Author.

Wright, C. (1985). Computer-aided nursing diagnosis for community health nurses. *Nursing Clinics of North America, 20*(3), 487-495.

SUGGESTED READINGS

American Nurses Association. (2007). *Public health nursing: Scope and standards of practice.* Silver Spring, MD: Author.

Anderson, E. T., & McFarlane, J. (2008). *Community as partner: Theory and practice in nursing.* Philadelphia: J. B. Lippincott.

Association for the Advancement of Health Education. (1992). PATCH: Planned approach to community health. *Journal of Health Education, 23*(3), 1-192.

Avila, M., & Smith, K. (2003). The reinvigoration of public health nursing: Methods and innovations. *Journal of Public Health Management Practice, 9*(1), 16-24.

Clark, H. M. (1986). A health planning simulation game. *Nurse Educator, 11*(4), 16-20.

Dever, G. E. A. (1997). *Improving outcomes in public health practice: Strategy and methods.* Boston, MA: Jones & Bartlett.

Flynn, B., Rider, M., & Ray, D. (1991). Healthy cities: The Indiana model of community development in public health. *Health Education Quarterly, 18,* 331-347.

Harris, E. (1992). Assessing community development research methodologies. *Canadian Journal of Public Health, 83*(suppl 1), S62-S66.

Lundeen, S. (1993). Comprehensive, collaborative, coordinated, community-based care: A community nursing center model. *Family and Community Health, 16*(2), 57-65.

McFarlane, J., Kelly, E., Rodriguez, R., et al. (1994). De Madres a Madres: Women building community coalitions for health. *Health Care for Women International, 15*(5), 465-476.

Minnesota Department of Health, Divison of Community Health. (2001). *Public health interventions: Applications for public health nursing practice.* St. Paul: Author.

Miskelly, S. (1995). A parish nursing model: Applying the community health nursing process in a church community. *Journal of Community Health Nursing, 12*(1), 1-14.

National Association of County and City Health Officials. (2000). *Mobilizing for Action through Planning and Partnerships* (MAPP). Washington, DC: Author. Retrieved October 8, 2007, at *http://mapp.naccho.org/mapp_introduction.asp*.

Phillips, L. (1995). Chattanooga Creek: Case study of the public health nursing role in environmental health. *Public Health Nursing, 12*(5), 335-340.

Riner, M., Cunningham, C., & Johnson, A. (2004). Public health education and practice using geographic information system technology. *Public Health Nursing, 21*(1), 57-65.

U.S. Department of Health and Human Services. (2000). *Healthy People 2010 objectives* (2nd ed.). Washington, DC: U.S. Government Printing Office.

U.S. Department of Health and Human Services. (2006). *Healthy People 2010: Midterm*.

Washington, DC: U.S. Government Printing Office.

Wallerstein, N. (1992). Powerlessness, empowerment, and health: Implications for health promotion programs. *American Journal of Health Promotion, 6,* 197-205.

FOCUS QUESTIONS

What are the responsibilities of a baccalaureate-prepared community/public health nurse in evaluation of nursing care with communities?

What are the steps in evaluation?

What questions can be answered by evaluation?

What outcomes are indicators of the effectiveness of nursing interventions with communities?

How does evaluation of nursing care with communities compare with evaluation of care with families and individuals?

How can evaluation of process be used to improve the operation of nursing programs?

How is evaluation used to modify nursing care with communities?

What methods and tools are used in evaluation?

CHAPTER OUTLINE

Responsibilities in Evaluation of Nursing Care with Communities
Responsibilities of Baccalaureate-Prepared Community/Public Health Nurses
Formative and Summative Evaluations
Community Involvement
Standards for a Good Evaluation
Steps in Evaluation
Questions Answered by Evaluation
Evaluation of Outcome Attainment

Evaluation of Appropriateness
Evaluation of Adequacy
Evaluation of Efficiency
Evaluation of Process
Uniqueness in Evaluation of Nursing Care with Communities
Criteria for Effectiveness
Sources of Evaluation Data
Recording Evaluations
Analyzing Evaluation Data

Modification of Nursing Care with Communities
Evaluation Methods and Tools
Designs for Evaluation of Effectiveness
Tools for Evaluation of Effectiveness
Efficiency Analysis

KEY TERMS

Adequate
Affective learning
Appropriate
Effective

Efficiency
Evaluation
Formative evaluation
Outcome measures

Result
Satisfaction
Summative evaluation

Evaluation of care with communities seeks to determine whether health has improved. Were the desired health goals reached? How much progress was made toward the goals? What themes, patterns, and results emerged? What side effects were evident? Evaluation provides information to help community/public health nurses improve their nursing practice.

RESPONSIBILITIES IN EVALUATION OF NURSING CARE WITH COMMUNITIES

Evaluation is the process by which a nurse *judges the value of nursing care* that has been *provided*. As with any type of

nursing care, the community/public health nurse seeks to determine the degree to which planned goals were achieved and to describe any unplanned results.

The purpose of the evaluation is to facilitate additional decision making. An evaluation might conclude that what had been done could not have been done better, that the goals were reached, and that the goals were mutually desirable to the nurse and the community members. This conclusion would be cause for celebration. As a result of another evaluation, the conclusion might be that alterations are needed in the plan of care to reach the desired outcomes more effectively; or possibly that, although goals were reached, the cost in money, time, or other resources was too expensive for the nurse or the community members.

Evaluation is based on several assumptions: first, that nursing actions have results, both intended and unintended; second, that nurses are accountable for their own actions and care provided; and third, that different sets of actions result in resources being used differently (i.e., some nursing interventions use more resources than others).

Evaluation involves two parts: measurement and interpretation. Many different schemes or models exist for organizing ideas about evaluation, which may result in confusion among people who use different terminology for similar concepts.

Basic to the nursing process, however, is the idea of measuring whether planned goals were achieved. Synonyms for this activity and its **result** are *outcome attainment* (Donabedian, 1980), *performance evaluation* (Suchman, 1967), *results of effort,* and *evaluation of effectiveness* (Deniston & Rosenstock, 1970). The question that the nurse attempts to answer is, "Were the planned goals achieved?"

Another basic idea addresses the quality of the results and the process that contributed to the results. Some terms used to express this idea are as follows:
- **Appropriate**—suitable for a particular occasion or use; fitting
- **Adequate**—able to fill a requirement; sufficient or satisfactory
- **Effective**—producing an expected result; productive

Each of these terms describes different aspects of measuring quality. The following are some questions that may be asked about quality. How and why did the interventions work? Were the nurses' actions ethical? Did the nurses address the most important goals? Did the nurses involve community members and recipients as participants (American Nurses Association [ANA], 2007)? Were resources used wisely? How many needs and goals did the plan actually address?

RESPONSIBILITIES OF BACCALAUREATE-PREPARED COMMUNITY/PUBLIC HEALTH NURSES

According to the ANA (2007), community/public health nurses with bachelor's degrees in nursing are expected to work with advanced practice public health nurses (masters prepared) and community members in evaluating *responses of the community* to nursing interventions.

The responsibilities of community/public health nurses for evaluating nursing care with communities vary, depending on the size and complexity of the community and whether the community is geopolitical or phenomenological (see Chapter 15).

Baccalaureate-prepared community/public health nurses are expected to work with community members, advanced public health nurses, and multidisciplinary teams to evaluate nursing care with geopolitical communities. Community/public health nurses may also work with multidisciplinary teams and nurses who engage in quality assurance and accreditation reviews (ANA, 2007). Baccalaureate-prepared community/public health nurses will be more capable members of evaluating teams if they have been introduced in their education to ideas and skills in evaluating nursing care with communities.

In some instances, a baccalaureate-prepared community/public health nurse will work with a small phenomenological community, such as a senior center or school; in this case, the nurse is likely to evaluate his or her own performance with minimal assistance from a supervisor and peers. Either independently or with help from supervisors, community/public health nurses are expected to evaluate the effectiveness of intervention programs that involve teaching, direct care, and screening and referral.

Regardless of the type or size of community, the members themselves should, when possible, be involved in planning and conducting the evaluation (ANA, 2007). The measurement of many health outcomes requires the judgment of the community members themselves.

FORMATIVE AND SUMMATIVE EVALUATIONS

When is nursing care with communities evaluated? Evaluation of the effectiveness of care that takes place after the interventions have been performed is known as **summative evaluation** because the nurse is evaluating the *sum,* the *bottom line,* the end results. Summative evaluation involves measurement of community responses to nursing care and interpretation of the degree to which planned goals were met. Summative evaluation usually consists of measurement of *outcomes* and goal attainment.

> After assessing the members of a senior retirement community, Ridge Center Retirement Community, a community/public nurse designed a program with the goal of increasing the walking regimen for obese and hypertensive seniors living in Ridge Center. She developed an intervention plan consisting of a health-education program and personal consultation with a sports fitness expert. All senior participants received a health clearance from their personal physician. A summative evaluation statement for the intervention was as follows: the target group will increase their walking regimen from an average of 15 minutes three times a week (data from the assessment) to 30 minutes three times per week.

Summative evaluation may also take place several months or years after nursing care has been provided. This evaluation seeks to determine whether a long-term impact was made on the health status and the health responses of the community.

Formative evaluation is evaluation that occurs throughout the nursing process but before evaluation of the outcomes of care. This evaluation occurs during the *formation* of the nursing care and during the process of its actual delivery. In other words, formative evaluation considers the day-to-day provision of programs of nursing care. Formative evaluation allows ongoing modification of nursing practices.

> In the intervention program discussed earlier, the program goal remains the same. Several formative evaluation statements for the interactive portion of the health-education program are as follows:
> - *The discussion portion of the program was longer because of technical difficulties.* Originally planned for ½ hour, it was 30 minutes longer because the room was locked and printed handouts were delivered late.
> - *Some senior participants were unable to hear the speaker. Planning did not account for hearing loss in some of the participants.* The room was large, and although the group was small ($n = 15$), they were initially spread out over the entire room.

In the formative example just mentioned, the nurse can take action to remediate some of the problems identified during the intervention process. For example, the nurse might take the names of participants and deliver the printed material to them at some later date. The nurse had the seniors move into a small group in the room and found and used a microphone to help with the presentation.

COMMUNITY INVOLVEMENT

Because the community members are involved in evaluation, at least part of the evaluation must occur in the clients' community. Mutuality is an important aspect of evaluation. Because much of the impact of the community/public health nurse is indicated by self-care and lifestyle changes of community members, a nurse must document and validate outcomes directly with community members. Additionally, although goals have been achieved, some negative or unexpected results might also have occurred. The nurse must explore the perceptions of community members to discover and validate the meaning of the experience. Determining how satisfied community members are with both the outcomes and the nursing interventions is important.

Stakeholders are individuals who have expectations about nursing care but who are not directly involved in its delivery. For example, there are individuals whose approval was necessary, those who contributed money or supplies, those who volunteered to assist, and those (such as competitors) for whom the presence of nursing services had an impact. Stakeholders in a community immunization campaign might be the county health officer, a retail pharmacist who donates syringes, a local pediatrician who is concerned about financial competition, and parents of persons who were immunized. Community health/public nurses need to identify the stakeholders and invite them to participate in evaluation.

STANDARDS FOR A GOOD EVALUATION

Standards for evaluation of nursing care with communities have been formulated by the Quad Council of Public Health Nursing Organizations and published by the ANA (2007):

- The employing agency is to provide supervision, consultation, and general evaluation plans for the baccalaureate-prepared community/public health nurse.
- The community members are to participate in the evaluation.
- The nursing care is to be revised based on the evaluation.
- Evaluation is to be documented and disseminated so that the record can strengthen nursing practice and knowledge.

STEPS IN EVALUATION

Evaluation is a process that includes several steps: planning, collecting the data, analyzing and interpreting the data, providing recommendations, reporting the results, and implementing the recommendations (McKenzie & Smeltzer, 2000). Box 17-1 identifies evaluation activities in greater detail related to each of the major steps.

QUESTIONS ANSWERED BY EVALUATION

Evaluation of nursing care with communities involves evaluation of programs of care for populations. Program evaluation includes evaluation of outcomes (program goals and outcome objectives), as well as evaluation of the structures and processes used to achieve the outcomes (Ervin, 2002). The ANA considers *outcomes, structures,* and *processes* as the primary categories of criteria to be used to measure the quality of nursing care. *Outcomes* are the end results; *structures* are the social and physical resources; and *processes* are the "sequence of

---

Box 17-1   Steps in Evaluation

Plan the Evaluation
1. Review goals and objectives.
2. Meet with stakeholders to identify which evaluation questions should be answered.
3. Develop a budget for evaluation.
4. Determine who will conduct the evaluation.
5. Develop the evaluation design: What will be done?
6. Decide which evaluation instruments will be used to collect information.
7. Analyze how the evaluation questions relate to the goals and objectives.
8. Analyze whether the questions of stakeholders are addressed.
9. Determine when the evaluation will be conducted; develop a time line.

Collect Evaluation Data
10. Develop specific processes for collecting data through questionnaires, review of records or documents, personal interviews, telephone interviews, and observation.
11. Determine who will collect the data.
12. Pilot the data-collection instruments.
13. Refine the instruments based on data from the pilot.

14. Identify the sample of persons from whom evaluation data will be collected.
15. Collect the data.

Analyze the Data
16. Determine how the data will be analyzed.
17. Determine who will analyze the data.
18. Analyze the data, generate several interpretations, and make recommendations.

Report the Evaluation
19. Determine who will receive results.
20. Determine who will report the findings.
21. Determine format for the report, including an executive summary.
22. Discuss how the findings will affect the program.
23. Determine which findings will be included in the report.
24. Distribute the report.

Implement the Results
25. Plan how the results will be implemented.
26. Identify who will implement the results.
27. Determine when the results will be implemented; develop a time line.

From McKenzie, J. F., & Smeltzer, J. L. (1997). *Planning, implementing, and evaluating health promotion programs: A primer* (2nd ed.; pp. 276-277). Boston: Allyn and Bacon. Copyright 1997 by Allyn and Bacon. Adapted by permission.

events and activities" (ANA, 1986, p. 18) used by the nurse during the delivery of care. For example, evaluation of a health program designed to identify adults with high cholesterol levels would include the following:

- Structure standard: Cholesterol screening will be available to all adults, regardless of whether they can pay for testing.
- Process standard: Cholesterol screening will be performed on all adults who come to the health screening event.
- Outcome standards:
  - (a) One hundred percent of the adults will be given their test results.
  - (b) Eighty percent of adults with cholesterol levels above the recommended norm will follow up with a physician's visit for evaluation.

Table 17-1 describes the following five categories of questions that can be answered by evaluation: (1) outcome attainment, also called effectiveness; (2) appropriateness of care; (3) adequacy of care in relation to the scope of the problem; (4) relationship of resources to results, also called efficiency; and (5) process. This set of questions includes the criteria of outcome, structure, and process evaluation and adds appropriateness and adequacy. Questions of appropriateness and adequacy evaluate the nursing care program in relation to the community health needs. Efficiency addresses the relationship of outcomes to structures and processes. Each of these sets of evaluation questions is discussed in more detail.

EVALUATION OF OUTCOME ATTAINMENT

Evaluation of outcome attainment, also called *effectiveness,* addresses the results of nursing interventions. Change toward predetermined goals, as well as unplanned effects, may have occurred (see Table 17-1). Frequently, large health programs are evaluated as a total intervention, without distinguishing the effects of nursing interventions from the effects of other health disciplines and program components. Therefore nursing care may be lumped into a single evaluation for the whole program rather than being evaluated as a separate intervention. Devising evaluation strategies and criteria for each component of a program is more useful because evaluators are given a better idea of which strategies are effective and which might need to be revised or eliminated. This is also true for multifaceted community/public health nursing programs; knowing which nursing intervention is contributing to which outcome is more helpful.

Evaluation of outcome attainment evaluates changes in the population, the health care system within the community, or the environment. Box 17-2 identifies several variables that can be used as **outcome measures** of community health. Changes can occur in the population's knowledge, behavior and skills, attitudes, emotional well-being, and health status.

When evaluating the health of a community, more than the outcomes of the population must be considered. Because the interaction of people in their environment facilitates or hinders

TABLE 17-1	Questions Answered by Evaluation	
Variable	**Questions**	**Examples of Measurement**
1. Outcome attainment	Did change occur?	Numbers and rates of children immunized
	To what degree was progress made toward the goal?	Numbers of cases of cancer found on Papanicolaou smears
	What are actual effects on clients?	Changes in attitudes regarding people with acquired immunodeficiency syndrome (AIDS)
	What unintended outcomes occurred?	Reduction in teenage pregnancy rate
2. Appropriateness	Did the goals fit the need?	Plan of care compared with clinical nursing knowledge
	Are the goals and plans acceptable to the community?	Community preferences
		Plan of care is evidence-based
	Are the plans likely to achieve the goals?	
	Does the plan duplicate existing efforts?	
3. Adequacy	To what degree does the intervention meet the total amount of need?	Rate of effectiveness multiplied by number of people exposed to service
	Were some people not served?	Outcomes relative to total needs in population
		Degree to which need was a priority
4. Efficiency	What resources were used?	Relation of effort to outcome
Cost-effectiveness	Can a better way be found to attain the same results?	Output and input:
		Money
	What resources were necessary to attain results?	Time
		Personnel
		Client convenience
Benefit-cost analysis	Do the benefits justify the use of resources?	
5. Process	What did nurses do? When? Where?	Number of clinics/or encounters/week or month
	How many people were reached?	Number of home visits
	What were the reasons for the successes or failures?	Amount of money spent
	What contributed to the results?	Education content taught and strategies used
	What methods were used?	Numbers of people attending screening sessions

Data from Deniston, O., & Rosenstock, I. (1970). Evaluating health programs. *Public Health Reports, 85,* 835-840; Donabedian, A. (1980). *The definition of quality and approaches to its assessment* (Vol. 1). Ann Arbor, MI: Health Administration Press; Freeman, R. (1963). *Public health nursing practice* (3rd ed.). Philadelphia: W. B. Saunders; Suchman, E. (1967). *Evaluative research: Principles and practice in public service and social action programs.* New York: Russell Sage Foundation.

Box 17-2 **Possible Outcome Measures**

1. Knowledge
2. Behaviors, skills
3. Attitudes, commitment to action
4. Emotional well-being
5. Health status (epidemiologic measures)
6. Presence of health care system services and components
7. Satisfaction or acceptance regarding the program interventions
8. Presence of policy that allows, mandates, or funds
9. Altered relationship with physical environment

health, variables such as the presence of health services, the satisfaction and acceptance of such programs, the presence of policies, and a harmonious balance with the environment must also be considered. Each of these variables, which are used as an outcome measure of the health of populations or communities, is discussed in more detail. Each of these variables can be used as a measure of the effectiveness of specific community/public health nursing interventions.

Knowledge

A great deal of client teaching and health education is evaluated by measuring the health-related information that the individual, group, or population has obtained. Although information alone does not result in behavior changes, having information will often increase the possibility of behavior changes. For example, just because a father knows how to prepare infant formula in the proper concentration and with adequate asepsis does not ensure that he will actually do so. However, if he does not have that information, the only way he can prepare the formula would be by trial and error or by chance. Having the information increases the probability that the formula will be prepared properly.

In response to an increased incidence of syphilis in an urban, Hispanic population, public health nurses and other professionals provided a 10-week outreach project to more than 2800 individuals through street and business outreach (Endyke-Doran and colleagues, 2007). The project evaluation measured knowledge changes in the population. Health education addressed knowledge and prevention of syphilis, and location of testing sites. Before and after levels of knowledge were based on interviews with different individuals. At the beginning of the project, only 4% could identify prevention measures or locations for testing. Near the end of the project 50% of those encountered had knowledge of prevention and transmission and 64% knew of available testing services. Additional surveillance data from the local health department showed that the number of Hispanics who sought testing for syphilis also increased.

When evaluating populations, surveys may be used to determine knowledge about specific health-related topics. These surveys may be conducted as interviews or through written questionnaires (Polit & Hungler, 2005). When working with populations, the community/public health nurse is interested in the proportion of the population that the teaching reached and the proportion that retained the information presented. Having information is not sufficient for healthy living; the information must be put to use.

Behaviors and Skills

Integrating health-related behaviors and skills into daily living affects health status—raising children, caring for an elderly bed-bound family member, seeking a prostate examination, and preparing nutritious foods require action. These actions are labeled *competent* or *skilled* if they are consistent with existing knowledge and if they are performed in an effective and efficient manner.

Health behaviors may change as a result of interventions performed by community/public health nurses (see Chapters 18 and 20 for more details regarding health promotion and health teaching).

When evaluating health behaviors of populations, the nurse's interest is in the proportion of the population who engage in such behaviors. The usual way to collect information about health behaviors is to ask people what they do. However, people do not always provide accurate reports because they may have forgotten information or want to look good to the surveyor.

Some data on health behaviors, such as use of a specific health service, can also be collected from client health records and health care information systems. For example, immunization rates can be determined for populations of preschool children receiving Medicaid or enrolled in a specific managed care organization by monitoring whether immunizations have been received.

Adherence to drug treatment for latent tuberculosis infection (LTBI) was one of the behavioral outcomes evaluated in a tuberculosis control and prevention program among a homeless population in Baltimore (Lashley, 2007). Nursing students and faculty partnered with a faith-based, inner-city mission and the local health department. Interventions included education, tracking persons who missed appointments, monthly appointment reminders, and incentives. The desired outcome was that 65% of those in treatment for LTBI would complete a 9-month course of therapy. Although only 33% completed at least 6 months of medication therapy, this far surpassed the city's 11% completion rate among the homeless.

Time and money often limit the degree to which behavior change can be measured. Observing the behavior of populations helps confirm the accuracy of what is reported; however, this process takes much more time and money. Asking people to make a contract with themselves to make a commitment to specific actions has been shown to increase the likelihood that the actions will be performed (Sloan & Schommer, 1991). Therefore when measuring actual behavioral changes of populations is not possible, community/public health nurses can measure the degree to which people commit to specific actions.

Attitudes

Attitudes include opinions and preferences about ideas, people, and things. Persons have attitudes about the concept of health and the ways in which health may be attained and maintained. Because attitudes predispose the selection of some actions over others, attitudes are a health-related measure. For example, if a population generally views health as the ability to perform work, people may take cold medication to allow them to feel well enough to go to work. However, a group may not alter their high-cholesterol diets because their current diets do not interfere with their immediate ability to work.

Community attitudes also predispose the population to support or work against various policies and services. For example, if the dominant community attitude toward criminals is that they should be punished and live stark lives, there may be little support for prison health services. If the predominant community attitude is that health prevention can reduce human suffering and dollars spent for care of the ill, there may be more support for prison health services.

Attitudes toward health and health behavior can be changed through planned or spontaneous experiences. Attitudinal change is also called *emotional learning* or **affective learning.** Attitudes of populations can be measured before and after an intervention to determine whether affective learning has occurred. Changes in attitude may predispose people to change their behaviors. For example, as more members of a population adopt the attitude that smoking is undesirable, smoking rates decrease. In some neighborhoods, volunteer or paid members of the community are trained by community/public health nurses to address attitudes of community members about obtaining health care services such as mammography screening, prenatal care, and treatment for substance abuse.

Emotional Well-Being and Empowerment

Emotional well-being in a population can be measured by the proportion of members who experience self-esteem and satisfaction with their lives. Emotional well-being of a community can be measured also by assessing the existing structures and processes to strengthen human development and connectedness.

A group of nursing students initiated a reminiscence group in which residents of a nursing home were able to reflect on and share their life experiences. The students' initial assessment indicated that the residents rarely communicated with each other (even when in the same room), had few visitors, and reported that they did not "feel at home." After several weekly meetings, the nursing students observed that the participants initiated conversation more with each other, and several of the residents reported "feeling at home."

Improved quality of life is another outcome related to human well-being.

In an evaluation of a community-based outreach worker program for children with asthma, one of the outcomes was quality of life of the children's caregivers (Primomo et al., 2006). Using an existing questionnaire, postintervention phone interviews were conducted 1 month after services were completed. Compared with before the program, caregivers reported an improvement in their quality of life, especially because they did not have to change their plans as frequently because of their child's asthma. They felt less helpless and frightened, and they got more sleep.

Criteria for emotional well-being of a community also include the degree of acceptance and cohesion among members and patterns of support, socialization, and decision making. When community members participate in the decision making that leads to goal achievement, perceptions of self-efficacy are enhanced. *Self-efficacy* is the belief that an individual can influence his or her environment and circumstances. Self-efficacy contributes to self-concept and is necessary if community members are to have an impact on their health.

Health Status

The ultimate measure of the effectiveness of health services and programs is the health status of the population. Community/public health programs seek to reduce premature deaths, disabilities, and injuries. Health status is measured using epidemiologic statistics about morbidity and mortality (see Chapter 7). Epidemiologic statistics that are collected for geopolitical communities do not distinguish the effects of nursing interventions from the effects of other health disciplines and programs. However, epidemiologic statistics can be used to evaluate changes in health status that result from nursing interventions.

Community/public health nurses in Lincoln-Lancaster County Health Department were concerned about the incidence of low-birth-weight babies born to high-risk mothers. The intervention plan they developed consisted of an intensive home visitation schedule to educate and support the high-risk women.

To measure outcomes, a care pathway tool was used to track the 55 clients' progress during and after pregnancy. The evaluation outcome revealed that five to nine home visits by a community/public nurse improved health outcomes for mothers and babies. Mothers had higher hemoglobin levels during pregnancy. No low-birth-weight babies were born to the mothers in the home-visit group. Program evaluation of outcome measures demonstrated the effectiveness of nursing interventions (Fetrick et al., 2003).

Epidemiologic measures can also be used to measure changes in health disparities.

The Omaha Healthy Start program in Nebraska was "designed to reduce local racial disparities in birth outcomes" (Cramer et al., 2007, p. 329). Birth and death certificate data provided by the state health department were used to track low birth weights and infant mortality rates among infants of three groups of mothers during 2002 and 2003. Birth outcomes improved during the second year among minority women and the evaluation is being extended to document long-term trends.

More recently, attempts have been made to measure increases in positive health (an outcome measure) that occur after nursing interventions. To measure positive health, the community/public health nurse focuses on what is desirable rather than on the reduction of health problems. Two examples of these measurements are the percentage of the population with normal blood pressure and the percentage of the population engaging in safer sex. In the previous clinical example of the Lincoln-Lancaster group, a positive health outcome measure was identified. Mothers with the more intense home-visit schedules chose breast-feeding as their feeding option more often than did comparable mothers without the nursing intervention (Fetrick et al., 2003).

Presence of Health-Related Services

Community/public health nursing interventions may be directed toward establishing new services and programs or strengthening the continuity of care among existing services. These interventions may be measured by the presence of new health services and by the increased numbers of people receiving care. For example, in one senior center, the community/public health nursing students noted that the population was not engaging in physical exercise. Knowing that nursing students were unable to be assigned permanently at that site, the students developed a videotape of exercises for older adults. Copies were made for all of the senior centers in the suburban county. This action resulted in multiple senior centers having access to professionally led, appropriate exercises. As a result of the nursing interventions, a new service was available for senior citizens.

The purpose of establishing new services is to fill gaps in health care that exist within the community, not to duplicate existing services. Therefore new services should result in an increased number of people receiving care. Establishing nurse-managed health centers targeted to underserved and vulnerable populations is one way to improve access to health care.

Not all new services are maintained. Evaluation can identify activities that may help maintain new services.

Phone interviews were conducted 6 months after instructor-training workshops to determine whether trainees had actually adopted and maintained exercise programs for people with arthritis (Gyurcsik & Brittain, 2006). The specific program is offered by the Arthritis Foundation in the United States. Results showed that 8 out of 11 trainees initiated a program in their community; however, within 6 months only 3 programs continued. Reported barriers were recruitment of participants and finding a common time for the exercise sessions. These barriers would need to be addressed in order to establish and maintain effective physical activity programs.

Satisfaction and Acceptance

Health-related services may exist in a community but be ineffective because the people within the community do not accept the service. The perceived quality of interpersonal relationships is an important factor in strengthening client satisfaction. For example, if the members of the community do not believe that they are treated with dignity when they attend a clinic, they are likely to stop attending; they will transfer to another service if one exists, or they may even forgo care to avoid the negative experiences. Even when the care provided through a nursing program is effective, more people may be reached if the program is also tailored to strive for the **satisfaction** of participants.

Geographic accessibility, waiting time, and cost are other factors that contribute to a population's satisfaction with nursing programs. When nurses are aware of the culture of the population, clients are likely to be more satisfied (Kim et al., 2002).

Satisfaction with services can be measured through interviews and questionnaires. Interviews may be conducted via phone or in person—one-on-one or in focus groups. Questionnaires have the advantage of being anonymous. Questions may be as simple as the following: "What do you like about this health service? What would you change?"

Nurses in Nebraska used 13 focus groups to evaluate the satisfaction of 113 newly arrived immigrants with a public health nursing program designed for the Medicaid managed care population (Kaiser et al., 2002). Results revealed that the diverse language groups did not understand the health system well, there were inadequate translation services, and cultural beliefs affected health-seeking behaviors and participation in the focus groups themselves. Results were used to strengthen population-focused public health nursing interventions.

Policies

Policies are expressions of goals and rules that exist within a community; they are expressions of values (Diers, 1985). Policies may be decided by persons within governments, formal organizations (e.g., ANA, the American Heart Association, nonprofit volunteer clinics), businesses, and informal groups. Interpersonal and political power influences the creation and maintenance of policies.

Community/public health nurses, often in collaboration with others, can use the existence of health and social policy as one measure of the effectiveness of interpersonal and political power. A new policy may be created, or an existing policy may be defended or changed. Policy may mandate, allow, or initiate actions that affect a community's health. For example, a New Jersey state law required the development of a school policy for delegation of epinephrine adminstration in nonpublic schools by unlicensed assistive personnel (Truglio-Londrigan et al., 2002). Public health nurses from the local health department used site visits, discussions, and focus groups to evaluate the development and implementation of the policy.

In state X, a budget crisis threatened reduction and discontinuation of health care services to poor and disabled persons served by state-funded programs. The nurses' association convention for state X debated the issue during its annual meeting. The association membership voted to pass a resolution opposing budget cuts in health care programs serving poor and vulnerable populations. The goal was to maintain services for at-risk populations.

This organizational policy acted as a guide for all nurses, both convention attendees and nonattendees. Many nurses and nurse specialty organizations in the state used this policy direction to take action. Individually and in groups, the nurses lobbied their state legislators to disallow funding cuts to medical assistance and primary health care programs for low-income and disabled persons. The nurses advocated maintaining all school nurse positions. Some of the nurses used the opportunity to lobby for universal health care for state residents. In addition to lobbying efforts, nurses took the initiative to attract media attention to the problem.

Evaluation of the newly adopted policy of the nurses' association for state X showed success. Some funding reductions did occur, but they were small in comparison to the proposed cuts. No programs were eliminated.

Altered Relationships with the Environment

Elimination or reduction of environmental hazards is one measure of the effectiveness of programs directed toward providing a safer environment. For example, the removal of trash in a vacant lot reduces breeding grounds for rats and other wild animals while also removing physical and chemical hazards. Additionally, the effectiveness of a community educational program about environmental hazards may result in reduced dumping. Reductions in environmental hazards result in fewer accidents and injuries.

The reduction of environmental hazards can also reduce illness. For example, public health nursing interventions can control asthma triggers, thereby improving asthma management and reducing hospitalizations.

> Perceived ability to control asthma triggers was one outcome used to evaluate the effectiveness of a home-based education program by outreach workers (Primomo et al., 2006). Preintervention and postintervention interview surveys were conducted in person or by phone with caregivers of children with asthma. All families reported making changes to reduce household asthma triggers. There was a significant reduction in hospitalization at follow-up, compared with the baseline.

When hazards cannot be removed immediately, the desired outcome may be avoidance of the hazard. For example, age-appropriate health-education lessons were developed for elementary school children to teach them to avoid swimming and fishing in the polluted Chattanooga (Tennessee) Creek (Phillips, 1995).

Reductions in consumption and waste are other measures of environmental health. More efficient use of resources is the goal. For example, increasing the number of people who weatherize their homes or participate in recycling demonstrates the effectiveness of conservation programs. Community/public health nurses may be instrumental in collaborating to establish programs or in referring people to existing programs.

Because the basic standard of living is associated with health behaviors and health status, the level of poverty in a community can be used as one measure of the community's health. The level of poverty directly relates to both the physical and the social environments (Haan et al., 1987). Therefore changes in the level of poverty can be used as a measure of the effectiveness of public health activities to improve the basic standard of living within the community.

EVALUATION OF APPROPRIATENESS

Appropriateness may be defined as how well the nursing planning and interventions fit the assessed health need. The community/public health nurse considers the appropriateness of both the goals and the interventions. Table 17-1 includes some questions used in the evaluation of the appropriateness of nursing care.

Goals are usually more appropriate when the community/public health nurse has accurately assessed health needs of the population, readiness to change, and resources available. The *Healthy People 2010* objectives (U.S. Department of Health and Human Services, 2000) are targets that guide local communities in selecting specific goals and objectives for health programs. When the assessment and planning have been conducted in partnership with the community members, the nursing care is more likely to be appropriate. Occasionally, the community/public health nurse must wait

until after the intervention has been accomplished to evaluate whether the specific goals and objectives were realistic for a given community. Just as each individual is unique, so is each community.

Interventions are usually more appropriate when they are evidence-based and the community health nurse researches literature that describes what has worked well with similar populations. Nursing case studies and experimental research are helpful in suggesting ideas for interventions within a specific community. For example, strengthening the decision-making skills of adolescents is helpful in preventing drug use and unprotected sex. Exercise has been shown to slow the progression of osteoporosis in postmenopausal women. Consequently, each of these interventions would be evaluated as appropriate with their respective populations.

EVALUATION OF ADEQUACY

The community/public health nurse also evaluates the adequacy of both the goals and the interventions. Adequacy addresses the degree to which goals and interventions are sufficient to achieve the desired change. Table 17-1 includes some questions related to adequacy.

Even when care is appropriate, it may be inadequate. Nursing care is inadequate when not enough of the care is available to meet the total population need. For example, community/public health nurses who provide outreach to identify pregnant women, refer them for prenatal care and nutrition programs, and teach them about the importance of nutrition are engaged in appropriate nursing care. Prenatal care and improved nutrition are ways to increase the birth weights of infants. However, this care may be inadequate if the number of pregnant women is greater than those who can be reached by the number of community/public health nurses. This care may also be inadequate if the women are *found,* but the prenatal and nutrition services have long waiting lists. When nursing services are appropriate but inadequate to meet the need, nurses should consider other interventions, such as creating community awareness that additional services are needed.

EVALUATION OF EFFICIENCY

Efficiency is related to evaluation of structure because it is a measure of the relationship of resources to outcomes. Resources may include the nurses themselves, equipment, supplies, facilities, policies or legal authority, organizational features, and environmental features (ANA, 1986). Money, time, and emotional energy are other resources.

Table 17-1 also includes some questions to ask when considering efficiency. For example, when evaluating the efficiency of an immunization clinic, the community/public health nurse might ask whether equipment exists that is not used, how many doses of immunizations were wasted, whether the layout of the clinic prevents privacy, or whether heat escapes out the door each time it is opened.

The money, time, and other resources of the population must also be considered. Interventions may be efficient for nurses but inefficient for individuals and their families. Are parents tired when they reach the clinic because they were unable to afford a sitter for the other children? Are parents dissatisfied with the information they receive because the language of the nurses and pamphlets is "over their heads"?

EVALUATION OF PROCESS

Process evaluation focuses on how well the health-related program is operating and is linked to the original plan (Ervin, 2002). The questions included in Box 17-3 help analyze how well the planned program is actually being implemented. Answering the questions helps the community/public health nurse refine and manage the program. Process evaluation is concerned with clinical nursing care, but it also focuses on administrative and fiscal issues (Kennedy-Malone, 1996). Evaluation of the process of implementing the program is formative because it occurs throughout the life of the program.

UNIQUENESS IN EVALUATION OF NURSING CARE WITH COMMUNITIES

CRITERIA FOR EFFECTIVENESS

In goal-based evaluation of populations, criteria for success are written in terms of *percentage of population,* not an individual or a family. Because more than one individual is being evaluated, the population must often be sampled. In large populations, a random sample of at least 10% to 20% of persons will be useful. With small populations, the nurse can obtain information from all members, or as many as possible. One hundred percent participation is rare, however.

More time and personnel may be needed to evaluate the care provided to populations or communities. Because of the numbers of people in the population, more than one person may be needed to collect the information for evaluation. More time may also be required to ensure that the evaluators are following the same procedures, which increases interobserver reliability (Polit & Hungler, 2005).

BOX 17-3 **Questions to Ask in Process Evaluation of Health Programs**

- Is the target population being reached? If not, what outreach or publicity may be needed? What evidence exists that the program is acceptable to the target population?
- How many people have been served? How does this compare with projections of desired utilization? What should be done if the demand for services exceeds the current capacity?
- Are the program activities being phased in on time? If not, what modifications in the time line are needed?
- What are the staff development needs of the nurses and other personnel? What aspects of the intervention are difficult to implement and require further education?
- Are the planned resources being received? Have the budget revenues continued as planned? Are the program expenditures within the proposed budget? Have equipment and materials been received? Have interested persons volunteered as they said they would?
- Have the planned interventions been carried out? If so, to what degree do they meet professional standards?
- Have any of the planned interventions not been implemented? If so, what are the barriers? Can these interventions be omitted because the objectives are being achieved without the interventions, or should the interventions still be initiated?
- What concerns have emerged regarding communication, decision making, and participation? Are all interested parties still involved and informed about the program's progress? How do they perceive the program?

For care provided to individuals and families, the evaluation is documented on the legal record of the respective client. When evaluating care provided to populations, the results are usually reported as statistics for the aggregate or as a case study (without identifying the specific participants).

Because populations include many individuals or families, the criteria for measuring goal achievement may compare the population with another population; measurements must be available for both populations to make the comparison. This process is called *normative referencing.* The population may be compared with itself before and after the implementation. If change occurred, the nurse would expect to see an increase or decrease in one or more outcome measures. The population also may be compared with an entirely different population, such as the average for the United States. For example, if the incidence of prostate cancer in a population was higher than the average rate in the United States, the goal might be to reduce the incidence of prostate cancer to the national rate.

Maryland has a tuberculosis case rate that has remained historically above the national average case rate. One of their program goals in the tuberculosis program is to decrease the case rate to the national norm. In 2002 the national case rate was 5.2 cases of tuberculosis per 100,000 people. For that same year, Maryland reported a case rate of 5.7 per 100,000. Progress has been made; in 2006 the Maryland case rate for tuberculosis was slightly below the national rate. In 2006 the national case rate was 4.6 cases of tuberculosis per 100,000 people compared with Maryland's case rate of 4.5 per 100,000 people.

Criterion-referenced evaluation measures the extent to which specific objectives are reached at the level desired by the planner. Many of the *Healthy People 2010* objectives are criterion-referenced objectives. The following is a criterion-referenced objective targeted toward mothers of infants and preschool children: in a smoking-modification program, at least 30% of the mothers will devise and implement a contract to modify their smoking habits by the fifth week of the program. If 30% of the mothers do so, the objective will have been achieved. The mothers are not compared with other populations. (Chapter 16 provides more examples of normative-referenced and criterion-referenced objectives.)

Determining what the criteria should be is not easy. If the desired behavior is essential for safety, the criteria are high. For example, 100% of participants will hold the infant with the head higher than the stomach and burp the infant during feeding to prevent choking. If a nurse believes that all of the participants should know how to demonstrate a skill, then the behaviors should be as clear as possible. The criteria for proper holding need to be explicit in this objective.

However, expecting 100% of the participants to reach the objectives is usually unrealistic. In group-education sessions, a few people are not interested, not feeling well, or distracted so that they do not participate fully. Even when the participants are interested in learning, the teaching may not be sufficient for them to learn; they may need different learning strategies or more time. If the desired learning is complex or requires a change in lifestyle, a lower percentage of the population should be expected to achieve the objective. For example, between 14% and 45% of smokers who quit are able to abstain from smoking for 12 months. Smoking cessation is a difficult process. Only approximately 2.5% of current smokers stop permanently each year (United States Department of Health and Human Services [USDHHS], 2000).

Criteria for desirable outcomes can be selected because they reflect the clients' interests. For example, elementary school children were given an interest inventory to determine what they most wanted to learn related to drugs (Box 17-4). The answers helped nursing students establish both the objectives of and the content for the teaching sessions.

Criteria for desirable outcomes also can be selected because they constitute the next logical step. For example, after parents have learned to take the temperature of their infant, they should know which temperatures to report to the pediatrician, clinic, or nurse practitioner.

SOURCES OF EVALUATION DATA

The nursing process is to be mutual with the entire population or its representatives. Consequently, evaluation of community/public health nursing practice involves participants from the community (ANA, 2007). As part of the planning for evaluation, decisions must be made regarding who will be involved in the evaluation.

Some evaluation questions can be answered by the nurse alone, and some questions can be answered best when others' perspectives are solicited. When measuring effectiveness, the community/public health nurse ensures that the relevant outcome measures are collected from the target population. In some instances, collecting information from others who are close to the target population will also be helpful. For example, in a smoking-cessation program, the community/public health nurse may also collect information about smoking habits from other members of the participants' households (with the participants' permission).

Epidemiologic mortality and morbidity data are often obtained from other health care team members who collected the information. If the goal is a health system change, such as establishing a clinic, a visit to the new clinic and interviews with both the health providers and the population receiving care will be useful.

The community/public health nurse can evaluate efficiency with information from both the nurses implementing the health care program and the population who received care. Nurses can best describe the effort that they contributed: Who did what? How many times? With how many people? The participants themselves can best describe their efforts in terms of time, money, and physical and emotional energy. To evaluate efficiency, both effort and outcomes must be measured and considered together.

Dissatisfaction occurs most frequently when expectations are not met. Nurses should expect dissatisfaction to be expressed by persons who perceive that care is inappropriate, inadequate, inefficient, or ineffective. Occasionally, the care provided by community/public health nurses may be both effective and relatively efficient yet contributes to the dissatisfaction of some. Many stakeholders have expectations about nursing care yet are not directly involved in its delivery. The more the community/public health nurse is aware of stakeholders' expectations during the planning phase, the fewer surprises there will be. Intermittent contact with all interested parties throughout the process will allow early identification of misunderstandings, negotiation, and revision of the process to balance the interests of many. Satisfying everyone is impossible.

RECORDING EVALUATIONS

Box 17-5 identifies data that are to be included in a written record of the evaluation of nursing care with communities. This documentation describes what actually occurred, provides a historic record from which to study trends, and provides a basis for deciding whether programs should be continued and how they might be modified.

Evaluation reports may need to be written in different formats for different audiences. For example, an evaluation report written to gain funding might have different content and focus than a report to be shared with the service participants. Evaluation reports to be delivered orally in small groups or public meetings should be written in a more conversational style.

When writing an evaluation report, the community/public health nurse should be politically and culturally sensitive. Negative realities can be addressed using positive words. Always imagine that the most powerful and influential persons in the community will read the report and word it in a way that they can accept. Similarly, consider the perspectives of the

---

BOX 17-4   Sample Tool to Assess Clients' Interests

Put a check mark (✓) by the three things about which you want to learn most.
_____ What is the difference between medicine and street drugs?
_____ What can street drugs do to my body?
_____ How can I say no to drugs?
_____ What can I do to feel good without using drugs?
_____ Why do people use drugs?
_____ Other: _____

BOX 17-5   Data in a Written Evaluation Report

1. Indicate baseline health status or behaviors of client population.
2. Indicate baseline resources and methods currently being used to address the health problem.
3. List the health-related goals and desired outcomes.
4. Describe the nursing interventions (effort). Enumerate what actions were completed. If an educational strategy is being evaluated, include both the actions completed and the content taught.
5. Indicate tasks that were planned but not done or completed.
6. Specify other changes in the environment that might have affected the health outcomes, such as changes in funding, a television health-education campaign, or the closing of a clinic.
7. Describe what behaviors indicate goal achievement and the degree to which the need is resolved.
8. Describe the level of satisfaction of persons involved, and identify actual and potential resistance.
9. Indicate any modifications that were made in the goals.
10. Discuss the relationship of effort to outcomes—efficiency.
11. Include interpretations and judgments.
12. Make recommendations.

service participants and write in a way that does not reinforce cultural stereotypes or blaming.

When written reports are long, writing an executive summary is helpful for the persons or groups who will not be able to read the whole document. An *executive summary* is a brief summary of the report that includes major findings and recommendations.

ANALYZING EVALUATION DATA

Distinctions should be made among facts, interpretations, judgments, and recommendations when discussing and presenting the results of an evaluation (Patton, 1982). Results are both factual and interpretive. Factual findings include data (e.g., the program has served 50 clients during the first 2 months). Interpretations are statements about interrelationships, reasons, and meanings (e.g., the clients have shown up because of the public service announcements on the radio). Judgments are evaluations made in the context of values and include statements about the desirability or undesirability or goodness or badness of the data and interpretations (e.g., "I'm really disappointed that we haven't reached 100 clients already"). Recommendations are suggested actions based on the facts, interpretations, and judgments. A recommendation in this situation might be to increase the publicity to double the numbers of clients served in the next 3 months.

MODIFICATION OF NURSING CARE WITH COMMUNITIES

Communities are dynamic and complex. Each human being exists within a community and is an agent of his or her own needs, desires, and self-expression. Social interaction among *multiple* human beings is even more complex. Consequently, because nursing care is created through the processes of human interaction, it must be continuously evaluated and revised. As the membership of the population changes, so do health status, health risks, health needs, and interests.

Community/public health nursing practice occurs within physical, political, economic, cultural, and social contexts. A change in any one of these contexts results in changes in all other aspects of the community system. While nurses implement the planned care, a multitude of changes occur simultaneously in their environments. Therefore formative evaluation helps community/public health nurses modify all steps of the nursing process.

EVALUATION METHODS AND TOOLS

DESIGNS FOR EVALUATION OF EFFECTIVENESS

Case descriptions and quasiexperimental designs may be used to evaluate the effectiveness of community/public health nursing interventions with communities (Kosecoff & Fink, 1982). A case description examines the community, health goals, community/public health nursing interventions, and outcomes. The evaluation described in this chapter can be used to develop a case description. The case-evaluation design allows a thorough description of the situation and is especially helpful in creating a history of the process, communicating information about a

new program or a demonstration program to others, and documenting both formative and summative evaluations. With a case description, the community/public health nurses cannot prove that the nursing intervention led to the specific health outcomes. However, ways to evaluate the likelihood that the outcomes were the result of the nursing interventions include the following: (1) the implementation can occur shortly after assessment so that developmental maturation does not account for the change; (2) the population members can be asked whether they participated in other activities from the time of assessment until the time of evaluation; and (3) the nurse can be alert to other community changes that might have contributed simultaneously to the health outcomes (Kosecoff & Fink, 1982).

The time-series design is a quasiexperimental method in which information is collected about the same population more than once (Kosecoff & Fink, 1982). The steps of the nursing process include assessment, pretest, implementation, evaluation (posttest), and later evaluation. This design allows pretest and posttest results to be compared to demonstrate that change did occur. Additionally, the later evaluation indicates whether the change was lasting; this evaluation considers permanency of results, also called *impact*. A time-series design was used to evaluate the effectiveness of the home-visit health-promotion and risk-reduction program previously discussed in this chapter (Fetrick et al., 2003).

Evaluation research attempts to discover links between implementations and health results, including the meaning of the experience to the participants. The goal of empirical-evaluation research is to establish that interventions are causally linked to desired outcomes. The knowledge can be generalized to similar situations and can assist community/public health nurses in selecting which intervention strategies are likely to work best. This information also helps persuade funding sources that their money will be well spent. Beneficial outcomes of home-based community/public health nursing interventions have been demonstrated; a major focus of future research efforts should be "rigorous outcome evaluation of community-level nursing strategies" (Deal, 1997, p. 125).

Because human beings are diverse, evaluation research also seeks to find what works best with different populations. How are the results different with women and men or with young and old? For example, empirical research indicates that young children learn best through participation. Interpretive evaluation research seeks to describe the meaning of the experience to the participants. When nurses understand the perceptual and cultural meanings that the nursing care has for the participants, nurses are better able to modify care. The care can become more beneficial and satisfying for the recipients.

TOOLS FOR EVALUATION OF EFFECTIVENESS

The category of health outcome that is being measured will help determine the tools that will be used. The tools are often the same ones that are used to measure change with individuals; however, the community/public health nurse is now collecting the information from a large number of people.

Behavior change is best measured through observation. Some parenting programs, for example, have used videotapes of parent-child interactions to collect information about aspects of parenting; the tapes are then given to the parents as a reward for participation. Criteria used to interpret parenting skills can take several forms. Box 17-6 includes a sample

BOX 17-6   Sample Checklist Tool for Evaluating Behaviors Related to Infant Formula Feeding

This tool can be used to observe parent or caregiver behavior related to infant formula feeding. An item is checked when the behavior is observed during a feeding session.

_____ Responds to hunger cues almost always
_____ Uses clean bottle, nipple, formula
_____ Changes or washes nipple if contaminated
_____ Holds infant
_____ Holds bottle so that air is not allowed in nipple or uses collapsible bag bottles
_____ Burps infant
_____ Stops at _____ ounces or sooner if infant is full

BOX 17-7   Examples of Questions Modified to Measure Knowledge and Attitude

Knowledge
For each item, circle either True or False.
1. True or False: Using condoms during sexual intercourse can help prevent HIV infection.
2. True or False: Environmental tobacco smoke can reach a fetus during the mother's pregnancy.

Attitude
For each item, circle Yes if you agree with the statement and circle No if you disagree with the statement.
1. Yes or No: Condoms should be used by sexually active individuals to prevent HIV infections.
2. Yes or No: Pregnant women should be encouraged to avoid environmental tobacco smoke.

Alternative Attitude Format
Circle the response that indicates the intensity with which you agree or disagree with each item.
1. Condoms should be used by sexually active individuals to prevent HIV infections.
   Strongly Agree Agree Uncertain Disagree Strongly Disagree
2. Pregnant women should be encouraged to avoid environmental tobacco smoke.
   Strongly Agree Agree Uncertain Disagree Strongly Disagree

checklist that can be used to record the presence or absence of specific parenting actions. Table 17-2 addresses similar actions and rates the quality of the parenting based on grouped behaviors.

Oral or written questions are usually used to collect information on factual knowledge and attitudinal learning. The same questions can be used to measure both aspects, but the scoring is different. Box 17-7 provides examples of questions that are modified to measure factual knowledge or attitudes. When developing questions to measure factual knowledge, the nurse needs to develop a key of right and wrong answers to use in scoring the tool. Note that when measuring attitudes, no right or wrong answers exist.

EFFICIENCY ANALYSIS
The efficiency of programs can be evaluated using cost-effectiveness and benefit-cost analyses. Both methods consider the resources used in relation to outcomes.

In cost-effectiveness, the cost per unit of outcome is determined. For example, in a home health agency, the average cost per home visit can be determined if costs and number of home visits are recorded. Similarly, the average cost per maternity clinic visit or the average cost of providing prenatal nursing care can also be computed. The costs must be computed, and the value of the outcomes must be estimated (Ervin, 2002). To compare the cost-effectiveness of programs accurately, the acuity of client problems must be similar for the two programs. Cost-effectiveness analysis is often used

to address the question, "Can similar outcomes be achieved with less cost?"

An excellent randomized study has demonstrated the cost-effectiveness of home-visit follow-up by expert neonatal nurses for infants with very low birth weights compared with continued hospital care (Brooten et al., 1986). Even though costs were incurred for the home-based nursing care, the hospital and physician costs were much less for those cared for at home. For persons who are cared for at home, better health outcomes were achieved at a net savings of $18,560 per infant.

Benefit-cost analysis also considers the resources used in relation to the resulting outcomes. However, benefit-cost analysis asks, "Are the outcomes achieved worth the cost incurred?" A significant number of difficulties are encountered

TABLE 17-2   Sample Rating Tool for Evaluating Behaviors Related to Infant Formula Feeding

Client demonstrates proper infant feeding by responding to infant hunger cues, preparing clean bottle/nipple/formula, holding infant, preventing sucking of air, and feeding no more than _____ ounces.

Score 1	Score 3	Score 5
Sometimes responds to cry	Usually responds to hunger cues	Always responds to hunger cues
Often uses contaminated nipples and dirty bottles	Occasionally uses contaminated nipples and dirty bottles	Uses clean equipment; changes nipple if contaminated
Usually props infant	Usually holds infant	Never props bottle; holds infant
Allows sucking of air	Usually does not allow air in nipple	Prevents air in nipple
Feeds continuously	Stops at _____ oz to burp infant	Stops at _____ oz to burp infant

in completing a benefit-cost analysis (Ervin, 2002). First, the analysis is difficult to do because it requires that a dollar value be placed on the benefits (outcomes), and health programs often produce some intangible effects. Not all outcomes can be quantified in terms of dollars. For example, what is the dollar value of improved self-esteem? Second, to provide justice (i.e., to correct unequal access to health care), the provision of care may be more important than whether it is efficient. Third, the value of benefits must be considered from several perspectives. For example, the provision of home visits to families with infants can benefit the infant, the parent, and society. If only the cost of care versus the immediate health outcomes is considered (e.g., having up-to-date childhood immunizations), the benefits may not seem worth the cost. However, if the long-term benefit of preventing hospitalization and disability from measles and the benefit of high immunization levels in the community are considered, the benefits are greater.

Olds and colleagues (1993) asked whether the outcomes of a prenatal and infancy nurse home-visit program were worth the financial cost of the program. Although there were positive outcomes for both the mothers and the infants, the dollar value of these benefits was not known. The researchers estimated that costs were saved by outcomes such as fewer hospital days at birth, fewer infant emergency department visits for accidents, lower incidence of child abuse and neglect, and reduced maternal dependence on welfare. When government cost savings for medical and social services were calculated, the savings were greater than the cost of the nursing interventions. The benefits (outcomes) were worth more than the costs.

Costs of programs include the direct costs of services, administrative costs, and the costs of increased demand on related services. For example, costs of an immunization program include direct costs of nursing services, supplies, educational material, and biologic agents; indirect costs include record keeping, utilities and building maintenance, salaries of administrative personnel, and publicity. Health care costs related to identification, referral, and treatment of health problems among the children who come for immunizations may also be increased.

The costs that clients incur in terms of time, energy, and money should be considered in benefit-cost analyses. However, current methods of benefit-cost analysis often ignore this human impact, especially for families with ill members. For example, care of ill persons in the home costs the health care system less than care in a hospital or nursing home. However, for some families, the cost of caring for their family member at home is expensive in terms of lost wages or emotional stress or both.

Evaluation of efficiency helps community/public health nurses refine programs so that more services are provided with the same dollars, or the same services are provided at a lower cost. Dollars saved can be channeled to serve more people or to fund other health programs. Because community/

public health nurses directly provide the care in many health programs, they are likely to have evidence of the less tangible benefits of the services. Nurses should contribute this information to any benefit-cost analysis. Because no precise estimation of the benefits can be made, community/public health nurses can help expand the discussion to include quality-of-life issues.

KEY IDEAS

1. The responsibilities of community/public health nurses include the evaluation of nursing care provided to communities. Evaluation enables the improvement of nursing care with communities.
2. Evaluation involves several steps, including planning the evaluation, collecting the data, analyzing and interpreting the data, reporting the evaluation, and implementing suggestions.
3. Evaluations are conducted to demonstrate that goals and desired outcomes are being achieved; to make decisions about continuing, expanding, or ending specific programs of nursing interventions; to improve nursing care so that goals and outcomes are achieved efficiently; and to improve nursing care so that it is acceptable to the community.
4. Health-related programs have goals, outcome objectives, process objectives, and management objectives.
5. Formative evaluation is conducted during the process of nursing care delivery to modify and improve the program. Summative evaluation occurs at the end of the program to determine whether goals and desired outcomes were achieved.
6. Community members are to be involved in evaluation. Stakeholders are individuals who may be affected by the nursing interventions, including those who contribute resources and those who receive the care.
7. An essential part of evaluation is determining effectiveness: whether the goals and desired outcomes have been achieved. Indicators of the effectiveness of nursing care include knowledge, behavior and skills, attitudes, emotional well-being and empowerment, morbidity and mortality rates, the presence of services or health policies, client satisfaction, and human-environment relationships.
8. Programs of nursing care should be appropriate to the assessed community needs and should be efficient; the resources need to be used wisely to achieve the desired outcomes.
9. Community/public health nurses seek to develop programs of nursing care that are adequate to the scope of community needs.
10. Evaluation of process objectives helps monitor and improve programs of nursing care. Process evaluation addresses the degree to which the program of interventions is being carried out as planned.

Evaluation at Northview High School

The following evaluation is based on the program of nursing care for Northview High School described in the Nursing Process in Practice feature in Chapter 16.

PHASE I: A SEX EDUCATION PROGRAM
NURSING DIAGNOSES OR PROBLEMS

1. Population at risk for health problems as evidenced by a high rate of sexual activity
2. Knowledge deficit related to the risks of pregnancy during sexual activity
3. Inconsistent use of birth control
4. Knowledge deficit related to functioning of various birth-control mechanisms
5. Knowledge deficit related to signs, symptoms, and potential consequences of untreated sexually transmitted diseases

PROGRAM GOALS

- Provide students with the skills needed to explore the pros and cons of engaging in sexual activity during adolescence.
- Increase the knowledge level of students about sexually related information so that students can make informed choices about behavior.

    Problem 1 Outcome Objective. Consistent with the *Healthy People 2010* objectives, reduce the number of students who begin sexual activity or increase the number of students who postpone beginning sexual activity until they are older.

    Problem 2 Outcome Objective. Increase student knowledge about the process of conception.

    Problems 3 and 4 Outcome Objective. Increase student knowledge about birth-control methods.

    Problem 5 Outcome Objective. Increase student knowledge of sexually transmitted disease.

    Process Objective. Seventy-five percent of students will participate in the instructional program during spring semester.

EVALUATION PLAN

Ms. Fields is responsible for formulating an evaluation plan. In consultation with other individuals who are involved in implementing the program (teachers, psychologist, social worker), an evaluation plan is developed. A student representative is also included on the committee. A series of four evaluation methods are decided on to measure the outcomes (effectiveness) of the program:

1. Observations and interviews with participants in the seminar discussion and peer network programs to evaluate problem 1
2. A posttest to measure knowledge levels to evaluate problems 2, 3, 4, and 5
3. A survey to measure sexual activity and practices to evaluate problem 1
4. A summary evaluation of the effectiveness of the entire sex education program

COLLECTION OF EVALUATION DATA

1. Ms. Fields attended two of the seminar discussions led by the social worker to observe student-leader interactions and student responses. Additionally, the students were asked to evaluate the seminars using a five-question evaluation survey to measure satisfaction, with room provided for additional comments. Ms. Fields and the psychologist devised an interview tool to guide the evaluation process of the peer-support program.
2. Ms. Fields and the other 2 teachers in the sex education program developed a 20-question posttest. The posttest measured knowledge in the area of pregnancy risks, appropriate use of birth control, and the signs, symptoms, and potential consequences of untreated sexually transmitted disease.
3. A random sampling survey was conducted of the student population who received the intervention program and measured sexual behavior 3 months after the program.
4. Summary evaluation of the program included evaluation steps 1, 2, and 3 as mentioned, as well as interviews with the principal, teaching staff, and counselors; an assessment of the number of students affected; and the time and materials necessary to accomplish the program.

ANALYSIS OF THE DATA

1. Evaluation of the seminar discussion group indicated that approximately 70% of the students in attendance were actively engaged in the guided discussion. Students asked and answered questions and raised issues during the discussion. The student evaluation of the seminars indicated that 80% believed the seminars were informative, and 65% said the discussions were helpful in aiding their decision-making process related to initiating or continuing sexual activity, in analyzing the role of peer pressure in the decision-making process, and in clarifying their position on the issues. Approximately 10% of students thought the discussions were useless, and 12% reported that they did not feel comfortable engaging in the discussion process. The peer-support program was intended to support students in their decision to remain celibate or to postpone sexual activity. Students were happy with the peer program; they reported a variety of responses from other students, including inquiry and ridicule. The members believed that the program helped them to be comfortable with their decisions. The peer group continues to meet, and the number of new members increased by 5%.
2. The posttest results indicated that students were able to differentiate between pregnancy-risk situations and situations that had less risk of pregnancy, and they were able to identify birth-control methods, pros and cons of various methods, and failure rates. Students improved in the area of knowledge about sexually transmitted disease but were unable to link specific health complications with selected diseases.
3. The survey of a random sample of students administered 3 months after the program revealed that students were using condoms with greater frequency during sexual activity and that the use of a concurrent birth-control method had increased approximately 10%. Essentially, no change was found in the numbers of students reporting sexual activity.

Continued

4. Summary evaluation indicated that the peer program was working well for students who had joined. The seminar discussion and teaching intervention reached all intended students (sophomores, juniors, and seniors), or 75% of the high school enrollment. Teachers reported that they were pleased with the instructional portion of the program but thought that adding audiovisual materials, including a film, would be useful to the learning process. Students were still uncomfortable leading the seminar discussions. Overall, the planned interventions had worked well. Recommendations: (1) Continue the program for all grades, with an emphasis on the incoming freshman class and the new sophomores who had missed the intervention during this school year; (2) add to audiovisual budget to upgrade available instructional media; (3) continue the peer-support program and encourage expanded enrollment in the program; and (4) provide a summer in-service program to increase teacher expertise with seminar discussion of sexual issues.

REPORT EVALUATION RESULTS

Ms. Fields prepared a written report of the evaluation results, including an executive summary, which she presented to the principal in a personal meeting. The principal reviewed the report, concurred with the results, and presented the report and recommendations to meetings of the parent-teacher association (PTA) and the school board. Ms. Fields was asked to attend both meetings and participated in the discussion.

IMPLEMENT RECOMMENDATIONS

The PTA was satisfied with progress in the sex education program and voted to provide funding support to improve audiovisual materials and contribute to a teacher in-service program. The school board has taken the report under advisement and is expected to decide on a course of action by the end of the summer, which will be too late to provide a summer in-service for interested teachers.

PHASE II: IMPROVE STUDENT ACCESS TO HEALTH SERVICES, INCLUDING SERVICES TO ADDRESS RISKY SEXUAL BEHAVIOR
NURSING DIAGNOSES OR PROBLEMS

1. Inadequate services to provide adolescent health care
2. Inadequate services to address primary prevention with respect to pregnancy and sexually transmitted diseases
3. Inadequate support services for teenage mothers with respect to daycare, parenting skills, and continuation of their educational program

PROGRAM GOAL

Improve health services for adolescents and improve support services for teenage parents, especially teenage mothers.

Problems 1 and 2 Outcome Objective. Provide adequate health care services to students within 24 months.

Problem 3 Outcome Objective. Develop support services for teenage parents that will facilitate their educational progress and the well-being of their children within 18 months.

Process Objectives. Several process objectives were developed for phase II consistent with the community standards suggested by the American Public Health Association (1991):

1. By 2 years from inception of the adolescent health program, 75% of Northview High School students who are referred to the program will receive services at the health center or be referred to other community-based services to meet their needs.
2. Within 2 years, all adolescent parents will have access to affordable certified child care.
3. Within 2 years, all adolescent parents who remain in school will be encouraged to attend a school-based parenting-skills program.

EVALUATION PLAN

To address problems 1 and 2, Ms. Fields and the committee proposed and received funding to improve adolescent health services situated within the local health center and to develop a community referral mechanism for students seen in the school health suite who need further medical care. To address problem 3, Ms. Fields received input from interested parties (teachers, school staff, teenage parents) and intends to convene a committee to develop a proposal for support services.

The formative evaluation plan consists of reviewing the progress on these two efforts with individuals involved in the process.

COLLECTION OF EVALUATION DATA

Ms. Fields met with the staff of adolescent services to review progress. She, health department personnel, and the principal reviewed her written plan for implementing referrals from the health suite. Ms. Fields and the vice-principal reviewed her progress on convening the committee to address support services for teenage parents.

ANALYSIS OF THE DATA

Adolescent health services will be operational in 2 weeks. The staff is in place, and all the requested supplies have been ordered. The existing equipment provided by the health department is in place and is operational. The service center originally planned to begin providing care in March, but implementation was delayed because of late-arriving equipment and the health department's delay in designating a nurse to staff the service. Ms. Fields does have an adequate plan for community referrals, which includes all agencies and professional personnel who are willing to provide care for free or at a reduced rate. Unfortunately, the two general practitioners in the community are unwilling to assume care for any more clients at reduced fees at this time. Ms. Fields has enlisted the help of other professionals in an effort to identify other physicians who might be willing to assist with the project. Ms. Fields has been only partially successful in gathering her committee to look at teenage parent support services. She has consulted with local community leaders (an alderman, three church pastors, and two local business owners) and enlisted their help in recruiting volunteers. She is hoping to have a complete committee in place in 1 month.

REPORT EVALUATION RESULTS

At this point, the individuals who need to know the results of the efforts are involved in the review of progress and are informed about the status of the efforts.

LEARNING BY EXPERIENCE AND REFLECTION

1. Based on the plan of nursing care that you developed for census tract 1 using the first guidelines for learning in Chapter 15, design an evaluation plan. Who are the stakeholders who need to be involved in the evaluation process? How will you evaluate program effectiveness? What will you include in your formative process evaluation?

2. Reflect on your own experience with a health program (e.g., health education, screening, clinical care). Why did you seek care from that program? What were your goals? What was helpful to achievement of your goals? What contributed to your satisfaction or dissatisfaction? How would you modify the program if you were the nurse involved?

3. Based on the incidence of teenage pregnancy and sexually transmitted diseases, including human immunodeficiency virus (HIV) infection, a school system has decided to permit the distribution of condoms to high school students who request them. The school board has voted for the policy, and its meetings were open to the public. A vocal minority of parents is upset by the policy because they believe sexual abstinence should be the school's policy; they also believe that the home (family) is the place for sex education. What point of view do you hold on this ethical question? What alternative courses of action would be possible if you were the school health nurse? What would you choose to do, and why?

4. Interview a community/public health nurse to determine how immunization or other clinic programs are evaluated. What data are routinely collected, and what questions are answered? To what degree does the nurse participate in collecting and interpreting the evaluation data? How are the data used to modify the program?

STUDY AIDS   http://evolve.elsevier.com/Maurer/community/

Visit the Evolve website for this book to find the following study and assessment materials:

- Quiz
- Web Scenario
- Critical Thinking Questions and Answers for Case Studies

- Care Plans
- *Healthy People* Updates
- Glossary

REFERENCES

American Nurses Association. (1986). *Standards of community health nursing practice.* Washington, DC: Author.

American Nurses Association. (2007). *Public health nursing: Scope and standards of practice.* Silver Spring, MD: Author.

American Public Health Association. (1991). *Healthy communities 2000—model standards: Guidelines for community attainment of the year 2000 national health objectives.* Washington, DC: Author.

Brooten, D., Kumar, S., Brown, L., et al. (1986). A randomized clinical trial of early hospital discharge and home follow-up of very-low-birth-weight infants. *New England Journal of Medicine, 315*(15), 934-938.

Cramer, M., Chen, L.-W., Roberts, S., et al. (2007). Evaluating the social and economic impact of community-based prenatal care. *Public Health Nursing, 24*(4), 329-336.

Deal, L. (1997). The effectiveness of community health interventions: A literature review. In B. Spradley J. Allender (Eds.), *Readings in community health nursing* (5th ed.; pp. 121-134). Philadelphia: J. B. Lippincott.

Deniston, O., & Rosenstock, I. (1970). Evaluating health programs. *Public Health Reports, 85,* 835-840.

Diers, D. (1985). Policy and politics. In D. Mason & S. Talbott (Eds.), *Political action handbook for nurses* (pp. 53-59). Menlo Park, CA: Addison-Wesley.

Donabedian, A. (1980). *The definition of quality and approaches to its assessment* (Vol. 1). Ann Arbor, MI: Health Administration Press.

Endyke-Doran, C., Gonzalez, R., Trujillo, M., et al. (2007). The Syphilis Elimination Project: Targeting the Hispanic community of Baltimore City. *Public Health Nursing, 24*(1), 40-47.

Ervin, N. E. (2002). *Advanced community health nursing practice.* Upper Saddle River, NJ: Prentice Hall.

Fetrick, A., Christensen, M., & Mitchell, C. (2003). Does public health home visitation make a difference in the health outcomes of pregnant clients and their offspring? *Public Health Nursing, 20*(3), 184-189.

Freeman, R. (1963). Public health nursing practice (3rd ed.). Philadelphia: W.B. Saunders.

Gyurcsik, N., & Brittain, D. (2006). Partial examination of the public health impact of the People with Arthritis Can Exercise (PACE®) Program: Reach, adoption, and maintenance. *Public Health Nursing, 23*(6), 485-567.

Haan, M., Kaplan, G., & Comacho, T. (1987). Poverty and health: Prospective evidence from the Alameda County study. *American Journal of Epidemiology, 125,* 989-998.

Kaiser, M., Barry, T., & Kaiser, K. (2002). Using focus groups to evaluate and strengthen public health nursing population-focused interventions. *Journal of Transcultural Nursing, 13*(4), 303-310.

Kennedy-Malone, L. (1996). Evaluation strategies for CNSs: Application of an evaluation model. *Clinical Nurse Specialists, 4*(10), 195-198.

Kim, J. J., Cho, H., Cheon-Klessig, Y. S., et al. (2002). Primary health care for Korean immigrants: Sustaining a culturally sensitive model. *Public Health Nursing, 19*(3), 191-200.

Kosecoff, J., & Fink, A. (1982). *Evaluation basics: A practitioner's manual.* Beverly Hills, CA: Sage Publication.

Lashley, M. (2007). A targeted testing program for tuberculosis control and prevention among Baltimore City's homeless population. *Public Health Nursing, 24*(1), 34-39.

McKenzie, J. F., & Smeltzer, J. L. (2000). *Planning, implementing, and evaluating health promotion programs: A primer* (3rd ed.). Upper Saddle River, NJ: Allyn and Bacon.

Olds, D., Henderson, C., Phelps, C., et al. (1993). Effect of prenatal and infancy nurse home visitation on government spending. *Medical Care, 31*(2), 155-174.

Patton, M. (1982). *Practical evaluation.* Newbury Park, CA: Sage Publications.

Phillips, L. (1995). Chattanooga Creek: Case study of the public health nursing role in environmental health. *Public Health Nursing, 12*(5), 335-340.

Polit, D., & Hungler, B. (2005). *Essentials of nursing research: Methods, appraisal, and utilization* (6th ed.). Philadelphia: J. B. Lippincott.

Primomo, J., Johnston, S., DiBiase, F., et al. (2006). Evaluation of a community-based outreach worker program for children with asthma. *Public Health Nursing, 23*(3), 234-241.

Sloan, M., & Schommer, B. (1991). The process of contracting in community health nursing. In B. Spradley (Ed.), *Readings in community health*

nursing (4th ed.; pp. 304-312). Philadelphia: J. B. Lippincott.

Suchman, E. (1967). *Evaluative research: Principles and practice in public service and social action programs.* New York: Russell Sage Foundation.

Truglio-Londrigan, M., Macali, M., Bernstein, M., et al. (2002). A plan for the delegation of epinephrine administration in nonpublic schools

to unlicensed assistive personnel. *Public Health Nursing, 19*(6), 412-422.

U.S. Department of Health and Human Services. (2000). *Healthy People 2010 objectives: Understanding and improving health* (2nd ed.). Washington, DC: U.S. Government Printing Office.

SUGGESTED READINGS

American Nurses Association. (2007). *Public health nursing: Scope and standards of practice.* Silver Spring, MD: Author.

Anderson, E., & McFarlane, J. (2008). *Community as partner: Theory and practice in nursing.* Philadelphia: Lippincott Williams and Wilkins.

Archer, S. E. (1974, September-October). PERT: A tool for nurse-administrators. *Journal of Nursing Administration, 4,* 26-32.

Deal, L. (1997). The effectiveness of community health interventions: A literature review. In B. Spradley & J. Allender (Eds.), *Readings in*

community health nursing (5th ed.; pp. 121-134). Philadelphia: J. B. Lippincott.

Donabedian, A. (1985). *The methods and findings of quality assessment and monitoring: An illustrated analysis.* Ann Arbor, MI: Health Administration Press.

Fryer, G., Igoe, J., & Miyoshi, T. (1997). Considering school health program screening services as a cost offset: A comparison of existing reimbursements in one state. *Journal of School Nursing, 13*(2), 18-21.

Gonzalez-Calvo, J., Jackson, J., Hansford, C., et al. (1997). Nursing case management and its role

in perinatal risk reduction: Development, implementation, and evaluation of a culturally competent model for African American women. *Public Health Nursing, 14*(4), 190-206.

Patton, M. (1990). *Qualitative evaluation and research methods* (2nd ed.). Newbury Park, CA: Sage Publications.

U.S. Department of Health and Human Services. (2006). *Healthy People 2010 objectives: Midcourse revisions.* Washington, DC: U.S. Government Printing Office.

Tools for Practice

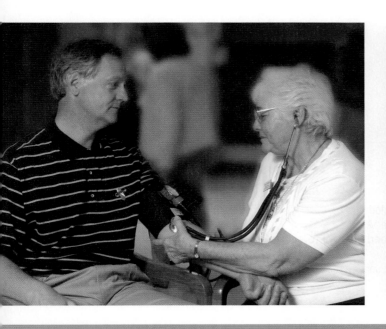

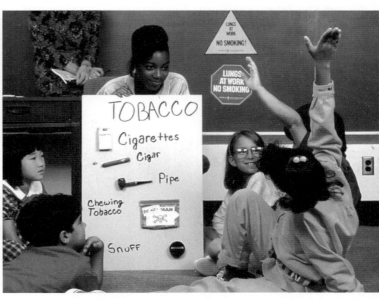

18 Health Promotion and Risk Reduction in the Community

Gail L. Heiss*

FOCUS QUESTIONS

What does being healthy mean?

What is the difference between promoting health and preventing illness?

What models help explain health-related behaviors?

What influences the health of a society?

What are the major national policies for health promotion?

What are the responsibilities of the community/public health nurse in promoting health and preventing illness in the community?

CHAPTER OUTLINE

KEY TERMS

Health information assaults our senses daily. Advertisements and articles about healthy living, healthy diets, health clubs, new vitamins, new medications, and new exercise programs are on the television, the radio, the Internet, magazine racks, and newspapers everywhere. Americans are trying and buying and moving toward health—or are they? A review of the *Healthy People 2010* objectives and the most recent *Healthy People 2010 Midcourse Review* will provide perspective on the current state of the nation's health and movement toward health for all (U.S. Department of Health and Human Services [USDHHS], 2000, 2006).

Healthy People 2010 is the most current plan to improve the nation's health and is designed to achieve two goals: (1) to help individuals of all ages increase life expectancy and improve their quality of life and (2) to eliminate health disparities among different segments of the population. The

Healthy People 2010 plan includes 28 focus areas that contribute to the achievement of these 2 overarching goals. In addition, a set of 10 leading health indicators will be used to measure the health of the nation over the next 10 years. Each of the 10 indicators also has 1 or more objectives associated with it (USDHHS, 2000). (See the *Healthy People 2010* box on page 473.) For the objectives to be achieved, renewed prevention efforts and commitment by individuals, groups, health care providers, and local, state, and federal government agencies are necessary.

Trends reported in the midcourse review of the *Healthy People 2010* objectives indicate that progress is evident for 70% of the objectives in *Healthy People 2010*. Greater numbers of objectives are moving toward the target for all population groups except for native Hawaiian and other Pacific Islanders. Relating to the two overarching goals in *Healthy*

---

*This chapter incorporates material written for the first edition by Mary Ellen Lashley.

■ HEALTHY PEOPLE 2010 ■
Leading Health Indicators

1. Physical activity
2. Overweight and obesity
3. Tobacco use
4. Substance abuse
5. Responsible sexual behavior
6. Mental health
7. Injury and violence
8. Environmental quality
9. Immunization
10. Access to health care

Data from U.S. Department of Health and Human Services. (2000). *Healthy People 2010: Understanding and improving health and objectives for improving health* (2nd ed.). Washington, DC: U.S. Government Printing Office; and U.S. Department of Health and Human Services. (2006). *Healthy People 2010: Midcourse review.* Accessed July 31, 2007, at *http://www.healthypeople.gov/data/midcourse/.*

People 2010, the midcourse review of the data reveals that years of life, measured as life expectancy, continue to increase; however, there are still disparities associated with gender, race, and ethnicity. Related to the second overarching goal of eliminating health disparities, there have been mixed results with improvements in some areas related to social and demographic characteristics, but increases in disparity related to racial and ethnic groups for other goals and objectives. The midcourse review presents a challenge to continue to measure the interactions between health promotion and disease prevention, which affect life expectancy and productivity for multiple population groups, and presents opportunity for efforts and initiatives to improve the quality of life and health for all. The *Healthy People 2010 Midcourse Review* executive summary, available in the Community Resources for Practice at the end of the chapter, provides additional details and future directions for national health promotions and disease prevention efforts.

Specific examples of focus areas that require continued efforts to improve the health of the nation are evidenced in the summary of progress related to two of the focus areas: (1) physical activity and fitness and (2) nutrition and overweight.

In the focus area of physical activity, none of the objectives met their target, but several objectives for adults and adolescents moved toward the target. For the focus area nutrition and overweight, again, no objectives met or exceeded their targets. Some measures for overweight adults and children actually moved away from their targets. Lack of progress toward goals requires action. An example of cooperative efforts between federal and state and local groups related to these two goals can be found in the *HealthierUS* initiative and the *Steps to a Healthier US Initiative* (USDHHS, 2007), both discussed later in this chapter and available in the Community Resources for Practice.

Funding for prevention efforts such as those mentioned previously is meant to help decrease the cost of chronic disease such as cardiovascular disease, which is directly related to obesity and lack of physical activity. Estimated costs for cardiovascular disease and stroke in 2005 were $394 billion and the estimated health costs attributed to obesity in 2003 were $75 billion. Notable also are the hospital costs for overweight

children and adolescents, which have more than tripled over the past 2 decades (Centers for Disease Control and Prevention [CDC], 2007). These data highlight the importance of health-promotion programs and the need for individual and community commitment to health-promoting lifestyle changes.

Health promotion is a major goal of community/public health nursing practice. Community/public health nurses facilitate health in the population through direct nursing interventions for health promotion and disease prevention with individuals, families, groups, and populations. The American Nurses Association (ANA, 1996) position statement on health promotion and disease prevention suggests specific nursing activities to influence comprehensive health-promotion services (Box 18-1).

In this chapter, the concept of health is explored in depth, and major influences on health are examined. Theoretical models are presented that attempt to explain health-related behaviors. National policies related to health promotion and risk reduction are reviewed, and types of health-promotion and risk-reduction/health-protection programs are examined. Finally, the responsibilities of the community/public health nurse in facilitating health promotion are explored using the nursing process.

MEANING OF HEALTH

The concept of health has been defined in a variety of ways. Historically, health and illness were viewed as extremes on a continuum, with the absence of clinically recognizable disease being equated with the presence of health. In 1947 the World Health Organization defined health in terms of total well-being and discouraged the conceptualization of health as simply the absence of disease. In 1995 the World Health Organization launched a process known as "Health For All," which is aimed at preparing countries to meet the challenges of the twenty-first

---

BOX 18-1   Nursing's Role in Prevention

The American Nurses Association supports efforts to do the following:

- Increase nurses' knowledge and skill in providing preventive services.
- Encourage partnerships with consumers and other disciplines to identify needs, set priorities, develop strategies, and evaluate progress in promoting health.
- Support health care legislation that holds health insurance plans accountable for preventive care.
- Become involved in research to evaluate the extent to which specific preventive interventions at the individual, family, group, and community levels improve health; affect access, use, cost, and desired outcomes; and prevent disease, injury, or disability.
- Encourage using multidisciplinary efforts to call consumers' attention to health-promoting behaviors and environments and developing community-focused primary prevention models for care.
- Influence local and national economic and political options toward reconceptualizing health care in preventive and health-promoting models.
- Continue to advance nursing's concern that prevention and health promotion be central to reformed health care.
- Educate the public to promote the health of the population through a broader definition of health and its relationship to behavior.

Reprinted with permission from American Nurses Association. *American Nurses Association position statement on health promotion and disease prevention.* Copyright 1995 by American Nurses Association, Silver Springs, MD.

century and emphasizes the need to see health as central to human development and societal growth. In the United States, an initiative from the USDHHS, known as *Steps to a Healthier US Initiative* was launched in 2003 to improve the lives of Americans through community-based chronic disease-prevention programs. Special emphasis is devoted to diabetes mellitus, obesity, and asthma. Recent updates to the *Steps* initiative include interactive health risk appraisals, practical consumer information for multiple population groups, and user-friendly links to other reliable health information websites.

More contemporary definitions of health have emphasized the relationship between health and wellness and health promotion. Although health may be viewed as a static state of being at any given point in time, wellness is the process of moving toward integrating human functioning and maximizing human potential. **Health promotion** is the process of helping people enhance their well-being and maximize their human potential. The focus of health promotion is on changing patterns of behavior to promote health rather than simply to avoid illness. The goal of health promotion is to enable people to exercise control over their well-being and ultimately improve their health. Health promotion involves focusing on persons and populations as a whole and not solely on people who are at risk for specific diseases. Health promotion combines education, organizational involvement, economics, and political influences to bring about changes in behaviors of individuals and groups related to improved health and well-being (O'Donnell, 1986). The terms wellness and health promotion are frequently used interchangeably, with both terms having elements of physical, mental, and social well-being for both the individual and the community.

INFLUENCES ON HEALTH

Many factors, including lifestyle, genetics, and the environment, influence health. *Lifestyle* refers to the way people live their lives and involves patterns of working, playing, eating, sleeping, and communicating. A healthy lifestyle is easier to maintain when healthful patterns of behavior are learned early in life. Therefore the family plays a critical role in developing health beliefs and behaviors, such as exercise patterns, sound nutritional practices, regular use of seat belts, avoidance of harmful substances (e.g., tobacco, alcohol, drugs), stress management, and routine medical and dental evaluations.

BIOLOGIC INFLUENCES

Genetic endowment influences susceptibility to illness. Familial tendencies toward diseases such as diabetes and heart disease are well established. However, illnesses related to genetics may also be influenced by cultural and environmental factors. Similarly, genetic features such as height and weight may be environmentally influenced. Thus, because many of these factors exist or operate simultaneously, determining the relative influence of genetics and the environment on the risk of developing disease is often difficult.

ENVIRONMENTAL INFLUENCES

Environmental influences also contribute to or detract from the ability of people to develop to their optimal potential. When examining environmental influences on health, the physical and sociocultural environments must be considered. Factors in

the *physical* environment that influence health include weather and climatic conditions, noise, light, air, food, water, and exposure to toxic substances. According to *Healthy People 2010,* an estimated 25% of preventable illnesses worldwide can be attributed to poor environmental quality (see Chapter 9).

Factors in the *sociocultural* environment that influence health include the historic era in which one lives, values of family and significant others, social institutions (e.g., governments, schools, faith communities), socioeconomic class, occupation, and social roles that encourage or diminish the importance of preventive health practices. For example, an industrial worker may be exposed to toxic or carcinogenic substances that render him susceptible to different types of illness. In addition, health resources may be available only in more affluent communities, which diminish access to services by persons of lower socioeconomic status. In the United States, higher education and higher socioeconomic class are associated with greater participation in health-promotion activities (see Chapter 10).

The *health care system* is another important aspect of the environment that must be considered when determining the health potential of a society. Health care systems focus (in varying degrees) on prevention, cure, and rehabilitation in an effort to improve the health of society. Examination of the *Healthy People 2010* leading health indicator "Access to Care" reveals that a strong predictor of access to care includes having health insurance, a higher income level, and a regular primary care provider or other source of ongoing health care. People with health insurance are more likely to have appropriate preventive health care, such as a Papanicolaou (Pap) test, immunizations, or early prenatal care. The target for *Healthy People 2010* is for 100% of persons under age 65 to have health care coverage, and for 90% of all persons to have a specific source of ongoing primary care (USDHHS, 2000). *The Healthy People 2010 Midcourse Review* indicates that there has been no change in the percent of persons with health insurance. However, community health center programs such as those funded by the federal Health Resources and Services Administration (HRSA) have produced movement toward the target for all age groups to have an ongoing source of care and reduced difficulties and delays in accessing health care. A lack of health care and primary preventive services has a tremendous impact on the health of a society (see Chapter 21). For this reason, current emphasis is on creating public and private partnerships to bridge the gap in service availability.

Health services may be directed toward primary, secondary, or tertiary levels of prevention. *Primary prevention* is aimed at preventing the onset of disease or disability by reducing risks to health, decreasing vulnerability to illness, and promoting health and well-being. *Secondary prevention* is aimed at diagnosis and treatment of illness at an early stage, thereby halting further progression of disease and assisting persons to return to normal functioning. Secondary prevention includes case finding and screening of high-risk groups for the presence of disease. *Tertiary prevention* focuses on the restoration of optimal functioning once a condition becomes irreversible by limiting the extent of disability that may occur and by assisting clients to function at an optimal level within the constraints of their existing disabilities. The focus of this chapter is on primary prevention to promote health and prevent illness in an individual, family, or community. Chapter 7 provides additional detail on levels of prevention.

NATIONAL POLICY

Health promotion is a social project, not solely a medical enterprise. Societies have a political responsibility to strengthen the link between health and social well-being. An integration of government, major interest groups (environmental, industrial, medical, labor, educational), and community forces is needed to establish and maintain public policy and community action that promotes the health of individuals, families, and communities in society. The ability of the health care system to engage in health promotion is often determined by national legislation and policies that provide economic and political support for health-promotion services in the community.

FOCUS ON HEALTH PROMOTION

Healthy People, the first U.S. Surgeon General's report on health promotion and disease prevention, was instrumental in identifying major health problems of the nation and in setting national goals for reducing death and disability. The central message of this report was that the health of the nation can be improved by individual and collective action in public and private sectors and by promoting a safe, healthy environment for all Americans (U.S. Department of Health, Education, and Welfare, 1979).

In 1980 the USDHHS published a second document entitled *Promoting Health/Preventing Disease: Objectives for the Nation.* This document set forth specific objectives for meeting the national health care priorities established in the Surgeon General's report. Subsequent reports leading up to the most current publication, *Healthy People 2010 Midcourse Review,* included priorities such as reduction in hypertension, decrease in chronic disease such as cardiovascular disease and diabetes, increase in immunizations, reduction in sexually transmitted diseases, improved access to preventive health services, accident prevention, and reduction in smoking and alcohol and drug abuse. The *Healthy People* reports and objectives are designed to improve the health of the nation through a management-by-objective planning process.

Healthy People 2010 builds on the accomplishments of previous decades and includes specific health objectives for the year 2010 (USDHHS, 2000). These 2 overall goals are supported by 467 objectives, each of which includes a statement of intent, a baseline value, and a target to be achieved. The objectives are organized into 28 focus areas. Data are collected and reported within the framework of 10 leading health indicators and can be accessed on the Internet at the website for the National Center for Health Statistics DATA2010 Database (National Center for Health Statistics, 2007). (See the Community Resources for Practice box at the end of this chapter for access to this site through the book's website.) New to the 2010 document are focus areas that include disability, chronic diseases, people with low income, and public health infrastructure. *Healthy People 2010* objectives identify target populations and activities for health promotion, health protection, clinical preventive services, and priorities for system-wide improvements in surveillance and data systems. The *Healthy People 2010* box presents objectives targeting selected health-promotion activities.

■ HEALTHY PEOPLE 2010 ■
Sample Objectives for Selected Health-Promotion Activities

Physical Activities and Fitness

1. Reduce the proportion of adults who engage in no leisure time physical activity. (Baseline 2000: 40%. Target: 20%. **Midcourse review: 15% of targeted change achieved.**)

2. Increase the proportion of adults who engage in vigorous physical activity that promotes development and maintenance of cardiorespiratory fitness 3 or more days per week for 20 minutes per occasion. (Baseline 1997: 23%. Target: 30%. **Midcourse review: 6% of targeted change achieved.**)

3. Increase the proportion of adolescents who engage in moderate physical activity for at least 30 minutes on 5 or more of the previous 7 days. (Baseline 1999: 27%. Target: 35%. **Midcourse review: moved away from the target and decreased from the baseline to 25% in 2003.**)

4. Increase to at least 75% the proportion of work sites offering employer-sponsored physical activity and fitness programs. (Baseline 1999: 46% of work sites offered physical activity or fitness programs [or both] at the work site or through health plans. **Midcourse review: trend data not available but alternate data sources identified; trends expected by the end of the decade.**)

5. Increase the proportion of physicians and dentists who routinely assess and counsel their clients about tobacco use cessation, physical activity practices, and cancer screening. (Baseline 1995: for physical activity 22%. Target: 85%. **Midcourse review: no data available on counseling.**)

Nutrition

1. Increase the proportion of adults who are at a healthy weight. (Baseline 1994: 42% of all people age 20 or older were at a healthy weight [body mass index ≥18.5 and <25]. Target: 60%. **Midcourse review: 50% movement away from target. Survey period 1999-2002, 33% of adults were at a healthy weight.**)

2. Reduce the proportion of children and adolescents who are overweight or obese. (Baseline 1994: children 6 to 11 years, 11%; adolescents 12 to 19 years, 11%. Target: children 6 to 11 years, 5%; adolescents 12 to 19 years, 5%. **Midcourse review: increase in number of overweight and obese children from 11% to 16%, representing an 83% move away from the target.**)

3. Reduce the proportion of adults who are obese. (Baseline 1994: 23%. Target: 15%. **Midcourse review: movement away from target; 2002 survey, 33% of adults are obese.**)

4. Increase the proportion of people ages 2 and older who meet the dietary recommendations for calcium. (Baseline 1994: 46% of people ages 2 and older. Target: 75%. **Midcourse review: data not available but expected by the end of the decade.**)

Continued

■ HEALTHY PEOPLE 2010 ■
Sample Objectives for Selected Health-Promotion Activities—cont'd

Nutrition—cont'd

5. Reduce the proportion of adults with osteoporosis. (Baseline 1994: 10%. Target: 8%. **Midcourse review: 88% movement away from the target; increase of baseline to 33% in 2002.**)

6. Reduce iron deficiency among young children and women of childbearing age. (Baseline 1994: children 1 to 2 years, 9%; 3 to 4 years, 4%; nonpregnant women 12 to 49, 11%. Target: children 1 to 2 years, 5%; 3 to 4 years, 1%; nonpregnant women, 7%. **Midcourse review: data not available on iron deficiency in children. Movement away from the target for nonpregnant women. Data expected to be available for final review.**)

7. Increase the proportion of pregnancies begun with an optimum folic acid level (defined as consumption of at least 400 mcg of folic acid each day from fortified foods or dietary supplements by nonpregnant women ages 15 to 44). (Baseline 1994: 21%. Target: 80%. **Midcourse review: data not available but expected for final review.**)

Tobacco

1. Reduce tobacco use by adults. (Baseline 1998: cigarette smoking: 24%, target: 12%; spit tobacco: 2.6%, target: 0.4%; cigars: 2.5%, target: 1.2%. **Midcourse review: movement toward target for reduction in all forms of tobacco use. Cigarette smoking current rate 21%, a 25% movement toward the target. Spit tobacco and cigar use also moved toward target 10% and 17%, respectively.**)

2. Increase the average age of first use of tobacco products by adolescents and young adults. (Baseline 1997: adolescents ages 12 to 17, 12 years at first use. Target: 14 years. Young adults ages 18 to 25, 15 years at first use. Target: 17 years. **Midcourse review: data not available for first use.**)

3. Reduce tobacco use by adolescents (students in grades 9 through 12). (**Midcourse review: general movement toward goal. Overall 68% achievement of targeted change.**)

Tobacco Product	1999 Baseline	2020 Goal	Midcourse Review Data
Any product (previous month)	40%	21%	Not available
Cigarettes (previous month)	35%	16%	22%
Spit tobacco (previous month)	8%	1%	7%
Cigars (previous month)	18%	8%	15%

4. Increase smoke-free and tobacco-free environments in schools, including all school facilities, property, vehicles, and school events. (Baseline 1994: 37% of middle, junior high, and senior high schools were smoke and tobacco free. Target: 100%. **Midcourse review: 45% of schools are smoke free, movement toward target.**)

5. Eliminate laws that preempt stronger tobacco control laws. (Baseline 1998: 30 states had preemptive tobacco control laws in the areas of clean indoor air, minors' access laws, or marketing. Target: 100%. **Midcourse review: movement toward target for seven measurable areas including public and private workplace, restaurants, daycare centers, and public transportation.**)

6. Reduce the proportion of children who are regularly exposed to tobacco smoke at home. (Baseline 1994: 27% of children ages 6 years and under lived in a household in which someone smoked inside the house at least 4 days per week. Target: 10%. **Midcourse review: data not available.**)

7. Increase insurance coverage of evidence-based treatment for nicotine dependency. (Baseline 1998: managed care organizations with coverage: 75%. Target: 100%. Medicaid programs: 24%. Target: 51%. **Midcourse review: data not available.**)

Data from U.S. Department of Health and Human Services. (2000). *Healthy People 2010: Understanding and improving health and objectives for improving health* (2nd ed.). Washington, DC: U.S. Government Printing Office; and U.S. Department of Health and Human Services. (2006). *Healthy People 2010: Midcourse review.* Accessed July 31, 2007, at *http://www.healthypeople.gov/data/midcourse/.*

NATIONAL HEALTH CARE SURVEYS

Numerous federal resources are available to obtain information on health care statistics and health surveys. The most comprehensive collection of data that relates to *Healthy People 2010* is DATA2010. The site is easily accessed through CDC Wonder, an interactive internet system that provides access to many statistical health reports, guidelines, and databases. The surveys and data reported on this website include data from the National Center for Health Statistics (NCHS), the nation's primary health statistics site, and data from other surveys including the National Health and Nutrition Examination Survey (NHANES) and the National Health Care Survey (NHCS), which includes data from a group of surveys, including information about health care services and characteristics of the clients served and other national vital statistics, including morbidity and mortality data (see Chapter 7). Additionally, the Centers for Disease Control and Prevention (CDC) provides statistical data on chronic health problems (e.g., cardiovascular health) and preventable problems (e.g., tobacco-related disease). (See Community Resources for Practice at the end of this chapter for access to this website.) Most notable in the chronic disease overview on this website is information related to the costs of chronic disease and the cost-effectiveness of prevention. The U.S. Public Health Service Office of Disease Prevention and Health Promotion (ODPHP) coordinates the efforts of public and private sectors to reduce the risks of disease and promote the nation's health. This office publishes general public information, health policy papers, and conference proceedings. The best way to access ODPHP is via the Internet (the Community Resources for Practice box explains how to access this site). These government reports represent a national trend toward making prevention of disease and promotion of health higher health care priorities. Federal government initiatives have stressed health care cost containment, improved quality of care, and improved access to care.

HEALTH MODELS

Biologic, environmental, and sociocultural factors can influence health status. These multiple influences on health ultimately determine the type and extent of personal health behaviors. A variety of conceptual models have been proposed in an attempt to describe, explain, or predict preventive health behaviors.

HEALTH-BELIEF MODEL

The **health-belief model,** which has been widely used to explain wellness and illness behaviors, was created in the 1950s and has since been revised and tested extensively (Becker, 1974; Becker et al., 1977; Hochbaum, 1956; Rosenstock, 1974). Proponents of the health-belief model contend that individuals will take action to avoid disease states. Actions are motivated by (1) the sense of personal *susceptibility* to a disease, (2) the perceived *severity* of a disease, (3) the perceived *benefits* of preventive health behaviors, and (4) the perceived *barriers* to taking actions to prevent a disease. Potential barriers include fear, pain, cost, inconvenience, and embarrassment (Rosenstock, 1974).

The client's perception of health status and the value placed on taking preventive action may also be affected by *demographic* variables (e.g., age, gender, race, ethnicity), *sociopsychologic* variables (e.g., social class, peer pressure, attitude toward medical authorities), and *structural* variables (e.g., personal experience with disease, knowledge of disease). *Internal cues* (e.g., detecting a breast lump) or *external cues* (e.g., advice from significant others, exposure to a media campaign) can also serve to motivate healthful behaviors (Figure 18-1).

Empirical research demonstrates that the attitude and belief dimensions of the health-belief model do predict individuals' health-related behavior. When an illness or injury is perceived to be serious and barriers are low, individuals are more likely to seek medical care and follow the suggested treatment. In addition, individuals are more likely to engage in preventive health behavior when barriers to care are low and when people perceive that they are susceptible to an illness or injury (Janz & Becker, 1984). These two components of the model, *perceived barriers* and *perceived susceptibility,* appear to be the most important variables for health-promotion intervention. Additional study of the model led to a proposal to include

self-efficacy in the health-belief model as a way to help explain health-protective behaviors (Rosenstock et al., 1988).

A study of older adults (Easom, 2003) supports the concept that limited self-efficacy can be seen as a barrier to participating in health-promotion activities. The goal of the project was to increase older adult participation in health-promotion activities, such as following an exercise program and eliminating unhealthy behaviors. The older adults who perceived themselves as unable or incapable of participating in physical activities because of various disabilities related to aging may have the barrier of a lowered sense of self-efficacy. Another barrier identified was the loss of satisfaction when giving up an unhealthy habit, such as smoking. Additional barriers related to self-efficacy for these older adults include lack of spousal or family support, lack of willpower, powerless attitude about disease progression, and fear of overexertion. Another recent study of long-term married couples identified the importance of spousal support and self-efficacy as a predictor of participation in health-promotion behaviors (Padula & Sullivan, 2006). Implications for nursing practice include the importance of providing additional verbal encouragement to decrease fear and anxiety about performing certain tasks and including the spouse in planning and implementation of the health-promotion intervention. Other interventions to eliminate barriers include education, exposure to role models and others who have been successful in accomplishing health behaviors, and decreasing unpleasant situations, such as pain from chronic disease.

In addition to helping clients decrease barriers to health promotion, nurses can also use the health-belief model to identify the need for specific programs for at-risk groups. Two recent studies related to nursing interventions to reduce the risk of osteoporosis included the importance of health beliefs as a component of the nursing intervention (Sadler & Huff, 2007; Sedlak

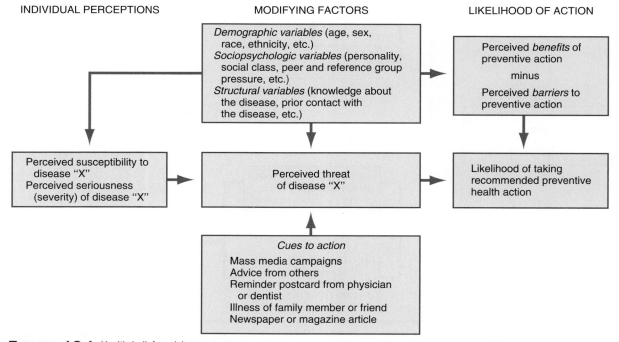

FIGURE 18-1 Health-belief model. (From Becker, M. [1974]. *The health belief model and personal health behavior.* Thorofare, NJ: Charles B. Slack.)

et al., 2005). In both studies, the intervention to reduce perceived barriers to calcium intake and exercise was an educational intervention that incorporated cultural differences and health beliefs as a method to change behavior to reduce osteoporosis risk. The importance of the nursing responsibility to address health beliefs is emphasized as a health-protecting behavior.

The health-belief model is driven more by health-protecting behaviors than it is health-promoting behaviors. **Health-protecting behaviors** are those that protect people from problems that jeopardize their health and well-being such as in the osteoporosis examples previously provided. **Health-promoting behaviors** are those that improve health by fostering personal development or self-actualization. Immunizing the population against infectious diseases and reducing exposure to environmental health hazards are examples of health-protecting behaviors. Many health behaviors, such as managing dietary intake, exercise, and stress management, serve a dual function by being both health-promoting and health-protecting.

HEALTH-PROMOTION MODEL

Whereas the health-belief model may account for actions taken to prevent disease, Pender et al. (2006) propose a revised **health-promotion model** that attempts to account for behaviors that improve well-being and develop human potential, *health-promoting* behaviors. Pender and associates (2006) contend that health-promotion behaviors are determined by the following factors:

- Individual characteristics and experiences (including prior related behavior and personal factors characterized as biologic, psychologic, and sociocultural)
- Behavior-specific cognitions and affect (including perceived benefits and barriers to action, perceived self-efficacy, activity-related affect, interpersonal influences, and situational influences)
- Behavioral outcomes (including the commitment to a plan of action and immediate competing demands such as family or work commitments)

Pender's model represents a multitude of factors affecting health-promotion behavior, which is the end point, or outcome, of the health-promotion model (Figure 18-2).

A clinical example of the importance of eliminating barriers is examined in a study of healthy eating behaviors in women underserved by the health care system (Timmerman, 2007). In this population, the barriers to healthy eating included individual characteristics, experience, and culture. The barriers

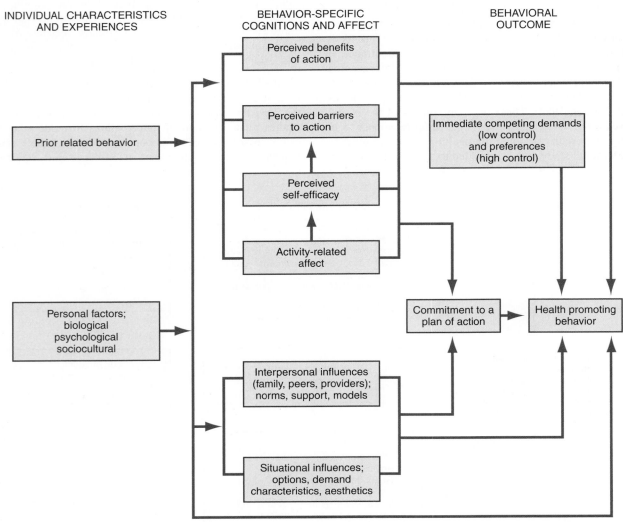

FIGURE 18-2 Pender's revised health-promotion model. (From Pender, N. J., Murdaugh, C., & Parsons, M. A. [2006]. *Health promotion in nursing practice* [5th ed.]. Upper Saddle River, NJ: Prentice-Hall Health, Inc.)

were internal, interpersonal, and environmental and were seen to overlap to impede healthy eating. Interventions to improve health-promoting behaviors included individualizing the interventions *(removal of internal barriers)* while working with the community *(removal of environmental barriers)* to develop a plan of action that is broad enough to be applicable to the larger population. Additional interventions included facilitating changes in public policy to eliminate barriers faced by underserved women (Timmerman, 2007).

PRIMARY HEALTH CARE MODEL

Another way to view health and its relationship to individuals is the **primary health care model** proposed by Shoultz and Hatcher (1997) (Figure 18-3). The focus of the model is health care for all members of the community, with a multisectoral approach. The model should not be confused with primary care or with personal health services, which address health care for individuals. Primary care services may be delivered in a community setting (e.g., clinic, school) but do not necessarily influence the health of the community. The primary health care model embodies the principles of community participation and a multisectoral approach with an emphasis on prevention. The six key elements of environment, health services, education and communication, politics, economics, and agriculture and nutrition surrounding the health of the community are interlinked, and each element has an impact on health. Important to note is that the delivery of personal health care to individuals is a component of health services. The model for primary health care provides a format for community/public health nurses to promote health and health education related to community influences and the environment. The model may also be adapted if necessary to add other sectors to the influences on health, such as the impact of spirituality on community health.

The models used to explain preventive health behaviors tend to be action oriented. People evaluate and respond to their perceived needs and subsequently act by taking preventive action or adopting health-promoting behaviors. Even so, because the models have as their end point a change in behavior, actual health outcomes or documented improvements in health are not directly addressed in the models presented.

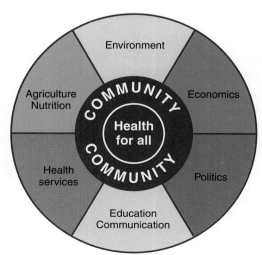

FIGURE 18-3 Primary health care model. (Copyright 1997 Hatcher, P. A., Shoultz, J., & Patrick, W. K. Used with permission.)

A woman believes that she is personally susceptible to developing breast cancer, owing to risk factors such as age and family history. She may realize that the disease is serious and appreciate the benefit of routine mammography and breast self-examination. In response to a media campaign in her community (external cue) or to palpating a breast lump (internal cue), she acts by seeking mammography screening. As a result of this behavior, the disease may be detected early and treated, and hopefully the woman will go on to live an active and healthy life. In this case, the theoretical model would need to take into account the possible health outcomes as a result of adopting preventive health behaviors.

Continuing work on theoretical models and their application to research is needed to better understand the relationship between changes in behavior and the actual effects of behavior modification on health status.

HEALTH-PROMOTION AND HEALTH-PROTECTION PROGRAMS

Many different types of programs have been implemented to reduce the risk of disease for individuals and groups in communities. *Health-promotion programs* attempt to increase the level of well-being and self-actualization of individuals and groups by promoting behaviors that expand the potential for health and personal development. The *goal* of health-promotion programming is to enable people to act positively in their environment by creating conditions that encourage and nurture health. *Health-protection,* also known as **risk reduction,** programs are aimed toward facilitating behaviors that enable people to react to threats to health through early identification and avoidance of risks (Pender et al., 2006). Thus health-protection programs are more reactive in their intent and are directed toward preventing illness by identifying, avoiding, and reducing risks to health or by detecting illness early, before the onset of symptoms. (See Chapters 19 and 9 for in-depth discussions on health protection and environmental influences.) The benefits of community approaches to prevention are summarized in Box 18-2.

The community/public health nurse develops, implements, and evaluates health-promotion and health-protection programs for individuals, families, and groups in schools, work sites, hospitals, faith communities, prisons, and community settings. When planning programs for wellness in the community, an important task is to develop partnerships with people who are most likely to be affected by the program and to promote a sense of cooperation, collaboration, and teamwork among groups. The development of partnerships is especially important in the design of culturally sensitive and effective prevention materials, as well as problem-prevention campaigns or educational programs.

PROGRAMS FOR INDIVIDUALS

Health-promotion and health-protection programs may be successfully implemented for individuals in many settings. Individual health-promotion programs depend on an accurate assessment of individual needs and risks to health

BOX 18-2   Benefits of Community Prevention Programs

1. Opportunity to reach the masses and effect widespread changes in social norms
2. Increased public awareness of and commitment to health-promotion programming
3. Increased cost efficiency of group intervention compared with one-to-one contacts
4. Ability of the program to serve as an environmental cue, triggering healthful behaviors
5. Ability of the program to promote the development of an environment of social support for health promotion
6. Opportunity to evaluate the effectiveness of health-promotion programs and to generalize findings to a wide range of demographic characteristics
7. Enhanced approach toward promoting health in large populations
8. Additional resources for information exchange and social support for members of the target population

Data from Pender, N. J., et al. (2006). *Health promotion in nursing practice* (5th ed.). Upper Saddle River NJ, Prentice-Hall Health.

based on genetic, biologic, psychologic, social, cultural, environmental, developmental, and situational variables. **Clinical practice guidelines** are a useful blueprint for providing health-promotion and disease-prevention services to individuals in primary care and public health settings. The National Guideline Clearinghouse (NGC) is a publicly available database of evidence-based clinical practice guidelines and is available to Internet users. NGC is updated weekly and is a sponsored by the Agency for Healthcare Research and Quality (AHRQ) in partnership with the American Medical Association. The Internet site provides the opportunity to search for clinical guidelines by disease condition, treatments, and interventions or measures. For consumers the site includes links to patient education and resources. The clinical practice guidelines can also be accessed directly through the AHRQ website,

which also provides numerous links to consumer resources, patient safety information, information targeted for specific populations, and research findings. Table 18-1 provides community/public health nurses with some examples of clinical practice guidelines that can be researched from the National Guideline Clearinghouse (NGC) site.

PROGRAMS FOR FAMILIES

The community/public health nurse works with families to promote health and prevent disease. Families are often the basis for developing positive lifestyles because parents can encourage their children to practice healthy personal habits. Educating parents on home safety hazards, use of child safety seats, immunizations, and injury prevention can ensure a safer environment for children through parental intervention in hazard reduction and reinforcing lifelong health practices (Figure 18-4). Clinical practice guidelines also include counseling topics for parents, many of which are geared toward parents to help them promote health and safety in the home (see Table 18-1).

PROGRAMS FOR POPULATIONS IN COMMUNITIES

The community/public health nurse may also develop and implement programs that reach larger groups in the community. Major types of community health-promotion programs include school, workplace, faith community, hospital, senior center, and community-wide programs. These populations may be viewed as phenomenological communities or aggregates or target groups.

School-Based Health Promotion

School-based health-promotion programs can facilitate health-promotion behaviors by encouraging the development of health-promoting habits early in life that, in turn, foster long-term healthy lifestyle behaviors (Figure 18-5). Successful school health-promotion programs are based on an understanding of human behavior and developing partnerships with people who will be most affected by the program (e.g., students, families, peers, faculty and staff, affiliating

TABLE 18-1   Sample Clinical Practice Guidelines

Client Population	Target Disease	Health-Promotion Strategies (Screening/Counseling/Immunization)
All clients	Obesity	Measure height and weight periodically.
Children ages 3 to 4 years	Visual difficulties	Screen for amblyopla and strabismus.
All clients of 21 years of age	Hypertension	Measure blood pressure periodically.
Men ages 35 and older and women ages 45 and older	Lipid disorders	Either a fasting lipid profile or a nonfasting total cholesterol and hi-density lipoprotein (HDL) cholesterol.
Smoking parents with children in the house	Otitis media, allergies, asthma, etc.	Counsel regarding the harmful effects of smoking on children's health.
All tobacco users	Complications of tobacco use	Counsel to encourage tobacco cessation on a regular basis.
Girls and women ages 11 and older	Osteoporosis	Counsel to maintain adequate calcium intake.
Healthy infants ages 12 to 18 months	Varicella	Immunize using American Academy of Pediatrics recommendations.
Adults	Tetanus	Complete tetanus-diphtheria (Td) vaccine series if the subject has not received primary series. Boosters every 10 yr or at least at age 50.

Data from National Guideline Clearinghouse, (2007). Available online at *www.guideline.gov*.

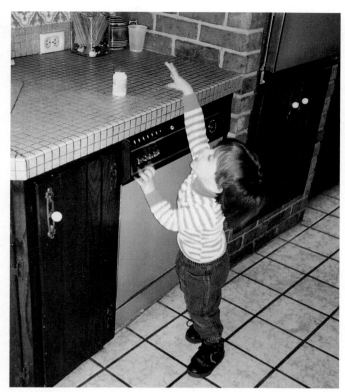

FIGURE 18-4 Health-promotion programs for families include teaching parents how to properly store medications and harmful chemicals so that they are not within the reach of young children. (From Hockenberry, M. J., Wilson, D., Winkelstein, M. L., et al. [2003]. *Wong's nursing care of infants and children* [7th ed.]. St. Louis: Mosby.)

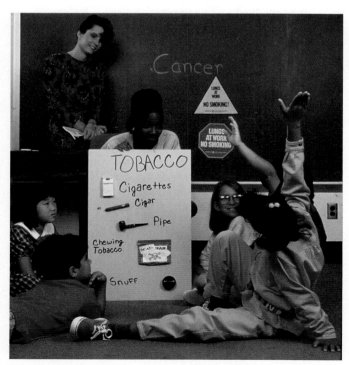

FIGURE 18-5 A school health-promotion program teaching about tobacco products and the harmful results of using them.

agencies). These programs contribute to overall community health-promotion efforts by developing a sense of individual and social responsibility for health, promoting an understanding of health and disease, reinforcing positive attitudes toward wellness, encouraging informed decision making in matters of health, and structuring the environment and social influences to support health-promotion behaviors (Pender et al., 2006).

Traditionally, school health programs included health-education curricula, health-promotion strategies, and the delivery of health services, including immunizations, physical health requirements, screening, and first aid. Currently, these dimensions have been expanded to include food services and nutrition, physical education, and guidance and counseling, as well as school psychology services. Chapter 30 provides an in-depth discussion of school health nursing.

Workplace Health Promotion

The workplace has become a major channel for health-promotion activities and, as such, has received national attention. One of the nation's objectives for the year 2010 is to provide employee health-promotion activities in at least 75% of workplaces with 50 or more employees (USDHHS, 2000). The 1999 baseline for this objective was 34% but has not been updated for the *Midcourse Review*. Another 2010 goal is to increase the number of employees who access employer-sponsored health-promotion programs to a target of 75%. With the 1994 baseline at 61%, at the time of the *Midcourse Review* this objective for employee participation has actually moved away from the target by 38% of the goal. A resource designed to increase health-promotion activities in the workplace is *Healthy Workforce 2010: An Essential Health Promotion Sourcebook for Employers, Large and Small* (Partnership for Prevention, 2001). The publication provides information on the advantages of work site health-promotion programs and strategies for developing and maintaining programs.

Numerous positive outcomes act as incentives for employer and employee participation in health-promotion activities. Incentives for employers include reduced rates of employee absenteeism because of improved health status, increased employee productivity, decreased use of medical insurance benefits and workers' compensation for illness and accidents, decreased employee turnover, decreased accidents, and decreased premature morbidity and mortality. Incentives for employee participation include promoting a safe work environment, improving access to services, providing a convenient service location, receiving company payment for services, and providing availability of services on company time. A review of research literature related to factors that influence employee participation in work site health-promotion programs returns to the concepts previously discussed in the health-promotion model (Kaewthummanukul & Brown, 2006). This review cites self-efficacy and perceived benefits as the strongest predictors of employee participation. For the occupational health nurse, implications of the review of literature combined with the data from the *Healthy People 2010 Midcourse Review* should guide clinical practice to create programs that address employee perception of self-efficacy and benefits of health-promotion activities.

Health-Promotion Programs in Faith Communities

Faith communities are ideal locations for reaching groups with health-promotion programs. Faith communities emphasize the spiritual dimension of health. When combined with programs that promote physical and mental health, faith communities truly serve to promote the total spectrum of health and well-being. According to the standards of faith community nursing practice (American Nurses Association & Health Ministries Association, 2005), **faith community nursing** (formerly called **parish nursing**) intentionally focuses on the care of the spirit as part of the process of promoting holistic health and preventing illness in a faith community.

In a review of the literature, Peterson and colleagues (2002) identify seven key elements for successful church-based health-promotion programs: partnerships, positive health values, availability of services, access to facilities, community-focused intervention, health-behavior change, and supportive relationships. Faith community nurses are also seen as health advocates performing roles such as helping to access care, assisting as a navigator in the health care system, and working with the faith group to acquire needed health services in the community (Peterson, 2007). Activities common to faith community nurses include organizing health fairs, making home visits, conducting blood pressure screening clinics, and providing counseling and referral services.

Hospital-Based Health-Promotion Programs

Hospital-based health-promotion programs are now focused on a variety of populations. Health-promotion and risk-reduction programs are offered not only to hospital employees and clients, but also to various groups in the community. Partnerships between hospitals and businesses, schools, faith communities, senior centers, and community organizations not only have facilitated a large increase in providing health-promotion services to the community, but also have served as a financial incentive for hospitals as they improve their ability to attract new physicians, clients, and the media.

Health Promotion in Geopolitical Communities

Community-wide health-promotion and disease-prevention programs use health care, educational, recreational, social, and governmental resources to develop and implement programs that enhance the well-being of large population groups. Community-centered programs have been credited with enhancing opportunities for social support and information exchange in the community and for exerting a significant impact on social policy. Goals for health promotion in geopolitical communities include decreasing morbidity and mortality in the community, achieving widespread community health protection, promoting cost-effective community-wide health promotion, and promoting and sustaining health-promotion efforts in the organizational network of the community. Interventions in these large-scale health-promotion projects may include using mass media and community health-education programs to increase public awareness of health risks and prevention practices, counseling, lifestyle assessments, faith community and social group involvement, training of health professionals, and reorganization of public services to target high-risk populations. One such example of a community-wide project is presented as an interactive internet guide to quitting smoking by the American Cancer Society (2007) titled *American Cancer Society Guide to Quitting Smoking.* Tools to help plan a quit date, telephone numbers and ideas for support, quizzes, on-line registration, and general information and statistics on smoking and cancer are available. This information is presented in the steps of the nursing process for planning a community-wide intervention in Box 18-3. Similar smoking cessation information and interactive materials with video presentation of the Surgeon General's report on the effects of smoking on various organs has also been developed on the Centers for Disease Control and Prevention (CDC) website. The CDC website also includes program materials for health care providers.

Another large-scale community-wide project that reaches a large and diverse population group is *WISEWOMAN: Well-Integrated Screening and Evaluation for Women Across the Nation: A Crosscutting Program to Improve the Health of Uninsured Women.* The project is part of the Centers for Disease Control and Prevention, Division for Heart Disease and Stroke Prevention (CDC, Division for Heart Disease and Stroke Prevention, 2007; *http://www.cdc.gov/wisewoman*). The mission of the project is to provide low-income and underinsured or uninsured women of all races and ethnic groups knowledge and skills to improve their health through lifestyle modification with the ultimate goal of reducing cardiovascular and chronic disease. The site provides health information, interactive health-risk assessments, and personal success stories designed to empower women to stop smoking, increase physical activity, achieve a healthy weight, and manage stress. The site is geared toward multicultural groups such as African Americans, Latinos, Native Americans, and others and includes recipes and prevention information in numerous languages. The site also includes links to other reliable health information resources.

HEALTH PROMOTION AND NURSING PRACTICE

The community/public health nurse uses the nursing process to assist people and groups to become more-self directed and motivated in taking actions that promote and maintain health and prevent disease. The community/public health nurse can be seen as an advocate for health, assisting individuals and groups in collaborative efforts to assess their level of wellness and access health resources. The community/public health nurse also provides health education and options for health care and helps clients establish goals for lifestyle changes.

APPRAISAL AND ASSESSMENT

The first step of the nursing process is assessment. The community/public health nurse must assess the client's (individual, group, aggregate, or population) health care needs and health-promotion behaviors to determine the major health risks that can potentially affect the client's overall health and well-being. In assessing needs, the community/public health nurse must also examine social, environmental, and cultural influences on health behaviors of families and communities.

A comprehensive health-promotion and health-protection assessment of an individual should include a complete health history and periodic routine health maintenance examinations. Physical fitness evaluations and nutrition assessments provide valuable data to assess overall health status. Health-risk appraisals may be used to collect data on individual health risks and health behaviors and to determine an individual's risk of developing certain illnesses over his or her lifetime.

Box 18-3   Community-Wide Smoking Cessation: Using the Nursing Process to Plan a Community-Wide Intervention

Assessment of the Problem
- An estimated 48 million people in the United States continue to smoke. Tobacco use is a serious risk for health problems and early death caused by lung disease, health disease, and cancers, including cancer of the mouth, bladder, kidney, cervix, and others.
- Smoking in the home is hazardous to children and is related to otitis media, allergies, and asthma.
- Women who smoke while pregnant risk having low-birth-weight babies or miscarriage.

Plan for Community Participation
- Form partnerships and establish support from schools, work sites, faith communities, and hospitals.
- Develop or adopt public-education campaigns (e.g., pubic service announcements, "Smoke-Out" dates) and public visual-media opportunities (e.g., advertisements in newspapers, on billboards, or on public transportation).
- Identify funding sources.
- Identify and publicize possible incentives for individuals and businesses to become involved, such as reduced insurance premiums or healthier employees with decreased absentee rates.
- Gather resources and materials.

Implement Programs for Individuals and Groups
Smoking cessation suggestions—four important factors:
1. Make the decision to quit.
2. Set a quit date and choose a quit plan.
   - Get rid of all cigarettes, lighters, and ashtrays.
   - Keep active.
   - Drink plenty of water.
   - Use nicotine replacement if that is your choice.
   - Avoid high-risk activities or situations in which the urge to smoke is strong.
3. Deal with withdrawal.
   - Use alternatives such as gum or hard candy, vegetables, or sunflower seeds.
   - Relax and perform deep-breathing exercises.
   - Delay the urge to light up.
4. Maintain or stay smoke free.
   - Renew and review your reasons for quitting.
   - Remind yourself that there is no such thing as just one cigarette.

Identify Benefits and Barriers
Benefits
- Damage to appearance, including stained teeth, bad breath, wrinkled skin, and yellowed fingernails, is reduced.
- Food tastes better, and the sense of smell returns.
- Ordinary activity no longer leaves you short of breath.
- Social acceptance is increased.
- Money spent on tobacco is saved.

Barriers
- Nicotine is an addictive drug, leaving the smoker physically and psychologically dependent.
- Withdrawal symptoms such as depression, irritability, headache, or increased appetite are increased.
- Not all health care providers counsel smokers on quitting, which provides the message that it is "OK" to smoke.

Evaluate the Success of Your Community-Wide Program
- Has a change occurred in policies about smoking in public places, such as restaurants?
- Are employees participating in workplace smoking-cessation programs? Are community members attending smoking-cessation group activities?
- Do the health care providers in your area counsel smokers on the benefits of stopping at every clinical visit?

From American Cancer Society. (2007). *American Cancer Society guide to quitting smoking*. Accessed at *www.cancer.org*.

Health-Risk Appraisal

The **health-risk appraisal** (HRA) (also termed the *health-hazard appraisal*) is a method for estimating an individual's health threats because of demographic, behavioral, and personal characteristics (Pender et al., 2006). Personal risk profiles are developed based on information provided by the client and information from laboratory data or other assessments.

HRAs have both assessment and motivational purposes. One goal of the HRA is to collect and organize personal health data to provide an accurate, individualized assessment of risk factors that may lead to health promotion. A second major goal of the HRA is to stimulate the necessary behavioral changes that may reduce health risks. The assumption holds that each person, having his or her own set of risk factors, can be compared with others with similar factors to establish morbidity and mortality estimates. Also assumed is that, armed with this knowledge, the client will be motivated to change high-risk behaviors (Pender et al., 2006).

The HRA, when first developed in the early 1970s, focused on assessing risk for specific disease entities and was primarily intended for physician use. However, since that time, a significant number of HRA tools have been published that reflect broader interests, such as health attitudes, social supports, stressful life events, and coping strategies. In addition, special versions of HRAs have been developed for different age groups.

HRAs enable the community/public health nurse to individualize assessment of risks and to recommend behavior changes that are compatible with a healthier lifestyle. In addition, HRAs can be administered to large groups and can be generated and processed by computers.

Appraisals usually begin with a questionnaire that identifies factors contributing most directly to individual risk. HRA instruments include questions regarding age, gender, ethnic background, personal and family history of disease, and lifestyle factors (e.g., smoking, drinking, exercise, driving practices, seat belt use, and job stress). Physical measures such as blood pressure and weight may be assessed, and blood tests may be obtained. In addition, risk factors for diseases that are amenable to early detection efforts, such as breast and colon cancer, are noted (see Chapter 19).

Personal data are compared with mortality data from cohort groups who share similar characteristics. Risk factors are weighted to determine the magnitude of the risks using

(1) statistical formulas based on professional, medical, or actuarial judgment; (2) average risks for the population; and (3) established epidemiologic and mathematic rules and assumptions. The magnitude of these risks is then shared with the client.

An example of an HRA, which includes recommendations on improvements to health, is available through the website of the U.S. Department of Health and Human Services, ODPHP, and is known as *Healthfinder* (USDHHS, ODPHP, 2007; *http://www. healthfinder.gov*). Navigation on the prevention and wellness part of the *Healthfinder* site leads to the Health Risk Appraisal link and the *Your Disease Risk Page* developed by the Harvard School of Public Health *(http://www.yourdiseaserisk.harvard.edu)*. The risk assessment identifies the five most important diseases in the United States, calculates personal risk of disease, and identifies prevention activities to reduce risk. The site is interactive and is based on personal health history and statistical data.

Community/public health nurses have an ethical responsibility to provide feedback, education, and appropriate follow-up for identified risks. The follow-up must be planned into community health-promotion programs that use HRA instruments. Individuals may be notified in writing or through follow-up counseling sessions on the findings of their HRAs. Recommendations for lifestyle changes or for seeking follow-up medical evaluation should be explained to each participant.

Stress-Risk Assessment
The Social Readjustment Rating Scale developed by Holmes and Rahe (1967) is a classic well-known tool used to assess the stressful effects of significant life events on persons. The scale is based on the assumption that stressful events may precipitate illness or have an additive effect in contributing to illness. The scale has also been used to identify links between stressful life events during the previous year and the development of illness; high scores on the tool have been found to predict the occurrence of illness. Stressful life events require a significant lifestyle adaptation or coping behavior on the part of the individual.

Although *The Social Readjustment Rating Scale* was originally developed for adults, in 1972, Coddington developed several stress measurement tools for use with children of various ages. An interesting note is that many of the life events for children are similar to those for the adult. Nurses working with families to teach coping skills need to recognize the impact of family events on the children. Both the Holmes and Rahe "Social Readjustment Rating Scale for Adults" and the Coddington "Life Change Unit Values for Children" are available on the book's website as **Website Resources 18A** and **18B.**

The nurse should critically analyze the social readjustment scale to determine how to interpret results for the client. Some cultural and community values might affect the meaning of the value of the life change event. For example, in some communities, an unwed pregnancy or fathering an unwed pregnancy will necessitate more life adjustments than it would in other communities. Additionally, the scale does not account for factors that mediate the degree of distress a person experiences in a stressful situation. Factors such as receiving support or counseling to deal with a painful divorce or the death of a spouse may help individuals cope more effectively with a potentially devastating life experience.

In addition to the classic Holmes and Rahe scale, interactive risk assessments related to stress including work site stress,

stress as a result of a disaster, the stresses related to caregiving, and stress in children related to holidays can also be found on the previously mentioned healthfinder.gov website through the prevention and wellness links.

Lifestyle Assessments and Wellness Inventories
Lifestyle assessments and *wellness inventories* are wellness-focused appraisals that place greater emphasis on promoting health rather than identifying risk factors for specific diseases. Lifestyle assessments focus on daily patterns of behavior that affect health and over which the individual has some control. Through the AHRQ Internet site and the *putting prevention into practice* area of the website, individuals can access a lifestyle assessment for men or women called *Stay Healthy at Any Age* (AHRQ, 2007). The assessment includes information on recommended screening tests, immunizations, and healthy lifestyle choices such as maintaining a healthy weight and increasing physical activity *(http://www.ahrq.gov/clinic/ppipix.htm)*.

Other lifestyle assessments may take a more focused approach to specific problems. For example, The National Heart, Lung, and Blood Institute (NHLBI) sponsors another lifestyle assessment related to healthy weight. The program is called "Aim for a Healthy Weight" and encourages individuals to calculate their body mass index, obtain a waist circumference, and examine other lifestyle risk factors (National Institutes of Health, NHLBI, 2007). Assistance in menu planning and lifestyle changes is also provided. This lifestyle assessment can be accessed through the NHLBI website *(http://www.nhlbi.nih. gov/health/public/heart/obesity/lose_wt/index.htm)*.

DEVELOPING A HEALTH-PROMOTION PLAN OF CARE
After a comprehensive assessment of lifestyle, health behaviors, and specific risks to health, the community/public health nurse develops a health-promotion plan of care with clients in the community. A plan for health promotion and health protection should be targeted to specific clients. The health planning process should involve both the nurse and the client using the following steps (Pender et al., 2006):
- Summarization and review of the information collected in the assessment
- Identification and reinforcement of strengths
- Development of health goals and appropriate lifestyle change options
- Identification of desired health and behavior outcomes that would signify a successful outcome from the clients' perspective
- Design of a behavior change plan that takes into consideration the clients' preferences and current stage of change
- Creation of a reward system for reinforcement of behavior
- Review of environmental and interpersonal facilitators and barriers to behavior change
- Development of an implementation time frame
- Commitment to the proposed behavior change goals and the support needed to accomplish them

This process of care planning is appropriate for both individuals and populations. However, when planning care for populations, of particular importance is to develop partnerships with community members, achieve consensus on health goals that are appropriate to the community, and gain commitment from key community leaders in supporting health-promotion efforts (see Unit IV).

INTERVENTION STRATEGIES

The community/public health nurse should consider the following strategies when assisting individuals and communities in recognizing patterns and adaptation of healthy practices:

- Dissemination of health-related information to inform and educate
- Encouragement and enhancement of client self-efficacy through lifestyle modification
- Development of environments that are conducive to health and healing practices
- Use of partnerships in health promotion to strengthen social networks and support and influence policy

Information Dissemination

Information dissemination refers to mass communication of health-promotion information to the community in the most effective and efficient manner. Information may be disseminated by using mass media, billboards, brochures, posters, or exhibits; information is often disseminated through a health fair or exposition. A *health fair* is a community event offering health screenings, information, resources, and counseling and referral services in a location that is convenient and accessible to community members (see Chapter 19).

The goal of information-dissemination programs is to inform the community of ways to promote health and prevent disease. Information dissemination is a consciousness-raising activity that alerts the community to health damaging behaviors and attempts to motivate the community to adopt healthier lifestyles. The presentation format of the information must be appropriate for the intended recipients of the health message. In a recent study on health messages for adolescents designed to promote responsible sexual behaviors, it was found that mass media communication such as television, Internet, and computer-assisted instruction were all effective for increasing knowledge and changing attitudes (Delgado & Austin, 2007). Other examples of information-dissemination programs include posters and commercial announcements, articles in local newspapers, and billboards and bumper stickers such as those that encourage seat belt use. Although information-dissemination programs are a helpful approach to promoting health in the community, information alone is insufficient to effect large scale, community-wide behavioral change. For example, despite widespread dissemination of literature on the health risks of obesity, overweight and obesity continues to increase (see *Healthy People 2010* sample objectives and *Midcourse Review*).

Lifestyle Modification

Lifestyle modification is a more comprehensive approach to effecting changes in health-promotion behaviors. *Lifestyle-modification programs* encourage self-responsibility for health and represent the action phase of health behavior. Assisting clients in implementing lifestyle changes often necessitates frequent contacts between the health professional and the client so the health professional can serve as a change agent, suggesting alternative behaviors and referring the client to resources in the community to facilitate positive lifestyle changes. Also during these contacts, the community/public health nurse should assess the client's motivation and readiness to change behaviors to a more positive lifestyle. A useful model for assessment of the readiness to change is the **transtheoretical model of behavioral change** developed by Prochaska and DiClemente (1983). The model identified five stages of change, which can allow for tailoring of support and interventions based on the client's needs and stage of change (Table 18-2).

TABLE 18-2   Stages of Change: The Transtheoretical Model and Sample Client Behaviors and Nursing Interventions Related to Health-Promotion Goal of Increasing Physical Activity and Exercise

Stage of Change	Client Behavior	Typical Client Comment	Nursing Intervention to Assist Client to Next Stage
1. Precontemplation	Client has no interest in change and is comfortable with current behavior.	Client: "I don't like to exercise when I get home from work; I enjoy relaxing on the sofa."	Raise client awareness about personal risks and alternative behaviors; discuss success rates, not failure rates, of behavioral change.
2. Contemplation	Client is considering behavior change.	Client: "I might like to start exercising when the weather is warm in a few months."	Elicit and address decision-making; encourage client to attempt an alternative behavior; explore motivators and client's perspective of perceived costs and benefits; identify client's time line; focus on short-term possibilities; provide ongoing counseling.
3. Preparation	Client is planning to change behavior.	Client: "I intend to start walking three days per week to improve my physical appearance and reduce stress."	Reinforce new behavior; help client restructure environment and social group to reenforce new behavior; set realistic goals.
4. Action	Behavior change is initiated.	Client: "I bought walking shoes and walked for 20 minutes yesterday."	Help overcome setbacks; encourage client self-evaluation and monitoring; build in rewards.
5. Maintenance	Behavior change has been initiated and maintained for 6 months.	Client: "I have been walking since the Spring and my clothing fits better and I feel more energized. I seldom skip a day of walking."	Acknowledge that relapse occurs; extend goals; monitor progress.

Adapted from Croghan, E. (2005). Assessing motivation and readiness to alter lifestyle behavior. *Nursing Standard, 19*(31), 50-52; and data from Maibach, E., & Cotton, D. (1995). Moving people to behavioral change: A staged social cognitive approach to message design. In E. Maibach & R. L. Parrott (Eds.), *Designing health messages: Approaches from communication theory and public health practice* (pp. 41-64). Thousand Oaks, CA: Sage Publications.

Environmental Restructuring

Environmental restructuring is an approach that facilitates healthful lifestyles and creates environments that are conducive to information dissemination, health appraisal and assessment, and lifestyle modification. Environments are restructured to optimize the healthful conditions existing in the environment. Restructuring may also mean increasing the availability of healthful options in the community by providing greater opportunities and resources to engage in health-promoting behaviors (Pender et al., 2006).

The community/public health nurse can educate communities on potentially harmful agents in the physical environment and on ways to eliminate, reduce, or minimize threats to health. For example, the community/public health nurse may be involved in restructuring the physical environment to *protect* health by promoting smoking cessation and helping to establish smoking guidelines in public buildings.

The environment may also be improved aesthetically, socially, and economically to *promote* or enhance health. For example, overcrowding may contribute to physical (infectious disease) and psychologic (anxiety) disturbances. Work environments can be monitored for noise and dust levels, temperature variations, and levels of toxicants. Chapter 9 provides a more in-depth discussion of environmental health concerns.

Strengthening Social Support. The sociocultural environment may also contribute to health promotion and community wellness. **Social support** refers to the supportive value of the interactions within relationships that encourage behavioral change. In 2005 the CDC National Center for Health Marketing conducted a systematic review of nine studies on the use of social support to increase physical activity (CDC, National Center for Health Marketing, 2005). The review indicated that social support interventions were effective in getting people to be more physically active. The review indicated that social support interventions can result in a 44% increase in time spent being physically active and a 20% increase in the frequency of physical activity. Some of the social support interventions included setting up a buddy system, making a contract with others to specify levels of physical activity, or setting up groups to provide friendship and support.

Public and Private Partnerships for Political Action

Creating a community environment of support for health promotion also requires partnerships between the public and private sectors. The community health nurse should advocate and promote legislation that provides the funding and resources needed to conduct community health-risk assessment and health-education programs, promote environmental health and safety, enhance existing support systems in the community, and promote research on health promotion and health protection/risk reduction. The community/public health nurse may mobilize consumer interest groups, businesses, community agencies, and other organizations to influence lawmakers and private policymakers to develop and support policies that result in the adoption of laws and programs that foster health promotion.

EVALUATION

The evaluation of health-promotion and health-protection program outcomes involves a process of systematic data collection, analysis, and interpretation to make informed decisions regarding program effectiveness, continuation, or revision (also see Chapter 17). Evaluating preventive programs for individuals, families, and communities is imperative to determine whether program goals have been met and whether the program has been effective in meeting the health needs of the targeted group. Evaluation may be ongoing and continuous with the assessment and intervention phases. Health-promotion or health-protection programs may be evaluated while they are in operation and after the program is complete. The previously mentioned National Center for Health Statistics (2007) provides a wealth of data sources that evaluate existing programs and suggestions for measurement of other health-promotion programs.

Although individuals, families, and the community as a whole may benefit from preventive programs, the criteria for evaluating the success of programs differ depending on the client focus. Individuals and families, for example, may experience more direct and readily applicable benefits (e.g., better health and increased life satisfaction) from participating in preventive programs. (Box 18-4 gives criteria for evaluation of health-promotion and risk-reduction programs that focus on individuals and families.) Perceived life satisfaction, self-esteem, social support, and life stress may be measured using published instruments and scales available in social science and health literature. Evaluation of health-promotion programs on a community level is based on an epidemiologic model. (Box 18-5 gives criteria for evaluation of health-promotion programs in the community.)

Evaluation data may be collected from analyzing vital statistics, observations, questionnaires, and other records. Evaluating health-promotion and health-protection programs allows the community and community/public health nurse to determine whether the benefits of the program outweigh the costs of time, money, and resources devoted to the project and to rate how the program compares with alternative programs and interventions that may be equally feasible and cost-effective.

The effectiveness of a health-promotion or health-protection intervention in a particular group may be measured by comparing that group with a control group that did not receive the intervention to determine whether the goals of the program would have been achieved in the absence of the intervention. Based on evaluation of the program's effectiveness, implications for changes in social and health policy may be made.

BOX 18-4   Criteria for Evaluating Health-Promotion Programs for the Individual or Family

1. Improved health status
2. Improved communication among members
3. Increased income owing to increased employment
4. Higher levels of work productivity
5. Decreased personal expenditures for health
6. Reported increases in life, work, and family satisfaction
7. Satisfying use of leisure time
8. Reduced dependency on family members
9. Improved self-esteem
10. Decreased reported life stress
11. Increased awareness and use of supportive social networks

Data from Borus, M., Buntz, C., & Tash, W. (1982). *Evaluating the impact of health programs: A primer.* Cambridge, MA: MIT Press.

BOX 18-5   Criteria for Evaluating Health-Promotion Programs in the Community

1. Reduced community-wide morbidity and mortality rates
2. Decreased number of days (on an aggregate level) missed from work owing to disability or illness
3. Decreased incidence of preventable communicable diseases
4. Decreased disability days, insurance usage, and unemployment owing to health reasons
5. Increased social satisfaction, quality of life, and self-esteem on an aggregate level
6. Decreased health care costs and reported hospitalizations
7. Decreased antisocial behaviors (e.g., arrests, driving while intoxicated)
8. Decreased monies spent on alcohol, drugs, and cigarettes in community
9. Decreased rates of divorce and domestic violence
10. Reported increases in exercise, fitness, nutrition, and other health-promotion behaviors

Data from Borus, M., Buntz, C., & Tash, W. (1982). *Evaluating the impact of health programs: A primer.* Cambridge, MA: MIT Press.

KEY IDEAS

1. Controlling risk factors related to lifestyle and health habits (e.g., poor diet, lack of exercise, smoking, drug and alcohol abuse) can increase the span of a healthy life.
2. Health promotion involves focusing on individuals and populations as a whole and not solely on people who are at risk for specific diseases.
3. Health promotion is a social project and not solely a medical enterprise.
4. The ability of the health care system to engage in health promotion is determined by national legislation and policies that provide economic and political support for health-promotion services in the community.
5. Continuing work on health models and their application to research is needed to better understand the relationship between changes in behavior and the actual effects of behavior modification on health status.
6. The community/public health nurse applies the nursing process in developing and sustaining health-promotion and risk-reduction programs throughout the community to promote community/public health and well-being.

THE NURSING PROCESS IN PRACTICE ▶ Initiating a Workplace Health-Promotion Program

Karen is an occupational health nurse working in a steel plant. Over the years, she noted a high incidence of hypertension; heart disease; cancer of the larynx, throat, and lung; and substance abuse in her client population. Karen grew increasingly concerned about these statistics. Although a few screening programs were available in the facility (e.g., blood pressure screening, chest radiographs) to detect disease at an early stage, Karen believed that a need existed for a comprehensive program that intervened before the onset of disease.

ASSESSMENT

After securing agreement and support from the plant management, Karen worked in partnership with her employer to assess her clients' health risks, perceptions of need, and receptivity to a workplace health-promotion program. She developed a questionnaire to assess employee health perceptions, determinants, and behaviors. She discovered that the majority of her clients defined health in terms of role performance. As one steel worker noted, "I feel I'm healthy as long as I can work." She also found that 70% of respondents did not routinely engage in health-promotion activities because of cost, poor access, lack of knowledge, or inconvenience of health-promotion services. Karen also administered an HRA tool to all employees who frequented the workplace clinic.

She analyzed the data and identified risk factors, such as an increased risk of morbidity and mortality based on age, family history, smoking, drug and alcohol use, stress, and poor nutrition and fitness patterns. In addition, individuals lacked knowledge of health-promotion behaviors and risks to health. Identified environmental hazards included concerns over exposure to air pollutants and chemicals in the workplace, lack of

access to affordable workplace health-promotion services, and lack of supportive social networks to encourage healthful behaviors. Based on these findings a plan was developed.

PLANNING

Karen presented the findings of her study to the administration. Company executives viewed the cost of funding a health-promotion program as a barrier to implementation. Karen provided information about the benefits of a workplace health-promotion program, including evidence from other studies that health promotion in the workplace has been found to reduce rates of employee absenteeism, improve worker productivity, decrease the use of medical insurance and workers' compensation claims, and improve employee morale and company image.

Karen formed a committee consisting of steel worker employees and administrative and support personnel at different levels of the corporation. The committee agreed that priority should be placed on addressing smoking cessation, alcohol and drug abuse, stress management, exercise and fitness, nutrition, accident prevention, and reduction of environmental hazards. The committee also decided that services would be offered on site and on company time as an incentive for participation. The following goals were developed for the program:

- Six months after initiation of the program, the number of days missed from work owing to disability or illness will decrease by 20%.
- In 6 months, at least 70% of employees participating in the program will report improvements in job satisfaction, self-esteem, and feelings of well-being.
- In 12 months, employee health care costs and hospitalizations will have decreased by at least 25%.

Continued

IMPLEMENTATION

Under Karen's direction and coordination, the committee developed a workplace health-promotion program. Information about the program was disseminated throughout the corporation through brochures, posters, and mass mailings. The program included educational programs on fitness, nutrition, stress management, accident prevention, and reduction of environmental hazards (e.g., toxins, air pollutants, noise). Smoking-cessation programs were offered at convenient times during the day and evening. Support groups were developed for employees to share concerns, discuss work-related issues, and promote supportive social relationships. Monthly activities (e.g., ballgames, picnics) were planned for employees and their families to provide opportunities for meaningful social interaction and to promote a spirit of community. Mental health counseling services were offered on site to assist clients who were experiencing marital, family, or occupational stress. Supervisors and executive personnel met to discuss ways to restructure the environment to optimize health and enhance the aesthetics of the workplace.

EVALUATION

After the program was in operation for 6 months, the committee began to analyze data to evaluate the program's effectiveness. Evaluation occurred at 6 month intervals while the program was in operation. Data revealed the following:

- A 25% decrease in number of days missed from work as a result of disability or illness
- A 30% increase in reports of job satisfaction, self-esteem, and feelings of well-being
- A 25% decrease in reported health care costs and hospitalizations
- A 30% decrease in reported antisocial behaviors (e.g., arrests, driving while intoxicated, incidents of domestic violence)

Employees also reported a 15% decrease in tobacco use (chewing and smoking) and a 10% reduction in alcohol and drug use. In addition, 30% of employees reported maintaining a nutrition and fitness regimen 1 year after the program was in operation. Karen also noted a 20% decrease in the number of clinic visits resulting from on-the-job accidents and a decreased incidence of hypertensive episodes during blood pressure screening clinics.

Less progress was reported in the area of environmental restructuring. Although standards of safety were reportedly more closely followed, lack of fiscal resources was cited as a major deterrent to securing improvements in lighting, temperature, and workspace to produce a more comfort, attractive, and aesthetically pleasing environment. Nonetheless, measurable improvements in employee health, well-being, and productivity were substantial enough to justify continued employer support of the program.

LEARNING BY EXPERIENCE AND REFLECTION

1. Develop a health-promotion plan for a client using one of the models of health presented in this chapter. Compare your plan with that of a fellow classmate who has chosen another model of health. What similarities or differences do you notice between the plans of care? To what extent are differences related to factors in the specific client? How does the model influence development of your care plan?

2. Talk with an individual client, family member, and colleague, exploring their ideas about health. Ask them to describe what being healthy means to them. Have them relate a personal experience in which they felt "better than ever" or "on top of the world." What was this experience like for them? What might have influenced their perceptions of health?

3. Explore conceptions of wellness and illness with people from different socioeconomic, occupational, or cultural groups. What similarities or differences exist among these persons? What influences the meaning of wellness or illness to different populations?

4. Reflect in writing on your perception of what being healthy means. Share your reflections with an individual who is experiencing acute or chronic illness.

5. Complete a wellness assessment or HRA tool. What risks to health are you able to identify in your own attitudes and behaviors? Identify one personal high-risk behavior in which you routinely engage, and attempt to modify your lifestyle in this area for 1 week. For this behavior, identify what stage of change you are in (see Table 18-2). What was this experience like for you? What facilitated or hindered your ability to effect a healthful behavior change?

6. As an occupational health nurse working in a textile factory, you are responsible for planning and implementing health care programs in your facility. Major health needs of your client population include substance abuse, respiratory problems, hypertension, cancer, and back injuries. Although you would like to develop programs reflecting primary, secondary, and tertiary levels of prevention for all the major health needs, inadequate fiscal and human resources prevent you from doing so. Given the scarcity of resources, what health needs would you address first, and why? What level of prevention would your program target? What are the positive and negative implications of your decisions? What additional information do you need to gather to prioritize health needs effectively?

COMMUNITY RESOURCES FOR PRACTICE

Information about each organization listed here is found on its website, which can be accessed through the **WebLinks** section of the book's website at *http://evolve.elsevier.com/Maurer/community/*.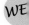

Agency for Healthcare Research and Quality

Agency for Healthcare Research and Quality, *Stay Healthy at Any Age,* for men and women (accessed through the Tools and Resources on the menu)

American Cancer Society, *Guide for Quitting Smoking*

Centers for Disease Control and Prevention

Centers for Disease Control and Prevention, Tobacco Cessation Program

Centers for Disease Control and Prevention, *WISEWOMAN*

Centers for Disease Control and Prevention Healthy Living

Centers for Disease Control and Prevention Wonder

Healthfinder

HealthierUS

Healthy People 2010

Healthy People 2010 Midcourse Review

Healthy People 2010 Executive Summary

Office of Disease Prevention and Health Promotion

National Center for Chronic Disease Prevention and Health Promotion

National Center for Health Statistics
  DATA2010 Database

National Guideline Clearinghouse

Steps to a HealthierUS Initiative

National Heart, Lung, and Blood Institute

National Heart, Lung, and Blood Institute *Aim for a Healthier Weight*

Your Disease Risk Page, Harvard School of Public Health

STUDY AIDS   http://evolve.elsevier.com/Maurer/community/

Visit the Evolve website for this book to find the following study and assessment materials:

- Quiz
- Web Scenario
- Critical Thinking Questions and Answers for Case Studies
- Care Plans
- *Healthy People* Updates
- Glossary

WEBSITE RESOURCES

EB *These items supplement the chapter's topics and are also found on the Evolve site:*

18A: Social Readjustment Rating Scale for Adults

18B: Life Change Unit Values for Children

REFERENCES

Agency for Healthcare Research and Quality. (2007) *Stay healthy at any age.* Accessed July 30, 2007, at *http://www.ahrq.gov/ppip/healthymen.htm* and *http://www.ahrq.gov/ppip/healthywom.htm.*

American Cancer Society. (2007). *American Cancer Society guide to quitting smoking.* Accessed July 30, 2007, at *http://www.cancer.org/docroot/PED/content/PED_10_13X_Guide_for_Quitting_Smoking.asp.*

American Nurses Association. (1996). *American Nurses Association position statement on health promotion and disease prevention.* Washington, DC: Author.

American Nurses Association & Health Ministries Association. (2005). *Faith community nursing: Scope and standards of practice.* Silver Spring, MD: American Nurses Association.

Becker, M. (Ed.). (1974). *The health belief model and personal health behavior.* Thorofare, NJ: Charles B. Slack.

Becker, M., Haefner, D., Kasl, S., et al. (1977). Selected psychosocial correlates of individual health related behaviors. *Medical Care, 15*(5), 24.

Borus, M., Buntz, C., & Tash, W. (1982). *Evaluating the impact of health programs: A primer.* Cambridge, MA: Massachusetts Institute of Technology Press.

Centers for Disease Control and Prevention, Division for Heart Disease and Stroke Prevention. (2007). *WISEWOMAN: Well-integrated screening and evaluation for women across the nation.* Accessed July 2007 at *http://www.cdc.gov/wisewoman/.*

Centers for Disease Control and Prevention, National Center for Health Marketing. (2005). *Providing social support in community settings is recommended to promote physical activity.* Accessed July 31, 2007, at *http://www.thecommunityguide.org/.*

Centers for Disease Control and Prevention, National Center for Chronic Disease Prevention and Health Promotion. (2007). *Quick facts: Economic and health burden of chronic disease.* Accessed July 31, 2007 at *http://www.cdc.gov/nccdphp/press/#3.*

Coddington, R. (1972). The significance of life events as etiologic factors in the diseases of children—A survey of professional workers. *Journal of Psychosomatic Research, 16*(1), 13-16.

Croghan, E. (2005). Assessing motivation and readiness to alter lifestyle behavior. *Nursing Standard, 19*(31), 50-52.

Delgado, H., & Austin, S. B. (2007). Can media promote responsible sexual behaviors among adolescents and young adults? *Current Opinion in Pediatrics, 19*(4), 405-410.

Easom, L. (2003). Concepts in health promotion, perceived self-efficacy and barriers in older adults. *Journal of Gerontological Nursing, 29*(5), 11-19.

Hochbaum, G. (1956). Why people seek diagnostic x-rays. *Public Health Reports, 71,* 377-380.

Hockenberry, M. J., Wilson, D., Winkelstein, M. L., et al. (2003). *Wong's nursing care of infants and children* (7th ed.). St. Louis: Mosby.

Holmes, T., & Rahe, H. (1967). The social readjustment rating scale. *Journal of Psychosomatic Research, 11,* 213-218.

Janz, N., & Becker, M. (1984). The health belief model: A decade later. *Health Education Quarterly, 11*(1), 1-47.

Kaewthummanukul, T., & Brown, K. C. (2006). Determinants of employee participation in physical activity: Critical review of the literature. *American Association of Occupational Health Nursing Journal, 54*(6), 249-261.

Maibach, E., & Cotton, D. (1995). Moving people to behavioral change: A staged social cognitive approach to message design. In E. Maibach & R. L. Parrott (Eds.), *Designing health messages: Approaches from communication theory and public health practice* (pp. 41-64). Thousand Oaks, CA: Sage Publications.

National Center for Health Statistics. (2007). *DATA2010: The Healthy People 2010 database.* Hyattsville, MD. Accessed July 2007 at *http://wonder.cdc.gov/data2010.*

National Institutes of Health, National Heart, Lung, and Blood Institute. (2007). Obesity education initiative: Aim for a healthy weight. Accessed July 2007 at *http://www.nhlbi.nih.gov/health/public/heart/obesity/lose_wt/.*

O'Donnell, M. (1986). Definition of health promotion. *American Journal of Health Promotion, 1*(2), 6-9.

Padula, C. A., & Sullivan, M. (2006). Long-term married couples' health promotion behaviors: Identifying factors that impact decision-making. *Journal of Gerontological Nursing, 32*(10), 37-47.

Partnership for Prevention. (2001). *Healthy workforce 2010: An essential health promotion sourcebook for employers, large and small.* Washington, DC: Partnership for Prevention.

Pender, N. J., Murdaugh, C., & Parsons, M. A. (2006). *Health promotion in nursing practice* (5th ed.). Upper Saddle River, NJ: Prentice-Hall Health, Inc.

Peterson, D. (2007). Eight advocacy roles for parish nurses. *Journal of Christian Nursing, 24*(1), 33-35.

Peterson, J., Atwood, J., & Yates, B. (2002). Key elements for church-based health promotion programs: Outcome-based literature review. *Public Health Nursing, 19*(6), 410-411.

Prochaska, J. O., & DiClemente, C. C. (1983). Stages and processes of self-change of smoking:

Toward an integrative model of change. *Journal of Consulting and Clinical Psychology, 51*(3), 390-395.

Rosenstock, I. (1974). The health belief model and preventive health behavior. *Health Education Monographs, 2*, 354-385.

Rosenstock, M., Strecher, V. J., & Becker, M. H. (1988). Social learning theory and the health belief model. *Health Education Quarterly, 15*(2), 175-183.

Sadler, C., & Huff, M. (2007). African-American women: Health beliefs, lifestyle and osteoporosis. *Orthopaedic Nursing, 26*(2), 96-101.

Sedlak, C. A., Doheny, M. O., Estok, P. J., et al. (2005). Tailored interventions to enhance osteoporosis prevention in women. *Orthopaedic Nursing, 24*(4), 270-276.

Shoultz, J. E., & Hatcher, P. A. (1997). Primary health care goes beyond primary care: An approach to community-based action. *Nursing Outlook, 45*(1), 23-26.

Timmerman, G. (2007). Addressing barriers to health promotion in underserved women. *Family and Community Health, 30*(suppl. 1), S34-S42.

U.S. Department of Health, Education, and Welfare. (1979). *Healthy People: The Surgeon General's report on health promotion and disease prevention* (DHEW Publ. No. [PHS] 79 55071). Washington, DC: U.S. Government Printing Office.

U.S. Department of Health and Human Services. (2000). *Healthy People 2010: Understanding and improving health and objectives for improving health* (2nd ed.). Washington, DC: U.S. Government Printing Office. Also accessed July 2007 at *www.healthypeople.gov.*

U.S. Department of Health and Human Services. (2006). *Healthy People 2010: Midcourse review.* Accessed July 31, 2007, at *http://www.healthypeople.gov/data/midcourse/.*

U.S. Department of Health and Human Services. (2007). *Steps to a healthier US initiative: 2007: A program and policy perspective.* Accessed July 2007 at *http://www.healthierus.gov/STEPS/.*

U.S. Department of Health and Human Services, Office of Disease Prevention and Health Promotion. (2007). *Healthfinder.gov.* Accessed July 30, 2007, at *http://www.healthfinder.gov/.*

SUGGESTED READINGS

Croghan, E. (2005). Assessing motivation and readiness to alter lifestyle behavior. *Nursing Standard, 19*(31), 50-52.

Croghan, E. (2005). Supporting lifestyle and health-related behavior change. *Nursing Standard, 19*(37), 52-53.

Fahrenwald, N., & Sharma, M. (2002). Development and expert evaluation of "moms on the move": A physical activity intervention for WIC mothers. *Public Health Nursing, 19*(6), 423-439.

McNabb, W., Quinn, M., Kerver, J., et al. (1997). The PATHWAYS church-based weight loss program for urban African-American women at risk for diabetes. *Diabetes Care, 20*(10), 1518-1523.

Nunez, D., Armbruster, C., Phillips, W., et al. (2003). Community-based senior health

promotion program using a collaborative practice model: The Escalante Health Partnerships. *Public Health Nursing, 20*(1), 25-32.

Peterson, J., Atwood, J. & Yates, B. (2002). Key elements for church-based health promotion programs: Outcome-based literature review. *Public Health Nursing, 19*(6), 410-411.

Raymond, D. M., & Lusk, S. L. (2006). Staging workers' use of hearing protection devices: Application of the transtheoretical model. *American Association of Occupational Health Nursing Journal, 54*(4), 165-172.

Resnick, B. (2000). Health promotion practices of the older adult. *Public Health Nursing, 17*(3), 160-168.

Robbins, L. B., Gretebeck, K. A., Kazanis, A. S., et al. (2006). Girls on the move program to

increase physical activity participation. *Nursing Research, 55*(3), 206-216.

Salmond, S., & Ropis, P. E. (2005). Job stress and general well-being: A comparative study of medical-surgical and home care nurses. *Medsurg Nursing, 14*(5), 301-309.

Speck, B. J., Hines-Martin, V., Stetson, B. A., et al. (2007). An environmental intervention aimed at increasing physical activity levels in low-income women. *Cardiovascular Nursing, 22*(4), 263-271.

The Transtheoretical Model of Behavioral Change (TTM). Retrieved September 12, 2007, from *http://www.umbc.edu/psyc//habits/content/the_model/index.html.*

C
H
A
P
T
E
R

19 Screening and Referral

Gail L. Heiss

FOCUS QUESTIONS

What is the value of screening in maintaining the health of people in the community?

How is screening linked to health promotion and maintenance?

What principles guide the selection, development, and targeting of screening programs?

What are the responsibilities of the community/public health nurse in selecting, establishing, implementing, and evaluating screening programs?

What is the relationship between screening and referral?

What are the responsibilities of the community/public health nurse in the referral process?

CHAPTER OUTLINE

KEY TERMS

Case finding	Presumptive identification	Screening
Health fair	of disease	Secondary prevention
Mass screening	Process evaluation	Sensitivity
Multiphasic screening	Referral	Specificity
Outcome evaluation	Reliability	Validity

An essential component in maintaining the health of a community is early detection of disease. Although, ideally, the hope is to prevent disease, not all diseases are completely preventable. For example, although some risk factors associated with the development of heart disease are known and can be avoided (e.g., high-fat diet, smoking, sedentary lifestyle), others are unmodifiable (e.g., age, sex, family history). For this reason, diseases that cannot be completely prevented must be detected early in their natural history when they are more amenable to treatment. Early detection and treatment of disease complements one of the overall goals of *Healthy People 2010* to increase the quality and years of healthy life (U.S. Department of Health and Human Services [USDHHS], 2000). Progress toward this goal is monitored on a regular basis and reported in *Health People 2010 Midcourse Review* (USDHHS, 2006).

Secondary prevention is aimed at the early detection and treatment of illness. *Screening* is a major secondary-prevention strategy. When previously unrecognized illnesses are identified through screening, referrals must be made for follow-up diagnosis and treatment. This chapter explores the concept of screening and the responsibilities of the community health nurse in the screening and referral process.

DEFINITION OF SCREENING

Screening is the process of using clinical tests and/or examinations to identify patients who require additional health-related interventions. The goal of screening is to differentiate correctly between persons who have a previously unrecognized illness, developmental delay, or other health alteration and those who do not. Screening recommendations for health screening events and routine health care appointments are often based on the clinical research and evidence-based preventive care presented by the U.S. Preventive Services Task Force (USPSTF). The Preventive Services Task Force is sponsored by the Agency for Healthcare Research and Quality (AHRQ) and is recognized as the leader in prevention and screening recommendations (USPSTF, 2006).

Screening involves several key terms. Screening is aimed at the **presumptive identification of disease.** In other words, if a screening test is positive (abnormal), one can only *presume* that the disease *may* be present. A screening test, in itself, is not sufficient to establish a positive diagnosis of disease because a single screening test, taken in isolation, is not always 100% accurate. For example, inaccuracies in test measurement can lead to false-positive or false-negative test results. For this reason, when a screening test is positive, a referral is made for follow-up diagnostic testing to confirm whether, in fact, the disease is present.

Screening tests detect previously *unrecognized* disease, meaning that screening tests are often conducted on seemingly healthy populations. Persons who undergo screening tests may be asymptomatic of disease and unaware that a problem potentially exists. Herein lies the value of screening. The goal of a screening test is to detect disease in an earlier stage than it would be if the client waited for clinical symptoms to develop before seeking help.

Screening is conducted by applying *tests and procedures.* These tests can be applied *rapidly* and *inexpensively* to *populations.* In other words, these tests should be appropriate for administration to a large group of people. To screen large groups in a timely manner, a test must be able to be administered rapidly and with ease. Tests should be relatively inexpensive so they are accessible to more economically diverse populations.

Mass screening is used to denote the application of screening tests to large populations. These groups may be typical of the general population or be selectively at a higher risk for certain problems. Because mass screening of the general population is often costly and does not necessarily detect enough new cases of disease to balance the cost of screening, some institutions and organizations believe that money may be better spent on targeting selected populations known to be at high risk for certain illnesses. For example, in a large city in which elevated lead levels in children are a potential problem because of inadequate housing, the community/public health nurse might suggest targeting screening toward minority and low-income children living in impoverished neighborhoods.

Case finding is screening that occurs on an individual or a one-on-one basis. Case finding attempts to use screening tests to identify previously unrecognized disease in *individuals* who may present to the health care provider for health maintenance checks or for an unrelated complaint. A good example is when the community/public health nurse makes a home visit and checks the blood pressure of each member of the family. In this instance, the nurse may detect previously unrecognized disease in family members who are unaware that a problem even exists. Another example is an individual who obtains a new job and has a preemployment physical; an elevated cholesterol level may be detected in this manner.

Multiphasic screening is used to denote the application of multiple screening tests on the same occasion. A health fair held at a church or synagogue, for example, may include screening for blood pressure, depression, colorectal cancer, and diabetes. Persons may present to different stations or providers and receive several screening tests during a single visit. Table 19-1 presents some suggestions on selecting screening tests when planning a multiphasic health fair.

CRITERIA FOR SELECTING SCREENING TESTS: VALIDITY AND RELIABILITY

VALIDITY, SENSITIVITY, AND SPECIFICITY

Validity is defined as the ability of the screening test to distinguish correctly between persons with and those without the disease. If a screening test were 100% valid, it would never have a *false-positive* or *false-negative* reading. The result would always be positive in people who had the disease and negative in people who did not. The validity of a screening test is measured using sensitivity and specificity.

TABLE 19-1	Planning a Multiphasic Health Fair
Nursing Process	**Explanation**
Assess: The diseases being screened should be significant health problems in the community.	Select screening tests based on demographic data and relevance of the problem to the community. For example, it would be appropriate to conduct a screening for osteoporosis at a community center serving primarily white women.
Plan: Gather support from the community and consider all the details.	Issues such as available dates and times, space, volunteers, funding for screening tests, advertising, and cultural issues must be considered from the beginning. For example, it would not be appropriate to conduct a hypertension screening at the Jewish Community Center during the Jewish New Year in September.
Implement: The screening tests should be safe, simple to administer, cost-effective, and acceptable to the client population.	Tests to consider might include screening for hypertension, diabetes, elevated cholesterol levels, and cancer. Some cancer screenings such as colon and rectal screening may be done with noninvasive fecal occult blood stool cards that the patient takes home. Invasive procedures should be avoided in mass screening settings.
Evaluate: Follow-up diagnosis and treatment of persons with positive test results is important.	A screening program should not be conducted unless adequate community resources are available to deal with the outcome of positive test results. If no resources exist in the community, the community/public health nurse has a responsibility to advocate for funding for such resources and to mobilize needed resources so that community health and well-being are protected.

Sensitivity is the ability of a screening test to identify correctly persons who have the disease. When the disease is correctly identified, this result is known as a *true-positive test*. A test with poor sensitivity will miss cases and will produce a large proportion of *false-negative test* results; people will be incorrectly told they are free of disease. The statistical formula for calculating sensitivity is the following:

$$\frac{\text{Number of true-positive test results}}{\text{Number of people with disease}}$$
$$\text{(Number of true-positives + false-negatives)}$$

Notice that the *denominator* in the formula is *all* persons with the disease. After a screening test, *persons with the disease* might have a screening result that is either true-positive (i.e., they do, in fact, have the disease) or false-negative (i.e., the screening test is normal, but they do actually have the disease). The greater the number of false-negative test results, *meaning the larger the number of persons with disease who have not been identified,* the lower the sensitivity of the screening test.

Specificity is the ability of the screening test to identify persons who are normal or without disease and who correctly test negative when screened. The formula for specificity is as follows:

$$\frac{\text{Number of true-negative results}}{\text{All persons without disease}}$$
$$\text{(Number of true-negatives + false-positives)}$$

In this case, persons *who are healthy* may have one of two test results. They may have either a *true-negative* finding (i.e., they do not have the disease, and the test findings are normal) or a *false-positive* finding (i.e., they do not have the disease, but their screening test result is positive for disease). The greater the number of false-positive test results, the lower the specificity of the screening test. Table 19-2 summarizes sensitivity and specificity.

Ideally, a screening test would be 100% sensitive and 100% specific. However, because this combination of perfect accuracy and precision in measurement is not likely, screening tests are not used to confirm a diagnosis positively and are not considered to be diagnostic.

A nurse is working in her community to help reach the *Healthy People 2010* goals of preventing diabetes and help reach the 2010 target of 80% of persons with diabetes whose condition has been diagnosed. She decides to implement a screening day for diabetes at the local pharmacy. The pharmacy owner has agreed to donate the supplies for the screening. Participants are requested to have fasted for 10 to 12 hours before arriving at the screening.

If the normal blood glucose level ranges from 70 to 100 mg/dl and for this screening event any level greater than 70 mg/dl were considered abnormal (that is, diabetes potentially present), what would happen to the sensitivity and specificity of the screening test? Because it is highly unlikely that anyone with diabetes would have a blood glucose level lower than 70 mg/dl, sensitivity would approach 100%. However, normal individuals with blood glucose levels between 70 and 100 mg/dl would be considered to potentially have diabetes; their positive test result would give a false picture of the presence of diabetes. There would be a large number of false-positive results. Specificity would then decrease, and the nurse would be making many, many referrals for potential diabetes. Therefore the relationship between sensitivity and specificity is inverse. The greater the sensitivity is, the lower the specificity will be, and vice versa. The more sensitive a test is made, the less specific it becomes. The nurse, in this case, would be wise to use the screening criteria suggested by the American Diabetes Association (ADA, 2007). Clients with a fasting blood glucose level between 100 and 126 mg/dl would be instructed to receive another screening test. Clients who have a fasting blood glucose level of greater than 126 mg/dl would be instructed to see their health care provider as soon as possible. In addition, the nurse might want to target the screening event for patients at high risk for diabetes, such as adults older than age 45 who also have a body mass index (BMI) greater than 25 kg/m², or screening individuals younger than age 45 if they have a high BMI and other risk factors such as a family history of diabetes or if they are from a high-risk population (Standards of Medical Care in Diabetes, 2007).

Is having a high sensitivity and a moderate or low specificity better, or should attempts be made to improve specificity, even though sensitivity may be compromised? The answer to these questions depends on the disease for which the individual is being screened and the physical, psychologic, and financial impact of false-positive versus false-negative test results. In the case of diseases that are potentially fatal if not detected early, sensitivity may be more important. However, the psychologic

---

TABLE 19-2   Sensitivity and Specificity

Sensitivity is the ability of the test to correctly identify persons *who have a disease*.

High sensitivity	Numerous **true-positive** results. People who actually have the disease correctly test positive.
Low sensitivity	Numerous **false-negative** results. People have a normal screening, but actually have the disease.

Specificity is the ability of the test to identify persons *who do not have disease* who correctly test negative.

High specificity	Numerous **true-negative** results. People who do not have disease correctly test negative.
Low specificity	Numerous **false-positive** results. People have an abnormal screening, but they do not have the disease.

trauma and financial cost of being labeled incorrectly as having a disease can be devastating. For example, if a client receives news that she or he is human immunodeficiency virus (HIV) positive and later commits suicide, a false-positive reading has had significant and even fatal consequences. In this case, high specificity is as important as high sensitivity.

An interesting discussion of sensitivity and specificity relating to school nurse screening for scoliosis is found on the scoliosis website (*http://www.iscoliosis.com/symptoms-screening. html*) and in **Website Resource 19A.** The screening of adolescents for scoliosis occurs in schools in all 50 states. The purpose of the screening is to detect scoliosis at an early stage. The test is described as *sensitive (always detects the presence of scoliosis versus a normal back)* and has a low false-negative rate *(does not miss kids that need treatment)*. The test is also determined to be *specific (finding scoliosis as opposed to other problems)*. A figure of the test and additional information on this screening test are also located in **Website Resource 19A.**

RELIABILITY OF SCREENING TESTS

Reliability refers to the consistency or reproducibility of test results over time and between examiners. A test is reliable when it gives consistent results when administered at different times and by different persons.

In a community, a blood pressure screening event is held at the entrance to the shopping mall every first Friday of the month. The event is well publicized on the radio and with flyers at the senior center and places of worship. The screening is easy to find, given that the entrance is a well-known location and is advertised as being the "mall entrance near the merry-go-round." At the screening, the community/public health nurse obtains a blood pressure reading of 190/110 mm Hg on a health fair participant. She seeks another nurse to recheck the findings. The second nurse obtains a reading of 120/80 mm Hg. This difference indicates poor reliability; the results were not consistent. The skill level of the nurses, degree of sensory impairment, or condition of the equipment may have affected *reliability*. As a solution, checking equipment, monitoring the correct procedure of the nurses working at the health fair, or altering environmental noise level might improve the reliability of this screening test. The nurses may want to consider moving the blood pressure screening to a location in the mall that is quiet—perhaps near a different entrance that does not have the merry-go-round. As an alternative solution when conducting blood pressure screening in an environment that is frequently noisy, or frequently uses multiple screeners, using automated blood pressure monitoring equipment might improve reliability.

CONTEXTS FOR SCREENING

Screening programs may be targeted to individuals (i.e., case finding) or to populations (i.e., mass screening). For individuals, selecting screening tests may be guided by the provider's knowledge of the client's personal history and risk factors. Population-based screenings can be offered in conjunction with national screening days, such as skin cancer screening or depression screening, or they may be selected based on demographic and epidemiologic data.

SCREENING OF INDIVIDUALS

A routine health-maintenance examination is one example of a multiphasic, case-finding intervention. Periodic health checkups include a comprehensive health history, physical examination, and relevant laboratory and diagnostic studies. Many health care providers and organizations follow the screening guidelines available through the National Guideline Clearinghouse (NGC). The NGC is sponsored by the Agency for Healthcare Research and Quality (AHRQ) of the USDHHS and provides recommendations based on evidence-based clinical practice. Recommendations for periodic screening of adults in the general population include hypertension, lipid disorders, obesity, colorectal cancer, and others (NGC, 2002) and are presented in Table 19-3.

In addition to screening guidelines, the nurse and the patient may use family history to determine which screening tests are most appropriate. Several useful tools for documenting family health history are located on the Centers for Disease Control and Prevention (CDC) website (CDC, 2007a) and may be found by accessing the main site and navigating to family history. The site includes general family history as well as a family cancer history tool.

Another health tool of interest to the community/public health nurse for use with families at risk for cardiovascular disease and diabetes is an American Heart Association (AHA) downloadable family history tree, which specifically illustrates familial tendencies for heart disease, diabetes, hypertension, obesity, and stroke (AHA, 2007a). The tool is user friendly and may be used as a health history tool or a discussion starter for lifestyle modification.

SCREENING OF POPULATIONS

On a population level, choice of screening tests is based on general sociodemographic rather than individual risk factors. To determine what screening tests should be administered, the community/public health nurse must assess the risks inherent in the target population. What diseases is the target population most at risk of developing? Are these diseases easily screened?

Age, gender, and ethnicity factors have an impact on the risk status of a population. A nurse planning a health fair in a local women's center, for example, may include screening for breast cancer. An individual attending the health fair may not be at an increased risk of developing breast cancer based on age or personal and family history. Nevertheless, because the population group as a whole has been determined to be at risk, screening mammograms are made available.

African American men are at a higher risk of developing malignant hypertension than are women or white men; therefore advertisements for some health fairs might be targeted to the African American community. Osteoporosis is more common in white and Asian postmenopausal women than it is in other population groups; thus a women's event might be a good place for this screening. Population data are an important consideration for nurses planning mass screenings.

MAJOR HEALTH THREATS IN THE GENERAL POPULATION

The leading causes of death in the general adult population are heart disease, stroke, and cancer. More than 927,000

TABLE 19-3   Recommendations for Selected Adult Health Screenings

Screening Method	Recommendation
Breast self-examination*	Indicated once a month for women older than 20 years
Clinical breast examination*	Women younger than 40 years: every 3 years
	Women 40 years and older: every year
Mammography*	Annually ages 40 and older
Digital rectal examination for colon cancer*	Every year after age 50 years
Stool for occult blood*	Every year after age 50 years
Sigmoidoscopy*	Every 5 years after age 50 years
Colonoscopy*	Instead of sigmoidoscopy, every 10 years after 50 years
Papanicolaou test and pelvic examination*	Annually for women 18 years and older or for all women who are sexually active; after three or more consecutive normal examinations, Papanicolaou test may be performed less frequently at discretion of provider
Testicular self-examination*	Monthly for postpubertal males
Prostate examination*	Prostate-specific antigen (PSA) blood screening test and digital rectal exam recommended annually for men beginning at age 50 years
	Men at high risk (African American and close family member diagnosed at early age) should start at age 45 years
Blood pressure and classification of hypertension[†]	**Recommendations for referral to a source of medical care**
Normal: Systolic less than 120 mm Hg; diastolic less than 80 mm Hg	**Normal**
	Recheck in 2 years
Prehypertensive: Systolic 120-139 mm Hg; diastolic 80-89 mm Hg	**Prehypertensive**
	Recheck in 1 year; provide advice about lifestyle modifications
Hypertensive	**Hypertensive**
Stage 1: Systolic 140-159 mm Hg; diastolic 90-99 mm Hg	**Stage 1**
	Confirm within 2 months; provide advice about lifestyle modifications
Stage 2: Systolic $\geqq$160 mm Hg; diastolic $\geqq$100 mm Hg	**Stage 2**
	Evaluate or refer to source of care within 1 month; for those with pressures $\geqq$180/110 mm Hg, evaluate and treat immediately or within 1 week, depending on clinical situation
Cholesterol[‡]	Check once every 5 years or more frequently if indicated
Desirable values:	
Total cholesterol: less than 200 mg/dl	
Low-density lipoprotein (LDL) "bad" cholesterol: less than 100 mg/dl optimal	
High-density lipoprotein (HDL) "good" cholesterol: 40-60 mg/dl	
Triglycerides: less than 150 mg/dl	
Diabetes screening[§]	Annually for high-risk individuals (e.g., family history, personal history of glucose intolerance, obesity, minority races, older than age 45 years); otherwise during routine medical examinations
	Screening may be verbal or written; only individuals with high risk or physical symptoms should be referred for blood testing
Skin cancer screening[¶]	Complete body skin examination every 3 years ages 20-40 years, annually ages 40 and older
Mantoux test with purified protein derivative— tuberculin (PPD) skin test[**]	Annually for high-risk groups (e.g., HIV-positive persons, known contact with tuberculosis patient, immunosuppressed persons, persons who live or work in long-term care facilities or work in hospitals or schools, foreign-born persons from countries with high tuberculosis rates); otherwise as indicated

*American Cancer Society. (2007). *Cancer facts and figures. Screening guidelines.* Available online at *www.cancer.org.*
[†]National Heart, Lung, and Blood Institute, National Institutes of Health. (2004). *The seventh report of the Joint National Committee on Detection, Evaluation, and Treatment of High Blood Pressure.* Washington, DC: Author. Available at *www.nhlbi.nih.gov/guidelines.*
[‡]National Cholesterol Education Program. (2007). *Guidelines for clinical preventive services.* Washington, DC: National Heart, Lung, and Blood Institute. Available at *www.nhlbi.nih.gov/guidelines.*
[§]American Diabetes Association. (2007). *Facts and figures.* Available at *www.diabetes.org.*
[¶]American Academy of Dermatology. (2007) *Skin cancer fact sheet.* Available at *www.aad.org.*
[**]U.S. Department of Health and Human Services. (1993). *TB facts for health care workers.* Washington, DC: U.S. Government Printing Office.
CDC, Heart Disease and Stroke Prevention.

Americans die of cardiovascular disease or stroke each year, which amounts to 1 death every 34 seconds (CDC, 2007b). Cancer, the second leading cause of death, is responsible for the death of more than 1500 people every day in the United States (CDC, 2007b). The cost of chronic disease is also dramatic. It is estimated that the direct and indirect (such as loss of productivity) costs of cardiovascular disease and stroke in the United States in 2007 were $431.8 billion. The cost of smoking-related illness was greater than $155 billion, including direct and indirect costs, and the direct medical costs associated with obesity were more than $75 billion in 2003 (CDC, 2007b).

Mental illnesses are also major threats to the health of the general population. In addition to screening for physical problems, community/public health nurses can also screen for depression, anxiety, and substance abuse.

Cardiovascular Disease, Stroke, and Hypertension

The principal risk factors for heart disease and stroke include hypertension (blood pressure reading of 140/90 mm Hg or higher), elevated serum cholesterol level (greater than 200 mg/dl), tobacco use, overweight and obesity, family history of atherosclerotic disease, advancing age, and physical inactivity (CDC, 2007c). A surprising fact for some health care consumers is that although cardiovascular disease is frequently considered a male health problem, more than half of the deaths each year from heart disease occur in women. Hypertension has the highest prevalence of any cardiovascular disease in the United States. In 2004, nearly one in three adults had hypertension and nearly 40% had prehypertension (systolic pressure 120 to 139 mm Hg, or diastolic pressure of 80 to 89 mm Hg) (CDC, 2007c).

Many of the risk factors related to cardiovascular disease are modifiable, and therefore cardiovascular disease is highly amenable to prevention efforts. Selected *Healthy People 2010* objectives for reducing the risk of cardiovascular disease through secondary prevention measures are presented in the *Healthy People 2010* box on this page. In addition to the initiatives related to *Healthy People,* in 2006 the CDC created the division for Heart Disease and Stroke Prevention (DHDSP), which provides national leadership and research to reduce the burden of disease, disability, and death from heart disease. That website can be found at the end of this chapter.

Hypertension. Screening programs aimed at the early identification of hypertension contribute greatly to the early diagnosis and treatment of this potentially fatal condition by making people aware of their blood pressure status and by referring those with elevated readings for follow-up diagnosis and treatment. A committee representing the National Heart, Lung, and Blood Institute (NHLBI) publishes guidelines every few years to guide the diagnosis and clinical treatment of hypertension. In May 2004 the *Seventh Report of the Joint National Committee on Prevention, Detection, Evaluation and Treatment of High Blood Pressure (JNC-7)* published new guidelines, which are reflected in Table 19-3. In addition to the guidelines, the report indicated that nearly 30% of adults in the United States remain unaware of their blood pressure, and the report discussed the strain that undiagnosed and untreated hypertension places on the health care system (NHLBI, 2004). It is estimated that an

■ HEALTHY PEOPLE 2010 ■
Selected National Health-Promotion Objectives to Reduce the Risk of Cardiovascular Disease

Hypertension

1. Increase the proportion of adults with high blood pressure whose blood pressure is under control. (Baseline 1994: 25%. Target: 68%.)
2. Increase the proportion of people with high blood pressure who are taking action (e.g., losing weight, increasing physical activity, reducing sodium intake) to help control their blood pressure. (Baseline 1998: 84%. Target: 98%.)
3. Increase the proportion of adults who have had their blood pressure measured within the preceding 2 years and can state whether their blood pressure was normal or high. (Baseline 1998: 90%. Target: 95%.)

Serum Cholesterol

1. Reduce the proportion of adults with high total blood cholesterol level. (Baseline 1994: 21% of adults ages 20 years and older had total blood cholesterol of 240 mg/dl or greater. Target: 17%.)
2. Reduce the mean total blood cholesterol level among adults. (Baseline 1994: 206 mg/dl was the mean total blood cholesterol for adults ages 20 and older. Target: 199 mg/dl mean.)
3. Increase the proportion of adults who have had their blood cholesterol checked within the preceding 5 years. (Baseline 1998: 67% of people ages 18 and older had their blood cholesterol checked within the preceding 5 years. Target: 80%.)

From U.S. Department of Health and Human Services. (2000). *Healthy People 2010.* Washington, DC: U.S. Government Printing Office; and U.S. Department of Health and Human Services. (2006). *Healthy People 2010: Midcourse review.* Washington, DC: U.S. Government Printing Office.

average reduction of 12-13 mm Hg of systolic pressure over 4 years can reduce the total cardiovascular disease deaths in the United States by 25% (CDC, 2005).

Serum Cholesterol. An estimated 105 million American adults have total blood cholesterol levels of 200 milligrams per deciliter (mg/dl), which is above desirable levels. Of these, 36.6 million adults have total blood cholesterol levels of 240 mg/dl or higher. In adults, 240 mg/dl is considered high, and a blood cholesterol level of 200 to 239 mg/dl is borderline high (AHA, 2007b).

In 1985 the NHLBI initiated the "National Cholesterol Education Program" to increase public awareness of the relationship between cholesterol level and heart disease. The program continues to update detailed guidelines for identifying and treating individuals with elevated serum cholesterol levels. The clinical guidelines for cholesterol health known as the ATP III Guidelines are available on-line *(http://www.nhlbi. nih.gov).* Initiating cholesterol screening programs in the community may assist in preventing heart disease through early identification of at-risk persons and counseling and referral of high-risk individuals for further intervention aimed at modifying dietary fat consumption, instituting exercise programs, or initiating pharmacotherapy, if indicated, to reduce blood lipid levels. Figure 19-1 shows a screening for cholesterol and glucose. In addition, efforts are being made to include children

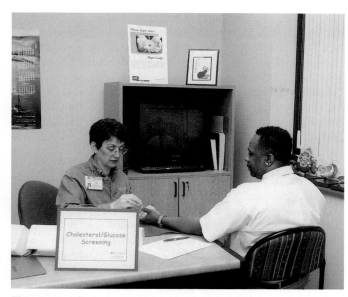

FIGURE 19-1 A screening for cholesterol and glucose. (Photograph taken at St. Luke's Hospital, Chesterfield, Missouri.)

and families in healthy lifestyle choices as a way to promote heart health. On-line education and self-risk tests for adults and children are found on the American Heart Association and the National Heart, Lung, and Blood Institute websites listed at the end of this chapter.

Obesity. Obesity is increasing and is present in approximately 30% of the adult population of the United States (CDC, 2007b). Among children and adolescents, overweight rates have doubled since 1980 so that one in every six children is overweight. The CDC estimates that about 112,000 deaths are attributed to obesity annually. Overweight and obesity contribute to the cardiovascular burden of the nation, costing nearly $75 billion in 2003. The annual hospital costs associated with obese children and adolescents have more than tripled over the past 2 decades. Overweight and obesity are also associated with increased risk of hypertension, diabetes, stroke, gallbladder disease, sleep apnea, arthritis, and other chronic diseases. Using screening tests that include percentage of body fat measurements, triceps skinfold test, computerized analyses, and body mass index (BMI), people who are overweight may be identified and referred for nutritional and fitness counseling (NHLBI, 2007).

Smoking. An estimated 45.8 million Americans smoke, even though this single behavior will result in disability or death for half of the regular tobacco users (CDC, 2007b). Pulmonary function studies are conducted to measure damage to respiratory function that may be caused by smoking or by other lung diseases. A peak flowmeter can be used to screen for compromised respiratory functioning. Screening for pulmonary dysfunction with prompt referral to smoking-cessation programs and medical providers for follow-up may halt progression of heart and lung disease caused by the harmful effects of tobacco. Even without the use of pulmonary function screening, persons who smoke should be referred to smoking-cessation programs regardless of their pulmonary status. Nursing involvement in tobacco cessation intervention is essential and is supported by the American Nurses Association. Research has demonstrated that nurse-delivered stop smoking interventions are effective in

achieving smoking abstinence for 6 months or longer (Wewers et al., 2006).

Cancer

Cancer is the second leading cause of death in the United States, exceeded only by heart disease. Approximately one in four of all deaths are from cancer (American Cancer Society [ACS], 2006). Screening examinations conducted regularly by a health care professional can result in the detection of many cancers, including cancer of the breast, colon, rectum, cervix, prostate, testes, and skin, at earlier stages when treatment is more likely to be successful. The relative survival rate for all cancers is approximately 66%. The *Healthy People 2010* box on this page lists selected national health objectives for the early detection and treatment of cancer.

Lung Cancer. Lung cancer is the leading cause of cancer deaths and the most prevalent form of cancer in both men and women. Lung cancer causes 29% of all cancer-related deaths (ACS, 2006). Approximately 87% of lung cancers are attributed to cigarette smoking. Since 1987 more women have died each year from lung cancer than from breast cancer. The lung cancer rates for men are slowly declining and the rates for women reached a plateau in 1998, due largely to the stop smoking efforts and decline in smoking over the past few decades. There is no early screening test available for lung cancer. Most often,

---

■ **HEALTHY PEOPLE 2010** ■
Selected National Health Objectives for Early Cancer Detection

1. Increase the proportion of physicians and dentists who counsel their at-risk clients about tobacco use cessation, physical activity, and cancer screening. (Baseline 1998 set by behavior: 50% of internists counseled about smoking. Target: 85%. Primary care providers who counseled about stool tests: 56%. Target: 85%.)
2. Increase the proportion of women ages 40 and older who have received a mammogram within the preceding 2 years. (Baseline 1998: 67%. Target: 70%.)
3. Increase the proportion of women age 18 or older who receive a Papanicolaou (Pap) test. (Baseline 1998: 92%. Target: 97%.)
4. Increase the proportion of adults 50 years or older who receive a colorectal screening examination. (Baseline 1998: 37% of adults ages 50 years and older have fecal occult blood test within the preceding 2 years. Target: 50%.)
5. Increase the proportion of persons who use at least one of the following protective measures that may reduce the risk of skin cancer: avoid the sun between 10:00 AM and 4:00 PM, wear sun-protective clothing when exposed to sunlight, use sunscreen with a sun-protective factor (SPF) of 15 or higher, and avoid artificial sources of ultraviolet light. (Baseline 2000: 59% of adults used at least one of the protective measures. Target: 85% of adults 18 years or older.)
6. Reduce the overall cancer death rate. (Baseline 1999: 200.8 cancer deaths per 100,000. Target: 158.6 deaths per 100,000 per population.)

From U.S. Department of Health and Human Services. (2000). *Healthy People 2010.* Washington, DC: U.S. Government Printing Office; and U.S. Department of Health and Human Services. (2006). *Healthy People 2010: Midcourse review.* Washington, DC: U.S. Government Printing Office.

a patient has symptoms and the cancer has spread to other organs before diagnosis. A national health objective for the year 2010 is to slow the rise in lung cancer deaths to achieve a rate of no higher than 33 per 100,000 population (USDHHS, 2000). Progress has been made toward this goal; the death rate from lung cancer is decreasing among white and black men and slowing among women.

Breast Cancer. Except for skin cancer, breast cancer is the most commonly diagnosed type of cancer for females and the second most common cause of cancer death in women (second only to lung cancer). Age is the most significant risk factor for developing breast cancer. Other risk factors include family history, early menarche, late menopause, late or no childbearing, lengthy exposure to postmenopausal estrogen, and use of oral contraceptives. Some breast cancer risk factors can be modified, including obesity, physical inactivity, use of hormones after menopause, and consumption of one or more alcoholic beverages per day (ACS, 2006). Early diagnosis is essential to breast cancer survival. Screening efforts aimed at the early detection of breast cancer include breast self-examination, breast examination by a health professional, and mammography. In Figure 19-2, a community/public health nurse is demonstrating the correct procedure for breast self-examination to a client. Mammography is the best way of detecting breast cancer in its earliest, most treatable stage—by about 1 to 3 years before a woman would notice a lump. Timely mammography for women older than age 40 could reduce breast cancer mortality by 20% to 35%. Use of screening mammography increased rapidly between 1980 and 2000, and by the year 2000, 70% of women reported having a recent mammogram. This rate remained steady until 2003, when mammography

rates for women over age 50 began to decline. The cause of this decline has not been identified but there is concern that lack of screening could eventually lead to an increase in breast cancer mortality because fewer cancers are detected at an early stage (ACS, 2006).

Colorectal Cancer. Following lung cancer, colorectal cancer is the third leading cause of cancer deaths in the United States for both sexes, accounting for 10% of all cancer deaths (ACS, 2006). The number of new cases (incidence) has decreased steadily since 1985 and mortality from colorectal cancer has also declined. The overall national decline may be a result of greater use of screening methods and removal of polyps before they become cancer. For patients who are diagnosed early in the disease process, the 5-year survival rate is 90%. Annual fecal occult blood testing is recommended beginning at age 50 years. Also beginning at age 50, flexible sigmoidoscopic examinations are recommended every 5 years and a colonoscopy every 10 years (ACS, 2006). A national health objective for the year 2010 is to increase the proportion of adults who receive a colorectal cancer screening examination (USDHHS, 2000).

A recent development in screening for colon cancer is the use of computed tomographic (CT) colonoscopy. Known in many communities as virtual colonoscopy, the procedure involves some of the same elements of traditional colonoscopy, including a bowel prep and insertion of air into the colon for visualization. However, in the new CT colonoscopy, the client is not sedated for insertion of the endoscope but is alert for the CT scan. Because of lack of sedation, some clients report more discomfort with the new procedure (resulting from air inserted into the colon for visualization), but others prefer it, and it may be useful for clients who cannot tolerate sedation. However, an advantage of the traditional colonoscopy is being able to identify and remove small growths such as polyps, which cannot be performed with the virtual colonoscopy.

Skin Cancer. More than 1 million new cases of skin cancer occur annually, primarily in white persons. Almost 90% of these skin cancers are caused by exposure to sunlight. White males have the highest death rate from skin cancer (ACS, 2006). Early detection of skin cancer is critical. Adults should be taught how to do monthly skin self-examinations and how to examine their children and significant others. Throughout the year, organizations are asked to participate in a national skin cancer-screening program sponsored by the American Academy of Dermatology (AAD). Dermatologists volunteer their time to perform the screenings. The AAD regularly updates the website with locations of local skin cancer screening. Education on prevention including use of sunscreen and protective clothing and limited exposure to ultraviolet rays is an important component of the screening program (AAD, 2007).

Cancer and Ethnicity in the United States. The incidence and death rates from cancer are disproportionately higher in African Americans than in any other racial or ethnic group in the United States (Table 19-4). The death rate from cancer among African American males is 38% higher than among white males; for African American females, it is about 17% higher. African Americans have a higher death rate than whites for each of the major cancer sites (colorectal, male lung, female breast, and prostate) as well as a higher incidence rate for all of these cancers except female breast (ACS, 2006).

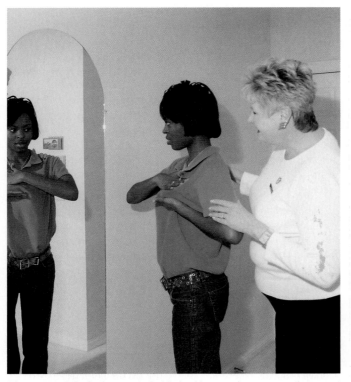

FIGURE 19-2 Community/public health nurse demonstrates the correct procedure for a breast self-examination to a client.

TABLE 19-4 Comparison of Cancer in Various Ethnic Groups		
Ethnic Group	Incidence of Cancer (All Sites) per 100,000: 1999-2003	Deaths from Cancer (All Sites) per 100,000: 1999-2003
African American	Male 640 Female 384	Male 331 Female 192
White	Male 555 Female 421	Male 239 Female 163
Asian American and Pacific Islander	Male 386 Female 303	Male 145 Female 99
American Indian and Alaskan native	Male 360 Female 305	Male 153 Female 112
Hispanic	Male 444 Female 327	Male 166 Female 109

Data from American Cancer Society. (2006). *Cancer facts and figures 2006.* Atlanta: Author. Accessed at *www.cancer.org.*

The causes of these inequalities are thought to be related to disparities in income, education, housing, and overall standard of living, and to barriers to high-quality cancer prevention, early detection, and treatment (ACS, 2006). In response to the increased incidence of cancer in this minority group, since 1987 the third week of April has been designated national "Minority Cancer Awareness Week" by the National Cancer Institute. The purpose of this event is to provide focus on minority cancer issues with an emphasis on early detection and early treatment to improve overall survival rates.

Mental Health Screening

In addition to screening for physical problems, providing screening for mental health issues is an important role for the community/public health nurse. National Depression Screening Day (NDSD), usually held in the Fall, is a cooperative national effort to provide in-person and on-line depression screening tests to identify patients with depression and to identify patients with suicidal thoughts and intentions *(http://www.mentalhealthscreening.org/).* Mental health volunteers such as psychiatrists, psychologists, nurses, and counselors meet individually with participants to administer and interpret nationally accepted screening questionnaires. Depression is prevalent among older adults but is often not recognized. Symptoms such as loneliness, sleeplessness, lethargy, and lack of interest in activities are frequently attributed to aging but may be undiagnosed as depression. Depression screening and appropriate treatment can enhance the quality of life for all age groups. The National Institute for Mental Health (NIMH) is another resource for patients experiencing other mental health problems, including anxiety, posttraumatic stress disorders, and substance abuse problems. To obtain information on National Depression Screening Day and other mental health screening, refer to the Community Resources for Practice box at the end of this chapter. Substance abuse screening is discussed in Chapter 25.

National Objectives and Recommendations

Table 19-3 presents national guidelines with parameters and times for screening common health problems in the general adult population. Box 19-1 lists screening tests that may be appropriate to administer to selected target populations based on an analysis of age and other sociodemographic risk factors.

SETTINGS FOR SCREENING

The places where screening programs are conducted vary. Individual case finding may occur in the home, clinic, or office. To access groups and populations, screening programs are frequently held in public places, such as in schools, churches, businesses, hospitals, shopping malls, community centers, apartment complexes, and mobile home parks. Such accessibility helps provide essential screening services to people where they live and work. Key to the selection of the setting should be considerations of space needed, confidentiality, equipment, and privacy. A **health fair** is a type of screening program that usually includes a large number of exhibits, resources, and services, including screening tests that are specific to the targeted population, general health information, booths and exhibits from health-related community organizations, and counseling and referral services.

For example, a community/public health nurse could plan a health fair at a local senior center. With general knowledge of the population, the nurse plans for age and culturally appropriate screenings such as blood pressure, vision, hearing, tobacco use, and depression. The nurse will need to partner with local health care organizations for referrals. The setting for the screening, the senior citizen center, would provide a familiar and accessible setting for the participants. Additionally, based on population outcomes, the nurse could target future health promotion and other healthy lifestyle events to meet the needs of the senior citizen group.

COMMUNITY/PUBLIC HEALTH NURSE'S ROLE IN SCREENING

Using the nursing process, the community/public health nurse is able to plan and implement screening programs that benefit the community being served. A process *similar* to the nursing process for community planning and health promotion is outlined on-line via the *Guide to Community Preventive Services* (Community Guide, 2007). The Community Guide is developed by a task force with members appointed by the Centers for Disease Control and Prevention who analyze scientific literature and the effectiveness and feasibility of interventions to improve community health and prevent disease.

ASSESSMENT

Initially, the community/public health nurse must determine the need for a screening program by identifying the at-risk population. Determining risk status of an individual or community is based on an analysis of sociodemographic characteristics such as age, ethnicity, cultural practices, and environmental hazards. When the community/public health nurse determines the risk status of the community, she or he is performing a community assessment to determine the needs and risks of the targeted population (see Chapter 15).

In addition to considering risks, the community/public health nurse should determine the resources available in the community. For example, what screening programs are already in place in local hospitals, senior centers, work

Box 19-1 Screening Tests for Selected Populations*

General Adult Population
Blood pressure
Lipid screening
Tobacco use screening
Colorectal cancer (stool for occult blood)
Breast cancer (breast self-examination, mammography)
Glaucoma
Visual acuity
Hearing
Diabetes (type 2 blood glucose level)
Cervical cancer (Papanicolaou smear)
Prostate cancer
Testicular cancer (testicular self-examination)
Height/weight and obesity
Dentition
Podiatry assessment (elderly population)
Mental status assessment (e.g., depression)
Skin check
Tuberculosis (Mantoux skin test with purified protein derivative [PPD])

Adolescents and Young Adults
Sexually transmitted diseases
Papanicolaou smear
Breast self-examination
Testicular self-examination
Blood pressure
Vision (ages 12, 15, and 18)
Hearing
Height/weight; body mass index
Dental health
Alcohol and drug use
Mental health (e.g., depression, schizophrenia, eating disorders)
Tuberculosis (Mantoux skin test with PPD based on risk)
Lipidemia screening (18 to 20 years or earlier if at risk)
Hematocrit or hemoglobin (based on risk)

School-Age Children
Vision

Hearing
Developmental surveillance
Blood pressure
Psychosocial/behavioral assessment
Scoliosis
Height/weight; body mass index
Tuberculosis (Mantoux skin test with PPD for patients at risk)
Dental health
Lipidemia screening (for patients at risk)
Hematocrit or hemoglobin (for patients at risk)

Preschool Children
Vision
Hearing (at 4 years or earlier if at risk)
Growth and development (e.g., Denver Developmental Screening Test [DDST], speech and language, head circumference up to age 2 years)
Psychosocial/behavioral assessment
Height/weight; body mass index (initially at 2 years)
Tuberculosis (Mantoux skin test with PPD; skin test at 1 year or earlier if at risk)
Blood pressure initially at age 3 years
Initial dental referral at age 3 years (or earlier if at risk)
Lipidemia screening (for patients at risk)
Hematocrit or hemoglobin (initially at 1 year)
Blood lead level (if at risk)
Autism screening (18 and 24 months)

Infant/Neonate
Height/weight
Growth and development (e.g., DDST, head circumference)
Psychosocial/behavioral assessment
Urinalysis
Hematocrit or hemoglobin
Phenylketonuria (PKU) test, usually indicated shortly after birth and at 2 to 4 weeks of age; testing guidelines are dictated by state law
Blood lead level at 6 to 12 months, then annually based on risk
Newborn hearing screening

Data from American Academy of Pediatrics. (2007). *Recommendations for preventive pediatric health care. AAP Policy Statement 2007-2008.* Accessed at *http://www.aap.org/visit/ prevent.htm*; and U.S. Preventive Services Task Force. (2006). *Guide to clinical preventive services, 2006.* Rockville, MD: Agency for Healthcare Research and Quality. Accessed at *http://www.ahrq.gov/clinic/pocketgd.htm.*
*In all population groups, periodic age-appropriate physical examinations are indicated.

sites, schools, faith communities, or other locations in the community? The community/public health nurse should avoid replicating existing screening programs in the community, provided that they are culturally acceptable and physically and financially accessible. If screening programs in the community are insufficient, the nurse then investigates resources for establishing new programs. (Box 19-2 lists specific questions to ask to assess community resources to support screening programs.)

Finally, assessing the appropriate time and site for conducting a screening program is important. When and where will the community/public health nurse have the most access to the target population? For example, a school would be a good place to screen for scoliosis (see **Website Resource 19A**), or a senior

housing site would be a good place to screen for hypertension. When screening large populations, estimating the number of people who will likely participate and having the necessary space and personnel to accommodate the anticipated numbers are important. If possible, requesting preregistration for specific screening tests allows more accurate arrangements for personnel, equipment, and space. In addition, clients are better prepared to participate (e.g., they would fast if registering for blood work), and the client waiting time can be reduced.

PLANNING

After assessing the community's health needs and resources, the community/public health nurse is ready to plan a screening program. Program priorities and goals need to be established

Box 19-2 Assessing Resources to Support Screening Programs

Consider the following questions when assessing resources to support a screening program:

1. Is funding available to support a health fair or a wellness program in the local community?
2. What is the cost of implementing such a program?
3. What are the personnel and equipment needs to run screening booths or health-education exhibits?
4. Is volunteer support available in the health care community to provide needed services or to loan screening equipment?
5. Are diagnostic and treatment services available to refer clients in whom presumed illness is detected?
6. What facilities are available for follow-up of persons who receive abnormal screening results?
7. Are key community leaders supportive of the program?

at the outset. To identify problems accurately and set goals that are meaningful to the community, people who are most likely to be influenced by the program should have a voice in program development. Key persons who will help secure needed resources or implement the program need to have input in the planning process, including health care personnel, volunteers, and community leaders. Persons who can help identify and overcome cultural and other barriers to accessing the program are also valuable assets.

The community/public health nurse must also design easy-to-use forms for documenting screening data. An appropriate form to obtain consent for screening is essential. A written form that documents screening test results, normal parameters, and counseling and referral information should be developed and given to the participant for use in the screening program. Figure 19-3 shows a sample form. This form should also include biographic data on the participant. Additional information such as health history data and participant health goals may also be included. The form provides the written documentation of test results and health instructions for both the participant and the provider and is important for subsequent participant follow-up and for program evaluation. The Agency for Healthcare Research and Quality (AHRQ, 2007) has developed a pocket guide for adults designed to help patients track their family history, checkups, screenings, test results, and immunizations. Any parts of this guide may be used or modified for a community health fair.

Additionally, the family health history tools previously mentioned in the discussion of screening of individuals could also be used during the health fair to collect health history data. If available at the health fair, the nurse could use a computer with Web access and collaborate with the patient to complete the form electronically, and then print the form for continued use during the health fair event, giving a copy to the patient for future reference. If the patient has e-mail at home, the nurse could also send the patient a link to the health history resource or provide the Web address for the patient to access the site independently.

National screening programs may have forms that are ready to use and based on national criteria, such as skin cancer screening, anxiety screening, or depression screening. In addition to necessary forms, procedure manuals are available for download or may be sent to the community/public nurse who is organizing a screening. These manuals include planning guidelines, sample materials, publicity materials, and follow-up information.

An occupational health nurse wants to develop a screening program for a large manufacturer. The nurse establishes a task force that consists of representation from administration, employees at all levels of the industry, and health care providers in the employee health suite.

Assess. The task force assesses the perceived health care needs of the target population, the extent of interest in conducting a workplace screening program, and the resources available to conduct the program. Health care personnel note a high incidence of hypertension in their employee health population. Workers express concern that they do not have the time to attend a screening program. The committee considers alternatives to holding a 1-day health fair during a designated time period. Management officials note that limited space and funding are available to conduct the program but that the administration is willing to schedule all employees on a rotating basis through the employee health suite for hypertension screening. Open hours are held in conjunction with the rotating schedule provided by the managers to maximize convenience and accessibility of the screening program to all interested employees. Volunteer support is solicited from outside agencies to assist in implementing the program.

Plan. The next step is to establish program goals and objectives. In this example, the task force establishes the following goal: to improve the health status of employees through early detection and treatment of hypertension. The following specific objectives are included: (1) One month following the screening program, all participants who received abnormal test results will have received follow-up diagnostic testing and treatment, if indicated. (2) In 6 months, the incidence and prevalence of hypertension will have *increased* by 5% in the target population. Note here that if a screening program is effective, the incidence and prevalence of the disease being screened for will increase because screening results in the early detection of previously unrecognized illness. (3) In 1 year, the number of days of absenteeism, number of disability days, and rate of hospitalization for illnesses resulting from complications of hypertension will decrease by 20%.

IMPLEMENTATION

After assessing the secondary prevention needs of a target population and planning a screening program to address these needs, the community/public health nurse is ready to implement a program plan. Some of the steps to implement a community screening are outlined in italic.

- *Advertise the program:* To implement a successful mass screening program, using media resources to disseminate information about the program to the community is often

Biographic Information

Date:

Participant name:

Address:

Telephone number (home, cell, work):

E-mail address:

Health History

Have you or anyone in your family ever had (circle answer):

Heart disease:	Yes	No
Cancer:	Yes	No
Anemia:	Yes	No
High blood pressure:	Yes	No
Lung disease:	Yes	No
Do you smoke?	Yes	No
(Amount:)		
Do you drink alcohol?	Yes	No
(Amount:)		

Screenings	Normal Range	Participant Result
Blood pressure	120/80 or less	(Ex: 142/88
Weight or BMI	Provide a height/BMI chart	200 lb
Cholesterol	Less than 200 mg/dl	230 mg/dl)

Participant health goals: _____

_____

_____

Recommendations and/or referrals: _____

Signature of health screener: _____

FIGURE 19-3 Sample screening form.

helpful. Flyers, mass mailings, notices on community websites, and local advertisements in newspapers or on radio and television help inform the target population of the program's existence. Press releases should be done at least several weeks in advance to ensure that information about the program is disseminated throughout the community. Information provided to the media should include the location, dates, and times of the program; services offered through the program; fees, if any, that may be required from the participant for obtaining selected screening tests or services; and any additional preparatory instructions that the client may need. For example, if blood tests are offered in the screening program, participants may need to be informed that they should fast at least 8 to 12 hours before receiving the blood test. Box 19-3 gives an example of a public service announcement.

• Another method to advertise a program or to encourage attendance is to invite participants electronically. A message about the health fair or screening event can be sent via e-mail to groups of patients. The Centers for Disease Control and Prevention (CDC, 2007d) has free e-cards on their website that can be used as reminders of health behav-

Box 19-3 Public Service Announcement

Public service announcements are messages on behalf of nonprofit groups presented like advertisements.

Advantages
Aired free by radio or television
Reach mass audience
Identify sponsoring group(s)
On television, visual aids can be used

Disadvantages
Station determines if and when message is aired
Must be presented to station several weeks before airing
Each station may have specific requirements:
   Must be brief: 30-second spot = 75 words

Content
Discuss how listeners will benefit
Give next step
Name sponsoring groups
Tell listeners to call for more information

Example of 45-Second Announcement
Would you like to know what your blood pressure is? Has it been a while since you had your vision checked? If so, come to the health fair on Saturday, April 18, Valley View Mall from 1:00 to 8:30 PM. The health department and the Junior Chamber of Commerce are sponsoring this health fair for you, your friends, and your family. Representatives from many health groups will be on hand to conduct screening tests and teach you how to improve your health! For more information call (123) 123-4567.

---

iors or invitations to health screening events. The cards may be customized with personal greetings to remind high-risk individuals of health events, or may provide specific health information.

- *Identify and train screeners:* Partnerships may be formed with volunteer and community organizations, health care providers, and other interested persons to assist with program implementation. For example, members of organizations whose goal is to do community service can be trained in clinical services and assist in ongoing programs. Other good resources are retired nurses who wish to remain active in the community and nursing students from local schools of nursing. Persons who administer selected screening tests may need to be trained in test administration. A training session may need to be conducted with persons who will be administering selected screening tests to ensure accuracy in test measurement and to improve reliability of test findings. Training may occur at a time separate from the actual program date, or persons may be asked to arrive an hour or two earlier on the date of the program to review procedures.

- *Set up the site:* The site where the program is to be held will often need to be set up to accommodate the anticipated number of participants and to provide tables, chairs, or other equipment for service providers. A good practice for morning screenings is to set up the evening before. Consideration must also be given to persons with disabilities to ensure access to all stations. Booths may be set up so that persons can move in a logical manner from station to station as they make their way toward the exit. A public-address system may be used to direct the flow of traffic. When the program begins, the community/public health nurse should be available to circulate among stations and to address any last-minute problems, such as screeners or providers who do not attend as planned. In this instance, the community/public health nurse may need to reorganize service providers to fill in gaps and to run selected stations during peak service times.

- *Consider space needs:* The facility in which the program is conducted should be capable of accommodating a large number of people in terms of both space and restroom facilities. An exception to this rule is the use of mobile vans, which bring screening services directly to neighborhoods, schools, or work sites. Although schools, places for worship, workplaces, malls, and community centers are usually equipped to deal with large aggregates, remember that the program may draw more people than some facilities can accommodate.

- *Be ready for case finding:* Another potential problem is the discovery of a severely abnormal test result. Also important is to have established protocols for emergency intervention—such as finding a blood pressure of 240/130 mm Hg in a participant—so it is clear to all providers when immediate referral to another care source is indicated. Referral guidelines may be based on national criteria, such as those listed in Table 19-3. Participants should not leave the screening until they have secured the telephone number of a health provider who is appropriate to handle their identified problems.

- *Feed the workers and the participants:* Nutrition is an important consideration when conducting a mass screening program. If the program is scheduled for the entire day, persons working in the program will need meals and rest breaks. Local businesses or restaurants may provide free lunches as a community service or in exchange for advertising. If blood tests are part of the screening program, participants may be required to fast the night before; and afterward, orange juice, graham crackers, or healthy snacks should be provided.

- *Plan to follow up:* At the completion of the program, the community/public health nurse may wish to tally the number of forms received (indicating the number of participants attending). Forms may be numbered ahead of time for ease in counting. At times, participants leave with their forms, making a tally of participants difficult. One way to overcome this problem is to have the consent for screening form signed and retained at the registration table. This action serves the purpose of a tally of participants and also is a legally responsible practice. Forms should be sorted so that persons with abnormal test results are placed in a separate file for subsequent follow-up. In a case in which screening test results are not known at the completion of the program (e.g., laboratory blood tests that may take several days or weeks to process), a mechanism for follow-up is needed to ensure that participants receive the screening results. One idea may be to ask the participant to self-address an envelope at the registration table. Laboratory results with a letter of explanation are sent to the participant as soon as possible.

EVALUATION

Evaluation, an essential component of screening programs, is conducted to justify continued program operation and funding from outside parties, to improve service delivery, or to determine the impact of the program on community health. Program evaluation enables the community/public health nurse to determine whether the benefits of the program outweigh the cost of time, money, and resources devoted to the program and will help the nurse plan or change (or both) the screening for the next implementation date. Evaluation includes both *process* and *outcome* dimensions (see Chapter 17).

Outcome evaluation refers to the actual end results of the program. Were program objectives achieved? Common outcome criteria for screening programs reflect epidemiologic trends such as an increased incidence and prevalence of disease (note that a secondary prevention measure, when effective, actually increases the number of reported cases of disease), increased numbers of persons receiving medical care, decreased mortality from disease, reduced disability and decreased incidence of advanced disease complications, and decreased health care costs for treatment of advanced disease.

Process evaluation focuses on actual program performance, regardless of whether the goals that have been set for the program are achieved. Process evaluation may include the number of people served by the program, number of volunteer hours needed to conduct the program, reliability and validity of screening tests, efficiency in test administration and reporting of results to participants, and choice of appropriate location and timing of program in terms of community interest and convenience to community members. The community/public health nurse may also consider a follow-up survey of participants, feedback from service providers who worked the screening program, and feedback from community agencies to which referrals from the screening program were made.

SCREENING AND THE REFERRAL PROCESS

Referral, an essential component of any screening program, is the process of directing persons to resources to meet needs. Clients who participate in a screening program must obtain appropriate counseling and referral for follow-up of any abnormal test results. *It is considered unethical to obtain data indicating an individual might be ill and then do nothing about it.* A separate counseling and referral station is often provided in a health fair setting, and participants are required to move through this station before leaving the health fair. At the counseling and referral station, trained volunteers review all the findings from the health fair with the participant, reinforcing appropriate health-maintenance activities and ensuring that the participant understands the meaning of his or her test results, including the need for follow-up evaluation, if indicated. An alternative method for referral and counseling is to have these activities completed at each health fair station by the personnel performing the screening. For example, a nurse screening

for hypertension can use national guidelines to counsel and refer clients to a medical care provider and can provide health-education materials.

Participants must be advised that a screening program is not a substitute for receiving ongoing health supervision from a health care provider. In many screening programs, participants are given written information that highlights this fact. Believing that they have been checked over and found healthy is not uncommon for persons who participate in screening programs.

ESTABLISHING CRITERIA FOR REFERRAL

The community/public health nurse uses outcome-based clinical evidence to establish guidelines for initiating referrals. Screening test results that fall outside of normal parameters and require follow-up evaluation indicate the need for referral. For example, any participant with a blood pressure reading of 140/90 mm Hg or higher, or a serum cholesterol level of 200 mg/dl or higher, should be referred for follow-up. A good practice for clients with results that are significantly outside acceptable parameters is for the nurse to place a follow-up telephone call in addition to the initial referral. Mechanisms for this quality level of follow-up should be part of the planning process.

ESTABLISHING A RESOURCE DIRECTORY

Participants who have identified needs that require further intervention are referred to organizations and programs in the community that provide the needed services. When possible, clients should be given a choice of providers if more than one exists. The community/public health nurse planning a mass screening program should maintain a list of community health organizations and programs for referral. Information on community resources may be obtained through local and state health departments, local and state medical societies, national organizations, local information and referral centers, police and fire departments, libraries, local government offices, or the local chamber of commerce. A community/public health nurse may want to keep her or his own personal directory, which may be as simple as a pocket-sized personal telephone book or a notebook or as sophisticated as a palm-sized personal electronic organizer.

The nurse's directory should be kept up to date and include (1) the name, address, and telephone number of the agency; (2) hours of operation; (3) major services provided; (4) eligibility requirements for utilization of services; (5) procedure for activating services; (6) source of funding for the program and payment mechanisms; (7) the name of the director or head of the agency and names of other important contact persons; and (8) a statement reflecting the general impressions received when interacting with the agency.

When possible, health information from local resources should be available at the health screening. Table 19-5 presents a possible way to organize and present community resource information to participants of a health screening.

INVESTIGATING PROCEDURE FOR INITIATING REFERRAL

Whether it is in the context of case finding or a mass screening program, the community/public health nurse should be aware

TABLE 19-5　Presenting Community Resource Information to Participants of a Health Screening

Agency name	Community Heart Health	Family Mission Care	Health Care for the Homeless
Location	1 West Street	Mobile van parked at various locations; schedule available	Lost Souls Outreach Center
Phone	(800) 222-1234	Call location announced for details	(330) 678-0000
Hours	M-F, 8 AM to 2 PM	M, W, F, 3 PM to 8 PM	Fri, Sat, Sun, 10 AM to 4 PM
Services provided	Wellness, prevention, diet counseling, exercise groups	Prevention, counseling, family planning, stop smoking group classes	Urgent care
How to initiate referral	Self-referral accepted	Must be referred by community health nurse or church leader	No referral needed
Service eligibility	WIC recipients, family income at or below poverty level	Residents of Cook or Baker Counties unable to purchase health insurance; services designed for working poor	Homeless
Payment mechanisms	$5 per individual visit, $2 per exercise class or counseling group	Donations accepted	Medical assistance, Medicare
Name of contact person	Ms. Carly Vessel	Mr. Kindly	Ms. Outreach Worker

of the procedure for initiating referrals to a recipient agency or organization. For example, can the client or the health care provider make a referral over the telephone? Does the referral need to be in writing? Must specific forms be completed? Ideally, a helpful practice is to give the client the name of a contact person in the agency that may be able to direct the client appropriately through the correct procedures for obtaining needed services.

DETERMINING CRITERIA FOR SERVICE ELIGIBILITY

The criteria for service eligibility should be assessed before initiating a referral because some agencies have specific criteria for accepting clients. For example, local health departments will often serve only the residents of a particular locale or region. Local departments of aging provide services to elderly residents. Some government programs, such as medical assistance, are provided only to clients who meet specific eligibility criteria, such as income level, verification of need, age, or other health criteria.

INVESTIGATING PAYMENT MECHANISMS

The community/public health nurse should also be aware of payment mechanisms that referral agencies require. For example, does the agency accept Medicare or medical assistance as payment in full? Do fees need to be paid immediately on delivery of the service? A working knowledge of the policies and procedures of the agency to which the client is being referred can assist the community/public health nurse in making more appropriate referrals based on the client's unique needs and resources. The client is also better informed of the agency's practices and is more likely to have realistic expectations of what services the agency is capable of providing. If the client is not eligible for services owing to an inability to pay, the nurse may need to seek out other resources in the community, such as philanthropic or service organizations, to assist with payment. Civic groups

such as the Lions Club, Rotary, or Knights of Columbus may provide donations or financial support to a client in need.

ASSESSING CLIENT RECEPTIVITY

The community/public health nurse also needs to assess the client's receptivity to the referral. Is the referral acceptable to the client and likely to be followed up? Has the client had a previous negative experience with the agency to which she or he is being referred? What has the client been told about her or his role in the referral? Does the client have particular beliefs, values, or cultural biases that prevent her or him from using the services of the agency? Additional barriers to acceptance of a referral may include differences in perception of needs between client and health care provider, lack of transportation to access the program or service, competing demands and responsibilities (e.g., childcare, working hours) that make it difficult for the client to establish contact and keep appointments with the agency, or inadequate finances to pay for needed services.

EVALUATING EFFECTIVENESS OF REFERRAL

People who are referred for additional services should be contacted after the screening program to see whether they followed through with the referral. The nurse can call the client referred to discuss her or his satisfaction with the referral agency. To assist the community/public health nurse in establishing and maintaining a resource directory, if this is the first time the nurse has referred a client to the agency or service, a follow-up call to the agency is also useful. The nurse calls to discuss the appropriateness of the referral and suggestions for the future. Of special concern during this call is client privacy. The nurse must be careful to discuss the referral process without compromising confidentiality. Information gathered about the referral process will enhance future referral practices (Table 19-6).

TABLE 19-6	Evaluating the Effectiveness of a Referral

Name of Agency: _____

Questions	Yes	No	Comments
To Ask the Patient:			
Were you able to access care? If not, what barriers did you experience?			
Did you have problems with payment?			
Did the services provided meet your expectations?			
Were you treated with dignity and respect?			
Did you need additional services not offered by this agency?			
Would you return to this agency for additional services?			
To Ask the Agency:			
Did the patient bring enough background information from the health fair to assist with establishing service?			
Was the referral appropriate? If not, why not?			
Were additional needs identified that this agency was not able to meet? What were they?			
Do you have any recommendations for future processing of referrals?			

KEY IDEAS

1. Screening is an important secondary prevention strategy. The purpose of screening is to detect diseases in an early stage of development when they are more amenable to treatment.
2. The settings for administering screening interventions are diverse and variable and depend on the client focus. Screening programs may be geared toward individuals or populations.
3. Case finding is the application of screening tests to individuals on a one-on-one basis.
4. Mass screening is the application of screening tests to large groups or populations.
5. Consider the following questions when selecting screening tests:
   - How significant is the disease being screened for?
   - What is the cost versus benefit of screening?
   - How acceptable is the test to participants?
   - What is the test's reliability and validity?
   - Is the test easy to administer?
   - Does the test detect disease at an early stage?
   - Is treatment available for the disease being screened for?

6. To determine what diseases should be screened for in a community, the community/public health nurse assesses the major health risks in the target population and the available constraints to and resources for implementing a screening program. Goals and objectives that specify desired outcome criteria for the screening program are developed.
7. The community/public health nurse implements the screening program in partnership with community members, volunteers, and health care providers.
8. Evaluation of the effectiveness of a screening program is based on analysis of epidemiologic data and feedback from participants and collaborating agencies.
9. Every screening program must include counseling and referral services. The community/public health nurse coordinating a screening program must provide for participant follow-up to ensure that referrals were followed up and that the client received the appropriate therapeutic intervention.
10. In making referrals, the community/public health nurse must investigate the procedure for initiating referrals, determine criteria for service eligibility, assess client receptivity, investigate payment mechanisms, and evaluate the effectiveness of the referral.

THE NURSING PROCESS IN PRACTICE ▶ Organizing a Health Fair and Case Finding

ORGANIZING A HEALTH FAIR

A community/public health nurse is assigned to a geographic district in which a large elderly population resides. Her experience with home visits to clients reveals that many of the elderly residents in the community regularly attend the local senior center and are very interested in maintaining personal health and fitness. However, because they live on a fixed income, these elderly residents are having difficulty meeting their basic living expenses. Because of financial constraints, many clients hesitate to see their personal health care providers unless they become ill; they also cite difficulty

with transportation as a major deterrent to seeking routine preventive health care.

Based on an analysis of sociodemographic risk factors, the community/public health nurse determines that this population is at risk of illness from chronic diseases, such as hypertension, heart disease, stroke, and cancer. Because many of these diseases can be prevented or treated effectively if diagnosed early, the community health nurse decides to conduct a health fair. She selects the local senior center as the desirable location for the fair because it is highly accessible and well used by the target population.

PLANNING

In planning the fair, the nurse obtains the help of key community leaders, the director of the senior center, and senior residents in the community who will likely benefit from the program. These individuals meet as a planning committee and identify program goals, resources, and constraints. The general goal for the screening program is to promote and maintain the health of elderly residents in the community through early detection and treatment of disease.

The director of the senior center indicates that members of the center would be willing to volunteer their services to assist with implementing the program. The community/public health nurse investigates the extent of support from others in the health care community and requests the help of local nursing students. The community/public health nurse selects appropriate screening tests to administer based on cost factors, client acceptance, availability, and reliability. She decides to conduct screenings for hypertension, diabetes, glaucoma, vision, hearing, podiatry, colorectal cancer, height and weight, and cholesterol level. In addition, volunteers from the local chapters of the ACS and the AHA are asked to participate and run booths with information on heart disease, hypertension, brain attack, nutrition and cholesterol, breast self-examination, mammography, and prostate and colon cancers.

Other local community and health organizations are invited to participate and to distribute information. The local chapter of the American Association of Retired Persons and the local department of aging are asked to explain their programs, services, and resources. Equipment for vision examinations is provided by the Society for the Prevention of Blindness. A local audiologist agrees to conduct hearing screenings. A local medical laboratory agrees to administer blood tests for cholesterol level and diabetes. The local chapter of the American Diabetes Association is also asked to participate and provide health-education literature.

The community/public health nurse establishes a list of community resources and guidelines for counseling and referring participants in the screening program who have abnormal screening test results. Guidelines for referral are based on nationally established criteria for normal test results. Nursing students at the local university are asked to conduct blood pressure screening and to run the counseling and referral station. Criteria are established for the students to make urgent referrals to health care providers.

IMPLEMENTATION

The community/public health nurse asks that health fair workers arrive early on the day of the fair for a general orientation. At this time, the discovery is made that the representative from the local chapter of the department of aging is ill and will be unable to attend. The community/public health nurse modifies her original plan; she provides persons at the counseling and referral station with the address and telephone number for general information on the department of aging for distribution to interested residents. She also calls the department of aging and investigates the possibility of obtaining some literature to be delivered via courier before the health fair begins.

EVALUATION

During the health fair, the community/public health nurse circulates between stations to assess progress and address any problems that may develop. At the completion of the health fair, participants are asked to complete an evaluation form, indicating their satisfaction with the health fair.

After the health fair, the community/public health nurse compiles a list of participants with abnormal test results and conducts follow-up telephone calls 2 to 3 weeks later to determine whether individuals have followed through with counseling and referral recommendations. For individuals who have not followed through, she makes an effort to identify barriers to care and then attempts to empower the client to overcome these barriers.

Six months after the health fair, the community/public health nurse surveys all participants to gather data on the impact of the screening program on health status. She notes that participants report greater awareness of the need for early detection. Several participants indicate that because of the screenings, previously unrecognized diseases such as hypertension, diabetes, and glaucoma were detected and treated early. These participants report no complications from advanced disease and believe that early detection greatly improved their current health status. In addition, the community/public health nurse surveys the nurse practitioner in the senior center's medical clinic to obtain feedback on perceived helpfulness of the mass screening program. The nurse practitioner reports an increased incidence of hypertension and diabetes owing to early detection but a decrease in mortality and disability from complications of advanced disease states. Based on the positive evaluation findings, the community/public health nurse recommends that the local department of aging hold health fairs for the elderly population in the community at convenient and accessible locations on an annual basis.

CASE FINDING

A nurse practitioner works in an employee health clinic at a steel plant. A 52-year-old African American male client comes in for an employee health physical. The client states that he is in good health and denies symptoms of illness, but his family has a history of stroke, heart disease, and diabetes. He acknowledges smoking three packs of cigarettes a day for 20 years. Based on an analysis of individual risk factors, the nurse practitioner performs a comprehensive physical examination, with special emphasis on blood pressure status and cardiac, respiratory, and peripheral vascular assessments. In addition, she monitors blood glucose and serum lipid levels and performs an electrocardiogram. Based on these screening tests, the nurse practitioner finds that the client is overweight and has elevated blood pressure and serum cholesterol and serum glucose levels. The electrocardiogram is within normal limits. The client is counseled regarding his risk factors and is referred to his medical provider for follow-up diagnosis and treatment.

The nurse practitioner contacts the client 1 week later to assess whether the client has followed through in seeking medical evaluation. The client reports that he returned to his medical provider and was placed on a low-fat diabetic diet and an exercise program. In addition, he reports being referred to a smoking-cessation program.

Three months later, the nurse practitioner sees the client for a follow-up employee health check. The client reports adhering to his prescribed regimen and feeling more energetic and less fatigued. With the client's permission, the nurse practitioner contacts the client's provider, who reports that the client's blood glucose and serum cholesterol levels and blood pressure have all returned to normal limits and that the client has lost 10 pounds. He continues to smoke but has reduced his consumption to one pack of cigarettes per day.

LEARNING BY EXPERIENCE AND REFLECTION

1. Select a family member, client, or group in your community (e.g., members of a faith community, members of an organization to which you belong). Assess the risk factors in the chosen individual or group. Identify screening tests that would be appropriate to administer to this individual or group based on the criteria for selecting screening tests outlined in the chapter.

2. Interview a friend or family member on her or his perception of the meaning and value of screening and early diagnosis of disease in personal health. To what extent does this individual engage in secondary prevention? When was the last time she or he had a physical examination or other recommended screening tests, considering individual risk factors? What motivates the individual to take advantage of health screenings? What barriers prevent her or him from complying with general recommendations for health screening?

3. Compare perceptions of the value of screening between individuals from different socioeconomic or cultural backgrounds. Do similarities or differences exist? What do you think accounts for the differences?

4. Analyze your own personal risk factors for developing illnesses that are amenable to early detection and treatment (e.g., heart disease, cancer, diabetes). Consider demographic variables and personal and family health history in your risk assessment. What screening recommendations are applicable to you? To what extent are you compliant with these screening recommendations? What factors have an impact on your decision to seek screening services?

5. Reflect on a time when you were referred for assistance in meeting an unmet need. What was the nature of the referral? What was it like for you to be referred? To what extent did you follow through on the referral? What affected your decision making and behavior related to your acceptance of the referral? What was the outcome of the referral?

6. A community/public health nurse working in a hypertension screening clinic discovers a client with dramatically high blood pressure. In attempting to make a referral for follow-up care, the nurse discovers that the client has no financial access to treatment. In what way does this situation constitute an ethical dilemma for the nurse? What can the nurse do to resolve this dilemma?

7. Select an article from the nursing literature that discussed the evaluation of a screening program. Identify the methods used to evaluate the program, the desired outcomes, and the actual outcomes. In what ways would you have evaluated the program differently?

COMMUNITY RESOURCES FOR PRACTICE

Information about each organization listed here is found on its website, which can be accessed through the **WebLinks** section of the book's website at *http://evolve.elsevier.com/Maurer/community/*.

Agency for Healthcare Research and Quality (AHRQ)
American Heart Association
Centers for Disease Control and Prevention
   Electronic health cards
   Family history tool
Centers for Disease Control and Prevention, National Center for Chronic Disease Prevention and Health Promotion
Guide to Community Preventive Services
National Heart, Lung, and Blood Institute
National Institute of Mental Health
National Scoliosis Foundation
Screening for Mental Health
U.S. Preventive Services Task Force

STUDY AIDS   http://evolve.elsevier.com/Maurer/community/

Visit the Evolve website for this book to find the following study and assessment materials:

- Quiz
- Web Scenario
- Critical Thinking Questions and Answers for Case Studies
- Care Plans
- *Healthy People* Updates
- Glossary

WEBSITE RESOURCES

These items supplement the chapter's topics and are also found on the Evolve site:

19A: What Is Scoliosis?

REFERENCES

Agency for Healthcare Research and Quality. (2007). *Pocket guide for adults.* Retrieved August 29, 2007, from *http://www.ahrq.gov/clinic/ppipix.htm*.

American Academy of Dermatology. (2007). *Skin cancer fact sheet.* Retrieved August 2007 from *www.aad.org*.

American Academy of Pediatrics. (2000). *Recommendations for preventive pediatric health care. AAP Policy Statement 2000.* Accessed at *http://www.aap.org/visit/prevent.htm*.

American Academy of Pediatrics. (2007). *Recommendations for preventive pediatric health care. AAP Policy Statement 2007-2008.* Retrieved March 28, 2008, from *http://www.aap.org/visit/prevent.htm*.

American Cancer Society. (2006). *Cancer facts and figures 2006.* Atlanta: Author. Retrieved August 2007 from *www.cancer.org*.

American Cancer Society. (2007). *Cancer facts and figures. Screening guidelines.* Available online at *www.cancer.org*.

American Diabetes Association. (2007). *All about diabetes.* Available at *www.diabetes.org*.

American Heart Association. (2007a). *Family history tree.* Retrieved March 28, 2008, from *http://www.americanheart.org/presenter.jhtml?identifier=3044888*.

American Heart Association. (2007b). *High blood cholesterol and other lipids—Statistics. 2007 update.* Accessed August 21, 2007, from *http://jamielangley.com/High%20Blood%20Pressure%20and%20High%20Cholesterol.pdf.*

Centers for Disease Control and Prevention. (2005). *Preventing chronic diseases: Investing wisely in health. Preventing heart disease and stroke.* Accessed August 21, 2007, at *www.cdc.gov/nccdphp.*

Centers for Disease Control and Prevention. (2007a). Tools to use for documenting family health history. Retrieved August 21, 2007, from *www.cdc.gov/genomics/public/famhist.htm.*

Centers for Disease Control and Prevention. (2007b). *Quick facts: Economic and health burden of chronic disease.* Accessed August 21, 2007, at *http://cdc.gov/nccdphp/press/.*

Centers for Disease Control and Prevention. (2007c). *Division for Heart Disease and Stroke Prevention. Addressing the nation's leading killers. At a glance 2007.* Accessed August 21, 2007, at *http://cdc.gov/nccdphp/publications/AAG/dhdsp.htm.*

Centers for Disease Control and Prevention. (2007d). *Electronic card reminders.* Retrieved August 21, 2007, from *www.2a.cdc.gov/ecards/.*

Community Guide. (2007). *Guide to community preventive services.* Accessed August 21, 2007, from *www.thecommunityguide.org/.*

National Cholesterol Education Program. (2007). *Guidelines for clinical preventive services.* Washington, DC: National Heart, Lung and Blood Institute, National Institutes of Health. Accessed August 2007 at *www.nhlbi.nih.gov/guidelines.*

National Guideline Clearinghouse. (2002). *Summary of policy recommendations for periodic health examinations.* Rockville, MD: Agency for Healthcare Research and Quality, U.S. Department of Health and Human Services. Retrieved March 28, 2008, from *http://www.guideline.gov/browse/guideline_index.aspx.*

National Heart, Lung and Blood Institute. (2004). *The seventh report of the Joint National Committee on detection, evaluation, and treatment of high blood pressure.* Accessed August 2007 at *http://www.nhlbi.nih.gov/guidelines/hypertension/jnc7full.pdf.*

National Heart, Lung and Blood Institute. (2007). *Obesity education initiative: AIM for a healthy weight.* Bethesda, MD: National Institutes of Health. Accessed August 29, 2007, at *www.nhlbi.nih.gov.*

Standards of Medical Care in Diabetes, American Diabetes Association. (2007). *Diabetes Care, 30,* S4-41. Accessed August 2007 at *http://care.diabetesjournals.org.*

U.S. Department of Health and Human Services. (1993). *TB facts for health care workers.* Washington, DC: U.S. Government Printing Office.

U.S. Department of Health and Human Services. (2000). *Healthy People 2010.* Washington, DC: U.S. Government Printing Office. Accessed August 2007 at *www.healthypeople.gov.*

U.S. Department of Health and Human Services. (2006). *Healthy People 2010: Midcourse review.* Accessed August 2007 at *www.healthypeople.gov/data/midcourse.*

U.S. Preventive Services Task Force. (2006). *Guide to clinical preventive services, 2006.* Accessed August 2007 at *http://www.ahrq.gov/clinic.*

Wewers, M. E., Sarna, L., & Rice, V. H. (2006). Nursing research and treatment of tobacco dependence: State of the science. *Nursing Research, 55*(4, Suppl. 1), S11-S15.

SUGGESTED READINGS

Loerzel, V. W., & Bushy, A. (2005). Interventions that address cancer health disparities in women. *Family and Community Health, 28*(1), 79-89.

McClellan, L., & Schlundt, D. (2006). Overview of Nashville REACH 2010's approach to eliminating disparities in diabetes and cardiovascular disease. *The Journal of Ambulatory Care Management, 29*(2), 106-111.

Phillips, K. A., Liang, S., Ladabaum, U., et al. (2007). Trends in colonoscopy for colorectal cancer screening. *Medical Care, 45*(2), 160-167.

Wilensky, S., & Roby, D. H. (2005). Health centers and health insurance: Complements, not alternatives. *The Journal of Ambulatory Care Management, 28*(4), 348-356.

20 Health Teaching

Gail L. Heiss

FOCUS QUESTIONS

What is the distinction between patient education and health education?

How do the *Healthy People 2010* objectives and the *Midcourse Review* data affect the role of the community/public health nurse?

How does the community/public health nurse identify health education needs?

What impact do the community environment and culture have on these learning needs?

What teaching strategies should the nurse use with the identified target group for education?

How does the nurse determine the appropriateness of educational aids such as print, audiovisual, or Internet materials for the learners?

How will the nurse know whether the teaching strategies have been effective?

What community resources are available to enhance health education?

CHAPTER OUTLINE

KEY TERMS

Andragogy
Behavioral objectives
Health education
Health literacy

Low literacy
Outcome evaluation
Patient education
PRECEDE model

Self-efficacy
SMOG
Teaching-learning process

The concept and practice of teaching clients in the community have been evolving since the days of Lillian Wald and continue to change with the profession of nursing. Today, individuals and families expect to be more involved in decisions about health care, and they want to learn about illness prevention and behavioral changes required to maintain health and an active lifestyle.

This chapter provides the community/public health nurse with the concepts and tools needed to develop and implement community health education programs. With the opportunity for health education, members of the community will have the resources and support to strive for personal, family, and community health.

HEALTH TEACHING PROCESS

DEFINITIONS
Patient Education

Differentiating between patient education and health education is helpful. The term **patient education** is normally used to describe a series of planned teaching-learning activities designed for individuals, families, or groups who have an identified alteration in health. The nurse uses a systematic process to assess patient learning needs that relate to the health problem and then implements the teaching plan to accomplish changes in attitude or behavior (Redman, 1997).

Health Education

Health education focuses on health promotion and disease prevention. The role of the community/public health nurse includes educating and empowering people to avoid disease, to make lifestyle changes, and to improve health for themselves, their families, the environment, and their community. The difference between patient education and health education is that health education is directed toward individuals or populations who are *not* experiencing an acute alteration in health. Community assessment identifies individuals, families, groups, and populations who would benefit from additional information on healthy behaviors and healthy lifestyles. The effectiveness of health education as it relates to the population of the United States is measured in the *Healthy People 2010* report (U.S. Department of Health and Human Services [USDHHS], 2000) and monitored through regular data collection and review as in the *Healthy People 2010 Midcourse Review* (USDHHS, 2006). Changes seen in the midcourse review are based on data collected through an interactive database known as DATA2010. DATA2010 was developed by the Health Promotion Statistics Branch of the National Center for Health Statistics and contains national and state data (USDHHS, 2000, 2006). See the *Healthy People 2010* box on this page.

POLICIES
Quad Council of Public Health Nursing Organizations

The Quad Council of Public Health Nursing Organizations collaborated to produce *Public Health Nursing: Scope and Standards of Practice* (American Nurses Association [ANA], 2007), which outlines health education and the provision of teaching-learning opportunities as a distinct intervention by the community/public health nurse. Health education interventions may be conducted with individuals, families, and groups in health care institutions, homes, schools, communities, and the workplace. Health education nursing interventions are often implemented in partnership with community members, community leaders, and other health care providers.

Financial Reimbursement

Nurses quite possibly have the greatest opportunity to implement educational programs because of the extensive amount of time they spend with individuals and families in the community. Currently, the structure of insurance companies in the United States is based on reimbursement for illness care rather than for wellness promotion. Reimbursement is available for physician-ordered education relating to existing illness such as diabetes management. A disappointing note is that, in many instances, no method exists for direct reimbursement of the nurse who provides health promotion education to the community. However, current practices in primary care settings provide opportunities for nurses to combine health promotion education with required health screenings to detect or prevent disease.

■ HEALTHY PEOPLE 2010 ■
Objectives Relevant to Health Education

Physical Activity and Fitness
1. Increase to 75% the proportion of work sites offering employer-sponsored activity and fitness programs. (Baseline, 1999: 46% of work sites offered physical activity or fitness programs at the work site or through health plans.)

Nutrition
2. Increase to at least 85% the proportion of work sites with 50 or more employees that offer nutrition education or weight-management programs. (Baseline, 1999: 55% offered nutrition or weight management classes. Midcourse trends show that adults who are overweight or obese increased from 23% to 30%.)

Tobacco Use
3. Increase the number of tribes, territories, and states and the District of Columbia with comprehensive evidence-based tobacco-control programs. (No baseline available. Midcourse data available demonstrate the improved availability of a network of national quit lines and other smoking cessation tools.)

Family Planning
4. Increase the proportion of young adults who have received formal instruction before turning 18 years of age on reproductive health issues, including all of the following topics: birth control methods, safer sex to prevent human immunodeficiency virus infection, prevention of sexually transmitted diseases, and abstinence. (Baseline, 1995: 64% of women had received instruction. Target: 90%. No data for men.)

Educational and Community-Based Programs
5. Increase the proportion of all employees who participate in employer-sponsored health promotion activities. (Baseline, 1994: 61%. Target: 75%. Midcourse review [−38%] showed movement away from the target.)
6. Increase the proportion of older adults who have participated during the preceding year in at least one organized health promotion program. (Baseline, 1998: 12%. Target: 90%.)
7. Increase the proportion of tribal and local health service areas and jurisdictions that have established a community health promotion initiative that addresses multiple *Healthy People 2010* focus areas. (No current baseline.)
8. Increase the proportion of local health departments that have established culturally appropriate and linguistically competent community health promotion and disease prevention programs for racial and ethnic minority populations. (Measurement based on various program topics [i.e., for tobacco cessation]. Baseline, 1997: 24%. Target for culturally appropriate tobacco cessation programs: 50%.)

Adapted from U.S. Department of Health and Human Services. (2000). *Healthy people 2010*. Washington, DC: U.S. Government Printing Office; and U.S. Department of Health and Human Services. (2006). *Healthy people 2010: Midcourse review*. Retrieved July 31, 2007 from *http://www.healthypeople.gov/data/midcourse/*.

Community educational programs are sometimes offered to the community for a fee. Individuals who value self-care and health will often pay out of pocket for educational programs such as weight management or childbirth education. In this case, the nurse does receive payment for teaching and preparation time. Unfortunately, people who cannot afford to pay for educational services are excluded.

Some nurses provide health education as a part of their jobs, such as nurses working for managed care organizations, and are reimbursed with a salary. This group may also include occupational health nurses, school nurses, and nurses in the traditional public health setting. In addition to planning group education, public health nurses often have a caseload of families and individuals who need direct care and home visits. Careful time management is required for planning and implementing health education.

EXPANDING OPPORTUNITIES

In today's health care delivery system, the community/public health nurse has unique opportunities to shape the future. A growing emphasis has been placed on the allocation of resources to consumer health education for health promotion and disease prevention and nursing opportunities outside of the traditional hospital roles. Nurse entrepreneurs can use the public demand for health education to develop and market educational programs that meet population needs. Nurses who work in community health agencies can use the health education trends to expand their job descriptions and advance professionally. Nurses can also work politically to influence public policy regarding development and funding of health education programs.

Health promotion through health education and utilization of resources is also of interest to the nurse in the occupational setting. The occupational nurse can work with distinct groups to assess health needs and provide education on topics such as stress management, smoking cessation, nutrition, exercise, and weight management. The nurse is also an important link between employees and community resources.

RESEARCH RESULTS: WHAT WORKS IN CLIENT HEALTH EDUCATION?

Research on health education has been extensive. Some of the most prominent public health research regarding individuals' adherence to health promotion activities was initiated in the 1950s by Becker, Hochbaum, Kegeles, and Rosenstock (see Rosenstock, 1974; see also Chapter 18). According to the research of these authors, participation in prevention activities such as educational programs will influence health behaviors.

MULTIPLE TOOLS AND METHODS

No doubt, health education works, and actual changes in behavior and attitudes occur after health education interventions. Health education includes a variety of strategies, such as lecturing, storytelling, modeling, and providing printed or audiovisual materials. Also available are technology-based educational opportunities including telehealth conferencing and counseling of inidividuals on how to identify reliable health-related Internet sites. All of these methods are effective in increasing skills or knowledge level.

Continued research is needed concerning the effectiveness of group versus individual instruction and the effectiveness of technology-based learning. Cost-saving efforts in health care delivery are a priority. A meta-analysis of web-based versus non–web-based interventions (Wantland et al., 2004) and an article on the effectiveness of videoconferencing as a method of providing patient education (Winters & Winters, 2007) indicated that the use of technology both is cost effective and leads to favorable patient health outcomes.

INDIVIDUALIZATION AND THE ADULT LEARNER

Individual characteristics such as age, social status, cultural attributes, and educational level influence teaching effectiveness and long-term health behaviors. Standard lecture methods that do not consider these or other individual differences may be ineffective in teaching health promotion and self-care. Therefore, the educational program should be individualized to meet the learner's needs.

The nurse needs to assess the learner's teaching-learning style. Clients may prefer to learn by reading, watching videotapes, viewing a demonstration, or listening and then attempting new behaviors. The match between learning style and the nurse's ability to meet the learner's needs will affect how well people learn. Assessment of **andragogy,** or the teaching-learning style, is most important in the process of teaching adults.

Adults learn best when they are actively involved, when the information is repeated, when prompt feedback is received, and when the adult attaches importance to the topic (Knowles, 1980) (Table 20-1). Learners remember best what is taught first, so the use of focusing activities early in the education session is important. Other strategies that are useful when teaching adults include the following:

- Relate the content to life experiences
- Focus on real-world problems
- Relate the activities to learner-focused goals
- Teach what the learner wants to know before you continue (the learner will not be able to focus on instruction if his question is not answered when asked)
- Listen to and respect the opinions of the learner
- Encourage the learner to share resources with you and other learners

SUPPORT SYSTEMS

The presence of a peer group can enhance learning by providing encouragement to learners as they try new behaviors and by giving positive reinforcement when goals are met. In addition, teaching a supportive family instead of just one family member is more effective in achieving learning objectives and modifying behavior. For groups of community learners,

TABLE 20-1	Characteristics of Adult Learners	
Children (Pedagogy)	**Adults (Andragogy)**
Others decide what is important	Decide for themselves what they want to learn
Accept information as you teach it	Validate and evaluate information based on life experiences and beliefs
Have limited past experience	Have a lifetime of experience
Expect to use information in the future	Want the information to be immediately useful
Focus on the facts	Focus on *application* of the facts
Teacher is the authority	Teacher and learners collaborate
Teacher plans the lesson	Planning of content is shared
Passive recipient of information	Active participant in the learning process

Data from Knowles, M. S. (1980). *The modern process of adult education: From pedagogy to andragogy.* New York: Cambridge Books.

special efforts to include culturally appropriate information and the use of culturally sensitive materials may enhance participation and learning. For example, provision of culturally appropriate instruction, support group interaction, and behavioral contracting were methods used to enhance adherence to a walking program among postmenopausal African American women (Williams et al., 2005).

NURSING ASSESSMENT OF HEALTH-RELATED LEARNING NEEDS

The development of content, strategies for teaching, and evaluation of the effectiveness of the health education program should be carried out in a systematic manner to achieve the most effective results. This systematic method is the **teaching-learning process.** The teaching-learning process parallels the nursing process (Figure 20-1). The nurse will use both the nursing process and the teaching-learning process to intervene for community health promotion.

ASSESSMENT OF COMMUNITY LEARNING NEEDS

To create a health education program for a community, both the needs of the community and the learning needs of the individual participants should be assessed. Assessment of the community is based on epidemiologic and demographic data, observations of health care personnel in the community, results of surveys, and conversations with community members (see Chapter 15). The need for community education can be assessed using the four classifications of educational needs as originally described by Atwood and Ellis (1971):

- A *real need* is one that is based on a deficiency that actually exists.
- An *educational need* is one that can be met by a learning experience.
- A *real educational need* indicates that specific skills, knowledge, and attitudes are required to assist the client in attaining a more desirable condition.
- A *felt need* is recognized as important by the learner.

The combined community assessment and educational needs assessment provide the impetus for planning a health education program.

A model that combines community assessment and educational planning is the **PRECEDE model.** PRECEDE is an acronym for *p*redisposing, *r*einforcing, and *e*nabling *c*auses in *e*ducational *d*iagnosis and *e*valuation (Green & Kreuter, 1991). *Predisposing* factors are characteristics of the learner; these include knowledge, attitudes, and perceptions that motivate health-related behavior. *Enabling* factors are environmental resources and learner skills that facilitate or hinder attainment of health behaviors. *Reinforcing* factors are the actual or expected rewards and feedback a learner receives after engaging in a health behavior. These three types of factors influence health-related behavior, which, in turn, contributes to the presence or absence of health problems that are linked with quality of life.

The phases of the PRECEDE model are similar to the steps of the nursing process. Phases 1 through 4 involve assessment, phase 5 is priority setting and planning, phase 6 is implementation, and phase 7 is evaluation (Table 20-2).

Most of the seven phases of the PRECEDE model begin with a diagnosis. In each phase, the health educator looks to the preceding cause and factors that influence the diagnosis. The educator answers *why* a situation is occurring before planning the educational intervention. Analysis of the causes of the health problem helps eliminate the risk of planning ineffective interventions based on guesswork.

ASSESSMENT OF THE LEARNER

Assessment of the learner is essential to planning the educational program. Assessment of the learner also helps facilitate the learner's acceptance and use of the information being offered. Within the community, the learner may be an individual, family, or group. Initial assessment of the learner is often referred to as assessment of the learner's readiness to learn. In an early publication, which continues to have relevance, Redman (1984) described two aspects of readiness: emotional and experiential.

Emotional Readiness

Emotional readiness is the learner's motivation, or the willingness to put forth the effort needed to learn. Motivation to learn is based on attitudes and beliefs about health-related behaviors.

Motivation may be internally or externally reinforced. Internal motivation is more self-directive and longer lasting and involves satisfaction in health-promoting activities based on the belief that the action is useful or enjoyable. External motivation must be constantly reinforced by rewards or praise. For example, an individual who joins a weight-loss group is more likely to achieve and maintain a weight loss if he or she joins the group to satisfy his or her own need for health, wellness, and self-esteem (internal motivation). If he or she joins the group to receive the rewards of buying new clothes or garnering the praise of others (external motivation), the person is less likely to maintain the weight loss.

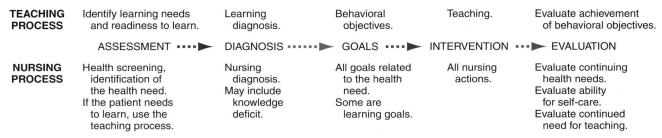

FIGURE 20-1 Relationship of the teaching and the nursing processes.

TABLE 20-2   Phases of the PRECEDE Model: Sample Community Educational Plan

Phase	Questions	Example
Assess		
Phase I: Social diagnosis	What are the general concerns of the population?	Teenagers hang out at local stores where alcohol and cigarettes are available.
Phase II: Epidemiologic diagnosis	What are the specific health problems?	Alcoholism and drug abuse Car accidents related to intoxication Asthma
Phase III: Behavioral diagnosis	What are health-related behaviors?	Underage drinking Illegal drug use Smoking
Phase IV: Educational diagnosis	What are predisposing, enabling, and reinforcing factors?	*Predisposing:* Teenagers desire to belong to peer groups. *Enabling:* Cigarettes, alcohol, and drugs can be purchased. *Reinforcing:* Teenagers who do not use substances are excluded by other teenagers.
Plan		
Phase V: Analysis of educational diagnosis	Which of the priority factors will be focused on during education?	Teenagers' desire to belong to a group; teen needs for activities Belief that substance use is necessary to belong Community accessibility of substances in local teen meeting places
Implement		
Phase VI: Administrative diagnosis	What specific objectives and resources are needed for health education?	**For teenagers:** *Objective:* Adolescents will explore alternative ways of being together. *Resources:* Young adult small group facilitators needed. *Action:* Youth meetings and recreational activities at drug and substance-free sites. **For community:** *Objective:* Community leaders will provide substance-free recreation sites and programs. *Resources:* Community education at civic associations and local government meetings regarding adolescent needs. *Action:* Dedicated funding and resources for teen activities.
Evaluate		
Phase VII: Evaluation	What are the results of education?	Civic club sponsors sports and games in substance-free site within 3 months. Thirty percent of teenagers attend and report reduced smoking and drug use.

Data from Green, L., & Kreuter, M. (1991). *Health promotion planning: An educational and environmental approach.* Mountain View, CA: Mayfield Publishing.
PRECEDE, Predisposing, reinforcing, and enabling causes in educational diagnosis and evaluation.

Experiential Readiness

Experiential readiness includes the client's background, skill, and ability to learn (Redman, 1984). Assessment of the client's background examines cultural factors, the home environment, and socioeconomic status. This background information is useful in describing current health behaviors and the learner's ability to use education to change behavior.

Client skills and self-perception of skills are part of experiential readiness. A client who is learning to bathe a newborn needs both coordination and the belief that he or she can learn. It is also useful to assess how clients prefer to learn procedures or skills. Based on experience, do clients prefer to try themselves, correcting their own mistakes, or do they prefer to be led through the process step by step several times until they feel confident?

Developmental stages of both the individual and the family present another aspect of experiential readiness. Educational content should be developmentally appropriate. For example, a class on the dangers of teenagers' drinking and driving would have similar content on the dangers of drinking and tips to prevent or resist alcohol use whether delivered to a group of teens or to a group of their parents, but the material would be presented differently to the two groups.

Finally, in determining experiential readiness, the client's ability to learn should be assessed. Most pertinent is determining the client's educational level. Direct questioning related to years of formal education is useful but does not always provide complete and accurate information. For example, although a client may have completed college, if the client did not study medicine or nursing, he or she may not understand complex medical terminology. In addition, reading ability and learning disabilities should be considered (Box 20-1).

Barriers to Learning

Assessment of the learner also requires assessment of barriers to learning. Barriers may be cultural, language, or physical barriers. One of the primary goals of *Healthy People 2010* is to eliminate health disparities; eliminating cultural barriers, including those inherent in health education programs, will help movement toward this goal. Inclusion of culturally appropriate teaching materials and a culturally sensitive approach to individual and family education is required. Culturally appropriate teaching materials for minority groups are available through the National Institutes of Health and through the U.S. Department of Health and Human Services, HealthFinder *(http://www.healthfinder.gov/)*, and Office of Minority Health *(http://www.omhrc.gov/)* by searching the special populations areas on these websites. In addition, the community/public health nurse should establish partnerships with leaders of the community. These partners can help the nurse develop understanding of the population(s) and interpret their acceptance (or lack of acceptance) of health recommendations.

Physical barriers are also important in assessing the learner. Some physical barriers are obvious, such as the use of mobility aids, and the nurse will be able to help clients with such difficulty access the learning environment. Less obvious are physical barriers such as vision or hearing problems. The nurse should make sure that the setting accommodates learners with these problems so that they do not become frustrated with health education. Large-print materials, good lighting, reduction of background noise, and appropriate seating are a few easy modifications that can reduce or eliminate physical barriers to learning.

WORKING WITH GROUPS OF LEARNERS

The community/public health nurse frequently implements health education programs with groups of learners. The group may come from within the community to participate in an advertised education program; the group may also be formed as a result of screening and identification of families with a health need (Boxes 20-2 and 20-3).

In a group, background, skills, abilities, and motivation are different for each group member. An assessment of each learner's readiness to learn before the first group meeting is useful for determining group composition. If performing an individual assessment before the group meeting is not possible, some introductory time during the first meeting might be used to assess readiness to learn and the learners' needs and motivations for behavioral change. The nurse may want to ask a colleague to record the information about learning needs and abilities so the task of taking notes will not distract from the important task of establishing rapport. An easy technique to use during the first group meeting to assess learners' needs is a flip chart and markers. Each member of the group may

---

BOX 20-1   Assessment of Readiness to Learn: Questions for the Nurse to Ask the Learner

Emotional Readiness

What sorts of things do you currently do or try to do to keep healthy?
> *Assesses attitudes about health promotion and disease prevention, sense of control over the ability to stay healthy, and self-satisfaction in health-seeking behaviors*

What things in your life make keeping healthy difficult?
> *Assesses perceptions of stressors or barriers to health promotion activities and cost of healthy behaviors*

Why did you join this health education group?
> *Assesses internal or external motivation to learn*

About what would you like to know more?
> *Assesses priorities*

What personal health goals do you hope to achieve by the end of the experience?
> *Assesses expectations for the future and client's interest in learning*

Experiential Readiness

Background

Tell me about yourself, your family, and your lifestyle; include your ethnic or cultural origins and your cultural beliefs about health and illness.
> *Describes current health behaviors and cultural traditions that may influence adherence to health promotion behaviors*

Skills

Learning a Manual Skill

How would you describe your ability to learn this skill?
How would you describe your manual dexterity at the present?
How much practice do you usually need to master a new skill?
> *Assesses the learner's actual and perceived manual dexterity and coordination*

Learning a Concept

How do you feel about learning these new ideas?
How often do you need something repeated before you feel comfortable with a new idea?
How do you think you learn best: by hearing? by seeing? by doing? by a combination of these?

Ability to Learn

What is your level of education? What did you study in school?
What subjects did you enjoy the most?
> *Assessment of formal level of education is not always sufficient; ability to read should be assessed using a readability formula.*

How is your sense of sight? hearing? speech?

Do you trust your memory? What things, if any, do you find difficult to remember? What do you do when you cannot remember?
> *Assesses ability to memorize information*

To what degree do the surroundings (e.g., noise, people) influence your ability to concentrate?
> *Assesses adequacy of the educational environment*

How long can you concentrate before getting tired?
> *Assesses the need for short or long teaching sessions and the need for periodic breaks*

Which of the following things have you said about yourself: "I heard it, but it just didn't register." "I heard it, but my mind went blank." "I can tune everything else out."
> *Assesses the ability of the learner to listen carefully and attentively*

Box 20-2   Factors in a Group of Learners

Type of Membership
Homogeneous Membership
- Members have similar learning needs, abilities, and learning style.
- Some homogeneity is needed so that members feel they belong (e.g., age, sex, background).
- No one member should stand out as different.
- Planning of educational strategies may be easier for the nurse.

Heterogeneous Membership
- Variation exists between members regarding learning needs, abilities, and learning style.
- Differences between members may enhance learning by allowing members to listen and understand the experiences of others.

- Very large groups can be divided into smaller learning clusters based on learning needs. Clusters can reconvene for large-group sharing.
- Small clusters can prevent members from being bored or overwhelmed (either of which can decrease motivation to attend group).

Stability of Membership
- Assessment of learning needs, and selection of members, provides less dissatisfaction and more stability of group.
- Time-limited behavioral change groups have a more stable membership than do continuing community groups, such as Weight Watchers, La Leche League, or Parents Without Partners.

Box 20-3   Tips and Tricks for Working with Groups

Be prepared: Having materials and supplies on hand will lower your anxiety, keep you feeling good, and enhance learning
- Keep a teacher's kit full of markers (water soluble and dry erase), chalk, pens and pencils, masking tape, Scotch tape, paperclips, rubber bands, Post-It notes, push pins, scissors, and a bell or whistle.
- Keep an emergency "repair anything" toolkit ready, including a screwdriver, hammer, pliers, string, duct tape, extension cords, and extra light/projector bulbs if you carry your own audiovisual equipment.
- Make a kit for yourself with mints, bottled water, lip balm, and a first aid kit, including bandages and something for a headache.
- Keep a supply of various colored index cards available. Use them for recording ideas, asking questions, etc.
- Zip-lock bags are good for storing everything!

Presentation tips: A great presentation makes the day *fly by* for you and your learners
- Know your subject backward and forward and inside out. Your learners will see you as the expert on the subject.
- If someone asks a question and you do not know the answer, say so and remark "what a great question." Work to find the answer at break time.
- As you are speaking, if you think of a new idea, use the index cards or Post-It notes to write it down so you can continue to improve your presentation next time.
- Drink the water from your kit above; water at room temperature is best for your voice.
- Be positive! Your nonverbal messages come through loud and clear.
- If you make a mistake, fix it and move on. Most groups are forgiving.
- Start your own library of articles on adult learners and presentation techniques.

Group activities: Adult learners remember experiences when they are actively involved
- Divide, mix, and move the group before you give instructions. People often forget the instructions during the shuffle.

- Before starting the activity, set up a clear refocus signal to allow you to get control of the group without shouting. A whistle or bell (in your kit) or a raised hand will work for this process.
- Use the format of a game show that many people know how to play. Using this format will cut down on explanation time and give your group more time for the activity.
- Wait to give handouts or materials for the group activity until after you have given the instructions; otherwise people will be reading instead of listening to you.
- Arrange seating so members participating in small-group activities can see each other and maintain eye contact.
- Have your game props counted and ready, which makes you look relaxed and prepared.

Audiovisual tips: Confidence in using equipment will help you concentrate on the learning experience
Flip Charts
- Use the broad side of the marker when writing to make big, bold letters.
- Print in upper and lowercase letters, do not use cursive script.
- Use deep-colored markers that are easy to read; blue, green, and black are best.
- Tape notes for yourself on the back of the easel.
- Cut some pieces of masking tape and put these on the back of the easel for quick access.

Slides or Liquid Crystal Display (LCD) Computer Projection
- If your participants need to take notes, check to see if you can still get a clear image if you merely dim the lights.
- Keep your visuals simple, with limited words on each slide.
- Do not read to the audience from your visuals; elaborate on the main points and face the audience.
- Forward to a blank screen or slide when you need to make a point; this technique helps you make eye contact with the audience.
- To help you avoid walking in front of the image when you move about the room, consider putting the screen in a corner or making a barrier so you do not walk around the projector.

From Gail L. Heiss, MSN, RN, BC, Nursing Education Specialist, VA MD HealthCare System; and Backer, L., Deck, M., & McCallum, D. (1995). *The presenter's survival kit—It's a jungle out there*. St. Louis: Mosby.

be asked simple questions during introduction time, such as, "What brought you to the meeting today?" "What would you like to learn?" or "How do you like to learn new things?"

CONSTRUCTION OF HEALTH EDUCATION LESSON PLANS

The next step in the teaching-learning process is the construction of the health education lesson plan. In the initial phase of the teaching-learning process, the nurse assesses *what* the learner wants or needs or is able to accomplish. The next step, creating the lesson plan, begins with statements of the results the nurse wants the learner to achieve. Each statement is a *behavioral objective*. The result of the education may be a change in attitude, skill, behavior, or knowledge, but it must be stated *before* the actual teaching begins.

CREATING BEHAVIORAL OBJECTIVES

Behavioral objectives reflect changes in the learner that are observable or measurable. If the behavioral objectives are properly written, they will be useful tools in evaluating educational outcomes. An important point to remember is that behavioral objectives are statements of what the learner achieves, not statements of the teacher's activities. A classic resource on the writing of behavioral objectives (Grolund, 1970) identifies the use of behavioral objectives to accomplish the following:

- Provide direction for the teacher and indicate to others the *instructional intent*
- Guide the selection of course content, teaching strategies, and teaching materials
- Facilitate evaluation of the educational program (evaluation measures the achievement of the objectives)
- Guide the student's learning by specifying what she or he is expected to do at the conclusion of the program

When behavioral objectives are written, an acceptable practice is to state a main objective in behavioral terms that guides large segments of learning. This main objective can be followed by more specific supporting objectives. The supporting objectives should represent all of the actions necessary to accomplish the main objective (Redman, 1997). Main objectives in the community may closely parallel the *Healthy People 2010* objectives, with supporting objectives specific to the community in which the program is implemented. Some guidelines and examples of behavioral objectives are given in Box 20-4 and Table 20-3.

BOX 20-4   Guidelines for Writing Behavioral Objectives

1. Begin each objective with an active verb (e.g., *discuss, name, compare, describe, predict*).
2. State the objective as a learner outcome, not as a teacher outcome or intent.
3. Include only one outcome per objective to facilitate evaluation of outcomes.
4. Be sure the stated objectives are appropriate for the learners' needs and abilities.

From Grolund, N. E. (1970). *Stating behavioral objectives for classroom instruction.* New York: Macmillan.

TABLE 20-3   Sample Behavioral Objectives

After attending the health education program entitled "Low-Fat Meals for Your Family," the participant will:

Poorly Phrased Behavioral Objectives	Well-Phrased Behavioral Objectives
Cognitive Domain	
Understand the importance of a healthy diet	Describe the health benefits of a low-fat diet
Know what high-fat foods the family eats	Name at least three foods or recipes enjoyed by the family that are high in fat
Psychomotor Domain	
Cook meals without as much fat	Rewrite the "family favorite" recipe using low-fat ingredients
Buy low-fat foods	When shopping, compare nutrition labels of popular snack foods (such as cookies and chips)
	Increase the percentage of purchased foods that are low in fat
Affective Domain	
Adjust successfully to the new family eating patterns	Predict the family reactions to low-fat meals and snacks
Appreciate the relationship between food and comfort	Discuss possible solutions to family resistance to change

Behavioral objectives are classified into three *domains* of learning: cognitive (intellectual), psychomotor (motor skills), and affective (attitudes and emotions) (Bloom, 1984). All behavioral objectives fit into one of these domains of learning.

By assessing learning needs, the nurse can evaluate the need for behavioral objectives in the cognitive, affective, or psychomotor domain. All three domains of learning are usually necessary to incorporate a new health behavior into the learner's life. Nurses generally want learners to do the following:

- *Cognitively* apply information
- Perform *skills* with some guidance and, eventually, independently
- *Value* the learning enough to use it

SELECTING CONTENT

Selection of the content of the health education program depends on the following:

- The needs identified by the target group of learners
- The nurse's determination of what the group needs to know
- The health care delivery system's constraints on the nurse

Needs of the learners lead to the development of the behavioral objectives. Behavioral objectives lead to development of the content of the health teaching program. When developing the content of the program, the nurse consistently refers to the behavioral objectives for guidance. Behavioral objectives that were carefully developed from the needs assessment and that include learning in all three domains will lead to the development of a teaching plan that is tailored to the needs of the target group (Box 20-5).

When the nurse is planning the educational program, recommendations suggest starting with the information that the group is seeking, even if this information is not the most important

| BOX 20-5 | Sample Health Education Lesson Plan |

Preparing Your Family for the Flu Season

This health education topic may be identified through community needs assessment, may be based on *Healthy People 2010* or community goals, may be derived through careful attention to national health care issues, or may be selected by health care organizations to promote cost savings.

Behavioral Objectives	Content Outline	Instructional Methods and Materials	Time Allotted and Evaluation Methods
Cognitive *At the conclusion of the program, the learner will be able to:* • Identify the symptoms of the flu • Compare the flu and a cold • Describe methods to reduce exposure to the flu virus	Symptoms of the flu and a cold Methods of acquiring the flu virus, including airborne (sneezing, coughing) and through contact such as handshaking Importance of reducing exposure of at-risk family members, such as the elderly, to other potentially ill persons Use of hand-washing as a method of prevention	**Methods:** Lecture presentation; group discussion **Materials:** Flip chart Posters PowerPoint presentation Prepared handout with comparison of flu and cold symptoms	30 minutes Observe participation in group discussion; note questions asked Return demonstration
Psychomotor *Using the equipment and materials provided by the health department, the learner will be able to:* • Create a list of items needed in the home to care for a family member with the flu • Demonstrate how to use a thermometer • Wash hands using hand gel	How to select and use of over-the-counter medications and other items to provide comfort care for persons with the flu Use of a thermometer and recommendation on when to use medication and when to call the doctor for a fever Use of hand gel to prevent flu transmission when caring for a family member	**Methods:** Group brainstorming activity to create a culturally appropriate "flu list" for each family Demonstration and return demonstration of thermometer and hand gel use **Materials:** Paper and pencils Instructor master list of recommended items for flu care Thermometers Prepared thermometer instructions Hand gel	1 hour (20 minutes for small-group brainstorming; 10 minutes for large-group sharing; 30 minutes for demonstration and return demonstration)
Affective *At the conclusion of the program, the learner will be able to:* • Discuss the importance of the flu vaccine for high-risk groups • Evaluate the advantages and disadvantages of immunization for members of the family • Decide whether or not the learner and family members will receive the flu vaccine	Purpose of vaccination for prevention of flu Myths and beliefs about vaccine and illness CDC recommendations for immunization	**Methods:** Lecture presentation Group discussion **Materials:** Posters CDC handouts	30 minutes Observe participation in group discussion Have each participant identify which members of his/her family should receive flu vaccine

CDC, Centers for Disease Control and Prevention.

component of the health education. After the group introductions and brief learning needs assessment, the nurse might need to modify his or her lesson plan to address the immediate desire to know certain information. For example, in the sample flu lesson plan in Box 20-5, the nurse could begin the session by discussing the flu vaccine if the group has identified fear of the vaccine as a priority learning need. By meeting this immediate need to know, the nurse captures interest and motivates group members for further learning. In addition, if the information the group is seeking is not addressed, the learners may not be able to concentrate on other information being taught.

The nurse independently determines some of the content of the health education program. Although the learners' or group members' assessments of their own learning needs has been expressed, their list of learning needs may not be comprehensive.

The nurse's expertise is useful in identifying information and attitudes needed for behavioral change that members of the group did not identify.

A nurse conducts a group for pregnant adolescents, with the overall goal of decreasing child abuse and neglect by adolescent parents. Group-identified learning needs may focus on the psychomotor aspects of new infant care and attitudinal changes necessary to becoming responsible parents. The group might not identify the need for information on the relationship between infant crying, development of infant self-comforting behaviors, and abusive behaviors such as shaking exhibited by some parents in reaction to infant crying. The nurse's responsibility is to include these concepts and positive health behaviors in the educational plan.

The health care delivery system and the insurance industry place constraints on health education programs. Time and money are limited resources and often influence the length of a program. The nurse also needs to plan on using educational materials within the constraints of a budget. Although use of purchased print and audiovisual materials may enhance the program, content may still be effectively taught using less expensive teaching aids prepared by the nurse or the institution (the preparation of teaching aids is discussed later in the chapter). In addition, the nurse must remember that some educational programs are reimbursed by third-party payers only if the content is approved by the insurer or is ordered by a physician. Alteration of content is sometimes required for compliance with these limitations.

SELECTING TEACHING STRATEGIES

Selection of the teaching strategy or technique to achieve the behavioral objectives is the next step in planning the health education program. Teaching techniques must be suitable to the size, composition, and learning abilities of the group. Consideration of cultural differences, barriers to learning, and community values is necessary. Differences in learning needs that were assessed influence the selection of the teaching strategy. Strategies should be suitable to the subject matter. Numerous teaching strategies that are useful in group education and factors that influence their selection are presented in Table 20-4.

SELECTING EVALUATION STRATEGIES

Evaluation and revision of health education programs is required for the community/public health nurse to adhere to the ANA's *Public Health Nursing: Scope and Standards* (2007). The evaluation should lead to the development of new databases for community planning. A prime example of continued evaluation and revision is the periodic modification of the *Healthy People 2010* health goals for the nation as seen in the midcourse review (USDHHS, 2006).

To evaluate health education, two types of evaluation are necessary: outcome evaluation and evaluation of teacher performance. **Outcome evaluation,** or evaluation of the learner, is further divided into short- and long-term evaluation and the evaluation of self-efficacy.

TABLE 20-4 Teaching Techniques for Use in Groups of Learners

Technique	Advantage	Disadvantage
Lecture: Traditional presentation	Effective in large groups; good for lower-level cognitive learning	Students are passive; students with increased intellectual ability may be bored
Use of examples: Begin with simple examples and progress; select examples based on common life experiences of the group	Useful for clarification; students may be able to provide examples to verify learning	Failure to relate the example to principles being taught results in learners' remembering only the example
Discussion: Often used to achieve objectives in the affective domain	Engages active participation of the learner; assists learner to focus, analyze, generalize	Not as effective in large groups; students in certain settings such as a lecture hall may not be able to hear the peer discussion
Role modeling: Provides members with model for learning; also known as *identification*	Learner is able to observe someone with desirable traits	Need to carefully select nurse leader who possesses the desirable traits
Positive reinforcement: Useful when teaching a group with high anxiety level	Increases participation in discussion because members feel valued	Reinforcement must be related to learner accomplishment, not the learner
Demonstration and guided practice: Effective for learning psychomotor skills	Encourages involvement; safe place to make mistakes	Difficult for left-handed learners
Simulation: Applies previously learned knowledge; useful for psychomotor skills practice and affective learning	Involves active participation; increases motivation and interest	Limited use for cognitive learning
Role playing: Provides exploration of attitudes and problem-solving skills	Involves active participation, comparison of own beliefs to those of others	Time consuming; experienced leader needed to focus the discussion
Support groups: Highly effective for attitude and behavioral change when used with cognitive teaching	Decreases sense of "aloneness"; member differences provide model for new behaviors	Group can become "stuck" in self-pity
Contracting: Written or verbal; emphasizes outcomes	Allows for differences in learner needs; can monitor change over time	Learners with limited self-discipline will have difficulty adhering to contract
Stress-reduction exercises: Reducing anxiety increases cognitive and affective learning	Applicable to most learning situations; can become part of regular mental health	Nurse needs to be comfortable with technique
Computer-assisted instruction: Individualizes learning needs	Useful for cognitive and affective learning; voice-generated instruction useful to overcome reading disabilities	Equipment costly; initially, highly individualized instructor time may be needed
Team teaching: Enhances teaching by using knowledge of more than one teacher; also provides backup in case of schedule conflicts for programs that have numerous sessions	Presents different points of view to the learner; teachers learn from each other and can provide ongoing peer review	Requires additional planning time and additional use of staff, may lack continuity

Data from Babcock, D. E., & Miller, M. A. (1994). *Client education theory and practice.* St. Louis: Mosby; and Redman, B. (1997). *The process of patient education* (8th ed.). St. Louis: Mosby–Year Book.

Outcome Evaluation

Assessment of learner outcomes has traditionally been based on achievement of the behavioral objectives. If the objectives are properly written, each objective is measurable. Actual performance of the desired behavior provides the evaluation data. The overall goal of community health education programs typically is to teach a health-promoting activity that is incorporated into the learner's lifestyle over a long period.

Short-Term Evaluation. Measurement of cognitive knowledge is the most common type of short-term outcome evaluation and is best achieved by using questionnaires or standardized testing. Although this method of evaluation yields usable data for comparison of groups, it is not always recommended. Questionnaires and standardized tests can be time consuming, have limitations for learners who cannot read, and may remind adult learners of their childhood schooldays. A negative experience with the use of a questionnaire or test might prevent adult learners from seeking out health education groups in the future. An example of a more positive method of evaluation is the use of a game-show format with groups. Learners are divided into teams that earn points for answering questions correctly.

In a small-group environment, an appropriate practice is to evaluate behavioral outcomes by interviewing each member of the group. A structured interview can be used to collect data about personal behavioral successes. These data would be uniform and provide for a simple analysis. If a structured interview is used, however, some of the personal successes and benefits of the instruction might not be revealed.

If, instead of using a structured interview, the nurse interviews each group member informally, the member might share more personal behavioral successes. Personal successes shared informally during group meetings provide motivation for other group members. Informal sharing about achievement of behavioral objectives also provides information about difficulties the learners are having and their satisfaction with the learning experience. The nurse is able to determine which objectives are difficult for the participants to achieve and can revise the educational strategies appropriately.

Long-Term Evaluation. Direct observation by the nurse provides some indication of success, but the participant often does actual measurement of the lifestyle change.

In the case of a health education intervention to increase exercise for promotion of cardiovascular health, the nurse may not be able to observe changes in the individual's pulse rate, blood pressure, weight, or cholesterol level before the end of a time-limited program. For example, only the learner knows whether he or she actually meets the behavioral objective of walking daily for 30 minutes. The participant can provide subjective reports of lifestyle changes by keeping a personal journal documenting exercise and activity over time. Long-term evaluation by the nurse is possible, but cardiovascular changes over time may also be influenced by other factors, such as the use of cholesterol-lowering or blood pressure medications.

Long-term evaluation also considers the effectiveness of the intervention for the community over time.

The "Crosswalk Campaign" is an example of community education and the effectiveness of partnerships over time. In a busy community in which there is a high incidence of pedestrian accidents that occur when people cross the street without using the crosswalk, the health department and other civic groups could collaborate to implement a crosswalk safety education program. Public partners such as health care providers, emergency management groups, public works agencies, and elected officials should be included. A media campaign to provide education via radio and local television and a contest for schoolchildren to design posters are examples of some possible efforts to educate the community. In addition, visual cues about the program may be provided to the community with new signage at crosswalks using the safety campaign slogan and logo. Evidence of implementation by public officials includes funding for new crosswalk lines on the streets and larger, brighter crosswalk lights at intersections. A long-term indicator of the effectiveness of the program would be a measured decrease in the incidence of pedestrian and motor vehicle accidents.

Self-Efficacy. Self-efficacy is the motivational factor that determines if an individual participates in self-care activities and to what extent (Bandura, 1977). Self-efficacy is an important attitude for learners. For example, living with chronic disease involves more than knowing what to do; it is the ability to organize and integrate cognitive, social, and behavioral skills into daily living to produce desired outcomes. As an evaluation measure, self-efficacy goes beyond cognitively knowing what to do. Self-efficacy provides a measure of the belief of the learner that he or she is capable of developing and performing skills that will improve his or her health.

Self-efficacy can be fostered through the learner's experiences of success; vicarious successful experiences of others, including teachers as models; and persuasion. Self-efficacy in older adults was part of a health teaching program presented by Easom (2003). The study found that fostering self-efficacy can improve health behaviors among participants in a health promotion program. The learner outcomes in this program were based on the long-term performance of self-care activities, such as exercise, range-of-motion activities, rest, and relaxation. Similar findings were demonstrated by Loeb (2004) in a study of older men's health motivations and participation in health-promoting behaviors. The success of the self-efficacy approach to health promotion may change the traditional approach to providing health education and lead to an increased emphasis on encouragement and motivational factors. The older adults in whom the nurse fostered higher self-efficacy were more likely to continue with health self-care activities.

Teacher Performance Evaluation

Process evaluation includes evaluating both the content of the lesson and the teacher as the lesson is being presented. The performance of the teacher influences the achievement of behavioral outcomes by the learners. Teacher performance can be evaluated through observation by a peer, review of videotapes of the teaching session, or feedback from the participants. Participant feedback on teacher performance can include nonverbal cues such as disinterest or confused expressions. An observant instructor will not ignore these nonverbal cues and will make brief pauses in the educational session to assess understanding. Evaluation of the lesson frequently includes learners' self-assessment of their achievement of objectives.

When working with groups, teacher performance can be enhanced using co-leaders. Co-leaders who have mutual trust

TABLE 20-5 **Sample Combined Teacher and Lesson Evaluation Tool for the Health Education Program "Low-Fat Meals for Your Family"**

Please evaluate the nurse who presented the lesson.
Circle the appropriate number.

	Strongly Agree	Agree	Cannot Decide	Disagree	Strongly Disagree
The nurse listened to my concerns.	5	4	3	2	1
The nurse understood what I needed to learn.	5	4	3	2	1
I was able to ask questions.	5	4	3	2	1
The nurse used language I could understand.	5	4	3	2	1
The nurse used examples that were familiar to me.	5	4	3	2	1
I had the opportunity to participate.	5	4	3	2	1

Please evaluate your ability to achieve the objectives.
Circle the appropriate number.

	Strongly Agree	Agree	Cannot Decide	Disagree	Strongly Disagree
I am able to describe the benefits of a low-fat diet.	5	4	3	2	1
I can name three foods or recipes enjoyed by my family that are high in fat.	5	4	3	2	1
I am able to rewrite a family recipe substituting low-fat ingredients.	5	4	3	2	1
I am able to read a food label to identify fat content.	5	4	3	2	1

and respect can learn from one another as they use various teaching strategies. Particularly useful is to pair a novice teacher with one who is more experienced.

Teacher effectiveness and achievement of learning objectives may be evaluated using the same feedback tool (Table 20-5). Feedback is most helpful when the learner feels free to give an honest opinion; therefore, the evaluation should be anonymous, or the inclusion of a name should be optional. Collection of feedback is less intimidating if the nurse places an envelope or folder on a table to collect feedback forms instead of having learners hand them to her.

HEALTH-RELATED EDUCATIONAL MATERIALS

PRINT MATERIALS
Problems of Low Literacy

Health literacy is the ability of individuals to obtain, process, and understand basic health information to make health decisions (USDHHS, 2000). Over 90 million Americans, however, have low health literacy and experience difficulty acting on health information provided to them (Institute of Medicine, 2004). The link between low health literacy and negative patient outcomes was highlighted in 2004 by the Institute of Medicine and the Agency for Healthcare Quality and Research. Learners often need to have the teaching experience supplemented with print materials that can serve to reinforce teaching and provide reminders about new behaviors after the learner has left the educational setting. Studies of reading abilities indicate that approximately 50% of health care clients have difficulty reading educational materials written at the fifth-grade level (Doak et al., 1996).

Clients frequently attempt to hide their inability to read, and problems with reading comprehension are often overlooked. Client-reported years of education often are not a good indicator of reading ability. Clients may self-report completing high school, but they may have graduated with only an elementary school reading ability.

Low literacy not only indicates a client's lack of reading ability, but it also affects his or her ability to understand oral instructions. In many instances, when clients are questioned about understanding, they will indicate that they do understand, even if they do not. When confronted with a fast-paced educational program, low-literacy clients will sometimes withdraw from the situation, appearing to have low motivation to participate (Doak et al., 1996). When asked to participate in instruction, they may show poor eye contact or comment that they do not have their reading glasses with them. Clients with low reading and comprehension skills and limited vocabulary are not able to express what is not understood and therefore may choose to conceal their illiteracy.

According to Doak and colleagues (1996), people who are able to read at a higher level are not offended by easy-to-read materials. This finding has practical implications for the community/public health nurse, who should consider using only health education materials written at a sixth-grade level or lower. In addition, the nurse should include follow-up after providing health information and education to determine understanding.

Predicting Readability of Materials

The challenge for nurses who are preparing health education programs is to select or create print materials that the learners can understand. The nurse should remember that, although some individuals in the group may have advanced literacy, it is easier for a good reader to read down than it is for a low-literacy learner to read up. A suggested method to improve readability (Houts et al., 2006) is to include pictures in the print material. Pictures can improve comprehension when they show relationships between ideas or when they have simply worded captions. To improve readability of text, use simple sentences with one noun and verb and words with only one or two syllables when possible. Medical terms may be used, but they should be defined when first introduced.

Existing print materials can be analyzed for actual readability of the text. Readability formulas, such as the SMOG readability formula (McLaughlin, 1969), Fry readability graph (Fry, 1977), or Flesch readability graph (Flesch, 1949), are useful in determining the appropriateness of health education materials. The **SMOG** readability formula has been chosen for inclusion in this text because it is easy to use and the formula can be applied to print materials of varying lengths, including pamphlets with fewer than 30 sentences. The nurse should practice using the SMOG formula until it becomes a natural part of his or her practice (Box 20-6 and Figure 20-2).

Another method of determining the readability of materials, particularly those on the Internet, is to use a computerized formula such as those available in WordPerfect or Microsoft Word. The easiest way to accomplish this task is to highlight the document for which you want to assess readability and copy it into a blank word-processing document. Then, use the Word program's spelling and grammar check option to obtain a reading level. If thr SMOG formula is being used, be certain to check at least 30 sentences of the online document.

The inability to read can have dangerous implications if the client does not understand instructions for medications and treatments. For clinical situations, the American Medical Association has four suggestions for health care providers to alleviate some of the problems of low literacy (Box 20-7).

Selecting Materials

In addition to readability, other factors should be considered when choosing print material. The selection process should include analysis of the content, format, and appropriateness of the print material for the target group.

Content. The content of the print material should be assessed to determine whether the material is accurate, is up to date, and presents all of the information a learner needs to know to change behavior. The nurse should discern whether too much unnecessary information is presented that might confuse the learner. (Remember, print materials are a supplement to, not a substitute for, education.) The material should be organized in a logical manner, and resources for more information should be included.

Format. The nurse should assess the format of the print material. The type style and size of print are important, especially when working with groups such as older adults whose visual acuity may be decreased. Although words written in all capital letters may appear larger and clearer, using all capital letters actually makes the print more difficult to read. Because capital letters do not vary in size and shape, the eye has difficulty differentiating

---

Box 20-6   The SMOG Readability Formula

Method A

To calculate the SMOG reading grade level, begin with the entire written work that is being assessed and follow these four steps:

1. Count off 10 consecutive sentences near the beginning, in the middle, and near the end of the text.
2. In this sample of 30 sentences, circle all of the words containing three or more syllables (polysyllabic words), including repetitions of the same word, and total the number of words circled.
3. Estimate the square root of the total number of polysyllabic words counted. This can be done by finding the nearest perfect square and taking its square root.
4. Finally, add a constant of 3 to the square root. The resulting number is the SMOG grade, or the reading grade level that a person must have achieved if he or she is to fully understand the text being assessed.

A few additional guidelines can help to clarify these directions:

- A sentence is defined as a string of words punctuated with a period (.), an exclamation point (!), or a question mark (?).
- Hyphenated words are considered as one word.
- Numbers that are written out should also be considered; if the numbers are in numerical form in the text, they should be pronounced to determine whether they are polysyllabic.
- Proper nouns, if polysyllabic, should also be counted.
- Abbreviations should be read as if they were spelled out to determine if they are polysyllabic.

Method B

Not all pamphlets, fact sheets, or other printed materials contain 30 sentences. To test a text that has fewer than 30 sentences, do the following:

1. Count all of the polysyllabic words in the text.
2. Count the number of sentences.
3. Find the average number of polysyllabic words per sentence as follows:

   Average = Total no. of polysyllabic words/Total no. of sentences

4. Multiply this average by the number of sentences by which the material is short of 30 (i.e., if the material has 20 sentences, multiply the average by 10).
5. Add the resulting figure to the total count of polysyllabic words in the material.
6. Find the square root of the number obtained in step 5 and add a constant of 3.

Method C

Perhaps the quickest way to perform the SMOG grading test is to use the SMOG conversion table. Simply count the number of polysyllabic words in your set of 30 sentences and look up the approximate reading grade level on the following chart.

SMOG Conversion Table

Total Polysyllabic Word Count	Approximate Grade Level (±1.5)
0-2	4
3-6	5
7-12	6
13-20	7
21-30	8
31-42	9
43-56	10
57-72	11
73-90	12
91-110	13
111-132	14
133-156	15
157-182	16
183-210	17
211-240	18

SMOG conversion table developed by Harold C. McGraw, Office of Educational Research, Baltimore County Schools, Towson, MD.

Sample Text: Tips to Stay Motivated with a Walking Plan
- Ask other people to walk with you. Find a partner or a group. When you know someone else is waiting for you, it keeps you going.
- Wear (comfortable) shoes and good socks to help cushion your feet.
- Wear clothes that are right for the season. Try using layers of clothing in the cold weather to keep you warm, and cotton clothes in the summer to keep you cool.
- Drink plenty of water. It doesn't have to be that fancy bottled stuff—get your own (container) and keep it filled with plenty of (regular) water. Carry it with you if you can.
- Don't forget to stretch before you walk. Try to start off slowly.
- Be safe—pay (attention) to your (surroundings.)
- Walk in a safe place that has plenty of lights in the (evening.) Try walking around a local school's parking lot, or going to the mall.
- Try to walk at least three times a week. It may seem like a lot at first, but you will (gradually) build up.
- Try to think of your walk in three parts. (Imagine) a warm-up period at the (beginning,) challenge yourself with a brisk pace in the middle, and (finally) picture a cool-down. You can feel success when you finish each part.

Calculating the Smog Readability Formula (for this Sample)

$$\frac{\text{Number of polysyllabic words} = 10}{\text{Number of sentences} = 19}$$

$$10/19 = 0.53 \times 11 \text{ (number of sentences short of 30)} = 5.8$$

$$5.8 + 10 = 15.8$$

$$\text{Square root of } 16 = 4 + \text{constant of } 3 = \text{seventh-grade reading level}$$

FIGURE 20-2 Sample use of the SMOG formula for evaluating print materials: using method B for health material with fewer than 30 sentences. (Health education print material from National Institutes of Health. *Your guide to lowering high blood pressure: Tips to stay motivated with a walking plan.* Retrieved August 13, 2007 from *http://www.nhlbi.nih.gov/hbp/prevent/p_active/tips.htm.*)

between letters. Many researchers recommend using **bold** print to highlight important elements and using uppercase and lowercase letters for text. Serif-style type is also preferred over sans serif because serif type uses additional details on the ends of some letters, making them easier to read.

Box 20-7   Four Steps for Helping Low-Literacy Learners in a Health Care Setting

1. **Create a shame-free environment.**
   Offer to help, especially with paperwork. Many clients begin their health care experience in a negative manner when they are handed a clipboard to complete a health history. If you see an incomplete form, ask the questions yourself and fill in the answers without impatience or annoyance.
   Let the client know that many people have difficulty reading and learning new information and that you can help.
2. **Use simple and direct language, and give examples.**
   Speak in simple and direct language. Avoid medical jargon. Cover only two or three points at a time. Read written material to the client and emphasize the key points. Make sure your written material is written at a fifth- or sixth-grade reading level.
3. **Use the teach-back technique.**
   Instead of asking the client if he or she understands, try to phrase the question so you get more than a yes or no answer. Ask the client to explain how to take his or her medications or to show you a procedure as he or she will do it at home. Consider that noncompliance might really be lack of understanding.
4. **Invite a family member or friend.**
   Ask the client if he or she would like to have a family member present during the counseling part of the visit.

Modified from Schwartzberg, J., & Lagay, F. (2001, June). *Health literacy: What patients know when they leave your office or clinic.* American Medical Association, AMA Ethics. Retrieved August 13, 2007, from *http://www.ama-assn.org.*

Reading materials with a right margin that is "ragged" (i.e., with equal space between all words so that lines are of varying lengths) are easier to read than materials in which the space between words is adjusted to ensure that all lines are the same length. Headings should be used for paragraphs. Each paragraph should present one idea and be about four sentences long. Enough space should be inserted between paragraphs or sections of the print material so that it does not appear crowded. Using white space is pleasing to the eye and can also be helpful for emphasis.

A consideration specific to health-related materials is the inclusion of medical jargon and abbreviations. Even though the nurse understands these terms, the general public needs definitions of words that are not in everyday use.

Selection of Materials for Target Groups. Selecting print materials that are appropriate for ethnic and cultural groups is of particular concern to the community/public health nurse. Photographs or sketches of people should represent the ethnicity of the community. For example, a booklet on new baby care with photographs of only white, middle-class families is not likely to be effective in a community of low-income African American single mothers. Simply substituting ethnic faces, however, is not enough. Culture also includes the values, traditions, norms, and customs of a community. The results of a clinical study on literacy and cultural barriers to the use of anticoagulant therapy among African Americans supports the inclusion of culturally sensitive content in patient education materials (Wilson et al., 2003). The assistance of a member of the target group is useful in selecting materials that are appropriate for the community.

The nurse must determine whether resources or commodities mentioned in the material are readily available in the community. For example, a nutrition pamphlet emphasizing eating fresh fruits and vegetables is not useful if these foods are too expensive or are not available in the community. A better choice of pamphlet might be one that compares the nutritional values of affordable and available frozen and canned foods.

NONPRINT MATERIALS
Purpose of Audiovisual Materials

Nonprint materials, often called *audiovisuals,* can take a variety of forms, including a simple diagram or picture, audiotape, record, film, slides, transparencies, videotape, radio, television, computer-assisted learning (CAL), or interactive websites. Audiovisuals enhance learning through clarification and reinforcement and are convenient and cost effective because they can be used over and over without using the nurse's time. Audiovisual materials can often be adjusted to the learner's own educational pace to meet individual learning needs.

Audiovisuals can be used to provide experiences that might not be possible otherwise. These experiences include bringing an expert into the community via videotape, transporting the learner to a new community and culture, or allowing the learner to experience a life event—such as what happens during a heart attack or the birth of a baby—without actually being there.

Selection of Audiovisual Materials

The nurse should preview the audiovisual aid and determine if use of the audiovisual aid is necessary to meet the learning objectives. All audiovisuals cost money. With current trends to limit health care costs, the nurse should consider the cost of renting or purchasing the audiovisual aid.

The nurse also needs to consider the cost of nursing time. For example, creating an interactive CD about dietary fat and cholesterol may be expensive in both staff time and production costs, and it may be too expensive to purchase commercial materials. The nurse could probably teach the same information using less expensive charts or pictures. However, if a learning objective is for each learner to plan low-fat meals for a week while keeping within the family budget, then investing in a CAL program might provide individual learner feedback while saving nursing time.

The nurse should determine the appropriateness of the audiovisual aid based on the reading and comprehension abilities of the target group. A DVD or television program is not useful if the language is too difficult for the group to comprehend. The inclusion of spoken medical jargon is often a problem.

Use of Audiovisual Materials

Use of audiovisual materials also depends on the equipment available. Nurses should practice using the equipment. When practicing, the nurse should move about the room to be sure the audiovisual material can be seen and heard. Using audiovisual equipment is not difficult, but the nurse should feel comfortable doing so and should be able to solve minor technical problems. An essential point to remember is to bring an extra projector bulb, an extension cord, and a backup disk or flash drive to the presentation. Some of the advantages, disadvantages, and uses of audiovisual aids are listed in Box 20-8.

SOURCES OF EDUCATIONAL MATERIALS

Community/public health nurses who prepare educational programs need to locate sources for class materials. The first place to start is the nurse's own agency. Most community/public

---

BOX 20-8   Audiovisual Teaching Aids

Overhead Transparencies (old but reliable)

Advantages
1. Simple to plan and design
2. Darkened room not usually required
3. Simple-to-operate projector

Disadvantages
1. Bulky projector
2. Presentation may appear "out of date" even though the content is current

Flip Charts

Advantages
1. Very inexpensive
2. Encourages audience involvement and feedback
3. Provides degree of informality
4. Useful for small- to medium-sized groups in informal settings

Disadvantages
1. Less dynamic and more limited in presenting information
2. Cannot be seen in large rooms
3. Impractical in terms of portability and storage

Videotape/DVD

Advantages
1. Allows for easy replay
2. Equipment generally available

3. Usually feasible to do some local production of reasonably high quality
4. Very useful with small groups
5. Materials portable and easy to store

Disadvantages
1. Trained support personnel required to create a local production
2. Not suitable for large auditorium presentations unless several monitors or a projection system is used

Liquid Crystal Display (LCD) Computer Projection

Advantages
1. Does not require darkened room
2. Seamless presentation of ideas with rate controlled by presenter
3. A variety of computer-aided design programs such as PowerPoint can be used to add visual interest
4. Presenter able to face audience

Disadvantages
1. Needs detailed instruction on setup and operation
2. May be transported, but presentation site must be equipped with electricity, screen, etc.
3. Use of "busy" pictures can distract from presentation; training in development of presentations highly recommended
4. Equipment is expensive

health agencies keep collections of resource materials, often compiled by the nurses themselves. Other possible sources are distributors of educational materials, catalogues, and community agencies. Businesses and agencies are often able to supply or can suggest how to obtain materials.

Time on the telephone can bring great results. A telephone directory of community services is often on a bookshelf in the nurse's own agency. The regular telephone book should not be overlooked as a resource for finding educational materials. The front of the book may provide listings of governmental or private agencies that offer health services. Other places to look in the telephone book are in the government section or listings under "health services" or "health care."

A special tip for the nurse using the telephone is to create a personal resource telephone book. When a call is productive, make a brief note of the agency telephone number, services and materials available, and the name of the contact person. *Networking* with colleagues is a valuable tool for all aspects of nursing care delivery.

Opportunities are available to locate educational materials from private sources. Businesses in the community such as pharmaceutical companies or manufacturers of medical devices sometimes supply materials. However, caution must be exercised before adopting these materials for use. These materials are often beautifully illustrated, with photographs of people using specific products, and free samples such as diapers or coupons are sometimes provided. The nurse should review the materials for appropriateness. The educational message must not depend on using a specific product. For example, cooking with a nonfat cooking spray is healthier than frying, regardless of the brand of cooking spray. When reviewing the pamphlet, the nurse should try to determine if the client is receiving the message to buy only one brand of cooking spray. Good judgment is necessary in selecting educational materials.

The nurse should also visit the community library and the local video store. The library usually keeps catalogues of community resources. Many libraries and video stores loan videotapes or DVDs with health information at minimal or no cost. Again, the nurse must review these materials before recommending them to learners.

INTERNET RESOURCES

Use of the Internet by nurses and their clients is changing the delivery of health care and health education. Via the World Wide Web, nurses and clients have easy access to a wide variety of health education materials. A client may bring new or conflicting information that was downloaded from the Internet to the health education setting. The nurse has the responsibility to help the client determine the quality of Internet materials (Box 20-9).

Some specific sources of health education information are listed in Community Resources for Practice at the end of the chapter. This list is not meant to be exhaustive, but it can be used as a starting point for nurses who are planning health education in the community. One of the sources included in the list is an interactive site called MedlinePlus accessible through the National Library of Medicine and the National Institutes of Health (*http://www.nlm.nih.gov/medlineplus/*). The site includes interactive tutorials that meet the criteria for patient education materials discussed in this chapter (Box 20-9). The patient education tutorials are easy to access and navigate, appropriate for diverse populations, and

---

Box 20-9   Criteria for Evaluating Internet Resources

Authorship
- Are the author's name and credentials on the site?
- What is the author's clinical reputation?
- Can the author be contacted? Can you give feedback to the site administrator?
- Is a peer review process available?

Nature of Information and Resources
- What is the purpose of the site? Is a mission statement provided?
- From where does the information originate? Is it a reputable organization?
- Are health care journals cited?
- Is the information up to date? Does a date indicate recent updates?

Content Accuracy
- Is the content complete? Is the information based on research?
- Does an advertiser sponsor the site? If yes, is the content presented as an advertisement?
- Does the site appear to be biased?
- Is the owner of the site trying to sell a product?

Navigation, Links, and User Friendliness
- Is the site easy to use?
- Is the presentation logical?
- Does the site have a site map?
- Does the site have links to other sites? Do they work? Are the linked sites credible and relevant?
- Does the site download and print without difficulty?
- Is client privacy protected?

Readability
- What is the reading level of the material?
- Is the site designed for clients or for professionals?
- Can the font be enlarged for use by visually impaired persons?

Data from Brooks, B. (2001). Using the Internet for patient education. *Orthopaedic Nursing, 20*(5), 69-77; and Cader, R., Campbell, S., & Watson, D. (2003). Criteria used by nurses to evaluate practice-related information on the World Wide Web. *Computers, Informatics, Nursing: CIN, 21*(2), 97-102.

---

easy to read, and come from reliable sources. The Web page includes a site map, is clearly intended for consumer health information, and has no advertising. The site is updated regularly; the sponsoring organization can be contacted with comments and suggestions.

PREPARATION OF TEACHING AIDS

If nurses cannot find appropriate teaching materials, they can design some. An advantage to designing teaching aids is the ability to make the teaching aid specific to the community. Nurses may choose to rewrite teaching aids that are too difficult for the target group to read or to supplement existing materials with culture-specific information.

Community/public health nurses also use various methods to develop their own resource files. Suggestions include cutting and saving articles and pictures from newspapers, magazines, professional journals, and pamphlets, being careful to note the source of each. These materials do not have to be from professional publications. A simple picture with an easy-to-read caption found in a lay magazine can be effective. However, specific health information should be consistent with the most recent professional standards. To organize these clippings, the nurse should develop a filing system. Categorization can be by disease, by nursing diagnoses, or by health-related topic. These clippings should be filed periodically and the file reviewed to discard information that is out of date. Using this file when looking for an educational aid or when the need exists to create an educational aid will save time and energy. As a note of caution, the nurse should be aware of copyright issues, taking care not to reproduce materials that have been copyrighted without permission from the author. Fortunately, federal government health-related resources are abundant, and these materials are not copyrighted and are in the public domain for use by anyone.

PRINCIPLES OF TEACHING

We can now consider the teaching principles that the nurse can use throughout the health education process. The nurse can think of these principles as an umbrella covering the entire teaching-learning process. A little bit of coverage can make the experience more comfortable for the nurse and the learners (Figure 20-3).

PHYSICAL ENVIRONMENT

The location of the meeting is the initial consideration. A convenient location prevents transportation problems that prohibit attendance. Health education often occurs in health centers or in public facilities, such as schools, libraries, senior centers, or fire halls. In areas with public transportation, these places are generally accessible during the day but may not be as accessible during the evening, especially if bus routes change after business hours. In rural areas or areas with no public transportation, educational programs may be offered in conjunction with other events, such as meetings of faith communities. The nurse also needs to assess the location and make sure it is accessible and appropriate for persons with disabilities or health problems. For example, conducting an arthritis group-educational session on the upper floors of a building without an elevator or conducting a session for clients who have hearing problems in a building in which renovation or construction is causing environmental noise would be inappropriate.

Another consideration is the safety of the neighborhood and available lighting if the educational session is held in the evening. The nurse might be able to make some security arrangements at the facility if problems exist. Encouraging participants to "come with a friend" is another good suggestion to promote safety.

The nurse should preview the physical environment to assess the size of the room and ensure adequate seating for the number of people expected. The nurse should arrange seating to suit the educational plan before the group arrives. If small-group discussion is planned, chairs around a circular table are ideal. For larger groups, just a circle of chairs is appropriate. If lecture and demonstration are planned, placement of chairs in a semicircle allows everyone to see the demonstration. With very large groups, using several semicircular rows is still effective if the chairs are not directly behind one another.

Two comfort factors are the lighting and temperature of the room. The ability to adjust the lighting is particularly important when using projected visuals. The nurse should practice lighting adjustments before the group arrives. Temperature is important, because learners who are too cold or too warm may have difficulty concentrating.

EDUCATIONAL ENVIRONMENT

In addition to assessing and altering the physical environment, the nurse should adjust the educational environment to promote the optimal learning experience. Using the following principles, the nurse can improve the response of the participants to the educational program.

Communication and Rapport

Learning should be a shared experience. The nurse's communication skills and ability to develop rapport with the learners enhance education. When the nurse offers some initial information about credentials and experience, the group's confidence in the nurse as a resource is increased. The nurse should encourage group participation and communicate willingness to support the learners until objectives are met. The nurse may want to increase the learners' comfort by ensuring the freedom to ask questions and make mistakes within the group.

The nurse needs to be flexible. Even when a lecture is planned, the nurse needs to allow time for audience participation, especially with adult learners who expect to share. The nurse needs to develop the ability to reinforce and clarify health information for the group. Rapport is enhanced as the nurse values member contributions to the group.

The nurse might not be able to answer all discussion questions. A candid statement such as, "I don't know the answer to that, but I can look for it" or "Let me tell you some of the resources we could both use to find the answer" supports the learner's needs and creates a climate of shared responsibility for learning. This response also reinforces for adult learners that asking for help and using community resources to meet learning needs is acceptable.

Nonverbal communication is of special importance when providing health education. Only a fraction of the meaning

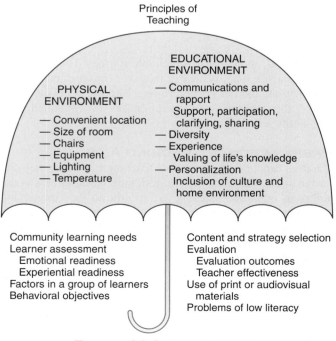

FIGURE 20-3 Principles of teaching.

of communication is transmitted through the spoken word; the rest is conveyed through nonverbal cues such as body language, facial expression, and tone and pitch of voice.

Awareness of nonverbal communication is important when working with clients who have hearing impairments, such as older adults. In this situation, the nurse must establish and maintain eye contact with the client and speak slowly so the client can use lip patterns and facial expression to help with comprehension. Good lighting is important for the client to obtain nonverbal cues. If a window is available, the hearing-impaired person should sit with his or her back to the window and the nurse should face the learner. With this arrangement, the light is on the face of the professional and not shining in the client's eyes. In addition, the nurse should be aware of daylight that provides an uncomfortable glare or exceptionally bright electric lights that put a glare on the nurse's face or shine in the client's eyes.

Diverse Strategies

The nurse should plan the health education program to provide a variety of learning experiences. Based on the assessment of learner needs, teaching strategies should be matched to learning styles. Some people learn by doing, some by hearing, others by reading. Use of a variety of teaching strategies will retain learner interest and meet group needs. The opportunity exists to choose a strategy (see Table 20-4) that meets the objectives and also meets the needs of adult learners (see Table 20-1) for self-direction and control over the learning environment.

Experience

Each learner brings his or her experiences, positive or negative, into the educational setting. The nurse needs to consider individual experiences when planning the content and strategies for health education. Listening carefully to the experiences of the group gives the nurse the needed information. The learner who has had a negative experience with health education might be reluctant to participate. The nurse must not pressure learners into a setting or activity in which they are uncomfortable. The nurse may need to have alternate activities or roles available for the reluctant participant. For example, if a person is unwilling to participate in a role-playing exercise, the client might be the designated note taker or observer of the exercise.

Personalization

Learners will have differences in age, gender, experience, socioeconomic status, culture, and other factors. Using cultural examples in the content can be useful for personalization. Culturally appropriate teaching materials are essential, and the nurse should have a list of resources that may help overcome cultural barriers, such as a resource list for persons who speak English as a second language. Learning can also be personalized by using individual learning contracts and individually negotiated behavioral modifications.

Another way to personalize teaching is to ask the learners how they will apply the knowledge at home. Sharing application ideas in the group provides reinforcement of content and also stimulates learning by encouraging others to try new ideas.

KEY IDEAS

1. Delivery of health education is an increasingly important role of the community/public health nurse. The current public and professional emphasis on health and wellness provides the perfect opportunity for community/public health nurses to use their teaching skills.
2. Promoting a healthy lifestyle through health education is a vital aspect of community/public health nursing.
3. To plan and implement health education programs, the nurse must have an awareness of the teaching-learning process and how it can be applied in a variety of community settings with individuals, families, and groups.
4. Assessing the community and the learners is necessary before the content and strategies for health education are planned.

5. Behavioral objectives are a useful tool for planning and evaluating learning experiences.
6. Content and strategies of the educational program should be tailored to the needs of the community or group.
7. Evaluating the learner outcomes, the nurse, and the educational session are necessary to maximize the value of the health education program.
8. Print, audiovisual, and Internet materials need to be carefully analyzed before use.
9. A variety of teaching techniques, personalized instruction, and interpersonal support promote lifestyle changes.
10. Principles of teaching can be used to enhance the teaching-learning process.

CASE STUDY   Planning a Health Education Program

Ginny is a community health nurse who has spent most of her career working in ambulatory care clinics. She decided she needed a change and moved to a new community. She quickly found a challenging job as an occupational health nurse in an electronics plant. Part of the job description for her new job includes planning and implementing health education programs.

After spending a few months in her new office, Ginny has begun to see some trends in the type of assistance being sought and the

individuals who are seeking it. Many of these people are young men, 25 to 35 years old, who request blood pressure checkups. Most of the men have normal blood pressure, and Ginny is not sure why they continue to come to her office. Ginny enjoys talking and begins to conduct informal assessments on the workers as they come to see her. Many of them have young families to support and fear losing their jobs. Some workers talk with her about the inability to cope with problems at home and the inability to sleep at night.

Continued

CASE STUDY Planning a Health Education Program—cont'd

Few of them engage in any regular cardiovascular exercise, and when she sees them in the cafeteria, Ginny observes them eating high-fat foods with little nutritional value. When their weight and height are assessed, more than two thirds of the men are found to be overweight. Ginny wants to begin her health teaching programs but cannot decide what content to include. She is not sure whether she needs to do any more assessment of the group, given that she may already have more health teaching to do than she can handle.

Where should Ginny begin? Is her needs assessment complete? How should she prioritize the content of the teaching program? Does she know enough about the learners to plan teaching strategies? Will anyone be interested in participating in a health education program?

Needs Assessment and Learning Diagnosis

Ginny recognizes the need for health education on cardiovascular health, diet, and stress reduction. She also recognizes the importance of continuing the establishment of rapport. To begin her health education series, Ginny plans to combine a continued needs assessment with a brief health teaching session.

The needs assessment will help Ginny clarify the priorities of the learning needs. A brief teaching will help establish rapport and identify her as a resource to the workers.

The health teaching will be "You Are Too Busy to Exercise." Ginny has chosen exercise because daily exercise can positively affect each of the identified health problems.

Ginny makes sure that the health education session is held at a convenient time and that all workers are given paid time to attend if they desire. The needs assessment is accomplished by briefly sharing her observations and requesting a show of hands to indicate interest in the cardiovascular health topics. Ginny is also open to discussion and suggestions for future topics and writes these on the overhead. Two index cards and a pencil are also given to each participant to write additional ideas anonymously and put them in a suggestion box. She also invites another nurse educator whom she knows professionally to attend and assist with the initial session.

Constructing the Lesson Plans
Overall Goal

The learners will participate in daily physical activities that promote health and well-being.

Behavioral Objectives (Samples)

1. Ninety percent of the learners will identify two times during the workday when they might walk instead of using the elevator or shuttle bus.
2. Ninety percent of the learners will identify two enjoyable physical activities that can be integrated into the family lifestyle.

3. Sixty percent of the learners will engage in physical activity for 30 minutes three times during the week.
4. Ninety percent of the learners will explore their feelings about starting an exercise program.

Content

- Health benefits of a regular exercise program
- Safety considerations for beginners (e.g., existing health problems)
- Examples of how to fit exercise into daily life
- Popular family activities that promote exercise and family togetherness
- How to choose an activity program that the individual will continue
- Examples of common excuses for not exercising
- Benefits of support from others
- List of community resources for low-cost activities

Teaching Strategies

- Lecture
- Small-group discussion for generating more ideas and examples
- Overhead projector for listing group ideas
- A "buddy system" to offer support
- Role-playing of the sedentary worker and his or her support buddy offering encouragement
- Continued intervention by giving each participant a hang tag for his or her car's rear-view mirror with a reminder to park far away and walk to work
- Pamphlets and brochures from community groups that offer organized activities

Evaluation Methods and Results

- Evaluation methods were planned when a lesson plan was developed.
- Game-show–style questions were used to evaluate objectives 1 and 2; all of the participants were able to meet the objectives during the class.
- Objective 4 was measured by observing the participants verbally sharing ideas in class and in small groups. All of the participants were able to meet this objective.
- To evaluate objective 3, participants were asked to report their exercise patterns at 1 month. Seventy percent of the participants reported increasing exercise to 30 minutes three times per week.

Additional Evaluation

- Evaluation of teacher effectiveness was accomplished by using (1) an evaluation tool (see Table 20-5) and (2) peer evaluation.
- Evaluation of the need for additional health education sessions was based on requests to repeat the session by workers who were unable to attend and on attendance at subsequent sessions.

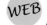 See **Critical Thinking Questions** for this Case Study on the book's website.

LEARNING BY EXPERIENCE AND REFLECTION

1. Select a teaching aid such as a booklet or pamphlet that you have used in the past for health education of a family or group. Analyze the teaching aid for readability, content, and format. Noting your results, will you use the material again or look for different material?

2. Talk with a community/public health nurse about some completed group health education sessions. Did the nurse consider the education to be successful? What criteria were used to measure success? What would the nurse do differently if he or she were repeating the program? Was the nurse reimbursed specifically for teaching or was it considered part of the job?

3. Working with a peer group, develop a health education plan for implementation either with actual clients or with a group of peers. Videotape the implementation of the program. With the group, review the videotape and offer constructive suggestions to one another on improving your teaching techniques.

4. Participate as a learner in a nurse-coordinated health education group in your community. How did you choose the group that you attended? Were your learning needs met? Did you experience a change in behavior? What made the experience a positive or a negative one?

5. Call some providers of health education in your area and inquire about their registration procedures for health education classes. Is requiring participants to register for the program a confidentiality issue, especially if the program deals with a sensitive topic or chronic illness? Should attendance at educational programs be monitored and reported to case managers for clients who participate in a managed care organization? Should attendance be mandatory for clients diagnosed with a controllable illness such as high blood pressure?

COMMUNITY RESOURCES FOR PRACTICE

WEB Information about each of the following organizations is on its website, which can be accessed through the **WebLinks** section of this book's website at *http://evolve.elsevier.com/Maurer/community/*.

Health-Oriented National Organizations
American Cancer Society
American Diabetes Association
American Heart Association
American Lung Association
American Academy of Pediatrics
National Safety Council

Selected Federal Government Resources
Agency for Healthcare Research and Quality
Centers for Disease Control and Prevention
Child Welfare Information Gateway
Consumer Product Safety Commission
HealthFinder
MedlinePlus
National Heart, Lung, and Blood Institute
National Health Information Center
National Institutes of Health
National Institute for Occupational Safety and Health
Office of Disease Prevention and Health Promotion
Office of Minority Health Resource Center
Office on Smoking and Health
President's Council on Physical Fitness and Sports
National Clearinghouse for Alcohol and Drug Information of the Substance Abuse and Mental Health Services Administration (SAMHSA)

STUDY AIDS   http://evolve.elsevier.com/Maurer/community/

Visit the Evolve website for this book to find the following study and assessment materials:

- Quiz
- Web Scenario
- Critical Thinking Questions and Answers for Case Studies
- Care Plans
- *Healthy People* Updates
- Glossary

REFERENCES

Agency for Healthcare Research and Quality. (2004). *New evidence report illustrates links between health literacy and health care use and outcomes.* Retrieved June 30, 2007 from *http://www.ahrq.gov/news/press/pr2004/litpr.htm*.

American Nurses Association. (2007). *Public health nursing: Scope and standards of practice.* Washington, DC: Author.

Atwood, H., & Ellis, J. (1971). Concept of need: An analysis for adult education. *Adult Leadership, 19,* 210-212.

Babcock, D. E., & Miller, M. A. (1994). *Client education theory and practice.* St. Louis: Mosby.

Backer, L., Deck, M., & McCallum, D. (1995). *The presenter's survival kit—It's a jungle out there.* St. Louis: Mosby.

Bandura, A. (1977). Self-efficacy: Toward a unifying theory of behavioral change. *Psychological Review, 84*(2), 191-215.

Bloom, B. S. (Ed.). (1984). *Taxonomy of educational objectives: The classification of educational goals.* New York: David McKay.

Brooks, B. (2001). Using the Internet for patient education. *Orthopaedic Nursing, 20*(5), 69-77.

Cader, R., Campbell, S., & Watson, D. (2003). Criteria used by nurses to evaluate practice-related information on the World Wide Web. *Computers, Informatics, Nursing: CIN, 21*(2), 97-102.

Doak, C., Doak, L., & Root, J. (1996). *Teaching patients with low literacy skills* (2nd ed.). Philadelphia: J. B. Lippincott. Retrieved August 9, 2007 from *http://www.hsph.harvard.edu/healthliteracy/doak.html*.

Easom, L. (2003). Concepts in health promotion perceived self-efficacy and barriers in older adults. *Journal of Gerontological Nursing, 29*(5), 11-19.

Flesch, R. (1949). *The art of readable writing.* New York: Harper & Row.

Fry, E. (1977). Fry's readability graph: Clarification, validity, and extension to level 17. *Journal of Reading, 21,* 242-252.

Green, L., & Kreuter, M. (1991). *Health promotion planning: An educational and environmen-*

tal approach. Mountain View, CA: Mayfield Publishing.

Grolund, N. E. (1970). *Stating behavioral objectives for classroom instruction.* New York: Macmillan.

Houts, P. S., Doak, C. C., Doak, L. G., et al. (2006). The role of pictures in improving health communication: A review of research on attention, comprehension, recall and adherence. *Patient Education Counseling, 61*(2), 173-190.

Institute of Medicine. (2004). *Health literacy: A prescription to end confusion.* Retrieved June 30, 2007 from *http://www.iom.edu/CMS/3775/3827/19723.aspx*.

Knowles, M. S. (1980). *The modern process of adult education:* From pedagogy to andragogy. New York: Cambridge Books.

Loeb, S. J. (2004). Older men's health: Motivation, self-rating, and behaviors. *Nursing Research, 53*(3), 198-206.

McLaughlin, G. H. (1969). SMOG grading: A new readability formula. *Journal of Reading, 12,* 639-646.

Redman, B. K. (1984). *The process of patient education* (5th ed.). St. Louis: Mosby.

Redman, B. K. (1997). *The process of patient education* (8th ed.). St. Louis: Mosby.

Rosenstock, I. M. (1974). Historical origins of the health belief model. In M. Becker (Ed.), *The health belief model and personal behavior.* Thorofare, NJ: Slack.

Schwartzberg, J., & Lagay, F. (2001, June). *Health literacy: What patients know when they leave your office or clinic.* American Medical Association, AMA Ethics. Retrieved 2001 from *http://www.ama-assn.org.*

U.S. Department of Health and Human Services. (2000). *Healthy People 2010.* Washington, DC: U.S. Government Printing Office.

U.S. Department of Health and Human Services. (2006). *Healthy People 2010 Midcourse Review.* Retrieved June 26, 2007 from *http://www.healthypeople.gov/data/midcourse.*

Wantland, D. J., Portillo, C. J., Holzemer, W. L., (2004). The effectiveness of Web-based vs. non–Web-based interventions: A meta-analysis of behavioral change outcomes. *Journal of Medical Internet Research, 6*(4), 40-47.

Williams, B. R., Bezner, J., Chesbro, S. B., et al. (2005). The effect of a behavioral contract on adherence to a walking program in postmenopausal African American women. *Topics in Geriatric Rehabilitation, 21*(4), 332-342.

Wilson, F. L., Racine, E., Tekieli, V., et al. (2003). Literacy, readability and cultural barriers: Critical factors to consider when educating older African Americans about anticoagulation therapy. *Journal of Clinical Nursing, 12*(2), 275-282.

Winters, J. M., & Winters, J. M. (2007). Videoconferencing and telehealth technologies can provide a reliable approach to remote assessment and teaching without compromising quality. *Journal of Cardiovascular Nursing, 22*(1), 51-57.

SUGGESTED READINGS

Billek-Sawhney, B., & Reicherter, E. A. (2005). Literacy and the older adult: Educational considerations for health professionals. *Topics in Geriatric Rehabilitation, 21*(4), 2275-2281.

Dornan, B., & Oermann, M. H. (2006). Evaluation of breastfeeding web sites for patient education. *American Journal of Maternal and Child Health, 31*(1), 18-23.

Huffman, M. (2007). Health coaching: A new and exciting technique to enhance patient self-management and improve outcomes. *Home Healthcare, 25*(4), 271-274.

Lee, C. A., Anderson, M. A., & Hill, P. D. (2006). Cultural sensitivity education for nurses: A pilot study. *Journal of Continuing Education in Nursing, 37*(3), 137-141.

Lewis, D. (2003). Computers in patient education. *Computers, Informatics, Nursing: CIN, 21*(2), 88-96.

McHenry, D. M. (2007). A growing challenge: Patient education in a diverse America. *Journal for Nurses in Staff Development, 23*(2), 83-88.

Redman, B. (2006). *The practice of patient education: A case study approach.* St. Louis: Mosby.

Thomas, C. (2007). Bulletin boards: A teaching strategy for older audiences. *Gerontological Nursing, 33*(3), 45-52.

U.S. Department of Health and Human Services. (2005). *Aim for a healthy weight (Publication No. 05-5213).* Washington, DC: U.S. Government Printing Office.

Contemporary Problems in Community/ Public Health Nursing

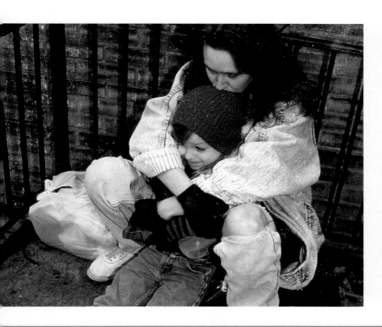

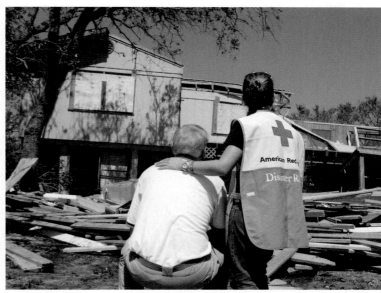

21 Vulnerable Populations

Frances A. Maurer

Focus Questions

Are there groups that are at greater risk for diminished or no access to health care services?

What predisposing factors make some people more vulnerable than others?

What are some of the risks associated with vulnerable groups?

What are some of the most common health problems for vulnerable groups?

What impact does lack of health insurance have on people?

What types of social services are available for vulnerable groups?

Has cost containment affected services? If so, in what ways?

How can community/public health nurses help vulnerable groups access services?

What actions can a community/public health nurse take to reduce health problems associated with poverty and other risk factors?

Chapter Outline

Key Terms

VULNERABLE POPULATIONS

Within the population of the United States, there are aggregates or groups that run a disproportionately greater risk for poor health than the remainder of the population. These groups have certain characteristics, traits, or experiences that increase their vulnerability. All health care professionals, especially community health nurses, come in frequent contact with individuals and families at great risk.

DEFINITION OF VULNERABLE POPULATION

A **vulnerable population** is a group or groups that are more likely to develop health-related problems, have more difficulty accessing health care to address those health problems, and are more likely to experience a poor outcome or shorter life span because of those health conditions. There are a number of characteristics, traits, or circumstances that enhance the potential for poor health. *Healthy People 2010* (U.S. Department of Health and Human Services [USDHHS], 2000) has identified certain groups as more vulnerable to health risks, including the poor, the homeless, the disabled, the severely mentally ill, the very young, and the very old. See the *Healthy People 2010* box on this page for more information.

Not all people who are at risk for poor health would be considered vulnerable. To be considered vulnerable, a person or group generally has aggravating factors that place them at *greater* risk for *ongoing* poor health status than other at-risk persons. For example, a middle-aged obese man with a sedentary lifestyle and hypertension would be considered at risk for cardiac problems. If that man also had an income below the poverty level, no health insurance, and stressors related to living conditions, he would be more likely to be vulnerable to ongoing poor health status than a man with similar risk factors but with an adequate income and health insurance. The man in poverty would be more likely to experience difficulties obtaining and maintaining a relationship with a primary care provider, would have problems accessing tests and procedures for diagnosis and ongoing monitoring, and would have difficulty obtaining and paying for the appropriate medications.

MULTIPLE FACTORS INCREASE VULNERABILITY

The more risk factors for poor health a person or group has, the more likely that person or group will be vulnerable. Figure 21-1 illustrates the interrelationships among multiple factors that affect health status. Some of these factors include lower socioeconomic status, lifestyle behaviors, the psychologic impact of poverty, genetic inheritance, race, ethnicity, and gender, as well as those factors previously mentioned in the discussion. As noted in Chapter 7, a person or group can alter some but not all factors associated with health risks. For example, a person who smokes can stop smoking and reduce his or her risk for lung cancer and heart disease, but a person cannot alter his or her genetic heritage. Some lifestyle situations are more resistant to change and are not easily overcome. For example, someone living in poverty might be there as a result of multigenerational poverty, poor education, poor health, or sudden change in financial situation. Persons with sudden changes in financial situation (e.g., as a result of a loss of employment or a downturn in the economy) are more likely to easily improve their financial situations. Others in poverty face years of struggle and many roadblocks to improving their economic situations.

■ **HEALTHY PEOPLE 2010** ■
Objectives Relevant to Vulnerable Populations— Improve Access to Care

1. Increase to 100% the proportion of persons with health insurance (baseline, 83% of persons under 65 years had health insurance in 1997).
2. Increase the proportion of persons who have a specific source of ongoing care.

Age Group	1998 Baseline	2010 Target
Children under 17 years	93%	97%
Adults 18 years and older	85%	96%

3. Increase to 85% the proportion of people with a usual primary care provider (baseline, 77% in 1996).
4. Reduce hospitalization rates for three ambulatory care–sensitive conditions.

Condition	1996 Baseline (per 10,000 Admissions)	2010 Target (per 10,000 Admissions)
Pediatric asthma	23	17.3
Uncontrolled diabetes in adults 18-64 years	7.2	5.4
Immunization-preventable pneumonia or influenza in adults 65 years or older	10.6	8.0

5. Reduce the proportion of persons who delay or have difficulty in getting emergency medical care to 1.5% (baseline, 2.4% delayed or had difficulty getting emergency care in 2001).
6. Increase the proportion of persons with long-term care needs who have access to the continuum of long-term services.

Care Need	Baseline 2001	2010 Objective
Home care	9.6%	7.7%
Adult daycare	2.9%	2.3%
Assisted living	3.3%	1.8%
Nursing home care	1.1%	0.8%

7. Increase food security among U.S. households to 94% and in so doing reduce hunger (baseline, 88% of households in 1995).

Data from U.S. Department of Health and Human Services. (2000). *Healthy people 2010: Understanding and improving health* (2nd ed.). Washington, DC: U.S. Government Printing Office.; and U.S. Department of Health and Human Services. (2006). *Healthy people 2010: Midcourse review.* Washington, DC: U.S. Government Printing Office.
Refer to Chapters 7, 8, 10, 23, 24, 25, 27, 28, 31, 32, and 33 for specific objectives related to specific vulnerable populations.

Nurses are accustomed to identifying risks associated with poor health and devising interventions to improve health status. Working with vulnerable populations, nurses must become adept at identifying risks that are amenable to intervention as well as those that require greater effort to overcome and those that are not alterable. This chapter identifies some of the most important factors associated with increased

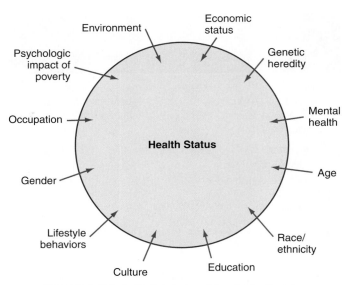

FIGURE 21-1 Multiple factors determine health status.

TABLE 21-1	Poverty Threshold in 2006 by Family Size and Number of Related Children under 18 Years

Family Unit* Size	Poverty Threshold
1	$10,488
2	$13,896
3	$16,242
4	$20,516
5	$23,691
6	$26,434
7	$28,985
8	$32,890
9 or more	$38,975

From U.S. Bureau of the Census. (2007). *Poverty threshold 2006*. Washington, DC: Author. Retrieved June 28, 2007 from *http://www.census.gov/hhes/www/poverty/threshold/thresh06.html*.
*One or more adults and all related children.

vulnerability and their relationship to poor health. Other chapters in this book address specific vulnerable groups, including children (Chapter 27), the elderly (Chapter 28), sexually active adolescents (Chapter 24), individuals exposed to violence (Chapter 23), addicted individuals (Chapter 25), and the mentally ill (Chapter 33), and these groups are not discussed in detail in this chapter.

POVERTY

The most important factor associated with health status is economic status. Poverty drastically increases a person's or group's vulnerability to poor health status.

POVERTY DEFINED

When we think of the poor, we think of people living in **poverty.** People who are poor have difficulty providing the basic necessities of food, clothing, and shelter for themselves and their families. The United States has chosen to set a living standard it considers "adequate," and persons who fall below this income are considered poor. This standard is called the **poverty index** or threshold.

The poverty index is derived by determining the costs of purchasing specific goods and services. It incorporates the cost of food for a minimum adequate diet (called the *Economy Food Plan*) and multiplies that cost by a factor of three to arrive at a *basic subsistence standard*. Adjustments are made to that figure for family size and age of household members (Table 21-1). In 2006, the poverty index for a family of four was $20,516. Any family of four whose income falls below this figure is considered to be poor, and any family whose income is above this level is considered not poor. However, the income standards used to set the poverty index are in dispute. Criticism of the income standards centers around conceptual and measurement issues.

Criticisms of the Poverty Index

There are many specific concerns with the criteria used to determine the poverty index (Citro & Michael, 1995; Short et al., 1999). **Website Resource 21A** provides a summary of specific criticisms of poverty measurements. The major

criticism of the current poverty index is that it is an inadequate measure of poverty. This concern was voiced as early as 1967 in testimony before the U.S. House of Representatives.

Newer criticisms center on the issue of **in-kind payments.** In-kind payments are government subsidies such as food stamps, public housing assistance, and vouchers provided by the Women, Infants, and Children (WIC) program that are not counted as income. Were these benefits counted as income, critics contend, the number of poor in the United States would be substantially lower (Lewit, Terman, & Behrman, 1997). The National Research Council performed an extensive review of the poverty index in 1995. The council found that including certain omitted items (such as in-kind payments) would have lowered the number of people categorized as living in poverty, but considering other factors (such as adequate adjustment for inflation of basic goods, work-related expenses, child care expenses) would have raised the poverty threshold. They recommended that a new poverty measure be adopted, one that better reflects the actual value of benefits and income and is more easily adjustable for changes in inflation and the cost of living (Citro & Michael, 1995).

No action was ever taken on the National Research Council recommendations. The U.S. Bureau of the Census has continued to conduct periodic studies to improve the poverty measures, but no decisions have been reached (U.S. Bureau of the Census, 2003). Current figures indicate that the incomes of 12.6% of all persons in the United States fall below the poverty level. This translates into 37 million, an increase of 2.4 million from 2003. Of that group, 16 million (43%) had incomes of *less than 50% of the poverty level*. People with incomes at 50% or less of the poverty level are considered the **extremely poor.**

Fluctuations in the Poverty Level

The poverty level remained relatively stable from the 1970s through the mid-1980s. Since then, however, this country has experienced at least one period of high inflation, three episodes of substantial economic recession, and high unemployment, which have pushed a large number of families closer to the poverty index ceiling. Figure 21-2 provides an illustration of the fluctuations in poverty level and shows the impact of

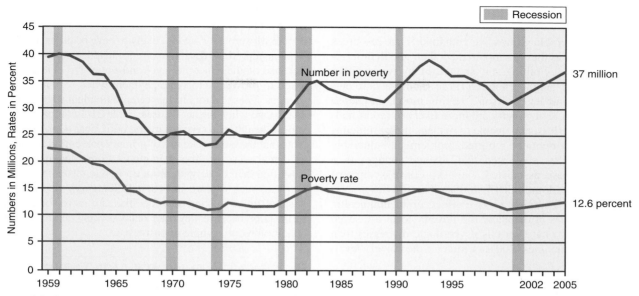

FIGURE 21-2 Number in poverty and poverty rate: 1959 to 2005. (Data from U.S. Bureau of the Census. [2003]. *Poverty in the United States: 2002* [Current Population Reports, P60-222]. Washington, DC: U.S. Government Printing Office; and DeNavas-Walt, C., Proctor, B., & Lee, C. [2006]. *Income, poverty, and health insurance coverage in the United States: 2005* [Current Population Reports, P60-231]. Washington, DC: U.S. Government Printing Office.)

recession on the poverty level. According to the U.S. Bureau of the Census (2006), there are approximately 49.3 million people whose income is *less than the poverty level* or *no more than 25% above the poverty level.*

Proponents of changing the poverty index measures believe that the government's reluctance to revise them is tied to the political implications of such a move. If the newer measures were adopted or inflation adjustments were done yearly, a substantial number of people might be added to the poverty rolls (Betson & Michael, 1997). No one in government wants to be held responsible for policies that could increase the size of the impoverished population.

Shrinking Middle Class at Risk for Poverty

The gap between rich and poor is widening, which leaves the poor relatively poorer in general terms. The middle class is shrinking, and some middle-class families have lost ground and slipped into a lower economic level. Although most Americans do not live in poverty, the trend toward increasing numbers of poor is a matter of concern. Americans who are relatively well off (median family income, $46,326) have become uneasy about their future status. In fact, the Bureau of the Census reports that the distribution of income has become more unequal over time. In 2005, the average after-tax income of those in the top 20% was 37 times greater than the income of families in the lowest 20%. That same year the top 20% of households earned as much as the combined income of the other 80% of households (U.S. Bureau of the Census, 2006). The nation's experience with economic slumps or recessions and the growing government budget deficit serve as uneasy reminders that many more American families could easily suffer economic reversals and join the poor.

EFFECTS OF SOCIOECONOMIC STATUS ON HEALTH

Socioeconomic status influences health status in many different ways. It is not sufficient to consider only access to health

care; the general standard of living is also an important influence on a person's level of health. Poor families have a harder time acquiring the basic necessities of food, clothing, shelter, and transportation. Diet, living conditions, and occupational hazards, as well as access to health care and the time frame in which medical care is sought, are all affected by income and, in turn, affect an individual's health. Because of cost, the poor often have to make choices between medical care and other basic needs. Persons at or below the poverty level are 5 times more likely than those better off to delay seeking care because of cost and 3.5 times more likely not to get care at all (USDHHS, 2006a). People below the poverty level are twice as likely to use the emergency room as those who are better off. Public health care practitioners must be aware of all the risks associated with poverty if they want to improve health status in poor populations.

HEALTH STATUS INDICATORS AND POVERTY

Mortality figures are used as one means of measuring health status. The effects of income on mortality are measured directly and indirectly. Studies suggest a link between very poor economic status and early death (Hadley, 2005; Institute of Medicine [IOM], 2001).

Certain illnesses have been identified as being more common among people living in poverty than in middle-income and high-income groups (USDHHS, 2002, 2006a). These include anemia, arthritis, asthma, diabetes, hearing impairments, influenza, pneumonia, tuberculosis, and certain eye abnormalities (National Health Care for the Homeless Council, 2004; USDHHS, 2006a). Adults 45 to 64 years of age who are below the poverty level are two to three times more likely to have three or more chronic conditions than are people with incomes of 200% or more above the poverty level. They are also more likely to experience severe headaches, migraines, low back pain, neck pain, and joint pain than are people in better economic circumstances (USDHHS, 2006a).

Impact on Health of Multiple Stressors Associated with Poverty

The poor and vulnerable groups live with inadequate resources and ongoing crises as they attempt to meet their and their families' needs for food, clothing, and shelter. Many worry about the safety of their neighborhoods. These multiple unrelenting stressors can impact a person's health, mood, and sense of well-being. People in poverty are more likely to report feeling hopeless, powerless, and unable to manage their problems. Depression is a commonly reported problem in vulnerable people. Research has suggested that adverse changes in a woman's income are associated with depressive symptoms (Children's Defense Fund [CDF], 2005a). The stresses associated with poverty have other adverse effects on mental health. Adults with incomes at or below the poverty level are seven times more likely to have serious psychologic distresses than those with higher incomes (200% or more of the poverty level) (USDHHS, 2006a).

Personal Perceptions of Individual Health

The poor are more likely than the nonpoor to see themselves as physically unwell. Health interview surveys are used to measure an individual's perception of health status. In these surveys lower-income persons have consistently reported greater disability in terms of impairment of activities or confinement to bed, more worry and discomfort from illness, and higher dissatisfaction with their health status (Brooks-Gunn & Duncan, 1997; Cantor et al., 1998; Haan & Kaplan, 1985). About 23% of the poor report a limitation in activity caused by chronic illness, whereas only 9.2% of the nonpoor report a similar limitation. The poor perceive their health as poor or fair (21.3%) at three times the rate reported by the nonpoor (6.3%) (USDHHS, 2002, 2006a).

INCOME LEVEL AND ACCESS TO HEALTH CARE

People who are poor are less likely to have health insurance, even if employed. Many do not qualify for health assistance programs. Because of their income level and uninsured status, many are asked to provide immediate payment when seeking health care services. These factors influence an individual's ability to obtain health care when the need arises. Table 21-2 compares the use of various health care services by the poor, near poor, and nonpoor. Note that the poor make use of primary prevention services, such as dental care, childhood immunizations, and mammograms, less often than those with more economic resources. Acute care services, such as care in hospital emergency departments and hospitalization in short-stay facilities, are more commonly used by the poor, because they often delay seeking treatment until their condition requires more intensive care.

RACE AND ETHNICITY AND THEIR RELATIONSHIP TO INCOME AND HEALTH STATUS

In the United States, ethnic and racial minorities are more vulnerable to poor health status than is the remainder of the population. They are also more likely to be poor, which illustrates the relationship between poverty and health. One of the main goals of *Healthy People 2010* is the reduction of health disparities between subgroups of the U.S. population.

MORTALITY AND MORBIDITY

Two important indirect measures of the influence of income on health are (1) comparison of mortality rates for white and minority populations in the United States and (2) examination of the total mortality rates from illnesses that affect the

---

TABLE 21-2 **Types of Health Care Services Used by Socioeconomic Status**

	Poor	Near Poor	Nonpoor
One to three health care visits to doctor's office or emergency department, or home visits	37.7%	42.5%	48.1%
No health care visits to office or clinic (children under 18 years)	15.9%	15.7%	9.4%
Vaccination rate, combined series (children 19-35 months)	78%	85%*	*
No usual source of health care (children under 18 years)	10.6%	7.7%	3.0%
No usual source of health care (adults 18-64 years)	28%	26%	13.7%
One emergency department visit during past 12 months (children under 18 years)	32.3%	23.8%	18.3%
One or more emergency department visits during past 12 months (adults 18 years or older)	29.3%	23.6%	18.7%
Dental visits in past year (children 2-17 years)	65.5%	69%	82.2%
Dental visits in past year (adults 18-64 years)	44.5%	47.6%	71.3%
Untreated dental caries			
Children 2-17 years	32.1%	28.8%	12.7%
Adults 18-64 years	40.1%	36.1%	16.1%
Mammogram (women over 40 years)	55.4%	60.8%	74.3%
One or more hospital stays in the past year	9.2%	6.9%	5.2%

Data from U.S. Department of Health and Human Services. (2006). *Health, United States, 2006.* Washington, DC: U.S. Government Printing Office.
"Poor" is defined as having an income below 100% of the poverty level.
"Near poor" is defined as having an income of more than 100% but less than 200% of the poverty level.
"Nonpoor" is defined as having an income of 200% or more of the poverty level.
*Combined data for near poor and nonpoor in these categories.

poor to a greater degree than other income groups. Examining the differences between whites and minorities is an appropriate indirect measure of the effect of income on health because minorities are at greater risk for poverty. Approximately 12.6% of the population is classified as poor. When this group is broken down by racial composition, white Americans are found to bear less risk for poverty than other racial and ethnic groups (Figure 21-3). Blacks, Hispanics, and American Indians have a three times greater risk for poverty than white Americans (U.S. Bureau of the Census, 2006).

The mortality rate for blacks is approximately 29% higher than that for whites (USDHHS, 2006a). The death rate is 10.8 per 1000 persons for blacks and 8.2 per 1000 for whites (USDHHS, 2006a). Mortality rates for the three leading causes of death show the same trend in racial disparity. Deaths from heart disease, stroke, and cancer are all higher in blacks than in whites. The severity of illness is also different. Blacks have a greater chance of high health care expenditures, a measure of more severe illness (see Chapter 10).

Some other racial/ethnic groups also have greater rates of poverty than the white population, and most experience health disparities. The life expectancy of American Indians is 7 years less than that of white Americans (Indian Health Service, 2002). Blacks, Mexican Americans, and American Indians have a higher rate of diabetes than the white population (see Figure 7-5). Other, more affluent racial/ethnic groups, for example, Chinese Americans and Japanese Americans, experience less health disparity and sometimes exhibit more favorable scores on health status measures than do white Americans (see Chapter 8).

Infant mortality is another indicator of health status. Infant death rates are higher for blacks and some other minorities (Figure 21-4). In 2003, the black infant mortality rate was 13.5 per 1000 live births, which is 2.5 times higher than the white infant mortality rate (5.7 per 1000) (USDHHS, 2006a). Note that Figure 21-4 illustrates different infant mortality rates for subsets within a certain racial/ethnic minority. For example, Puerto Ricans have a higher infant mortality rate, whereas Mexicans have a lower infant mortality rate.

OTHER FACTORS THAT IMPACT RACIAL/ETHNIC HEALTH DISPARITIES

Many factors contribute to health disparities. Poverty is perhaps the most important factor, but other factors also play a role. Discrimination, the health care environment, and the specific health behaviors and beliefs of individuals and groups also affect health status. Research indicates that racial and ethnic minorities receive a lower quality of health care than nonminorities, even when conditions are comparable (insurance status, income, age, and severity of condition) (Smedley et al., 2002). Health behaviors and beliefs influence health because, among other things, they dictate how and when a person seeks health care services, what health practices they employ, and their diet and exercise behaviors.

DIET, HEALTH, SOCIOECONOMIC STATUS, AND RACIAL/ETHNIC INFLUENCES

Income and nutritional status are positively correlated. Studies indicate that American Indians, Alaska Natives, Mexican Americans, and African Americans—all populations with greater levels of poverty than whites—have a significantly greater risk for nutritionally related diseases. Although some dietary choices are the result of cultural influences, income-related restrictions on diet choices play a greater role in nutritional deficiencies in all groups, especially minorities.

In studies of minority children, vitamin and mineral deficiencies are found to be relatively commonplace. Growth retardation in preschool children is a health indicator and might reflect the inadequacy of a child's diet (USDHHS, 2000). In American Indian and Hispanic children, there is an increased incidence of linear growth stunting (Lewit & Kerrebrock, 1997; Trowbridge, 1984). Diet and weight relationships in minority children indicate greater deviation from average weights, either above or below the norm. Classic studies of minority populations in America found that many more children were either underweight or overweight with unbalanced diets (Jacob et al., 1976; USDHHS, 2000; Yanochik-Owen & White, 1977). In 2004 the obesity rate for black and Mexican children was higher than for white children, and those children at or below the poverty level had a higher rate of obesity than

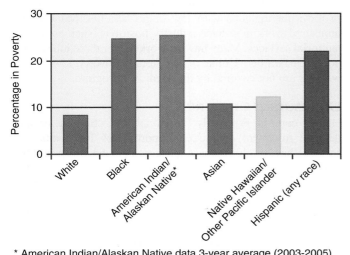

* American Indian/Alaskan Native data 3-year average (2003-2005)

FIGURE 21-3 Percentage in poverty by race and ethnic origin. (Data from DeNavas-Walt, C., Proctor, B., & Lee, C. [2006]. *Income, poverty, and health insurance coverage in the United States: 2005* [Current Population Reports, P60-231]. Washington, DC: U.S. Government Printing Office.)

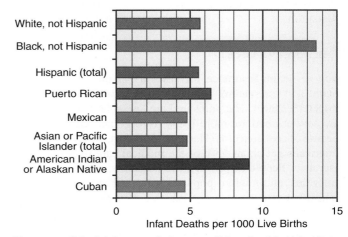

FIGURE 21-4 Infant mortality by race and Hispanic origin: United States, 2001 to 2003. (Data from U.S. Department of Health and Human Services. [2006]. *Health, United States, 2006* [Table 23, pp. 167-169]. Washington, DC: U.S. Government Printing Office.)

children whose families had more income (USDHHS, 2006a). Some studies find that all children in poverty show a greater incidence of growth stunting than do children from other economic environments (Brooks-Gunn & Duncan, 1997; Rutter, 1994; USDHHS, 2000).

Obesity is more common among Hispanic, black, American Indian, and Pacific Islander women (USDHHS, 2006a). Each of these racial/ethnic groups has higher rates of poverty than the general population. Obesity is at epidemic proportions in the United States. Old studies indicated that people whose family income was less than 130% of the poverty index were more likely to be obese than people with higher incomes (USDHHS, 2000). Newer data indicate that adults of all economic levels have a similar risk for obesity (USDHHS, 2006a).

Diet-related health issues are more common in the poor. Adults below the poverty level have a greater risk of having high serum cholesterol levels than those whose income is above the poverty level (USDHHS, 2006a). Anemia is a frequent health problem in low-income persons. Studies have found anemia to be especially prevalent in blacks, American Indians, and Mexican American children (USDHHS, 2000). The incidence in American Indians is triple the national rate (USDHHS, 1997). Anemia and concomitant low weight gain in pregnancy are also more prevalent in minorities (Schneck et al., 1990; USDHHS, 2000). About 44% of all pregnant black women have a hemoglobin level below 11 g/dL (USDHHS, 2000). The prevalence of third-trimester anemia among low-income pregnant women persists (Centers for Disease Control and Prevention, 1996). Several government programs have been designed specifically to support the health and diet needs of poor pregnant women and their children (see Chapter 24).

Poverty is correlated with food scarcity and hunger. Some people in this country still experience hunger and lack access to needed food. The federal government uses the term **food insecurity** to describe the condition of people who do not consistently have access to enough food to allow for active and healthy living (CDF, 2005a, p. 18). In 2005, 12.6 million people were food insecure. Thirty-three percent of people with incomes below 130% of the poverty index experience food scarcity compared with only 6.7% with incomes at or above 185% of the poverty index (Nord et al., 2006). *Healthy People 2010* is committed to eliminating hunger in the American population.

THE UNINSURED

Lack of health insurance increases a person's risk for poor health and premature death (Hadley, 2005; IOM, 2001; USDHHS, 2000). The uninsured are less able to access health care services and are more likely to forgo needed health care because of cost concerns (Hadley & Holahan, 2004). Uninsured Americans get about 55% of the medical care of people with insurance. People in poverty, the homeless, racial and ethnic minorities, and migrant populations are all at greater risk for no health insurance coverage, which increases their vulnerability to poor health.

NUMBER OF UNINSURED

More than 46.6 million people, or 15.9% of the population, do not have health insurance (U.S. Bureau of the Census, 2006). Others are without health insurance for some time during the

calendar year. For example, new college graduates who have not found employment might lose coverage under their parents' plan, which stops after college graduation, if not before. The United States Department of Health and Human Services (USDHHS, 2006a) reports that 25% of the population younger than 65 years of age is uninsured at some point during a given year.

The number of uninsured has increased since 2000, when 14% of the population was without health insurance. An economy with large numbers of low-level entry jobs and fewer blue collar high-paying job opportunities has left more people unemployed or underemployed and without employer-provided insurance. Even workers with health insurance plans are vulnerable to loss of coverage. An increasing number of employers are eliminating or reducing health insurance coverage to employees and their families (see Chapter 4). Workers who are between jobs and workers whose employers do not offer health insurance coverage are also at risk for having no insurance coverage. The Consolidated Omnibus Budget Reconciliation Act (COBRA) provided health insurance portability for workers who changed jobs, but many find the premiums too costly. Only approximately 20% of eligible workers participate in the COBRA program (Kapur & Marquis, 2003). Individuals with no health insurance who try to find individual insurance plans find the costs too high. In 2001, the estimated cost of COBRA family health insurance was between $7000 and $8000 (Lambrew, 2001; Scandlen, 2001). No newer data are available, although the cost of insurance has continued to rise every year since that report. About 53% of adults who do not have health insurance cite cost as the major reason they are uninsured (Insurance Information Institute, 2007).

EMPLOYMENT STATUS AND HEALTH INSURANCE

It is a misconception that most of the uninsured are unemployed (Figure 21-5). Most of the uninsured are workers or the dependents of employed persons. Low-income workers are four times less likely to have health insurance (24.4%) than those with higher incomes (8.5% of those with incomes over $75,000). Most workers without health insurance are employed in lower-paying jobs with few or no benefits. Many of the uninsured work in service industry positions, such as food or janitorial services. Many have to work two or three jobs to support their families. Unlike nonworkers in poverty, low-income workers are not covered by the Medicaid program.

UNINSURED CHILDREN

Health care is especially important for children because delayed treatment or missed opportunities for health care services have lifelong consequences. Poor health in children also affects their educational progress. There are 8.3 million uninsured children in the United States (U.S. Bureau of the Census, 2006). Expansion of health insurance for children has been a major goal of government. In fact, the uninsured rate among children dropped from 25% in 1997 to 12% in 2000 and has remained relatively steady since then. Today, the rate of noninsurance among children is 11.2% (U.S. Bureau of the Census, 2006). The rate decline is attributed to the State Children's Health Insurance Program (SCHIP) begun in 1997 (see Chapters 4 and 27). Despite the success of SCHIP, eligible children have been missed. Approximately 20% to 50%

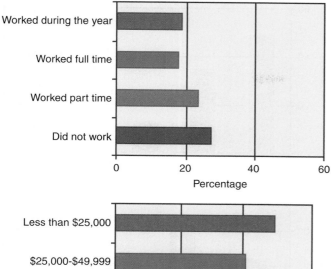

FIGURE 21-5 People without health insurance by work experience and income level. (Data from DeNavas-Walt, C., Proctor, B., & Lee, C. [2006]. *Income, poverty, and health insurance coverage in the United States: 2005* [P60-231]. Washington, DC: U.S. Government Printing Office.)

of the 8.3 million uninsured children are eligible for SCHIP (Congressional Budget Office [CBO], 2007; Freking, 2007).

IMPACT OF NO HEALTH INSURANCE ON HEALTH

The uninsured are more likely to be hospitalized for preventable conditions (Hadley & Holahan, 2004; Kozak et al., 2001). Because of delays in seeking health care, the uninsured are sicker when they seek treatment (Hadley, 2005; IOM, 2002a). Women with breast cancer who are uninsured have a 30% to 50% greater risk of dying than women with health insurance (IOM, 2007). The uninsured are less likely to receive early treatment for heart disease and diabetes. Even when diagnosed with heart disease or diabetes, they are less likely to use appropriate medications and follow-up services. Delayed care is expensive care. The estimated cost of uncompensated care provided to the uninsured by hospitals and other service providers is between $28.8 and $40.7 billion per year (American Hospital Association, 2006; Hadley & Holahan, 2004). The Institute of Medicine (IOM, 2003) estimated the actual economic costs of not having health insurance to be between $65 and $130 billion per year in health care costs, lost wages, and increased spending burdens on other public welfare programs. Hadley and Holahan (2004) argue that money would be better spent in providing some kind of insurance coverage for the uninsured. That strategy would improve the health status of a vulnerable group and have an added benefit in reducing costs associated with delayed care.

HOMELESSNESS

Homeless people include persons from all walks of life: very poor men, women, and children, unskilled workers, farmers, housewives, social workers, health care professionals, and scientists. Some become homeless because of poverty or a failure of their family support systems. Others become homeless through loss of employment, abandonment, domestic violence, alcoholism, mental illness, social deviance, mental retardation, physical illness, or disability. Whatever the cause, the homeless are more vulnerable to health problems and reduced access to health care services.

DEFINITION OF HOMELESSNESS

Homelessness describes the existence of a person who has no fixed nighttime residence or who has a nighttime residence that is designed to provide temporary shelter or is a public or private place not intended to provide sleeping accommodations for human beings. This definition encompasses those persons who are literally homeless but does not include those who are living with relatives or in substandard housing. Homeless families who have had to move in with relatives or friends and rural homeless persons are not nearly as visible and are more likely to be omitted from federal programs designed to address issues relating to homelessness.

There is great variation in the characteristics of homeless people, the length of homelessness, and the extent of disability. Belcher and colleagues (1991) identified three stages of homelessness:

- Stage 1 *(episodic homelessness)* includes persons who are vulnerable to homelessness and might be homeless from time to time.
- Stage 2 *(temporary homelessness)* includes homeless persons who continue to identify with mainstream society.
- Stage 3 *(chronic homelessness)* includes persons for whom homelessness has become normative.

NUMBER OF HOMELESS

Estimates are that between 2.3 and 3.5 million people are homeless in a given year (National Law Center on Homelessness and Poverty, 2004). Homelessness is not a permanent situation for most people. A national study reported that as many as 13.5 million adults have been homeless at some time in their lives (U.S. Department of Housing and Urban Development [HUD], 2007). The growing shortage of affordable housing, declines in public assistance, and increase in poverty are largely responsible for increases in homelessness (National Coalition for the Homeless, 2006a).

CHARACTERISTICS OF THE HOMELESS

Homelessness is both an urban and a rural problem, but rural homelessness is harder to document. In rural areas, white single or married women and their children are the largest groups of homeless (Fisher, 2005; Vissing, 1996). In urban areas, single men and families with children are the two largest groups of homeless persons (Figure 21-6). It is always difficult to categorize homeless people, because each person might have several characteristics that place them in more than one risk group. For example, a veteran with a history of substance abuse and mental illness could be included in at least three subgroups of the homeless.

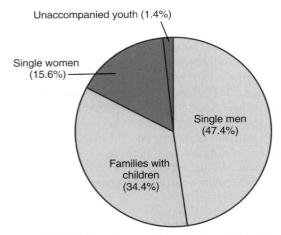

A homeless man who has lived on the streets for several years. What sort of life does this man experience? How does he feel about his situation?

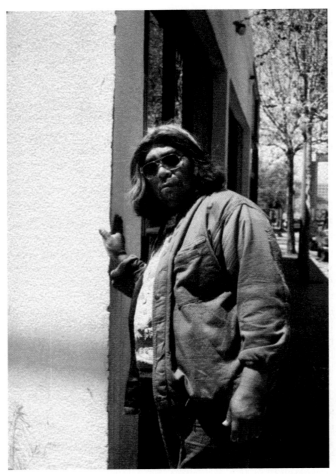

FIGURE 21-6 Estimated composition of urban sheltered homeless: United States. (Data from U.S. Department of Housing and Urban Development. [2007]. *The annual homeless assessment report to Congress.* Washington DC: Author.)

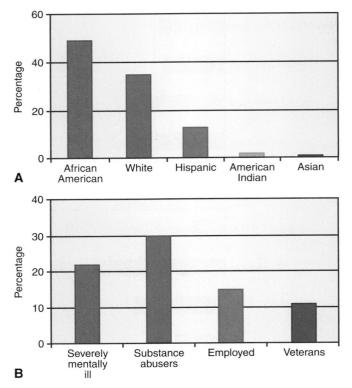

Note: Categories are not mutually exclusive.

FIGURE 21-7 **A,** Estimated racial composition of urban homeless, United States. **B,** Estimated subgroups of the urban homeless, United States. (Data from U.S. Conference of Mayors. [2004]. *Hunger and homelessness in America's cities 2004.* Washington, DC: Author; and U.S. Conference of Mayors. [2005]. *Hunger and homelessness in America's cities 2005.* Washington, DC: Author.)

The racial and ethnic makeup of the homeless varies according to geographic location. Approximately 50% of urban homeless people are black (HUD, 2007) (Figure 21-7). Rural homeless people are more likely to be white, American Indian, or migrant workers (National American Indian Housing Council, 2007; U.S. Department of Agriculture, 1996). People in poverty, people with serious mental illness, and substance abusers are more likely to be homeless.

The Poor

Persons living at or below the poverty level are more vulnerable and more likely to become homeless than are those living above the poverty level. *Between 7% and 9% of all poor people are homeless, but nearly all homeless people are poor.* Any financial emergency, major illness, or job loss may result in homelessness.

Because African American, Hispanic, and American Indian populations are at greater risk for poverty, they are also at greater risk for homelessness. The National American Indian Housing Council (2007) reports that more than 90,000 American Indian families are homeless or in extremely poor living arrangements. The council states that there is an immediate need for 200,000 housing units. The council estimates that American Indians have a rate of substandard housing that is six times that of the general population. Many families live in cars, tents, or makeshift shelters. Overcrowding is a major issue. American Indians live in overcrowded homes at a rate three times that of the general population. Some homes have as many as 25 people living in one dwelling.

Homeless Men

Single homeless men still make up the largest and most visible subgroup of the homeless population. Veterans comprise at least 17% of the urban homeless population (HUD, 2007). For some, homelessness becomes a long-term condition, with a few men reporting that they have been homeless for 30 to 50 years. Older homeless men are more likely to have been married at some time in their lives, whereas many younger homeless men have never been married.

Homeless Women

Homeless women are not as visible and are more difficult to count than men. There are many types of homeless women, including the following:

- Single women with a history of drug and alcohol abuse or domestic violence (HUD, 2007)
- Women known as *bag ladies*
- Women with dependent children (the largest group) (HUD, 2007; Lowe et al., 2002).

Bag ladies are alienated from the mainstream of society and use few resources. They are *psychologically decompensated* (emotionally and mentally separated from society) and *socially decompensated* (unable to interact with other people).

Homeless Families and Children

An increase in the number of homeless families has been reported in all areas of the United States. *Families with children are the fastest growing group among the homeless population* (U.S. Conference of Mayors, 2005). Families comprise the largest group of homeless in rural areas. Although some homeless families are two-parent units, most consist of one parent with an average of two or three young children.

Homeless mothers tend to be young, have less education, and have low employment rates. More than 80% of single homeless women with children are nonwhite (Bassuk et al., 1997; Smith & North, 1994). *Domestic abuse* has been cited as the primary cause of homelessness for mothers with children. The U.S. Conference of Mayors (2005) reports that half of the cities surveyed cited domestic violence as the primary cause of homelessness in that population. In San Diego, 50% of homeless women are victims of domestic violence (ACLU, 2004). Pregnant homeless women are especially vulnerable to multiple risk factors. They lack prenatal care, adequate nutrition, and basic necessities of life, which places both themselves and their unborn children at risk.

Homeless families tend to seek shelter, and women with small children receive priority for temporary housing. Two-parent families might "double up" with other families, live in tents in parks, or live in the family car. Once homeless, families have a difficult time finding a place to live because of the lack of available housing and the substantial down payments demanded for rental units. One or both parents might be employed on a full- or part-time basis, but their income is not sufficient to meet the minimal needs of their family members.

Data on homelessness indicate that 39% of the total homeless population are youths under the age of 18. Most homeless children are preschoolers between infancy and 5 years of age (National Coalition for the Homeless, 2006b). Developmental testing of preschool children indicates that preschool homeless children exhibit significant developmental delay in all areas (National Coalition for the Homeless, 2006c). Many homeless children have attended preschool and school programs on a sporadic basis. They often have deficiencies in learning readiness and social interaction skills, and they experience long intervals between school attendance. This lost school time results in academic underachievement and gaps in learning and experience.

Homeless Teenagers

Between 500,000 and 1.3 million teenagers are homeless (National Coalition for the Homeless, 2006d). The National Law Center on Homelessness and Poverty (2004) reports that unaccompanied minors comprise 5% of the urban homeless population. Some are **runaways**, and others are **"throwaways."** *Runaway* teens have significant psychologic disturbances and a higher rate of drug abuse and contacts with the legal system than other youths. Studies of runaway youths reveal a high incidence of family violence and physical abuse. These homeless teenagers reported being victims of chronic, severe abuse, both physical and sexual, beginning at an early age (Tyler & Cauce, 2002). *Throwaway* children have parents who have severed all relationships with them; usually, rejection is preceded by months or years of failed relationships. Divorce, incestuous behaviors, or scapegoating might contribute to the desertion of the child.

Some homeless youths are separated from their families because shelter policies prohibit the admission of teenagers, especially older boys, in family shelters. In 2005 over 57% of families had to break up to enter emergency shelters (U.S. Conference of Mayors, 2005). Some youth are homeless because they have been discharged from residential or institutional placements or have become too old for foster care (National Coalition for the Homeless, 2006d).

Homeless youths adapt quickly to life on the street, where they are subject to criminal victimization, such as learning to solicit money and drugs through prostitution. They gravitate toward neighborhoods where they are tolerated, such as areas frequented by intravenous drug users and prostitutes. They engage in substance abuse and risky sexual practices (Steele et al., 2003).

Homeless youths have more serious and complex health problems but are the most difficult population to reach. Their distrust and fear of persons in authority make it harder to provide health care and other services. They often have poor hygiene practices, receive inadequate nutrition, and are vulnerable to poor health, human immunodeficiency virus (HIV) infection and acquired immunodeficiency syndrome (AIDS), other sexually transmitted diseases, and premature death (Rew, 2003; Woods et al., 2003).

SHELTERS AND FOOD ASSISTANCE

Many religious organizations and advocacy groups have worked to help homeless people, but these efforts have not kept pace with the growing numbers and changing needs. Despite a dramatic increase in shelter beds during the 1980s and 1990s, there are not enough shelters and transitional housing spaces for the homeless population (National Coalition for the Homeless, 2006a). In almost all major cities, the estimated number of homeless people exceeds the available spaces. Thirty-two percent of homeless families are turned away from shelters because there is no space. The majority of surveyed cities (88%) report that they have to turn away homeless families due to lack of resources (U.S. Conference of Mayors, 2005). Although rates of homelessness in rural areas are similar to or higher than rates in urban areas, there are few or no shelters in rural communities (Aron & Fitchen, 1996; National Coalition for the Homeless, 2006e).

In 2006, the requests for emergency food assistance increased by 12%. More than 43% of cities report that they have to turn away people due to lack of adequate food supplies (U.S. Conference of Mayors, 2005). Cities report that the resources and budgets to meet those needs decreased at the same time that the need for food supplies increased. More than 83% of the cities polled reported that they had to decrease the quantity of food provided and/or limit the number of times people could come for food assistance (U.S. Conference of Mayors, 2005).

MEDICAL PROBLEMS ASSOCIATED WITH HOMELESSNESS

Homelessness has a severe impact on a person's health and well-being. Rates of acute and chronic health problems among the homeless are high (Box 21-1).

Physical Health Problems

Homeless people are exposed to extreme weather conditions, the common cold and influenza, and minor injuries, as well as diseases such as tuberculosis and HIV/AIDS. Chronic diseases are often exacerbated because health care services are not consistently available. Colds and influenza are the most common acute health problem. The second most common acute problem is accidents or trauma. Scabies and lice infestations not only are troublesome but also can contribute to dangerous secondary infections.

Hypertension, diabetes, respiratory illnesses, and cardiovascular diseases are the most common chronic medical problems among the homeless population (National Coalition for the Homeless, 2006f; National Health Care for the Homeless Council, 2004). Chronic alcoholics are subject to gastrointestinal disorders, esophageal hemorrhage, pancreatitis, and cirrhosis. Cancer is not generally detected until the disease is advanced and the person is debilitated. Homeless women have the same illnesses as homeless men, may be subjected to rape, and may have one or more sexually transmitted diseases.

Homeless children are more likely to have a variety of physical illnesses, including higher rates of asthma, anemia, diarrhea, and poor nutrition (National Coalition for the Homeless, 2006c; National Health Care for the Homeless Council, 2004). Homeless children have ear infection rates that are 50% higher than the national average (Redlener & Johnson, 1999). Many homeless children are subjected to physical abuse. Immunizations might not be started or may be incomplete, which places children at risk for preventable communicable diseases. In New York City, 61% of children without housing have not completed the recommended immunization series for their age. Homeless children are more vulnerable to mental health problems, such as anxiety, depression, and withdrawal (National Coalition for the Homeless, 2006c; National Health Care for the Homeless Council, 2004).

Mental Illness and Substance Abuse

Mental illness, low self-esteem related to past neglect or abuse, and substance abuse are some of the intrinsic factors that predispose people to homelessness. Approximately 23% of the homeless are mentally ill, and 32% are substance abusers (National Institute of Mental Health, 2005; U.S. Conference of Mayors, 2005). Severely mentally ill persons have difficulty carrying out activities of daily living, managing themselves, engaging in interpersonal relationships, and going to work. The mentally ill homeless are homeless for longer periods than are homeless persons who are not mentally ill. The chances for the severely mentally ill to escape homelessness are limited because of the disruption they experience in personal judgment, motivation, and social skills (National Coalition for the Homeless, 2006g; McQuistion et al., 2003).

BOX 21-1 **Health Problems of the Homeless**

Acute Physical Disorders
- Upper respiratory tract conditions
- Trauma, including major and minor injuries
- Minor skin ailments
- Infestations (mites and lice)
- Nutritional deficiencies
- Tuberculosis

Chronic Physical Disorders
- Alcoholism and other substance addictions
- Hypertension
- Gastrointestinal disorders
- Peripheral vascular disorders
- Dental problems
- Diabetes
- Human immunodeficiency virus infection/acquired immunodeficiency syndrome
- Neurologic disorders

Problems Associated with Pregnancy
- Lack of prenatal care
- Inadequate nutrition
- Obstetric complications

Mental Health Problems
- Schizophrenia
- Bipolar disorder
- Depression
- Panic disorder
- Borderline personality disorder
- Antisocial personality disorder

Health Problems in Children
- Anxiety
- Incomplete or no immunizations
- Speech and language problems
- Upper respiratory tract illnesses and asthma
- Minor skin ailments
- Ear infections
- Gastrointestinal disorders
- Trauma
- Eye disorders
- Lice infestations

Data from Lindsey, A. (1995). Physical health of homeless adults. *Annual Review of Nursing Research, 13,* 31-61; Wright, J. D., & Weber, E. (1987). *Homelessness and health.* New York: McGraw-Hill; Better Homes Fund. (1999). *Homeless children: America's new outcasts.* Newton Centre, MA: Author; and National Health Care for the Homeless Council. (2004). *People need health care.* Retrieved January 9, 2004 from *http://www.nationalhomeless.org/facts/health.html.*

Only 5% to 7% of the homeless with mental illness need to be institutionalized (see Chapter 33). Most can live in the community with appropriate support services (National Coalition for the Homeless, 2006g). The problem is that the chronically mentally ill often do not seek help.

Substance abuse is a significant risk for homeless populations. The U.S. Conference of Mayors (2005) reported that approximately 30% of homeless urban adults are substance abusers. Of homeless substance abusers, many are alcoholics (see Chapter 25). A review of studies of homeless populations indicated that alcoholism is six to seven times more prevalent in homeless men than in the general population; the rate of alcoholism among homeless women might be even higher than the rate among homeless men (Reardon et al., 2003).

Drug addiction includes dependence on drugs such as cocaine, crack, heroin, and a variety of prescription medications and inhalants. Runaway and homeless youths who live on the streets have higher rates of illicit drug use than do youths living in shelters or households (Woods et al., 2003). Many of the people with substance abuse problems might also have one or more mental disorders (see Chapter 25).

Depression is one of the most frequent and most serious mood disorders among homeless individuals. One study of homeless and low-income women with families found that both groups have higher rates of depression than the overall female population (National Coalition for the Homeless, 2001). Community health nurses working with the homeless should routinely evaluate clients for signs of depression. Approximately 33% of homeless mothers have made at least one suicide attempt (Bassuk et al., 1997). Nurses working in clinics that serve the homeless population should assess clients for depression and suicidal ideation. Some clients might freely tell the nurse that they are depressed; others might withhold the information unless they are asked.

Willie came to the walk-in health clinic in an inner-city soup kitchen. It was past time to see clients, and the nurses were preparing to leave. A community health nurse asked Willie why he had come to the clinic. He said, "I'm going to kill myself today." When the nurse asked if he had a plan, he told her that he had a loaded gun under his mattress. When he left the clinic, he was going to go to his room and shoot himself in the head at 4:00 PM. When asked why he planned to kill himself, he said that he was so depressed he could not stand it anymore. "I'm an alcoholic. I'm all alone. I have no friends, and my family won't speak to me. I haven't had a job in over 10 years. What's the point? Life is just not worth living." The nurse told Willie that arrangements had been made for an emergency evaluation at a psychiatric hospital. He was transported to the hospital and arrived at the emergency department within an hour after he had come to the clinic.

MIGRANT/SEASONAL WORKERS

Migrant and seasonal workers are vulnerable to health risks, and many lack access to health care services. A **migrant worker** is someone who moves from state to state with the seasons in search of employment. A **seasonal worker** is someone who lives and works in one geographic area. Seasonal workers might travel to work, but they usually limit that travel to a single state or area. Some workers travel with their families,

and the whole family, including children, might work. Other workers travel without families in small groups. For example, a group of men might travel from job to job together and send money home to their families, rather than have their families travel with them.

Most migrant/seasonal workers are employed in agricultural work in nurseries, orchards, canneries, or farm fields. For example, they may do planting, potting, or trimming in nurseries; pick apples or oranges in orchards; prepare and pack fruits, vegetables, and fish in canneries; or harvest corn or wheat in the field.

CHARACTERISTICS OF MIGRANT/SEASONAL WORKERS

Estimates of the number of migrant/seasonal workers vary and might not be very accurate. Migratory populations are difficult to count. Undocumented workers, those without visas or work papers, do not cooperate with data collectors. Many are involved in agriculture and other seasonal work. An estimated 11 to 12 million undocumented migrants live in the United States (Pew Hispanic Center, 2006). An estimated 1 million migrant/seasonal workers are in California alone (Villarejo et al., 2000). Approximately 60% of the migrant workers in California are undocumented workers (University of California, 2005). Many more work in states such as Texas, Arizona, Florida, Georgia, Washington, Oregon, and other states with agricultural businesses.

Most agricultural workers are foreign born. They are predominantly Hispanic of Mexican origin, but include people from Central America, blacks, American Indians, and Asians. The most recent surveys indicate that migrant/seasonal workers are mostly young males (median age 31), who are married (59%) and have little schooling (6 or fewer years of school). Most do not speak English well, cannot read Spanish well, and have a very low income (University of California, 2005; Villarejo et al., 2000).

VULNERABILITY OF MIGRANT/SEASONAL WORKERS

Agricultural workers have multiple risk factors, which increases their chances of poor health and premature death. Their low wages place them at the very bottom of the impoverished population. Seventy-five percent of farmworkers earn less than $10,000 per year and 60% have incomes below the poverty level (National Center for Farmworker Health, 2007a). Most do not have health insurance. Seventy percent of migrant/seasonal workers in one sample had no health insurance, and only 7% were covered by any government-funded program for low-income people (Villarejo et al., 2000). Because they have no health insurance and low income, they are subject to the health problems and risks associated with these two conditions, as identified earlier in this chapter.

Many migrant/seasonal workers are undocumented and therefore at special risk. Because they risk discovery and deportation, these workers have little recourse when working conditions and housing are not adequate. Workers are often housed in overcrowded barracks, trailers, buses, or sheds with poor sanitation. One study found that 30% of California farmworkers lived in such situations (National Center for Farmworker Health, 2007b). Heating and cooling, utilities, and plumbing are substandard or not available (Holden, 2001; National Center for Farmworker Health, 2007a). Many use communal bathing and toilet facilities.

Working conditions are poor. Agricultural workers in general are exposed to pesticides and have a high rate of work-related injuries (see Chapters 9 and 32). The Environmental Protection Agency (EPA) estimates that 300,000 farmworkers have pesticide-related health problems each year (National Center for Farmworker Health, 2007b). Agricultural workers are excluded from the protections of the Fair Standards Act and the National Labor Relations Act, and workers on small farms are excluded from the protections of the Occupational Health and Safety Administration (OSHA) (National Center for Farmworker Health, 2007a). They are exempt from overtime pay provisions and have no collective bargaining rights. Children as young as 12 are allowed to work in agriculture, and there are no age restrictions for children working on family farms (National Center for Farmworker Health, 2007b; Villarejo et al., 2000). Oversight of what few protections the law provides is sporadic and ineffective. For example, the EPA and OSHA mandate that workers be educated and trained regarding the safe handling and application of pesticides. However, a large number of migrant workers are still without that training (National Center for Farmworker Health, 2007a).

Jason and José are migrant workers who travel with several other men to different states seeking work. They have contracted with a crew boss to work in the fields of a Mr. Samuels. The farmer owns 700 acres of orchards and employs 22 workers, and his enterprise is therefore covered by OSHA regulations. Today the two men are picking and packing peaches. They have been working for 8 hours and are expected to continue for another 2 to 4 hours or longer. The crew boss supplied them with sandwiches and soda at lunchtime. The temperature is over 90 degrees. Both men are suffering from dehydration. Today, representatives of the local health department are visiting Mr. Samuels because there have been complaints in the past. The health department personnel note that there are no toilets or water sources in the fields. In the past, they have reminded the farmer that he is required by OSHA regulations to provide sanitation and fresh water to workers. Mr. Samuels has responded by spacing his workers in the fields in such a way that they are not concentrated enough to be covered by OSHA regulations. Today the health department personnel notice that the workers are concentrated enough to be covered by OSHA regulations and, after a half hour of dispute, Mr. Samuels agrees to provide water and toilet facilities. Jason and José note that this pattern of compliance/noncompliance is a regular occurrence and have no faith that their working conditions will improve.

SPECIAL HEALTH CONCERNS OF MIGRANT/ SEASONAL WORKERS

For many migrant/seasonal workers, English is a second language, and others speak little or no English. This makes it doubly hard for them to negotiate the health care system when they are ill (see Chapter 10). Many feel uncomfortable seeking care in the United States (Mines et al., 2001). Workers feel intimidated by health care professionals and have different expectations of service. For example, many expect their problems to be treated immediately. They do not expect to have to come to the clinic several times before the problem is pinpointed and dealt with. Those with undocumented immigration status are less likely to attempt to see a health care worker. Forty-three percent of undocumented workers have never visited a doc-

tor or clinic since entering the United States (Lighthall, 2004). Many are reluctant to seek care because they run the risk of losing their jobs.

Extreme poverty, lack of insurance, and difficulty accessing health care create additional risks above and beyond the normal risks associated with language barriers, immigration issues, and the other factors discussed earlier. Migrant workers' health problems include the following (Mines et al., 2001; University of California, 2005; Villarejo et al., 2000):

- Twenty-five percent have a diagnosed chronic condition (e.g., high blood pressure, diabetes).
- Eighty percent report that they suffer from stress and anxiety.
- More than 75% of men and women are overweight.
- Rates of iron deficiency anemia, leukemia, high serum cholesterol level, and stomach, uterine, and cervical cancer are higher than in the general population.
- Twenty-seven percent have had a work-related injury.
- Prenatal care is delayed, with 30% of pregnant women waiting till the second trimester and 14% waiting until the third trimester to seek care.
- The infant mortality rate is 25% higher than the national average.
- Rates of infectious diseases, including tuberculosis, are higher than in the general population.

More than 40% of farmworkers who visit migrant health clinics have multiple and complex health problems. They also experience the usual problems associated with vulnerable populations: poor nutrition, poor dental care, poor vision care, and lack of, or little, prenatal care. Children of migrant farmworkers receive little preventive health care, have poor schooling, and experience exposure to environmental pesticides. All family members are exposed to the problems associated with poor housing conditions, such as lice, rats, roaches, lead paint, poor sanitation, no heat, and poor ventilation (National Center for Farmworker Health, 2007a, 2007b).

THE PRISON POPULATION

Vulnerable populations are overrepresented in the juvenile justice and adult prison systems. Prisoners are more likely to come from poverty. They have lower levels of education than the general public. They are more likely to come from single-parent homes (see Chapter 24). They are more likely to have been exposed to drug trafficking, weapons, and gang violence in their neighborhoods (CDF, 2005a).

There is a disproportionate representation of racial minorities in the prison population. For example, minority youths comprise 62% of the population in the juvenile justice system (CDF, 2005a). In 2004 the adult population in jails and state and federal prisons was 2.13 million, most of whom were males. Females comprised only 8.5% of the total prison population (USDHHS, 2006a). Racial minorities are at significantly greater risk of imprisonment than are whites. Blacks are 7 times more likely and Hispanics 2.5 times more likely to be incarcerated than are whites (USDHHS, 2006a).

Racial minorities comprise a larger portion of the adult prison population that would be expected from their numbers in the general U.S. population. For example, whites comprise 31%, blacks 42%, and Hispanics 19% of the prison population. However, whites are 67%, blacks are 12.7%, and Hispanics are 11.2% of the total U.S. population

(U.S. Bureau of the Census, 2007b). Prisoners have more health risks and poorer health status than members of the general population. This is to be expected given the characteristics of the prisoner population with regard to poverty, minority status, poor education, exposure to violence and substance abuse, and single-parent home environments, all of which have been noted previously in this chapter or in Chapter 24 to be risks for poor health.

HEALTH ISSUES IN THE PRISON POPULATION

Prisoners report more, and more chronic, health problems than would be expected in their age group. Approximately 20% consider themselves disabled and 40% of inmates 45 years or older reported a physical impairment (Maruschak, 2006a). The U.S. Department of Justice (2006) reported that 64% of inmates were found to have a mental problem. Inmates are at risk of injury because of their exposure to violence within the prison system. Approximately 13% report being injured, and the risk of injury increases with time served. One in three inmates who served 1 year or more reports being injured while in prison.

Prisoners are more likely to be substance dependent or substance abusers. Half of all federal inmates were using drugs before incarceration (Mumola & Karberg, 2006). Histories of drug use have increased among prisoners over the past 20 years. Marijuana is the most commonly used substance, followed by crack cocaine, heroin, depressants, methamphetamine, hallucinogens, and inhalants. Many committed crimes to pay for drugs. The U.S. Department of Justice reported that 25% of violent offenders (those convicted of homicide, sexual assault, or physical assault) committed their crimes while using drugs (Mumola & Karberg, 2006). Inmates do have access to some drug treatment programs. The most common methods are peer counseling, drug education, and self-help programs. Only 14% of inmates are in a treatment program run by a trained professional.

Because prisoners have a higher rate of risky behaviors, they have a greater risk of HIV/AIDS. In 2004, 23,046 state and federal prisoners were HIV positive, more than three times the rate in the U.S. population (Maruschak, 2006b). Testing for HIV is sporadic. Twenty states test all inmates on admission. Almost all states will test an inmate if the inmate has potentially HIV-related symptoms or requests testing. A more uniform HIV testing policy is appropriate given the higher risk of the prison population.

SERVICES AVAILABLE FOR VULNERABLE POPULATIONS

There are a number of government and private assistance programs that help selected vulnerable groups (Box 21-2). The two largest federal-state programs, Temporary Assistance to

---

Box 21-2 Programs Providing Assistance to Vulnerable Populations

Temporary Assistance to Needy Families (TANF)
Replaced Aid to Families with Dependent Children (AFDC) in 1996. Provides temporary financial assistance to needy families with dependent children. Places a time limit on benefits; most recipients must have a job within 2 years of starting the program. Monthly payment of $300 to $500 per month intended to pay for low-cost rental housing, food, and clothing. Persons enrolled in the TANF program generally qualify for Medicaid.

Medicaid
Federal and state-funded assistance program to provide health care services to certain people in need (see Chapter 4). Medicaid increasingly relies on managed care programs to provide care to qualified individuals and families.

State Children's Health Insurance Program (SCHIP)
Designed to enroll children who would not be covered under the Medicaid program, for example, children in one- or two-parent families whose income is more than the qualifying income for Medicaid but who are still needy (see Chapter 27).

Women, Infants, and Children (WIC) Program
Provides supplemental food and formula for infants, young children, and pregnant and new mothers (see Chapters 3 and 27).

Food Stamp Program
Provides redeemable coupons that can be used to purchase a restricted list of groceries and food items at participating food stores.

**Section 8 Rental Assistance Program/
Voucher Programs**
Provide rental subsidies designed to help low-income people pay for low-rent housing. Recipients pay 30% of their income and the federal government pays 70% (Turner, 2003).

Low-Income Housing Units
Also known as public housing. These units are built with government funding, and persons who qualify based on income may live in the units.

Supplemental Security Income (SSI)
Provides cash supplements for qualified individuals who cannot work because of physical or mental problems, including the blind, aged, and disabled. Persons receiving SSI benefits qualify for Medicare after a selected period of SSI eligibility.

Migrant Health Centers
Established as part of the Migrant Health Act of 1962. The centers provide primary and selected preventive health care to migrant/seasonal workers and their families. In 2001 the centers served 600,000 people at 120 cites (Hawkins, 2001). Rural health centers (see Chapter 32) also provide selected health care services to migrants, the homeless, and other vulnerable groups.

McKinney Homeless Assistance Act, 1987
Provided for outpatient health care services and attempted to ensure homeless children access to the same educational opportunities as children living in homes. Services of 16 federal agencies are coordinated under the act.

USDHHS-Funded Nurse-Managed Clinics
Certain nurse-managed health centers are funded under grants from the U.S. Department of Health and Human Services (USDHHS) to provide health care services to vulnerable populations, including the homeless.

Voluntary Organizations
Church programs, charitable organizations, and foundations offer selected programs in selected geographic areas. These include soup kitchens, overnight shelters, temporary housing, medical care either in clinics or on site, transportation, translation assistance, and advocates to assist persons attempting to navigate the governmental assistance programs.

Needy Families (TANF) and Supplemental Security Income (SSI), covered 11.5 million people in 2005 and had a combined budget of $63.9 billion (U.S. Bureau of the Census, 2007b). Both programs covered only 34% of the 37 million people below the poverty line in 2005. Voluntary and charitable organizations also provide assistance to needy groups. Services are sporadic, are seldom comprehensive, and are not available in every area of the country.

WELFARE REFORM—TANF/MEDICAID

In 1996, Congress passed the Personal Responsibility and Work Opportunity Reconciliation Act, known as *welfare reform*. This act, and related legislation designed to balance the budget, disproportionately affected the poorest and most vulnerable groups in this country. The act created TANF, which put tight limitations on the length of time a family could receive welfare assistance (5-year lifetime limit). Each family had to develop a plan to improve its independence. Families could be punished for noncompliance, including having health benefits canceled. Benefits are very meager. The current median TANF benefit and food stamp allotment combined provide the equivalent of approximately 29% of the poverty-level income (Nickelson, 2004). Consequently, families on these two programs do not receive adequate relief. The eligibility requirements for Medicaid were also altered.

> Edith Wilson and her four children are newly enrolled in the TANF and food stamp programs. Sally Haines, a community health nurse, visits with Edith to review her children's eligibility for SCHIP or Medicaid. Edith reports that she receives $539 per month in TANF benefits. She is paying 30% ($159) of her TANF allotment for rent. She is being asked to participate in a welfare-to-work program to improve her chances of employment. Edith reports that she has no one to watch her two preschool children for free during the day. Her neighbor will watch her two youngest children for $200 a month ($50 a week). That leaves her with $200 to see her four children through all other expenses for the month. She receives food stamp assistance, but despite very hard budgeting, she is unable to stretch the food stamps to pay for all her groceries and other subsistence products (soap, food wrap, etc.) for the month. Edith shares with Sally her frustration at the demands of the program. She feels that the program administrators do not understand her predicament and have done nothing to help her with her situation.

At the same time, the WIC program was sharply curtailed. Homeless mothers housed with others can use the supplemental feeding program to feed their children for only 1 year. Women in prison or teenaged mothers in detention centers are denied benefits for their children. Adults without children can use the program for 3 months over a period of 3 years. Children and elderly adults enrolled in daycare are not permitted to receive federally funded snacks during the hours they are away from home (National Coalition for the Homeless, 2001).

Effects of Welfare Reform on Immigrants

Welfare reform had a particularly strong effect on immigrants. Legal immigrants who entered the country after August 22, 1996, were barred from receiving benefits from SSI, Medicaid, TANF, or state block grants. Medicaid coverage was provided only in emergencies. For example, prenatal care is not considered an emergency, but labor and delivery are. States have the option to resume services to immigrants after they have been in the United States for 5 years. If immigrants become U.S. citizens, they are eligible for services. Undocumented or illegal immigrants are barred from all federal public benefits, and all states are required to bar illegal immigrants from state and locally funded programs. This has created a dilemma for health care workers, who feel that they have been asked to operate as agents of the Immigration Service. Many facilities simply do not ask immigration status when providing care to individuals and families.

In 2006, Congress required states to demand proof of citizenship for all Medicaid recipients. This has resulted in an additional administrative burden for states and a delay in Medicaid coverage for families. For example, in 2006 the state of Maryland spend $12 million dollars in administrative costs to comply with the new regulation (Epstein, 2007). A passport or two types of identification, including a driver's license, are required for proof of citizenship. This requirement places additional burdens on poor people, many of whom do not have passports and/or driver's licenses. A smaller but significant number do not have birth certificates. In Virginia, 6 out of 10 legitimately eligible children went without Medicaid coverage for weeks to months because their parents had difficulty providing the necessary documentation (Jenkins, 2007). In 1997, Congress created SCHIP. That program has similar but less restrictive criteria than Medicaid. Children who have been in this country for fewer than 5 years are prohibited from coverage under federal funding, but states can use their own funds to provide care. After 5 years of residency, children are mandated care under SCHIP with both federal and state monies (Guttmacher Institute, 2003).

Effects of Welfare Reform on Families

One of the effects of welfare reform is a drop in the number of households receiving welfare assistance. In 1991 over half of all low-income families received benefits under Aid to Families with Dependent Children (AFDC), the precursor to TANF. In 2005, only 20% of families received TANF assistance (CBO, 2007). In addition, the average TANF payment ($4100 in 2005) is less than the payment under AFDC more than 10 years ago ($6500 in 1991). To make up for these deficits, the federal government is using the Earned Income Tax Credit (EITC), which is a tax credit for low-income households that pay taxes on wages. The tax credits make up approximately 11% of the income of eligible low-income households (CBO, 2007).

The impact of these changes is just now starting to emerge. Early findings suggest that approximately 60% of families who have moved off welfare have improved their economic situations, but 40% of families are not doing well (CBO, 2007). Most individuals, including those who are doing all right, are employed in low-wage jobs that pay below the poverty level and have no health care benefits. In 1997, 675,000 people, including 400,000 children, lost health insurance because of welfare reform (Families USA, 1999). The TANF time limitations (5 years) started to impact families in 2001, when a quarter of a million families lost benefits (Bloom et al., 2002). Research studies suggest that one third of those who leave the TANF program each year do so because they have reached the specified time limits (CDF, 2005a).

If families leave the TANF program before they have reached the time limit, they are more likely to stay out of the program if they receive other types of support. For example, families who have housing subsidies are more likely to stay off TANF benefits than those who do not (CDF, 2005a). Most families leaving welfare do not receive subsidized housing. Only 25% of TANF families live in public housing or receive housing vouchers (National Coalition for the Homeless, 2006a). A study sponsored by the Urban Institute found that families that had child care assistance were less likely (19.5%) than families that did not (27.7%) to return to TANF. Families that were able to continue with government health insurance were less likely (21.7%) than families that could not (32.8%) to return to TANF (Loprest, 2003).

TANF imposed new limitations on the number of welfare recipients eligible to continue schooling. Before welfare reform, educational pursuits were considered a work activity. Under TANF states may have only 20% of their caseloads in educational activities, which leaves 80% at a disadvantage (CDF, 2005a). Forty-one percent of TANF recipients do not have a high school diploma, and 76% are considered to have low literacy levels (Tally, 2005). Further education would have beneficial results on individuals' earning capacity and job attainment, and assist them in gaining employment stability with the possibility of advancement into better-paying jobs.

Limitations in state budgets (see Chapter 4) have eroded the ability of states to provide TANF families with support services such as child care and transportation (CDF, 2005b). These limitations, coupled with the TANF term limits, have created a pool of people who are at great risk. The subset of extremely poor is increasing. Nearly 60% of children in poverty and 250,000 families are in extreme poverty (CDF, 2005a; U.S. Bureau of the Census, 2006). Without changes to the current welfare program, the expectation is that an increasing number of vulnerable families and individuals might experience a loss of benefits, work at poorly paying jobs, or remain unemployed. For individuals and families in such circumstances, there will be an even greater risk for poor health and limited access to health care services.

MEDICAL CARE

In addition to the services provided under the Medicaid program, medical services are available for free or at a reduced rate from various private and publicly funded health care services. For example, many metropolitan cities allocate public monies to provide part of the budgets for medical clinics for the homeless. These clinics may receive other funds through private charities or fund raising. These services are erratically located and often are not available to some vulnerable people.

The most numerous sources of medical services are community health centers (CHCs). CHCs originated in the 1960s and offer medical care in both urban and rural areas. There are over 1000 CHCs providing services at 5000 sites in the United States. CHCs serve approximately 15 million people per year (Sardell, 2007). Their clients are poor, may be uninsured or on Medicaid, and are usually sicker, often chronically ill, and comprised of more minorities than the general population (National Association of Community Health Centers, 2005; Sardell, 2007). Almost all CHC patients have incomes at or below 200% of the poverty level; 40% are uninsured,

with most of the remainder on Medicaid. CHCs rely heavily on nurse practitioners and other nursing staff to provide much of the care (Health Resources and Services Administration, 2004). President George W. Bush has supported CHCs by increasing the federal funds available for these centers.

HOUSING

This country's lack of affordable housing and limited availability of housing assistance places many in poverty at risk for homelessness (National Coalition for the Homeless, 2006a). Rent increases and availability of only a few units have exacerbated the situation. The estimated shortage is at least 4.9 million units (National Coalition for the Homeless, 2006a). By 2007, rent had increased 28% faster than inflation or wages (Pelletiere et al., 2006). Federal housing subsidies for low-income families have decreased by 49% since 1980, and the average wait for Section 8 vouchers is 3 years (National Coalition for the Homeless, 2006c; U.S. Conference of Mayors, 2005). Because of this backlog, families spend more time in shelters or remain homeless for longer periods, which creates further stress on the available shelter spaces.

In almost every locality, the minimum wage is not adequate to afford an unsubsidized one- or two-bedroom apartment. The combined earnings of two full-time minimum-wage workers will not pay the rent in most parts of the United States (National Low Income Housing Coalition, 2004). Figure 21-8 shows the difference between minimum wage income and the actual income (national housing wage) needed to afford the rent for one- or two-bedroom units. The **national housing wage** assumes that individuals will use 30% of their total income for housing costs. An estimated 5 million households earn less than the lowest median income and spend more than 50% of their income on housing with no help from public assistance housing programs (CDF, 2005a). All of these households are one paycheck away from being homeless.

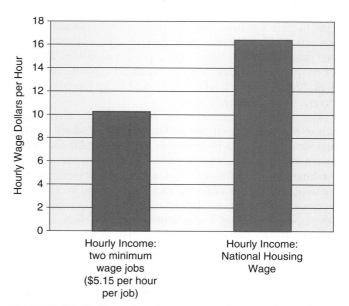

FIGURE 21-8 Comparison of minimum-wage income and national housing wage (income needed to afford rent for a one- or two-bedroom unit). (Data from Pelletiere, D., Wardrip, K., & Crowley, S. [2006]. *Out of reach 2006*. Washington, DC: National Low Income Coalition.)

GOVERNMENT BUDGET CRISIS AND AVAILABILITY OF SERVICES

The current fiscal crisis impacts funding for programs at both the national and state levels. States are especially stressed because they have borne increasing responsibility for publicly funded programs as a result of the federal change to a block grant system (see Chapter 4). Starting in 2002, states have had to contend with shrinking revenues and increased program responsibilities. No states have responded by raising income taxes. Some states have made efforts to increase fees, such as the cost for renewing driver's licenses or car registrations. Others have or are in the process of increasing property taxes, tuition at state-funded colleges and universities, sales taxes, cigarette taxes, and other revenue sources.

Many states have used program cuts as the primary method for balancing the budget. Funding cuts have been especially heavy in programs serving low-income families—for example, TANF, SCHIP, Medicaid, and other welfare programs (CDF, 2002; Smith et al., 2005). The following are some examples of these cuts (Parrott & Wu, 2003; Smith et al., 2005):

- Fifteen states made cuts in welfare-to-work programs.
- Eleven states have cut assistance to poor families with the most severe problems.
- Eight states have cut transportation assistance.
- Ten states have cut basic cash assistance benefits.
- Forty-three states initiated additional pharmacy cost controls to the Medicaid program.
- Three states and the District of Columbia have reduced or eliminated teen pregnancy prevention efforts.
- Thirty-two states have reduced the income level for eligibility for child care programs.

These cuts have affected an estimated 1.2 to 1.6 million low-income people (Ku & Nimalendran, 2003). Funding cuts are expected to continue and to be more comprehensive. States are experiencing shortfalls (revenues lower than expenditures) of approximately $40 billion (Smith et al., 2005). These shortfalls will require additional cuts in programs for vulnerable populations, and the cuts might extend to other programs as well. Some states have made changes to the Medicaid application process that requires more reverifications at shorter time intervals. This requirement may create an additional difficulty for recipients, resulting in lower Medicaid enrollments (Smith et al., 2005). The effects will be added hardships for low-income individuals and families.

The federal government has been reducing the proportion of the budget spent on welfare programs. Many of these cuts have been made by changing to block grants for federal contributions to state-run programs. Current efforts involve a combination of continuing block grants and/or reduced funding to programs. For example, President George W. Bush first proposed converting the Department of Housing and Urban Development housing voucher program into block grants to states (Turner, 2003). The proposal met stiff resistance, and therefore an alternative proposal for the 2004 fiscal year budget called for funding cuts to the voucher program. The allocation of federal funds for housing assistance has not kept pace with inflation, which resulted in an actual decrease of 2.4% in the housing assistance budget in 2007 (Harvard University, 2007). Currently the federal government provides rental assistance to only 25% of eligible renters. In addition, the portion of federal funds provided to the states for their Medicaid and SCHIP programs is planned to be reduced by $98 billion during the next 10 years (Ku & Nimalendran, 2003).

Current funding levels do not allow adequate coverage of all those in need of the services provided by the programs. With additional stresses on state and federal budgets, little effort will be made to expand those programs to include persons already eligible for their services. For example, funding and services are a critical issue for migrant health centers. Service expansion is not possible without additional funding. Currently migrant clinics serve fewer than 20% of the migrant farmworker population (National Center for Farmworker Health, 2002). With the current budget crisis, there is little hope that additional funding will be available. SCHIP is another program that does not provide services to all eligible children. The current federal funding proposal is for $5 billion per year. State officials are lobbying for funding at three times the current level (Freking, 2007). Without these additional funds, states will be hard pressed to continue services or to increase the number of eligible needy children enrolled in the program. Between 2 and 5.5 million eligible children are not enrolled in SCHIP (CBO, 2007; Freking, 2007). States have no incentive to continue outreach enrollment efforts when their budgets are already stressed and they have considered or are considering cuts to the SCHIP program. In 2004, six states stopped enrolling children in the SCHIP program, and by 2005, 39 states had added cost-sharing co-pays to the SCHIP program (CBO, 2007; Ross & Cox, 2004).

NURSING CONSIDERATIONS FOR VULNERABLE POPULATIONS

Community/public health nurses frequently care for individuals and families with many health risks and limited access to care. The health needs of these individuals are often complex and linked to social and financial conditions. Nurses need to develop expertise in a broad range of areas to best serve this population.

KNOWLEDGE OF AVAILABLE PROGRAMS

For vulnerable individuals, poor health is often exacerbated by the lack or limited availability of health care services. Knowledge of the primary assistance programs, their benefits, and their scope of coverage is important to community health nursing. Nurses need this information so that they can refer families to these programs and assist them in applying for the benefits for which they are eligible. Nurses should become familiar with additional programs and services that might be unique in their communities. They should develop contacts at each agency and be aware of the eligibility criteria to avoid sending clients on futile appointments.

An extensive application process is required for most government assistance programs. Clients often require help in gathering the necessary data (proof of income, bills, etc.) and filling out the forms. Nurses can either help with the application process or refer clients to others they know who are capable of performing that task.

People enrolled in many of these programs must undergo periodic review of their cases to renew their eligibility. If their financial situation has changed, there is always the possibility that payments will not continue. If they fail to attend a review appointment, their benefits or cash payments might be stopped.

Nurses should be familiar with the renewal criteria for programs and be prepared to remind clients and encourage compliance with the schedule. It is also possible to find assistance for people having trouble with transportation to appointments or problems with completing paperwork.

ASSISTANCE WITH LANGUAGE BARRIERS AND CULTURAL CONCERNS

Many migrant/seasonal workers have difficulty reading or speaking English. Other minorities might have similar problems. Interpreter services should be available so that every effort is made to interpret their concerns accurately. Sensitivity to differences in cultural values and health care practices should also be part of quality care (see Chapter 10).

PRIMARY AND SECONDARY PREVENTION

Nurses should take every opportunity to screen for potential problems and provide health education on appropriate health issues. Because many vulnerable children and adults have incomplete vaccination records, all should be screened for immunization status. Areas such as adequate nutrition, the importance of prenatal care and vitamins, the need for dental and eye examinations, good dental hygiene, safe food storage, and the importance of ensuring safe water supplies are all appropriate to address in health education.

Screening to identify health problems and reduce further complications is also a concern. This chapter has identified numerous health problems that tend to occur in vulnerable populations. Nurses should be aware of and screen for these health conditions. They include hypertension, diabetes, obesity, poor foot care, infectious diseases, anemia, high cholesterol level, dental caries, and substance abuse. Every encounter should be used as an opportunity to check for other health problems or concerns. This is not only good nursing care but is cost effective. For example, people in poor health are less able to work and provide for their families (Hadley & Holahan, 2003). If early screening and treatment improve a person's health so that the person can work, not only is the cost of care reduced (delayed care is more expensive), but the family's financial resources are also improved.

CASE FINDING

Nurses should consider every client contact as an opportunity to search for other family members in need of health services.

Karen Boggs is a community health nurse doing prenatal home visiting. She visits Jackie Allen, a 16-year-old expecting her first baby. Jackie lives with her mother (Doris Jones), her mother's boyfriend, several siblings, and her grandmother (Sammy Allen). During the visit, Karen reviews the usual prenatal concerns and addresses Jackie's questions about dieting during pregnancy. She notices that Jackie's grandmother, Sammy, is sitting in a chair with her right foot propped up on two pillows. After Karen has completed her visit with Jackie, she asks Sammy about her foot. Sammy tells the nurse that she has diabetes and her foot is causing her problems. Karen examines Sammy's foot and finds it swollen, hot to the touch, and with reduced pain sensation. The nurse discovers that Sammy has no primary care provider and has not been taking her prescribed medication because she cannot afford it. The nurse, with Sammy's permission, arranges for an appointment that afternoon at the local nurse-centered clinic. During subsequent visits to her primary client, she continues to monitor Sammy's health and assist her in acquiring needed services, including a source of prescription medication.

In this case, the nurse could have ignored other family members and simply done the job she was sent to do, which is perform a prenatal check on Jackie. Instead, she took the time to discover another family member in need. Although the program in which she was employed could provide services only to Jackie, the nurse was knowledgeable about other types of community services that would fit the needs of the grandmother, Sammy Allen. She took the time to initiate care, and in so doing, reduced Sammy's chances of additional complications.

ADVOCACY FOR IMPROVED SERVICES

Community nurses are in a position to know the problems associated with specific service programs. They have a unique body of information to share with others in efforts to improve funding and program effectiveness. Nurses can advocate by becoming involved as members of special interest groups, testifying before governmental agencies, advocating changes from within their current employing agencies, and providing information to other community groups and organizations. Many people are truly not aware of the problems experienced by vulnerable groups. Speaking out helps put an issue in the forefront of public consciousness. The IOM (2004) recently determined that the best means of improving health status for vulnerable populations is to adopt some type of universal health insurance (see Chapter 4).

PARTNERSHIP WITH COMMUNITY GROUPS

One of the recommendations of the IOM (2002b) is that public health organizations partner with other community groups to provide needed services. This is a relatively new role for community health nurses, but one that could improve services to needy populations. Nurses should become active in identifying potential community partners to help address specific health needs for at-risk groups. For example, a community might have a high rate of HIV/AIDS among the teenaged population. The community health nurse could form a work group to coordinate a response. Community participants might include representatives of the nurse's employer (the local health agency), leaders of youth groups (e.g., Boy Scouts or Girl Scouts), local area church leaders, leaders of local sports associations, and representatives of the local HIV/AIDS activist group (if present in the community).

DATA COLLECTION AND RESEARCH

One of the most important ways nurses can help improve services for vulnerable populations is to document the effects of poor, improved, or good service. To do this, nurses must develop accurate data collection systems. They must conduct well-designed research studies with established outcome measures. Different types of intervention programs can be tested for effectiveness. Collaboration with other health professionals should strengthen these research endeavors.

In the current climate of economic retrenchment, cost concerns must be addressed as part of any intervention strategy. All studies should include cost-benefit measures as part of the research design. All nurses involved in research study and design need to remember that interventions that produce improved health results and save money or cost no more than current services are more likely to be favorably received by decision makers.

ETHICS IN PRACTICE

Refusing to Provide Care

Gail A. DeLuca Havens, PhD, RN

The emergency department (ED) is remarkably quiet for a Friday evening. As Maureen, the registered nurse manager for the evening shift, passes the doorway to the waiting room, she catches a glimpse of a dusky face and hands; a man is huddled in a corner at the far end of the room. She wonders why the person is not in one of the examining rooms being evaluated. However, before she has the opportunity to find out why this man is in the waiting room, she is called to assist in calming down an 8-year-old.

Two hours later, activity has increased in the ED. Maureen is headed down the hallway adjacent to the waiting room to retrieve some supplies from a seldom-used cabinet. Her attention is drawn to the same figure in the corner of the waiting room. He doesn't seem to have moved since she noticed him earlier. There is something vaguely familiar about the huddled figure, but what draws Maureen into the waiting room and to the corner is her intuition that something is amiss here. She realizes that the person in the waiting room is experiencing respiratory distress at about the same time that she recognizes the person as Horace, a homeless alcoholic who is a frequent visitor to the ED.

"Thanks for finally coming to get me, Miss Maureen. I was beginning to feel mighty poorly."

"No problem, Horace," replies Maureen, as she starts to wheel him from the waiting room into the treatment area. "What seems to be the problem?"

"Trouble breathing. When I take a deep breath it hurts right around where the doctors listen to my heart."

"How long have you been waiting to see the doctor, Horace?"

"Since one o'clock."

Maureen notes that was 8 hours ago. "Horace, did the admitting clerk register you when you arrived?"

"It seemed like she did," he replied.

Maureen situates Horace on a gurney in an examining bay and goes to retrieve his chart from the admitting clerk's area while the physician is evaluating him. Maureen is summoned back into the treatment area by a code call. Returning, she finds that Horace has stopped breathing, and the physician is slow to respond. She notices that no one but herself seems particularly committed to responding appropriately in this emergency situation. She says, "Folks, you'd better move quickly and effectively, because if this man dies it will be your fault!"

Horace is swiftly and competently resuscitated and several minutes later is responding appropriately to verbal cues. His assessment reveals bilateral pneumonia that is compromising respiratory functions. Horace is admitted and placed on mechanical ventilation for a brief period so that he can be oxygenated properly and suctioned as needed. Horace recovers from his pneumonia without complications and is discharged in several days.

Meanwhile, Maureen questions why she didn't anticipate this kind of reaction to Horace from the ED staff. She had observed and been informed about the growing reluctance of the staff to treat Horace, yet she never considered the possibility that nurses and physicians would collectively refuse to care for a patient. What alternatives do you perceive as responses to this problem?

Over the next several days after Horace's admission, Maureen meets with each of the nurses, physicians, and support personnel on duty the evening that Horace experienced respiratory arrest. Their anger and frustration overwhelm her at times. They no longer feel obliged to care for Horace. He doesn't care for himself, so why should they feel any moral obligation to care for him? He consumes precious resources with each almost weekly visit to the ED. Even when he agrees to be admitted to the detoxification unit, he signs himself out before he gives the treatment a chance to work. The ED care providers on duty that evening express bitter resentment at having to continue to provide services to someone who, judging from his behavior, really doesn't want to be well.

Do health care providers have a right to refuse to provide care to an individual who continuously consumes health care resources by knowingly and repeatedly placing himself or herself at risk for disease and injury? What should be Maureen's course of action? How much of the response of the center personnel is attributable to a difference between their values and Horace's values as a homeless person? In developing a health care clinic for homeless men in the community, Wilde and colleagues (2004) demonstrated that value differences between homeless men and the dominant American culture need to be acknowledged and reconciled to achieve desired outcomes.

One approach to the dilemma is simply to consider the staff's reaction that evening as a manifestation of their job-related stress and frustration and to believe that it was a single aberrant incident that will not be repeated. However, this strategy would not acknowledge Horace's right to be treated with respect as a person. This is the fundamental principle of the *Code of Ethics for Nurses* (American Nurses Association, 2001), which was breached the evening in question. This strategy also does not address the underlying reason for the staff's refusal to treat Horace. Thus, there remains the potential for an incident of this nature to be repeated. The potential to inflict grave harm—namely, to act with maleficence—in the process is a real possibility as well. Finally, Maureen recalls that the ED was relatively quiet the evening of the incident involving Horace, so it is doubtful that situation-induced stress was a factor.

Maureen completes an incident report. This process will lead to notification of all appropriate nursing and medical administrative personnel, who will be responsible for follow-up with the individuals involved. Still, Maureen is left with grave concern. Nursing and medicine have a covenant with society to provide competent care to its members. Personnel are bound by the principle of fidelity to remain faithful to the trust and responsibility placed on nursing (and medicine) by society to provide care that is not limited by personal beliefs and attitudes (American Nurses Association, 2001).

Maureen is particularly concerned about the nurses involved in this incident. Conflicting obligations of fidelity have been characterized as more pervasive and morally troubling in nursing than they are in any other area of health care. This is due primarily to the

Continued

role of nursing in health care, which means that a nurse often must choose between responsibilities to the employing institution, on the one hand, and responsibilities to patients, on the other (Beauchamp & Childress, 2001).

Maureen decides to convene a consultant's group comprised of peers, a social worker, a representative from the institution's ethics committee, and a psychiatrist who specializes in problems professionals encounter in their practice. Her goal is to have the group meet with the ED nurses and physicians on duty the evening of the incident with Horace to engage them in ongoing dialogue and to offer continuing support for future problems of this nature.

REFERENCES

American Nurses Association. (2001). *Code of ethics for nurses with interpretive statements*. Washington, DC: American Nurses Publishing.

Beauchamp, T. L., & Childress, J. F. (2001). *Principles of biomedical ethics* (5th ed.). New York: Oxford University Press.

Wilde, M. H., Albanese, E. P., Rennells, R., et al. (2004). Development of a student nurses clinic for homeless men. *Public Health Nursing, 21*, 354-360.

KEY IDEAS

1. Poverty is linked to poor health, limited access to health care services, and delay in seeking such services.
2. Certain groups are at greater risk for limited access to health care services because of cost. Groups at greatest risk include people in poverty, the uninsured, low-income children, the homeless, migrant/seasonal workers, and the elderly.
3. Multiple factors contribute to vulnerability. Some factors are easily rectified; many others are not.
4. The homeless, migrant/seasonal workers, their families, and others in poverty live in desolate conditions in cities, towns, and rural areas across the United States.
5. Cost containment measures that result in less access are not cost effective. Acute and delayed care is ultimately more costly than preventive services and immediate treatment.
6. The community/public health nurse can serve as a vital link to resources and health care services for vulnerable groups.
7. Community/public health nurses can help break down the barriers to health care through public and professional education and research in effective intervention strategies.
8. Community/public health nurses can advocate on behalf of vulnerable groups by writing and calling government representatives and speaking to professional and community organizations about the problems and needs of high-risk groups.

THE NURSING PROCESS IN PRACTICE — A Homeless Man at Risk for Acquired Immunodeficiency Syndrome (by Jennifer Maurer Kliphouse)

Mr. J. is a 37-year-old man who has been homeless for 2 years in a large city. He completed the tenth grade in school and has worked episodically in food service occupations. He has come to the health care clinic on several occasions for treatment of a cold or to "have my blood pressure checked." He was dependent on intravenous cocaine before he was imprisoned 5 years ago for drug-related activities. He did not use drugs for 3 years, but since his release from prison, he says he has "gotten high every chance I get. I don't have much money, so I only use cocaine about once a week. If I have a little money I may drink beer. When I don't have any money, I do without. It's too embarrassing to beg." Mr. J. has expressed interest in a drug treatment program, but there is a long waiting period for inpatient programs that accept persons without any insurance.

Mr. J. states that he is aware of behaviors that place him at risk for human immunodeficiency virus (HIV) infection. He carries condoms with him and says that he uses them. He is not as careful with his needles. Sometimes he forgets and borrows a friend's needle when using cocaine. Mr. J. has no steady relationships but stays with girlfriends for a few weeks at a time. He has a 10-year-old son whom he has not seen in 2 years. Two years ago, Mr. J. tested negative for HIV and tuberculosis. He has refused tests since that time.

Mr. J.'s blood pressure is 160/94 mm Hg. He reports that his grandmother died of a stroke 2 years ago. He has refused a complete physical examination, insisting, "What you don't know can't hurt you." On his last two visits, Mr. J. expressed concern about whether his situation will ever get better. He said, "This is a terrible way to live. No place to call your own. No one wants to look at me or talk to me. I just don't see the point in going on. One way or another, this has got to stop. Life hurts too much to keep going on."

During this visit, Mr. J. tells the nurse that his cold does not seem to be getting better, saying, "I cough at night, and lately it seems that I wake up in the night sweating a lot. I don't really understand it, because the mission is pretty cold." As the nurse continues to talk with him, she learns that he has begun having diarrhea in the past week. Mr. J. also asks about a change of clothes, because the clothes he is wearing seem to be getting too big for him.

Based on a thorough assessment of the client, the nurse might begin to develop a mutually acceptable plan of care for Mr. J.

ASSESSMENT

- Assess the physical, psychologic, social, spiritual, and environmental needs of the client.
- Assess for the presence of depression, suicidal intentions, social isolation, ability to meet nutritional needs, self-care behaviors, and compliance with health regimen.
- Assess the degree of family and social supports available to assist the client through prolonged homelessness (i.e., shelter, legal assistance, transportation, job training, advocacy, financial aid).

- Assess for neglect because of ineffective individual coping.
- Assess the potential for injury because of the client's lifestyle and exposure to multiple risk factors.
- Assess the potential need for legal services.

NURSING DIAGNOSES

- Hopelessness related to long-term stress of homelessness as evidenced by despondent mood of conversation, i.e., "This is a terrible way to live"; "I don't see the point in going on."
- Risk for suicide related to depression as evidenced by his statement, "One way or another, this has got to stop. Life hurts too much to keep going on."
- Diarrhea related to undetermined process as evidenced by loose stools lasting at least 1 week.
- Deficient fluid volume related to loss of body fluids, as evidenced by diarrhea, concentrated urine, and night sweats.
- Imbalanced nutrition: less than body requirements related to inability to absorb nutrients as evidenced by clothes that have become too big.
- Ineffective health maintenance related to ineffective individual coping as evidenced by hypertension and absence of HIV and tuberculosis testing.

- Deficient knowledge of HIV and associated symptoms related to lack of interest in learning HIV status by refusal of HIV testing and statement "What you don't know can't hurt you."
- Risk for infection related to lack of knowledge about the modes of transmission of HIV as evidenced by sharing of intravenous needles.
- Ineffective individual coping related to situational crises as evidenced by substance abuse (cocaine and alcohol abuse).
- Powerlessness related to homelessness as evidenced by inability to get a job.
- Social isolation related to unacceptable social behavior as evidenced by exclusion from his family and perceived rejection by others.
- Chronic low self-esteem as evidenced by denial of problems, self-neglect, and self-destructive behaviors.
- Ineffective sexual patterns related to ineffective individual coping as evidenced by short-term relationships.
- Ineffective denial related to lack of control of life situation as evidenced by refusal to have a medical evaluation.
- Spiritual distress related to homelessness as manifested by questioning the meaning of life.

Nursing Diagnosis	Nursing Goals	Nursing Interventions	Outcomes and Evaluation
Hopelessness related to long-term stress of homelessness as evidenced by despondent mood of conversation (see above for detail)	Client will describe an improved sense of well-being and control over his personal circumstances.	Arrange referral for psychiatric evaluation for antidepressant therapy and psychotherapy	Mr. J. missed the first scheduled appointment with a psychiatrist. A second appointment was made, which he kept. The clinic provides free weekly dispensing of the medication, and at each dispensing, Mr. J. attends a 1-hour therapy session.
		Explore available self-help options, such as psychiatric outpatient groups	Mr. J. states that it is hard enough to attend one weekly session and shows no interest in group therapy.
Risk for suicide related to depression as evidenced by his statement, "One way or another, this has got to stop. Life hurts too much to keep going on."	Client will verbalize a decreased level of hopelessness and despair.	Make a verbal contract with the client that he will not harm himself	Mr. J. completes the verbal contract, which is renewed with each weekly session. He states that he has still thought of "ending it," but he has not created a plan to harm himself.
		Support the client through this period of distress by accepting his behavior, avoiding judgmental evaluations, and reinforcing positive statements and behaviors	The nurse continues to offer Mr. J. a chance to voice his feelings with each visit. He is thankful, stating, "It's nice to know there is someone to listen to me."
Diarrhea related to undetermined process as evidenced by loose stools lasting at least 1 week.	Client will report less diarrhea.	Consult with a primary care provider about the use of antidiarrheal medication	A prescription is written for atropine/diphenoxylate (Lomotil), which is provided free to Mr. J. He reports no further episodes of diarrhea at this time.
		Explain the effects of diarrhea on hydration	Mr. J. verbalizes dehydration as a possible effect of diarrhea. "I've been trying to drink more water, but I forget sometimes." As diarrhea is absent after treatment, there is a decreased risk of dehydration.

WEB   Find additional **Care Plans** for this client on the book's website.

LEARNING BY EXPERIENCE AND REFLECTION

1. Determine your state's income cap for Medicaid eligibility for a family of three. What percentage of the current poverty level is your state's eligibility cap—30%, 50%, 70%, or some other percentage? Plan a 1-month budget for a family of three for minimally adequate food, clothing, and safe shelter. Include the cost of a telephone, electricity, and fuel. Compare your state's Medicaid cap for this fictional family with your monthly budget. Is the capped income more or less than your expected monthly costs? If less, consider what you might be willing to forego paying for or purchasing. What if you had additional expenses, including medical costs? How would you restructure your budget to meet these unexpected expenses? Is this achievable?

2. Research the starting salary for registered nurses in your geographic area. Look up the monetary payments under TANF in your state. Does the TANF allotment received by anyone match the nurse starting salary amount? If so, how many people does TANF expect you to support on that allotment? Look up the current poverty index and compare that with the nurse starting salary. How many people are you expected to support on the starting salary before that amount would put you below the poverty index (if it ever would).

3. For 2 weeks, clip items from newspapers and magazines concerning poverty, homelessness, and vulnerable groups, and federal and state policies that directly or indirectly affect the very poor. What examples, if any, relate to inequities of access to health care? What examples, if any, relate to injustices of health status or health care based on race or income level?

4. Volunteer to work in a soup kitchen or shelter for at least 4 hours. What did you feel when you first arrived? How approachable were you to the clients you encountered? What was significant for you in this experience?

5. Visit an emergency department and interview staff nurses about methods of working with vulnerable populations. Observe the pattern of interaction with patients in the waiting room or treatment room. Do you note differences that might be related to the patient's condition? How do nurses respond when you ask them about caring for the poor, the homeless, migrants/seasonal workers, and those without health insurance? What problems do they perceive and how do they deal with them?

COMMUNITY RESOURCES FOR PRACTICE   WEB

Information about most of the following organizations is found on their websites, which can be accessed through the **WebLinks** section of this book's website at *http://evolve.elsevier.com/Maurer/community/.*

Children's Defense Fund
Coalition for the Homeless
Homeless Initiative Office, Department of Veterans Affairs
Interagency Council on Homelessness
National Center for Children in Poverty
National Center for Farmworker Health
National Coalition for the Homeless
National Health Care for the Homeless Council
National Law Center for Homelessness and Poverty
National Low Income Housing Coalition
National Resource Center on Homelessness and Mental Illness
National Runaway Switchboard
Salvation Army National Headquarters
Streetkid-L Resource Page (a global discussion list about the plight of homeless children)
University of California at San Francisco student-run Students' Homeless Clinic
Local agencies (check the local phone book for specific organizations)
Local food and clothing banks
Church-sponsored health and social services
Local public health agencies
Community mental health centers
Local shelters
Many states have a Coalition for the Homeless or similar organization. Check websites for the selected state and request information about homeless programs in that state.

STUDY AIDS   http://evolve.elsevier.com/Maurer/community/

Visit the Evolve website for this book to find the following study and assessment materials:

- Quiz
- Web Scenario
- Critical Thinking Questions and Answers for Case Studies
- Care Plans
- *Healthy People* Updates
- Glossary

WEBSITE RESOURCES

The following items supplement the chapter's topics and are also found on the Evolve site:

21A: Criticisms of the Poverty Index

REFERENCES

American Civil Liberties Union. (2004). *Domestic violence and homelessness*. Washington DC: ACLU, Women's Rights Project.

American Hospital Association. (2006). *Uncompensated hospital care cost: fact sheet*. Retrieved July 5, 2007 from *http://www.aha.org/aha/content/2006/pdf/uncompensatedcarefs2006.pdf*.

Aron, L. Y., & Fitchen, J. M. (1996). Rural homelessness: A synopsis. In J. Baumohl (Ed.), *Homelessness in America* (pp. 81-85). Phoenix: Oryx Press.

Bassuk, E. L., Buckner, J. C., Perloff, J. N., et al. (1997). Prevalence of mental health and substance abuse disorders among homeless and low-income housed mothers. *American Journal of Psychiatry, 155*(11), 1561-1564.

Belcher, J. R., Scholler-Jaquish, A., & Drummond, M. (1991). Three stages of homelessness: A conceptual model for social workers in health care. *Health and Social Work, 16*(2), 87-93.

Betson, D. M., & Michael, R. T. (1997). Why so many children are poor. *Future of Children, 7*(2), 25-39.

Bloom, D., Farrell, M., Fink, B., et al. (2002). *Welfare time limits: State policies, implementation, and effects on families*. Washington, DC: MDRC.

Brooks-Gunn, J., & Duncan, G. J. (1997). The effects of poverty on children. *Future of Children, 7*(2), 55-71.

Cantor, J. C., Long, S. H., & Marquis, M. S. (1998). Challenges of state health reform: Variations in ten states. *Health Affairs, 17*(1), 191-200.

Centers for Disease Control and Prevention. (1996). *Pregnancy nutrition surveillance, 1996*. Atlanta: Author.

Children's Defense Fund. (2002). *Low-income families bear the burden of state child care setbacks*. Washington, DC: Author.

Children's Defense Fund. (2005a). *The state of America's children: 2005*. Washington, DC: Author.

Children's Defense Fund. (2005b). *Testimony of the Children's Defense Fund on the impact on children of the welfare reauthorization proposals*. Washington, DC: Author.

Citro, C. F., & Michael, R. T. (1995). *Measuring poverty: A new approach*. Washington, DC: National Academy Press.

Congressional Budget Office. (2007). *The State Children's Health Insurance program*. Washington, DC: Author.

DeNavas-Walt, C., Proctor, B., & Lee, C. (2006). *Income, poverty, and health insurance coverage in the United States: 2005* (Current Population Reports, P60-231). Washington, DC: U.S. Government Printing Office.

Epstein, G. A. (2007, June 17). Requiring documents for Medicaid hurts poor, advocates say. *Sun*, pp. A1&A8.

Families USA. (1999). *Losing health insurance: The unintended consequences of welfare reform*. Washington, DC: Author.

Fisher, M. (2005). *Why is the U.S. poverty rate higher in nonmetropolitan than metropolitan areas?* Corvallis, OR: Rural Poverty Research Center.

Freking, K. (2007, June 18). States, feds split on kids' health insurance. *USA Today*. Retrieved June 18, 2007 from *http://www.healthdecisions.org/News/default.aspx?doc_id=123049&print=true*.

Guttmacher Institute. (2003). Immigrants and Medicaid after welfare reform. *Guttmacher Report on Public Policy, 6*(2), 1-7.

Haan, M. N., & Kaplan, G. A. (1985, August). The contribution of socioeconomic position to minority health. In U.S. Department of Health and Human Services, *Report of the Secretary's Task Force on Black and Minority Health* (vol. 2). Washington, DC: U.S. Government Printing Office.

Hadley, J. (2005). *Consequences of the lack of health insurance on health and earnings*. Washington, DC: Urban Institute.

Hadley, J., & Holahan, J. (2003, February 12). How much medical care do the uninsured use and who pays for it? *Health Affairs*, Web Exclusives. Retrieved June 10, 2008 from *http://content.healthaffairs.org/cgi/reprint/hlthaff.w3.66v1.pdf*.

Hadley, J., & Holahan, J. (2004). *The cost of care for the uninsured: What do we spend, who pays, and what would full coverage add to medical spending* (Issue Update). Washington, DC: Kaiser Commission on Medicaid and the Uninsured.

Harvard University. (2007). *Fact sheet: The state of the nation's housing*. Cambridge, MA: Harvard University Joint Center for Housing Studies.

Hawkins, D. (2001). *Migrant health issues: Introduction*. Buda, TX: National Center for Farmworker Health.

Health Resources and Services Administration. (2004). *Health care providers in CHCs*. Bureau of Primary Health Care, Uniform Data System Section 330. Retrieved August 12, 2007 from *http://www.bphc.hrsa.gov/uds/data.htm*.

Holden, C. (2001). Monograph No. 8: Housing. In National Center for Farmworker Health, *Migrant health issues* (pp. 40-44). Buda, TX: National Center for Farmworker Health.

Indian Health Service. (2002). *Facts about Indian health disparities*. Washington, DC: Author. Retrieved December 19, 2003 from *http://www.info.ihn.gov/Health/Health11.pdf*.

Institute of Medicine. (2001). *Coverage matters: Insurance and health care*. Washington, DC: Author.

Institute of Medicine. (2002a). *Care without coverage, too little, too late*. Washington, DC: Author.

Institute of Medicine. (2002b). *The future of public health in the twenty-first century*. Washington, DC: Author.

Institute of Medicine. (2003). *Hidden costs, value lost*. Washington, DC: Author.

Institute of Medicine. (2004). *Insuring America's health: Principles and recommendations*. Washington, DC: Author.

Institute of Medicine. (2007). *Fact sheet 5: Uninsurance facts and figures: The uninsured are sicker and die sooner*. Retrieved July 5, 2007 from *http://www.ion.edu/CMS/17645.aspx*.

Insurance Information Institute. (2007). *Health insurance*. Retrieved July 3, 2007 from *http://www.iii.org/media/facts/statsbyissue/health/?printerfriendly=yes*.

Jacob, J., Hunt, I. F., Dirige, O., et al. (1976). Biochemical assessment of the nutritional status of low-income pregnant females of Mexican descent. *American Journal of Clinical Nutrition, 29*, 650-660.

Jenkins, C. L. (2007, June 7). Medicaid wait rising for Va. Children, study says. *Washington Post*, pp. B1, B5.

Kapur, K., & Marquis, S. S. (2003). Health insurance for workers who lose jobs: Implications for various subsidy schemes. *Health Affairs, 22*(3), 203-213.

Kozak, L. J., Hall, M. J., & Owings, M. F. (2001). Trends in avoidable hospitalizations. *Health Affairs, 20*(2), 225-232.

Ku, L., & Nimalendran, S. (2003). *An illustration of how much each state might lose in federal Medicaid and SCHIP matching funds under the House Budget Resolution*. Washington, DC: Center on Budget and Policy Priorities.

Lambrew, J. (2001). *How the slowing U.S. economy threatens employer-based health insurance*. New York: Commonwealth Fund.

Lewit, E. M., & Kerrebrock, N. (1997). Population-based growth stunting. *Future of Children, 7*(2), 149-156.

Lewit, E. M., Terman, D. L., & Behrman, R. E. (1997). Children and poverty: Analysis and recommendations. *Future of Children, 7*(2), 4-21.

Lighthall, D. (2004). *Confronting the challenge of farmworker health and housing: A food system perspective*. Davis, CA: California Institute for Rural Studies.

Lindsey, A. (1995). Physical health of homeless adults. *Annual Review of Nursing Research, 13*, 31-61

Loprest, P. (2003). *Use of government benefits increases among families leaving welfare* (Snapshots of American Families, No. 7). Washington DC: Urban Institute.

Lowe, E. T., Slater, A., Welfley, J., et al. (2002). *A status report on hunger and homelessness in America's cities*. Washington, DC: U.S. Conference of Mayors.

Maruschak, L. M. (2006a). *Medical problems of jail inmates* (Special Report NCJ 210696). Washington DC: U.S. Department of Justice.

Maruschak, L. M. (2006b). *HIV in prisons, 2004* (Special Report NCJ 213897). Washington DC: U.S. Department of Justice.

McQuistion, H. L., Finnerty, M., Hirschowitz, J., et al. (2003). Challenges for psychiatry in serving homeless people with psychiatric disorders. *Psychiatric Services, 54*(5), 669-676.

Mines, R., Mullenax, N., & Saca, L. (2001). *The binational farmworker health survey.* Davis, CA: California Institute for Rural Studies.

Mumola, C. J., & Karberg, J. C. (2006). *Drug use and dependence, state and federal prisoners, 2004* (Special Report NCJ 213530). Washington, DC: U.S. Department of Justice.

National American Indian Housing Council. (2007). *Indian housing fact sheet.* Washington, DC: Author.

National Association of Community Health Centers. (2005). *The safety net on the edge.* Washington, DC: Author.

National Center for Farmworker Health. (2002). *Profile of a population with complex health problems: Fact sheet about farmworkers.* Buda, TX: Author.

National Center for Farmworker Health. (2007a). *Facts about farmworkers.* Buda, TX: Author.

National Center for Farmworker Health. (2007b). *Occupational safety.* Buda, TX: Author.

National Coalition for the Homeless. (2001). *Homeless families with children* (NCH Fact Sheet No. 7). Washington, DC: Author.

National Coalition for the Homeless. (2006a). *Why are people homeless?* Washington, DC: Author.

National Coalition for the Homeless. (2006b). *Who is homelessness?* Washington, DC: Author.

National Coalition for the Homeless. (2006c). *Homeless families with children.* Washington, DC: Author.

National Coalition for the Homeless. (2006d). *Homeless youth.* Washington, DC: Author.

National Coalition for the Homeless. (2006e). *Rural homelessness.* Washington, DC: Author.

National Coalition for the Homeless. (2006f). *Health care and homelessness.* Washington, DC: Author.

National Coalition for the Homeless. (2006g). *Mental illness and homelessness.* Washington, DC: Author.

National Health Care for the Homeless Council. (2004). *People need health care.* Retrieved January 9, 2004 from *http://www.nationalhomeless.org/facts/health.htm.*

National Institute of Mental Health. (2005). *The numbers count.* Washington, DC: Author.

National Law Center on Homelessness and Poverty. (2004). *Homelessness in the United States and the human right to housing.* Washington DC: The Author.

National Low Income Housing Coalition. (2004). *Out of reach 2004: America's housing wage climbs.* Washington, DC: Author.

Nickelson, I. (2004). *The district should use its upcoming TANF bonus to increase cash assistance and remove barriers to work.* Washington, DC: Fiscal Policy Institute.

Nord, M., Andrews, M., & Carlson, S. (2006). *Household food security in the United States, 2005.* Washington, DC: U.S. Department of Agriculture, Food Assistance and Nutrition Research Program.

Parrott, S., & Wu, N. (2003). *States are cutting TANF and child care programs: Supports for low-income working families and welfare-to-work programs are particularly hard hit.* Washington, DC: Center on Budget and Policy Priorities.

Pelletiere, D., Wardrip, K., & Crowley, S. (2006). *Out of reach 2006.* Washington, DC: National Low Income Coalition.

Pew Hispanic Center. (2006). *Estimates of the unauthorized migrant population for states based on the March 2005 CPS.* Washington DC: Author.

Reardon, M. L., Burns, A. P., Preist, R., et al. (2003). Alcohol use and other psychiatric disorders in the formerly homeless and never homeless: prevalence, age of onset, comorbidity, temporal sequencing, and service utilization. *Substance Use and Misuse, 38*(3-6), 601-644.

Redlener, I., & Johnson D. (1999). *Still in crisis: The health status of New York's homeless children.* New York: Children's Health Fund.

Rew, L. (2003). A theory of taking care of oneself grounded in experiences of homeless youth. *Nursing Research, 52*(4), 234-239.

Ross, D. C., & Cox, L. (2004). *Out in the cold: Enrollment freezes in six State Children's Health Insurance Programs withhold coverage for eligible children.* Washington, DC: Center on Budget and Policy Priorities.

Rutter, M. (1994). Beyond longitudinal data: Causes, consequences, changes, and continuity. *Journal of Clinical Psychology, 65*(5), 928-990.

Sardell, A. (2007). Taking action: Community Health Centers: A successful strategy for improving health care access. In D. J. Mason, J. K. Leavitt, & M. W. Chaffee (Eds.), *Policy and politics in nursing and health care* (5th ed.; pp. 286-295). St. Louis: Saunders.

Scandlen, G. (2001). *Helping laid-off workers keep insurance* (Brief Analysis No. 373). Washington DC: National Center for Policy Analysis.

Schneck, M. E., Sideras, K. A., Fox, R. A., et al. (1990). Low-income pregnant adolescents and their infants: Dietary findings and health outcomes. *Journal of the American Dietetic Association, 90*(4), 555-558.

Short, K., Garner, T., Johnson, D., et al. (1999). *Experimental poverty measures: 1990-1997.* (Current Population Reports, P60-205). U.S. Bureau of the Census. Washington, DC: U.S. Government Printing Office.

Smedley, B. D., Stith, A. Y., & Nelson, A. R. (2002). *Unequal treatment: Confronting racial and ethnic disparities in healthcare.* Washington, DC: National Academy Press.

Smith, E. M., & North, C. S. (1994). Not all homeless women are alike: Effects of motherhood and the presence of children. *Community Mental Health Journal, 30*(6), 601-610.

Smith, V., Rudowitz, R., & O'Malley, M. (2005). *The continuing Medicaid budget challenge: State Medicaid spending growth and cost containment in fiscal years 2004 and 2005. Results from a 50-state survey.* Washington DC: Kaiser Commission on Medicaid and the Uninsured.

Steele, R. W., Ramgoolam, A., & Evans, J. (2003). Health services for homeless children. *Seminars in Pediatric Infectious Diseases, 14*(1), 38-42.

Tally, M. K. (2005). *Job training and education fight poverty* (Fact Sheet D444). Washington, DC: Institute for Women's Policy Research.

Trowbridge, F. L. (1984). Malnutrition in industrialized North America. In P. L. White & N. Selvey (Eds.), *Malnutrition determinants and consequences* (pp. 45-60). New York: Alan R. Liss.

Turner, M. A. (2003). *Strengths and weaknesses of the housing voucher program. Testimony prepared for the Committee on Financial Services, Subcommittee on Housing and Community Opportunity, United States House of Representatives.* Washington, DC: Urban Institute.

Tyler, K. A., & Cauce, A. M. (2002). Perspectives of early psychological and sexual abuse among homeless and runaway children. *Child Abuse and Neglect, 269*(12), 1261-1274.

University of California. (2005). *Health policy fact sheet: Agricultural workers.* Berkley, CA: University of California, California Policy Research Center.

U.S. Bureau of the Census. (2003). Poverty in the United States: 2002. *Population Reports* (P60-222). Washington, DC: U.S. Government Printing Office.

U.S. Bureau of the Census. (2006). Income, poverty, and health insurance in the United States: 2005. *Population Reports* (P60-231). Washington, DC: U.S. Government Printing Office.

U.S. Bureau of the Census. (2007a). *Poverty threshold 2006.* Washington, DC: Author. Retrieved June 28, 2007 from *http://www.census.gov/hhes/www/poverty/threshold/thresh06.html.*

U.S. Bureau of the Census. (2007b). *Statistical abstract of the United States, 2007: The national data book* (126th ed.). Washington, DC: U.S. Government Printing Office.

U.S. Conference of Mayors. (2005). *Hunger and homelessness survey: A status report on hunger and homelessness in America's cities.* Washington DC: Author.

U.S. Department of Agriculture. (1996). *Rural homelessness: Focusing on the needs of the rural homeless.* Washington, DC: U.S. Department of Agriculture, Rural Housing Service, Rural Economic and Community Development.

U.S. Department of Health and Human Services. (1997). *Healthy people 2000 review 1997.* Washington, DC: U.S. Government Printing Office.

U.S. Department of Health and Human Services. (2000). *Healthy people 2010: Understanding and improving health* (2nd ed.). Washington, DC: U.S. Government Printing Office.

U.S. Department of Health and Human Services. (2002). *Health, United States, 2002.* Washington, DC: U.S. Government Printing Office.

U.S. Department of Health and Human Services. (2006a). *Health, United States, 2006.* Washington, DC: U.S. Government Printing Office.

U.S. Department of Health and Human Services. (2006b). *Healthy people 2010: Midcourse Review.* Washington, DC: U.S. Government Printing Office.

U.S. Department of Housing and Urban Development. (2007). *The annual homeless assessment report to Congress.* Washington, DC: Author.

U.S. Department of Justice. (2006). *Study finds more than half of all prison and jail inmates have mental health problems.* Retrieved March 18, 2008 from *http://www.ojp.usdoj.gov/newsroom/ pressreleases/2006/BJS06064.htm.*

Villarejo, D., Lighthall, D., Williams, D., et al. (2000). *Suffering in silence: A report on the health of California's agricultural workers.* Davis, CA: California Institute for Rural Studies.

Vissing, Y. (1996). *Out of sight, out of mind: Homeless children and families in small town America.* Lexington, KY: University of Kentucky Press.

Woods, E. R., Samples, C. L., Melchione, M. W., et al. (2003). Boston HAPPENS Program: HIV-positive, homeless, and at-risk youth can access care through youth-orientated HIV services. *Seminars in Pediatric Infectious Diseases, 14*(1), 43-53.

Wright, J. D., & Weber, E. (1987). *Homelessness and health.* New York: McGraw-Hill.

Yanochik-Owen, A., & White, M. (1977). Nutrition surveillance in Arizona: Selected anthropometric and laboratory observations among Mexican children. *American Journal of Public Health, 67,* 151-154.

SUGGESTED READINGS

Children's Defense Fund. (2005). *The state of America's children: 2005.* Washington, DC: Author.

Institute of Medicine. (2002a). *Care without coverage, too little, too late.* Washington, DC: Author.

Harrington, C., & Estes, C. L. (2008). *Health policy: Crisis and reform in the U.S. health care delivery system* (5th ed.). Sudbury, MA: Jones & Bartlett.

Nord, M., Andrews, M., & Carlson, S. (2006). *Household food security in the United States, 2005.* Washington, DC: U.S. Department of Agriculture, Food Assistance and Nutrition Research Program.

Patel, K., & Rushefsky, M. (2006). *Health care politics and policy in America.* Armonk, NY: M. E. Sharpe.

U.S. Bureau of the Census. (2003). *Poverty in the United States: 2002* (Current Population Reports, P60-222). Washington, DC: U.S. Government Printing Office.

U.S. Conference of Mayors. (2005). *Hunger and homelessness survey: A status report on hunger and homelessness in America's cities.* Washington DC: Author.

Disaster Management: Caring for Communities in an Emergency

Mary L. Beachley and John W. Young

FOCUS QUESTIONS

What are the different types of disasters?

What happens when a disaster occurs? Who is in charge?

What are the common physical and psychosocial effects on disaster victims and workers?

What are the agencies that might be involved in predisaster planning?

What impact has terrorism had on disaster planning efforts?

What are the responsibilities of community/public health nurses in disaster nursing?

What is your emergency preparedness plan? Your family's plan?

CHAPTER OUTLINE

KEY TERMS

Disaster has many forms: floods, wind, fire, explosions, extreme range of environmental temperatures, epidemics, multiple car crashes with many casualties, school shootings, and environmental contamination from chemical agents and/or bioterrorism. The Iraqi invasion of Kuwait and the resulting deliberate environmental damage is one example of disaster. In the past 10 years, there have been many natural and man-made disasters in the United States (Table 22-1). Flooding is the most common natural disaster worldwide and is the third leading cause of weather-related deaths in the United States (National Oceanic and Atmospheric Administration [NOAA], 2007). Major floods in the Northwest, the Midwest, North Dakota, and the Southeast cost billions of dollars in lost homes, businesses, and crops and created long-term shelter needs for thousands of people. Hurricane Katrina in 2005 caused an estimated $200 billion in damages to personal property and public infrastructure (Wolk, 2005).

Frequently occurring natural and man-made disasters during the past 30 years have brought the need for emergency preparedness to the attention of the American public. Hurricanes, earthquakes, brush and forest fires, and terrorism have created a concern across the country for preparedness. In the 1990s and in 2001, Americans experienced terrorist acts that pointed to an urgent need for special planning, training, and organization to treat mass casualties and address the threat of chemical and biologic terrorism. These threats require more coordinated disaster planning and response from a broader team of emergency responders and agencies.

Worldwide, there has been an increase in terrorist activities. Deadly sarin gas was released in a subway in Tokyo, Japan. In the United States, bombings of public buildings have targeted abortion clinics, the World Trade Center in New York City, a federal building in Oklahoma City, and Olympic Park in Atlanta during the 1996 Summer Olympics. Over 14,000 incidents of terrorism occurred worldwide in 2006. This was a 28.5% increase over 2005, and the incidents claimed over 74,500 lives (U.S. Department of State, 2007). In the United States, the most egregious example of a man-made disaster was the terrorist attacks of September 11, 2001, that caused mass casualties and major property damage in New York City and at the Pentagon in Washington, DC. These attacks were followed by a bioterrorist act involving the mailing of anthrax-contaminated letters to locations on the East Coast.

Successful efforts to address these and other disaster situations demand sophisticated preplanning measures and a well-coordinated emergency response during the actual disaster situation. Comprehensive planning requires the combined efforts of all levels of government, academia, health care professionals, business, and voluntary organizations cooperating to develop contingency plans to meet situations that might arise during and after the occurrence of the actual disaster.

DEFINITION OF DISASTER

The American Red Cross (ARC) defines a **disaster** as "an occurrence," either natural or man-made, "that causes human suffering and creates human needs that victims cannot alleviate without assistance" (ARC, 2002). The Robert T. Stafford Disaster Relief and Emergency Assistance Act (Public Law 93-288) defines a major disaster as "any natural catastrophe (including any hurricane, tornado, storm, high water, winddriven water, tidal wave, tsunami, earthquake, volcanic eruption, landslide, mudslide, snowstorm, or drought), or, regardless of cause, any fire, flood, or explosion, in any part of the United States which in the determination of the President causes damage of sufficient severity and magnitude to warrant major disaster assistance under this Act to supplement the efforts and available resources of States, local governments, and disaster relief organizations in alleviating the damages, loss, hardship, or suffering caused thereby" (Federal Emergency Management Agency [FEMA], 2007, p. 2). There have been more than 1500 presidential disaster declarations since 1964. **Website Resource 22A** provides a map showing the types and distributions of these disasters.

A major disaster can create a *mass casualty incident* or a *multiple casualty incident*. A **multiple casualty incident** is one in which more than 2 but fewer than 100 persons are injured. Multiple casualties generally strain and, in some situations, might overwhelm the available emergency medical services and resources. A **mass casualty incident** is a situation

TABLE 22-1	Examples of Disasters—United States		
	Place	**Date**	**Casualties**
Man-Made Disasters			
Bombing of Murrah Federal Building	Oklahoma City, Oklahoma	April 19, 1995	168 deaths
Terrorist plane crashes	New York, New York (World Trade Center), Washington, DC (Pentagon), and Shanksville, Pennsylvania	September 11, 2001	3025 deaths
Anthrax mailings	United States	October-December 2001	5 deaths
Chlorine leak	Graniteville, South Carolina	January 2005	9 deaths
Natural Disasters			
Tornado	Tuscaloosa, Alabama	April 1998	32 deaths, 256 injuries
Tornadoes	Oklahoma	May 1999	41 deaths, 748 injuries
Hurricane Isabel	Virginia, North Carolina, Delaware, and Washington, DC	September 2003	40 deaths
Wildfires	Los Angeles and San Diego, California, area	October 2003	20 deaths
Hurricane Katrina	Gulf Coast	August 2005	1330 deaths, 2096 missing

in which there are a large number of casualties, usually 100 or more, that significantly overwhelm available emergency medical services, facilities, and resources.

When there are mass casualties, a community or region usually requires the assistance of emergency personnel and resources from surrounding communities or states. The Oklahoma City federal building bombing and the September 11, 2001, plane crashes in Manhattan, Washington, DC, and Pennsylvania are examples of mass casualty incidents in which the affected communities required outside assistance.

TYPES OF DISASTERS

Essentially, there are two types of disasters: *natural* and *man-made*. Both types vary in intensity, severity, and impact. **Natural disasters** include hurricanes, tornadoes, flash floods, blizzards, slow-rising floods, typhoons, earthquakes, avalanches, epidemics, and volcanic eruptions. **Man-made disasters** include war, chemical and biologic terrorism, transportation accidents, food or water contamination, and building collapse. Fire can be either man-made or naturally occurring. The Los Angeles fires of 1993 and the California fires of 2003 that destroyed many communities, including homes and businesses, resulted from a combination of man-made and natural causes: arson and weather conditions (i.e., a dry summer season and high winds).

AGENTS OF HARM OR DAMAGE IN A DISASTER

The *agent* is the physical entity that actually causes the injury or destruction. Primary agents include falling buildings, heat, wind, rising water, chemical and biologic agents, and smoke. Secondary agents include bacteria and viruses that produce contamination or infection after the primary agent has caused injury or destruction.

Primary and secondary agents vary according to the type of disaster. For example, a hurricane with rising water can cause flooding and high winds; these are primary agents. Secondary agents include damaged buildings and bacteria or viruses that thrive as a result of the disaster. In an epidemic, the bacteria or virus causing a disease is the primary agent rather than the secondary agent.

FACTORS AFFECTING THE SCOPE AND SEVERITY OF DISASTERS

A number of factors affect the degree of impact that disasters will have on individuals, families, and communities. These factors are addressed in the following section.

VULNERABILITY OF A POPULATION OR INDIVIDUAL

Certain characteristics of humans influence the severity of the disaster's effect on individuals and communities. For example, the age of a person, preexisting health problems, degree of mobility, and emotional stability all play a part in how someone responds in a disaster situation. Those most severely affected by a disaster are the physically handicapped who have limited mobility or are wheelchair dependent; people who are ventilator dependent or attached to other life-support equipment; the mentally challenged; elderly persons, who might have trouble leaving the area quickly; young children whose immune systems are not fully developed; and persons with

respiratory or cardiac problems. For example, a fire in a nursing home, a more vulnerable community, is potentially more lethal than a fire in a college dormitory. Nursing home residents are at greater risk because they are less physically fit and more susceptible to smoke and other consequences than are young college students.

ENVIRONMENTAL FACTORS AND TYPE OF IMPACT

In a disaster situation, physical, chemical, biologic, and social factors influence the scope and severity of the outcomes. Physical factors include the time when the disaster occurs, weather conditions, the availability of food and water, and the functioning of utilities, such as electricity and telephone service. For example, in the summer of 2003, parts of the Northeast and central Ohio suffered a failure of the power grid supplying electricity to those regions. Fifty million people were without electricity. As a result of Hurricane Katrina in 2005, residents of New Orleans were without drinking water due to broken water mains and approximately 3 million homes or facilities were without power (NOAA, 2005). Some communities were without power for a short period of time (1 to 2 days), whereas others were without power for weeks or months. In general, those without electricity for longer periods have a more difficult time coping with the disaster than those who are without power for a day or so.

Chemical, biologic, and social factors impact the scope and severity of a disaster. Leaks of stored chemicals into the air, soil, groundwater, or food supplies are examples of chemical factors. Biologic factors are those that occur or increase as a result of water contamination, improper waste disposal, insect or rodent proliferation, improper food storage, or lack of refrigeration owing to interrupted electrical service. Some social factors to consider are those related to an individual's support systems. Loss of family members, changes in roles, and the questioning of religious beliefs are social factors to be examined after a disaster. In general, individuals and families with ample social support do better in coping with emergencies than do individuals with little or no social support.

WARNING TIME AND PROXIMITY TO DISASTER

Demi and Miles (1983) have identified both situational and personal factors that influence an individual's response to a disaster. Situational variables include the amount of warning time before disaster occurs, the nature and severity of the disaster, physical proximity to the disaster, and the availability of emergency response systems. An individual's reaction to a disaster will be greater if there is little or no warning and the victim is in close physical proximity to the disaster site. For example, the loss of life in tornadoes is often affected by warning systems. When towns have warning sirens and a planned system of monitoring for potential tornadoes, more people are able to take shelter. In these instances, even with substantial damage to buildings and personal property, personal injuries and deaths are limited.

The closer an individual is to the actual site of the disaster and the longer the individual is exposed to the immediate site of the disaster, the greater the psychologic distress that the individual experiences. A research study of residents in Manhattan conducted 5 to 8 weeks after the September 11, 2001, terrorist attacks found a high risk for depression and posttraumatic stress disorder in this population (Galea et al., 2002).

INDIVIDUAL PERCEPTION AND RESPONSE

Personal variables influence an individual's reaction to a disaster. Psychologic proximity, coping ability, personal losses, role overload, and previous disaster experience all influence individual response. An individual's risk for developing severe psychologic consequences is greater if that person is emotionally close to the individuals affected, has compromised coping abilities, has experienced many losses, feels overloaded in her or his role, or has never before experienced a disaster. Psychologic reactions in the aftermath of disasters are addressed in greater detail later in this chapter.

An individual who perceives a disaster to be less severe than it is will probably have a less severe psychologic reaction than a person who perceives the situation as catastrophic (Richtsmeir & Miller, 1985). An individual's perception of an emergency or disaster might evolve over time as the person begins to acknowledge the full impact of the disaster. The human mind is capable of allowing perceptions to be only as disastrous as the mind can cope with at a given time.

Doris Jones is in her back yard when she hears her neighbor, Alice Alvarez, calling for help. She runs next door to find Alice holding her 3-year-old daughter, who is bleeding profusely from numerous large cuts on her left arm. Blood is all over the concrete patio and extends into the kitchen. Ms. Jones grabs the toddler and applies pressure to the cut area with kitchen towels. She has Ms. Alvarez call 911. After the paramedics arrive and transport the child and her mother to the hospital, Doris gathers with several neighbors and learns how the injury occurred. The toddler had climbed onto the kitchen counter, dislodging several glasses. The glasses fell to the floor and broke. The girl then fell from the counter into the pile of glasses. During the conversation, Doris starts to tremble and cry. Another neighbor takes her home and cares for her. Doris cannot understand why she got so upset after the emergency was over instead of during the emergency.

DIMENSIONS OF A DISASTER

Disasters can differ along a number of dimensions: predictability, frequency, controllability, time, and scope or intensity. These dimensions influence the nature and possibility of preparation planning, as well as response to the actual event.

PREDICTABILITY

Some events are more easily predicted than others. Advances in meteorology, for example, have made it more feasible to accurately predict the probability of certain types of natural, weather-related disasters (e.g., tornadoes, floods, and hurricanes), whereas other disasters, such as earthquakes, are not as easily predicted. Man-made disasters, such as explosions or vehicle crashes, are also less predictable. Authorities and emergency personnel have more time to prepare for the situation when an event is predictable than when an event is not foreseeable.

FREQUENCY

Although natural disasters are infrequent, they appear more often in certain geographic locations. Residents of the Gulf Coast of the United States live in what is commonly referred to as "hurricane alley." These people are at greater risk for experiencing a hurricane than someone who lives in Alaska. California residents are at greater risk for earthquakes, and people who live near large river systems are at greater risk for flooding than people who live elsewhere. The National Weather Service calculates that average annual fatalities for hurricanes and tornados have increased (Figure 22-1). The largest number of deaths are from heat-related causes, which were not calculated until recently. However, the greater frequency and intensity of natural disasters may or may not prepare citizens for their occurrence. Some citizens become immune to repeated warnings and are less likely to seek shelter to protect themselves and their property when warned. Other citizens take each warning seriously and regularly take appropriate safety precautions.

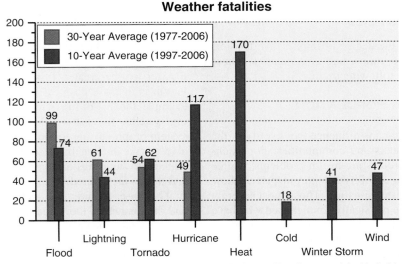

Weather fatalities

FIGURE 22-1 Average number of fatalities per weather-related incident in the U.S., Puerto Rico, Guam, and the Virgin Islands. (From National Weather Service. [2007]. *Natural hazard statistics: Weather fatalities.* Birmingham, AL: Author. Retrieved June 11, 2007 from *http://www.nws.noaa.gov/om/hazstats.shtml#.*)

CONTROLLABILITY

Some situations allow prewarning and control measures that can reduce the impact of the disaster; others do not. **Mitigation** is a term used in disaster planning that describes actions and/or processes that can be used to prevent or reduce the damage caused by a specific disaster event. In the Midwest floods of 1993, for example, some control and mitigating actions were possible. Emergency planners were able to control some of the effects of the flooding by sandbagging levees and riverbanks to reduce the effects of water damage and by deliberately blasting dikes and dams to divert floodwaters to less populated areas. The immediate impact on people was reduced by the ability of emergency personnel to organize evacuations and decrease the risk of injury and death. Sometimes the scope of a disaster can overwhelm resources available to mitigate the effects, as was the case with Hurricane Katrina (Figure 22-2). Many poor and disabled citizens of New Orleans were stranded because there were inadequate resources to aid with evacuation.

The Los Angeles earthquake of 1994 did not allow prewarning and immediate precautionary actions, but other types of control measures were available. Mitigating measures can be implemented well in advance of potential disasters. The enactment of building standards and codes intended to reduce the harmful effects of a disaster are one example. More stringent fire safety measures (e.g., smoke detectors, sprinkler systems, improved fire doors) have made more newly constructed buildings safer in the event of an actual fire. Newer buildings that complied with more stringent construction codes survived the most recent San Francisco earthquake with less structural damage than older buildings built before these codes were implemented. Los Angeles was in the process of retrofitting its freeway system to strengthen highway resistance to earthquake damage when the 1994 earthquake hit the area.

TIME

Time factors that relate to disaster impact include the speed of onset of the disaster, the time available for warning the population, and the actual length of time of the impact phase. It is more difficult to prepare for very sudden events. A flash flood, for instance, might catch many unaware, whereas gradual flooding allows more time for preparation. When there is a lengthy period of warning, more protective measures can be introduced. For example, several days' warning allows authorities in low coastal areas to evacuate vulnerable communities before a hurricane hits. Tornadoes do not offer such lengthy warning periods. The impact phase of the disaster might last for minutes, hours, or even days. The most damage is generally caused by the worst possible combination of time factors: a rapid onset, no opportunity for warning the populace, and a lengthy duration of the impact phase.

SCOPE AND INTENSITY

Scope refers to the geographic area and social space dimension impacted by the disaster agent. A disaster might be concentrated in a very small area or involve a very large geographic region. A disastrous event might affect a small segment or a large percentage of the population in a geographic area. *Intensity* refers to a disaster agent's ability to inflict damage and injury. A disaster can be very intense and highly destructive, causing many injuries and deaths and much property damage, or less intense, with relatively little damage done to property or individuals.

Scope and intensity should be considered separately in disaster planning. For example, in the case of a building explosion, the scope is small, with a limited area of a community affected, but the intensity is great. The explosive forces are highly destructive to the building and cause death and injury to people within the building and in the immediate vicinity. A tornado is another example of a high-intensity and small-scope disaster; in contrast, a hurricane can have a high intensity and a large scope of impact. The area of damage from a specific hurricane can cover several states and involve many communities. An explosion at a water-purifying plant might cause minimal injury to property and personnel at the plant but might reduce or eliminate the water supply for an entire community for days or even weeks.

PHASES OF A DISASTER

There are three phases to any disaster. The actions of emergency personnel and other health professionals depend on which phase of the disaster is at hand.

PREIMPACT PHASE

The preimpact phase is the phase before a disaster. This is the time for disaster planning and mitigation before the actual occurrence. Disaster planning activities have a critical influence on how a disaster will affect a region, state, and community. This is the time for assessment of probabilities and risks of occurrence of certain types of disasters. Based on risk assessment, specific action plans should be designed to reduce the effects of predicted disasters. Mitigation might involve legislating specific building codes and land-use restrictions. Assessment and inventory of resources for special equipment, supplies, and personnel necessary to support an emergency response is essential. Planning activities should be coordinated by the emergency management agency and should involve all appropriate government agencies, public safety organizations, private organizations, and health care entities. Disaster

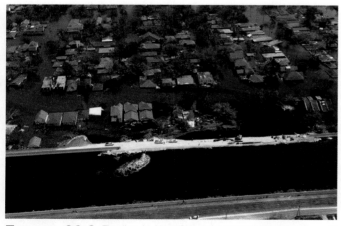

FIGURE 22-2 Flooding in New Orleans, Louisiana, in the aftermath of Hurricane Katrina in 2005. (From Federal Emergency Management Agency, Washington, DC. Available online at *http://www.photolibrary.fema.gov/photolibrary/photo_details.do?id=19208.*)

plans and personnel training must be reviewed and tested on a regular basis. A critical component of the predisaster phase preparation is education of the public to encourage individual preparedness. Examples of public education are the hurricane watch preparation and evacuation procedures for communities in the Southeast hurricane belt.

An important part of the preimpact phase is the warning opportunity. A warning is given to a community at the first possible sign of danger. For some disasters, no warning is possible. However, with the aid of weather networks, satellites, and new weather-monitoring technology, many meteorologic disasters can be predicted.

Giving the earliest possible warning is crucial to preventing loss of life and minimizing damage. This is the period when the emergency preparedness plan is put into effect. Emergency operations centers (EOCs) are opened by the state or local emergency management agency. Communication is a key factor during this phase. Disaster personnel will call on amateur radio operators, radio and television stations, and any other available sources to alert the community and keep citizens informed. The community must be educated to heed warnings and to recognize threats as serious. When communities experience several false alarms, members may not take future warnings very seriously.

The role of the nurse during the warning period will vary depending on her or his employer's role in disaster response. Nurses should be informed of their specific roles and responsibilities for disaster response. Community health nurses might be assigned to assist the ARC in preparing shelters, to assist with emergency aid stations, and to establish contact with other emergency service groups.

Nurses should establish their own family disaster response plans to protect their families and homes while still being able to respond to their communities' need. The nurse's personal plan should address options for emergency communication with family members and employer as well as child care and transportation options.

IMPACT PHASE

The impact phase occurs when the disaster actually happens. It is a time of enduring hardship or injury and of trying to survive. This is a time when individuals help neighbors and families at the scene, a time of holding on until outside help arrives. The impact phase might last for several minutes (e.g., during an earthquake, plane crash, or explosion) or for hours, days, or weeks (e.g., in a flood, famine, or epidemic).

During this phase, there should be a preliminary assessment of the nature, extent, and geographic area of the disaster. The number of persons requiring shelter, the type and number of anticipated disaster health services, and the general health status and needs of the community must be determined. It is important to have an estimate of the needed emergency resources as soon as possible after a disaster event to activate mutual aid plans and ensure a timely response from emergency medical services and other vital community support services.

The impact phase continues until the threat of further destruction has passed and the emergency plan is in effect. If there has been no warning, this is the time when the EOC is established and put in operation. The structure and functions of the EOC are addressed in more detail later in this chapter.

The ARC oversees the opening of shelters. Every shelter has a nurse as a member of the ARC disaster action team. The nurse is responsible for assessing health needs and providing physical and psychologic support to victims in the shelters. During the impact phase, injured persons undergo triage, morgue facilities are established and coordinated, and search and rescue activities are organized.

POSTIMPACT PHASE

The postimpact phase has two components: emergency and recovery. The *emergency phase* begins at the end of the impact phase and ends when there is no longer any immediate threat of injury or destruction. The emergency phase is the time of rescue and first aid. The incident command is established if it was not established in the warning phase. An assessment is made to establish the extent and types of emergency resources needed.

Recovery begins during the emergency phase and ends with the return of normal community order and functioning. The disaster planning cycle should begin again during the recovery phase. Evaluation of the current disaster plan and community response should be done based on the recent disaster. Debriefing should occur for all disaster response agencies and personnel. The disaster plans should be modified in keeping with the lessons learned from the most recent event. For survivors of a disaster, the impact phase might last a lifetime (e.g., victims of the September 11 terrorist attacks).

EFFECTS OF DISASTER ON THE COMMUNITY

Not only are individuals affected physically and emotionally by a disaster, but the entire community is also affected. Local and regional economies can be devastated by a disaster and require years of recovery. By 2006, the federal government had committed over $110 billion and citizens had donated almost $3.5 billion in cash and in-kind services to ongoing Gulf Coast rebuilding efforts (White House, 2006). The most important disruptions to the community are the following:

- Public service personnel are overworked.
- Lifelines are interrupted, including telephone systems, television and radio broadcasting, transportation, and water and sanitation services.
- Resources, such as food and medical supplies, are depleted.
- Rumors run rampant and are hard to check.
- Public and private buildings might be damaged.

In a disaster, the social and psychologic reactions of individuals are closely interwoven with those of the community. According to the ARC (1987), the four phases of a community's reaction to a disaster are as follows:

- *Heroic phase:* strong, direct emotions focusing on helping people to survive and recover
- *Honeymoon phase:* a drawing together of people who simultaneously experienced the catastrophic event
- *Disillusionment phase:* feelings of disappointment because of delays or failures when promises of aid are not fulfilled (people seek help to solve their own personal problems rather than community problems)
- *Reconstruction phase:* a reaffirmation of belief in the community when new buildings are constructed (delays in this phase might cause intense emotional response)

DISASTER MANAGEMENT: RESPONSIBILITIES OF AGENCIES AND ORGANIZATIONS

Governments bear the primary responsibility for designing and implementing disaster relief. Private and voluntary agencies contribute expertise and efforts to selected areas as designated by government plans. The key to effective disaster management is predisaster planning and preparation.

PLANNING

The purpose of disaster planning is to provide the policies, procedures, and guidelines necessary to protect lives, limit injury, and protect property immediately before, during, and after a disaster event. A comprehensive emergency management plan addresses four areas: mitigation, preparedness, response, and recovery.

A comprehensive plan demands a coordinated, cooperative effort among many different people, agencies, and levels of government. Planning should use valid assumptions about possible disaster agents based on previous community, state, and regional experiences, as well as experiences from other regions. The United Nations (UN) General Assembly has identified disaster events as a major threat to the global community and declared the 1990s as the International Decade of Natural Disaster Reduction. The UN called for a worldwide planning effort to reduce loss of life and property. As part of the UN effort, the World Health Organization (WHO) developed a planning guide for community emergency preparedness (WHO, 1999). The guide assists countries in preplanning efforts, personnel training, and postevent evaluation.

Planning requires technology to forecast events; engineering to reduce risks; public education about potential hazards; surveillance systems to detect environmental hazards; a coordinated emergency response; and a systematic assessment of the effects of a disaster to better prepare for future disasters. Responsibility for addressing these five areas of disaster planning is shared by federal, state, local, and voluntary agencies. Some of the organizations involved in disaster planning and relief are listed in Community Resources for Practice at the end of this chapter.

FEDERAL GOVERNMENT

The federal government generally enacts laws and provides funds to support state and local governments. The Public Disaster Act of 1974 (Public Law 93-288) provided for consolidation of federal disaster relief activities and funding under a single agency.

Federal Emergency Management Agency

The Federal Emergency Management Agency (FEMA) was established in 1979 as the coordinating agency for all available federal disaster assistance. The agency works closely with state and local governments by funding emergency programs and providing technical guidance and training. The scope and intensity of FEMA's response to a disaster is influenced by the severity of the disaster's impact on the community. If damage is limited and the existing local, state, and regional resources can handle the problems, FEMA's services might not be needed. FEMA responds to all moderate (level II) and massive (level I) disasters. FEMA provides both direct aid (supplies and personnel) and indirect services (funding and coordination efforts). In 2003 FEMA was downgraded from an independent agency and consolidated into the Department of Homeland Security (DHS). In 2005, as a result of poor response to Hurricane Katrina, some of the responsibilities for emergency preparedness were removed from FEMA and given to other agencies within DHS.

Department of Homeland Security

The President created the DHS as a response to the terrorist attacks in 2001. A Presidential Directive (HSPD-5) in 2003 ordered the creation of a National Response Plan (NRP). The NRP was periodically updated to incorporate lessons learned from exercises and real-world events. In 2008 the NRP was superseded by the National Response Framework (NRF). The NRF establishes a comprehensive, national, all-hazards approach to domestic incidence response. The Framework identifies the key response principles, as well as the roles and structures that organize a coordinated and effective national response by communities, states, the Federal Government, and private-sector and nongovernmental partners. In addition, it describes special circumstances in which the Federal Government exercises a larger role, including incidents in which Federal interests are involved and catastrophic incidents in which a state would require significant support. An important element of the NRF is the National Incident Management System (NIMS), a consistent nationwide system that standardizes incident management practices and procedures. Under the NRF, DHS is responsible for *mass care*; that is, the coordination of nonmedical services such as shelter, food, emergency first aid, search and rescue, and efforts to reunite displaced family members (Lister, 2006).

Department of Health and Human Services

The U.S. Department of Health and Human Services (USDHHS) partners with the Departments of Agriculture, Defense, Energy, Justice, and Transportation; the Environmental Protection Agency; the DHS; the National Communications System; and the U.S. Postal Service to serve as the lead federal agency for public health and medical services under the NRP. The USDHHS also directs and manages the National Disaster Medical System (NDMS). The NDMS is designed to deal with medical care needs in disasters of great intensity and scope that overwhelm the local health care system (Riley, 2003). It has three main objectives:

- Provide medical assistance to a disaster area in the form of medical assistance teams, medical supplies, and equipment
- Evacuate patients who cannot be cared for in the affected area to other predetermined locations
- Provide a national network of hospitals that are designated to accept patients in the event of a national emergency
  Other agencies supporting the NDMS include the DHS and the Departments of Defense and Veterans Affairs.

Centers for Disease Control and Prevention, Department of Health and Human Services

The emphasis in disaster planning at the Centers for Disease Control and Prevention (CDC) is prevention and/or mitigation of epidemics and biochemical hazards (both natural and deliberate terror). The CDC has updated and refined its surveillance system to rapidly identify health threats to the population.

Educating health professionals to recognize and treat biochemical hazards is a priority (CDC, 2003a). There is a concern that biologic agents, such as those causing smallpox, anthrax, and influenza, can be used as weapons. The CDC has developed recommendations for pre-event smallpox vaccinations and plans for mass immunization of health care workers and other emergency personnel if the need arises (CDC, 2003b). In 2003, the CDC mailed an informational packet about smallpox to all health care providers and encouraged health professionals to register online to receive updated information (CDC, 2003c). Other CDC activities are addressed later in the chapter.

The federal government has other agencies involved in disaster relief. **Website Resource 22B** lists most agencies and their responsibilities during disaster. A few examples are mentioned here. The National Guard provides transportation, assistance with evacuations, and police services when local or area police resources are strained or overwhelmed by disaster needs. The U.S. Department of Housing and Urban Development's temporary housing program helps families either relocate or repair their homes. The Small Business Administration has a disaster program that helps both businesses and families by providing government-guaranteed loans to assist in their recovery. The Individual Family Grant Program provides grants of up to $5000 to families to assist in their recovery.

STATE GOVERNMENTS

State governments coordinate the development of the state emergency operations plan and establish an emergency management agency to coordinate the state response to a disaster event. For disaster planning purposes, if the disaster involves more than one local jurisdiction, the state might coordinate response services.

Usually there is one state agency designated as the emergency management agency for all state-coordinated disaster efforts. When a disaster happens, the state governor will open the state's EOC, in which some state agencies (e.g., state police; National Guard; state emergency medical services; and state health, welfare, and social service agencies) will work together at the same location to direct their specific agency's functions for disaster relief (Figure 22-3). Most states also have a state coordinator to manage fire department resources and personnel.

The state emergency management agency advises the governor when the state has exhausted its resources or the disaster is predicted to be of such magnitude that the state does not have the resources to respond and manage the disaster event. The governor then notifies FEMA that federal disaster relief assistance is needed. Timely assessment and evaluation of the local and state resources and their ability to respond to any disaster event is critical to activate the appropriate communication channels to obtain federal assistance and mutual aid from surrounding states in a timely manner during a disaster event.

LOCAL GOVERNMENTS, COMMUNITIES, AND VOLUNTEER GROUPS

Local governments are responsible for the safety and welfare of their citizens. They act to protect the lives, health, and property of their citizens; carry out evacuation rescues; and maintain public works. Local disaster response organizations should include local area government agencies, such as fire departments, police departments, public health departments, public works departments, emergency services, and the local branch of the ARC.

Communities must have an emergency operations plan. Local planning efforts include contingency action plans for various types of disaster situations, designation of an overall incident commander, and identification of community resources that can be used in a disaster. The plan is developed and tested in mock-disaster exercises and then revised and refined. The local emergency management agency has communication links with the state's EOC and with FEMA and the DHS.

Area hospitals develop their own action plans for handling small community disasters, such as a school bus accident or

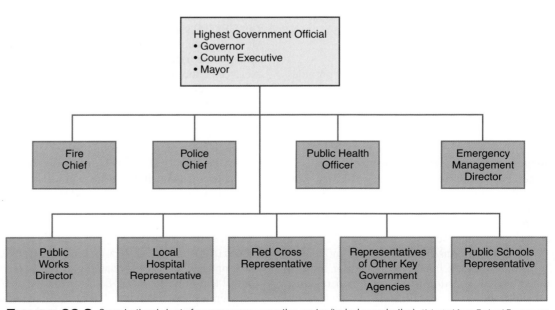

FIGURE 22-3 Organizational chart of an emergency operating center (typical organization). (Adapted from Federal Emergency Management Agency. [1981]. *Disaster operation: A handbook for local governments* [CPG16]. Washington, DC: Author.)

a large apartment fire. They are also involved in community planning preparation for larger-scale disasters that require a coordinated community effort. Local hospitals play an important role in the NRF. Local volunteer organizations, such as the Boy Scouts, Girl Scouts, Jaycees, veterans associations, and church groups, can be considered additional resources to be used as the need arises. Local health care professionals who do not participate in community organizations that are officially involved in disaster planning might be called on to volunteer their services during an emergency.

AMERICAN RED CROSS

The ARC was founded in 1881 by Clara Barton. It is a voluntary agency that was granted a charter on January 5, 1905, by the U.S. Congress. The charter gives the ARC the authority to act as the *primary voluntary* national disaster relief agency for the American people and to be ready for immediate action in every part of the United States. The federal statute allows the ARC to coordinate efforts with other federal agencies. This federal legislation applies only to those emergencies and major disasters that have been declared as such by the President. On a national level, and in many communities, the ARC acts to coordinate the disaster relief efforts of a variety of voluntary agencies. The ARC has created five programs to meet the human needs of a disaster (Box 22-1).

BOX 22-1   American Red Cross Programs for Disaster Relief

1. **Damage assessment:** The first task after a disaster strikes is to gather immediate and accurate information about the physical damage resulting from the disaster.
2. **Mass care:** Shelter and food are provided to the affected community or communities, including:
   Food provision: Food is provided at shelters or feeding stations or might be taken by mobile units to disaster areas.
   Shelter provision: Mass shelters are organized in schools, public buildings, hotels, motels, or churches.
   Supply provision: Personal hygiene articles, toilet articles, and/or cleaning supplies are provided.
3. **Health services:** Medical, nursing, and health care is provided in shelters and emergency aid stations. Services include provision of blood and blood products; provision of emergency medical and hospital supplies; assistance to public health officials; and assistance to families in finding available health services.
4. **Family services:** Emergency assistance helps families resume living by providing food, clothing, and shelter. Shelter assistance includes funding of temporary hotel stays, rent payments, security deposits, utility deposits, and temporary home repairs. Help in obtaining household items such as furniture, cooking and eating utensils, linens, and necessary appliances, and/or occupational supplies and equipment, such as tools or uniforms, is another potential area of assistance. ARC assistance is free and is provided through funds donated by the American people.
5. **Disaster welfare inquiry service:** Disasters frequently disrupt communication. The ARC disaster welfare inquiry service gathers information about the disaster area (what and who were affected, and individuals killed or injured) and makes this information available to concerned relatives through their local ARC chapters.

EMERGENCY RESPONSE NETWORK

The primary goals of disaster management are to prevent or minimize death, disability, suffering, and loss on the part of disaster victims. How these goals are achieved varies with the type of disaster and the type of rescue worker. Police officers and firefighters will have an entirely different focus than health care workers. It is vital that efforts be directed in a well-designed and coordinated manner to ensure the most efficient and timely response to disaster needs. Two strategies have been developed to facilitate coordination and reduce duplication of services. These two strategies are the incident command system and the EOC.

INCIDENT COMMAND SYSTEM

Established organizations provide many of the community services needed in a disaster (Table 22-2). The incident command system (ICS) was adopted by FEMA to coordinate responses to a disaster at the scene of the disaster. The most important feature of the ICS is a common organizational structure in which all community and local government agencies are represented (Figure 22-4). Each organization maintains its own autonomy while being integrated into the central organization. For example, emergency management personnel are not mixed with people from the public works department. Each organization can concentrate on its assignment and not be distracted by other responsibilities. For example, emergency medical system personnel do not have to be concerned with organizing shelters or providing care in the shelters. That responsibility belongs to the ARC.

EMERGENCY OPERATIONS CENTER AND EMERGENCY MEDICAL SYSTEM

The EOC is the *command* center for coordination of the community-wide response to a disaster. The EOC coordinates interactions among various response personnel involved in the *ICS* at the scene as well as services provided at other locations. It serves as *the* center for communication with other government agencies, local emergency medical services, the ARC,

---

TABLE 22-2   Existing Agencies Involved in Incident Command System

Agency	Resource/Function
American Red Cross	Shelter personnel, road signs, blockades, communication equipment
Electric company	Repair personnel, trucks, repair equipment, communications equipment
Emergency management	Emergency Operating Center, equipment
Fire	Firefighters, fire equipment
Law enforcement	Police officers, flares, blockades, communication equipment
Public health	Surveillance systems, public health personnel
Public works/highway department	Repair personnel and equipment, trucks, communication equipment

Data from Federal Emergency Management Agency. (1998). *Basic incident command system* (IS-195). Washington, DC: Author.

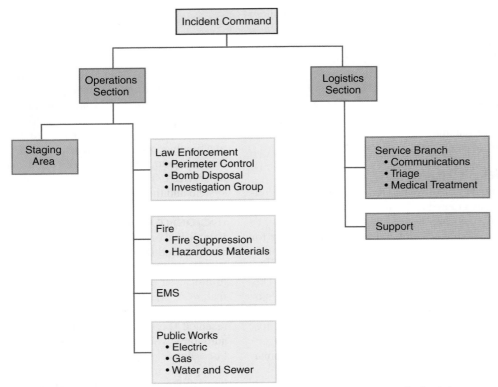

FIGURE 22-4 Sample organizational chart for an incident command system (at the scene of a disaster). (Adapted from Federal Emergency Management Agency. [1998]. *Basic incident command system* [IS-195]. Washington, DC: Author.)

and public safety agencies. In conjunction with other partners, the EOC forms an emergency management partnership. Figure 22-5 illustrates how the EOC operates with other agencies and organizations not under its authority. Each community determines the locale and personnel involved in its EOC. The EOC includes health personnel representing the local emergency medical system, public health department, and, usually, representatives from hospitals in the community.

PRINCIPLES OF DISASTER MANAGEMENT

According to Garb and Eng (1969), there are eight fundamental principles that should be followed by all who have a

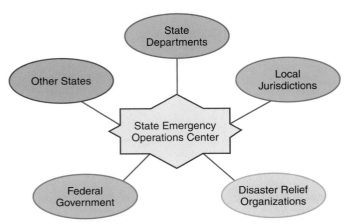

FIGURE 22-5 Emergency management partnership. (Redrawn from State of Maryland Emergency Operations Plan, March 20, 2002.)

responsibility for helping the victims of a disaster. It is critical that rescue workers apply these principles in proper sequence, or they will be ineffective and possibly detrimental to disaster victims. The eight basic principles are as follows:

1. Prevent the occurrence of the disaster whenever possible.
2. Minimize the number of casualties if the disaster cannot be prevented.
3. Prevent further casualties from occurring after the initial impact of the disaster.
4. Rescue the victims.
5. Provide first aid to the injured.
6. Evacuate the injured to medical facilities.
7. Provide definitive medical care.
8. Promote reconstruction of lives.

PREVENTION AND MITIGATION

The first three principles address prevention and mitigation of the impact of a disaster. Certain types of disasters, particularly man-made ones, might be preventable. Disasters have been prevented by the enforcement of good building codes or by proper land and water management. Other disasters are not preventable, but their impact might be mitigated. Public education can be used to reduce the impact of dangerous situations. In areas that are prone to certain types of disaster situations, public education can alert the community on how best to prepare for such situations *in advance* of an actual event. Community health nurses might be involved in such efforts, including providing instruction regarding proper safety precautions and proper storage of emergency supplies, and giving first aid courses to prepare the public to care for injuries in the event of an actual emergency. Public communication systems, such as radio and television, routinely broadcast information about how people can obtain information in the event of an actual disaster situation.

Early warning systems alert the public to the probability of immediate danger and help to reduce the impact of predictable disasters, such as hurricanes or tornadoes. They might also provide information on an evacuation plan or other immediate actions that improve the chance of survival and reduce the probability of injuries.

Preventing further casualties after initial impact depends on evaluating and lessening any unsafe conditions present *immediately* after the disaster. For example, access to unstable buildings and washed-out bridges must be prevented, and contamination of water and food supplies must be averted or corrected. Periodic physical assessments of the disaster scene are essential to make certain the area continues to be safe. These activities are generally carried out by local utility personnel, firemen, and other individuals trained in structural assessment.

RESCUE AND EMERGENCY MEDICAL CARE

Rescue involves locating and freeing trapped victims and then evacuating them to a safe place. In the event of a disaster, the EOC becomes operational. Disaster service personnel, including emergency medical service personnel, are called to respond. These personnel will be involved in treating people at the scene of the disaster as well as at other designated locations, including local hospitals.

Triage

There are several times during the emergency response at which triage might be necessary to best determine the needs of injured victims. *Triage* is a French word meaning "sorting" or "categorizing." During a disaster, the goal is to maximize the number of survivors by sorting the treatable from the untreatable victims. In a disaster, the potential for survival and the availability of resources are the primary criteria used to determine which clients receive immediate treatment. In a disaster situation, saving the greatest number of lives is the most important goal. Triage might take place during the rescue operation at the scene of the disaster and again at each stage of transport of the disaster victims. Many different personnel are involved in the triage operation. Each person must know her or his exact role. Nurses and other emergency personnel, rather than physicians, are often used as triage officers because physicians are administering emergency care to the more critical victims.

Prioritizing of victims for treatment can be done in many ways. Some communities use color coding. Probably the best and most easily understood is the category color-coding system. Colored tags quickly identified the priority of care. A new concern is the need to identify people who might be contaminated with biochemical agents (Christen & Maniscalco, 2002; Eckert, 2006). An example of a coding system is presented in Box 22-2.

Ideally, triage leads to appropriate and definitive care for all victims. However, this can occur only if the cause of the multiple casualties is quickly controlled so that rescue teams can care for the injured in an organized manner. If the disaster conditions continue or if secondary events, such as fires or building collapses, occur, the rescue effort will be disrupted, and the treatment of victims will be inhibited.

BOX 22-2 | **Five-Category Coding for Triage**

1. Red—Most urgent; first priority
First-priority patients have life-threatening injuries and are experiencing hypoxia or nearing hypoxia. Examples of injuries of patients in this category are shock, chest wounds, internal hemorrhage, head injuries producing increased loss of consciousness, partial- or full-thickness burns over 20% to 60% of the body surface, and chest pain.

2. Yellow—Urgent; second priority
Second-priority patients have injuries with systemic effects and complications but are not yet hypoxic or in shock. Patients appear stable enough to withstand up to a 2-hour wait without immediate risk. Examples of injuries of patients in this category are multiple fractures, open fractures, spinal injuries, large lacerations, partial- or full-thickness burns over 10% to 20% of the body surface, and medical emergencies such as diabetic coma, insulin shock, and epileptic seizure. Patients with second-priority status might need to be observed closely for signs of shock, at which time they would be recategorized to first priority.

3. Green—Third priority
Third-priority patients have minimal injuries unaccompanied by systemic complications. Usually these patients can wait longer than 2 hours for treatment without danger. Examples of injuries of patients in this category are closed fractures, minor burns, minor lacerations, sprains, contusions, and abrasions.

4. Black—Dying or dead
Dying or dead patients are hopelessly injured patients or dead victims. These patients have catastrophic injuries (e.g., crushing injuries to the head or chest) and would not survive under the best of circumstances. These patients present the greatest difficulty, because failure to treat patients conflicts with nursing philosophy. In a disaster, triage must give the chance of survival to the greatest number of victims rather than to one individual. Personnel and equipment must be reserved to treat the greatest number of viable patients.

5. Contaminated—Might have a color code or a hazardous material (hazmat) triangle tag
These patients are contaminated with hazardous bacteriologic or chemical substances. They will be routed to a decontamination sector to eliminate hazards before additional treatment is provided.

EVACUATION AND DEFINITIVE MEDICAL CARE

Evacuation of victims must be done in an orderly but timely fashion. Many factors will affect evacuation and must be considered by the nurse. These include availability of transport vehicles, current weather conditions, condition of the roads leading to advanced care facilities, and time between disaster impact and arrival at the hospital. Hospitals should receive advance notice of the impending emergency transports. Advance notification allows the hospital to mobilize staff and resources to meet the sudden increase of emergency patient admissions and to treat the more critically injured patients in a timely manner. If there is more than one hospital in a local community, patients should be triaged to each hospital based on the hospital's capabilities at that time. The EOC should establish communications with each hospital to determine the current capabilities and to advise the hospitals of the estimated number of patients being transported and the severity of their injuries.

Hospitals must have well-honed disaster plans to meet the needs of large groups of victims in a short time. These plans should be practiced at least twice each year. The plans should provide for disasters that occur internally as well as externally. An internal disaster is a catastrophic event occurring on the medical center grounds and resulting in multiple injuries, for example, an outbreak of severe acute respiratory syndrome (SARS) in a hospital. An external disaster is a catastrophic event occurring off the medical center grounds and resulting in multiple injured persons for whom the hospital would need to provide emergency care, for example, a building collapse in the community. To meet the accreditation requirements of the Joint Commission, all hospitals *must* have disaster plans, hold disaster drills, and regularly evaluate these plans and activities.

Sometimes the disaster is of such a massive scale that local medical services and facilities are unable to respond. In Hurricane Katrina, hospitals and other medical facilities in Alabama and Louisiana were destroyed or damaged and were unable to function. In such massive disasters, the federal government needs to step in to organize medical response teams to help with medical services and to evacuate health personnel and injured citizens.

RECONSTRUCTION AND RECOVERY

The reconstruction of the victim's life begins with initial care and continues until the victim has recovered. This might take days, months, or years. Victims, disaster workers, and volunteers must receive adequate psychologic counseling and emotional support to be able to return effectively to normal living.

STAGES OF EMOTIONAL RESPONSE

The victims of a disaster go through four stages of emotional response similar to the four-stage response to death and dying. These are the following (Richtsmeir & Miller, 1985):

- *Denial*—Victims might deny the magnitude of the problem or, more likely, will understand the problem but might seem unaffected emotionally. The victim might appear unusually unconcerned.
- *Strong emotional response*—People are aware of the problem but regard it as overwhelming and unbearable. Common reactions during this stage are trembling, tightening of the muscles, sweating, difficulty speaking, weeping, heightened sensitivity, restlessness, sadness, anger, and passivity. Victims might want to retell or relive the disaster experience over and over.
- *Acceptance*—Victims begin to accept the problems caused by the disaster and make a concentrated effort to solve them. They feel more hopeful and confident.
- *Recovery*—Victims feel they are back to normal and experience a sense of well-being. Routines become important again.

PSYCHOLOGIC REACTIONS AFTER DISASTER

Box 22-3 lists some common reactions to disaster. Psychologic reactions can be categorized along three dimensions: mild to severe, normal to pathologic, and immediate to delayed. A reaction might be severe but normal, or mild and yet abnormal. A few people will be so overwhelmed by the trauma that they will experience extreme psychologic distress immediately. Others, despite their intense involvement in the disaster, might

---

BOX 22-3   Common Reactions to a Disaster

Psychologic
Sadness or apathy
Guilt or shame
Disorientation
Difficulty concentrating
Difficulty with decision making
Feelings of helplessness or hopelessness
Moodiness, irritability
Withdrawal or disconnectedness
Fatigue
Nightmares and/or panic attacks
Anger
Feelings of loss or grief
Mood swings

Physical
Immediate
Shock symptoms, including difficulty breathing; chills; pale, cold, clammy skin
Hyperventilation
Chest pains, palpitations
Rapid heartbeat
Hypertension

Delayed
Skin rashes or disorders
Increased use of caffeine, alcohol, or drugs
Loss of or increase in appetite
Increased startle reflex
Headaches, fainting
Gastrointestinal problems, including nausea, vomiting, diarrhea, constipation
Teeth grinding
Insomnia
Hyperactivity

---

appear unaffected psychologically during both the impact and postimpact phases. These people might be using denial and repression as defenses to handle their thoughts and feelings. For example, one firefighter treated for an obviously painful eye injury during the 9/11 disaster denied he had a serious injury (Taintor, 2003). It should be noted that all disaster victims and workers might need critical stress debriefing and possible referral and follow-up with a mental health care professional to restore them to their predisaster mental health level.

Feelings of guilt might arise in survivors when many victims have died. Fear of death or occurrence of another disaster is a frequently seen reaction. For example, survivors of the 1993 World Trade Center bombing reported that they felt hypervigilant, just waiting for the next attack to occur (Taintor, 2003). Anger might be exhibited as general irritability or full-fledged rage and might be directed toward the cause of the disaster, displaced onto the support system, or directed inward. For example, after the 9/11 attack, there were assaults on foreign-looking persons including the following:

- A Sikh gas station owner killed in Mesa, Arizona
- A Pakistani Muslim grocery store owner killed in Dallas, Texas
- A Middle Eastern taxicab driver beaten by two passengers in Northridge, California

LONG-TERM EFFECTS OF THE DISASTER EXPERIENCE

The psychologic stress experienced as a result of a disaster might lead to long-term effects, such as interpersonal or social problems. Some individuals might turn to alcohol or drugs in an attempt to relieve their stress. Others might have difficulty resuming their usual routines and relationship patterns. Lingering health effects were reported by witnesses, survivors, and emergency personnel 1 year after 9/11 (Figure 22-6). Vlahov and colleagues (2002) report a substantial increase in substance use among Manhattan residents in the acute post-disaster period after the 9/11 attacks. Other problems include long-term respiratory syndromes, such as asthma and bronchitis, and mental health problems such as posttraumatic stress disorder and depression. Children are particularly vulnerable after a traumatic event. A survey of New York City schoolchildren reported that nearly all experienced some problems related to the disaster (Figure 22-7).

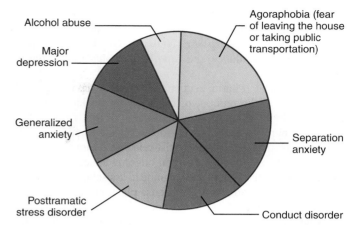

FIGURE 22-7 Children's reaction to September 11, 2001, as measured 6 months after the event. (Data from Ferri, R., & Sofer, D. [2002]. September 11: Health effects linger. *American Journal of Nursing, 102* [9], 18-19.)

Health officials estimate that over 400,000 people have lingering health effects from 9/11. Dust particles contained carcinogens, concrete, and other environmental hazards. Swallowing or breathing these toxins can create severe physical problems that might not be apparent for 15 to 20 years (Wielawski, 2006). A consortium of public health officials (federal, state, local, and others) are conducting long-term surveillance of survivors to identify and document illnesses caused by exposure to contaminants from the 9/11 disaster.

Posttraumatic stress disorder (PTSD) was first recognized in veterans of the Vietnam War. It is now known to occur after other traumatic events, including war, terrorism, kidnapping, and disasters. According to the American Psychiatric Association (APA, 2000), the following are three characteristics of the syndrome:

- The person is exposed to a traumatic event and experiences fear or horror related to the event.
- The trauma event is reexperienced through flashbacks, dreams, or triggering events.
- The person avoids things that remind him or her of the trauma.

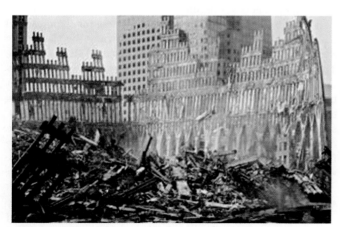

FIGURE 22-6 New York, NY, September 27, 2001. The remaining section of the World Trade Center is surrounded by a mountain of rubble following the September 11 terrorist attacks. (From Federal Emergency Management Agency, Washington, DC. Retrieved June 24, 2007 from *http://www.photolibrary.fema.gov/photolibrary/photodetails.do?id15691*.)

In addition, victims of PTSD experience two or more of the following symptoms: hyperalertness, exaggerated startle response, sleep disturbance, survival guilt, decreased concentration, impaired memory, and avoidance behavior. Reminders of the trauma increase the symptoms in victims of this syndrome (APA, 2000).

Community health nurses and others involved in treating clients should be aware that the symptoms of PTSD might not be evident for some time after the actual event. Several factors have been identified that will increase the likelihood of an individual's developing PTSD. These include witnessing a violent act, witnessing or experiencing a previous disaster event, lacking a social support network, and having a previous history of psychiatric illness (Mitchell et al., 2002).

NEW CHALLENGES FOR DISASTER PLANNING AND RESPONSE

The recent acts of **biologic terrorism (bioterrorism)** and **chemical terrorism** using biologic and chemical agents as weapons to inflict death, injuries, property damage, and disruption of public services have created the need to reexamine disaster plans at all levels of government and public health agencies. All public safety, public health, and health care organizations must work closely together to develop plans, train personnel, educate the professional responders and the public on the use of protective equipment, and develop communication models. Nurses practicing in all health care settings need to be involved in disaster planning and receive disaster response education and training (Eckert, 2006; Kennedy, 2001; Riley, 2003). Training must include strategies to protect health care workers from possible biologic or chemical agents. The Occupational Safety and Health Administration (OSHA, 2005) has published guidelines to assist hospitals with developing practice criteria for mass casualty incidents involving hazardous substances.

BIOTERRORISM

The CDC began planning for the public health response to bioterrorism with the possibility of anthrax attacks in 1998. Planning determined how to improve public health preparedness for possible acts of bioterrorism. One outcome was improvements by the CDC to the following:

- The Laboratory Response Network for Bioterrorism—improved surveillance and reporting of suspicious illness clusters
- The National Pharmaceutical Stockpile—updating and expansion of the number of medications available for dispensing in the event of an incident

These improvements allowed for an effective public health response to the 2001 bioterrorist-related anthrax outbreak (Perkins et al., 2002). As part of an ongoing educational effort on bioterrorism, the CDC issued a guide to assist health care professionals in preparedness and response planning (CDC, 2000).

The USDHHS (2007) is responsible for developing an implementation plan to address chemical, biologic, radiologic, and nuclear threats. Currently the USDHHS has identified 14 potential threat agents and medical countermeasures for these. The USDHHS began developing local metropolitan medical response systems (MMRS) in 1995. Now managed by FEMA, the program contracts with emergency management of existing emergency response systems, medical and mental health providers, public health departments, law enforcement agencies, fire departments, emergency medical services (EMS), and the National Guard (local MMRS) to provide an integrated, unified response to a mass casualty event (Thompson, 2001).

The USDHHS is responsible for planning upgrades to the public health infrastructure. The current priority is improvement in communication and responses in all types of disaster situations (see *Healthy People 2010* objectives in Chapter 29).

The National Institutes of Health has a bioterrorism research program lead by the National Institute of Allergy and Infectious Diseases. This research program includes both short-term and long-term research targeted at designing, developing, evaluating, and approving the diagnostic methods, therapies, and vaccines needed to control infections caused by microbes that have a potential for bioterrorist use (Thompson, 2001).

It is crucial that health care personnel be trained to immediately recognize bioterrorism agents and take steps to protect themselves and treat the victims. According to the CDC (2007), training for hospital emergency staff is progressing but still needs improvement. The CDC survey of hospital emergency response managers found a range of training levels depending on the toxic agent, with 86% of hospital staff trained to recognize smallpox (highest level) but only 52% of staff receiving training about hemorrhagic fever (lowest level).

There are special characteristics of biologic agents that are used by terrorists. The biologic agent must be capable of causing morbidity and possible mortality, and/or cause a disease that is difficult to diagnose and treat. The fear factor is important to the terrorist; the more severe the morbidity and mortality, the greater the fear factor. Other characteristics of the agent that must be considered by the terrorist are (1) accessibility, (2) reproducibility, (3) stability, and (4) dispersibility (Brachman, 2002). Potential biologic agents have been categorized based on their characteristics (Table 22-3).

An early, effective response to a bioterrorism act depends on the quality of health surveillance. There must be routine, mandatory, timely reporting of certain illnesses by laboratories, schools, hospitals, and other health care facilities. Routine reporting creates challenges. The routine reporting from medical laboratories is highly reliable; however, there are many weaknesses in timely reporting from public health agencies and health care providers. Methods for secondary surveillance that exist in some local communities and state health departments include monitoring sales of over-the-counter medicines, monitoring diseases in animals, and monitoring emergency department ambulance diversions; however, this information is not usually timely and may have a lag time of weeks to months. In planning an effective defense against bioterrorism, new models of surveillance that yield timely information must be developed, and ongoing continuing education of primary care and emergency care providers is crucial (Agency for Healthcare Research and Quality, 2005). Syndromic surveillance is one example of such a model and focuses on syndromes such as dyspnea, pneumonia, rash, nausea and/or vomiting, diarrhea, encephalitis, and other unexplained or unusual illnesses or causes of death (Brachman, 2002). This type of surveillance can be helpful because many potential bioterrorism agents cause similar symptoms. For example, fever, malaise, and cough are symptoms that can result from inhalational anthrax, pneumonic plague, and/or tularemia.

CHEMICAL AND HAZARDOUS MATERIALS

Today, in the United States, there is a high probability of accidental and/or deliberate environmental contamination with a hazardous substance. The Agency for Toxic Substances and Disease Registry (ATSDR), an agency of the USDHHS, protects the public from hazardous wastes and environmental spills of hazardous substances (see Chapter 9). ATSDR is the lead agency within the Public Health Service to help prevent or reduce further exposure to hazardous substances. Its functions include public health assessments of waste sites; health consultations concerning specific hazardous substances; health surveillance and maintenance of registries; and education and training concerning hazardous substances.

The ATSDR has prepared an education and training series, Managing Hazardous Material Incidents (MHMI), for rescue and health care workers. The MHMI books and video provide recommendations for on-scene (prehospital) and hospital medical management of patients exposed during a hazardous materials incident. This information is available on the ATSDR website (see Community Resources for Practice at the end of the chapter to access this site).

The ATSDR operates a surveillance system for chemical and hazardous substances. This system is known as the Hazardous Substances Emergency Events Surveillance (HSEES) system. The ATSDR works with states to collect and analyze information about releases of hazardous substances. This information is then used to develop strategies to prepare and respond to events involving hazardous substances and to assist federal, state, and local public health agencies in planning for any type of hazardous release. The HSEES system is used to do the following (HSEES, 2001):

- Describe the distribution and characteristics of hazardous substances emergencies
- Describe the morbidity and mortality experienced by employees, responders, and the general public as a result of hazardous substance releases
- Identify risk factors associated with morbidity and mortality
- Identify strategies that might reduce future morbidity and mortality resulting from the release of hazardous substances

TABLE 22-3	Critical Biologic Agents by Priority		
Category	Description	Agents	Disease
A	High-priority agents include organisms that pose a risk to national security because they can be easily disseminated or transmitted person-to-person; cause high mortality, with potential for major public health impact; might cause public panic and social disruption; and require special action for public health preparedness.	*Variola major* *Bacillus anthracis* *Yersinia pestis* *Clostridium botulinum toxin* *Francisella tularensis* Filoviruses 　*Ebola* 　*Marburg* Arenaviruses 　*Lassa* *Junin* and related viruses	Smallpox Anthrax Plague Botulism Tularemia Ebola hemorrhagic fever Marburg hemorrhagic fever Lassa fever Argentine hemorrhagic fever 　Q fever
B	Second-highest priority agents include those that are moderate morbidity and low mortality; and require specific enhancements of CDC's diagnostic capacity and enhanced disease surveillance.	*Coxiella burnetti* *Brucella* species *Burkholderia mallei* Alphaviruses Ricin toxin Epsilon toxin of *Clostridium perfringens* *Staphylococcus* enterotoxin B	Brucellosis Glanders Venezuelan encephalomyelitis and Eastern and Western equine encephalomyelitis Toxic shock
	Subset of B agents includes pathogens that are food or waterborne.	*Salmonella* species *Shigella dysenteriae* *Escherichia coli* 0157:H7 *Vibrio cholerae* *Cryptosporidium parvum*	
C	Third-highest priority agents include emerging pathogens that could be engineered for mass dissemination in the future because of availability; ease of production and dissemination; and potential for high morbidity and mortality and major health impact.	Nipah virus Hantaviruses Tickborne hemorrhagic viruses Tickborne encephalitis viruses Yellow fever Multidrug-resistant tuberculosis	

Data from Thompson, T. (2001, October 23). *Civilian preparedness for biological warfare and terrorism: HHS readiness and role in vaccine research and development.* Testimony before the Committee on Government Reform Subcommittee on National Security, Veterans Affairs and International Relations United States House of Representatives. *CDC*, Centers for Disease Control and Prevention.

An analysis of HSEES data for 2004 indicates that 7744 hazardous substance emergency events occurred. Most (88%) involved one substance (ATSDR, 2004). A relatively small number of events (620) accounted for 1838 victims and 42 deaths. Most hazardous events occurred at fixed facilities 5687 (73.4%); only 2057 (26.6%) were transportation related (ATSDR, 2004).

Health care providers must be aware of these chemical and hazardous substance threats and know how to access information on self-protection from contamination and the appropriate client decontamination and treatment measures for the specific contaminate. Planning for chemical and hazardous substance contamination must be part of all health care agencies' disaster planning and training.

NURSING'S RESPONSIBILITIES IN DISASTER MANAGEMENT

Disaster nursing can be defined as the adaptation of professional nursing skills to recognize and meet the nursing,

physical, and emotional needs resulting from a disaster. The goal of disaster nursing is to achieve the best possible level of health for the people and the community involved in the disaster.

Many nurses in various clinical specialties are involved in disaster management at some level, either in preplanning, immediate care, or recovery efforts. Some nurses are directly involved in providing disaster care. These include nurses belonging to the following groups:

- Community/public health nurses employed by state and local health departments. They are involved in preplanning, public education, and immediate disaster response. They are part of the first cadre of personnel alerted for disaster relief.
- Disaster medical assistance teams (DMATs), whose members are volunteers and include physicians, nurses, and other emergency personnel (Schwarz & Kennedy, 2003). These are rapid response teams. As part of the NDMS system, they can be deployed nationwide. For example, on September 11, 2001, DMAT teams from New England and

the mid-Atlantic region were deployed to New York, and in 2005 teams from all over the United States were deployed to Louisiana and Alabama to assist with the care of survivors and rescue workers.

- ARC disaster assistance teams (DATs). These teams, including nurses, are volunteers with ARC. DATs provide disaster response, damage assessments, mass care, and shelter care.
- U.S. Public Health Service Nurse Corps and U.S. Military Nurse Corps. These nurses, employed by the federal government, are the government first responders in the event of disaster.

Other nurses provide direct care in disaster situations. These include local emergency department and intensive care nurses. They might provide care in their institutions or be sent as a team to the disaster or a site in close proximity to the affected areas. Depending on the nature and duration of the disaster, other nurses in the community might be asked to volunteer, work overtime, or provide relief for the first responders. Many nurses are involved in other areas of disaster management.

PREPLANNING: DEVELOPING A RESPONSE PLAN

A response plan should be concerned with delivering emergency health care as efficiently and as quickly as possible. To that end, community nurses should know in advance all community medical and social agency resources that will be available during a disaster. They should know where equipment and supplies have been stored and their prearranged role and rendezvous site.

Most agencies have a disaster notification network to alert personnel. Staff must follow a protocol of notification so that all available personnel are alerted or called to duty when the need arises. A good notification network should include a contingency plan for cases in which some personnel might not be reachable. In that way, the communication network is not disabled. Nonresponders are simply bypassed, and the notification process continues. If possible, when disasters are predictable or probable, health care personnel should be prewarned or placed on alert. Having personnel on alert status reduces the response time during the actual disaster.

Another important element of a response plan is the designation of an alternative reporting site for health care workers. In the event of a major disaster, some designated sites might be destroyed or damaged. A good plan will include alternative response sites to which workers can report.

Emergency personnel should be *very familiar* with the equipment and supplies they will use in the event of an actual disaster. In addition to mock disaster drills, which allow personnel to practice procedures and set up equipment, a periodic check of equipment and supplies should be part of the response plan. Some supplies are perishable and need to be restocked at regular intervals. If supplies are not actually unpacked at regular intervals, health care personnel might be disconcerted during a disaster to find that a significant portion of their supplies are damaged, destroyed, or outdated.

Emergency personnel responding to a disaster site must have the appropriate personal protective equipment and have knowledge of how to use this equipment. In addition, the emergency responders need to have previous knowledge of and training in how to assess potential hazards at the disaster site, such as unstable building structures, possible explosive hazards, and chemical or other hazardous substances.

IMPACT OF DOMESTIC DISASTERS ON DISASTER PLANNING

All health care organizations should have disaster plans. The attacks of 9/11 and the hurricane season of 2005, in particular, spurred hospitals and other organizations to review, update, and revise preexisting plans to accommodate all types of potential hazards (Drenkard et al., 2002; Eckert, 2006; Williams, 2003). Agencies without plans developed them. These disasters also prompted some agencies to perform more realistic and frequent practice drills.

The 9/11 disaster prompted state nursing boards to update volunteer rosters or initiate new ones. For example, the Maryland Nursing Board sent a letter to all registered nurses asking them to volunteer for disaster relief. Nurses who responded were provided training and photo identification, and were placed on a state notification roster. Maryland used the system in 2005 to deploy over 160 nurses and other health care providers to the Gulf Coast in response to an Emergency Management Assistance Compact request from Louisiana's governor. Other states have started similar processes ("In the event of a disaster emergency," Schwarz & Kennedy, 2003).

COMMUNITY PREPAREDNESS

Community preparedness for disaster events should be part of the planning preparation. Community health nurses, the ARC, and other volunteer nurses provide education programs. Public education is directed toward safety, self-help, and first aid measures. A good education program should include information about proper storage of food and water, rotation of canned goods to ensure use before expiration dates, and safety precautions for water use (e.g., boiling water if equipment is available or using bottled water when plumbing is not working or tap water is not safe to drink).

A good first aid program should include information about the types of supplies needed in a home first aid kit (Box 22-4). First aid courses help the public become prepared to address trauma injuries, such as fractures, bleeding, and burns. Although the general public cannot be prepared to deal with sophisticated injuries, a sound knowledge of first aid will help most families cope with the most likely injuries in a disaster situation.

Every family in the community should be encouraged to develop a personal preparedness plan (Box 22-5). Family members should have a prearranged site at which to reassemble in case they are forced to evacuate a dwelling from different exits. This simple plan can save confusion and the unnecessary injuries that often occur when family members attempt to reenter a dwelling to look for others who have already evacuated. Every home should store the following items in a designated location:

- Emergency telephone numbers
- Battery-operated radio
- Working flashlight
- First aid kit
- Three-day supply of nonperishable food and water for drinking and sanitation
- Medical information (allergies, blood types, prescription medications)

Box 22-4 Items for First Aid Kit

- Aspirin or nonaspirin pain reliever, adult and child formulas
- Antibiotic ointment
- Antacid (low-sodium) tablets
- Cleansing agents (isopropyl alcohol, hydrogen peroxide)/soap/germicide
- Eye wash
- First aid manual
- Antidiarrheal agent (e.g., Kaopectate)
- Laxative
- Emetic agent (e.g., ipecac)
- Activated charcoal (for use if so advised by Poison Control Center)
- Moistened towelettes
- Gauze pads, assorted sizes
- Gauze rolls
- Adhesive tape
- Adhesive bandages
- Latex gloves
- Lubricant (e.g., petroleum jelly)
- Triangular bandages
- Scissors
- Tweezers
- Sewing needle and thread
- Safety razor blades
- Safety pins, assorted sizes
- Thermometer
- Tongue blades
- Sunscreen

Adapted from Federal Emergency Management Agency. (2003). *Are you ready: A guide to citizen preparedness.* Washington, DC: Author.

- Physicians' names, addresses, and telephone numbers
- Persons to be notified in an emergency

Prearranged supplies and personal information make it more likely that the items will be easily located in case of an emergency or evacuation.

Box 22-5 Family Disaster Plan

- Children know how to dial 911
- Emergency phone numbers posted by phone
- How and where to turn off utilities
- How to escape and where to go
- Where to meet with family members in case of separation (e.g., a neighbor's house or across the street from the front door)
- Establish point of contact outside immediate area in case of family separation
- Plans for care of pets (pets are not allowed in shelters)
- Safety precautions for various kinds of disasters (e.g., fire, hurricane)
- Practice and maintain plan
- A list of necessary items in the event of a disaster. The items on this list might include medications, dentures, or eyeglasses; special food or infant formula; sturdy shoes and clothing for cold or inclement weather; identification; checkbook, credit cards, driver's license, and other important papers; money in low-denomination bills and coins; blankets; favorite toys and extra clothing for children.

Adapted from Federal Emergency Management Agency. (2003). *Your family disaster plan.* Washington, DC: Author. Retrieved from *http://www.fema.gov/rrr/famplan.shtm.*

Residents should be alerted to the types of supplemental supplies that could ease shelter living in the event of an evacuation order. A survey of evacuees during Hurricane Elena indicated that having items such as food, blankets, pillows, prescription medication, personal grooming items, portable chairs, and a radio would have improved comfort in the shelter (Brown et al., 1988). Special care items for infant, elderly, or disabled family members (e.g., diapers, sanitary supplies, extra eyeglasses), a change of clothing, as well as diversionary recreational equipment for children and adults (e.g., crossword puzzles, card games, drawing materials, and toys) are helpful (FEMA, 2003a; Hayes et al., 1990).

EMERGENCY RESPONSE

During the impact phase of a disaster, nurses and other emergency personnel are usually advised to *remain in place* until the situation has stabilized before attempting to provide care. In weather-related or predictable disasters, such as hurricanes or tornadoes, emergency personnel might be asked to evacuate the site of the pending disaster as a safeguard so that they can render assistance after the disaster has struck.

Personal Concerns for Health Care Providers

Evacuation out of the danger area might be difficult for health care personnel. Many are torn between their duty and the real need to remain with family members. Having a personal disaster plan that includes advance arrangements for family members helps reduce anxiety.

Health care organizations need to consider the personal needs of their personnel when developing disaster response plans (Chaffee, 2006). Child care and family shelter should be part of the plan. Alternative transportation and modes of communication are essential. In certain circumstances, such as floods, earthquakes, and snowstorms, health care personnel might not be able to report to their assigned posts on their own. If telephone service is interrupted, telephones and beepers might not function. It is important to include local radio stations, ham radio operators, and telephone company representatives to assist in developing a realistic communication plan for the organization to allow for optimum communication between the organization, its personnel, and other community organizations during a disaster event.

Survey Assessments

After a severe disaster, survey teams are assigned to make a rapid assessment of the casualties and damage to infrastructure. Health personnel are assigned to survey teams, and often community health nurses function as health assessment personnel. Nurses who function on assessment teams are expected to perform casualty damage assessments, *not* render immediate first aid. This might also be problematic for some community health nurses, whose first instinct will be to render immediate care. The information obtained from survey assessments is crucial to help the EOC determine the emergency needs and plan for the appropriate equipment and personnel needs.

Determination of Immediacy of Care

In a shelter or emergency aid station, planning focuses on establishing the priority of care needs (triage) and deciding whether care can be provided at the station or only at an acute care hospital. Discharge planning begins when a victim enters the shelter or aid station. If victims are transferred to a regular community health care facility, the nurse needs to determine medical follow-up as needed in the community. Plans must also be made to deal with dead victims, notify and provide grief counseling for families, and arrange for burial.

Role at Emergency Aid Stations

According to the ARC disaster services regulations, at least one registered nurse must be present while the emergency aid station is open. The ARC (1989) defines the functions of the disaster health service nurse in charge as follows:

- Arranging with the volunteer medical consultant for initial and daily health checks based on the health needs of shelter residents
- Establishing nursing care priorities and planning for health care supervision
- Planning for appropriate transfer of clients to community health care facilities as necessary
- Evaluating health care needs
- Arranging for secure storage of supplies, equipment, records, and medications and periodically checking to see whether material goods must be ordered
- Requesting and assigning volunteer staff to appropriate duties and providing on-the-job training and supervision
- Consulting with the shelter manager on the health status of residents and workers and identifying potential problems and trends
- Consulting with the food supervisor regarding the preparation and distribution of special diets, including infant formulas
- Planning and recommending adequate staff and facilities when local health departments initiate an immunization program for shelter residents
- Establishing lines of communication with the health service officer
- Arranging with the mass care supervisor for the purchase and replacement of essential prescriptions for persons in the shelter

Major Health Concerns after a Disaster

After a major disaster producing severe disruption of community services and dislocation of citizens, a number of health-related concerns are present. Some of these can be anticipated and addressed in predisaster planning. In addition, any major disruption can expect to have repercussions that have health-related consequences, including potential overcrowding in shelters and other types of community-living arrangements, decreased personal hygiene and sanitation because of reduced services and privacy, increased personal injuries and malnutrition, potential contamination of food and water supplies, and disruption of public health services. Nurses working with a community disrupted by disaster can anticipate these types of problems and plan to reduce the health hazards associated with them by activating community resources, ensuring adequate sanitation facilities and on-the-spot health education to reduce health and sanitation hazards, initiating immunization programs to reduce the spread of communicable diseases, and overseeing nutritional and hydration programs to ensure adequate minimum standards for the population under care. During disaster situations, nurses must help individuals make the most of their health care, help maximize the population's health, and find ways to improve the environment.

Psychologic Needs of Victims

Disasters produce physical, social, and psychologic consequences that are exhibited to varying degrees in different people, families, communities, and cultures depending on past experiences, coping skills, and the scope and nature of the disaster (see Box 22-3). Health effects can linger for long periods, as noted after 9/11 (Ferri & Sofer, 2002; Wielawski, 2006). Because most people affected by a disaster pass through predictable stages of psychologic response, nurses and other health care professionals can anticipate and prepare for the needs of the victims. The following victims of a disaster are more likely than others to need crisis intervention:

- Those who have lost one or more family members
- Those who have suffered serious injury
- Those who have a history of a psychiatric disorder
- Those who have lost their home or possessions
- Those who have been previously institutionalized for a mental illness
- Those who have suffered a predisaster stress
- Those who are poor or on a fixed income
- Elderly individuals
- Members of minority groups
- Those who have not handled previous crises in a healthy way, especially those who have been hostile or self-destructive during a previous crisis
- Those without adequate support systems

After the 9/11 disaster, undocumented or illegal immigrant families were less likely to receive aid. Many feared they would be detected and deported, so they did not seek out assistance from volunteer and government agencies (Taintor, 2003).

Most victims will have some psychologic reaction to the disaster situation. These reactions are usually transient, and many victims recover on their own with support from volunteer workers and family members. The most important thing emergency personnel can do for victims is to recognize that they have a legitimate reason for their reactions and emotions and to work toward providing them with emotional support. A psychologic assessment by the nurse will aid in identifying those individuals more prone to severe psychologic distress.

It is critical that each survivor of a disaster be assessed for the level of psychologic stress she or he is suffering and the degree of impairment she or he is experiencing in physical and emotional health and productive functioning. Individuals suffering minimal distress usually need support only from family and friends. Those who experience a moderate amount of distress usually need the help of a support group or short-term counseling. Persons with severe distress might need extensive therapy.

At the disaster site or primary triage point, simple support measures can alleviate the psychologic trauma experienced by survivors. These measures include the following:

- Keeping families together, especially children and parents
- Assigning a companion to a frightened or injured victim or placing victims in groups in which they can help each other
- Giving survivors tasks to do to keep them busy and reduce trauma to their self-esteem
- Providing adequate shelter, food, and rest
- Establishing and maintaining a communication network to reduce rumors

- Encouraging individuals to share their feelings and support each other
- Isolating victims who demonstrate hysterical or panic behavior

Some persons will need more intensive support. Whenever possible, community mental health nurses will be an important asset to the health care team to assist in meeting the psychosocial needs of victims. A quick psychologic assessment guide is a useful tool to help emergency personnel determine the psychologic state of victims (Box 22-6). Individuals at risk for suffering psychologic crisis after disaster might not seek help, even if they need it. Therefore, it is essential that the nurse assess the stress level of victims, make other rescue team members aware of this, and refer those victims who need help to appropriate professional counselors. The nurse, as a member of the disaster team, participates in rescue operations and acts as a case finder for persons suffering psychologic stress, intervening to help the victims deal effectively with the stress.

BOX 22-6	**Disaster Stress Reaction Assessment**

1. Has client experienced a disastrous event?

            _____ Yes _____ No

2. Was this event generally outside the normal range of human experience? _____ Yes _____ No

3. Would this event evoke symptoms in almost everyone exposed to it, including those who were emotionally healthy previously?

            _____ Yes _____ No

If answer to first three questions is yes, client might be experiencing a disaster stress reaction. Continue assessment.

4. Does client have any of the following symptoms? (Place a check next to each symptom experienced.)
   - _____ a. Reexperiencing of disaster through recurrent intrusive recollections or dreams
   - _____ b. Reexperiencing of disaster in response to environmental triggers
   - _____ c. Feeling of unreality, numbness, or lack of responsiveness to events
   - _____ d. Decreased interest in previously significant people
   - _____ e. Decreased interest in previously meaningful activities
   - _____ f. Hyperalertness
   - _____ g. Increased startle response
   - _____ h. Guilt about surviving disaster or about behavior during disaster
   - _____ i. Difficulty concentrating and/or remembering
   - _____ j. Avoidance of activities or places that stimulate recollection of disaster
   - _____ k. Worsening of symptoms with exposure to events that symbolize or resemble disaster experience

The presence of three or more of the preceding symptoms indicates high likelihood that the client is having a disaster stress reaction.

Other symptoms that are not diagnostic of disaster stress reaction but that might accompany the reaction are the following:
- _____ Increased irritability
- _____ Unpredictable explosions of aggressive behavior
- _____ Impulsive behavior (if a change from previous pattern)
- _____ Overwhelming sadness

From Demi, A. S., & Miles, M. S. (1983). Understanding psychological reactions to disaster. *Journal of Emergency Nursing, 9*, 13-16.

RECOVERY

During the recovery phase of a disaster, nurses are involved in efforts to restore the community to normal. Referral of injured victims for rehabilitation and convalescence is important to reduce the chances of long-term disability. Ongoing psychosocial needs must be addressed. Victims need to be linked with support agencies to help with food, clothing, shelter, and long-term counseling needs. Depending on the extent of damage to the community and the injuries of victims, the recovery phase can be relatively quick or can extend over a long period of time. Community recovery from the hurricanes of 2005 is expected to take years. In New Orleans the recovery of health care facilities has been slow. Only 15 of the 22 preexisting hospitals are operational, and bed capacity has been cut in half (from 4400 to only 2000 beds) (Berggren & Curiel, 2006). The San Francisco area has still not completely recovered from the earthquake of 1989.

It is very important for all emergency response personnel to learn from each disaster to improve response to the next emergency situation. For this reason, evaluation is an essential element of any disaster plan. Evaluation should include assessment of the effectiveness of the immediate response, determination of the impact of the disaster on the community, follow-up of victims to determine how well victim needs were met by the services provided, and assessment of the impact of the disaster on response personnel. The evaluation might result in new priorities, goals, and care plans.

Nurses from Massachusetts General Hospital in Boston became part of a DMAT rapid response team dispatched to New York on 9/11. Eighty-nine nurses, doctors, and other health professionals were in New York 10 hours after the team was activated. They prepared to treat mass casualties, but there were few live victims. Team members were rerouted to provide relief for burn unit nurses and care of rescue workers at Ground Zero. After completing their mission and returning to Boston, the team met to evaluate their performance and recommend changes. Among their findings were the following (Forgione et al., 2003):

- Standard instrument kits were too heavy for workers to cart over the necessary distances without vehicle transportation. Recommended change: Kits were modified.
- Problems were encountered in sterilizing equipment and using cauteries because of lack of electricity. Recommended change: Battery-operated cauteries and waterless sterilization systems were identified and procured.
- Client documentation was deficient. Recommended change: There is an ongoing effort to improve the documentation process.

PERSONAL RESPONSE OF CARE PROVIDERS TO DISASTER

Disaster workers are often overlooked when those affected by a disaster are considered. Health care workers are subject to the same concerns and emotional traumas as other community residents. Many disaster workers report being overwhelmed by the devastation and the extent of personal injuries. They might feel unqualified to cope with some of the medical emergencies presented. In major disasters, many work without relief for 24 to 36 hours. If they are residents of the affected community, they must deal with personal losses and concerns for friends and relatives in addition to working with the people under their care.

Responders can become stressed because of understaffing in their work environment. They might be overwhelmed for days or even weeks after a disaster. As they reflect on the event, emergency personnel might second-guess their actions and question their competency (Landersman, 2001). They might "burn out" on the job, becoming detached or overinvolved. French and colleagues (2002) examined the responses of nurses during the aftermath of Hurricane Floyd in 1999. They reported that the nurses experienced conflict between family and work-related responsibilities. A 2005 study identified barriers that might prevent health care workers from reporting to work in an emergency (Qureshi, 2005). These include concerns about personal and family safety; transportation issues; child care, elder care, or pet care needs; and other work or volunteer obligations. For example, a health care worker might also be a disaster assistance response volunteer.

Postdisaster it is important that health care workers address stress issues. They may have feelings of anger, grief, and frustration about their personal losses. Supportive colleagues can ease the stress for health care workers. The ARC encourages disaster workers to go through a debriefing process after their disaster work is complete. This process might consist of one or several sessions and is designed to help health care workers recognize and deal with the personal impact of the disaster.

ETHICAL AND LEGAL IMPLICATIONS

There are no laws specifically defining the scope of practice for nurses during a disaster. There are guideline sources, however, including a state's Nurse Practice Act, professional organization standards, a state attorney's opinions, and current and common practice laws. All nurses should be familiar with the Nurse Practice Act in the state in which they live and work, not only for disaster purposes but also for the general practice of nursing.

Although it does not have standards specific to disaster nursing, the American Nurses Association (ANA) has standards for emergency nursing practice. These are professional, not legal, standards; however, compliance with standards-of-care criteria will protect the nurse working within these standards of practice. The ANA is currently developing a comprehensive guide for nurses working under disaster conditions (Trossman, 2007).

For nurses working with the ARC, protection is provided under the federal mandate. The authority vested in the ARC makes it unnecessary for state or local governments to issue special permission or a license for the ARC to activate or carry out its relief program. No state, territory, or local government can deny the right of the ARC to render its services in accordance with the congressional mandate and its own administrative policies.

As a volunteer during a disaster, a nurse is covered by the "Good Samaritan" act of the state in most situations. The purpose of Good Samaritan acts is to encourage medically trained persons to respond to medical emergencies by protecting them from liability through grants of immunity.

KEY IDEAS

1. Disasters can be naturally occurring or man-made.
2. Individuals respond in many different ways to the disaster experience, and emergency care providers are not immune to personal responses to the experience.

3. A critical component of disaster preparedness is preplanning and use of mock-disaster exercises to prepare response personnel for an actual event.
4. During the preimpact phase of a disaster, nurses and other designated disaster relief personnel can initiate shelter preparation if there is a significant warning interval; if there is minimal or no warning, they must respond to the community's emergency needs after the impact of the disaster event.
5. Local, state, federal, and voluntary agencies should be involved in community disaster planning efforts.
6. The ARC is responsible for resident relief during disasters, including shelter operations, health care, and relief supplies for workers in the field.
7. The 9/11 disaster heightened the country's awareness of the need for disaster preparedness. This has lead to increased efforts to monitor biochemical hazards, improvement in biologic surveillance systems, and upgrades and revisions to many organizations' disaster plans.
8. Community/public health nurses are an integral part of disaster planning and implementation efforts. They are involved as planners, educators, direct caregivers, and assessment supervisors. They might serve as community survey assessors or triage officers after the disaster has occurred.
9. Evaluation and reassessment of the actual disaster relief effort is a crucial part of disaster management efforts. The information gathered by a thorough evaluation should be used to strengthen the community's response plan to better meet the next emergency situation.

LEARNING BY EXPERIENCE AND REFLECTION

1. Call your local branch of the ARC and ask what kind of activities related to disaster relief the agency has undertaken in the past 5 years.
2. Identify your local emergency management agency and your local emergency operations center. If you are unsure about how to find this information, call your local police or fire department and ask for the information.
3. Ask other health personnel if they have had personal experiences taking care of victims in disaster or emergency situations.
4. Consider what your response might be in an emergency situation. What if you witnessed a car or bus wreck? If you were driving by, would you stop? If not, why not? If yes, what would you do first? If you were home and heard about the wreck on a radio news bulletin, would you report to work? Would you report to work if your supervisor called and asked you to come in? If you were not employed, would you call the ARC and volunteer your professional services? Would you go to the scene?
5. Research a major disaster that has occurred in the United States during the past 5 years. Identify the health needs of the population. According to your research sources, was the disaster handled efficiently by the disaster health personnel? Were any areas singled out as needing improved performance? Can you identify any areas for improvement based on your readings?

COMMUNITY RESOURCES FOR PRACTICE

Information about each of the following organizations is found on its website, which can be accessed through the **WebLinks** section of the book's website at *http://evolve.elsevier.com/Maurer/community/*.

Federal Agencies
Agency for Toxic Substances and Disease Registry
Federal Emergency Management Agency
Department of Homeland Security
Army Corps of Engineers
Department of Health and Human Services

International Disaster Relief Agencies
American Red Cross
Disaster Relief Organization

United Nations Headquarters
Pan American Health Organization

All national agencies have state and local offices that respond to disasters; the local group is the source of immediate response. If the disaster exceeds both local and state resources, including those of the private sector and volunteer organizations, the state might request aid from other states or the federal government.

Local Volunteer Organizations
Boy Scouts of America
Goodwill Industries
Mennonite Disaster Service
Volunteers of America
Seventh Day Adventists
Church of the Brethren

STUDY AIDS   http://evolve.elsevier.com/Maurer/community/

Visit the Evolve website for this book to find the following study and assessment materials:

- Quiz
- Web Scenario
- Critical Thinking Questions and Answers for Case Studies

- Care Plans
- *Healthy People* Updates
- Glossary

WEBSITE RESOURCES

The following items supplement the chapter's topics and are also found on the Evolve site:

22A: Historical Presidential Disaster Declarations
22B: National Emergency Support Functions and Agencies

REFERENCES

Agency for Healthcare Research and Quality. (2005). *Bioterrorism and other public health emergencies: Linkages with community providers* (AHRQ Publication No. 05-0032). Washington DC: Author.

Agency for Toxic Substances and Disease Registry. (2004). *Annual Report 2004*. Atlanta: U.S. Department of Health and Human Services, Agency for Toxic Substances and Disease Registry. Retrieved June 22, 2007 from *http://www.atsdr.cdc.gov/HS/HSEES/annual2004.html*.

American Psychiatric Association. (2000). *Diagnostic and statistical manual of mental health disorders* (4th ed.). Washington, DC: Author.

American Red Cross. (1987). *Disaster services, regulations, and procedures*. Washington, DC: Author.

American Red Cross. (1989). *Disaster services, regulations and procedures* (3076-1A). Washington, DC: Author.

American Red Cross. (2002). *Statement of understanding between the American Radio Relay League, Inc. and the American National Red Cross*. Retrieved March 24, 2008 from *http://www.arrl.org/fandES/field/mov/redcro.html*.

Berggren, R. E., & Curiel, T. J. (2006). After the storm—Health care infrastructure in post-Katrina New Orleans. *New England Journal of Medicine, 354*(15), 1549-1552.

Brachman, P. (2002). Bioterrorism: An update with a focus on anthrax. *American Journal of Epidemiology, 155*(11), 981-987.

Brown, S. T., Kurtz, A. W., Turley, J. P., et al. (1988). Sheltering and response to evacuation during Hurricane Elena. *Journal of Emergency Nursing, 14*(1), 23-26.

Centers for Disease Control and Prevention. (2000). Biological and chemical terrorism: Strategic plan for preparedness and response. *Morbidity and Mortality Weekly Report, Recommendations and Reports, 749*(RR-4).

Centers for Disease Control and Prevention. (2003a). Recognition of illness associated with expo-

sure to chemical agents—United States, 2003. *Morbidity and Mortality Weekly Report, 52*(39), 938-940.

Centers for Disease Control and Prevention. (2003b). Recommendations for using smallpox vaccine in a pre-event vaccination program: Supplemental recommendations of the Advisory Committee on Immunization Practice (ACIP) and the Healthcare Infection Control Practices Advisory Committee (HICPAC). *Morbidity and Mortality Weekly Report, Recommendations and Reports, 52*(RR-7).

Centers for Disease Control and Prevention. (2003c). *Smallpox vaccine information statement*. Retrieved January 16, 2003 from *http://www.cdc.gov./smallpox*.

Centers for Disease Control and Prevention. (2007). Quickstats: Percentage of hospitals with staff members trained to respond to selected terrorism-related diseases or exposures—National Hospital Ambulatory Medical Care

Survey, United States, 2003-2004. *Morbidity and Mortality Weekly Report, 56*(16), 401.

Chaffee, M. W. (2006). Making the decision to report to work in a disaster. *American Journal of Nursing, 106*(9), 54-57.

Christen, H., & Maniscalco, P. M. (2002). *Mass casualty and high-impact incidents: An operational guide.* Upper Saddle River, NJ: Prentice Hall.

Demi, A. S., & Miles, M. S. (1983). Understanding psychological reactions to disaster. *Journal of Emergency Nursing, 9*(1), 13-16.

Drenkard, K., Rigotti, G., Hanfling, D., et al. (2002). Healthcare system disaster preparedness. Part 1: Readiness planning. *Journal of Nursing Administration, 32*(9), 461-469.

Eckert, S. (2006). Preparing for disaster: How to plan for the unthinkable. *American Nurse Today, 1*(10), 34-37.

Federal Emergency Management Agency. (1981). *Disaster operation: A handbook for local governments* (CPG16). Washington, DC: Author.

Federal Emergency Management Agency. (1988). *Basic incident command system* (IS-195). Washington, DC: Author.

Federal Emergency Management Agency. (2003a). *Are you ready: A guide to citizen preparedness.* Washington, DC: Author. Retrieved November 23, 2003 from *http://www.fema.gov/doc/areyouready/areyouready.doc.*

Federal Emergency Management Agency. (2003b). *Your family disaster plan.* Washington, DC: Author. Retrieved from *http://www.fema.gov/rrr/famplan.shtm.*

Federal Emergency Management Agency. (2007, June). *The Robert T. Stafford Disaster Relief and Emergency Assistance Act (Public Law 93-288).* FEMA 592. Retrieved March 24, 2008 from *http://www.fema.gov/pdf/about/stafford_act.pdf.*

Ferri, R., & Sofer, D. (2002). September 11: Health effects linger. *American Journal of Nursing, 102*(9), 18-19.

Forgione, T., Owens, P. J., Lopes, J. P., et al. (2003). New horizons for OR nurses—Lessons learned from the World Trade Center attack. *AORN Journal, 78*(2), 240-245.

French, E. D., Sole, M. L., & Byers, J. F. (2002). A comparison of nurses' needs/concerns and hospital disaster plans following Florida's Hurricane Floyd. *Journal of Emergency Nursing, 28*(2), 111-117.

Galea, S., Ahern, J., Resnick, H., et al. (2002). Psychological sequelae of the September 11 terrorist attacks in New York City. *New England Journal of Medicine, 346*(13), 982-987.

Garb, S., & Eng, E. (1969). *Disaster handbook* (2nd ed.). New York: Springer.

Hayes, G., Goodwin, T., & Miars, B. (1990). After disaster: A crisis support team at work. *American Journal of Nursing, 90*(2), 61-64.

Hazardous Substances Emergency Events Surveillance. (2001). *Hazardous Substances Emergency Events Surveillance (HSEES) annual report 2001.* Retrieved November 20, 2003 from http://www. atsdr.cdc.gov/HS/HSEES.

In the event of a disaster emergency—We need all Utah nurses. (2003). *Utah Nurse, 12*(2), 17.

Kennedy, M. S. (2001). Disaster education and training are sorely needed. *American Journal of Nursing, 101*(11), 18-19.

Landersman, L. Y. (2001). *Public health management of disasters.* Washington, DC: American Public Health Association.

Lister, S. A. (2006). *The public health and medical response to disaster: Federal authority and funding: Congressional Research Report for Congress, July 28, 2006.* Washington, DC: Congressional Research Service, Library of Congress.

Mitchell, A. M., Sakraida, T. J., & Kameg, K. (2002). Overview of post-traumatic stress. *Disaster Management and Response.* Premier issue.

National Oceanic and Atmospheric Administration. (2005). *Climate of 2005: Summary of Hurricane Katrina.* Retrieved June 24, 2007 *http://www.ncdc. noaa.gov/oa/climate/research/2005/katrina.html.*

National Oceanic and Atmospheric Administration. (2007). *Storm data: Weather fatalities.* Retrieved June 22, 2007 from *http://www.nws.noaa.gov/om/hazstats/images/30-yer.gif.*

National Weather Service. (2007). *Natural hazard statistics: Weather fatalities.* Birmingham, AL: Author. Retrieved June 11, 2007 from *http://www.nws.noaa.gov/om/hazstats.shtml#.*

Occupational Safety and Health Administration. (2005). *OSHA best practices for hospital-based first receivers of victims from mass casualty incidents involving the release of hazardous substances.* Washington, DC: Author.

Perkins, B., Popovic, L. T., & Yeskey, K. (2002). Public health in the time of bioterrorism. *Emerging Infectious Diseases, 8*(10), 1015-1018.

Qureshi, K., Gershon, R. R. M., Straub, T., et al. (2005). Health care workers' ability and willingness to report to duty during catastrophic disasters. *Journal of Urban Health, 82*(3), 378-388.

Richtsmeir, J. L., & Miller, J. R. (1985). Psychological aspects of disaster situations. In L. M. Garcia (Ed.), *Disaster nursing.* Rockville, MD: Aspen.

Riley, J. (2003). Providing nursing care with federal disaster-relief teams. *Disaster Management and Response, 1*(3), 76-79.

Schwarz, T., & Kennedy, M. S. (2003). Disaster volunteer teams. *American Journal of Nursing, 103*(1), 64AA-64DD.

Taintor, Z. (2003). Addressing mental health needs. In V. W. Levy & B. S. Sidel (Eds.), *Terrorism and public health* (pp. 49-68). New York: Oxford University Press and the American Public Health Association.

Thompson, T. (2001, October 23). *Civilian preparedness for biological warfare and terrorism: HHS readiness and role in vaccine research and development.* Testimony before the Committee on Government Reform Subcommittee on National Security, Veterans Affairs and International Relations United States House of Representatives.

Trossman, S. (2007). Issues update: Care during crises. *American Nurse Today, 2*(3), 44-45.

U.S. Department of Health and Human Services. (2007). *HHS public health emergency medical countermeasure enterprise: Implementation plan for chemical, biological, radiological and nuclear threats.* Washington, DC: Author.

U.S. Department of State, National Counter-terrorism Center. (2007). *Country reports on terrorism: Annex of statistical information.* Retrieved June 1, 2007 from *http://www.state. gov/s/ct/rls/crt/2006/82739.htm.*

Vlahov, D., Galeas, S., Resnick, H., et al. (2002). Increased use of cigarettes, alcohol, and marijuana among Manhattan, New York, residents after the September 11th terrorist attacks. *American Journal of Epidemiology, 155*(11), 988-996.

White House. (2006). *Fact sheet: The one year anniversary of Hurricane Katrina.* Retrieved June 1, 2007 from *http://www.whitehouse.gov/news/releases/2006/20060824.html.*

Wielawski, I. M. (2006). The health legacy of September 11. *American Journal of Nursing, 106*(9), 27-28.

Williams, S. (2003). Be prepared: Unpredictability of Mother Nature—and human nature—prompts more hospitals to examine and upgrade their emergency response systems. *Nurseweek (South Central), 8*(3), 12-15.

Wolk, M. (2005, September 13). *How Hurricane Katrina's costs are adding up.* MSNBC News. Retrieved June 24, 2007 from *http://www.msnbc. com/id/9329293/.*

World Health Organization. (1999). *Community emergency preparedness: A manual for managers and policy-makers.* Geneva: Author.

SUGGESTED READINGS

American Hospital Association. (2000). *Hospital preparedness for mass casualties.* Washington, DC: Author.

American Public Health Association. *Resource guide: Federal assistance programs for terrorism preparedness.* Washington, DC: Author. Retrieved June 6, 2007 from *http://www.apha.org/*

advocacy/priorities/issues/rebuilding/legislative buildresourceguide.htm.

Centers for Disease Control and Prevention. (2000). Biological and chemical terrorism: Strategic plan for preparedness and response. *Morbidity and Mortality Weekly Report, Recommendations and Reports, 749*(RR-4).

Christen, H., & Maniscalco, P. M. (2002). *Mass casualty and high-impact incidents: An operational guide.* Upper Saddle River, NJ: Prentice Hall.

Demi, A. S., & Miles, M. S. (1983). Understanding psychological reactions to disaster. *Journal of Emergency Nursing, 9*(1), 13-16.

Downing, D. (2002). Learning as we go: Public health, one year later. *American Journal of Nursing, 102*(9), 76-77.

Federal Emergency Management Agency. (2003). *Are you ready: A guide to citizen preparedness.* Washington, DC: Author. Retrieved November 23, 2003 from *http://www.fema.gov/doc/areyouready/areyouready.doc.*

Friedman, E. (1994). Coping with calamity. *Journal of the American Medical Association, 272*(23), 1875-1879.

Jurkovich, T. (2003). September 11th—The Pentagon disaster response and lessons learned. *Critical Care Nursing Clinics of North America, 15,* 143-148.

Kennedy, M. S. (2001). Disaster education and training are sorely needed. *American Journal of Nursing, 101*(11), 18-19.

Landersman, L. Y. (2001). *Public health management of disasters.* Washington, DC: American Public Health Association.

Levy, V. W., & Sidel, B. S. (2003). *Terrorism and public health.* New York: Oxford University Press and the American Public Health Association.

Nursing resources: Bioterrorism resources on the web. (2002). *American Journal of Nursing, 102*(9), 86-88.

Perkins, B., Popovic, L. T., & Yeskey, K. (2002). Public health in the time of bioterrorism. *Emerging Infectious Diseases, 8*(10), 1015-1018.

Phreaner, D., Jacoby, I., Dreier, S., et al. (1994). Disaster preparedness of home health care agencies in San Diego County. *Journal of Emergency Medicine, 12*(6), 811-818.

Veenema, T. G. (Ed.). (2003). *Disaster nursing and emergency preparedness for chemical, biological, radiological terrorism and other hazards.* New York: Springer.

Ward, P. M., Eck, C. A., & Sanguino, T. F. (1990). Emergency nursing at the epicenter: The Loma Prieta earthquake. *Journal of Emergency Nursing, 16*(4), 49A-55A.

CHAPTER

23 Violence: A Social and Family Problem

David R. Langford

Focus Questions

What are some of the factors that contribute to family violence?

What criteria are useful in assessing for possible abusive or neglectful situations?

What are the responsibilities of the community/public health nurse as a health professional in abusive situations?

What are some primary, secondary, and tertiary prevention measures for the different forms of interpersonal violence?

What community resources are available to prevent abuse and to assist the victims and perpetrators in abusive situations?

Chapter Outline

Key Terms

Bullying

Child abuse

Child neglect

Child protective services

Cycle of violence

Elder abuse

Emotional abuse

Incest

Intergenerational transmission of violence

Intimate partner violence (IPV)

Mandatory reporting

Physical abuse

Sexual abuse

Social learning theory

Violence

Violence at home and in the community is an issue that generates enormous public concern and has become a focus of prevention in nursing and public health. **Violence** consists of nonaccidental acts that result in physical or emotional injury. Every day, local and national news reports are replete with examples of violent actions and their tragic consequences. In fact, violence has become so commonplace that it is unusual to find anyone who has not been exposed to violence either by personal experience or by acquaintance with a victim. In some communities, violence is so prevalent that residents are desensitized to it. Community members feel powerless to stop it and instead concentrate on efforts to ensure their safety and that of their family members.

EXTENT OF THE PROBLEM

Violence, like other community health problems, has patterns that, when identified, can help nurses to better understand the distribution of the problem and delineate those at risk and risk factors. What often appears or is reported as random violence is not. For example:

- Men are more likely victims of violent crimes by strangers, whereas women are more likely to be victimized by intimate partners, relatives, friends, or acquaintances.
- More than 6 in 10 sexual assaults are committed by intimates, relatives, friends, or acquaintances.
- Family members are most likely to murder a young child, whereas a friend or acquaintance is most likely to murder an older child (15 to 18 years old).
- About 44% of murder victims are related to or acquainted with their assailants.
- Intimate violence is the primary crime against women.
- Overall, violent crimes are more likely to occur during the day (6 AM to 6 PM). The exception is rape, which more often occurs at night (6 PM to 6 AM).

Based on these statistics from the Bureau of Justice Statistics (2003), care must be exercised in determining the real risks of victimization within a community. The myth and fear of stranger violence is often exaggerated, given that most individuals are at greater risk for victimization by family members or acquaintances.

Violent crime has been steadily decreasing since 1994 and reached its lowest recorded level in 2005 (Bureau of Justice Statistics, 2007). Adolescents and young adults are at especially high risk for being victims or perpetrators of violence, and minority young are at an exceptional risk. Figure 23-1 shows the rates of violence by age group. Teens and young adults have the highest rates of victimization, and the rates in these groups have demonstrated the most significant decline since the early 1990s. Young African American men are especially vulnerable, experiencing more overall violence than are their white male counterparts.

NATIONAL HEALTH PRIORITIES TO REDUCE VIOLENCE

Violence and injury prevention is a national health priority (U.S. Department of Health and Human Services [USDHHS], 2000).

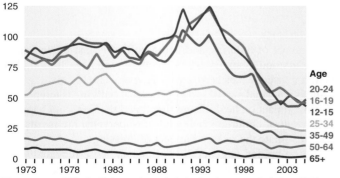

FIGURE 23-1 Violent crime victimization by age of victim, 1973 to 2003 (victimization rate per 1000 persons in age group). (From Bureau of Justice Statistics. [2006]. *Key facts at a glance: Trends in victimization rates by age.* Retrieved August 16, 2007 from *http://www.ojp.usdoj.gov/bjs/glance/tables/vagetab.htm*.)

Specific objectives in *Healthy People 2010* related to injury and violence prevention are aimed at reducing injuries, disabilities, and deaths due to unintentional injuries and violence. The *Healthy People 2010* box on this page outlines the objectives related to injury and violence for 2010 and progress in meeting those goals. As with many other community problems, there is a significant disparity among population groups in exposure to violence and abuse. For example, homicide is the leading cause of death in blacks aged 15 to 34 years and the second leading cause of death in black children aged 1 to 4 years (National Center for Injury Prevention and Control, 2007). The homicide rate for black men and women is well above the rate for their Hispanic and white non-Hispanic counterparts.

VIOLENCE IN THE COMMUNITY: TYPES AND RISK FACTORS

To date, there is no accurate method of predicting which individuals will engage in violent behaviors. Studies have identified factors that place individuals at greater risk for engaging in violence (Box 23-1). However, not everyone to whom these risk factors applies behaves violently. An individual's use of

---

■ HEALTHY PEOPLE 2010 ■
Violence and Abuse Prevention Objectives

1. Reduce homicides to 2.8 homicides per 100,000 population. (Baseline: 6.0 homicides per 100,000 population in 1998.)
2. Reduce maltreatment of children to 10.1 per 1000 children younger than age 18 years. (Baseline: 12.6 child victims of maltreatment per 1000 children younger than age 18 years in 1998.)
3. Reduce the rate of physical assault by current or former intimate partners to 3.3 physical assaults per 1000 persons aged 12 years and older. (Baseline: 4.4 physical assaults per 1000 persons aged 12 years and older by current or former intimate partners in 1998.)
4. Reduce the annual rate of rape or attempted rape to 0.7 rapes or attempted rapes per 1000 persons. (Baseline: 0.8 rapes or attempted rapes per 1000 persons aged 12 years and older in 1998.)
5. Reduce sexual assault other than rape to 0.4 sexual assaults other than rape per 1000 persons aged 12 years and older. (Baseline: 0.6 sexual assaults other than rape per 1000 persons aged 12 years and older in 1998.)
6. Reduce physical assaults to 13.6 physical assaults per 1000 persons aged 12 years and older. (Baseline: 31.1 physical assaults per 1000 persons aged 12 years and older in 1998.)
7. Reduce to 32% the proportion of adolescents engaging in physical fighting. (Baseline: 36% of adolescents in grades 9 through 12 engaged in physical fighting in the previous 12 months in 1999.)
8. Reduce to 4.9% the proportion of adolescents carrying weapons on school property. (Baseline: 6.9% of students in grades 9 through 12 carried weapons on school property during the past 30 days in 1999.)

From U.S. Department of Health and Human Services. (2000). *Healthy people 2010: Understanding and improving health.* Washington, DC: U.S. Government Printing Office; and U.S. Department of Health and Human Services. (2006). *Healthy people 2010: Midcourse review.* Washington, DC: U.S. Government Printing Office. Retrieved June 25, 2007 from *http://www.healthypeople.gov*.

Box 23-1 Factors Associated with Risk of Violence

Sociologic
Low socioeconomic status
Involvement with gangs
Drug dealing
Access to guns
Media exposure to violence
Community exposure to violence

Developmental/Psychologic
Alcohol or drug abuse
Rigid sex role expectations
Peer pressure, especially for adolescents
Poor impulse control
History of mental health problems
High individual stress level
Manual laborer, unemployed, or employed part-time
Younger than 30 years

Family
History of intergenerational abuse
Social isolation
Verbal threatening of children by parents
High levels of family stress
Two or more children

violence seems to be influenced by a variety of factors both external (family, society, and other environmental conditions) and internal (innate personality characteristics).

EXPOSURE AND SOCIAL CONDITIONING

One explanation for violence is that people learn to use violence when violence is condoned or is considered an acceptable strategy in solving problems. This view is based on the principles of **social learning theory,** according to which children learn to respond with acts of violence by observing role models and seeing violent problem solving as successful in the media (Warriner, 1994).

Many American cultural institutions model and even encourage violence and aggression. Aggressive actions are applauded in sports, movies, television, and video games. It is estimated that by the age of 18, the average television viewer has witnessed 200,000 acts of violence on television, not to mention in video games and through other media channels (Committee on Public Education, 2001). This exposure to media violence has a positive relationship to increases in aggressive behavior. Viewing violence on television, in movies, and in games has been linked to increased violence and aggression and increased risk taking in children and adolescents that carries over into adulthood (Carll, 2006; Huesmann et al., 2003). DuRant and colleagues (2006) report that teens who watch televised professional wrestling programs are more likely to engage in fighting and date fighting, and to carry weapons. In its policy statement on media violence, the American Psychological Association calls for physicians and other health care professionals to get more involved in working with families and the political system to reduce children's exposure to media violence (Carll, 2006). The American Academy of Pediatrics (2007) urges parents to limit media exposure and to be actively involved in the selections of materials viewed by children and teens.

ADOLESCENTS AND VIOLENCE

Adolescents are exposed to and particularly vulnerable to increasing violence at school and in the community. An alarming number of adolescents know victims of or have witnessed assaults, rapes, or other life-threatening violence. Inner-city youth have the greatest exposure risk (U.S. Department of Justice, 2005). One survey of inner-city 7-year-olds found that 75% had heard gunshots, 18% had seen a dead body on the street, and 10% had seen a shooting or stabbing in their home (Hurt et al., 2001). In 2005, 24% of all serious violent crime was committed by juveniles (Federal Interagency Forum on Child and Family Statistics, 2007). Some have suggested that teens with little to look forward to have less to risk and more to gain by using violence. Bollard and colleagues (2001) found that hopelessness was relatively rare in teens; however, when present, it was predictive of fighting and carrying weapons. Other predictors of adolescent violence are poor grades, deviant behavior, weak bonds in middle school, early drug use, and association with peers using drugs (Children's Defense Fund [CDF], 2005). The majority (80%) of juveniles involved in the court system are involved with drugs (National Center on Addictions and Substance Abuse, 2000).

The National Center for Injury Prevention and Control (2007) at the Centers for Disease Control and Prevention (CDC) reports the following:

- More than 780,000 young people aged 10 to 25 years were treated in emergency departments for injuries sustained through violence.
- Thirty-six percent of youth in grades 9 through 12 reported being in a physical fight in the past 12 months and 18.5% reported carrying a weapon on one or more occasions in the previous month.
- Six percent of students in grades 9 through 12 report not going to school on one or more days in the previous month because they felt unsafe at school or on their way to or from school.
- Homicide is the second leading cause of death for young people aged 10 to 24 years.
- Firearms are responsible for 82% of the homicides in young people aged 10 to 24 years.
- Homicide is the leading cause of death among black youth and the second leading cause of death among Hispanic youth aged 15 to 24 years.

BULLYING

The impact of bullying and being bullied is just beginning to be understood as an important aspect of violence. Bullying has health consequences across the life span. The beliefs that bullying is a normal part of growing up, that bullying is temporary, that its impact on health is minimal, and that bullying happens as a result of children's being left unsupervised are myths and underestimate the risk and impact of bullying.

Being bullied is generally defined as being repeatedly the target of negative actions by one's peers. **Bullying** is a pattern of physical, verbal, or other behaviors directed by one or more children toward another child that are intended to inflict physical, verbal, or emotional harm. Many children with preexisting health conditions or disabilities are at risk for victimization because they are different or act differently from their peers. Children who are overweight or have attention-deficit/hyperactivity disorder (ADHD) are more likely to be bullied (Blachman & Hinshaw, 2002; Janssen et al., 2004; Zalecki & Hinshaw, 2004).

The prevalence of bullying among middle and high school students is estimated to be 7% to 30% (DeVoe et al., 2004; Nansel et al., 2001). Male students report higher rates of bullying, and bullying is most prevalent in the sixth through eighth grades. Boys use more physical forms of bullying, whereas girls use more relational forms of bullying, such as exclusion, isolation, and initiation of rumors.

Bullying is a form of violence that has a significant impact on children's health. Many somatic and mental health complaints such as bedwetting, headaches and stomachaches, neck and shoulder pain, back pain, anxiety, fatigue, loneliness, short temper, depression, suicidal ideation, increased drug and alcohol use, aggression, and delinquency are related to being bullied (Fekkes et al., 2004; Kaltiala-Heino et al., 1999; Kim et al., 2005; Sullivan et al., 2006; van der Wal et al., 2003; Wolke et al., 2001). Bullying is also a risk factor for violent behavior and injury. Young people who bully or are bullied are more likely to be involved in fights, injured in fights, and carry weapons to school (Fox et al., 2003; Nansel et al., 2003). Being rejected and bullied by peers is a characteristic common to students who commit school shootings (Leary et al., 2003).

School nurses and nurses working with children and adolescents can screen for bullying during well and routine health care visits such as school physicals. Nurses should include parents when asking about bullying and encourage children to tell a parent or other adult when bullying occurs. Lyznicki and colleagues (2004) list questions the nurse can ask children to help identify bullying issues. They include the following:

- What do you do when others pick on you?
- Have you ever told a teacher or an adult what happened?
- What kinds of things do you get teased about?
- Do you get teased about your illness or handicap?

SCHOOL VIOLENCE
School violence takes many forms; for example, excessive teasing, pushing and shoving, bullying, intimidation, stalking, serious physical assault, and murder. In 2004 students were exposed to 1.4 million nonfatal crimes at school, including 583,000 violent crimes such as assault, rape, and robbery (National Center for Education Statistics, 2006). Many of these children showed signs of anxiety and depression, and 61% worried about their safety. Higher exposure to violence was associated with lower grade point average and more days absent from school. According to the U.S. Department of Education and Justice, approximately 5% of students skip school, avoid places within school, or avoid school activities because they are fearful (DeVoe et al., 2005). The presence of youth gangs in elementary and secondary schools increases the rate of serious crime in those schools. Approximately 17% of public schools report gang activity in their schools (National Center for Education Statistics, 2006). Howell and Lynch (2000) report that schools with gangs have more accessible drugs and double the risk of student violence compared to schools without gangs. When students are preoccupied with their safety and schools must divert energy and resources to deal with potential violence and violent behavior, the educational mission of the schools suffers.

GANG VIOLENCE
There were an estimated 760,000 gang members and 24,000 gangs active in the United States in 2004 (Egley & Ritz, 2006). Most gang members are male, but female membership is growing. Although most gang members are adolescents and young adults, gang members range in age from 8 to 55 years.

Gangs are flourishing in both rural and urban communities. Gangs can provide a sense of stability and family for many disenfranchised adolescents with unstable family situations (CDF, 2005). Gang members identify five reasons for joining gangs: (1) only option, no jobs available; (2) peer pressure; (3) protection; (4) companionship; and (5) excitement (Allender, 2001; Palm Bay Police Department, 2007). Having a previous conduct disorder and having friends who joined gangs or engaged in aggressive behaviors are predictive of joining a gang among adolescents (Palm Bay Police Department, 2007).

Violence is part of everyday life for gang members. Youth gang members are more likely to engage in drug use, drug trafficking, and violence than other youth and are three times more likely to be involved in violent activities than non–gang members (Battin-Pearson et al., 1998; Howell & Decker, 1999). Most gang members had engaged in illegal activities, including violence, before becoming a member of a gang (Howell & Decker, 1999). Violence is a part of their neighborhoods and families, and violence is an expected part of their role and individual status as gang members. Over half the homicides in Los Angeles and Chicago are gang related (Egley & Ritz, 2006). A sense of belonging, peer pressure, or the threat of retaliation makes it difficult for individuals to leave gangs.

Entire communities must come together to reduce gang membership and violence. Preventing young men and women from joining gangs should be the first priority. Strategies include preventing youth from dropping out of school and strengthening social institutions to better provide activities and legitimate economic opportunities for youth (CDF, 2005). Several cities, including Boston, Indianapolis, and Stockton, California, have initiated successful comprehensive gang violence reduction programs. These entail concentrated police enforcement, involvement of community leaders and pastors in violence reduction messages, and a network of support services for at-risk youth.

GUNS AND VIOLENCE
Firearms are the second leading cause of death among 10- to 19-year-olds (USDHHS, 2004). Over a 25-year period, 100,000 children were killed by firearms (CDF, 2005). In the United States, the rate of firearm-related deaths in children is higher than the *combined* rates of 25 other industrialized countries (CDF, 2005). Regulations regarding the manufacture and licensing of firearms are more lenient in the United States than in other developed countries, which makes them easily accessible. Higher rates of household ownership and accessibility of firearms are associated with disproportionately higher homicide rates (Miller et al., 2002).

A number of interventions have been tried to reduce firearm violence in the United States. An evaluation of the laws enacted to prevent firearm violence found inconclusive evidence that bans, restrictions and waiting periods, registration and licensing regulations, laws regulating the carrying of concealed weapons, child-access laws, and zero-tolerance laws in schools and other public places have had little if any impact in reducing firearm violence (CDC, 2003). Opponents of gun control, such as the National Rifle Association, argue that criminal assault and injury will continue despite gun control, and that assailants will simply switch to other weapons. Proponents argue that stricter gun control laws will help to bring murder and injury rates in line with those of other nations. The Expert Panel on Violence of the American Academy of Nursing (1993) recommends that nursing firmly support making handguns illegal. In 2004, Congress let the assault weapons ban expire. The effect had been an upswing in the sales of assault weapons.

ADDITIONAL RISK FACTORS

Poverty is an important risk factor associated with violence victimization. Individuals are at greater risk for being the victims of violent acts if they are poor (Bureau of Justice Statistics, 2007). Poverty and living in impoverished neighborhoods also increase the risk for intimate partner abuse (Cunradi et al., 2000; Fox & Benson, 2006). In addition, the increasing levels of drug, alcohol, and tobacco use among adolescents were associated with their increasing exposure to violence, not only in the United States but internationally (Vermeiren et al., 2003). Using drugs exposes adolescents to violent victimization, delinquent peers, and drug dealing. Adolescents subsequently develop favorable attitudes toward violence that continue even when they are not using drugs any longer (Kuhns, 2005).

IMPACT OF VIOLENCE ON THE COMMUNITY

Violence in the community creates a sense of fear and danger. The fear of violence has a tremendous impact, causing residents to be suspicious of one another and to become more isolated. Parents' increased concern and anxiety about safety in their neighborhoods (presence of gangs, child aggression, crime, violence, traffic) is related to lower levels of children's physical activity and outdoor play (Weir et al., 2006). The family is the first place in which acceptable social behavior is learned. Abusive behavior that starts within the family has an impact on the entire community, economically and emotionally.

Although community health nurses encounter violence and violence-related concerns in a number of situations, their most frequent professional contact is with individuals and families in clinics and homes. For this reason, the remainder of this chapter concentrates on family violence and the nursing role in prevention and intervention with the family.

VIOLENCE WITHIN THE FAMILY

Family violence involves the direct use of force, emotional battering, or neglect carried out by one family member against another. It is very difficult to determine with certainty the actual prevalence of family violence. Most cases go unreported. Family violence researchers use data from both small and national samples to estimate the extent of the problem. Much of the research has also been conducted on clinical populations, those who have already been identified, and therefore care must be taken when generalizing these findings to nonclinical populations.

GENERATIONAL PATTERNS OF ABUSE

A pattern of abusive behavior in families continuing one generation after another, also called the **intergenerational**

transmission of violence, has been widely documented. However, the relationship between being abused and witnessing abuse as a child and being abusive or victimized as an adult is complex. Not all children who grow up in violent homes become violent in later life. Lackey (2003) found that exposure to violence at home as an adolescent was strongly related to later partner violence in men but not in women. Heyman and Slep (2002) found that exposure to violence in the family of origin (parent-child and/or parent-parent) was related to parent-child abuse and partner abuse for both men and women. Exposure to violence in the family of origin does not necessarily predict gender- or role-specific patterns of abuse transmission such as men's use of violence or women's victimization (Kwong et al., 2003). Ernst and colleagues (2007) found that adults who witnessed intimate partner violence as children were no more likely than those who did not to be victims of ongoing partner violence as adults.

INEQUALITY OF FAMILY MEMBERS

Gelles and Straus (1988) contend that people abuse family members because there are few or no repercussions. There continues to be inequity in arrest or criminal prosecution for partner violence. Social attitudes, the private nature of family violence, and the structural inequalities in family relationships combine to create a climate in which violence is acceptable and tolerated. Violent acts against family members often go unpunished, although similar actions against other people would be criminally prosecuted. Parental use of physical punishment is widely practiced and often socially condoned. Increased visibility of family violence and national campaigns are slowly changing public attitudes and acceptance of family violence.

What happens within the family has been considered a private, "family matter." Because of the strong belief in family privacy, neighbors, family members, and authority figures such as teachers, health professionals, police, and prosecutors are often hesitant to intervene (Jecker, 1993). Culturally, the value of men, women, and children is unequal. Historically, this was supported by legal statutes under which women and children were considered property and had few rights under the law. Children could be sold into slavery, loaned to work for wages collected by the father, or bartered into marriage without legal recourse. In fact, it is still very difficult for minor children to establish rights independent of their parents. Common law identified husbands as the heads of households and wives were subordinate (Pleck, 1987). Since the late 1900s, women have slowly acquired the right to personal assets and property, independent of a spouse, on a state-by-state basis. It was 1929 before women in the United States were granted the right to vote nationwide. As recently as 1970, one Pennsylvania town still had a law that allowed wife beating during certain times and days (Williams-White, 1986). Despite the repeal of most such laws, the social inequality among family members persists, creating a climate in which violence continues.

CHILD ABUSE AND NEGLECT

The National Center for Injury Prevention and Control (2006) reports that the following:

- In 2004, 1490 children in the United States died as a result of abuse or neglect.

- Child protection services investigated 3.5 million reports of child abuse and neglect in 2004; this amounts to nearly 5% of all the children in the United States. In approximately 25% of cases (872,000) the children were classified as victims (60%, neglect; 7%, emotional abuse; 18%, physical abuse; and 10%, sexual abuse).
- Fourteen percent of U.S. children experience some form of child maltreatment.
- Women (58%) are more often the perpetrators of all forms of child maltreatment.
- Girls, accounting for 52% of cases, are at slightly higher risk than boys for all forms of child maltreatment.
- Children who have experienced abuse and neglect are at increased risk for adverse health effects and behaviors as adults, including smoking, alcoholism, drug abuse, physical inactivity, severe obesity, depression, suicide, sexual promiscuity, and certain chronic diseases.
- Infants are at greatest risk of dying from homicide during the first week of infancy, with the risk being highest on the first day of life. Children younger than 1 year account for 44% of child maltreatment fatalities.

Children encounter violence and abuse from caretakers other than parents. Daycare providers (especially unlicensed providers), family friends, and neighbors might also abuse children. However, the greatest risk is from family members and relatives.

FACTORS ASSOCIATED WITH ABUSE AND NEGLECT

Sometimes abuse is inflicted on all of the children in a family, but often one child is singled out or targeted to receive most or all of the abusive attention. A child who is considered different or has physical or emotional disability is at special risk of abuse (United Nations Children's Fund, 2005). Children with disabilities are nearly 3.5 times more likely to be abused than children without disabilities (Govindshenoy & Spencer, 2007; Sullivan & Knutson, 2000). In one study, Mandell and colleagues (2005) reported that 18.5% of children with autism had been physically abused. It is important to note that other siblings in the family, although spared the immediate abuse, are also affected. Removal of one child does not guarantee a solution to the problem. Another child in the household usually becomes the next target.

The nurse should exercise caution in generalizing from reported case data, because these data may be *biased*. Although child abuse and neglect occur across the socioeconomic spectrum, poverty seems to be a risk factor, whereas parental education is a poor predictor. The rate of abusive incidents is relatively stable across educational levels (CDF, 2005). Social expectations about race and poverty often influence who is reported as abusive.

Black children are at highest risk of substantiated maltreatment and Asian children have the lowest risk (Federal Interagency Forum on Child and Family Statistics, 2007). Children who live in homes at lower socioeconomic levels are at greater risk of substantiated maltreatment than those from higher-income homes. Large national family surveys do not show black families to be at greater risk for child abuse (Gelles & Cornell, 1990). The discrepancy between substantiated reported cases and family survey data might be explained by reporting bias. The larger number of reported cases of child abuse and neglect among the poor (more of whom are black families) is probably the result of those families' involvement with public social and health services and emergency departments (CDF, 2005). These care providers are more likely to report abuse and neglect. Family cultural practices might provide supports to reduce risks for abusive situations. For example, African American and Hispanic families tend to have greater extended family involvement and use family networks for emotional, financial, and child-rearing support. These characteristics might offset the stressors of higher unemployment and less socioeconomic power.

TYPES OF ABUSE

There are four major types of maltreatment or **child abuse.** Generally, *child abuse* applies to abuse of persons younger than 18 years of age. States' definitions might vary (National Clearinghouse on Child Abuse and Neglect [NCCAN], 2002).

Physical Abuse

Physical abuse of a child is characterized by the infliction of physical injury as a result of punching, beating, kicking, biting, burning, shaking, or otherwise harming a child. The parent or caretaker might not have intended to hurt the child; the injury might have resulted from overdiscipline or physical punishment (NCCAN, 2002). Box 23-2 provides examples of moderate and severe abuse as well as some injuries that might be indicative of child abuse. Because physical abuse is often not an isolated incident, evidence of past injuries might be present. The explanations for old or healing injuries should be carefully explored.

Child Neglect

Child neglect is characterized by failure to provide for the child's basic needs (USDHHS, 2007). Neglect can be physical, educational, or emotional. Physical neglect includes failure to provide adequate food, clothing, and shelter; refusal to seek or delay in seeking health care; abandonment, expulsion from the home, or refusal to allow a runaway to return home; and inadequate supervision. Educational neglect includes allowing chronic truancy, failing to enroll a child of mandatory school age in school, and failing to attend to special educational needs. Emotional neglect includes such actions as marked inattention to the child's needs for affection, failure to provide needed psychologic care, spousal abuse in the child's presence, and permitting of drug or alcohol use by the child. Assessment of child neglect requires consideration of cultural values and standards of care as well as recognition that the failure to provide the necessities of life might be related to poverty (NCCAN, 2002).

Neglect is a pattern of failure to provide care rather than a single instance of negligence. In neglect cases neighbors or relatives will frequently recall that they felt uneasy about a situation but did not report the parent or caretaker to the appropriate authorities. Substance abuse and addiction are frequently implicated in parental failure to provide an adequately nurturing environment.

Sexual Abuse

Sexual abuse includes fondling, intercourse, incest, rape, exhibitionism, and commercial exploitation through prostitution or the production of pornographic materials (USDHHS, 2007). Many experts believe that sexual abuse is the most underreported form of child maltreatment (NCCAN, 2002).

Box 23-2	Selected Examples of Physically Abusive Actions and Injuries

Physically Abusive Actions

Mild/Moderate	Severe
Pushing	Kicking
Throwing something	Biting
Grabbing	Hitting with fist
Spanking with bare hand	Spanking with an object
	Trying to hit with an object
	Beating up
	Threatening with a weapon
	Using a weapon
	Shaking

Physical Injuries Presented in Child Abuse Cases

Type	Very Suspicious	Inconclusive (Investigate)
Physical	Immersion burns	Subdural hematoma
	Whiplash syndrome in infants	Fractured skull
	Cauliflower ears	Injuries to face; black eye, loose or missing teeth, fractured jaw
	Spiral fractures of upper extremities	Fractures of extremities
	Radiologic evidence of healed or healing fractures with no history of treatment	Inexplicable scars
		Chest or abdominal injuries inconsistent with reason or trauma
	Identifiable marks on body, such as hand print, belt buckle, human bites, shoe print, cigarette burns	
	Severe cranial trauma in infants (shaken-baby syndrome)	
Sexual	Report of sexual conduct with adolescents or adults	Repeated urinary tract infections with negative urine culture results
	Evidence child posed for pornography	Genital itching or discharge, lacerations, bruises, or injury to genitals
	Sexually transmitted diseases	
	Enlarged/stretched vaginal opening	

It is important to note that sexual abuse of children can be committed by strangers, acquaintances, or trusted leaders of the community, as well as by family members. The sex abuse scandal involving priests in the Catholic Church in 2003 is a good example of how sexual abuse of children can be perpetrated by trusted members of a community and how it can stay hidden for many years. Widespread publicity and public outrage prompted changes and better oversight of priests within the Catholic Church. In approximately 80% of cases, however, the perpetrator of sexual abuse is a family member **(incest)**, family friend, neighbor, foster parent, or guardian (USDHHS, 2007).

Emotional Abuse

Emotional abuse includes acts or omissions by parents or other caregivers that cause, or could cause, serious behavioral, cognitive, emotional, or mental disorders. Emotional or psychologic abuse is very hard to detect, and the behavioral consequences might take years to develop. Acts that might not immediately harm a child can be sufficient to warrant reporting and investigation by child protective services. For example, the parents or caregivers might use extreme or bizarre forms of punishment, such as confinement of a child in a dark closet. Less severe acts, such as habitual scapegoating, belittling, or rejecting treatment, are often difficult to prove, and therefore child protective services might not be able to intervene without evidence of harm to the child (NCCAN, 2002).

Abuse and neglect are repetitive patterns of behavior. Approximately 30% of children named in reports of child abuse or neglect had been the subject of a report to child protective services at least once before in the previous 5 years (Fluke et al., 2005). In half the cases of child abuse–related deaths, a previous report of abuse or neglect had been filed with the state's child protective agency (Child Welfare League of America, 2004). Box 23-3 reviews behaviors and symptoms common in abuse and neglect.

Box 23-3	Selected Behaviors to Assess in Screening for Child Abuse and Neglect

Behaviors of Abusive Parents
- Do not volunteer information or are vague about cause of child's illness or injury
- Tell contradictory stories to explain injury
- Delay getting medical attention for child
- Respond inappropriately to child during treatment, such as ignoring, offering no comfort, or showing no concern, or, conversely, showing overinvolvement with attention
- Have record of "hospital shopping" or using different facilities for treatment of child
- Blame siblings or baby-sitters without substantiation or place blame on child's clumsiness
- Show obvious signs of drug or alcohol use

Behaviors of Abused Child
- Accepts injury as punishment
- Tells several stories of how injury occurred, which might appear rehearsed
- Looks to parent for behavioral cues or is excessively obedient
- Gives story inconsistent with observed injuries
- If confronted, often defends parent or refuses to cooperate with investigation
- Has psychosomatic complaints with no obvious organic cause
- Emotional abuse should be ruled out in withdrawn children, overeaters, truants, and runaways

Behaviors of Neglected Child
- Has vacant or frozen affect
- Does not cry, even if situation warrants
- Might be wary of physical contact or crave physical contact with virtual strangers
- Has delayed development physically, emotionally, cognitively
- Shows poor grooming of body, hair, and clothes on a regular basis
- Has behavior related to lack of supervision, including poor school performance and attendance
- Pregnancy in young females in both abuse and neglect situations

IMPACT OF CHILD ABUSE LAWS

Because of national concern, the federal government enacted the Child Abuse Prevention and Treatment Act (CAPTA) in 1974. It was most recently amended and reauthorized on June 25, 2003. The act sets established minimum definitions of child abuse and neglect. CAPTA provides federal funding to states for use in the prevention, investigation, prosecution, and treatment of child abuse and neglect. In addition, it establishes the Office on Child Abuse and Neglect and the National Clearinghouse on Child Abuse and Neglect Information.

Child abuse and neglect are crimes in all 50 states. All 50 states, plus the District of Columbia, have mandatory child abuse and neglect reporting laws that require certain professionals and institutions to report suspected cases of maltreatment to a designated child protection agency. More than half of all reports of alleged child abuse or neglect (55.8%) are made by professionals (USDHHS, 2007). These laws emerged from the moral concerns of protecting the vulnerable and promoting nurturing families (see the *Ethics in Practice* box). Each state has different criteria and procedures for reporting suspected cases. **Child protective services** is the agency assigned to investigate reports of child abuse or neglect. The emotional aspect of abuse is not clearly addressed in most laws and has been difficult to prosecute in practice. Physical neglect of a persistent nature with severe consequences is more likely to incur legal prosecution than are subtler forms of physical and emotional neglect.

To prove neglect, an adult's recognition that his or her actions have or could cause adverse consequences to the child is usually a legal requirement to show intent. Economic, emotional, and mental health factors might cloud the issue.

> A child was seen for an ear infection. An antibiotic was prescribed, but the prescription was never filled. The child developed complications and required hospitalization.

Does this constitute deliberate neglect? Are there cultural or religious factors that might impact parents' decisions to seek and follow medical care? Some of the issues the authorities would examine before deciding to prosecute include parental understanding of the risks of withholding medication, ability to pay for the prescription, and, finally, intent. Was the decision not to provide medication deliberate or the result of multiple stressors or poor coping skills?

FAMILY PRESERVATION ALTERNATIVE

The question of what should be done with the children who are victims of child abuse is a social policy challenge. Approximately 15% of child victims are removed from their homes by court order. Most are placed in foster care (USDHHS, 2005). Many of these children, an estimated 800,000 during any one year, will bounce between foster care and a parent before parental rights are terminated. Most will not be adopted and will remain in foster care until adulthood.

Family preservation programs are being tested as an alternative to parental punishment, jail time, or removal of children from their parents. It has been many experts' belief that abusive families can benefit from intense, long-term community support and supervision that addresses the myriad social and family issues that precipitated the abuse or neglect. Preservation programs stress intensive intervention with all family members and stringent supervision. The intent is to provide basic needs, educate, and build on family strengths to keep families together rather than to place children in foster care. Evaluation of such programs has shown disappointing results. Some studies have found fewer subsequent reports of child maltreatment, decreased frequency of out-of-home placements of children, and use of a broader array of community support services among families linked to a family preservation caseworker who provided strong collaboration in developing a treatment plan than among families without a family preservation caseworker (CDF, 2005; Littell, 2001; Walton, 2001). Others, however, have found no improvement in the level of family functioning, effectiveness in preventing future maltreatment, or risk of future foster home placement (Chaffin et al., 2001; Walton, 1996; Westat et al., 2002).

LONG-TERM CONSEQUENCES

Children who are abused or mistreated are at increased risk for learning disorders, mental retardation, and developmental delays, including delays in language development, speech, and gross motor activities. Abused and neglected children generally have lower IQ scores than children with similar characteristics who have not been abused and are much more likely to have academic difficulties in school (USDHHS, 2005). Physical abuse in childhood and the cumulative effects of experiencing maltreatment and witnessing family violence are also related to chronic physical and mental health problems throughout childhood and into adulthood (Thompson et al., 2004; Turner et al., 2006).

Initiating mutually satisfying interpersonal relationships with peers and adults is difficult for mistreated children. Their social skills and self-concept suffer. They have difficulty setting limits or boundaries with others. Classmates might describe them as socially withdrawn or as troublemakers. Physically abused individuals are more likely to be suicidal, use drugs, and exhibit aggressive behaviors (Rew, 2003). Children who are abused and/or neglected are at greater risk of involvement in juvenile or other criminal activity. Compared to children who were not maltreated, abused and neglected children are up to six times more likely to be involved in the juvenile justice system and up to three times more likely to be arrested as adults (CDF, 2005, p. 117).

Children who run away from home often do so because of sexual and other abuse in the home (Brandford et al., 2004). Girls run away more often than boys and also run away multiple times. This suggests that girls may be subject to more dysfunctional relationships or feel less able to protect themselves at home. Once on the street, runaways are vulnerable to predators, pimps, drug dealers, and those engaging in other types of exploitation (see Chapter 21). Girls and boys often engage in sex acts for money, which can lead to a lifetime of problems. Prostitution and promiscuous sexual activity are more prevalent in adults who were sexually assaulted as children. Victims of sexual abuse report lifelong difficulty in maintaining healthy adult relationships.

ETHICS IN PRACTICE

Protecting the Vulnerable

Gail A. DeLuca Havens, PhD, APRN, BC

"Victoria has become so introverted since the beginning of the school year. Her schoolwork is suffering terribly. She rarely engages in conversations or in play with classmates, and her absences have increased significantly. I know something is troubling her, but she has not shared anything with me when we have had the opportunity to talk. I came to see you today in the hope that, as our school nurse, you might be able to find out what is troubling her."

In response to the third-grade teacher's plea, Melissa, the community health nurse for the four Central City elementary schools, establishes a rapport with Victoria over the next several weeks. Today Melissa asks Victoria why she was absent from school all of the previous week. Tearfully, Victoria describes the beating she received from her mother a week earlier. She had not cleaned up the kitchen to her mother's satisfaction. Her mother had hit her so hard that it hurt to walk. She described her urine as having looked "like blood," as well. Melissa learns that Victoria has been receiving beatings from her mother since her father left the family last summer. Victoria has a sister and a brother, both younger than she. Melissa does not believe that they have been hurt by their mother.

This situation presents questions regarding the rights of children versus the rights of parents. When does a child cease to be the biologic offspring of two individuals and become, instead, a member of society with all of the rights, duties, and responsibilities accorded such individuals? Parents in our society are permitted a great deal of latitude in raising their children. To a great extent the process of child rearing is defined by the prevailing cultural norms of the particular family unit. It is presumed that the safety and well-being of the child will be preserved within that family unit. As in Victoria's situation, however, when a question of child abuse arises it becomes necessary to question the scope of parental authority. Child abuse is contrary to the societal norms that set the standards for moral parental behavior. A child has the right to be protected from harm. Being a parent, however, does not make one incapable of inflicting harm to one's child. Under what circumstances do others have a duty to protect children from their parents? Are there limits to parental authority, or do parents have inviolate rights to exercise their discretion in raising their children? What obligations, if any, do others have to the abuser?

Melissa believes that she is obliged to protect Victoria from further harm. She is also concerned for the future safety and well-being of Victoria's siblings. Finally, she is concerned about the changes in Victoria's mother's behavior and the underlying problems. Melissa is also aware that the law requires her to report any suspected cases of child abuse to the local child protection agency caseworker.

Melissa considers the courses of action that she perceives are options in this situation. She can ask Victoria's mother to come to school to discuss the child's problems in school with her. This might offer a means to reveal to Victoria's mother the harm she is doing to her daughter. It also might provide a catalyst for her to seek counseling and support. This action might serve to diminish the harm to Victoria, if her mother appears for the meeting. However, the mother has not kept appointments scheduled in the past by Victoria's teacher. If Victoria's mother does meet with Melissa, the concern remains that she will be angry at the nurse's interference in her private life and retaliate by becoming even more abusive of Victoria.

The other course of action that Melissa is obliged to take is to report Victoria's story and past behavior observed in school to the child protection agency that serves the neighborhood in which Victoria and her family live. This action has the advantage of involving individuals in the case who have expertise and accountability in addressing this type of family problem. It is an action that will better serve the interests of Victoria, her siblings, and her mother. The short-term consequences of the action involve the issue of trust, because Victoria confided in Melissa as the school nurse, not necessarily intending that others would become involved in the situation. Again, there is the fear of possible reprisal by Victoria's mother. Another consequence is the possibility of Victoria's being placed in a foster home.

The nurse's primary moral concern in this situation is the protection of Victoria from further harm. Nonmaleficence, or doing no harm, is one of the fundamental principles that guide nurses' clinical decision making (American Nurses Association, 2001). Beauchamp and Childress (2001) state that "Refraining from aiding another person, by not providing a good or by not preventing or removing a harm, can be devastating in its consequences, and as morally wrong as inflicting a harm." Even though Melissa is not harming Victoria directly, having knowledge of the harm she is experiencing and choosing not to intervene carries with it the same moral force as direct harm. There is an equally compelling moral principle operating here, however. By acting to protect Victoria from harm, Melissa acknowledges that the child is a distinct member of society and that she is not defined solely by her mother's identity. In essence, by her actions Melissa acknowledges Victoria's autonomy, her independence as a person with particular needs and rights, and her separate identity.

A second moral concern is that Victoria be a member of a safe, nurturing family unit. To protect her from further abuse and to ensure that her family becomes a safe haven for Victoria, it is necessary that her mother's needs be attended to. Melissa is aware that people usually attribute responsibility for an abusive incident to the parent. However, a characteristic that is common to abusing parents is a history of having been abused themselves (Adams, 2005). Victoria's mother must be "reparented" to effectively intervene in the child abuse cycle (Cerny & Inouye, 2001). As Melissa intervenes in this case, she acknowledges her professional and moral commitment to assist both Victoria and her mother.

REFERENCES

Adams, B. L. (2005). Assessment of child abuse risk factors by advanced practice nurses. *Pediatric Nursing, 31,* 498-502.

American Nurses Association. (2001). *Code of ethics for nurses with interpretive statements.* Washington, DC: Author.

Beauchamp, T. L., & Childress, J. F. (2001). *Principles of biomedical ethics* (5th ed.). New York: Oxford University Press.

Cerny, J. E., & Inouye, J. (2001). Utilizing the Child Abuse Potential Inventory in a community health nursing prevention program for child abuse. *Journal of Community Health Nursing, 18,* 199-211.

INTIMATE PARTNER VIOLENCE

Intimate partner violence (IPV) is also often referred to as *partner abuse, domestic violence,* or *woman battering.* IPV is the leading cause of injury for women. According to national crime statistics, battering is the single most common cause of injury to women, far exceeding accidental injuries and injuries caused by other criminal activities. Findings from the National Violence Against Women Survey reveal the following: (Tjaden & Thoennes, 2000).

- Nearly 25% of women and 7.6% of men surveyed reported being physically assaulted or raped by a former or current spouse or partner over their lifetimes.
- In the United States, estimates are that approximately 1.5 million women and 834,732 men are assaulted annually by the partners.
- Estimates are that approximately 503,485 women and 185,496 men are stalked annually in the United States.
- Rates of intimate partner abuse vary greatly among women of diverse ethnic backgrounds.
- Women experience more assaults and injuries from their intimate partners than men do.
- Of women reporting IPV, 41.5% reported being injured by their partners during the most recent assault, compared to 20% of men.
- Estimates are that approximately 2 million intimate partner rapes and assaults against women will result in injury and 552,192 will require medical treatment of the victim.
- Most IPV is not reported to the police. Only 20% of rapes, 25% of physical assaults, and 50% of stalkings perpetrated against intimate female partners were reported.

There is a growing body of research documenting the range of significant health problems and resulting disability experienced by victims of physical and sexual abuse. Battered women are less healthy and have a variety of battery-related health problems. These include traumatic injuries, chronic pain, bone and joint pain, headaches, sleep disorders, autoimmune disorders, urinary and vaginal infections, unplanned pregnancy, increased substance abuse, depression, and increased suicide attempts (Coker et al., 2002; Jackson et al., 2002; Plichta, 2004; Roberts et al., 2003). Adolescents who are the victims or perpetrators of severe dating violence report poorer quality of life, increased suicide ideation and attempts, substance use, and lower life satisfaction (CDC, 2006a; Coker et al., 2000).

Battered women use health care services nearly twice as much as women who have not been battered (Ulrich et al., 2003). Battering is predictive of more hospitalizations, clinic use, and mental health service use at an estimated mean cost of $2665 per year for each victim of battering (National Center for Injury Prevention and Control, 2003). The total health care costs of IPV exceed $8.3 billion each year, nearly $7.1 billion of which is for direct medical and mental health care services (Max et al., 2004).

Women are at increased risk for violence during pregnancy. Estimates vary widely, but between 8% and 21% of all pregnant women are battered (McFarlane et al., 1996). Surveys of women with a history of being battered indicate that 30% to 60% were abused during pregnancy, and approximately 50% needed medical care for a previous assault (McFarlane et al., 1992). Battering is also related to poor pregnancy outcomes, such as miscarriage, preterm labor, and low-birth-weight infants. However, women who were abused during and after pregnancy did not differ from nonabused women in their use of well-baby care (Martin et al., 2001). This suggests that pediatric offices might be an important place to screen for IPV.

DEFINITION

IPV entails a pattern of verbal and physical attacks by one intimate partner against the other. The definition of *abuse* includes violence between unmarried, cohabiting, separated or divorced, and dating partners as well. All abuse between partners, whether married, unmarried, or dating, is referred to as IPV in this chapter.

In this chapter, the assailant is referred to as male and the victim or survivor as female, because in 80% of IPV the assailant is male and the victim female (Rennison, 2003). The size and strength differences between men and women place women at higher risk of injury or death as a result of the violence. Women often strike back in self-defense (Sorenson & Wiebe, 2004). There is legitimacy to the claim that cases in which the woman is the aggressor are underreported because the male victims fear ridicule.

IPV includes physical, sexual, verbal, and emotional abuse. Physical assault ranges in degree from slapping to murder. Sexual abuse includes unwanted or forced sexual acts. All the abusive actions are aimed at controlling the other person, humiliating the person, and reducing the victim's self-esteem and identity. Verbal and emotional abuse breaks down women's self-esteem. A common theme of verbal abuse is criticism of the victim's ability to adequately perform her role of mother or wife. Verbal abuse convinces the victim that she deserves harsh treatment, and it serves to reinforce the abuser's belief that his actions are justified, even required, to ensure that the spouse acts appropriately.

The Domestic Abuse Intervention Project (also called the *Duluth Model*) has been a pioneer in intervening to prevent men's violence against their female partners. This treatment and education model is based on the theory that power and control are at the heart of partner violence. The power and control wheel (Figure 23-2) illustrates the variety of strategies used for controlling others' behaviors. These behaviors should serve as warning signs of potentially abusive relationships.

VIOLENCE IN DATING COUPLES

The definition of IPV has expanded to include violence in dating relationships. Based on data from the Youth Risk Behavior Survey, 9% of high school students report experiencing physical violence in their dating relationships (CDC, 2006a). The prevalence of victimization was about the same for young women and young men. In a large national survey of college women, 20% to 25% reported experiencing rape or attempted rape during their college years (Fisher et al., 2000). Ninety percent of the assailants were known to their victims. Thirteen percent of the college women in one survey and 20% in another survey reported being stalked by boyfriends, classmates, or someone at work (Fisher et al., 2000; Haugaard & Seri, 2004). Twelve percent of a sample of 5400 high school students reported being either the victim or the perpetrator of severe physical or sexual dating violence in the previous 12 months (Coker et al., 2000). In a longitudinal study of college women, Smith and colleagues (2003) found that 88% of the women reported at least one incident of physical or sexual violence during adolescence or their college years.

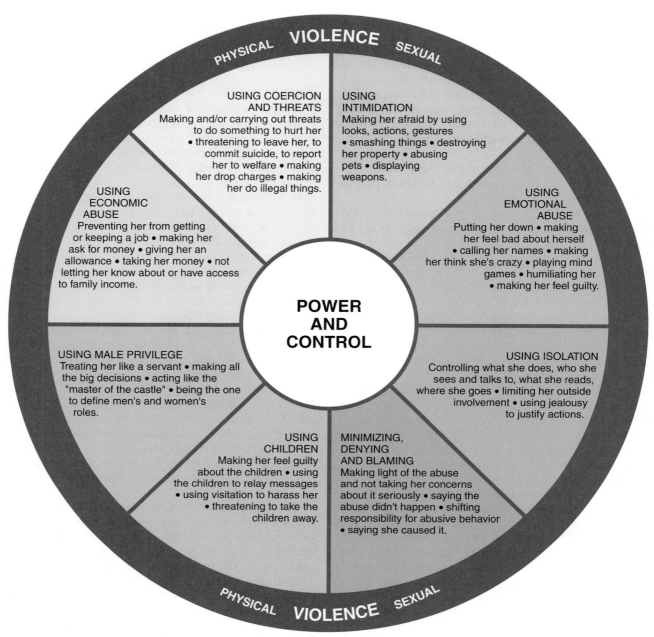

FIGURE 23-2 Relationship of violence to use of power and control. (From Domestic Abuse Intervention Project. [nd]. *Wheel gallery.* Retrieved August 17, 2007 from *http://www.duluth-model.org.*)

This study also found that young women who experienced dating violence in adolescence were at greater risk for experiencing dating violence in college.

CHARACTERISTICS OF ABUSERS AND VICTIMS

A number of important factors are associated with IPV. Families at or below the poverty level are at greater risk for IPV (CDC, 2006b). National family surveys indicate that socioeconomic status is a risk factor but that abuse is prevalent at all income levels.

Abusers characteristically are jealous, controlling, possessive, and emotionally dependent. Abusive partners might lack some social skills, such as communication skills, particularly in the context of problematic situations with their intimate partners (Center for Children and Families in the Justice System, 2004; Holtzworth-Munroe et al., 2000). Violent husbands report more

anger and hostility toward women than nonviolent husbands. Abusive men report more depression, lower self-esteem, and more aggression than nonviolent men. Some scientists suggest that violent intimate partners might be more likely to have personality disorders, such as borderline personality, antisocial or narcissistic behaviors, and dependency and attachment problems (Holtzworth-Munroe et al., 2000). Abusive men may be serial batterers; that is, they may engage in abusive behavior in each successive relationship (Center for Children and Families in the Justice System, 2004).

CYCLICAL PHASES OF ABUSE

Walker (1979) identified three general phases in a repeating **cycle of violence:** (1) the tension-building phase, (2) the battering phase, and (3) the apologetic phase (Figure 23-3). In

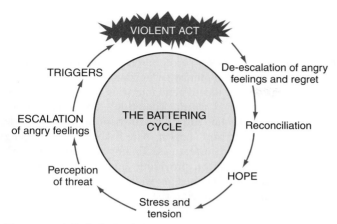

FIGURE 23-3 Cycle of violence. (From Browne, K., & Herbert, M. [1997]. *Preventing family violence.* New York: John Wiley & Sons. Reproduced by permission.)

the tension-building phase the batterer's levels of frustration, anger, and belittlement of the victim escalate. Women are able to identify cues of the increasing tension that are displayed by the abuser (Langford, 1996). The victim attempts to placate the abusive individual by being attentive, nurturing, and self-deprecating. Avoidance strategies are often unsuccessful, and tension continues to escalate into violence.

During the battering phase, the abuser physically and often sexually assaults his partner. The violence might last an hour or several days. The battering phase is followed by a contrite and apologetic phase during which the batterer is apologetic and loving and may shower his partner with gifts and promises. He assures his partner that the episode will not be repeated, perhaps blaming it on stress at work or consumption of too much alcohol. This is often referred to as "the honeymoon phase." Often the abusive partner will make an effort to please in other ways, such as helping with housework or planning activities that are sure to please family members. This honeymoon phase gives way to tension building, however, and the cycle is repeated.

BLAMING THE VICTIM

The batterer refuses to acknowledge responsibility for the abuse. In fact, he will blame his boss, alcohol, stress, and his partner for his violent behavior. The abuser's sincerity, coupled with the victim's willingness to accept responsibility for "fixing" problems and maintaining the relationship, lead to the victim's acceptance of blame for abusive behavior. "If only I had not gotten him mad" and "I know he hates me to fold his socks that way" are comments illustrating victims' internalization of the blame for their assailants' abusive behavior. Families of battered women often inadvertently support victim blaming by saying things such as, "What did you do to make him react so violently?" Many of the behaviors health care providers see in battered women, such as lack of focus and/or passivity, might not be personality characteristics leading to abuse or failure to leave a batterer, but might instead be a manifestation or coping mechanism resulting from the battering itself.

> Connie and her husband John are an upper-middle-class couple married for 20 years with three children. They have a violent relationship. Connie has some postsecondary education but has not worked outside the home since her marriage. John is a college graduate with a very successful, but stressful, career. John started hitting Connie during her first pregnancy. She tried to tell her mother about the situation, but her mother told her that all couples need time to adapt and that John was a wonderful person. Since that time, Connie has kept the violence and her injuries secret from family members, neighbors, and John's business acquaintances. Connie is very unhappy but says she cannot leave because she has no job prospects; she knows her husband will not cooperate with support, and her children deserve an intact home environment.

WHY SPOUSES STAY

One of the most difficult things nurses and other health care providers have to accept is the battered spouse's continued reluctance to end the relationship. The most frequently heard comment is, "Why doesn't she just leave?" The woman stays for a variety of realistic and unrealistic reasons, the most frequent of which are the following:

- She hopes her husband will reform.
- She thinks there is no place to go.
- Children make it difficult to leave, both for financial reasons and because it is harder to find alternative living arrangements.
- She has financial problems—she is unemployed or has no money.
- She is afraid of living alone.
- She is emotionally dependent on the abusive spouse.
- She believes that divorce is shameful.
- She fears reprisal from her husband.

Many battered women fear reprisal from their partner if they choose to leave. Their concern is very real. Women are at greater risk of being killed when they leave their abusive partner (American College of Emergency Physicians, 2006; Campbell et al., 2003). Abusive partners often go to great lengths to terrorize a partner who has left, including stalking (National Center for Victims of Crime, 2006). For this reason, shelters for battered women often do not publish their addresses. In rural areas, it is much more difficult to escape and hide from the abuser.

LEGAL EFFORTS TO COMBAT INTIMATE PARTNER VIOLENCE

Legal efforts to combat IPV are limited and inconsistent, although there has been substantial improvement in recent years. Penalties for abusive partners are still not consistent with penalties imposed on individuals convicted of similar offenses against strangers, friends, or acquaintances. There is a tendency to consider the relationship as a mitigating factor that provides some rationale explaining the perpetrator's behavior.

Restraining orders have been one legal avenue used to restrict access of an abuser to his partner. Although the news often reports the stories of women who have secured restraining orders that were subsequently violated by abusers with tragic results, there is evidence that restraining orders are effective in reducing contact, threats, violence, and injury from an abusive partner (Holt et al., 2003; McFarlane et al., 2004).

Stalking is a tremendous problem in abusive relationships. Data from the large National Violence against Women Survey showed that 5% of the women surveyed reported having been stalked by a current or former partner or date (Tjaden & Thoennes, 2000). Congress passed legislation making stalking a federal offense. Stalking is a crime in all 50 states. It remains to be seen whether elevating stalking to a federal crime will be effective in increasing arrests and prosecutions.

Perceptions of strong criminal justice policies have a direct effect on attitudes, leading to a favoring of criminal justice response and a decrease in blaming of the victim. This is hypothesized to lead to transformation of community attitudes and new social norms reducing acceptance and tolerance of IPV (Salazar et al., 2003).

A number of communities have developed comprehensive approaches aimed at reducing the number of repeat offenders. They have instituted specialized domestic violence units within the police department and domestic violence courts in the justice system that specialize in complex issue of IPV. Other legal interventions include mandatory arrest or counseling and, in some instances, jail time, even for first offenders. The intent is to penalize the offender, raising the cost of continuing his offensive behavior. The focus is on breaking the cycle of violence by concentrating on the offenders.

The greatest boost in combating domestic violence came in 1994 with the passage of the federal Violence against Women Act. The act was reauthorized in 2005. The Violence against Women Act of 2005 contains a number of new initiatives aimed at helping children exposed to violence, training health care providers, encouraging men to teach nonviolence to the next generation of men, and improving crisis services for victims of rape and sexual assault. The act also includes initiatives aimed at improving the legal system's response and improving supportive services, such as transitional housing, for women and children forced to leave their homes because of violence.

The ultimate decision to stay in an abusive situation or to leave is the victim's. Leaving a relationship is a difficult decision, and many choose to return to their partners. Health professionals must work hard to understand the reasons women return to their partners. Nurses should place their emphasis on ensuring women's safety and maintaining an accepting, supportive relationship with women experiencing abuse rather than focusing on whether a woman leaves the relationship or not. Over time, the nurse might see positive results from sustained support.

CONSEQUENCES FOR CHILDREN EXPOSED TO INTIMATE PARTNER VIOLENCE

Recently, there has been a growing recognition that IPV has long-term health and behavioral effects on children who witness the abuse (Rosewater, 2003). Between 3.3 and 10 million children are exposed to family violence each year (CDF, 2005). Although some children show no obvious effects, others show signs of distress, anxiety, depression, and poor self-esteem (CDF, 2005). Children might become very protective of their mothers and siblings and suspicious of outsiders. Many exhibit persistent academic or behavioral problems, or difficulty with conflict resolution and positive peer interactions (National Clearinghouse on Child Abuse and Neglect, 2005). Rhea and associates (1996) recommend incorporating standard questions about family violence into all mental health and school counseling interviews.

NURSING CARE IN ABUSIVE SITUATIONS: CHILD OR PARTNER ABUSE

Community health nurses see children and families in a variety of settings and community organizations. Nurses are in an important position to identify and intervene with persons experiencing violence and abuse. Their long-term relationships with clients and families allow them the opportunity to provide ongoing monitoring and support of at-risk families. Nursing efforts should be directed at case finding and assessing risk of abuse, ensuring safety, providing emotional support, and advocating for abuse victims, as well as performing primary prevention aimed at reducing risk and eliminating the intergenerational transmission of violence.

SECONDARY AND TERTIARY PREVENTION
Screening and Assessment

The community health nurse should always be alert to possible abuse or neglect. Some of the risk factors for abuse in families were identified earlier in the chapter (see Box 23-1). Documentation by the nurse of risk assessment, anticipatory guidance, and physical condition is essential.

Physical and Sexual Abuse. In assessing child abuse and neglect, the nurse should be suspicious of atypical or unusual injuries and ask for an explanation. The nurse should remain nonjudgmental and be accessible and open to parental concerns. Sometimes parents are troubled enough about their behavior to seek the nurse's opinion. They might attempt to justify their behavior or the behavior of another caregiver by presenting a list of complaints about the child.

The type of injury and the circumstances under which it occurred should always be evaluated. The nurse should question whether the explanation of the cause is consistent with the type of injury found. Serious injuries in children deserve special vigilance. Certain types of trauma are particularly suggestive of physical or sexual abuse (see Box 23-2). Most injuries are not easily classified as resulting from abuse. Children are very active, sometimes clumsy, and not often safety conscious. Bruising is common. Nurses must be sensitive to subtle signs of abuse or neglect. Reports by friends or neighbors, even if no observable injuries are present, should not be dismissed. It is particularly important to suspect any cases of repeated trauma to either a child or adult.

Victims of IPV might be ashamed or reluctant to volunteer information, but might provide information if asked. Emergency department nurses are in a position to identify IPV. Crandall and colleagues (2004) found that 93% of murdered women had at least one previous injury-related visit to the emergency department. Routine screening of women for IPV is recommended and is shown to increase identification (Poirier, 1997; Wiist & McFarlane, 1999). Adding four simple questions to a nursing history are effective in assessing a woman's abuse history (McFarlane et al., 1991, 1996). These questions are the following:

- Within the last year, have you ever been hit, slapped, kicked, or otherwise physically hurt by someone?
- Within the last year, has anyone forced you to engage in sexual activities?
- Are you afraid of anyone?
- Since you have been pregnant, have you been hit, slapped, kicked, or otherwise physically hurt by someone?

Many barriers exist to implementing widespread assessment of violence as part of client histories. Reasons cited by health care providers for not screening are lack of education, lack of time and effective interventions, and fear of offending clients (Waalen et al., 2000). Colleges and universities educating nurses, physicians, and other health care providers have started increasing the course content on IPV and other family violence.

Emotional Abuse. Assessing for emotional abuse is much more difficult than assessing for physical abuse. Emotional abuse is frequently overlooked by health professionals. Community health nurses are in a position to observe family dynamics and interactions more frequently than are other professionals. Consistent tension, anger, or demeaning remarks are cause for concern. Frequent episodes of yelling, cursing, or derogatory remarks aimed at a child are indicative of emotional abuse. Some children react to a nonsupportive and hostile environment by displaying behavioral problems at home or school. Some develop somatic complaints. If there is no obvious explanation for such behavior in a child, the possibility of abuse should be considered.

Increased stress might also result in numerous physical complaints in physically or emotionally abused spouses. Sometimes the only signs of abuse are emotional and stress related. Box 23-4 lists common health and behavioral indicators the nurse can use to screen for abuse. Both victims of domestic violence and those who witness abuse might show physical and emotional signs of posttraumatic stress disorder (CDF, 2005).

More often than not, the nurse is faced with situations that are not clearly abusive or neglectful, and can find making a decision about contacting local authorities very difficult.

> Jim is a 7-year-old boy whose school reports that he is often tardy, comes wearing dirty clothes, and is doing poorly academically. The community health nurse is visiting his mother and new sister for well-baby visits. Jim's mother says that she is exhausted caring for the infant and is doing the best she can.

Box 23-4 Emotional and Physical Problems Associated with Violence Victimization

Physical
Atypical chest pain
Asthma
Recurrent headaches
Somatic complaints with no identifiable cause
Eating disorders and other gastrointestinal tract complaints

Emotional
Anxiety, panic attacks
Depression
Drug overdose
Forgetfulness
Hopelessness/helplessness/suicide attempts
Guilt
Inability to solve problems or make decisions
Low self-esteem
Sleep disturbances

Is Jim being neglected? Does the nurse have enough evidence to warrant contacting protective service? Are the conditions in the home different from those in which many poor people live in the area? The nurse might want to look closely at issues such as (1) whether Jim has enough to eat, (2) whether he is adequately clothed for the weather, and (3) whether he has missed school days and, if so, how many. Most of the time, single episodes do not provide clear evidence of abuse or neglect. It is the accumulation of concerns, circumstances, and observations that points toward abuse or neglect. The community health nurse must examine the impact of his or her personal values and expectations on the assessment of the situation. The reasons for suspecting abuse or neglect cannot be based on differences in personal values.

> During a home visit with Joan D., the community health nurse finds Joan and her three children (18 months, 3 years, and 4 years old) still in sleepwear at 2 PM. They are having a breakfast of hamburgers, chips, and soda. Joan explains that they just got out of bed because they all were up late last night watching videotapes. The community health nurse is personally upset that Joan's children are up late at night and are not eating the usual breakfast-type foods.

In this instance, the community health nurse and the family have different sleep-wake patterns and dietary habits. Although the nurse might feel that the mother demonstrates neglectful behavior, the situation as presented does not justify her feelings. If the children are adequately fed and given sufficient sleep time, the mother is not neglectful. If this pattern continues, a problem might develop when the children are school age. A reassessment at that time would be in order to see how well the family has or has not adjusted the sleep-wake pattern to school demands.

Legal Responsibilities of the Community/Public Health Nurse in Cases of Child Abuse

Nurses are included in a class of designated professionals who are required to report suspected cases of child abuse and neglect. These laws require that all *suspected* cases be reported but do not expect health professionals to determine the validity of the claim. Nurses file a report to the designated local authorities (child protective services or the police), and the authorities conduct an investigation. The agencies that investigate child abuse are authorized to remove children who are in imminent danger of injury. In most reported child-abuse cases, there is no *immediate* danger, and the child remains in the home. The procedure for investigating reported cases varies among states. Box 23-5 illustrates a common procedure for reporting child abuse. Neighbors, friends, or relatives of the child might also take action but are not clearly required to do so by law.

Exemptions from Liability. One concern of those mandated to report suspected cases of abuse is the possibility of a legal suit should the investigation not result in charges against the parent or caregiver. In every state, the law protects health care professionals from legal action if the charges are unproved. The threat of legal action against an individual who reports suspicions can have an impact on the willingness to report. It is hoped that protection offered by law will encourage those who have concerns to feel more comfortable about reporting such incidents to the proper authorities.

BOX 23-5	Typical Procedure for Notification and Investigation in Child Abuse and Neglect Cases

Actions Taken by Community Health Nurse
- Identification of suspected case of abuse/neglect
- Verbal report to
  1. Child protection agency or
  2. Local law enforcement agency
- Report sent to child protection agency within 48 hours of initiating complaint and a copy sent to the state's attorney's office.

Actions Taken by Designated Child Protection Agency
- Prompt investigation within 24 hours if abuse; usually within longer period—perhaps as much as 5 days—if neglect
- Completion of investigation within 10 days and reporting of findings to state's attorney's office
- Dispensation of case:
  1. No evidence found
  2. Inconclusive; file kept open
  3. Evidence exists; action taken
- Possible actions include:
  1. Mandated supervision in home
  2. Imposition of conditions on parents to continue custody (e.g., attend parenting classes, drug rehabilitation)
  3. Temporary removal of child to foster care or other relatives' homes
  4. Permanent removal of child from home
  5. Court action to terminate parental rights to clear for adoption

Nurse's Legal Responsibilities in Partner Abuse

Unlike in cases of suspected child abuse, there are no national **mandatory reporting** requirements in cases or suspected cases of partner abuse. Currently, six states and the armed services require that health care providers, including nurses, report IPV to local authorities (Gupta, 2007). There is much controversy over these laws and whether they prevent women from getting the health care they need and increase the risk of violence (Gielen et al., 2000; Rodriguez et al., 2001). One of the arguments against reporting laws is that it takes the responsibility away from women who are adults and are capable of such reporting themselves.

The nurse should be aware of the resources available for survivors of IPV. The nurse's first step should be taking a history to assess for violence and carefully documenting specific injuries observed by the nurse. Nurses can assist victims with referrals to resources such as legal aid organizations for civil protection orders, domestic violence shelters for shelter, and often support groups or counseling.

Ensuring the Safety of the Abuse Victim

When the nurse suspects an abusive situation, the priority is to ensure the safety of the victim or victims. Efforts should be directed toward eliminating potential harm or reducing the risk of assault. Families may choose to stay with relatives or friends, or use the services of a shelter; some may consider it safer to return home. Many communities have shelters for battered women. Shelters are often overcrowded, however, and as many as 40% of those seeking shelter have to be turned away because of space limitations.

Nurses can work with women to develop a safety plan. The goal of a safety plan is to have a plan in place to maximize a woman's safety and minimize the potential for violence. A safety plan should include plans for leaving the abuser, returning home, being at work or school, and dealing with children's safety at school. Box 23-6 outlines basic elements of a safety plan.

Referral to Community Resources

One intervention is education and referral of survivors of IPV to the resources available in the community. Communities vary in the resources they offer. Smaller rural regions may have to

BOX 23-6	Personal Safety Plan

If you have left your abusive partner:
- Change the locks on doors and windows, increase outside lighting.
- Teach children to call the police.
- Talk to the school and child care providers about who has permission to pick up the children.
- Obtain a restraining order that includes home, work, children's school, and forms of electronic contact.
- Develop an escape plan.

If you are leaving your abusive partner:
- Decide whom you can trust to tell that you are leaving and whom you might rely on if you need somewhere safe to go.
- Plan how you will travel safely to and from work and school, and other routinely traveled routes.
- See also items in previous section.

If you are returning to your abusive partner:
- Decide whom you can call in a crisis. Do you have someone you trust about the abuse? Could you stay with that person if needed?
- Work out a signal with children and neighbors to tell them that they should call the police.
- Plan escape routes.
- Prepare a bag or suitcase with the following items you will need if you have to flee. Store it in a safe place such as a friend's house.
  Important papers, such as birth certificates, Social Security cards, marriage license, driver's license, insurance information, car title, credit cards and account numbers, immunization and health records
  Extra keys to the house or apartment and the car
  Prescription medicines for yourself and the children
  A change of clothing for yourself and the children
  A favorite toy or blanket for the children

Safety planning for you at the workplace:
- Save any threatening or harassing messages.
- Park close to the entrance, talk to security personnel, and have someone escort you to your car or other transportation after work.
- Have calls screened and remove your name from the office directories and website.
- Relocate your workstation to a more secure area.
- Secure a restraining order; keep it current and always carry it with you.
- Provide a photo of the abusive person to security personnel and receptionists, and plan a response if he contacts you at work.
- Review safety plans for the children and arrangements with schools and child care providers.
- Create and distribute to trusted persons an emergency contact list.

share resources across an entire county. Resources that are available in most communities are women's shelters, support groups for women who are survivors of abuse, batterer's treatment programs, treatment programs for child witnesses of partner violence, and victim assistance programs to help women obtain court orders and follow through in legal proceedings. Treatment for the partner's violence is essential and should precede other interventions to reconcile or work on family dynamics. Often batterers are referred to treatment programs through the courts after they have been arrested and charged. Some programs allow self or voluntary referrals.

The community health nurse should know of appropriate community resources available for families before, during, and after the occurrence of abuse. Nurses must be familiar with the specific resources available in their communities to ensure speedy referrals. They should invite agency representatives to speak to

nursing audiences at nursing association meetings or at work. In addition, it might be possible to visit or tour some agencies.

Community health nurses can address the health needs of women and children living in shelters. Formal health services are rarely provided in shelters. Stress and health issues related to the violence are not the only health needs to be considered. Many of the shelter residents will have had past difficulty arranging for health services and routine care, such as immunizations, as well as for immediate health needs related to children's developmental phases, such as those resulting from accidents (Hatton, 1997).

PRIMARY PREVENTION

Primary prevention measures should include public education efforts to transform attitudes about child and partner violence as well as to identify and assist individuals at risk. The equality wheel (Figure 23-4) outlines multifaceted strategies

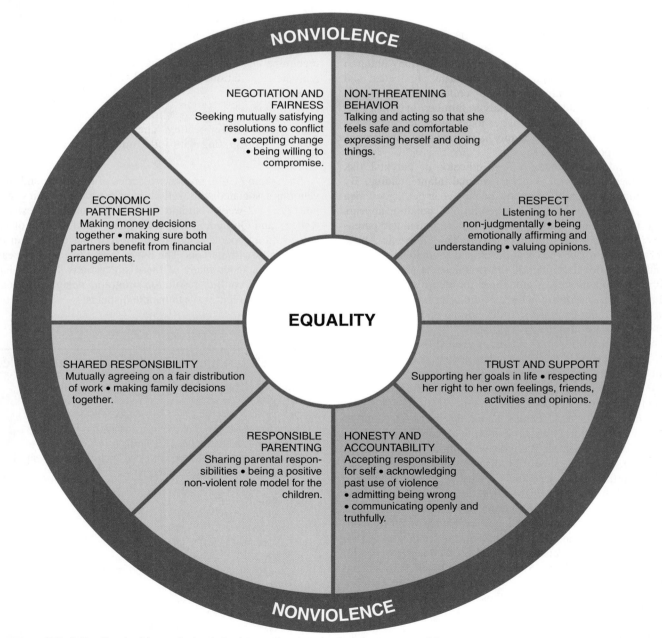

FIGURE 23-4 Equality wheel for use in developing intervention strategies for intimate partner violence. (From Domestic Abuse Intervention Project. [nd]. *Wheel gallery*. Retrieved August 17, 2007 from *http://www.duluth-model.org*.)

that health professionals can use when intervening with survivors of domestic violence. This model can be adjusted to guide intervention in other types of family violence cases.

Prevention for Families

Community health nurses often work as part of a team with other professionals in addressing family health needs, normal and abnormal child growth and development issues, and parenting styles. A report of the CDC (2003) reviewed the effectiveness of early childhood home visitation programs and found that they were effective in preventing child abuse and neglect. Home visitation programs commonly target high-risk families; low-income, young, less educated, first-time mothers; substance abusers; families with low-birth-weight infants; and other families at risk for child abuse or neglect. Although early-start home visitation programs may improve child outcomes, they have not been shown to improve family- or parent-related outcomes (Fergusson et al., 2006).

The presence of guns in the home is a clear risk. Nurses should assess families for the presence of firearms and, if they are owned, ensure that they are safely stored. Many children (1.7 million) live in homes where firearms are loaded and improperly stored and accessible to children (Okoro et al., 2005). Nurses should assess and advise families on proper firearm storage and the use of trigger locks to reduce the accessibility of firearms. If the family is willing, the family may consider disposing of the firearm.

Parent-Child Interactions. A key indicator of parental risk for neglectful behavior is poor maternal-infant bonding. By observing parent-child interplay, the nurse can get a good idea about parenting technique and bonding. If bonding appears weak, the nurse can work on increasing attachment and parental confidence in the role of caretaker. The Domestic Abuse Intervention Project (nd) has developed guidelines to assist health professionals in identifying troublesome parental/caregiver behaviors as well as guidelines for identifying nurturing behaviors. The nurturing behavior guide can be used to assist parents and other caretakers in developing and strengthening their positive nurturing behaviors.

Access to positive role models is crucial for at-risk families. One strategy is the foster grandmother program, which matches volunteer older women with young, at-risk mothers. Social support programs such as this can be expanded to include abusive as well as at-risk parents.

Family and cultural beliefs about discipline are another area for exploration and intervention. The community health nurse should encourage alternatives to hitting as a means of discipline. Spanking should be discouraged, because it role-models hitting as an acceptable means of teaching children how to act. In a review of the research on spanking over the past 62 years, Gershoff (2002) found substantial evidence that spanking is associated with a higher prevalence of abuse, more delinquency, more aggressive behavior, poorer mental health, poorer parent-child relationships, and other negative health consequences in children. Slade and Wissow (2004) found that spanking was associated with behavior problems in children from white families but not in those from black or Hispanic families.

Proactive anticipatory guidance by health care providers is essential for violence prevention. Community health nurses traditionally provide parental education about growth and developmental milestones, parenting stress, and effective parenting skills. Murry and colleagues (2000) suggest that the traditional child abuse screening protocols are not sensitive or concise enough to identify children under 3 years of age who are at risk for abuse or neglect. One suggested way of screening very young children is to include at least three nurse checks in the first 9 months of life (Browne, 1989). The first screening should include assessment for the risk factors associated with abuse and neglect. The next visit should explore parents' perceptions of their child and specific family stressors. The third visit should review infant behaviors and attachment. Box 23-7 offers a quick guide for assessment of parental behaviors to help identify parents who are experiencing difficulty in bonding and appropriate parent-child interactions.

Abusive parents often have unrealistic expectations of age-appropriate behavior for children. It is important to include a review of developmental milestones of infants and children, such as motor and cognitive abilities, during at least one home or clinic visit. This information helps parents to recognize age-appropriate behavior. The nurse can validate realistic expectations for the child with the parent and dispel unrealistic ones.

> An 8-month-old girl is admitted to the hospital for injuries sustained in a beating. The parent said that the baby was not cooperating with toilet training and needed to be disciplined.

Stringham (1998) proposes a series of questions and interventions associated with well-child primary care starting at the newborn or 2-week visit and continuing through adolescence. Roberts and Quillian (1992) have integrated the topic of violence into a general health teaching tool that nurses can use periodically with parents. The list of health teaching issues in Box 23-8 includes many of these suggestions. Schools have also initiated conflict resolution programs designed to teach children nonviolent ways to handle disputes.

BOX 23-7   Parental Behavior Assessment Guide

Good Behaviors
Makes good eye contact
Shows caring, gentle handling
Talks to infant/child in warm, accepting manner
Sets age-appropriate limits in a calm manner
Gives feedback that is mostly positive and involves praising remarks
Shows affection easily, hugs, smiles, pats

Risk Behaviors
Makes little or no eye contact
Shows rough or careless handling
Yells or screams at infant or child as primary communication technique
Sets no limits and/or sets age-inappropriate limits; might be accompanied by hitting or slapping
Gives no feedback or primarily negative feedback
Does not show affection; avoids physical contact
Leaves child alone when not appropriate

Box 23-8   Nurse/Parent Guide to Anticipatory Violence Counseling with Children

- Periodically review television and movie-viewing habits; encourage limits on viewing time and types of shows
- Stress the influence of peer pressure and recognize that it increases with the age of the child

For Elementary School Children:
- Teach coping techniques to avoid fights in school and neighborhood (e.g., walk away from situation)
- Review stranger danger and good touch/bad touch safety issues

For Children 10 to 12 Years Old:
- Teach the danger of alcohol and drugs; start no later than 10 years of age
- Identify high-risk situations in which drinking, drugs, or other problems are most likely to occur and role-play how to avoid or get out of them

For Children 13 to 19 Years Old:
- Review tobacco, alcohol, and drug use and the social and health consequences of each
- Reinforce the correlation between substance abuse and accidents
- Explore exposure to school violence
- Reinforce previous teaching related to avoidance of violent situations

Data from Roberts, C., & Quillian, J. (1992). Preventing violence through primary care intervention. *Nurse Practitioner, 17*(8), 62-64, 67-70.

Prevention of Intimate Partner Violence. Primary prevention of IPV consists of reducing the social belief that violence in relationships can be justified. Working with teens to develop equitable and healthy relationships is one way of preventing abuse. Teens, both young women and young men, can be helped to identify the warning signs of controlling behaviors and to set limits on intrusive or threatening behavior.

During a clinic appointment with Ashley, a pregnant 17-year-old who is moving in with her 24-year-old boyfriend, the community health nurse notices that Ashley's boyfriend repeatedly calls her on a cell phone and that she defers many of the assessment questions until she can ask her boyfriend if it is okay. On further assessment, the nurse discovers that although Ashley's boyfriend has not hit her, he does make derogatory comments about her personality, her intelligence, and her physical appearance. He also limits her association with friends and her family. During a conversation, the nurse determines that Ashley is hurt by her boyfriend's comments and frustrated with this part of the relationship. Ashley and the nurse explore the range of controlling behaviors in the context of abusive relationships and community resources that might be available. During subsequent visits, the nurse will monitor and encourage Ashley in her efforts. If the boyfriend's behavior remains the same, the nurse should explore other options, such as ascertaining Ashley's feelings about leaving the relationship, and encourage her to seek supportive relationships.

Community Efforts at Primary Prevention

The community health nurse can develop and assist with the delivery of community education and support programs aimed at reducing child and adult-partner abuse. The nurse can organize parent support groups and parenting classes. Civic and religious groups are often open to community guest speakers. The nurse can use these forums to educate about child and spouse abuse and the impact of exposure to violence on children.

Part of the role of the community health nurse is working to improve the overall health of communities as well as that of individuals and families. In that role, nurses should become politically active. Some of the ways the nurse can address child abuse and violence in the community include (1) advocating for inclusion of conflict resolution techniques in school curricula, (2) working with community groups to develop programs geared toward reducing exposure to violence and improving safety for communities at risk; and (3) communicating with legislators to increase funding for programs that supply economic, health, and other support services to communities and families.

Spouse abuse prevention should include public education designed to transform attitudes about IPV. Media awareness programs are designed to meet several goals:

- Assist women in recognizing their legal rights in abusive situations
- Enhance public awareness that IPV requires legal intervention and is not just a private matter between partners
- Recognize the need for improving the uneven application of legal restraints and prosecution of violent partners
- Encourage efforts designed to assist with behavioral changes in battering and battered individuals
- Discourage victim-blaming dialogue in public and private discussions about spousal violence
- Enhance public understanding of the need for long-term programs to support both victim and abuser to improve the chances of success
- Support policies that ensure equal opportunities for education and work for women, men, and minorities

Working to prevent or ameliorate child and partner abuse should be a commitment for every community health nurse. Social change takes a long time. The community health nurse cannot expect to see substantive change in a week or a month; rather, the nurse must be prepared for a sustained long-term effort. The National Advisory Council on Violence against Women has developed a checklist of community activities aimed at ending violence against women (see Community Resources for Practice at the end of the chapter). The checklist addresses 16 segments of community life, including health and mental health services, the workplace and college campuses, media and the entertainment industry, and churches. Box 23-9 highlights what the health care and mental health care systems can do. Although the checklist is aimed specifically at spousal abuse, the same activities can be used to address other forms of abuse as well.

The funding of prevention efforts is particularly challenging. A number of initiatives of the federal government have provided funding to support prevention. Many states have additional fees linked to marriage licenses and firearm registration that support shelters and other family violence prevention programs. In a study in California, two-thirds of those surveyed supported the use of surcharges and extra fees of up to

---

Box 23-9   What the Health and Mental Health Care Systems Can Do to Make a Difference

- Conduct public health campaigns
- Educate all health care providers about violence against women
- Create protocol and documentation guidelines for health care facilities, and disseminate widely
- Protect victim health records
- Ensure that mandatory reporting requirements protect the safety and health status of adult victims
- Create incentives for providers to respond to violence against women
- Create oversight and accreditation requirements for sexual assault and domestic violence care
- Establish health care outcome measures
- Dedicate increased federal, state, and local funds to improving the responses of the health and mental health care systems to violence against women

From National Advisory Council on Violence against Women & Violence against Women Office. (nd). *Toolkit to end violence against women.* Retrieved January 12, 2004 from *http://toolkit.ncjrs.org/default.htm.*

$5 to support domestic violence prevention (Sorenson, 2003). Although controversial, such fees remains an important means of funding prevention programs.

ELDER ABUSE

The Administration on Aging (2004) reports the following:
- Some 551,011 persons aged 60 and older experienced abuse, neglect, and/or self-neglect in a 1-year period.
- Almost four times as many new incidents of abuse, neglect, and/or self-neglect were *not* reported as were reported to and substantiated by adult protective services agencies.
- Persons aged 80 years and older suffered abuse and neglect at rates two to three times higher than their proportion in the older population.
- In 90% of cases in which the perpetrators of abuse and neglect were known, the perpetrator was a family member. Two-thirds of the perpetrators were adult children or spouses.

Elder abuse has received less media attention than child or spouse abuse. The research on elder abuse is also less developed than that on child and partner abuse. Definitions of abuse and neglect in the elderly are unclear and inconsistent (Fulmer, 2002). Many of the self-report methods for measuring abuse and neglect in other populations are more difficult to use in the elderly because of changes in memory and, in some cases, dementia. As individuals age, they require increased levels of caregiving that create a climate of stress and opportunity for the elderly to be abused, neglected, and exploited. Elder abuse is more common if the older adult lives with family members. Elders who live independently are at less risk.

A particular problem in gathering elder abuse data is the reluctance of elderly and caregivers to report suspected cases (Levine, 2003). As with other types of abuse, most cases are never reported. Elderly persons do not report because they or their spouses might be afraid of the caretakers, ashamed of the problem, or have limited alternatives for living arrangements. Health professionals do not report incidents because of ignorance of the problem, ignorance of their legal responsibilities in suspected cases, and lack of education about maltreatment that causes failure to adequately assess at-risk situations, and because of concern that alternative living arrangements might be less tolerable than the current one (Levine, 2003; Kahan & Paris, 2003).

DEFINITION

Elder abuse is defined as maltreatment of older persons (usually older than 65 years). The abuse can be physical, emotional, or financial. Failure to provide adequate care and comfort to seniors who are under the community health nurse's care would be considered neglect. Financial exploitation of vulnerable elders is a growing problem, recently identified as the single most common form of elder abuse. Common definitions of the types of abuse and neglect are as follows (Administration on Aging, 2004):
- *Physical abuse* is the willful infliction of physical pain or injury (e.g., slapping, bruising, restraining).
- *Sexual abuse* is the infliction of nonconsensual sexual contact of any kind.
- *Psychologic abuse* is the infliction of mental or emotional anguish (e.g., humiliating, intimidating, threatening).
- *Financial or material exploitation* is the improper action of an individual to use the resources of an older person without his or her consent for the benefit of someone else.
- *Neglect* is the failure of a caretaker to provide goods or services necessary to avoid physical harm, mental anguish, or mental illness (e.g., abandonment, denial of food or health-related services).

FACTORS ASSOCIATED WITH ABUSE BY FAMILY MEMBERS

Elder abuse is found in all socioeconomic groups and at all educational levels. Older adults are often abused by caregivers. An adult child is the most common source of abuse (32.6%), but elders may also be abused by other family members (21.5%) and spouses (11.3%) (National Committee for the Prevention of Elder Abuse & National Adult Protective Services Association, 2006). In 16% of cases, the abuser cannot be identified. Paid caregivers (including nurses and health care providers) often abuse or neglect the elderly in long-term care or housing facilities. Both sexes are equally at risk of being abusive. Elders suffering from confusion, incontinence, frailty, or severe physical and mental disabilities demand enormous amounts of time, energy, and patience from caregivers. Adults who have caregiving responsibilities for two generations—their parents and their children—are often referred to as the *sandwich generation*. For these individuals, the burden of working, raising children, and caring for an elderly parent can be overwhelming.

A review of the research on elder maltreatment revealed only a small number of risk factors associated with an increased risk of abuse (National Research Council, 2002). Elders who had a shared living arrangement were at greater risk than those living alone (Levine, 2003). This seems to be related not to disability but to opportunity. Other risk factors were social isolation, dementia, and certain characteristics of the abuser, such as the presence of mental illness and drug or alcohol abuse. In addition, abusers were more often emotionally and financially dependent on the older family member. There was little evidence that the elder's needs for assistance or caregiver stress led to a greater risk of abuse.

The prevalence of maltreatment in nursing homes is difficult to quantify. It is estimated that only 1 in 14 allegations of maltreatment is reported to authorities. Although allegations of maltreatment should be reported immediately, in 50% of cases the reports were submitted 2 or more days after the nursing home learned of the abuse (General Accounting Office, 2002). Delays in reporting severely compromise the ability of law enforcement agencies to investigate. When an employee in involved, many agencies simply dismiss the offending employee.

States must keep a registry of qualified nurse aides, the primary caregivers in nursing homes. Included in that registry are any substantiated findings that the aide has been abusive or neglectful to residents (Government Accountability Office, 2007). Any such finding effectively bans the aide from employment at nursing homes in that state. Screening of workers in nursing homes and home health agencies for criminal backgrounds and substance abuse is an attempt to reduce some of the risk factors for caregiver abuse. However, crimes committed in other states often are not revealed by such searches. In addition, many of the employees who work in nursing homes and who provide in-home services for home care agencies are minimally educated and minimally paid. These conditions make it difficult to retain well-qualified, competent employees.

NURSING CARE FOR ELDERS AND CAREGIVERS

Community health nurses are involved in primary, secondary, and tertiary prevention efforts for elders and caregivers. Four major areas in which nurses play an important role in addressing elder abuse are (1) identification of suspected cases; (2) reduction of risk and maintenance of independence; (3) oversight, supervision, and encouragement of caregivers; and (4) development of support groups for caretakers.

Identification of Suspected Cases

Early identification of at-risk elderly is important. To that end, the nurse should become proficient at identifying potential or probable abusive or neglectful situations. Box 23-10 briefly identifies areas to screen for the presence of elder maltreatment. Clearly, any unexplained bruises or injuries should be assessed and evaluated. Elders tend to bruise more easily than younger adults, but explanations that do not ring true and repeated incidents of bruising should arouse suspicion. As in other abusive situations, reporting and documenting injuries is an important part of the nursing process.

Currently, much research is focused on creating elder abuse screening tools to better identify elders and caregivers at risk for abuse, but these are still in the developmental stages (Cohen et al., 2006; Meeks-Sjostrom, 2004). A diminishing social network and poor social functioning are emerging as potential risk factors for abuse (Shugarman et al., 2003).

Brandl and Horan (2002) recommend use of the following questions as an initial screen for risk of abuse:
- Do you live alone?
- Who does your cooking?
- Who controls your finances?
- How often do you see or go out with friends?

Box 23-10	Screening for Elder Maltreatment
Physical abuse	Acts of violence, for example, force feeding, inappropriate use of restraints
	Physical signs (e.g., unexplained bruises, welts, fractures)
Emotional abuse	Verbal harassment, intimidation, threats, physical isolation from visitors
Financial abuse	Theft of money or possessions, coercion of older person into signing legal documents for power of attorney or turning over deeds, bank accounts, etc.
	Failure to contract for care when finances are available
Sexual abuse	Unexplained venereal disease or genital lacerations or infections
	Elder complaints of sexual assault
Neglect	Failure to provide clean environment or physical needs such as glasses, medication, false teeth
	Absence of safety precautions
	Signs in the elder of dehydration, malnourishment, pressure sores, poor hygiene

- Are you afraid of anyone?
- Does anyone slap you, pull your hair, hit you, or act rough with you?
- Does anyone threaten to do any of these things?
- Does anyone force you to do sexual acts you do not want to do?

When assessing for abuse or neglect, the nurse needs to be aware that some elderly persons have cognitive impairments that affect their ability to make decisions about their safety (Brandl & Horen, 2002). Depression and dementia to be significantly higher in the maltreated elderly (Levine, 2003). In one study Kahan and Paris (2003) found that half of all elders in reported elder abuse cases had diagnosed memory impairments. Depression, poor judgment, confusion, and the inability to communicate clearly are also common responses to abuse, and nurses should assess for maltreatment in elderly persons with these symptoms. Overmedicating or medicating to reduce an elderly person's activity is often done by caregivers. Sometimes caregivers consider the use of medication to be a humane way to control behavior and allow the elderly to remain in a familiar environment. Overmedication of an older adult is not to be condoned. The nurse should review medications during home or clinic visit to assess whether the existing supply of medication matches what would be expected if someone were taking the medication as prescribed. A groggy or disoriented elderly person might be overmedicated if there is no obvious organic cause for the condition.

Nurse as Threat or Advocate

It might be difficult for the nurse to decide whether there is sufficient reason to suspect abuse. Caregivers and the elderly might be reluctant to share information or to answer questions. The nurse might be viewed as a threat rather than an asset, especially if the family or elder person fears removal from the home.

> Mrs. E. is a 67-year-old woman with Parkinson's disease. She is recently widowed. Although she can walk with a walker, she requires help with activities of daily living and needs assistance to travel outside the home. On a monthly home check, the nurse finds that Mrs. E.'s much younger stepsister Mrs. T. (42 years old) and her husband have moved in to help. Since the nurse's last visit, the furniture has been replaced with modern black lacquered pieces, and Mrs. T. has a new car. Mrs. E. tells the nurse that she misses her old furniture, but her brother-in-law did not like it. The new car has been bought with Mrs. E.'s funds and is driven by Mrs. T. Mrs. E.'s old car is used by Mrs. T.'s son because Mrs. E. "did not need it any more." Mrs. E. tells the nurse she is afraid that she does not have much money left in her bank account but begs the nurse not to do anything about it because she wants to stay in her home.

Mrs. E.'s concern about institutionalization is valid. Almost 50% of the cases handled by adult protective services are resolved by placing the elderly person in a nursing home (Lachs et al., 2002).

The overriding principle guiding the nurse's decision should be the safety and well-being of the elder client. The example provided is not an uncommon situation encountered by the community health nurse. If reasonable evidence of abuse is present, the nurse should report the circumstances and let the designated authorities investigate the case.

Legal Responsibilities of the Nurse

Forty-one states and the District of Columbia have laws that require the reporting of elder abuse (Gupta, 2007). Because the mechanism for reporting cases varies among states, nurses need to be aware of the protocols and reporting agencies in their states. Elder abuse is commonly not reported. An estimated 84% of cases are not reported to adult protective services (Kahan & Paris, 2003). Nurses affiliated with agencies serving the elderly population need to work with providers to increase reporting rates. Three factors that have been associated with higher reporting rates are lower socioeconomic status of the elderly population, more education of community professionals about elder maltreatment, and higher community agency service ratings (Wolf, 1999). Nurses in community and hospital settings need to take responsibility to learn the warning signs and the procedure for reporting elder abuse. Physicians often do not know the warning signs or understand reporting mechanisms (Kennedy, 2005; Taylor et al., 2006).

State definitions of elder abuse vary; some do not include neglect, and very few include financial exploitation. The specific agency to which the nurse reports varies according to the state involved but is usually the state's social service agency (adult protective services) or an independent senior service agency (office on aging) that investigates suspected cases of abuse. As in reporting child abuse, the nurse must state the circumstances that have led to the belief that a problem exists, the name of the individual, the address, and the name of the caregiver if it is known.

Autonomy Versus Safety

One of the most difficult issues in elder care is what to do when an older adult chooses to remain with an abusive caregiver. In cases in which immediate danger to life is present, the state may act and mandate action to safeguard the individual. However, the family preservation model is sometimes being applied to address the problem of elder abuse and neglect.

> An elderly couple, 68-year-old Marie and 79-year-old Ryan M., were forcibly removed from their home and placed in a nursing home. Mr. M. was blind and diabetic, and had numerous open wounds on both legs. Mrs. M. was confused and frequently disoriented. Their home reeked of urine. The couple had not paid their electric, telephone, and water bills for over a year. They had no water because of plumbing problems. They were malnourished and seldom shopped for food, although money was available. Mr. M. was prescribed insulin injections, but the couple seldom remembered to administer them. Both vigorously resisted institutionalization. Six months after placement, both are still adamant that they want to return home.

Usually the state acts only in extreme cases because of the limited resources for alternative placement of the elderly. For the most part, the law recognizes an adult's right to self-determination. Community health nurses frequently come in contact with elders who choose to remain in abusive or neglectful situations. Accepting the personal rights of elders might be one of the most difficult situations a nurse can face.

Reduction of Risk through Community Resources

Because maintaining older individuals' financial and physical independence is the single most important factor in reducing elder abuse, a thorough knowledge of the community resources available for elders is important. Most communities have senior centers and services for the aging that can provide some resources and support for senior citizens. A variety of home-related services to assist in independent living are also available. Examples of these services are home repair and maintenance services, fuel assistance programs, home visiting programs, daily telephone call programs, meal delivery services, special transportation services, and medically related services such as visits by home aides, registered nurses, physical therapists, and physicians. Respite care is an important resource for supporting families caring for aging parents. In rural areas, the nurse might need to help create informal networks of friends and volunteers to address the variety of needs. Ombudsman programs show promise for improving abuse reporting and the protection of the elderly in nursing homes (Jogerst et al., 2005). Chapter 28 provides more information on working with the aging population.

Assistance to Caregivers

Nurses can act as counselors and resource directors to assist families at risk for elder abuse. Caregiving is demanding and stressful, and caregivers need respite. The following are warning signs common among stressed caregivers (Capstead, 1993):

- Early signs
  - Multiple complaints
  - Anxiety
  - Growing depersonalization (beginning to distance from elder)
  - Fatigue
- Late signs
  - Depression
  - Open hostility

- Avoidance or distancing
- Misappropriation of financial resources

Capstead's list is a valuable screening assessment tool for community health nurses involved with elderly people and their caregivers. Counseling families to recognize caregiver stress and its impact on both the elder and the caregiver is essential. The nurse can teach the family about a variety of stress-reduction techniques. The nurse also serves as a resource person recommending community resources to assist with care and support. Beyond hotlines, support groups, and some classes offered by social service or home care agencies, few resources exist for elders at risk of abuse or their caregivers.

Respite care is an option for many families. A variety of types of respite care are available, but they are often not reimbursed. Adult daycare offers a supervised structured setting during the day while the caregiver is at work. Some facilities have begun to offer weekend programs so that family members can do chores or engage in other activities without concern for the elder's safety. Another form of respite is 24-hour care for limited periods to allow caregivers a break from their duties. Caregivers often get little benefit from respite care because respite care episodes are too brief or infrequent (Strang & Haughey, 1999).

Not all communities offer respite services, and not all families can afford to pay for such care. Health insurance does not always cover care associated with long-term illness, home care, medications, and supplies (see Chapter 4). Low-income families, because of their limited incomes, might have access to state and federally subsidized medical care and resources that some middle-class families do not.

Nurse's Role in Community Education and Advocacy

Community health nurses should become involved in exploring service options for elderly individuals and in educating themselves and the public on the problem of abuse of older individuals. These goals can be partly accomplished by designing and delivering educational programs to community groups and organizations or by advocating for legislation designed to help elders remain independent and assist elder caregivers whenever possible. Public understanding of the aging process and safeguards to ensure a safe and secure environment for the senior members of our communities will go a long way toward reducing the problems of elder abuse.

Violence is preventable. Community health nurses are in a unique position to address the health needs related to violent behavior. Both the American Nurses Association (2000) and the American Association of Colleges of Nursing (AACN, 1999)

have position statements on violence as a nursing issue. The AACN recommends specific competencies for nursing in the areas of prevention and treatment of violence. See Community Resources for Practice at the end of the chapter for information on how to link to these position statements and other Internet resources. The very nature of community nursing directs community health nurses toward establishing long-term relationships with individuals, families, and communities.

New roles are emerging in nursing as the discipline gains a better understanding of the health consequences of violence, the needs of survivors, and the physical and biologic evidence necessary to convict assailants. Two such emerging roles in nursing are those of the forensic nurse and the sexual assault nurse examiner, who specialize in evidence collection and preservation, and care of survivors and witnesses to violence (Campbell et al., 2005; Sekula, 2005).

The causes and consequences of violence are not readily eliminated. They are the result of multiple social and family influences. Community health nurses are in an ideal position to case-find and provide primary, secondary, and tertiary interventions to address violence and prevent it from occurring.

KEY IDEAS

1. Violence is a major public health concern.
2. Violent behavior is the result of the complex relationship of many issues and is influenced by sociologic, environmental, and individual factors.
3. Certain individual and group characteristics place people at risk for being victims or perpetrators of abusive behavior, but not all persons with risk factors become victims or abusers.
4. Women, children, and older adults are at special risk for family violence, because society has been reluctant to breach the family structure and dictate behavior.
5. There is mounting evidence that education, social pressure, and mandatory punishment for abusive behavior are effective in reducing such behavior.
6. Primary prevention is the single most important method for reducing violent behavior among family members and in the society at large.
7. Accomplishing the behavioral and social changes needed to mitigate violent activity or risk of victimization is a long-term activity.
8. Community/public health nurses are uniquely qualified and well situated to work with victims and abusers and engage in primary prevention efforts with individuals and community groups.

THE NURSING PROCESS IN PRACTICE
A Violent Family (by Jennifer Maurer Kliphouse)

Ms. Jones, a community health nurse, has been asked to do a home assessment of the Charles family as part of an intensive home visiting program instituted by Child Protection Services. When Ms. Jones visits Mrs. Charles, she finds a 20-year-old woman living at home with three children, aged 3 years, 2 years, and 7 months. Mrs. Charles is attempting to correct the 3-year-old by threatening to beat her with a belt if she does not stop pulling her sister's arm. The home is unkempt and cluttered, with dried food and several days' worth of dishes piled in the sink. The children are in their nightwear and are

just eating breakfast at noon. Mrs. Jones notices that there is no heat in the home, there is no running water in the kitchen, and Mrs. Charles is using the gas oven as a heat source. During the conversation that follows, Mrs. Charles shares her concerns about money, her anxiety about having to care for the children by herself, and her problems with the landlord. She relates that Mr. Charles has been ordered by the court to remain outside the home and undergo therapy because he has been found to be responsible for a broken arm suffered by the 3-year-old. She says the landlord does not respond to telephone calls about the housing situation. She also tells the nurse that she has visited the social services office for an application for financial assistance but that she has not completed the application. Mrs. Charles has about $20 and 2 days' supply of food left in the house.

ASSESSMENT

- The nurse will perform a complete brief financial assessment, including identification of all immediate income sources and expenses, to determine aid eligibility. Also, the nurse will evaluate the status of the application for financial assistance from the Temporary Aid to Needy Families (TANF) program.
- The nurse will evaluate the current food supply for nutritional content and quality.
- The nurse will conduct a home environment and safety assessment, both physical and psychologic.
- The nurse will take a brief history and conduct a physical examination of both Mrs. Charles and her three children. A standard growth and developmental assessment, as well as determination of current immunization status, will be included in the children's physical examinations.
- The nurse will discuss with Mrs. Charles Mr. Charles's compliance with the judicial court's restraining order and directive to undergo counseling. Because Mr. Charles has continued to stay with the family, the nurse will assess the degree and quality of interaction Mrs. Charles and the children have with Mr. Charles and any safety concerns stemming from these interactions.
- The nurse will assess Mrs. Charles's knowledge of parenting techniques and current practice.
- The available social support network for both Mrs. Charles and her children will be evaluated.

NURSING DIAGNOSES

- Impaired home maintenance related to insufficient financial resources as evidenced by available monetary funds of $20 and 2-day food supply in house
- Impaired parenting related to changes in family structure and legal stress as evidenced by threats of physical abuse against her three children
- Risk for other-directed violence related to stress as evidenced by past abusive behaviors of Mr. Charles and mother's threats against the 3-year-old
- Disabled family coping related to a court restraining order against Mr. Charles as evidenced by statements of anxiety about being sole care provider for her children

Nursing Diagnosis	Nursing Goals	Nursing Interventions	Outcomes and Evaluation
Impaired home maintenance related to insufficient financial resources as evidenced by available monetary funds of $20 and 2-day food supply in house	Family's financial situation and food resources will improve.	Review the client's TANF application and help the client complete the application process as necessary.	The TANF application is completed that day.
		Arrange for emergency food assistance, including a TANF emergency grant for food and funds for living expenses. Include same-day transportation arrangements to the social services office and meet with the social worker to complete these applications.	Food supplies are provided immediately, so Mrs. Charles can feed her children and decrease anxiety regarding food availability. In addition, the acceptance process for long-term programs begins, which addresses long-term needs of the family.
		Review and help the client contact other potential sources of financial assistance, such as church organizations and social service agencies.	The Women, Infants, and Children (WIC) program provides additional food supplements. After initial familial crises have abated, Mrs. Charles becomes involved in a local program that provides skills training.
	The family's home environment will improve.	Explain the process of environmental bacterial growth and insect infestation to encourage Mrs. Charles to clean the apartment.	Mrs. Charles verbalizes understanding of simple bacterial growth and the fact that crumbs and foodstuffs provide an inviting environment for insects.
		Review with Mrs. Charles normal child and infant behaviors, which include but are not limited to putting objects in their mouths as they explore their environment. With knowledge, Mrs. Charles will understand that foodstuffs on the floor may pose potential harm to her children's health.	Mrs. Charles notes that her children do tend to put many objects into their mouths. "I've been so anxious lately that I really haven't kept the house like I would like." On subsequent visits the nurse notes that, although the house is cluttered, the sink is clear of dishes and the apartment is swept.
		Contact the health department to perform an inspection of the apartment building. The health inspection will direct the landlord to complete necessary maintenance to provide a safe living environment for all tenants. At this point it would be important to note that Mrs. Charles may have to explore other immediate housing options, because the landlord may be unwilling to make necessary repairs or illegally retaliate for health department notification through eviction.	The health department inspects the building and finds multiple code violations. Although Mrs. Charles expresses "worry" that the landlord will find out that "it was because of me," the landlord has made simple dwelling improvements and has not engaged in verbal intimidation or investigated the source of the report.

WEB

Find additional **Care Plans** for this client on the book's website.

LEARNING BY EXPERIENCE AND REFLECTION

1. Follow several reported family abuse cases in the newspaper to their conclusion in the court system. Review the life experiences of the individuals involved, both abusers and abused, and try to understand the family dynamics of each case.
2. Become familiar with attempts to change laws related to abuse. What are the proposed new provisions? Why were they proposed? What are the positions of advocates and opponents of the new law? Determine your position on the effort.
3. Consult with fellow students and health professionals about their experiences with abusive situations. How were the situations resolved? Were the individuals involved satisfied that the victims were adequately protected? What would you do under similar circumstances?
4. Explore community resources that might be valuable referrals for children, spouses, or elders in need. Review the funding of such resources. Are they adequate to meet the needs as identified by the agency personnel and persons assisted?
5. Review state and local funding for support programs for abuse victims and perpetrators. Correspond with your local state representative to determine his or her position on funding priorities for resources for these programs.
6. Discover whether your community has respite care for caregivers. If none is available, what actions could you take to encourage the community to provide such a resource?
7. Reflect on the meaning of family violence to you. What experiences with social, intimate, or family violence have you had? How do your experiences and background affect your reaction to violent situations and victims of family violence?

COMMUNITY RESOURCES FOR PRACTICE

Information about many of the following organizations is found on their websites, which can be accessed through the **WebLinks** section of this book's website at *http://evolve.elsevier.com/Maurer/community/*.

Local Organizations
The following resources are usually available in a local community. Check the local phone book or contact the local library for ways to contact these resources.

Child Abuse
Department of Social Services
Big Brother and Big Sister programs
Home care assistance program
Prenatal classes
Family preservation programs

Foster grandparent program
Young Women's Christian Association (YWCA)

Intimate Partner Violence
Department of Social Services
Local legal assistance organizations
Local legal defense fund
YWCA
Crisis telephone line
Shelters

Elder Mistreatment
Meal programs, such as Meals on Wheels
Senior centers
Senior daycare centers
Senior companion programs
State or local office on aging

National Organizations

Child Abuse
Children's Defense Fund
Child Welfare Information Gateway, U.S. Department of Health and Human Services
Domestic Abuse Intervention Project
Grassroots Shelter Directory—United States
National Center for Education in Maternal and Child Health
National Center for Missing and Exploited Children
National Runaway Switchboard
National Council on Child Abuse and Family Violence
Parents Anonymous

Intimate Partner Violence
Family Violence Prevention Fund
National Advisory Council on Violence against Women
National Coalition against Domestic Violence
Violence against Women, National Women's Health Information Center
VIOLET: Law and Abused Women (website)
Women's Law Initiative
Stalking Resource Center
Emerge: A Men's Counselling Service on Domestic Violence
National Domestic Violence Hotline

Elder Mistreatment
National Center on Elder Abuse
Administration on Aging, Elder Abuse Prevention
American Association of Retired Persons (AARP)
National Council of Senior Citizens
National Institute on Aging
Older Women's League

STUDY AIDS   http://evolve.elsevier.com/Maurer/community/

Visit the Evolve website for this book to find the following study and assessment materials:

- Quiz
- Web Scenario
- Critical Thinking Questions and Answers for Case Studies

- Care Plans
- *Healthy People* Updates
- Glossary

REFERENCES

Administration on Aging. (2004). *Fact sheets: Elder abuse prevention*. Washington, DC: Department of Health and Human Services. Retrieved June 20, 2007 from *http://www.aoa.gov/press/fact/alpha/fact_elder_abuse.asp*.

Allender, D. M. (2001). *Gangs in middle America* (FBI Law Enforcement Bulletin 70[12]1-15). Quantico, VA: FBI Academy.

American Academy of Nursing. (1993). AAN Expert Panel working paper: Violence as a nursing priority: Policy implications. *Nursing Outlook, 41*(2), 83-92.

American Academy of Pediatrics. (2007). *Understanding the impact of media on children and teens*. Retrieved July 19, 2007 from *http://www.aap.org/family/mediaimpact.htm*.

American Association of Colleges of Nursing. (1999). *AACN Position statement: Violence as a public health problem*. Retrieved June 25, 2007 from *http://www.aacn.nche.edu/Publications/positions/violence.htm*.

American College of Emergency Physicians. (2006). *Domestic violence*. Retrieved July 22, 2007 from *http://www.acep.org/webportal/PatientsConsumers/HealthSubjectsByTopic/Violence/domviolence.htm*.

American Nurses Association. (2000). *Position statement on violence against women*. Washington, DC: Author.

Battin-Pearson, S. R., Thornberry, T. P., & Hawkins, J. D. (1998, October). *Gang membership, delinquent peers and delinquent behavior* (Juvenile Justice Bulletin). Washington, DC: U.S. Department of Justice, Office of Justice Programs, Office of Juvenile Justice and Delinquency Prevention.

Blachman, D. R., & Hinshaw, S. P. (2002). Patterns of friendship among girls with and without attention-deficit/hyperactivity disorder. *Journal of Abnormal Child Psychology, 30*(6), 625-640.

Bollard, J. M., McCallum, D. M., Liam, B., et al. (2001). Hopelessness and violence among inner-city youths. *Maternal and Child Health Journal, 5*, 237-244.

Brandford, C., Brunnel, S., Moe, M., et al. (2004). Runaway behavior of children in Washington state DCFS custody. Seattle: Office of Children's Administration Research.

Brandl, B., & Horan, D. L. (2002). Domestic violence in later life: An overview for health care providers. *Women and Health, 35*(2/3), 41-54.

Browne, K. (1989). The health visitor's role in screening for child abuse. *Health Visitor, 62*(9), 275-277.

Bureau of Justice Statistics. (2003). *Statistics about—*. Retrieved June 14, 2007, from *http://www.ojp.usdoj.gov/bjs/welcome.html*.

Bureau of Justice Statistics. (2007). *Crime and the nation's households, 2005*. Retrieved June 25, 2007 from *http://www.ojp.usdoj.gov/bjs/abstract/cnh05.htm*.

Campbell, J. C., Webster, D., Koziol-McLain, J., et al. (2003). Risk factors for femicide in abusive relationship: Results from a multisite case control study. *American Journal of Public Health, 93*, 1089-1097.

Campbell, R., Patterson, D., & Lichty, L. F. (2005). The effectiveness of sexual assault nurse examiners (SANE) programs: A review of the psychological, medical, legal, and community outcomes. *Trauma, Violence, and Abuse, 6*(4), 313-329.

Capstead, L. (1993). Families of the elderly. In D. L. Carnevali & M.Patrick (Eds.), *Nursing management for the elderly* (3rd ed.; pp. 239-249). Philadelphia: J. B. Lippincott.

Carll, E. K. (2006, March 29). *Testimony on behalf of the American Psychological Association before the United States Senate Subcommittee on the Constitution, Civil Rights and Property Rights*. Washington, DC: American Psychological Association. Retrieved July 19, 2007 from *http://www.apa.org/ppo/childmedia/testimony2.html*.

Center for Children and Families in the Justice System. (2004). *Helping children thrive: Supporting woman abuse survivors as mothers*. Retrieved July 22, 2007 from *http://www.lfcc.on.ca/HCT_SWASM_4.html*.

Centers for Disease Control and Prevention. (2003). First reports evaluating the effectiveness of strategies for preventing violence: Early childhood home visitation and firearms laws. Findings from the Taskforce on Community Prevention Services. *Morbidity and Mortality Weekly Report, Recommendations and Reports, 52*(RR-14).

Centers for Disease Control and Prevention. (2006a). Physical dating violence among high school students—United States, 2003. *Mortality and Morbidity Weekly Report, 55*(19), 532-535.

Centers for Disease Control and Prevention. (2006b). *Intimate partner violence: Overview*. Retrieved July 22, 2007 from *http://www.cdc.gov/ncipc/factsheets/ipvfacts.htm*.

Chaffin, M., Bonner, B. L., & Hill, R. F. (2001). Family preservation and family support programs: Child maltreatment outcomes across client risk levels and program types. *Child Abuse and Neglect, 25*(10), 1269-1289.

Children's Defense Fund. (2005). *The state of America's children, 2005*. Washington, DC: Author.

Child Welfare League of America. (2004). *Number of child abuse and neglect fatalities (NCANDS), 2004*. Retrieved July 22, 2007 from *http://ndas.cwla.org/data_stats/access/predefined?Report.asp?PageMode=1&%ReportID=216&%20GUID+{4A2228E2-91F3*.

Cohen, M., Halevi-Levin, S., Gagin, R., et al. (2006). Development of a screening tool for identifying elderly people at risk of abuse by their caregivers. *Journal of Aging and Health, 18*(5), 660-685.

Coker, A. L., Davis, K. E., Arias, I., et al. (2002). Physical and mental health effects of intimate partner violence for men and women. *American Journal of Preventive Medicine, 23*, 260-268.

Coker, A. L., McKeown, R. E., Sanderson, M., et al. (2000). Severe dating violence and quality of life among South Carolina high school students. *American Journal of Preventive Medicine, 19*, 220-227.

Committee on Public Education. (2001). Policy statement, American Academy of Pediatrics: Media violence. *Pediatrics, 108*(5), 1222-1226.

Crandall, M., Nathens, A. B., Kernic, M. A., et al. (2004). Predicting future injury among women in abusive relationships. *Journal of Trauma, 56*(4), 906-912.

Cunradi, C. B., Caetano, R., Clark, C., et al. (2000). Neighborhood poverty as a predictor of intimate partner violence among white, black, and Hispanic couples in the United States: A multilevel analysis. *Annals of Epidemiology, 10*(5), 297-308.

DeVoe, J. F., Peter, K., Kaufman, P., et al. (2004). *Indicators of school crime and safety: 2004*. (No. NCES 2005–002/NCJ 205290). Washington, DC: U.S. Government Printing Office.

DeVoe, J. F., Peter, K., Noonan, M., et al. (2005). *Indicators of school crime and safety: 2005*. (No. NCES 2006–001/NCJ 210697). Washington, DC: U.S. Government Printing Office.

Domestic Abuse Intervention Project. (nd). *Wheel gallery*. Minnesota Program Development. Retrieved August 17, 2007 from *http://www.duluth-model.org*.

DuRant, R. H., Champion, H., & Wolfson, M. (2006). The relationship between watching professional wrestling on television and engaging in date fighting among high school students. *Pediatrics, 118*(2), 2005-2098.

Egley, A., & Ritz, C. E. (2006, April). *Highlights of the 2004 National Youth Gang Survey* [Fact sheet]. Washington, DC: U.S. Department of Justice, Office of Justice Programs, Office of Juvenile Justice and Delinquency Prevention.

Ernst, A. A., Weiss, S. J., Del Castillo, C., et al. (2007). Witnessing intimate partner violence as a child does not increase the likelihood of becoming an adult intimate partner violence victim. *Academic Emergency Medicine, 14*(5), 411-418.

Federal Interagency Forum on Child and Family Statistics. (2007). *America's children: Key national indicators of well-being, 2007*. Washington, DC: U.S. Government Printing Office.

Fekkes, M., Pijpers, F. I. M., & Verloove-Vanhorick, S. P. (2004). Bullying behavior and associations with psychosomatic complaints and depression in victims. *Journal of Pediatrics, 144*, 17-22.

Fergusson, D. M., Grant, H., Horwood, L. J., et al. (2006). Randomized trial of the Early Start program of home visitation: Parent and family outcomes. *Pediatrics, 117,* 781-786.

Fisher, B. S., Cullen, F. T., & Turner, M. G. (2000). *Sexual victimization of college women.* Washington, DC: U.S. Department of Justice, Office of Justice Programs.

Fluke, J. D., Shusterman, G. R., Hollinshead, D., et al. (2005). *Reporting and recurrence of child maltreatment: Findings from NCANDS.* Report submitted to the Office of the Assistant Secretary for Planning and Evaluation. Washington, DC: U.S. Department of Health and Human Services, Administration on Children, Youth and Families.

Fox, G. L., & Benson, M. L. (2006). Household and neighborhood contexts of intimate partner violence. *Health Reports, 121*(4), 419-427.

Fox, J., Elliot, D., Kerlikowske, R., et al. (2003). *Bully prevention is crime prevention.* Washington, DC: Fight Crime: Invest in Kids.

Fulmer, T. (2002). Elder mistreatment. *Annual Review of Nursing Research, 20,* 369-395.

Gelles, R. J., & Cornell, C. P. (1990). *Intimate violence in families* (2nd ed.). London: Sage.

Gelles, R. J., & Straus, M. A. (1988). *The definitive study of the causes and consequences of abuse in the American family.* New York: Simon & Schuster.

General Accounting Office. (March, 2002). *Nursing homes: More can be done to protect residents from abuse.* (Document GAO-02-312). Report to Congressional requesters. Washington, DC: U.S. Government Printing Office. Retrieved June 24, 2007 from *http://www.gao.gov/new.items/d02312.pdf.*

Gershoff, E. T. (2002). Corporal punishment by parents and associated child behaviors and experiences: A meta-analytic and theoretical review. *Psychological Bulletin, 128,* 534-579.

Gielen, A. C., O'Campo, P. J., Campbell, J. C., et al. (2000). Women's opinions about domestic violence screening and mandatory reporting. *American Journal of Preventive Medicine, 19,* 279-285.

Government Accountability Office. (2007). *Nursing home reform: Continued attention is needed to improve quality of care in small but significant share of homes. Testimony before the U.S. Senate Special Committee on Aging by Kathryn G. Allen, director of health care.* Washington, DC: Author.

Govindshenoy, M., & Spencer, N. (2007). Abuse of the disabled child: A systematic review of population-based studies. *Child: Care, Health and Development, 33*(5), 552-558. Retrieved March 20, 2008 from *http://www.blackwell-synergy.com/toc/cch/33/5.*

Gupta, M. (2007). Mandatory reporting laws and the emergency physician. *Annals of Emergency Medicine, 49*(3), 369-376.

Hatton, D. C. (1997). Managing health problems among homeless women with children in a transitional shelter. *Journal of Nursing Scholarship, 29*(1), 33-37.

Haugaard, J. J., & Seri, L. G. (2004). Stalking and other forms of intrusive contact among adolescents and young adults from the perspective of the person initiating the intrusive contact. *Criminal Justice and Behavior, 31*(1), 37-54.

Heyman, R. E., & Slep, A. M. S. (2002). Do child abuse and interpersonal violence lead to adulthood family violence? *Journal of Marriage and the Family, 64*(4), 864-870.

Holt, V. L., Kernic, M. A., Wolf, M. E., et al. (2003). Do protection orders affect the likelihood of future partner violence and injury? *American Journal Preventive Medicine, 24,* 16-21.

Holtzworth-Munroe, A., Meehan, J. C., Herron, K., et al. (2000). Testing the Holtzworth-Munroe & Stuart (1994) batterer typology. *Journal of Consultation and Clinical Psychology, 68,* 1000-1019.

Howell, J. C., & Decker, S. H. (1999). *The youth gangs, drugs, and violence connection* (Juvenile Justice Bulletin). Washington, DC: U.S. Department of Justice, Office of Justice Programs, Office of Juvenile Justice and Delinquency Prevention.

Howell, J. C., & Lynch, J. P. (2000). Youth gangs in school (Juvenile Justice Bulletin). National Youth Gang Survey trends from 1996-2000 [Fact sheet]. Washington, DC: U.S. Department of Justice, Office of Justice Programs, Office of Juvenile Justice and Delinquency Prevention.

Huesmann, L. R., Moise-Titus, J., & Podolski, C. L. (2003). Longitudinal relations between children's exposure to TV violence and their aggressive and violent behavior in young adulthood: 1977-1992. *Developmental Psychology, 39,* 201-221.

Hurt, H., Malmud, E., & Brodsky, J. (2001). Exposure to violence: Psychological and academic correlates to child witnesses. *Archives of Pediatric and Adolescent Medicine, 155,* 1351-1357.

Jackson, H., Philip, E., Nutall, R. L., et al. (2002). Traumatic brain injury: A hidden consequence for battered women. *Professional Psychology, 33*(1), 39-45.

Janssen, I., Craig, W. M., Boyce, W. F., et al. (2004). Associations between overweight and obesity with bullying behaviors in school-aged children. *Pediatrics, 113*(5), 1187-1194.

Jecker, N. S. (1993). Privacy beliefs and the violent family: Extending the ethical argument for physician intervention. *Journal of the American Medical Association, 269,* 776-780.

Jogerst, G., Daly, J., & Hartz, A. (2005). Ombudsman program characteristics related to nursing home abuse reporting. *Journal of Gerontological Social Work, 46*(1), 85-98.

Kahan, F. S., & Paris, E. C. (2003). Why elder abuse continues to elude the health care system. *Mount Sinai Journal of Medicine, 70*(1), 62-68.

Kaltiala-Heino, R., Rimpela, M., Marttunen, M., et al. (1999). Bullying, depression and suicidal ideation in Finnish adolescents: School survey. *British Medical Journal, 319,* 348-351.

Kennedy, R. D. (2005). Elder abuse and neglect: The experience, knowledge, and attitudes of primary care physicians. *Family Medicine, 37*(7), 481-485.

Kim, Y. S., Koh, Y., & Leventhal, B. (2005). School bullying and suicide risk in Korean middle school students. *Pediatrics, 115*(2), 357-363.

Kuhns, J. B. (2005). The dynamic nature of the drug use/serious violence relationship: A multi-causal approach. *Violence and Victims, 20*(4), 433-454.

Kwong, M. J., Bartholomew, K., Henderson, A. J., et al. (2003). The intergenerational transmission of relationship violence. *Journal Family Psychology, 17,* 288-301.

Lachs, M. S., Williams, C. S., O'Brien, S., et al. (2002). Adult protective service use and nursing home placement. *Gerontologist, 42,* 734-739.

Lackey, C. (2003). Violent family heritage, the transition to adulthood, and later partner violence. *Journal of Family Issues, 24,* 74-98.

Langford, D. R. (1996). Predicting unpredictability: A model of women's processes of predicting battering men's violence. *Scholarly Inquiry for Nursing Practice, 10*(4), 387-390.

Leary, M. R., Kowaleski, R. M., Smith, L., et al. (2003). Teasing, rejection, and violence: Case studies of the school shootings. *Aggressive Behavior, 29,* 202-214.

Levine, J. M. (2003, October). Elder neglect and abuse: A primer for primary care physicians. *Geriatrics, 58,* 37-44.

Littell, J. H. (2001). Client participation and outcomes of intensive family preservation services. *Social Work Research, 25,* 103-113.

Lyznicki, M. S., McCaffree, M. A., & Robinowitz, C. B. (2004). Childhood bullying: Implications for physicians. *American Family Physician, 70,* 1723-1730.

Mandell, D. S., Walrath, C. M., Manteuffel, B., et al. (2005). The prevalence and correlates of abuse among children with autism served in comprehensive community-based mental health settings. *Child Abuse and Neglect, 29*(12), 1359-1372.

Martin, S. L., Mackie, L., Kupper, L. L., et al. (2001). Physical abuse of women before, during, and after pregnancy. *Journal of the American Medical Association, 285,* 1581-1584.

Max, W., Rice, D. P., Finkelstein, E., et al. (2004). The economic toll of intimate partner violence against women in the United States. *Violence and Victims, 19*(3), 259-272.

McFarlane, J., Christoffel, K., Bateman, L., et al. (1991). Assessing for abuse: Self-report versus nurse interview. *Public Health Nursing, 8,* 245-250.

McFarlane, J., Malecha, A., Gist, J., et al. (2004). Protection orders and intimate partner violence: An 18-month study of 150 black, Hispanic, and white women. *American Journal of Public Health, 94*(4), 613-618.

McFarlane, J., Parker, B., & Soeken, K. (1996). Physical abuse, smoking, and substance use during pregnancy: Prevalence, interrelationships, and effects on birth weight. *Journal of*

Obstetric, Gynecologic and Neonatal Nursing, 25(4), 313-320.

McFarlane, J., Parker, B., Soeken, K., et al. (1992). Assessing for abuse during pregnancy: Severity and frequency of injuries and associated entry into prenatal care. *Journal of the American Medical Association, 267,* 3176-3178.

Meeks-Sjostrom, D. (2004). A comparison of three measures of elder abuse. *Journal of Nursing Scholarship, 36*(3), 247-250.

Miller, M., Azrael, D., & Hemenway, D. (2002). Rates of household firearm ownership and homicide across U.S. regions and states, 1988-1997. *American Journal of Public Health, 92*(12), 1988-1993.

Murry, S. K., Baker, A. W., & Lewin, L. (2000). Screening families with young children for child maltreatment potential. *Pediatric Nursing, 26,* 47-54.

Nansel, T. R., Overpeck, M. D., Haynie, D. L., et al. (2003). Relationships between bullying and violence among U.S. youth. *Archives of Pediatrics and Adolescent Medicine, 157,* 348-353.

Nansel, T. R., Overpeck, M., Pilla, R. S., et al. (2001). Bullying behaviors among U.S. youth: Prevalence and association with psychosocial adjustment. *Journal of the American Medical Association, 285*(16), 2094-2100.

National Advisory Council on Violence against Women & Violence against Women Office. (ND). *Toolkit to end violence against women.* Retrieved January 12, 2004 from *http://toolkit.ncjrs.org/default.htm.*

National Center on Addictions and Substance Abuse. (2000). *Analysis of the arrestee drug abuse monitoring program.* Washington, DC: U.S. Department of Justice, National Institute of Justice.

National Center for Education Statistics. (2006). *Indicators of school crime and safety: 2006.* Retrieved July 23, 2007 from *http://nces.ed.gov/programs/crimeindicators/.*

National Center for Injury Prevention and Control. (2003). *Cost of intimate partner violence against women in the United States.* Atlanta: Centers for Disease Control and Prevention.

National Center for Injury Prevention and Control. (2006). *Child maltreatment: Facts at a glance.* Atlanta: Centers for Disease Control and Prevention. Retrieved June 24, 2007 from *http://www.cdc.gov/ncipc/dvp/CM_Data_Sheet.pdf.*

National Center for Injury Prevention and Control. (2007). *Youth violence: Facts at a glance.* Atlanta: Centers for Disease Control and Prevention. Retrieved June 24, 2007 from *http://www.cdc.gov/ncipc/dvp/YV_DataSheet.pdf.*

National Center for Victims of Crime. (2006). *Stalking fact sheet.* Retrieved July 23, 2007 from *http://www.ncvc.org/src/AGP.net/components/DocumentViewer/download.aspxnz?dOCUMENTid=40616.*

National Clearinghouse on Child Abuse and Neglect. (2002). *What is child maltreatment?* (fact sheet). Washington, DC: U.S. Department of Health and Human Services, Administration for Children and Families. Retrieved November 24, 2003 from *http://nccanch.acf.hhs.gov/pubs/factsheets/childmal.cfm.*

National Clearinghouse on Child Abuse and Neglect. (2005). *Children and domestic violence: A bulletin for professionals.* Washington, DC: U.S. Department of Health and Human Services, Administration for Children and Families, Children's Bureau.

National Committee for the Prevention of Elder Abuse & National Adult Protective Services Association. (2006). *The 2004 survey of state adult protective services: Abuse of adults 60 years of age and older.* Prepared for the National Center on Elder Abuse. Retrieved June 25, 2007 from *http://www.elderabusecenter.org/pdf/2-14-06%20FINAL%2060+REPORT.pdf.*

National Research Council. (2002). *Elder mistreatment: Abuse, neglect, and exploitation in an aging America.* Washington, DC: National Academy Press.

Okoro, C. A., Nelson, D. E., Mercy, J. A., et al. (2005). Prevalence of household firearms and firearm-storage practices in the 50 states and the District of Columbia: Findings from the Behavioral Risk Factor Surveillance System, 2002. *Pediatrics, 116*(3), 370-376.

Palm Bay Police Department. (2007). *A parents' guide to gangs.* Palm Bay, FL: Palm Bay Police Department, Criminal Intelligence Unit. Retrieved July 20, 2007 from *http://www.palmbayflorida.org/police/public/gang_parents_guide.html.*

Pleck, E. (1987). *Domestic tyranny: The making of American social policy against family violence from Colonial times to the present.* New York: Oxford University Press.

Plichta, S. B. (2004). Intimate partner violence and physical health consequences: Policy and practice implications. *Journal of Interpersonal Violence, 19*(11), 1296-1323.

Poirier, L. (1997). The importance of screening for domestic violence in all women. *Nurse Practitioner: American Journal of Primary Health Care, 22*(5), 105-106, 108, 111-112.

Rennison, C. M. (2003). *Intimate partner violence, 1993-2001* (Publication NCJ197838). Washington, DC: U.S. Department of Justice, Bureau of Justice Statistics.

Rew, L. (2003). A theory of taking care of oneself grounded in experiences of homeless youth. *Nursing Research, 52*(4), 234-239.

Rhea, M. H., Chafey, K. H., Dohner, V. A., et al. (1996). The silent victims of domestic violence—Who will speak? *Journal of Child and Adolescent Psychiatric Nursing, 9*(3), 7-15.

Roberts, C., & Quillian, J. (1992). Preventing violence through primary care intervention. *Nurse Practitioner, 17*(8), 62-64, 67-70.

Roberts, T. A., Klein, J. D., & Fisher, S. (2003). Longitudinal effect of intimate partner abuse on high-risk behavior among adolescents. *Archives of Pediatrics and Adolescent Medicine, 157*(9), 875-881.

Rodriguez, M. A., McLoughlin, E., Nah, H., et al. (2001). Mandatory reporting of intimate partner violence to police: What do emergency department patients think? *Journal of the American Medical Association, 286*(5), 580-583.

Rosewater, A. (2003). *Promoting prevention, targeting teens: An emerging agenda to reduce domestic violence.* San Francisco: Family Violence Prevention Fund. Retrieved June 25, 2007 from *http://www.endabuse.org/field/PromotingPrevention1003.pdf.*

Salazar, C. F., Baker, C. K., Price, A. W., et al. (2003). Moving beyond the individual: Examining the effects of domestic violence policies on social norms. *American Journal of Community Psychology, 32*(3/4), 253-264.

Sekula, L. K. (2005). The advance practice forensic nurse in the emergency department. *Topics in Emergency Medicine, 27*(1), 5-14.

Shugarman, L. R., Fris, B. E., Wolf, R. S., et al. (2003). Identifying older people at risk of abuse during routine screening practices. *Journal of the American Geriatrics Society, 51,* 24-51.

Slade, E. P., & Wissow, L. S. (2004). Spanking in early childhood and later behavior problems: A prospective study of infants and young toddlers. *Pediatrics, 113*(5), 1321-1330.

Smith, P. H., White, J. W., & Holland, L. J. (2003). A longitudinal perspective on dating violence among adolescent and college-age women. *American Journal of Public Health, 93,* 1104-1109.

Sorenson, S. B. (2003). Funding public health: The public's willingness to pay for domestic violence prevention programming. *American Journal of Public Health, 93*(8), 1934-1938.

Sorenson, S. B., & Wiebe, D. J. (2004). Weapons in the lives of battered women. *American Journal of Public Health, 94*(8), 1412-1417.

Strang, V., & Haughey, M. (1999). Respite: A coping strategy for family caregivers. *Western Journal of Nursing Research, 21,* 450-470.

Stringham, P. (1998). Violence anticipatory guidance. *Pediatric Clinics of North America, 45,* 439-448.

Sullivan, P. M., & Knutson, J. F. (2000). Maltreatment and disability: A population-based epidemiological study. *Child Abuse and Neglect, 24,* 1257-1273.

Sullivan, T. N., Farrell, A. D., & Kliewer, W. (2006). Peer victimization in early adolescence: Association between physical and relational victimization and drug use, aggression, and delinquent behaviors among urban middle school students. *Development and Psychopathology, 18,* 119-137.

Taylor, D. K., Bachuwa, G., Evans, J., et al. (2006). Assessing barriers to the identification of elder abuse and neglect: A community-wide survey of primary care physicians. *Journal of the National Medical Association, 9*(3), 403-404.

Thompson, M. P., Kingree, J. B., & Desai, S. (2004). Gender differences in long-term health consequences of physical abuse of children:

Data from a nationally representative survey. *American Journal of Public Health, 94*(4), 599-604.

Tjaden, P., & Thoennes, N. (2000). *Extent, nature, and consequences of intimate partner violence: Findings from the National Violence against Women Survey.* Washington, DC: National Institute of Justice and Centers for Disease Control and Prevention.

Turner, H. A., Finkelhor, D., & Ormrod, R. (2006). The effect of lifetime victimization on the mental health of children and adolescents. *Social Science and Medicine, 62*(1), 13-27.

Ulrich, Y. C., Cain, K. C., Sugg, N. K., et al. (2003). Medical care utilization patterns in women with diagnosed domestic violence. *American Journal of Preventive Medicine, 24*, 9-15.

United Nations Children's Fund (UNICEF). (2005). *Summary report: Violence against disabled children.* New York: United Nations, UNICEF. Retrieved July 21, 2007 from *http://www. violencestudy.org/IMG/doc/UNICRF_- _Violence_Against_Disabled_Children_Report_ -_Submitted_Version.doc.*

U.S. Department of Health and Human Services. (2000). *Healthy people 2010: Understanding and improving health* (2nd ed.). Washington, DC: U.S. Government Printing Office. Retrieved June 24, 2007 from *http://www.healthypeople. gov/document.*

U.S. Department of Health and Human Services, Administration on Children, Youth and Families. (2005). *Child maltreatment 2003.* Washington, DC: U.S. Government Printing Office. Retrieved June 25, 2007 from *http://www. acf.hhs.gov/programs/cb/pubs/cm05/cm05.pdf.*

U.S. Department of Health and Human Services, Administration on Children, Youth and Families. (2007). *Child maltreatment 2005.* Washington, DC: U.S. Government Printing Office. Retrieved June 25, 2007 from *http://www. acf.hhs.gov/programs/cb/pubs/cm05/cm05.pdf.*

U.S. Department of Health and Human Services. (2004). *Firearms deaths of children and teens by age, manner, and race/Hispanic origin, 2002.* Washington, DC: National Center for Injury Control and Prevention. Retrieved June 24, 2007 from *http://www.cdc.gov/ncipc/wisqars.*

U.S. Department of Justice. (2005). *Highlights of the 2002-2003 National Youth Gang Surveys.* Washington, DC: Office of Justice Programs, Office of Juvenile Justice and Delinquency Prevention.

van der Wal, M. F., de Wit, C. A. M., & Hirasing, R. A. (2003). Psychosocial health among young victims and offenders of direct and indirect bullying. *Pediatrics, 111*(6), 1312-1317.

Vermeiren, R., Schwab-Stone, M., Deboutte, D., et al. (2003). Violence exposure and substance use in adolescents: Findings from three countries. *Pediatrics, 111*, 535-540.

Waalen, J., Goodwin, M. M., Spitz, A. M., et al. (2000). Screening for intimate partner violence by health care providers. *American Journal of Preventive Medicine, 19*, 230-237.

Walker, L. E. (1979). *The battered woman.* New York: Harper & Row.

Walton, E. (1996). Family functioning as a measure of success in intensive family preservation services. *Journal of Family Social Work, 1*(3), 67-82.

Walton, E. (2001). Combining abuse and neglect investigations with intensive family preservation services: An innovative approach to protecting children. *Research on Social Work Practice, 11*, 627-644.

Warriner, A. (1994). Zap! Pow! Biff! Social learning theory suggests a child may copy acts of aggression seen through the media. *Nursing Standard, 8*(4), 44-45.

Weir, L. A., Etelson, D., & Brand D. A. (2006). Parents' perceptions of neighborhood safety and children's physical activity. *Preventive Medicine, 43*(3), 212-217.

Westat, Chapin Hall Center for Children, & James Bell Associates. (2002). *Evaluation of family preservation and reunification programs: Final Report.* Submitted to Department of Health and Human Services, Assistant Secretary for Planning and Evaluation. Retrieved July 21, 2007 from *http://aspe.hhs.gov/hsp/evalfam-pres94/Final/index.htm.*

Wiist, W. H., & McFarlane, J. (1999). The effectiveness of an abuse assessment protocol in public health prenatal clinics. *American Journal of Public Health, 89*, 1217-1221.

Williams-White, D. (1986). Self help and advocacy: An alternative approach to helping battered women. In L. J. Dickstein & C. C. Nadelson (Eds.), *Family violence: Emerging issues of a national crisis* (pp. 45-60). Washington, DC: American Psychological Press.

Wolf, R. S. (1999). Factors affecting the rate of elder abuse reporting to a state protective services program. *Gerontologist, 39*, 222-228.

Wolke, D., Woods, S., Bloomfield, L., et al. (2001). Bullying involvement in primary school and common health problems. *Archives of Disease in Childhood, 85*, 197-201.

Zalecki, C. A., & Hinshaw, S. P. (2004). Overt and relational aggression in girls with attention deficit hyperactivity disorder. *Journal of Clinical Child and Adolescent Psychology, 33*(1), 125-137.

SUGGESTED READINGS

Centers for Disease Control and Prevention. (2006). *Intimate partner violence: Overview.* Retrieved July 22, 2007 from *http://www.cdc.gov/ncipc/ factsheets/ipvfacts.htm.*

Federal Interagency Forum on Child and Family Statistics. (2007). *America's children: Key national indicators of well-being, 2007.* Washington, DC: U.S. Government Printing Office.

Humphreys, J. C., & Campbell, J. C. (2003). *Family violence and nursing practice.* Philadelphia: Lippincott Williams & Wilkins.

Prothrow-Stith, D., & Spivak, H. R. (2004). *Murder is no accident: Understanding and preventing youth violence in America.* San Francisco: Jossey-Bass.

Renzetti, C. M., Edleson, J. L., & Bergen, R. K. (2000). *Sourcebook on violence against women.* Newbury Park, CA: Sage.

Thornton, T. N., Craft, C. A., Dahlberg, L. L., et al (2002). *Best practices of youth violence prevention: A sourcebook for community action* (rev. ed.). Atlanta: Centers for Disease Control and Prevention, National Center for Injury Prevention and Control.

Adolescent Sexual Activity and Teenage Pregnancy

Frances A. Maurer

FOCUS QUESTIONS

How prevalent is sexual activity among U.S. adolescents?

What are some of the factors that influence a teenager's decision to engage in sexual activity?

What are some of the risks associated with early sexual activity?

What are some of the reasons teenagers become pregnant?

What are some of the factors associated with increased risk for pregnancy for young girls?

What are some of the social costs of teenage pregnancy?

What are some of the personal costs associated with early parenting for adolescents and their infants?

How can community/public health nurses act to reduce the risks of teenage pregnancy?

What are the nurse's responsibilities as a health professional visiting an at-risk family?

What community programs are available to assist teenage parents and their children?

CHAPTER OUTLINE

KEY TERMS

Abstinence-only programs
Comprehensive sex education programs
Life options programs

Low birth weight
Risky behaviors
Teenage sexual activity

Unintended pregnancy
Unprotected intercourse
Virginity pledgers

Teenage sexual activity involves sexual intercourse and other sexual acts in adolescents younger than 20 years of age. Early sexual activity is very common and is accompanied by major public health concerns, such as increased risk for sexually transmitted diseases (STDs), pregnancy, and early parenthood. Adolescent parents are more likely to have substantial problems adjusting to parenthood and acquiring adequate parenting skills. Their children are often affected by their difficulties. Children born to younger teens are at greater risk for health problems than children born to mothers in other age groups (Martin et al., 2006; Menacker et al., 2004).

Although substantial progress has been made in educating teens and influencing sexual behaviors, much remains to be done. The teenage pregnancy rate is at its lowest since 1993, and as a result both the birth rate and the abortion rate among teenage girls have also declined. There is evidence to suggest that teens are delaying the start of sexual activity, but by age 18 to 19 years, the majority of both girls and boys have had a sexual experience.

TEENAGE SEXUAL ACTIVITY

Sexual intercourse, especially **unprotected intercourse** (sexual intercourse without the use of barriers or other contraceptives), carries the risk for pregnancy. The level of sexual activity among teenagers is extremely high (Alan Guttmacher Institute [AGI], 2006a; U.S. Department of Health and Human Services [USDHHS], 2007). Peer pressure, an adolescent's need to belong, and the sexual content of media messages make it difficult for teens to delay or abstain from sexual activity.

EXTENT OF SEXUAL ACTIVITY AMONG TEENAGERS

Sexual activity among adolescents continues to be a prevalent issue although some data suggest that there has been a decline in sexual activity among certain age groups (AGI, 2006a; Frost et al., 2001). Between 1971 and 1995, the number of teenagers who engaged in sexual intercourse increased by approximately 60% (AGI, 2000a; Ventura, 1995). For approximately 8 years starting in 1995, there was a 10% decline in the number of teens who had ever engaged in sexual intercourse (Eaton et al., 2006). After 2003, the decline in initial sexual activity among teens leveled off and current data suggest the rate has remained at approximately the same level through 2005 (Federal Interagency Forum on Child and Family Statistics, 2007). However, the rate of sexual intercourse increases with age. At age 15, only 13% of girls and 15% of boys have engaged in sexual activity; by the time they reach 18 to 19 years of age, 69% of girls and 64% of boys have engaged in sexual activity (Abma et al., 2004).

There is some evidence to suggest that teens are delaying the age of first intercourse, although a significant percentage of teens initiate sexual activity early. Among teens 15 to 17 years of age, 30% of girls and 31% of boys have engaged in sexual intercourse (Abma et al., 2004). Approximately 15% of girls and 13% of boys have had their first sexual encounter before the age of 15 (Abma et al., 2004; National Campaign to Prevent Teen Pregnancy [NCPTP], 2002). The *Healthy People 2010* objectives (USDHHS, 2000) have identified priorities associated with teen sexual activity, including the following (see also the *Healthy People 2010* box on page 610):

- Increasing the age at first intercourse
- Reducing the number of adolescents engaging in sexual activity
- Increasing the number of adolescents who use protective measures when engaging in sexual activity.

MIXED EMOTIONS ABOUT FIRST SEXUAL INTERCOURSE

Abma and colleagues (2004) reported on teens and their first sexual intercourse. Nine percent of girls reported that their first sexual intercourse was not voluntary. In addition, 13% of girls and 6% of boys reported that they did not want their first intercourse to happen when it did, and 52% of girls and 31% of boys had mixed feelings about the timing of their first intercourse. This suggests much ambivalence about initiation of sexual activity. Educational programs and counseling should continue to stress techniques to handle pressure from peers and potential partners related to initiation of sexual activity.

INCREASED FREQUENCY OF ORAL SEX

The practice of oral sex is now as common as intercourse in the teen population. Approximately 25% of teens use oral sex as a substitute for intercourse. In one survey, half the teens did not consider oral sex to be a sexual activity. Half of all college students who pledged to remain virgins reported that they engaged in oral sex (Dailard, 2003). One-third of teens reported having oral sex with someone who was not the right partner for intercourse or someone with whom they wished to delay initiation of intercourse (Dailard, 2006). Most were unaware of the risk for STDs associated with oral sex.

COMPARISON OF TEENAGE SEXUAL BEHAVIOR AMONG COUNTRIES

The most current comprehensive comparative study (AGI, 2001) shows little difference in sexual experience or age of initial sexual intercourse among teenagers in developed countries (Figure 24-1). There are, however, differences in contraceptive behaviors. Teenagers in the United States are less likely to be aware of contraceptive methods, to know or to explore how to obtain and use contraceptives, and to initiate action to protect themselves from unwanted pregnancies either before or just after their first sexual experience (AGI, 2001, 2002a, 2006b). The reason for such sexually risky behavior is at least partially the way in which sexuality and sexual behaviors are addressed in the United States.

In other developed countries, information about sexual intercourse and birth control is regularly provided to teenagers. Government-sponsored sex education programs in the school systems are common. Programs include health teaching on contraceptive methods, encouragement of responsible sexual activity, and easy access to contraceptives (AGI, 2006b). Service is generally provided in a nonjudgmental fashion. The United States provides little information on contraceptives, and contraception is not an important element of most school-based sex education programs (AGI, 2002b; Lindberg, Santelli, & Singh, 2006a). In contrast, sexuality and contraception education is mandatory in public schools in England, Wales, France, and Sweden and in most Canadian schools.

The United States has also been ambivalent about providing contraceptive services to teenagers. In some instances,

Sexual Activity

1. Increase the proportion of sexually active, unmarried adolescents aged 15 to 17 years who use contraception that both effectively prevents pregnancy and provides barrier protection against disease.

Method	1995 Baseline	2010 Target
Condom		
Males	72%	83%
Females	69%	75%
Condom plus hormonal method		
Males	8%	11%
Females	7%	9%

2. Increase to 88% the proportion of adolescents who have never engaged in sexual intercourse before the age of 15 years (baseline: 81% of females and 79% of males have never engaged in sexual intercourse by age 15 in 1995).

3. Increase the proportion of adolescents aged 15 to 17 years who have never engaged in sexual intercourse.

Sex	1995 Baseline	2010 Target
Females	62%	75%
Males	57%	75%

4. Reduce the proportion of adolescents and young adults with *Chlamydia trachomatis* infections.

Sex	1997 Baseline	2010 Target
Females aged 15 to 24 years attending STD clinics	12.2%	3%
Males aged 15 to 24 years attending STD clinics	15.7%	3%

5. Reduce the proportion of females with human papillomavirus (HPV) infection (developmental, no current baseline).

Family Planning
Health Status Objectives

1. Reduce teen pregnancies among adolescent females aged 15 to 17 years to no more than 43 per 1000 adolescents (baseline: 68 pregnancies per 1000 females in 1996; blacks, 124 per 1000; Hispanics, 105 per 1000).

2. Increase to 70% the proportion of all pregnancies that are intended (baseline: 51% of pregnancies intended among women aged 15 to 44 years in 1995).

Risk Reduction Objectives

1. Increase to 100% the proportion of females aged 15 to 44 (and their partners) at risk for unintended pregnancy who use contraception (baseline: 93% of females aged 15 to 44 years in 1995).

2. Increase male involvement in pregnancy prevention and family planning efforts.

	2002 Baseline	2010 Target
Unmarried males who have gone to family planning clinic with woman partner in last 12 months	21%	22%
Unmarried males aged 15 to 24 who received birth control counseling or methods from a family planning clinic in the last 12 months	31%	37%
Unmarried males aged 15 to 24 years who received advice from a doctor or other medical care provider about birth control methods, including condoms	21%	37%

Service and Protection Objectives

1. Increase the proportion of young adults who have received formal or informal instruction before turning age 18 years on reproductive health issues, including all of the following topics: abstinence, birth control methods, safer sex to prevent HIV infection, prevention of sexually transmitted diseases, and abstinence.

	2002 Baseline	2010 Target
Formal instruction		
Abstinence		
Females	86%	88%
Males	83%	85%
Birth control methods		
Females	70%	73%
Males	66%	70%
HIV/AIDS prevention		Developmental
STDs		Developmental

Note: For informal instruction targets and baselines, see U.S. Department of Health and Human Services. (2006). *Healthy People 2010: Midcourse Review*, Objectives 9-11. Washington, DC: U.S. Government Printing Office.

Maternal and Infant Health
Health Status Objectives

1. Reduce infant mortality (under 1 year of age) to no more than 4.5 deaths per 1000 births (baseline: 7.2 per 1000 in 1998; mothers aged 15 to 19 years, 10 per 1000; blacks, 13.8 per 1000; American Indians and Alaska Natives, 9.3 per 1000).

Risk Reduction Objectives

1. Reduce to 5% low-birth-weight newborns and to 0.9% very-low-birth-weight newborns (baseline: 7.6% for low-birth-weight newborns and 1.4% for very-low-birth-weight newborns in 1998).

2. Reduce to 24 per 100 deliveries the number of pregnant women who experience maternal complications during labor and delivery (baseline: 31.2 per 100 deliveries in 1998).

3. Increase abstinence from use of tobacco, cigarettes, and other illicit drugs among pregnant women.

Substance	2002-2003 Baseline	2010 Target
Alcohol	90 per 100	95 per 100
Binge drinking	96 per 100	100 per 100
Cigarette smoking	87 per 100 (in 1998)	99 per 100
Illicit drugs	96 per 100	100 per 100

Service and Protection Objectives

1. Increase to 90% the proportion of pregnant women who receive early and adequate prenatal care (baseline: 74% in 1998).

2. Increase first-trimester prenatal care to at least 90% of live births (baseline: 83%; blacks, 73%; Hispanics, 74%; American Indians and Alaska Natives, 69%; whites, 85%; all in 1998).

3. Increase to 77% the proportion of pregnant women who attend a series of prepared-childbirth classes (baseline: 66% in 2000).

4. Ensure appropriate newborn blood spot screening and follow-up testing (developmental, no current baseline).

5. Increase to 100% the proportion of children with special health needs who receive their care in family-centered, comprehensive, and coordinated systems (baseline: 35% of children in 2001).

6. Increase to 52% the proportion of preschool children aged 5 years and under who receive vision screening (baseline: 36% of children in 2002).

7. Increase to 90% the proportion of newborns who are screened for hearing loss by age 1 month (baseline: 66% of newborns in 2001).

From U.S. Department of Health and Human Services. (2000). *Healthy people 2010: Understanding and improving health* (2nd ed.). Washington, DC: U.S. Government printing office. *AIDS*, Acquired immunodeficiency syndrome; *HIV*, human immunodeficiency virus; *STD*, sexually transmitted disease.

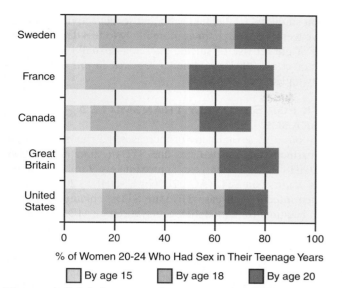

FIGURE 24-1 Percentage of women who engage in sexual activity during their teen years by age: comparison of selected countries. (*Note:* Data are for the mid-1990s.) (From Darroch J. E., Frost, J. J., Singh, S., et al. [2001]. *Teenage sexual and reproductive behavior in developed countries: Can more progress be made?* [Occasional Report No. 3]. New York: Alan Guttmacher Institute.)

federal or state funding for clinics serving large numbers of young disadvantaged females has been reduced or discontinued (see Chapter 4, 21 and 27). A significant number of U.S. teenagers and their families have no health insurance and find access to any kind of health care services (including contraceptive services) difficult (Lindberg, Frost, Sten et al., 2006). Some federal programs have actively attempted to restrict rather than increase access to reproductive services. Parental permission requirements and abstinence-only programs are two methods supported at the federal level. By 2007 approximately 80% of states that provide either sex education or STD/human immunodeficiency virus (HIV) education required parental consent for children to attend classes (AGI, 2007a). Federal funding for abstinence-only sex education programs increased by 157% between 1997 and 2005 (Lindberg, Santelli, & Singh, 2006a). No program that takes federal funds is allowed to provide information about the positive effects of contraceptive use.

FACTORS ASSOCIATED WITH DECISIONS TO ENGAGE IN SEXUAL ACTIVITY

An adolescent's decision to initiate sexual activity appears to be influenced by multiple factors. A brief discussion of the most important findings is presented here.

Peer and Intimacy Needs

Research suggests that one of the most important influences on a teenager's decision to begin sexual activity is the attitudes and behaviors of peers (Dowell & Vandestienne, 1996; NCPTP, 2002). Adolescent motives for sexual behavior are linked to the desire for intimacy, social status, and pleasure (Ott et al., 2006). Teenage girls listed intimacy as the most important motive for sexual activity, whereas teenage boys listed pleasure and social status as more important. Before 1980, race, socioeconomic status, type of neighborhood and dwelling, and religion were significantly related to age at first intercourse.

Although many of these factors still have an effect, they are diminishing in significance.

Racial/Ethnic Differences

Some differences are seen in the age of onset of sexual behavior among races. Blacks are sexually active at an earlier age, but white and Hispanic youths are rapidly catching up. About 52% of all black males report sexual activity between ages 15 to 17. About 31% of Hispanic males and 25% of white males engage in sexual activity in that same age range. Female teenagers of all races initiate sexual intercourse later than adolescent males. Between ages 15 and 17, 42% of black females, 25% of Hispanic females, and 30% of white females have had sexual intercourse (Abma et al., 2004). Approximately 69% of girls and 64% of boys of all races report beginning sexual activity by age 19.

Religious Influence on Sexual Activity

Religious upbringing has some impact on adolescent sexual activity, reducing the proportion of teens who are sexually active. The main reason given by teens who have not initiated sexual activity is religious or moral beliefs (Abma et al., 2004). Approximately 71% of adolescent females with no religious affiliation have engaged in sexual activity, whereas 50% of Roman Catholic and Protestant girls and boys have engaged in intercourse (Frost et al., 2001). Of those still abstaining, almost all have initiated sexual activity by 19 years of age. Whitehead and colleagues (2001) suggest that some of the statistical relationship between religious affiliation and the decision to postpone or never engage in sexual activity might be associated with other factors, such as socioeconomic status. Additional study in this area might help clarify those distinctions.

Socioeconomic Status, Family Composition, and Risky Behaviors

Family income and academic standing also influence the adolescent's decision making related to sexual activity. Poor and low-income teenagers are moderately more likely to be sexually active, and initiate sexual activity approximately 4 to 6 months earlier than adolescents from higher-income families. This is especially true for adolescent females. Teens whose family income is at or below the poverty level are more sexually active than are teens in families with mid to high income levels (Lammers et al., 2000).

Students who are academically motivated, progressing well in school, are future oriented, and have established goals generally delay sexual activity (Lammers et al., 2000; Manlove et al., 2004). Frost and colleagues (2001) reported that for girls, education seems to delay age of first intercourse. Thirty-three percent of girls who did not complete high school reported starting sexual activity before age 15. Only 17% of female high school graduates and only 9% of females with some college education initiated sexually activity before age 15. Differences linked to educational level remain constant when one looks at females who started sexual intercourse by age 18 or 20 (Frost et al., 2001). Lammers and colleagues (2000) reported that better school performance and parental expectations positively influenced the decisions of both boys and girls to postpone sexual activity.

Common opinion links single-parent families, poor parental communication on sexual matters, and school-based sex education with early sexual activity. Teens of both sexes who are from single-parent homes are more likely to have a child at a young age than children from two-parent families (NCPTP, 2002). Recent studies indicate that the absence of a father in the household increases a girl's risk for early sexual activity and pregnancy (Ellis et al., 2003). Girls in one-parent families and those in out-of-home placements are more likely to have fewer support sources (Carpenter et al., 2001; McLanahan & Carlson, 2002). Most studies find no relationship or only very weak correlations between school-based sex education and a teenager's decision to initiate sexual activity. There is some evidence to suggest that such education encourages sexually active teenagers to use contraceptives (Manlove et al., 2004).

Teenagers who engage in other **risky behaviors,** such as smoking, drinking, and drug use, are more likely to engage in sexual activity (Bruckner & Bearman, 2003; Eaton et al., 2006). This is especially true of younger teens. Those adolescents 14 and 15 years of age who engage in other risky health behaviors are twice as likely as their peers to be sexually active (Albert et al., 2003). For example, 24% of sexually active young teens drink or use drugs before having sex (Eaton et al., 2006). Children and adolescents who have been sexually abused are at greater risk for continued sexual activity (Brennan et al., 2007; Santelli et al., 2005) (see Chapter 21).

Initiation of sexual intercourse during the teen years tends to increase the risk for multiple partners (Abma et al., 2004; Eaton et al., 2006). The younger the adolescent at the start of sexual activity, the greater the risk for multiple partners. Women who initiated sexual experiences by age 15 report having more sexual partners than women who started sexual activity later in their teens (Abma et al., 2004; NCPTP, 2002). Abma and colleagues (2004) found that sexually active male and female adolescents are most likely to have had two or more partners in the previous year.

Other Factors Associated with Adolescent Sexual Activity

Early sexual maturation coupled with a prolonged transition to independence compounds the adolescent's journey toward responsible adulthood. The number of years youth are expected to spend in preparation for work or a career is longer than at any other time in history. Along the way, adolescents encounter mixed messages about sex, sexual activity, and responsible behavior (AGI, 2001; NCPTP, 2007). A longitudinal analysis of programming on four major television networks showed a steady increase in the amount of sexual activity and behavior (Frutkin, 1999; Kunkel et al., 1996). Fewer than 30% of sexual situations involved responsible sexual activity, such as waiting to have sex or attempting to reduce the risk for STDs, HIV infection, or unintended pregnancy (Kunkel et al., 1999). Teens report that TV shows which deal with teen pregnancy or health and social problems associated with sexual relations make them think more about the consequences of sexual activity (NCPTP, 2007).

Some teens have additional concerns that can affect their decision process and behavior. Poverty, family dysfunction, and poor school performance can influence the development of a healthy self-esteem, hinder long-term goal setting, and reduce future expectations (Klima, 2003). All these factors are associated with an early initiation into sexual activity and an increase in pregnancy rates (AGI, 2001; Boonstra, 2002). One recent study linked mental health and sexual activity. Sexually active teens were three times more likely to feel depressed and were at greater risk of suicide than non–sexually active teens (Rector et al., 2003). Additional research in this area is currently underway.

RISK FOR SEXUALLY TRANSMITTED DISEASES

Early onset of sexual activity increases the risk for multiple sex partners, unprotected sex, and STDs (Abma et al., 2004; USDHHS, 2000). Each year, approximately 9 million adolescents contract an STD (AGI, 2006b; USDHHS, 2000). Of the top ten infectious diseases, five are STDs: chlamydia, gonorrhea, acquired immunodeficiency syndrome (AIDS), syphilis, and hepatitis B. In 2008, a Centers for Disease Control and Prevention study reported that 26% of girls between the ages of 14 and 19 (3.2 million girls) were infected with at least one of the most common types of STD (human papilloma virus [HPV], chlamydia, genital herpes, trichomoniasis) (CDC, 2008). This study did not include syphilis, HIV, or gonorrhea, and it did not includes young males. Incidence rates can be expected to be higher if the excluded STDs and young males were included in the study.

The rates of chlamydia, gonorrhea, genital herpes, and syphilis among sexually active teens are higher than the rates in the general population (Table 24-1). HIV/AIDS is a growing problem in the adolescent population. Infections are often contracted in the teen years and go undetected until people reach their twenties or thirties (see Chapters 7 and 8). The rates of STDs are higher among racial and ethnic minorities and adolescents living in poverty than among adolescents in other racial groups or teens living in families with higher socioeconomic levels (see Chapters 7, 8, and 21). One reason for the differences in STD rates is the higher rates of sexual activity among these vulnerable groups of adolescents.

The rates of chlamydia and gonorrhea are higher among females than males. Much of that difference might be due to greater female exposure to screening and detection provided by reproductive health care services. Males, who are largely asymptomatic, do not generally seek reproductive health care services, and the infections are more likely to go undetected (Abma et al., 2004; Chesson et al., 2004). Females are also

TABLE 24-1   Sexually Transmitted Diseases among Adolescents

Disease	New Cases
HPV	4.6 million
Trichomoniasis	1.9 million
Chlamydia	1.5 million
Genital herpes	640,000
Gonorrhea	431,000
HIV	15,000
Syphilis	8200
Hepatitis B	7500
Total	**9.1 million**

Data from Weinstock, H., Berman, S., & Cates, W. (2004). Sexually transmitted diseases among American youth: Incidence and prevalence estimates: 2000. *Perspectives on Sexual and Reproductive Health, 36*(1), 6-10.

more likely to experience health complications from STDs, such as pelvic inflammatory disease, cervical cancer, infertility, and ectopic pregnancy (USDHHS, 2007).

CONTRACEPTIVE USE

Contraceptive use among teenagers has steadily increased since the 1980s. Nevertheless, approximately 20% of teens do not use protection during intercourse (AGI, 2006a; USDHHS, 2006). The young, poor, and poorly educated are less likely to use birth control regularly (Jones et al., 2002). Birth control use generally starts after sexual activity has already begun. Teenagers use birth control sporadically and tend to switch methods without taking the proper precautions (Santelli et al., 2006).

Condoms are the most common type of contraception used at first intercourse. More than 66% of sexually active teens report using condoms (Abma et al., 2004; AGI, 2006b). Teens who engage in ongoing sexual activity switch to more effective methods, such as birth control pills, injectable Depo-Provera, and intrauterine devices (AGI, 2006a; Frost et al., 2001). About 61% of adolescent females report using birth control pills. Concern about HIV and STDs have led to an increased use of barrier methods (condoms) *in conjunction with* other birth control measures. Although dual contraceptive use doubled between 1991 and 2002, only 25% of teens report using two methods of birth control (Abma et al., 2004).

Poverty is associated with less access to and successful use of reversible contraceptive measures. Poor people have difficulty obtaining contraceptive health care services and paying for birth control products (USDHHS, 2000). Frost and colleagues (2001) report that poor teens are less likely to use birth control pills than those who are more economically advantaged. The price of one cycle of pills averages $30 per month. Teens who are not well off must rely on public programs to obtain contraceptive services. Subsidized family planning services are stressed and can provide care for only approximately 50% of those estimated to need such care. By 2003, the number of agencies that waived fees for adolescents fell by 22% (Lindberg, Frost, Sten et al., 2006).

TEENAGE PREGNANCY

The United States has one of the highest teenage pregnancy rates in the developed world.
- Approximately 750,000 teenagers become pregnant each year.
- Eighty-seven percent of these pregnancies are unintended.
- Of pregnancies in 15- to 17-year-olds
  - 57% result in live births;
  - 30% result in abortion;
  - 14% end in miscarriage.
- More than 400,000 children are born to mothers younger than 19 years of age each year.
- One of every three adolescent girls becomes pregnant.
- Pregnant teenagers are more likely to drop out of high school, live in poverty, and have limited occupational choices than girls who do not become pregnant during the teenage years (AGI, 2006b, 2006c; Hamilton et al., 2006; Hoffman, 2006).

TRENDS IN PREGNANCY AND BIRTH RATES AMONG TEENS

Tabulation and publication of national data on pregnancy and birth rates among teens are delayed by 4 or more years. Preliminary figures through 2005 point to a sharp decline in pregnancy rates and a more moderate decline in birth and abortion rates among adolescents (Figure 24-2). In 1991, the birth rate for teens (15 to 19 years) was 62.1 per 1000. In 2005, the birth rate was 40.4 per 1000 (Hamilton et al., 2006). Approximately 14% of the decline in pregnancy rates is attributable to delaying sexual intercourse, and 86% is related to the use of highly effective contraceptive methods among sexually active adolescent girls (Santelli et al., 2007). Nevertheless, both the pregnancy rate and teen birth rate remain high.

INTENDED VERSUS UNINTENDED PREGNANCY

Most teen pregnancies (82%) are unintended (AGI, 2006b). Whether intended or unintended, adolescent girls who become pregnant and choose to continue the pregnancy are more likely to come from low socioeconomic circumstances, live on their own or with one parent, have lower educational and career aspirations, and have older sexual partners (Abma et al., 2004; Finer & Henshaw, 2006; Martin et al., 2006).

An **unintended pregnancy** is unplanned or accidental and is accompanied by increased risks for the pregnancy, the mother, and the baby. Unintended pregnancies are more likely to result in premature or low-birth-weight babies, little or no prenatal care, abortion and miscarriages, and pregnancy complications (Finer & Henshaw, 2006; Frost et al., 2001; USDHHS, 2000). Unintended pregnancies have a social cost to young mothers. These young women are at great risk for limited educational

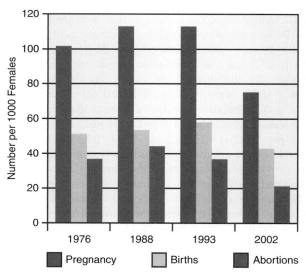

FIGURE 24-2 Pregnancies, births, and abortions in U.S. adolescents aged 15 to 19 years for selected years. Rates per 1000 females. (Data from Alan Guttmacher Institute. [2006]. *U.S. teenage pregnancy statistics: National and state trends and trends by race and ethnicity.* New York: Author; Centers for Disease Control and Prevention [CDC]. [2003]. Revised pregnancy rates, 1990-1997 and new rates for 1998-99: United States. *National Vital Statistics Reports, 52*[7]. Hyattsville, MD: National Center for Health Statistics; and CDC. [1999]. Highlights of trends in pregnancies and pregnancy rates by outcome: Estimates for the United States, 1976-1996. *National Vital Statistics Reports, 47*[29]. Hyattsville, MD: National Center for Health Statistics.)

and employment opportunities, the consequences of which can last a lifetime (Hoffman, 2006).

PREGNANCY OUTCOMES

Approximately two thirds of pregnancies result in birth, and one third of pregnancies end in abortion (see Figure 24-2). Most unwed mothers keep their infants rather than place them for adoption. Therefore, there is a greater demand for adoptions than there are infants placed for adoption.

CHARACTERISTICS ASSOCIATED WITH RISK FOR PREGNANCY

Some variations are seen in pregnancy and birth rates among adolescents. A teen's age and the age of her sexual partner, marital status, racial/ethnic group, and socioeconomic status influence the chance of pregnancy and childbirth.

Older teens have a higher pregnancy and birth rate than younger teens, perhaps because more older adolescents than younger teens engage in sexual intercourse. The pregnancy rate for females 15 to 17 years of age is 53.5 per 1000, and for females 18 to 19 years of age, it is 129.9 per 1000 (Abma et al., 2004). The older the teen's sexual partner, the more likely it is that an adolescent female will become pregnant.

Teens marry later but, in general, do not delay sexual activity or pregnancy until marriage. Marriage because of pregnancy used to be common; today, few teenagers opt for marriage if they become pregnant. Approximately 83% of pregnant adolescents remain unwed (Hamilton et al., 2006). Pregnancy is still the main reason for teen marriage, although fewer teens exercise this option. Among married females aged 15 to 19 years, the pregnancy rate is 283.6 per 1000 compared with a pregnancy rate of 35.4 per 1000 among unmarried females of the same age (Martin et al., 2003; National Center for Health Statistics, 2002).

There are differences in pregnancy and abortion rates among racial/ethnic groups. The highest rates of birth are among black and Hispanic adolescents, and the lowest are among Asian and Pacific Islander adolescents (Figure 24-3). The pregnancy rates in all racial and ethnic groups have declined in the past decade, with the sharpest decline in black pregnancy rates (AGI, 2006b). Abortion rates are lowest among white adolescents, perhaps because they have a lower pregnancy rate. Black adolescents chose abortion at twice the rate of Hispanic teens (49.4 per 1000 versus 28.5 per 1000). The pregnancy rates for other ethnic groups are not as widely published. Birth rate data provide some indication of pregnancy rates. American Indian and Alaska Native teens have a birth rate between those of Hispanics and blacks, and, therefore, their pregnancy rate should fall somewhere in between the rates of those two groups. Asians and Pacific Islanders have a birth rate just below that of white teens, so their pregnancy rates should reflect the lower birth rates.

A common public perception is that most pregnancies in and births to teenagers occur in racial minorities. *This is not true.* In 2005, white teenagers accounted for the largest percentage of pregnancies and births (45.5%), followed by Hispanics (24%) and blacks (11.6%) (Hamilton et al., 2006). Hispanic and black teenagers have a *higher proportional rate* of adolescent pregnancy, but because they are fewer in number, the *largest number* of teenage births is to white mothers.

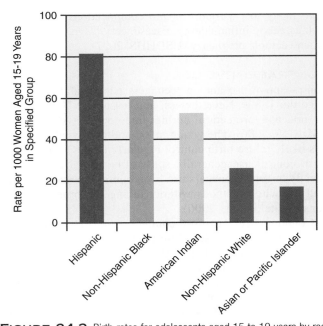

FIGURE 24-3 Birth rates for adolescents aged 15 to 19 years by race and/or Hispanic origin 2005. (Data from Alan Guttmacher Institute. [2006]. *U.S. teenage pregnancy statistics: National and state trends and trends by race and ethnicity.* New York: Author.)

Among adolescent females, there is a link between pregnancy rate and socioeconomic status. Teens from lower-income families start sexual intercourse at an earlier age, which increases their risk for pregnancy. Lower-income teens are more likely than middle- or upper-income teens to become pregnant and, once pregnant, to choose birth as their option (Young et al., 2004). Of teens aged 15 to 19 years, 19% of those with family incomes at or below 150% of the poverty level have a child, compared with 2% of teens with family incomes at or above 300% of the poverty level (Frost et al., 2001).

REASONS FOR PREGNANCY AMONG ADOLESCENTS

With advances in birth control, increased sexual activity does not necessarily mean an increased risk for pregnancy. Why, then, are teenage pregnancy rates so high? There is no single, clear-cut answer. Teenagers get pregnant for a variety of reasons. Any effort to reduce the rate of adolescent pregnancy must begin with a clear understanding of the conscious or unconscious reasons for and motives that affect teenage pregnancy. Knowledge about the motives and reasoning of sexually active teenagers helps the community health nurse identify teens at particular risk for pregnancy. Some of the factors associated with pregnancy in the teenage population are enumerated in Box 24-1. Many teens who become pregnant do not do well academically and have few expectations for the future (Manlove et al., 2004). In one study of pregnant teens in California, 44% dropped out of school prior to pregnancy, and many lived in chaotic family situations. Approximately 25% could not identify any future life goals. Many of the girls reported that in their social circles early childbearing was common, and almost 70% identified an adolescent friend or sibling who was either pregnant or already had a child (Frost & Oslake, 1999; Raneri & Wiemann, 2007).

BOX 24-1   Factors Associated with Teenage Pregnancy

Hormonal Changes, Awakening Sexual Awareness, and Peer Pressure

Adolescence is a period of heightened sexual awareness, curiosity, and experimentation (Kalmuss et al., 2003). Peer pressure influences some teens' decisions to engage in sexual intercourse (Ott et al., 2006). Many pregnant teens know someone or have a relative who was a pregnant teen (Manlove et al., 2004). In addition, teens who engage in sexual intercourse are more likely to have friends who do so.

Pervasive Sexual Messages in the Media

Adolescents are exposed to multiple messages about sex, sexual activity, and the importance of being attractive to the opposite sex.

Involuntary Sexual Activity

Adolescent sexual activity is not always voluntary. The younger the pregnant teen, the more likely she is to have engaged in coercive sex. Eighteen percent of girls who have sex before age 15 report that it was involuntary (Abma et al., 2004).

Inaccuracy or Lack of Knowledge about Sex and Conception

The increase in sexual activity among teenagers is not necessarily accompanied by increased knowledge about sexual function, procreation, or birth control. Misunderstandings abound related to risk periods and timing, including periods of susceptibility during the menstrual cycle, age-related susceptibility, and timing of male ejaculation.

Misuse or Nonuse of Contraceptives

Teenagers also lack accurate knowledge about specific birth control methods and the correct use of contraceptives. Inconsistent use of contraceptives is common. One in four girls discontinues the pill despite continued sexual activity (Kerns et al., 2003). Regular, effective contraceptive use increases with age. Older teens are more likely to use birth control pills or long-acting contraceptives and younger teens to use condoms.

Difficulty of Access to Birth Control

The most effective birth control methods (intrauterine device, birth control pills, injectable implants, and injections) require appointments and examinations by health care professionals. Cost is an issue, and most teens have never sought care without their parents' permission. Finer and Zabin (1998) found that the interval between first intercourse and the first visit to reproductive health services was 22 months. Public programs that provide contraceptives are underfunded and must limit services (Lindberg et al., 2006).

Destigmatization of Illegitimacy

Formerly, pregnancy out of wedlock resulted in severe social censure, especially for women. Today, unwed motherhood is common, and most young girls who are pregnant remain single (Hamilton et al., 2006).

Efforts at Independence

Adolescence is a turbulent period and a period of increasing independence. It is a time in which children complete the task of separation from their parents and further develop their own identities. It also is a period of uncertainty and conflict and a time of exploration. As the child explores and develops, conflicts arise with parents and other authority figures. If the child's attempts at independence are severely restricted, "acting out" behaviors may result. Pregnancy can be one means of acting out; others include running away, performing poorly in school, and engaging in substance abuse.

Need to Feel Special, Loved, and Wanted

Pregnancy can make a person feel special. The teenager receives extra attention from family, peers, and acquaintances. Sometimes, for the first time, she might be on "center stage" in the family unit. Some girls report that they got pregnant because they expect the infant to meet their need for love and attention.

Lack of Future Orientation and Maturity

Teenagers generally live in the present; future planning is minimal. Teenagers who are oriented to the present and just beginning to develop abstract reasoning often do not consider the future consequences of their current sexual activity. As adolescents become more developmentally mature and more proficient at identifying psychosocial costs, their use of contraceptives increases. Older girls are more likely to use birth control (Abma et al., 2004). Sexual abstinence is more common among academically achieving teens (Manlove et al., 2004).

Data from Abma, J. C., Martinez, G. M., Mosher, W. D., et al. (2004). *Teenagers in the United States: Sexual activity, contraceptive use, and childbearing* (Vital and Health Statistics Series 23, No. 24). Hyattsville, MD: National Center for Health Statistics; Finer, L. B., & Zabin, L. S. (1998). Does the timing of the first family planning visit still matter? *Family Planning Perspectives, 301*(1), 30-33, 42; Hamilton, B. E., Martin, J. A., & Ventura, S. J. (2006). *Births: Preliminary data for 2005*. Hyattsville, MD: National Center for Health Statistics; Kalmuss, D., Davidson, A., Cohall, A., et al. (2003). Preventing sexual risk behaviors and pregnancy among teenagers: Linking research and programs. *Perspectives on Sexual and Reproductive Health, 35*(2), 87-93; Kerns, J., Westhoff, C., Morroni, C., et al. (2003). Partner influence on early discontinuation of the pill in a predominantly Hispanic population. *Perspectives on Sexual and Reproductive Health, 35*(6), 256-260; Kirby, D. (2001). *Emerging answers: Research findings on progress to reduce teen pregnancy*. Washington, DC: National Campaign to Prevent Teen Pregnancy; Lindberg, L., Santelli, J. S., & Singh, S. (2006). Provisions of contraceptive and related services by publicly funded family planning clinics, 2003. *Perspectives on Sexual and Reproductive Health, 38*(3), 139-147; Lynch, C. O. (2001). Risk and protective factors associated with adolescent sexual activity. *Adolescence and Family Health, 2*(3), 99-107; Manlove, J., Papillio, A., & Ikramullah, E. (2004). *Not yet: Programs to delay first sex among teens*. Washington, DC: National Campaign to Prevent Teen Pregnancy; and Ott, M. A., Millstein, S. G., Ofner, S., et al. (2006). Greater expectations: Adolescents' positive motivations for sex. *Perspectives on Sexual and Reproductive Health, 38*(2), 84-89.

COMPARISON OF PREGNANCY-RELATED ISSUES IN OTHER COUNTRIES

Sexual activity among teenagers is commonplace in all developed countries (AGI, 2001, 2006b). Although the levels of teenage sexual activity are similar, developed countries differ in the ways they deal with sex education and sexually active teens. Experts suggest that the United States' methods are not as effective as those used by other developed countries, as evidenced by significantly higher rates of teenage pregnancy, birth, and abortion (AGI, 2006b; USDHHS, 2006).

PREGNANCY RATES IN SELECTED COUNTRIES

The United States leads most developed nations in the rate of teenage pregnancy (AGI, 1986, 1994, 2006b). The United States has a higher pregnancy rate than almost every industrialized nation. A comparison of five countries indicates that the

U.S. pregnancy rate is two or more times higher than the rates in four comparable countries (Figure 24-4).

Teenagers appear to run a greater risk for pregnancy at an earlier age in the United States than in other countries. Comparison of the five industrialized countries for which pregnancy data were given earlier shows that in all of them contraceptive services are more readily available and in greater use than in the United States (Figure 24-5). This disparity in availability and use can be explained partly by the different types of health insurance available in each country. The four other countries—France, Sweden, Great Britain, and Canada—all have national health care systems. In those countries, contraceptive services and supplies are provided free or at reduced cost; contraceptives are advertised in the media; and contraceptive methods are included in the sex education programs provided to adolescents (AGI, 2001, 2006b). In the United States, many teens and their families lack health insurance coverage (see Chapters 4 and 21). Furthermore, birth control supplies are not advertised in print or television media, and many sex education programs restrict information to abstinence-only approaches.

ABORTION RATES IN SELECTED COUNTRIES

As with pregnancy rates, the abortion rate is higher in the United States than in the four other industrialized countries with which it is compared in Figure 24-4. Although the abortion rate (per 1000 females) is highest in the United States, the actual selection of abortion as an outcome of pregnancy is common in all five countries. Once they are pregnant, many teenagers choose abortion, with some variations seen among countries. In Sweden, the rate at which pregnant teenagers opt for abortion as an alternative is higher than that for pregnant teenagers in the United States.

In all four of the other countries, access to abortion is less problematic, and there is little or no controversy about abortion compared with the United States. Abortion is provided by

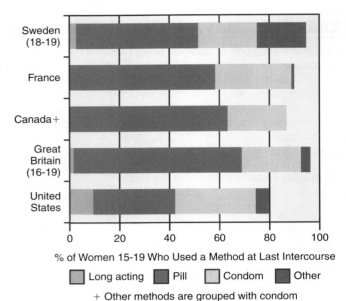

FIGURE 24-5 Contraceptive use in female adolescents aged 15 to 19 years: comparison of selected countries. (*Note:* Data are for the mid-1990s.) (From Darroch J. E., Frost, J. J., Singh, S., et al. [2001]. *Teenage sexual and reproductive behavior in developed countries: Can more progress be made?* [Occasional Report No. 3]. New York: Alan Guttmacher Institute.)

government health services or funded by national health insurance. In the United States, abortion might be covered under health insurance for those whose families have insurance, but some policies specifically deny coverage—for example, federal insurance programs and some state Medicaid programs (AGI, 2006b). Abortion services are provided by separate providers, not the teen's or family's regular physician or health care practice. Some states have made it more difficult for teens to have abortions, requiring parental consent, judicial reviews, waiting periods, and mandatory counseling sessions (see Chapter 6). Advocacy groups are attempting to further restrict service availability by boycotting or protest campaigns, and are attempting to secure the passage of state regulations or legislation that restricts clinic operations.

PUBLIC COSTS OF ADOLESCENT PREGNANCY AND CHILDBEARING

Teenage pregnancy has both short- and long-term effects on the national economy. Public funds pay for a significant amount of the care and consequences associated with teen pregnancy, and therefore all taxpayers ultimately contribute to the costs associated with teen pregnancy.

It is difficult to determine the exact health costs of teenage pregnancy and adolescent motherhood, but an estimate is $7 billion per year (Hoffman, 2006; NCPTP, 2002). The costs include medical care for pregnant adolescents without private health insurance and the higher costs of medical care for their infants, who are at greater risk for medical complications and death.

Young mothers and their families impact social welfare programs in ways other than medical costs. The need of young mothers to care for infants and children and their relatively low educational levels limit their ability to obtain and hold jobs

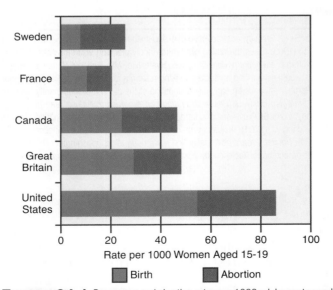

FIGURE 24-4 Pregnancy and abortion rates per 1000 adolescents aged 15 to 19 years: comparison of selected countries. (*Note:* Data are for the mid-1990s.) (From Darroch J. E., Frost, J. J., Singh, S., et al. [2001]. *Teenage sexual and reproductive behavior in developed countries: Can more progress be made?* [Occasional Report No. 3]. New York: Alan Guttmacher Institute.)

providing a living wage. As a result, adolescent mothers and their dependent children are at greater risk for needing welfare programs and for remaining in these programs for longer periods than are other welfare applicants. More than 50% of all teen mothers receive welfare assistance after the birth of their child (NCPTP, 2002). An estimated $23.6 billion in services was provided in 2004 to families headed by females who were teens when they had their first child (Hoffman, 2006). That amount includes funds for Temporary Assistance to Needy Families (TANF), food stamps, Women, Infants, and Children (WIC) program, social service block grants, foster care, and adoption services (see the *Ethics in Practice* box).

Starting in 1997, limitations were placed on the amount of time young mothers may receive public assistance and subsidized health benefits. The full impact of recent reforms in the welfare system at both the federal and state levels is not yet known. All able-bodied adults receiving TANF are expected to look for work. Persons are limited to 2 consecutive years of TANF benefits and a life-time maximum of 5 years. All states make some exemption for mothers with very young babies or children, but each state's definition of "very young" is different (Frost et al., 2001). For example, Oregon applies the term "very young" to children younger than 3 months of age, Texas to children younger than 4 years of age.

Because of the time limits, the impact of the 1997 changes is just now starting to become apparent. What is known is that families are moving off "welfare" programs. The preliminary data indicate that although the majority (60%) of families have improved their economic situations, many (40%) of these families have not made a successful entry to new jobs and financial independence (Congressional Budget Office, 2007) (see Chapters 4 and 21). The National Center on Family Homelessness (2005) reports that the number of families using homeless services has increased. Many are without health insurance, are either chronically underemployed or working minimum-wage jobs, and are less well off than when they were receiving TANF benefits. Some families are homeless and receiving TANF benefits. Philadelphia and New York City report that 40% to 70% of homeless families were receiving TANF benefits (Courtney et al., 2004; Jung et al., 2004). Changes in TANF and the medical relief programs Medicaid and State Children's Health Insurance Program (SCHIP), as well as the effects of economic retrenchment, have long-term impacts on social program recipients (see Chapter 21). Most states have announced cutbacks to Medicaid and SCHIP medical assistance programs.

Forcing mothers off TANF support and limiting or denying medical assistance might simply delay problems and increase public costs. When people do not have health insurance, they delay seeking care. Consequently, when they do go for care, their health problems are more serious, take longer to treat, and cost more to treat (see Chapter 21). The health status and quality of life of both mothers and infants who are affected by these program changes are an important factor that demands serious monitoring during the next few years.

CONSEQUENCES OF EARLY PREGNANCY FOR TEENAGERS AND INFANTS

To provide quality care for pregnant adolescents, the community health nurse must understand the scope of the problem and the needs, concerns, and health issues of pregnant teenagers. There are economic, medical, and emotional consequences of pregnancy and childbearing for young mothers and their children (Martin et al., 2006). Teen mothers and their infants are at greater risk for serious medical complications, infant **low birth weight,** and poorer outcomes than are older women and their infants (Martin et al., 2002; NCPTP, 2002). Teenagers who become pregnant jeopardize their educational progress and endanger their future expectations (Hoffman, 2006). Children born to adolescent mothers are at greater risk for poverty. Family members and significant others are also affected, because they are called on to provide physical, emotional, and financial support while burdened with their own responsibilities. Six million children live in grandparent-headed households, and 2.5 million of these children do not have a parent present in the home (Children's Defense Fund [CDF], 2005).

ROLE IN THE POVERTY CYCLE

Families headed by young females have a greater chance of being poor than do other families (Hoffman, 2006). Comparisons of poverty risk for teen mothers and for those who delay pregnancy indicate that teen mothers have a greater risk for poverty. Although only 38% of young females (15 to 19 years) are poor, 73% of pregnant adolescents are poor (Frost et al., 2001). More than 33% of single women with children live in poverty (Fields, 2003). Poverty is accompanied by many quality-of-life problems for mothers and children, including an increase in health problems and limited access to health care services (see Chapter 21). Teenage pregnancy is viewed as the hub of the poverty cycle in the United States, because teenage mothers are likely to rear children who repeat the cycle (Elfenbein & Felice, 2003; Hoffman, 2006).

EDUCATIONAL AND ECONOMIC CONSEQUENCES

Pregnancy affects educational achievement. Only 41% of women who become mothers in adolescence complete high school compared with 61% of women who delay childbirth until age 20 to 21 (NCPTP, 2002; Pfitzner et al., 2003). Many teenagers who became pregnant were not doing well in school and dropped out before they became pregnant. Shearer and colleagues (2002) compared adolescent females' test scores and found that teens with lower cognitive scores initiate sex earlier and have a higher rate of pregnancy than girls with higher test scores. Others drop out of school because of the demands of pregnancy and child rearing. The younger the teenager at the time of pregnancy, the greater the danger that she will not complete high school. Teen mothers are also less likely to attend college. Only 2% of women who become pregnant before 18 years of age go on to college (Hoffman, 2006).

It is important for the community health nurse and others involved with pregnant teens to encourage the girls to remain in school if possible. Lack of education hampers the mother's prospects in the job market. The income of young mothers is only half that of women who delay childbearing until after 25 years of age.

LESS PRENATAL CARE

A third of pregnant teens receive inadequate prenatal care (Chen et al., 2007). Many pregnant teenagers delay seeking prenatal care or do not receive regular care. Although the number of

ETHICS IN PRACTICE

Distributing Community Resources Fairly

Gail A. DeLuca Havens, PhD, APRN, BC

"It seems like coercion to me," says Eileen. "Like we are being vindictive and punishing a teenager for getting pregnant and electing to carry the baby to term. Teenagers are babies themselves in many respects. This doesn't solve the problem; it hides it so the community doesn't have to confront the underlying reasons for the high incidence of teenage pregnancy that prevails here. This proposed regulation is nothing more than a cop-out."

Cynthia disagrees. "In this day and age, getting pregnant is a choice. If a teenager with no means of financial support chooses to get pregnant, especially when she already has one child, then she should expect to have to decide whether she wishes to practice birth control in the future or have the aid for her dependents decreased if she has additional children. We can't afford to keep supporting all these young mothers and their babies in this city, particularly when so many of our other health and social services are significantly underfunded. Consider the dollars we spend per capita on programs for the learning disabled in our city, for example. Or the percentage of the city's budget allocated to programs for the elderly. Both are significantly underfunded in comparison to the dollars spent for similar programs in cities of comparable size throughout the state."

On the way home, Eileen and Cynthia continue the debate over the Department of Social Services' proposed regulation requiring that females in the community younger than 18 years of age who are receiving benefits under Temporary Assistance to Needy Families (TANF) must show evidence of practicing birth control to continue the aid. The proposal includes provision of free birth control counseling and products as well. Eileen and Cynthia are both community health clinical nurses employed by the community. Eileen practices in the Pediatric Service and Cynthia in the Council on Aging's Geriatric Intervention Program. They have just attended the last of the public hearings sponsored by a joint task force created by the Departments of Health and Social Services and the school board to hear opinions from members of the health care professions and the community at large regarding the proposal, which is intended to address the problem of teenage pregnancy in the community. Now the task force will deliberate on the issue and make recommendations to the departments and the board. If you were a member of the task force, how would you go about the decision-making process? What would be your decision? Why?

The problem appears to be just distribution of resources. The community has a finite budget allocated for multiple social services that serve many different populations. It is being argued that a disproportionate amount of the community's social services budget is being spent on aid to the dependent children of teenage mothers. A plan intended to ensure a more equitable distribution of social service resources across the community's populations has been proposed as a solution. Theoretically, limiting the number of people covered by the TANF program ought to make a greater percentage of the city's budget available for other social services programs targeted at underserved populations.

The plan's defenders believe that, although the solution does not include all the choices a teenage mother might be accustomed to, it does offer reasonable options considering the overall needs of the community. Detractors of the plan argue that it violates the autonomy of teenage mothers in the community because it coerces them into not becoming pregnant in order to have the means they need to care for the children they presently have. Coercion has been characterized as an extreme form of influence that entirely compromises one's autonomy (Beauchamp & Childress, 2001).

If the proposal is adopted, it would be a step toward a more equitable distribution of resources, and thus if the planning has been accurate, it ought to have some short- and long-term effects on the social services programs for the community. A plan such as this is grounded in the ethical theory of utilitarianism, which seeks to maximize the positive consequences of an action by achieving the greatest good for the greatest number (Beauchamp & Childress, 2001). Services in need of resources ought to be targeted, monitored, and measured to see if they benefit. Adopting the proposal has the potential to jeopardize the health and well-being of a population of children already at risk, namely, the children of teenage mothers.

If teenage females continue to have children, their ability to care for those children already dependent on them will be diminished because of a lack of resources. The short-term consequences might be a rising incidence of children who fail to thrive, are afflicted by disease, or are disabled by developmental and psychologic problems. The long-term consequences might be a generation of children who would overburden the community's social services. Such an action would contradict the ethical principle of nonmaleficence (i.e., avoiding harm), contained in the *Code of Ethics for Nurses* (American Nurses Association, 2001). In addition, it would go against the value of promoting autonomy and self-determination through the achievement of health and well-being, as expressed by the code.

Not adopting the proposal is an alternative. However, this changes nothing for the community and for its teenage mothers. Another alternative attempts to address the issue of teenage pregnancy in the community by seeking ways to discover the underlying causes of the increased incidence of teenage pregnancy. One strategy that has been successfully introduced in a growing number of communities is school-based clinics. Decreased fertility rates, decreased pregnancy rates, and later sexual activity are evidence of the success of school-based clinics. Outcomes directly attributable to school-based clinics include improvements in students' health, lowered birth rates, increased use of contraceptives, and improvements in school attendance (Santelli et al., 2006).

REFERENCES

American Nurses Association. (2001). *Code of ethics for nurses with interpretive statements.* Washington, DC: Author.

Beauchamp, T. L., & Childress, J. F. (2001). *Principles of biomedical ethics* (5th ed.). New York: Oxford University Press.

Santelli, J. S., Morrow, B., Anderson, J. E., et al. (2006). Contraceptive use and pregnancy risk among U.S. high school students, 1991-2003. *Perspectives on Sexual and Reproductive Health*, 38(2), 106-111.

young women who receive first-trimester care has increased over the past 10 years, more than 33% have had no prenatal care at the end of their first trimester (Philliber et al., 2003; Ventura et al., 2001). The same teenagers at greatest risk for pregnancy—those from poor families—are also at greatest risk for poor prenatal care. In general, this group tends to be more oriented to illness rather than prevention in its health practices (see Chapter 4). Delays in seeking prenatal care might also be influenced by denial of the pregnancy and an orientation toward concrete, present-centered reasoning.

SUBSTANCE USE AND EXPOSURE TO VIOLENCE

Pregnant adolescents are more likely to smoke than pregnant women over the age of 20 (Ventura et al., 2001). In fact, one study shows that cigarette smoking has actually increased among pregnant teens (Mathews, 2001). Alcohol consumption is also a concern. About 50% of all pregnant teens drink during their pregnancy (Wiemann & Berenson, 1998). Teens who continue to drink alcohol are also more likely to use other types of illegal drugs.

Pregnancy increases the risk for physical abuse by a woman's partner (see Chapter 23). Pregnant teens appear to be at greater risk than most pregnant women. Research suggests that the risk of being murdered is three times higher for pregnant teens than for other teens (Krulewitch et al., 2003).

PHYSICAL CONSEQUENCES FOR THE MOTHER

During adolescence, rapid growth patterns place considerable demands on the body. Pregnancy places additional demands. In general, adolescents experience greater health problems with pregnancy than do women older than 20 years of age (Scarr, 2002). The consequences are especially severe to the youngest adolescents, those 12 to 15 years of age (NCPTP, 2002). Older teenagers (16 to 19 years) are not as likely to experience serious difficulties.

Teenagers are at greater risk for developing pregnancy-induced hypertension and toxemia (Martin et al., 2003). The incidence of hypertension ranges from 10% to 35%, which is higher than in any other age group except women over the age of 40. Teenagers are also at increased risk for anemia, nutritional deficiencies, poor weight gain, and urinary tract infections (Koniak-Griffin & Turner-Pluta, 2001; Treffers et al., 2001). Studies indicate that 10% to 40% of pregnant teens are anemic, a condition exacerbated by the poor nutritional status of most teenagers. Good, consistent prenatal care reduces the risk for complications.

Young girls are more likely to deliver prematurely, undergo rapid or prolonged labor, experience eclampsia, and develop infections; fetal infections and the presence of moderate to heavy meconium at delivery are also more common in this age group (Martin et al., 2003; Scarr, 2002). Although some early studies suggested that teenagers are more likely to have cesarean section deliveries, current research shows little difference in cesarean rates for 15-year-olds and 30-year-olds (Martin et al., 2003).

CONSEQUENCES FOR THE NEWBORN AND CHILD

Infants born to teenagers are also at risk. Stillbirths are twice as common among teens, and the mortality rate is two to four times higher during the first year of life for infants born to

adolescents (Phipps et al., 2002). The highest risk is for infants born to mothers 15 years of age or younger. Babies born to young mothers are at greater risk for health problems and hospitalization during childhood than babies born to older mothers (Guevara et al., 2001). Teen mothers are more likely to have babies born with certain congenital anomalies, such as anencephalus, spina bifida/meningocele, hydrocephalus, microcephalus, and gastrointestinal anomalies (Martin et al., 2003). Child abuse and neglect are more common among young mothers, perhaps because young mothers have multiple factors associated with risk for abuse (Hoffman, 2006; Koniak-Griffin & Turner-Pluta, 2001). Reducing the rate of teen pregnancy and therefore the cost of care for abused or neglected children of teen mothers would lower welfare costs by about $3.6 billion per year (Hoffman, 2006).

Some studies suggest that infants of adolescent mothers are at risk for a lower level of cognitive development, a problem usually attributed to the mother's single-parent status and low educational achievement. Educational deficits persist with time. Therefore, children born to teen mothers do not perform as well in school as children born to older mothers (Hoffman, 2006; NCPTP, 2002). These children are more likely to be placed in special education programs and have higher rates of milder educational problems as well.

Low birth weight (birth weight under 5.5 lb [2500 g]) is associated with higher rates of infant mortality, birth injuries, neurologic defects, and mental retardation (Martin et al., 2005; NCPTP, 2003). Prematurity is a significant risk in teen births; the rate of premature births is 21% higher for adolescents than for women 20 to 24 years of age. In 2002, 13.5% of infants born to mothers under 15 years of age were of low birth weight, compared with 6.9% of infants born to mothers aged 25 to 29 years (Martin et al., 2003). Birth weights increase with the age of the mother, but all teenagers are at greater risk for having low-birth-weight infants than are those in other age groups (Philliber et al., 2003).

There are also long-term consequences for children born to teen mothers. These children are less likely to complete high school, and partly as a result of their lower educational levels, they earn less over their lifetimes (Maynard & Hoffman, 2007). The estimated total wages lost for children born to teen mothers in 2004 was $5.53 billion (Hoffman, 2006). This also translates into a corresponding shortfall to the government in lost taxes because of lower wages.

Daughters born to teen mothers are more likely to repeat the cycle of early pregnancy and childbirth. Approximately one third of the daughters of teen mothers have a first child as a teen compared with only 11% of teens whose mothers postponed pregnancy until their twenties (Hoffman & Scher, 2007).

The sons of teen mothers are 2.2 times more likely to be incarcerated than the sons of mothers who delay pregnancy until later. Hoffman (2006) estimated that the public sector cost of confinement would drop by $5.3 billion per year if the sons of teen mothers had an incarceration rate similar to the sons of older mothers.

PSYCHOSOCIAL CONSEQUENCES

Pregnancy can be a crisis that disrupts the adolescent's transition to independence. The pregnant teenager is abruptly thrust into the responsibilities of adulthood. She must learn to function as a parent while struggling to solidify her own identity, a daunting task. Social isolation is possible because she and her friends may no longer have the same interests and because she is less likely to attend school (Grady & Bloom, 2004). Only 4 of 10 teen mothers complete high school (Hoffman, 2006). If the pregnant teen's family is not supportive, there might be additional stress. Many report feeling depressed. Stress and isolation increase after delivery, when the adolescent must cope with demands of the infant and interactions with peers become even more limited (Holubet et al., 2007). Stress can lead to child abuse, neglect, or suicide attempts (Frost & Oslake, 1999; Hoffman, 2006; Olds et al., 1999).

Reba Jackson is 15 years old and a new mom. She tells her clinic nurse, Sally Arnold, that she has not been seeing her friends as much. Reba complains, "When they talk about the weekend's great party, I get mad and sad." She feels out of place because her mother makes her stay home to care for her new baby. "Don't get me wrong, I love Sam with all my heart, but I am so sorry when I hear my friends talk about where they are going on spring break." Reba reports that she is also worried about keeping her grades up and about what she would do if she had to move out of her mother's house.

EFFECTS OF PREGNANCY ON FAMILY DYNAMICS

Pregnancy affects both the teenager and the members of her family. Pregnancy represents added economic and emotional pressure and often is a burden with which the family is not equipped to deal. In some cases, grandparents become the infant's primary caregiver. Because of this, their usual pattern or routine might be drastically changed.

Reba Jackson's mother, Tania, is feeling stressed by the demands of the new baby in the house. She tells Sally Arnold, the nurse who is making a home visit, "My husband and I worked all our lives so that we could travel in our retirement. Instead, we are taking care of our grandson while my daughter finishes high school. We were lucky; our health insurance policy paid for some of Reba's expenses, but we have had to pay for some. Our savings are slowly sinking, and I'm looking at working for another 10 years, if my health holds up."

Siblings and other family members can become resentful. Siblings might feel they have to compete for attention. When the infant arrives, both siblings and other household members might have less privacy and might be forced to share sleeping space to accommodate the new arrival. Sometimes the extended family shares or assumes the economic costs of caring for the pregnant teenager and her child.

FATHERS OF BABIES BORN TO ADOLESCENT MOTHERS

Most pregnancies in adolescent girls are the result of relationships with young adult males (20-plus years) rather than teenage males. Only 1.9% of males 19 years of age or younger have a child, whereas 7.8% of females the same age have a child (Martinez et al., 2006). This means that men over age 19 must be responsible for most births to teen mothers. Fifty-three percent of men aged 20 to 24 years report that their female partner is younger, and 58% of men aged 25 to 29 years report younger female partners. In fact, 33% of men aged 25 to 29 years have female partners that are either 3 to 6 years younger or 7 or more years younger (Martinez et al.,

2006). A study of California teen mothers found that the fathers of their babies were an average of 3½ years older than the mothers (Frost & Oslake, 1999). This suggests that interventions aimed at fathers need to target a wider audience of males than current programs. When available, intervention programs are aimed primarily at adolescent fathers.

Teenage fathers, like teenage mothers, have monetary and educational problems. Although more teenage fathers than mothers complete high school, almost 50% drop out, which leaves them vulnerable to the same economic difficulties as teenage mothers (Martinez et al., 2006).

Teen fathers who do not graduate from high school usually have lower paying jobs than teens and young men who delay parenthood (NCPTP, 2002). Hoffman (2006) estimates the cost to the public sector as $3.1 billion per year in lost taxes as a result of those lower-paying jobs among young fathers.

There is a renewed interest in fathers and the role fathers play in child rearing. Because most fathers of babies born to teen mothers are young, they are less able psychologically and financially to contribute much to their children's upbringing (Elfenbein & Felice, 2003). Before delivery, most unwed fathers plan to contribute financially to the support of the mother and the child, but only a few follow through.

Fathers generally are available to the pregnant teenager before delivery, but their relationship with the mother and infant weakens over time. Studies indicate that most are still involved at delivery. Fathers of young babies see their infants regularly (daily or weekly) (Gavin et al., 2002; Rhein et al., 1997). By the time the child is 5 years old, however, only a handful have regular contact with their child, and absent teen fathers pay less than $800 per year in child support (NCPTP, 2002). Most teen fathers (80%) do not marry the mothers of their children (NCPTP, 2002).

The health care system has devoted most of its attention to caring for the adolescent mother, and the adolescent or young adult father has been largely ignored. Much work must be done to address adolescent male health, sexuality, and responsible sexual behavior, and the father's role in teenage pregnancy. The following initiatives appear promising:

- Primary prevention stressing male responsibilities in birth control
- Secondary prevention geared toward increasing the young fathers' role in pregnancy and child care
- Tertiary prevention directed at improving parenting skills and supporting lifestyle changes (e.g., education, job training) that increase the possibility of financial stability and independence.

LEGAL ISSUES AND TEEN ACCESS TO REPRODUCTIVE HEALTH SERVICES

With respect to the right to privacy and confidentiality, there are conflicting laws affecting minors. The Supreme Court has acknowledged a minor's right to privacy, including privacy in medical service needs. Nevertheless, a minor's access to reproductive health services is limited. Consent for medical care is governed primarily by state laws. Most states allow adolescents to obtain reproductive health services, such as contraceptives, sexual disease treatment, and pregnancy testing, without parental consent. Many states have passed explicit laws that allow access to certain medical services (Box 24-2). Some states

Box 24-2 State Laws Governing Adolescent Access to Reproductive Services

- Adolescents may obtain contraceptive services in 46 states and the District of Columbia (some restrictions may apply).
- Pregnant adolescents may obtain prenatal care and delivery services in 35 states and the District of Columbia.
- Teens may seek diagnosis and treatment of sexually transmitted diseases in all 50 states and the District of Columbia.
- Abortion services:
  - 35 states have some type of parental consent or parental notification requirement.
  - 22 states require parental consent; two of these require consent of both parents.
  - 11 states require parental notification.
  - 2 states require both parental consent and notification.
  - Most states that require parental involvement make exceptions for medical emergencies and teens who have been abused.

Adapted from Alan Guttmacher Institute. (2007). Selected fact sheets. Retrieved February 2, 2007 from http://www.guttmacher.org.

restrict the types of health care minors may receive without parental authorization. For example, treatment for STDs is allowed, but contraceptive services require parental approval.

EXCEPTIONS TO PARENTAL CONSENT REQUIREMENTS

Certain minors are considered legally "mature" for the purpose of making decisions, including obtaining medical services. States define these adolescents as "emancipated." Married minors, members of the armed forces, and teens who live apart from their parents are most often considered legally mature by state standards (see Chapter 6).

STATE AND FEDERAL EFFORTS AT INFLUENCING CONSENT LAWS

There have been efforts at both the state and federal levels to create legislation requiring parental consent for contraceptive and other medical services. Two states, Texas and Utah, passed legislation that limits a minor's access to birth control and STD treatment by refusing to pay for these services with state funds if the minor does not have parental consent (Jones & Boonstra 2005). Services provided with federal funds are not limited in this fashion.

RESTRICTIONS ON ABORTION CONSENT

Access to abortion services is treated differently than access to other reproductive health care. This is an area of continued and ongoing legislative effort. Currently, parental involvement in abortion decisions is mandated by 35 states (AGI, 2007b). Some states require parental notification, and others require parental consent. All states with parental consent laws are required by a Supreme Court decision to have some type of judicial bypass mechanism. Adolescents who are fearful of obtaining or unable to obtain parental consent may seek a judicial review and bypass parental consent, if they show adequate reasons.

LEGAL AMBIGUITY PREVAILS

Plan B (levonorgestrel, the medication to prevent conception) is currently approved for over-the-counter emergency contraceptive use in the United States. However, access to Plan B without a prescription is restricted to adults 18 years or older, who must provide proof of age to buy the medication. Plan B remains a prescription-only drug for girls age 17 and younger (Aschenbrenner, 2006).

Many states allow adolescents to make certain life decisions, such as leaving school or marrying, at a younger age than they can independently make certain medical decisions. In 40 states and the District of Columbia, a minor may place her child for adoption without parental consent (AGI, 2007c). Some states allow adolescent parents to consent to medical treatment for their child while restricting their ability to consent to medical services for themselves. It is important for community health nurses to be familiar with the laws in their states concerning adolescent health services and to be aware of any restrictions that would necessitate parental approval.

NURSING ROLE IN ADDRESSING TEENAGE SEXUAL ACTIVITY AND PREGNANCY

Community health nurses providing care to sexually active and pregnant teenagers should use a balanced approach. A comprehensive intervention program should address all prevention levels: primary, secondary, and tertiary. A strategy that encourages abstinence, delayed initiation to sexual activity, and responsible contraception for those who choose to be sexually active is part of a comprehensive approach to primary prevention. Primary prevention is a crucial component of any intervention program. If young girls become pregnant, however, it is imperative that they receive adequate prenatal care coupled with long-term postpartum follow-up to ensure a healthy outcome for both them and their children.

Community health nurses, because of their expertise in assessment, health teaching, and program development, are well suited to this task. Their accessibility to adolescent populations places them in a pivotal position to play a significant role in the delivery of care before initiation of sexual activity, during contraceptive use, during pregnancy, and during long-term follow-up with the parents and child. Community Resources for Practice at the end of this chapter can help nurses plan and provide care for all three prevention levels.

PRIMARY PREVENTION

It is apparent that pregnancy during the teen years presents some unique risks and special needs for the teen, her pregnancy, and her infant. The best choice for most young girls is to delay pregnancy until they are physically and emotionally mature. Primary prevention has three focuses:

1. To delay or stop participation in sexual activity
2. To provide access to contraceptives
3. To strengthen future life goals

Most experts believe that a comprehensive primary prevention program should include sex education, family life education, family planning, and some form of life planning program that stresses identification of future goals and steps to those goals (Lindberg, Santelli, & Singh, 2006a; NCPTP, 2002). A good sex education program encourages self-esteem and responsible decision making in addition to containing specific information on sexual matters. Most of the available primary prevention programs address one or two but not all aspects of a comprehensive program.

EDUCATIONAL PROGRAMS

Most educational efforts are school based. Sex education is provided by some private schools and by public schools in approximately 70% of the states (AGI, 2006d). Only 19 states and the District of Columbia require sex education in public schools (AGI, 2007a). Many programs are limited in the content they may present. For example, 35 states and the District of Columbia require STD/HIV education, but 70% of those states require that abstinence content be stressed if taught and 30% mandate that abstinence be included in content on STD/HIV. Only 18 states (half) of those that mandate STD/HIV education require those programs to include contraceptive education.

In 35 of the 38 states that provide some form of sex education, parents have the option to disenroll their children (AGI, 2007a). A typical sex education effort consists of fewer than 10 class periods scattered throughout a student's 12 years of education. Only 1 in 10 programs is a comprehensive sexuality education program (USDHHS, 1995). The National Campaign to Prevent Teen Pregnancy has identified 10 characteristics of effective sexual education programs (Box 24-3).

Sex and Contraception Content

Sex education contains, at the very least, information about the anatomy and physiology of reproduction in males and females. Beyond this narrow focus, there is little agreement and much controversy about appropriate content for sex education classes.

Box 24-3   Characteristics of Effective Sex and HIV Education Programs

- Focus on reducing one or more sexual behaviors that lead to unintended pregnancy or HIV/STD infection
- Are based on theoretic approaches that have been demonstrated to influence other health-related behavior and identify specific important sexual antecedents to be targeted
- Deliver and consistently reinforce a clear message about abstaining from sexual activity and/or using condoms or other forms of contraception*
- Provide basic, accurate information about the risks of teen sexual activity and about ways to avoid intercourse or use methods of protection against pregnancy and STDs
- Include activities that address social pressures that influence sexual behavior
- Provide examples of and practice with communication, negotiation, and refusal skills
- Employ teaching methods designed to involve participants and have them personalize the information
- Incorporate behavioral goals, teaching methods, and materials that are appropriate to the age, sexual experience, and culture of the students
- Last a sufficient length of time (i.e., more than a few hours)
- Select teachers or peer leaders who believe in the program and then provide them with adequate training

From Manlove, J., Papillio, A., & Ikramullah, E. (2004). *Not yet: Programs to delay first sex among teens.* Washington, DC: National Campaign to Prevent Teen Pregnancy; and Kirby, D. (2001). *Emerging answers: Research findings on programs to reduce teen pregnancy* [Summary]. Washington, DC: National Campaign to Prevent Teen Pregnancy.
HIV, Human immunodeficiency virus; *STD,* sexually transmitted disease.
*Appears to be one of the most important characteristics distinguishing effective from ineffective programs.

Some programs include information on sexual orientation, STDs, and contraception. These topics are the most contentious and engender public debate and opposition by parents or community groups. When faced with protest, school districts are reluctant to go against parental wishes. Of states with sex education content, 40% discourage or prohibit the inclusion of pregnancy prevention content (AGI, 2003a). Over the past decade, the proportion of teens who received formal education about birth control decreased by 10% (Lindberg, Santelli, & Singh, 2006a). School districts are also reluctant to improve or add to existing content because it might generate renewed public interest and opposition. Teachers feel constrained by community opposition, and some stick to a prepared script rather than risk discussion and exploration of sexual topics (Frost et al., 2001).

Most of the public appears to support sex education with content aimed at reducing teenage pregnancies (Albert, 2007; Bleakley et al., 2006; National Public Radio, Kaiser Family Foundation, & Kennedy School of Government, 2004). About 15% of those surveyed support abstinence-only programs. The remainder feel either that abstinence should be included in a comprehensive approach or that abstinence is not an important element of a sex education program.

The best way to reduce concern and increase community support of sex education is to expand the content to address community concerns whenever possible. Although a comprehensive sex education curriculum cannot ignore contraceptive information, there are legitimate issues related to abstinence, the advantages of delayed sexual activity, and the medical risks of teenage sexual conduct (e.g., exposure to STDs) that should be addressed. A program that provides such an approach is comprehensive and has the additional advantage of increasing community support.

Abstinence-Only Curriculum

Abstinence-only programs, sexual education programs that teach abstinence as the only option for the unmarried and adolescents, have the support of an active minority of Americans. Abstinence-only programs have received emphasis in federally funded projects. Federally funded abstinence programs do not allow mention of contraceptives, except to cite their failure rates (Bleakley et al., 2006). About 35% of public school districts require that abstinence be taught as the only option for teens (AGI, 2006e; Boonstra, 2002). In those districts, other methods of contraception are not discussed or content is limited to the ineffectiveness of such methods.

The federal government funded abstinence-only programs at the level of $176 million for 2006 (AGI, 2006e). To qualify for grant money, education programs must meet eight designated criteria, including teaching that sexual activity outside of marriage is likely to have harmful psychologic and physical effects (AGI, 2000b). In 2004, a congressional report outlined many errors in the current abstinence education programs. The report (United States House of Representatives, 2004) concluded that abstinence-only education programs

- Made false claims about the physical and psychologic risks of abortion;
- Provided misinformation on the incidence and transmission of STDs;
- Provided religious and moral views in place of scientific facts;
- Distorted medical evidence and basic scientific facts.

There is little evidence to suggest that abstinence-only programs are successful in curtailing sexual activity before marriage or in reducing STDs or pregnancy among adolescents (AGI, 2006e; Bleakley et al., 2006). Health and educational professionals have asked for stringent review of abstinence-only programs and comparison of their results with those of other types of sex education programs. One study of adolescent **virginity pledgers** (teens who committed to delay sexual activity until marriage) found that these teens did delay first sexual intercourse but had lower use of condoms at the time of first sexual activity and were less likely to seek care for STDs (Bruckner & Bearman, 2005). Virginity pledgers had the same rates of STDs as other teens and substituted anal or oral sex for sexual intercourse at higher rates than other teens. The Minnesota Department of Health evaluated an abstinence-only program and reported that there was an increase in the rate at which teens engaged in sexual activity 1 year after they attended the program ("Can abstinence programs lead to more sex?" 2004). In response to public concern, the USDHHS conducted a study of abstinence-only programs and released the results in April 2007. That study followed teens for 4 to 6 years after receiving abstinence-only education and found that those teens engaged in sexual activity, initiated sexual activity, had the same number of sexual partners, and engaged in unprotected sex as often as teens who received other types of sex education.

Comprehensive Sex Education—Most Effective

Data indicate that programs that provide a comprehensive sex education (discussion of abstinence, contraception, STDs) with a more balanced approach are more successful and do not encourage sexual activity (AGI, 2006e). Sex education teachers who teach the effectiveness of contraceptives in their programs are more likely to include information about preventing unintended pregnancies and STDs and the correct use of birth control methods (Landry et al., 2003). **Comprehensive sex education programs** delay the onset of sexual activity in teens, reduce the frequency of sex, reduce the frequency of unprotected sexual activity and increase the use of contraceptives among sexually active teens, reduce the teen pregnancy rate, and lower the number of sex partners (AGI, 2006e; Bleakley et al., 2006; Manlove et al., 2004; Satcher, 2002). Several such successful programs are listed in Box 24-4, which also gives some examples of other innovative primary and tertiary prevention efforts.

Family Life Programs

Family life programs offer information on family systems and the interactions and influences among family members. Topics include marriage, divorce, separation, and birth. Most family life programs are offered at the junior or senior high school level as an elective course, which means that they do not reach many teenagers and cannot target those at greatest risk. Family life programs use a variety of teaching techniques, including simulation and game playing, that help concrete thinkers consider the rigors as well as the delights of parenting. One popular technique requires students to assume full-time personal responsibility for the welfare of a baby simulator or raw egg for 1 week. Students must ensure that the baby substitute is always in the presence of a responsible person and comes to no harm. They are then graded on how well they accomplish this task.

Role of the Nurse in Education

In some school systems with school nurses, the nurse is involved in both sex and family life education. If family life courses are not available in the school system or are not reaching at-risk teenagers, nurses might consider implementing such a program with their community agency's support or in conjunction with other community organizations such as the Young Men's or Young Women's Christian Association.

Community health nurses can provide factual sex education to teenagers in class as they provide other health services. Most sex education teachers have little training in sex education. Many have asked for additional training in how to educate students about pregnancy, HIV infection, and other STDs (AGI, 2002b). Nurses make effective sex educators because they are equipped to provide sexual content in a factual and nonsensational approach. They are also proficient at encouraging and guiding client discussion, characteristics helpful in addressing sex education with teenagers.

SCREENING FOR RISK BEHAVIORS

Adolescents who use health care services should be screened for potential risky behaviors. Areas to access include sexual activity, symptoms of HIV infection and other STDs, and knowledge and use of barrier protection if sexually active. In one study, health care providers missed opportunities to counsel students on sexual health behaviors on more than 50% of the visits monitored during the study (Burnstein et al., 2003).

Adolescent Counseling

The aim of counseling and education for teens should be to delay the start of sexual activity and to provide accurate information to reduce the risk of STDs and pregnancy for sexually active teens. Most publically funded family planning clinics counsel new teen clients about the benefits of abstinence and encourage them to discuss sexual issues with their parents (Lindberg, Santelli, & Singh, 2006b). About half of these clinics also have education programs on related topics that are provided at the clinic or in schools and youth centers.

CONTRACEPTIVE SERVICES

Access to and regular use of birth control is the goal of contraceptive services for adolescents. Family planning clinics and private physicians are one source; school-based clinics are a more recent effort. Box 24-4 provides examples of school-based contraceptive programs.

Community health nurses can encourage clinic attendance, promote access to contraception, and provide referrals to appropriate contraceptive services when counseling individuals or teaching sex education classes. The nurse must emphasize the importance of contraceptive use by all sexually active adolescents.

The key to compliance with birth control methods by teenagers is regular, continued attendance at a clinic site and the use of long-acting contraceptives. Although much progress has been made, teens are still less likely to use contraception regularly and more likely to rely on condoms as their primary method of birth control (Santelli et al., 2007). Clinic programs should provide regular contact and monitor compliance; school-based programs have been particularly successful in this effort (Sidebottom et al., 2003). Community health nurses are adept at monitoring and improving adolescent compliance

Box 24-4   Selected Examples of Prevention Programs

Primary Prevention

Teen incentives program. A pregnancy prevention program using skill development to promote healthy behaviors and improve self-perception and decision-making behaviors, especially regarding sexual activity and pregnancy prevention. It showed statistically significant results in decreasing sexual activity and increasing contraceptive use (Smith, 1994).

Becoming a Responsible Teen (BART). A community-based program aimed at prevention of human immunodeficiency virus infection/acquired immunodeficiency syndrome that includes information about pregnancy prevention and abstinence. The program emphasizes decision-making skills and communication regarding sexual behavior. In a 1-year follow-up, participants had lower levels of sexual activity and were more likely to use condoms if sexually active than teens not in the program (St. Lawrence, 1998; Manlove et al., 2004).

School-based clinics contraceptive services—Minneapolis. A program that includes both school-based contraceptive services and a voucher system to provide students with contraceptives. The vouchers are given at school for community clinics. At schools, the program found there was a similar demand for contraceptives, but the on-site programs increased access and use of contraceptives (Sidebottom et al., 2003).

Life's Walk Program. A school-based sexuality abstinence-only education program taught in eighth and tenth grades. The program students were stronger advocates for abstinence than students who did not use the program. However, there was no difference with regard to level of sexual activity between those who used the program and those who did not (Barnett & Hurst, 2003).

Secondary Prevention

Teenage mothers–grandmothers program. A program for teens and their mothers that includes group meetings and counseling about parenting and other concerns of participants. Teens whose mothers participated were less likely to drop out of school and had better self-esteem than those whose mothers did not participate (Roye & Balk, 1996).

Pre- and post-pregnancy intervention programs. Programs developed for adolescent teens and those who have already given birth. Programs provide education to improve child health outcomes, lower repeat pregnancy risk, improve parenting skills, and support educational programs for young mothers (Harris & Franklin, 2003; Ford et al., 2002).

Comprehensive Programs

Safer choices intervention program. A comprehensive school-based program developed with teacher, parent, child, and community input. The program included use of peer educators, curriculum and staff development activities, and school and community links for activities and services (Coyle et al., 1996). It was implemented in California and Texas high schools. Teens in the program were 43% less likely to initiate sexual intercourse than nonprogram teens. Sexually active program teens were more likely to use contraceptives than nonprogram teens during a 3-year follow-up (Manlove et al., 2004).

California's Adolescent Sibling Pregnancy Prevention Program. A program targeting high-risk teens who have siblings who were adolescent parents (male or female). It provides comprehensive services, including case management, academic guidance, promotion of decision-making skills, job placement, self-esteem enhancement, contraceptive services, and sexual education. The results are promising: pregnancy rates are lower, there is delay in initiating or abstinence from sexual activity, contraceptive use is higher, and school truancy is lower than in a comparable peer group (East et al., 2003).

Children's Aid Society–Carrera Program. An intensive long-term after-school program for high-risk students in New York City that emphasizes planning for the future. Students stay in the program throughout high school. Components include employment and academic assistance, family life and sexuality education, performing arts participation, sports training, physical health, mentoring, and ongoing counseling. Females in the program were less likely to have sexual intercourse or become pregnant and two times more likely to use two types of contraceptives than were control teens. Males in the program were more likely to use two types of contraceptives than were control teens. The program is expanding to Nebraska, Florida, New York State, New Mexico, and Baltimore, MD (Philliber et al., 2001; Philliber et al., 2003).

Data from Barnett, J. E., & Hurst, C. S. (2003). Abstinence education for rural youth: An evaluation of the Life's Walk Program. *Journal of School Health, 73*(7), 264-268; Coyle, K., Kirby, D., Parcel, G., et al. (1996). Safer choices: A multicomponent school-based HIV/STD and pregnancy prevention program for adolescents. *Journal of School Health, 66*(3), 89-94; East, P., Kiernan, E., & Chavez, G. (2003). An evaluation of California's Sibling Pregnancy Prevention Program. *Perspectives on Sexual and Reproductive Health, 35*(20), 62-70; Ford, K., Weglicki, L., Kershaw, T., et al. (2002). Effects of a prenatal care intervention for adolescent mothers on birth weight, repeat pregnancy, and educational outcomes at one year postpartum. *Journal of Perinatal Education, 11*(1), 35-38; Harris, M. B., & Franklin, C. G. (2003). Effects of a cognitive-behavioral, school-based, group intervention with Mexican American pregnant and parenting adolescents. *Social Work Research, 27*(2), 71-83; Manlove, J., Papillio, A., & Ikramullah, E. (2004). *Not yet: Programs to delay first sex among teens.* Washington, DC: Campaign to Prevent Teen Pregnancy; Meadows, M., Sadler, L. S., & Reitmeyer, G. D. (2000). School-based support for urban adolescent mothers. *Journal of Pediatric Health Care, 14*(5), 221-227; Philliber, S., Kaye, J., & Herrling, S. (2001). *The national evaluation of the Children's Aid Society Carrera-model program to prevent teen pregnancy.* Accord, NY: Philliber Research Associates; Philliber, S., Brooks, L., Lehrer, L. P., et al. (2003). Outcomes of teen pregnancy programs in New Mexico. *Adolescents, 38*(151), 535-553; Roye, C. F., & Balk, S. J. (1996). Evaluation of an intergenerational program for pregnant and parenting adolescents. *Maternal-Child Nursing Journal, 24*(1), 32-40; Sidebottom, A., Birnbaum, A. S., & Nafstad, S. S. (2003). Decreasing barriers for teens: Evaluation of a new pregnancy prevention strategy in school-based clinics. *American Journal of Public Health, 93*(11), 1890-1892; St. Lawrence, J. S. (1998). *Becoming a responsible teen: An HIV risk reduction program for adolescents.* Santa Cruz, CA: ETR Associates; and Smith, M. A. B. (1994). Teen incentive program: Evaluation of a health promotion model for adolescent pregnancy prevention. *Journal of Health Education, 25*(1), 24-29.

with birth control measures because they provide clear, direct, and nonjudgmental guidance.

LIFE OPTIONS OR YOUTH DEVELOPMENT PROGRAMS

Life options programs are comprehensive programs that provide a broad range of support services for adolescents. These programs attempt to expand an adolescent's future goals and expectations by improving educational and employment prospects. The aim is to increase a teen's self-worth and ease the teen's transition to adulthood. Because future-oriented, goal-directed adolescents are less likely to become preg-

nant, the expected result is a reduction in the rate of teenage pregnancies.

Programs might be school or community based and target especially risky populations such as low-income teens. Efforts are directed toward reducing social factors associated with increased pregnancy rates (Klerman, 2002). Life option programs offer a variety of structures and strategies, including the following:

- One-on-one mentoring and role modeling by successful adults
- Community service participation
- Remedial education

- Tutoring services
- Counseling, by both professionals and peers
- Self-worth enhancement techniques
- Exposure to new experiences (e.g., concerts, museums, and travel) to expand life options

These are relatively new programs intended to provide long-term intensive support to targeted teenagers. The results take years to achieve. Some preliminary data suggest success in delaying sexual initiation, increasing condom use, and reducing rates of STDs (Lonczak et al., 2002).

SECONDARY PREVENTION: THE CARE OF PREGNANT TEENAGERS

Since 1995, there has been a renewed public effort to address the serious problem of teen pregnancy, which has resulted in a 33% decline in the pregnancy rate (Santelli et al., 2006). The National Campaign to Prevent Teen Pregnancy (NCPTP) has been instrumental in addressing the problem of teenage pregnancy in the United States. This nonprofit, nonpartisan, broad-based group of social and religious leaders, health professionals, researchers, politicians, and concerned citizens is supported by private donations. Its mission is the reduction of teen pregnancy in the United States.

Community health nurses have a unique opportunity to affect teenage pregnancy rates and reduce the health risks for both the pregnant adolescent and her infant. Care should be directed toward providing a satisfactory and healthy outcome. The critical elements of any program include the following:

- Early detection of pregnancy
- Pregnancy resolution services
- Prenatal health care
- Childbirth education
- Parenting education

EARLY DETECTION

Early detection provides more time to decide what to do about the pregnancy and a longer period of prenatal care if the adolescent decides to continue the pregnancy. Community health nurses can facilitate early detection by considering the possibility of pregnancy during the initial assessment of physical complaints by female adolescents. Complaints such as fatigue, appetite loss, nausea and vomiting, weight loss, or missed menstrual periods, coupled with a history of sexual activity and inadequate birth control, should be clues to pursue additional questioning.

Sensitive but direct questioning is important. The community health nurse must be accepting of the teenager or the teenager will be reluctant to share information, ask questions, and express concerns. It is not uncommon for a teenager to deny or attempt to hide a pregnancy. If the nurse is brusque, it is unlikely the teenager will feel comfortable seeking or volunteering information of an intimate nature (Montgomery, 2003). Previous experience with nurses and other health care providers has an impact on a teenager's willingness to seek care or to trust the nurse. All nurses should take care to ensure that young clients are treated with respect and dignity and receive culturally competent care (see Chapter 10).

PREGNANCY RESOLUTION SERVICES

Once pregnancy is confirmed, the teenager faces an important decision. The American College of Obstetrics and Gynecology,

Planned Parenthood, the American Nurses Association, and numerous other professional health care organizations take the position that a comprehensive program should include all possible pregnancy options: abortion, adoption, and keeping the baby.

- Approximately 6 of every 10 pregnant adolescents choose childbirth.
- Three in 10 teen pregnancies end in abortion.
- About 10% of adolescent pregnancies end in miscarriage.
- Choice of adoption is rare.

Abortion

Adolescents choose abortion more frequently than adults and wait longer to do so. Approximately 30% of adolescent pregnancies are terminated by abortion (AGI, 2006a). The most common reasons teenagers give for choosing abortion are the following (Andrews & Boyle, 2003; Finer et al., 2005):

- Too young to be a mother
- Cannot afford a child now
- Does not want others to know she is pregnant
- Parents want her to have an abortion
- Partner is unreliable

Abortion is a controversial issue. Both supporters and opponents are vocal and strident. For the past three decades, abortion opponents have attempted to reduce access to and availability of abortion services. Both federal and state efforts are aimed at reducing funding and tightening regulations for programs receiving public money. Federal funding for Medicaid abortion services was eliminated, although there are some exceptions, such as abortions in cases of rape or incest (AGI, 2007d). Any state that wanted to continue funding had to assume all the costs for abortion services. Some states (17) chose to continue funding, but most (33) chose not to do so (AGI, 2007d). Because many pregnant teenagers are served by publicly supported programs, their access to abortion services was directly affected by the changes.

In the 1980s federal regulations imposed a "gag" restriction on health professionals who counsel pregnant adolescents. This gag rule forbade health professionals from reviewing abortion as an option and from providing referrals for abortion services. President Clinton rescinded this order when he took office in 1993. Although there is no gag order currently in effect in the United States, President George H. W. Bush reauthorized a global gag order. Counselors cannot discuss abortion alternatives with women overseas who are served by family planning programs that receive U.S. government funds (Cohen, 2001). President George W. Bush continued this restriction on funding for foreign family planning services.

State efforts have targeted changes to the legal criteria for abortion services (e.g., parental notification and waiting periods). These restrictions are costly, and there is some question as to their effectiveness. The Supreme Court has upheld some but not all of the state initiatives on parental notification and waiting periods (AGI, 2003b). In general, state initiatives that allow teenagers an alternative to parental notification or do not impose an "undue burden" in waiting time have been upheld; the remainder have been struck down.

It is difficult to determine whether abortion restrictions have an impact on teenage abortion. Nationally, there has been a decline in the rate at which teenagers seek abortion services, but there has also been a decline in the rate of teenage pregnancies.

The unresolved question is whether abortion rates would be higher without the legal and financial obstacles. Some suggest that limited access to Medicaid funding increases the hardships for low-income women who choose the abortion option (Frost et al., 2001). Further studies are needed to determine the exact impact of funding reductions and legal limitations on abortion choices of adolescent females.

Adoption

Placement for adoption is less controversial but is an infrequent choice for teenagers. Few teenagers or other pregnant women choose this option (Finer et al., 2005). Adolescents who choose adoption are older, farther along in their schooling, and more future oriented with respect to educational goals than are teenagers who keep their infants. There is some evidence that parental support influences a teen's decision to place her child for adoption.

A federal effort directed by the Office of Adolescent Pregnancy Programs to encourage the adoption option among pregnant teenagers began in the 1980s. Research studies were funded that were intended to increase the likelihood of adoption and to identify factors that influenced the adoption choice. In 2000, legislation provided funding to support the training of family planning and other health providers in how to provide information on adoption to women reluctant to continue a pregnancy (Dailard, 2004). No appreciable change has occurred in the adoption rate, although efforts continue to increase the rate of adoption, especially as an alternative to abortion.

Teen Satisfaction with Choice

Adolescents appear satisfied with their pregnancy decisions. Despite assertions that teenagers who choose abortion or adoption suffer negative psychologic consequences, no evidence supports this position (Andrews & Boyle, 2003; Pope et al., 2001). In general, teenagers feel they made the best personal choice at the time.

PRENATAL HEALTH CARE

Once a teenager decides to continue the pregnancy, effort is directed toward ensuring a healthy outcome for the mother and infant. Early initiation and regular continuation of prenatal care significantly reduce the risk for both adolescents and their infants, although complication rates remain above those in other age groups (Klima, 2003; Martin et al., 2006; Mummert et al., 2007). Short gestation, low infant birth weight, and neonatal mortality are all reduced with regular prenatal care (Ford et al., 2002). Home visits by community health nurses improve pregnancy outcomes and infant health status (CDF, 2005; Olds et al., 1999, 2004). The Nurse-Family Partnership program started by David Olds, a community health nurse, has expanded to 263 counties in 20 states (CDF, 2005).

Special Needs of Pregnant Adolescents

An estimated 33% of adolescent mothers receive inadequate prenatal care (Ford et al., 2002; Philliber et al., 2003). A standard obstetrics text should serve as the basis for a prenatal plan of care. There are some special concerns of which the community health nurse must be aware when planning prenatal care for pregnant teenagers. As previously noted, adolescent mothers and their infants are at greater risk for serious medical problems than are older mothers and their infants. Age alone is not the problem. The risk associated with early pregnancy has been correlated with factors such as lower socioeconomic status, poor prenatal care, inadequate nutrition, and unhealthy lifestyle practices (Martin et al., 2003, 2006). When care is taken to reduce the associated risks, teenage pregnancy is less problematic.

The essential components of a prenatal program to reduce low birth weight in infants should include the following:
- Screening for harmful behaviors
- Ongoing risk assessment
- Individual care and case management
- Nutritional counseling
- Health education aimed at reducing poor health habits
- Social support services

Good prenatal programs also should include preparation for labor and delivery, introduction to newborn care, and exploration of birth control options for postdelivery use. Adolescents have some special health needs and concerns associated with pregnancy related to their developmental age, nutrition, and health habits. **Website Resource 24A** identifies for the nurse some important areas of concern for assessment and investigation.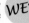

Prenatal Programs Available to Teenagers

Three types of programs offer prenatal care to adolescents: clinic programs, private medical services, and school-based programs. The choice of program depends on accessibility and the financial circumstances of the teenager and her family.

Private medical service is available only to people who are covered by a medical insurance plan or can afford to pay. Most family insurance plans limit coverage to children younger than 18 years of age, although some plans provide coverage until age 21 or 23 if the child is a full-time college student. Parents might be surprised to find that their child is not insured, and they are unprepared to meet the expenses of pregnancy when their child is not a full-time student.

For families without insurance or the financial resources to pay for prenatal care, there are several options:
- Medical assistance or public health insurance through Medicaid or SCHIP
- Prenatal and obstetric clinics associated with publicly funded hospitals that accept medical assistance clients and people with limited financial means, who are offered a sliding-scale fee program
- Prenatal clinic care provided through state and county health departments

Some hospitals and health departments operate satellite clinics in low-income neighborhoods with high rates of adolescent pregnancy. Because socioeconomic status has been associated with a greater number of potential complications, clinics serving low-income teenagers expect to have a larger number of clients requiring intense supervision. Recent reforms have limited care options for low-income pregnant teens. States require most medical assistance recipients to use managed care organizations. At the same time, many health departments have dropped or restricted prenatal programs (see Chapter 29).

Prenatal care services provided through comprehensive community-based programs achieve the best results with pregnant teens. These programs have a heavy outreach and educational emphasis, use multidisciplinary health care teams with an emphasis on community health nurse involvement, and do home visiting (Klima, 2003; Montgomery, 2003). The community health nurse acts as the broker or case manager for prenatal care and sees that clients are provided with needed services. The nurse is usually the team member who spends the most time with the adolescent, providing health screening, counseling, and education for pregnant clients.

School-based prenatal services are offered in conjunction with other school clinic services or in separate schools designed for the exclusive use of pregnant teenagers. Approximately 20% of school-based clinics offer prenatal care (AGI, 2002c). School-based prenatal services employ a comprehensive approach and are usually found in large school districts with high rates of adolescent pregnancy. School-based prenatal programs are associated with a high level of compliance with appointments and the care regimen, a reduction in the number of complications, and the secondary benefit of increased school attendance both before and after delivery (Meadows et al., 2000).

Support Systems and Nurse Home Visits

Adolescent pregnancy is often associated with or hastens a family crisis. During pregnancy, the expectant teenager looks for emotional, financial, and physical support from family members. The community health nurse and other caregivers should take care to assess the degree of support available from family and others. Most pregnant teens live with their parents. The amount of support (financial, physical, and psychologic) varies with families. Many adolescent mothers live in households in which poverty and other problems are common (AGI, 2002d). If families are unable or unwilling to provide support, the teenager will need help identifying other support sources. Examples of potential support include other relatives, the father of the infant and his family, church organizations, other community groups, and clubs and organizations in which the teenager has participated. If the teenager is separated from her family, social services can arrange financial assistance for housing or, for younger teenagers, foster care.

For adolescents, pregnancy often accompanies other personal problems or emotional issues. Failure to address related problems and issues in a supportive, caring atmosphere is equivalent to providing only partial care to the pregnant adolescent. Persistent home visitation by the community health nurse is one way to provide long-term support. Studies have demonstrated that pregnant adolescents who are visited at home by community health nurses have better employment records, have fewer pregnancies, and delay a second pregnancy longer, and their children have fewer hospitalizations and better immunizations, compared with adolescents who do not receive home visits (Koniak-Griffin et al., 1999; Olds et al., 1999, 2004).

The Adolescent and Young Adult Father

Secondary prevention efforts aim to improve parental participation in prenatal care, childbirth preparation, and parenting activities. Programs are intended to improve the quality and duration of the relationship between the father and the child. The more successful efforts have been those that engage fathers early, no later than the birth of the baby (McLanahan & Carlson, 2002). Community health nurses can assist in these efforts by encouraging the father's participation in prenatal visits. The community health nurse should invite the father to prenatal classes, encourage questions and participation in prenatal visits, and acknowledge the father's role as a partner in the birth process. Fathers can be encouraged, but not forced, to participate in the delivery process.

CHILDBIRTH EDUCATION

Teenagers are likely to get information about labor and delivery from their peers; much of which may be erroneous. Assessment of the teenager's knowledge base, correction of misconceptions, and reinforcement of valid information is key. If the adolescent's mother or other relative is involved, the nurse should include that person in the dialogue. The mother's knowledge base might be incorrect or outdated if it consists solely of her own personal experiences. Including the mother in the interview allows the nurse to correct misinformation, acknowledge the mother's contribution to her daughter's care, and facilitate the mother's cooperation with the prenatal and postpartum programs.

The delivery of a child usually represents a pregnant adolescent's first experience with hospitalization. Most hospitals or birthing centers provide tours and orientation prior to delivery. Whenever possible, teenagers should be encouraged to attend an orientation program. Most facilities allow a support person to remain with the teenager during delivery. The nurse might have to help the teenager choose her support person, especially if a number of persons are available. This decision should be made as soon as possible. If the teenager has opted for natural childbirth classes, the person who will support her in labor should attend classes with her if possible.

POSTPARTUM AND NEWBORN CARE

Changes in the delivery of health services have reduced the amount of in-hospital time mothers are allowed by their health insurance providers. These changes affect the amount of education and monitoring delivered by hospital staff and make it crucial that monitoring be provided in the home and community. Postdelivery care varies widely in scope and duration of services. All prenatal programs provide a postpartum check for the mother, and a well-baby check is included in most services. The most extensive postpartum care is delivered in community programs that rely heavily on nurses. These programs usually include the following:

- Health assessment of both the mother and infant
- Newborn care education and supervision
- Parental education on growth and development and parenting skills
- Review of role adjustments and available supports
- Sex education and birth control information

One valuable component of these programs is the emphasis on regular contact with the new mother, starting the first week after delivery. This is especially relevant for adolescent mothers, who have little experience in caring for a newborn and distinguishing between normal and abnormal physical conditions for both themselves and their new infants. Regular nurse visits reduce anxiety and increase infant health (Olds et al., 1999). Mothers experience many concerns or problems before the first scheduled clinic or physician visit. Earlier contacts allow the teenager and nurse to address these issues and reduce anxiety. Contact need not always be in person; some care can be provided by telephone monitoring of the new mother.

Health Status of the New Mother

At a minimum, the new mother should have a 6-week postpartum examination. Some community health programs start home visits at about 2 weeks postpartum. The physical assessment should focus on the standard postpartum areas as well as on specific concerns of the adolescent. Consistent with teenagers' concern about body image, they have frequent questions about weight loss and figure restoration.

Dorothea Collins is a new 16-year-old mother. When Tom Dresher, the community health nurse, made his first postpartum visit, he found that Dorothea was successfully coping with baby feedings and changes. However, the primary issue on Dorothea's mind was her prom dress, which she had purchased during her pregnancy and promptly tried on as soon as she left the hospital. Dorothea told Tom, "I'm going to have to crash diet because I don't fit into the dress. This is the dress size I wore before I became pregnant. I don't understand why it doesn't fit. I am only 5 pounds heavier than I was before I got pregnant." Tom spent some time helping Dorothea understand that her shape would continue to change for some time after delivery. He reviewed her eating habits, and together they worked on a balanced diet plan designed to help her lose about 1 pound per week. He also encouraged her to begin some moderate exercise, such as walking.

Role Adjustment and Emotional Support

Adjusting to the role of a parent during adolescence is particularly difficult. The adolescent mother needs support as she attempts to integrate her new responsibilities into her daily routine. The teenager might be juggling school and infant care. Fatigue and stress are common and can be exacerbated if the new mother attempts to resume her social activities in addition to her other obligations. The first task, and one that might best be accomplished on a home visit, is to assess the support systems available to the teenage mother. If the adolescent is involved in a comprehensive prenatal and postpartum program, health care professionals have already assessed available support. If not, the nurse should look at the immediate family, other relatives, significant others, and the father of the infant and his family. Even if support systems are adequate, the family might need some help in understanding and supporting the adolescent as a maturing individual.

Role conflict is a common problem in families. Family members might expect the teenager to instantly become an adult and mother, or expect the opposite, that she will remain a child and allow her parents to assume all the responsibilities. Neither situation is especially healthy for the adolescent or infant. Ideally, both parents should be encouraged to continue developing as individuals (e.g., continue their education, participate in some social activities, and explore relationships with peers) and at the same time increase their proficiency and confidence in parenting.

When support is minimal or lacking, the community health nurse might be able to refer the teenager to other possible resources, such as parenting programs, cooperative daycare, or programs that pair the new mother with an older adolescent mother who has had a successful experience. One such program, the Taking Charge Program, paired small groups of pregnant or parenting girls with young women who had been pregnant adolescents. They helped the teenagers improve parenting skills and problem solving (Harris & Franklin, 2003). A mother-grandmother program provides support and encouragement to both the teen mother and her mother, the baby's grandmother (Roye & Balk, 1997).

Adequate support is an important concern, because adolescent mothers have rates of child abuse and neglect twice as high as those of young mothers in their twenties (Hoffman, 2006). Adequate physical and emotional support, along with health teaching and realistic expectations for their children, successfully reduces the incidence of abuse and neglect in at-risk mothers (CDF, 2005; Olds et al., 1999, 2004) (see Chapter 23).

Health Status of the Newborn

In addition to performing the usual newborn assessment, the community health nurse should look for signs of adequate maternal and infant bonding. Evidence of attachment includes calling the child by its given name, cuddling the infant, talking to the infant, and demonstrating an interest in infant care and development. Sometimes teenagers demonstrate difficulty in bonding simply because they have had no previous experience with infants and are afraid to do anything. Sometimes another person has assumed the role of caregiver, and the teenager becomes an observer rather than caregiver. Bonding can be evaluated in clinic situations, but home visits allow the nurse a more accurate picture of the teen and infant relationship, because the nurse can observe for a longer time and evaluate the interaction among the infant, teenager, and other caregivers.

When another person assumes most of the responsibilities for infant care, the nurse should explore the adolescent's wishes. The teenager might want to care for her infant and might simply require encouragement, demonstration, and supervision to become confident in infant care. The nurse might have to suggest that family members help by supporting the teenager as she attempts to establish a relationship with her child.

Nancy Riley is making a home visit to Jamie Schult, who is 2 weeks postpartum. Jamie is 16 years old and lives with her mother, grandmother, and three siblings. She still is involved in a relationship with the father of her child, but he lives with his brother and his family. During the visit, Nancy asks Jamie how the baby is doing, and Jamie has little to say. Her mother, Delores, answers all the questions. She is also the one holding the baby, and she feeds the baby during the nurse's visit. When Nancy sees Jamie at the clinic for her postpartum check, she asks how things are going at home. Jamie says, "I don't take care of my baby. My mother thinks I can't do anything right. I want to feed her, but my mother says I just give her gas because I don't know how to hold the bottle."

Health Teaching Regarding Newborn Care

Most prenatal care includes basic information about child care, although the extent of the content varies. Adolescents will have more formalized classroom instruction if they participate in a school-based prenatal program. Even if the teenager received extensive preparation, she usually needs health teaching reinforced after delivery. The most common topics teenagers identify for review and reinforcement are listed in Box 24-5.

Because teenagers usually focus on the present, they frequently do not pay attention to information that has no immediate relevance. When the infant arrives, problems then

Box 24-5   Suggested Health Teaching Topics and Content for Teenage Mothers

Positioning and Handling of Infant

Nutrition: Breast- and bottle-feeding technique (encourage breast-feeding when possible), feeding schedule, dietary recommendations for the first 6 months, and vitamin and iron supplements

Hygiene: Skin care and bathing, care of diaper rash, nail care, and umbilical and circumcision care

Elimination: Diapering and frequency of changes, bowel movements (frequency and appearance), constipation, and recognition of problems

Growth and development: Normal growth and development, chart of developmental milestones, and suggested techniques to encourage development

Appropriate Discipline Techniques

Immunization schedule: Recommended schedule, rationale for administration, and possible side effects

Health care issues: Behaviors that signal distress or discomfort, thermometer reading and normal versus abnormal readings, common symptoms (e.g., upper respiratory tract infection, dehydration, and diarrhea), teenager's health coverage, and selection of a clinic or private physician

---

develop. It is very frightening to be caring for a tiny infant and be presented with a crisis. Under these circumstances, the teenage mother becomes very receptive to reviewing and discussing child care issues. Community health nurses should take advantage of the adolescent's concern to teach healthy infant care and distinguish between normal and abnormal infant behavior.

> When Maria Gomez makes her first home visit to Karena Hernandez after her delivery, she finds Karena crying. Karena reports, "My baby won't eat anything. I've tried everything, including formula, toast soaked in milk, and oatmeal. She just won't eat." Maria sits down to talk with Karena and help her to position the baby for a formula feed. The baby is fussy but slowly takes the formula. During the visit, Maria takes the opportunity to find out why Karena felt that toast or oatmeal would be appropriate for a 1-week-old infant. She discovers that Karena's grandmother had suggested she start the infant right away on more substantial food so she would sleep through the night. Maria spends some time reviewing the appropriate age-related food schedule and leaves several pamphlets with Karena. She also suggests that Karena call the clinic if she runs into other problems that won't wait until the next home visit.

An important point to remember is that people vary in child care customs and practices. Child care techniques common to a culture or family tradition need not be discouraged or eliminated if they do no harm. For example, some families swaddle (tightly wrap) infants, whereas others do not; some introduce solid foods early, and others do not; some use an umbilical band, and others do not; some pierce the infant's ears, but others do not. When the nurse sees child care practices contrary to his or her agency's standard protocol or teaching plan, or to her or his own personal habits or values, the practices should be evaluated in terms of harmfulness. Any health care professional who discourages or disapproves of practices that pose no harm runs an unnecessary risk of altering the family-provider

relationship or alienating the family. An important question to ask is, "Is this care issue worth jeopardizing my ability to continue to provide health care to this mother and her infant?" If the answer is "No," then clearly the nurse is better off not running the risk.

TERTIARY PREVENTION

Tertiary prevention is rehabilitative. With respect to teenage pregnancy, prevention should be designed to improve the chances of self-sufficiency for adolescent mothers and fathers while ensuring a healthy, supportive environment for their children. None of the interventions are unique to tertiary prevention, aside from those aimed at enhancing child welfare.

BIRTH CONTROL

Ideally, contraception should be addressed as part of the prenatal program. After delivery, the adolescent must decide if she will continue sexual activity. If so, the nurse should review her contraceptive options. Some girls are opposed to contraception on religious grounds. If this is the case, the nurse should accept the adolescent's decision but caution her about the risks involved in unprotected sexual activity. Even if there is no immediate need, contraception should be reviewed. If the adolescent has already used birth control, it is helpful to identify what the method was, how it was used, and why it was discontinued. Such a review helps to determine whether contraception was used properly and to correct any misconceptions or faulty technique. The nurse should ensure that the teenager is aware of community resources (family planning clinics) where she may be supplied with contraceptives.

Preventing or delaying another pregnancy is a priority. Statistics show that teenagers (both boys and girls) who are parents run a significant risk for having another child while they are still teenagers (Pfitzner et al., 2003; Raneri & Wiemann, 2007). The same strategies employed in primary prevention to avoid pregnancy can be used to prevent repeat pregnancy. Accurate information, accessible contraceptive services, regular clinic visits, and monitored compliance with contraceptive use are effective in reducing the incidence of a second or third pregnancy in adolescent parents.

PARENTING SKILLS

Parenting support, ideally started during and immediately after delivery, is continued long term, sometimes for 2 or 3 years. Parenting classes, individual counseling, and peer support groups are all successful interventions. Home visits by community health nurses and trained community parent aides provide young mothers and fathers (when present) with encouragement and monitoring (Olds et al., 1999, 2004). School-based infant and child care programs are beneficial to young mothers and their children. They increase the likelihood that the mother will complete high school while providing support and guidance for her parenting efforts (Key et al., 2001; Meadows et al., 2000). Infants and children are ensured quality child care, educational companionship, and a head start on learning opportunities.

COMPREHENSIVE PROGRAMS

A number of innovative interventions have combined various strategies into comprehensive support programs (see

Box 24-4). Sex education, birth control support, life options guidance, parenting support, and child care services are all parts of comprehensive programs. Most evaluation efforts have been short term and have appraised selected segments rather than a total program. Some success has been noted. For example, one study found reduced adolescent pregnancy rates among participants in life options programs targeting at-risk teens (Tabi, 2002). Evaluation efforts need to continue and to focus on long-term results. One long-term study, the Seattle Social Development Project, followed children from fifth grade through age 21. When evaluated at age 21, children enrolled in that project were found to have delayed initiation of sexual activity, to have had fewer sexual partners, to use contraceptives more frequently, and to be less likely to have had an STD than a comparison group of peers.

Olds and colleagues (1999) reported on the effects over time (20 years) of the Nurse Home Visiting Program. The intervention was short term, only from prenatal care through an infant's second birthday; however, the results appeared to continue long term. Women who participated in the program deferred subsequent pregnancies and improved their workforce participation, and their children were less likely to experience childhood injuries or learning delays (Olds et al., 2002). A follow-up study at 4 years indicated that study participants increased the interval between pregnancies, experienced less domestic violence, and continued to show improvement in maternal-child relationships and the early childhood development of their children (Olds et al., 2004). At age 15, the children of the teen mothers in the study had fewer arrests and convictions, smoked and drank less, and had fewer sexual partners than their peers. Continued long-term studies are needed to determine what strategies are the most effective. It might be that regular, consistent support of any type is beneficial and effective.

KEY IDEAS

1. The pregnancy, abortion, and birth rates for adolescents are higher in the United States than in other developed countries, although the rate of sexual activity is approximately the same.

2. Adolescents who participate in sexual activity at an early age are more likely to have multiple sex partners and a higher risk for contracting STDs.

3. Many teens substitute oral sex for intercourse and often don't view oral sex as "real" sexual activity.

4. The pregnancy rate is higher among racial and ethnic minorities, but the largest number of babies are born to white adolescents.

5. There is no single cause of teenage pregnancies; instead, a combination of social and personal factors is responsible.

6. Adolescents who have children are more likely to discontinue education, need public assistance, continue on public assistance for a longer period, and have a poorer work history over time than are adolescents who postpone childbearing to later years.

7. Pregnant teenagers and their infants are at greater risk for medical complications (e.g., hypertension, toxemia, anemia, low birth weight, stillbirth, and infant mortality) than older women and their infants.

8. Government funding and policy changes affect services provided to sexually active and pregnant teens.

9. Primary prevention programs that include sex education, contraceptive information, and access to contraceptive services can delay sexual activity and increase contraceptive use in sexually active teenagers. The evidence suggests that abstinence-only programs are not successful when used as the sole method of primary prevention.

10. Secondary prevention programs that include early initiation of adequate, regular prenatal care have been proven to reduce medical complications and improve the health status of both pregnant teenagers and their newborn infants.

11. Tertiary prevention programs that provide a variety of support services for new mothers and their infants reduce health risks for both the mother and child and increase the chances that the mother will continue her education.

12. Community/public health nurses have an enormous opportunity to affect teens by doing the following:
    • Encouraging abstinence or delay of sexual activity
    • Providing factual information on sex education, contraception, and STDs
    • Assisting pregnant teens with health care and parenting skills.

THE NURSING PROCESS IN PRACTICE ▶ A Pregnant Adolescent (by Jennifer Maurer Kliphouse)

Ann Jones is a 16-year-old girl who comes to the family planning clinic for a pregnancy test. She is 5 months pregnant. She tells the community health nurse that she delayed coming to the clinic because she was afraid her mother would talk her into an abortion. In the initial interview, the nurse learns that Ann:
• Is happy she is pregnant and wants to keep her infant;
• Feels fine;
• Does not need maternity clothes because "I am watching my weight and have not gained one pound yet";
• Is not sure she can continue to live with her mother because her mother is "mad I got knocked up and is not talking to me right now";
• Is one grade behind but is doing "okay" in school.

She also tells the nurse that the father of the infant, Bob, is a sophomore in high school, lives with his parents, and is willing to help with finances. Bob works 15 hours per week at a fast-food restaurant after school. His parents are not yet aware that Ann is pregnant, but Bob thinks they will be very angry with both him and Ann.

ASSESSMENT
• Compare actual weight gain with expected weight gain for 20 weeks of pregnancy
• Review dietary intake
• Ascertain what financial assets and health insurance, if any, are available to the client

- Determine the presence of risk factors associated with poor maternal and infant outcomes
- Ascertain the client's knowledge level related to pregnancy, childbirth, and child care

ADDITIONAL AREAS FOR FURTHER ASSESSMENT

Progress and satisfaction with school, including expected schedule for graduation

- Experience with birth control, birth control plans after delivery, and accuracy of sexual knowledge
- Experience with child care, accuracy of information, skill level, and education related to deficient areas
- Knowledge of growth and development
- Use of community support referrals or resources to provide ongoing support after delivery

NURSING DIAGNOSES

- Imbalanced nutrition: less than body requirement related to growing fetus, lack of knowledge, and body-image concerns as evidenced by Ann's weight watching and lack of weight gain
- Disabled family coping related to situational crises of teen pregnancy and lack of parental support as evidenced by lack of communication between Ann and her mother
- Ineffective health maintenance related to young maternal age and delay in initiation of prenatal care as evidenced by first prenatal medical visit at 5 months
- Supplemental Food Programs Division
- Deficient knowledge related to pregnancy, infant growth and development, and parenting as evidenced by expressed weight watching and avoidance of medical attention

Nursing Diagnosis	Nursing Goals	Nursing Interventions	Outcomes and Evaluation
Imbalanced nutrition: less than body requirement related to lack of knowledge and body image concerns as evidenced by Ann's weight watching and lack of weight gain	Adequate dietary intake for a pregnant woman Normal weight gain during pregnancy	The nurse provided teaching on normal weight gain and its relationship to positive infant outcome. The nurse contracted with Ann to gain at least 1 lb per week during pregnancy. Since she registered late, Ann was scheduled for weekly visits to monitor weight gain progression during her pregnancy.	Normal weight gain during pregnancy is 30 to 35 lb. Ann's initial weight was 110 lb, and her weight increased by 1 lb per week during the remainder of her pregnancy.
		The nurse performed routine prenatal blood tests.	Blood laboratory results determined Ann's blood type, O positive, and indicated that she was anemic.
		The nurse provided prenatal vitamins. The nurse asked Ann to perform a 72-hour diet recall.	Prenatal vitamins were provided free of charge by the clinic. Ann verbalized understanding of nutritional changes during pregnancy and reported with each subsequent visit, "I always take my vitamins." The 72-hour diet recall revealed deficiencies in caloric intake and intake of fruits and vegetables and dairy products.
		The nurse arranged for nutritional consultation with a registered dietitian.	Together with the dietitian Ann modified her diet to increase the amount of fresh fruits and vegetables as well as drink four glasses of whole milk a day. Ann reported that she was able to stick to the diet for a few weeks, but at her fifth appointment, she stated, "It's hard to remember to drink so much milk." The dietitian listed other sources of calcium, such as broccoli and other green, leafy vegetables.

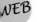

Find additional **Care Plans** for this client on the book's website.

LEARNING BY EXPERIENCE AND REFLECTION

1. Discuss with adolescents their feelings about sexual activity, perception of risks, and educational and future goals. Encourage them to share their personal experiences related to how they acquired sexual information and conversations they might have had with others regarding sexual activity or risky behavior.

2. Identify a client who is a teenage mother in your clinical area and explore with her what she finds rewarding and what is difficult about her situation. Review her educational progress, her child care, and her living arrangements.

3. Become familiar with a specific community's values regarding sex education and contraceptive services for adolescents. Identify the proponents and opponents of these measures, their arguments, and their stated goals. Identify your own values and positions.

4. Review the sex education and family life lesson plans in your school district, if they exist. Describe the content and teaching strategies. Do you think they are adequate? When was the last time the content was changed or upgraded? What are the qualifications of the teachers? Do teachers use a prepared script? Are teachers comfortable allowing discussion and statements of views by children or adolescents in class?

COMMUNITY RESOURCES FOR PRACTICE

Information about each of the following organizations is found on its website, which can be accessed through the **WebLinks** section of this book's website at *http://evolve.elsevier.com/Maurer/community/*.

Advocates for Youth
Commodity Food Programs
Food and Nutrition Service
Goodwill Industries International
March of Dimes Birth Defects Foundation
National Campaign to Prevent Teen Pregnancy
Planned Parenthood Federation of America
Office of Public Health and Science (Office of Population Affairs, Office of Adolescent Pregnancy Programs, Office of Family Planning and Reproductive Health)
Salvation Army National Headquarters
U.S. Department of Agriculture
Women, Infants, and Children Program

STUDY AIDS   http://evolve.elsevier.com/Maurer/community/

Visit the Evolve website for this book to find the following study and assessment materials:

- Quiz
- Web Scenario
- Critical Thinking Questions and Answers for Case Studies
- Care Plans
- *Healthy People* Updates
- Glossary

WEBSITE RESOURCES

The following items supplement the chapter's topics and are also found on the Evolve site:

24A: Nutrition and Health Habits: Special Importance in Adolescent Pregnancy

REFERENCES

Abma, J. C., Martinez, G. M., Mosher, W. D., et al. (2004). *Teenagers in the United States: Sexual activity, contraceptive use, and childbearing* (Vital and Health Statistics Series 23, No. 24). Hyattsville, MD: U.S. Department of Health and Human Services.

Alan Guttmacher Institute. (1994). *Sex and America's teenagers*. New York: Author.

Alan Guttmacher Institute. (1986). *Teenage pregnancy in industrialized countries*. New Haven, CT: Yale University Press.

Alan Guttmacher Institute. (2000a). *Fulfilling the promise: Public policy and U.S. family planning clinics*. New York: Author.

Alan Guttmacher Institute. (2000b). *Issues in brief: Welfare law and the drive to reduce "illegitimacy."* New York: Author.

Alan Guttmacher Institute. (2002a). *Facts in brief: Sexuality education*. New York: Author.

Alan Guttmacher Institute. (2002b). *Issues in brief: Sex education: Politicians, parents, teachers, and teens*. New York: Author.

Alan Guttmacher Institute. (2002c). *Issues in brief: Teen pregnancy: Trends and lessons learned*. New York: Author.

Alan Guttmacher Institute. (2002d). *Issues in brief: School-based health centers and the birth control debate*. New York: Author.

Alan Guttmacher Institute. (2001). *Can more progress be made? Teenage sexual and reproductive behavior in developed countries [Executive summary]*. New York: Author.

Alan Guttmacher Institute. (2003a, October 1). *State policies in brief: Minors' rights as parents (fact sheet)*. New York: Author.

Alan Guttmacher Institute. (2003b, October 1). *State policies in brief: Parental involvement in minors' abortions* [Fact sheet]. New York: Author.

Alan Guttmacher Institute. (2006a). *In brief: Facts on American teens' sexual and reproductive health*. Retrieved February 2, 2007 from *http://www.guttmacher.org/pubs/fb_ATSRH.html*.

Alan Guttmacher Institute. (2006b). *U.S. teenage pregnancy statistics: Nation and state trends and trends by race and ethnicity*. New York: Author.

Alan Guttmacher Institute. (2006c). *In brief: Facts on sex education in the United States*. Retrieved February 2, 2007 from *http://www.guttmacher.org/pubs/fb_sexEd2006.html*.

Alan Guttmacher Institute. (2006d). *Sexuality education, state policies in brief*. Retrieved February 2, 2007 from *http://www.guttmacher.org/statecenter/spibs/spib_SE.pdf*.

Alan Guttmacher Institute. (2006e). *Sex education: Needs, programs and politics*. Retrieved February 2, 2007 from *http://www.guttmacher.org/presentations/ed_slides.html*.

Alan Guttmacher Institute. (2007a). *State policies in brief: Sex and STD/HIV education*. New York: Author.

Alan Guttmacher Institute. (2007b). *State policies in brief: Parental involvement in minors' abortions*. New York: Author.

Alan Guttmacher Institute. (2007c). *State policies in brief: Minors' rights as parents*. New York: Author.

Alan Guttmacher Institute. (2007d). *State policies in brief: State funding of abortion under Medicaid*. New York: Author.

Albert, B. (2007). *With one voice: America's adults and teens sound off about teen pregnancy*. Washington, DC: National Campaign to Prevent Teen Pregnancy.

Albert, B., Brown, S., & Flanigan, C. M. (Eds.). (2003). *14 and younger: The sexual behavior of young adolescents*. Washington, DC: National Campaign to Prevent Teen Pregnancy.

Andrews, J. L., & Boyle, J. S. (2003). African American adolescents' experiences with unplanned pregnancy and elective abortion. *Health Care for Women International, 24*(5), 414-433.

Aschenbrenner, D. S. (2006). Over-the-counter access to emergency contraception. *American Journal of Nursing, 106*(11), 34-36.

Barnett, J. E., & Hurst, C. S. (2003). Abstinence education for rural youth: An evaluation of the Life's Walk Program. *Journal of School Health, 73*(7), 264-268.

Bleakley, A., Hennessy, M., & Fishbein. (2006). Public opinion on sex education in U.S. schools. *Archives of Pediatric Medicine, 160*(11), 1151-1156.

Boonstra, H. (2002). Teen pregnancy: Trends and lessons learned. *Guttmacher Report on Public Policy, 5*(1), 1-9.

Brennan, D. J., Hellerstedt, W. L, Rose, M. W., et al. (2007). History of childhood sexual abuse and HIV risk behaviors in homosexual and bisexual men. *American Journal of Public Health, 97*(6), 1107-1112.

Bruckner, H., & Bearman, P. (2003). Selected aspects of adolescent health. In B. Albert, S. Brown, & C. M. Flanigan (Eds.), *14 and younger: The sexual behavior of young adolescents*. Washington, DC: National Campaign to Prevent Teen Pregnancy.

Bruckner, H., & Bearman, P. (2005). After the promise: The STD consequences of adolescent virginity pledges. *Journal of Adolescent Health, 36*(4), 271-278.

Burnstein, G. R., Lowry, R., Klein, J. D., et al. (2003). Missed opportunities for sexually transmitted diseases, human immunodeficiency virus, and pregnancy prevention services during adolescent health supervision visits. *Pediatrics, 111*(5, pt 1), 996-1001.

Can abstinence programs lead to more sex? (2004). *American Journal of Nursing, 104*(4), 22.

Carpenter, S. C., Clyman, R. B., Davidson, A. J., et al. (2001). The association of foster care or kinship care with adolescent sexual behavior and first pregnancy. *Pediatrics, 108*(3), E46.

Centers for Disease Control and Prevention. (2008). *2008 National STD Prevention Conference*. Retrieved March 26, 2008 from http://www.cdc.gov/stdconference/2008/media/release-11March2008.pdf.

Chen X. K., Wen, S. W., Fleming, N., et al. (2007). Teenage pregnancy and adverse birth outcomes: A large population based retrospective cohort study. *International Journal of Epidemiology, 36*(2), 368-373.

Chesson, H. W., Blandford, J. M., Gift, T. L., et al. (2004). The estimated direct medical cost of sexually transmitted diseases among American youth, 2000. *Perspectives on Sexual and Reproductive Health, 23*(1), 11-19.

Children's Defense Fund. (2005). *The state of America's children: 2005*. Washington, DC: Author.

Cohen, S. A. (2001). Global gag rule: Exporting antiabortion ideology at the expense of American values. *Guttmacher Report, 4*(3), 1-6.

Congressional Budget Office. (2007, May). *Changes in the economic resources of low-income households with children*. Washington, DC: Congress of the United States, Congressional Budget Office.

Courtney, M., McMurray, S. L., & Zinn, A. (2004), September/October. Housing problems experienced by recipients of child welfare services. *Child Welfare*, special issue: Housing and Homelessness.

Coyle, K., Kirby, D., Parcel, G., et al. (1996). Safer choices: A multicomponent school-based HIV/STD and pregnancy prevention program for adolescents. *Journal of School Health, 66*(3), 89-94.

Dailard, C. (2003). Understanding "abstinence": Implications for individuals, programs, and policies. *Guttmacher Report on Public Policy, 6*(5), 1-6.

Dailard, C. (2004). Out of compliance? Implementing the infant adoption awareness act. *Guttmacher Report on Public Policy, 7*(3), 1-7.

Dailard, C. (2006). *Legislating against arousal: The growing divide between federal policy and teenage sexual behavior*. Guttmacher Policy Review, *9*(3), 1-7.

Dowell, W. M., & Vandestienne, G. (1996). The use of focus groups to examine pubertal concerns in preteen girls: Initial findings and implications for practice and research. *Issues in Comprehensive Pediatric Nursing, 19*(2), 103-120.

East, P., Kiernan, E., & Chavez, G. (2003). An evaluation of California's Sibling Pregnancy Prevention Program. *Perspectives on Sexual and Reproductive Health, 35*(20), 62-70.

Eaton, D. K., Kann, L., Kinchen, S., et al. (2006). Youth risk behavior surveillance—United States, 2005. *Morbidity and Mortality Weekly Report, Surveillance Summaries, 55*(SS-5), 1-102.

Elfenbein, D. S., & Felice, M. E. (2003). Adolescent pregnancy. *Pediatric Clinics of North America, 50*(4), 781-800, viii.

Ellis, B. J., Bates, J. E., Dodge, K. A., et al. (2003). Does father absence place daughters at special risk for early sexual activity and teenage pregnancy? *Child Development, 74*(3), 801-821.

Federal Interagency Forum on Child and Family Statistics. (2007). *America's children: Key national indicators of well-being, 2007*. Washington, DC: U.S. Government Printing Office.

Fields, J. (2003). *Children's living arrangements and characteristics: March 2002* (Current Population Reports, P20-547). Washington, DC: U.S. Bureau of the Census.

Finer, L. B., Frohwith, L. F., Dauphinee, L. A., et al. (2005). Reasons U.S. women have abortions: Quantitative and qualitative perspectives. *Perspectives on Sexual and Reproductive Health, 37*(3), 110-118.

Finer, L. B., & Henshaw, S. K. (2006). Disparities in rates of unintended pregnancy in the United States, 1994 and 2001. *Perspectives on Sexual and Reproductive Health, 38*(2), 90-96.

Finer, L. B., & Zabin, L. S. (1998). Does the timing of the first family planning visit still matter? *Family Planning Perspectives, 301*(1), 30-33, 42.

Ford, K., Weglicki, L., Kershaw, T., et al. (2002). Effects of prenatal care interventions for adolescent mothers on birth weight, repeat pregnancy, and educational outcomes one year postpartum. *Journal of Perinatal Education, 11*(1), 35-38.

Frost, J. J., Jones, R. K., Wong, V., et al. (2001). *Teenage sexual and reproductive behavior in developed countries: Country report for the United States* (Occasional Report No. 8). New York: Alan Guttmacher Institute.

Frost, J. J., & Oslake, S. (1999). *Teenagers' pregnancy intentions and decisions: A study of young women in California choosing to give birth*. New York: Alan Guttmacher Institute.

Frutkin, A. (1999, July 19). Is sex getting hotter? *Mediaweek*.

Gavin, L. E., Black, M. M., Minor, S., et al. (2002). Young disadvantaged fathers' involvement with their infants: An ecological perspective. *Journal of Adolescent Health, 31*(3), 266-276.

Grady, M. A., & Bloom, K. C. (2004). Pregnancy outcomes of adolescents enrolled in a Centering Pregnancy program. *Journal of Midwifery and Women's Health, 49*(5), 412-420.

Guevara, J. P., Young, J. C., & Mueller, B. A. (2001). Do protective factors reduce the risk for hospitalization in infants of teenage mothers? *Archives of Pediatric and Adolescent Medicine, 155*(1), 66-72.

Hamilton, B. E., Martin, J. A., & Ventura, S. J. (2006). *Births: preliminary data for 2005*. Hyattsville, MD: National Center for Health Statistics.

Harris, M. B., & Franklin, C. G. (2003). Effects of a cognitive-behavioral, school-based, group intervention with Mexican American pregnant and parenting adolescents. *Social Work Research, 27*(2), 71-83.

Hoffman, S. D. (2006). *By the numbers: The public costs of teen childbearing*. Washington, DC: National Campaign to Prevent Teen Pregnancy.

Hoffman, S. D., & Scher, L. S. (2007). Children of early childbearers as young adults—Updated estimates. In R. A. Maynard & S. Hoffman (Eds.), Kids having kids (rev. ed.). Washington, DC: Urban Institute.

Holubet, C. T., Kershaw, T. S., Ethier, K. A., et al. (2007). Prenatal and parenting stress on adolescent maternal adjustment: Identifying a high risk subgroup. *Maternal and Child Health Journal, 119*(2), 153-157.

Jones, R. K., & Boonstra, H. (2005). Confidential reproductive health care for adolescents. *Current Opinion in Obstetrics and Gynecology, 17*(5), 456-460.

Jones, R. K., Darroch, J. E., & Henshaw, S. K. (2002). Contraceptive use among U.S. women having abortions in 2000-2001. *Perspectives on Sexual and Reproductive Health, 34*(6), 294-303.

Jung, M. P., Metraux, S., Brodbar, G., et al. (2004). Child welfare involvement among children in homeless families. *Child Welfare*, special Issue: Housing and Homelessness.

Kalmuss, D., Davidson, A., Cohall, A., et al. (2003). Preventing sexual risk behaviors and pregnancy among teenagers: Linking research and programs. *Perspectives on Sexual and Reproductive Health, 35*(2), 87-93.

Kerns, J., Westhoff, C., Morroni, C., et al. (2003). Partner influence on early discontinuation of the pill in a predominantly Hispanic population. *Perspectives on Sexual and Reproductive Health, 35*(6), 256-260.

Key, J. D., Barbosa, G. A., & Owens, V. J. (2001). The Second Chance Club: Repeat adolescent pregnancy prevention with a school-based intervention. *Journal of Adolescent Health, 28*(3), 167-169.

Kirby, D. (2001). *Emerging answers: Research findings on progress to reduce teen pregnancy*. Washington, DC: National Campaign to Prevent Teen Pregnancy.

Klerman, L. V. (2002). Adolescent pregnancy in the United States. *International Journal of Adolescent Medicine and Health, 14*(2), 91-96.

Klima, C. S. (2003). Centering pregnancy: A model for pregnant adolescents. *Journal of Midwifery and Women's Health, 48*(3), 220-225.

Koniak-Griffin, D., Mothenge, C., Anderson, N. L. R., et al. (1999). An early intervention program for adolescent mothers: A nursing demonstration project. *Journal of Obstetrics and Gynecologic Neonatal Nursing, 28*(1), 51-59.

Koniak-Griffin, D., & Turner-Pluta, C. (2001). Health risks and psychosocial outcomes of early childbearing: A review of the literature. *Journal of Perinatal and Neonatal Nursing, 15*(2), 1-17.

Krulewitch, C. J., Roberts, D. W., & Thompson, L. S. (2003). Adolescent pregnancy and homicide: Findings from the Maryland Office of the Chief Medical Examiner. *Child Maltreatment, 8*(2), 122-128.

Kunkel, D., Cope, K. M., & Beilyu, E. (1999). Sexual messages on television: Comparing findings from three studies. *Journal of Sex Research, 36*(3), 230-236.

Kunkel, D., Cope, K. M., & Colvin, C. (1996). *Sexual messages on family hour television: Content and context*. Prepared for Children Now and the Kaiser Family Foundation. Menlo Park, CA: Kaiser Family Foundation.

Lammers C., Ireland, M., Resnick, M., et al. (2000). Influences on adolescents' decision to postpone onset of sexual intercourse: A survival analysis of virginity among youths aged 13 to 18 years. *Journal of Adolescent Health, 26*(1), 42-48.

Landry, D. J., Darroch, J. E., Singh, S., et al. (2003). Factors associated with the content of sex education in U.S. public secondary schools. *Perspectives on Sexual and Reproductive Health, 35*(6), 261-269.

Lindberg, L., Santelli, J. S., & Singh, S. (2006a). Changes in formal sex education: 1995-2002. *Perspectives on Sexual and Reproductive Health, 38*(4), 182-189.

Lindberg, L., Santelli, J. S., & Singh, S. (2006b). Provisions of contraceptive and related services by publicly funded family planning clinics, 2003. *Perspectives on Sexual and Reproductive Health, 38*(3), 139-147.

Lindberg, L. D., Frost, J. J., Sten, C., et al. (2006). The provision and funding of contraceptive services at publicly funded family planning agencies: 1995-2003. *Perspectives on Sexual Reproductive Health, 38*(1), 37-45.

Lonczak, H. S., Abbott, R. D., Hawkins, J. D., et al. (2002). Effects of the Seattle social development project on sexual behavior, pregnancy, birth, and sexually transmitted disease outcomes by age 21 years. *Archives of Pediatrics and Adolescent Medicine, 156*(5), 438-447.

Lynch, C. O. (2001). Risk and protective factors associated with adolescent sexual activity. *Adolescence and Family Health, 2*(3), 99-107.

Manlove, J., Papillio, A., & Ikramullah, E. (2004). *Not yet: Programs to delay first sex among teens*. Washington, DC: National Campaign to Prevent Teen Pregnancy.

Marshall, E., Buckner, E., Perkins, J., et al. (1996). Effects of a child abuse prevention unit in health classes in four schools. *Journal of Community Health Nursing, 13*(2), 107-122.

Martin, J. A., Hamilton, B. E., Sutton, P. D., et al. (2003). Births: Final data for 2002. *National Vital Statistics Reports, 52*(10). Hyattsville, MD: National Center for Health Statistics.

Martin, J. A., Hamilton, B. E., Sutton, P. D., et al. (2006). Births: Final data for 2004. *National Vital Statistics Reports, 55*(1). Hyattsville, MD: National Center for Health Statistics.

Martin, J. A., Hamilton, B. E., Ventura, S. J., et al. (2002). Births: Final data for 2001. *National Vital Statistics Reports, 51*(2). Hyattsville, MD: National Center for Health Statistics.

Martin, J. A., Hamilton, B. E., Ventura, S. J., et al. (2005). Births: Final data for 2004. *National Vital Statistics Reports, 54*(1). Hyattsville, MD: National Center for Health Statistics.

Martinez, G. M., Chandra, A., Abma, J. C., et al. (2006). *Fertility, contraception, and fatherhood: Data on men and women from Cycle 6 (2002) of the National Survey of Family Growth (Vital and Health Statistics Series 23, No. 26)*. Washington, DC: National Center for Health Statistics.

Mathews, T. J. (2001). Smoking during pregnancy in the 1990s. *National Vital Statistics Reports,* 49(7). Hyattsville, MD: National Center for Health Statistics.

Maynard, R. A., & Hoffman, S. D. (2007). The costs of adolescent childbearing. In R. A. Maynard & S. D. Hoffman (Eds.), *Kids having kids* (rev. ed.). Washington, DC: Urban Institute.

McLanahan, S. S., & Carlson, M. J. (2002). Welfare reform, fertility, and father involvement. *Future of Children, 12*(1), 146-165.

Meadows, M., Sadler, L. S., & Reitmeyer, G. D. (2000). School-based support for urban adolescent mothers. *Journal of Pediatric Health Care, 14*(5), 221-227.

Menacker, F., Martin, J. A., MacDorman, M. F., et al. (2004). Births to 10-14 year-old mothers, 1990-2002: Trends and health outcomes. *National Vital Statistics Reports, 53*(7). Hyattsville, MD: National Center for Health Statistics.

Montgomery, K. S. (2003). Nursing care for pregnant adolescents. *Journal of Obstetric, Gynecologic, and Neonatal Nursing, 32*(2), 249-257.

Mummert, A., Nagamine, M., & Myers, M. (2007). *Childbirth-related hospitalizations among adolescent girls, 2004* (Statistical Brief No. 31). Washington, DC: Agency for Healthcare Research and Quality.

National Campaign to Prevent Teen Pregnancy. (2002). *14 and younger: Sexual behavior of adolescents* [Report highlights]. Retrieved February 1, 2007 from *http://www.teenpregnancy.org/resources/reading/pdf/14summary.pdf*.

National Campaign to Prevent Teen Pregnancy. (2003). *Teen pregnancy: So what?* Washington, DC: Author.

National Campaign to Prevent Teen Pregnancy. (2007). *One in three: The case for wanted and welcomed pregnancy*. Washington, DC: Author.

National Center on Family Homelessness. (2005). *Homeless children: America's new outcasts*. Newton Centre, MA: Author.

National Center for Health Statistics. (2002). *Birth rates for married women by age, race, and Hispanic origin: United States, 2002*. Hyattsville, MD: National Center for Health Statistics, Division of Vital Statistics.

National Public Radio, Kaiser Family Foundation, & Kennedy School of Government. (2004). *Sex education in America: General public/parent survey*. Washington, DC: National Public Radio.

Olds, D. L., Henderson, C. R., Kitzman, H. J., et al. (1999). Prenatal and infancy home visitation by nurses: Recent findings. *Future of Children, 9*(1), 44-65.

Olds, D. L., Robinson, K., O'Brien, R., et al. (2002). Home visiting by paraprofessionals and by nurses: A randomized controlled trial. *Pediatrics, 110*(3), 486-496.

Olds, D. L., Robinson, K., Pettitt, L. M., et al. (2004). Effects of home visits by paraprofessionals and by nurses: Follow-up results of a randomized controlled trial. *Pediatrics, 114*(6), 1560-1568.

Ott, M. A., Millstein, S. G., Ofner, S., et al. (2006). Greater expectations: Adolescents' positive motivations for sex. *Perspectives on Sexual and Reproductive Health, 38*(2), 84-89.

Pfitzner, M. A., Hoff, C., & McElligott, K. (2003). Predictors of repeat pregnancy in a program for pregnant teens. *Journal of Pediatric and Adolescent Gynecology, 16*(2), 77-81.

Philliber, S., Kaye, J., & Herrling, S. (2001). *The national evaluation of the Children's Aid Society Carrera-model program to prevent teen pregnancy.* Accord, NY: Philliber Research Associates.

Philliber, S., Brooks, L., Lehrer, L. P., et al. (2003). Outcomes of teen pregnancy programs in New Mexico. *Adolescents, 38*(151), 535-553.

Phipps, M. G., Sowers, M., & DeMonner, S. M. (2002). The risk for infant mortality among adolescent childbearing groups. *Journal of Women's Health, 11*(10), 889-897.

Pope, L. M., Adler, N. E., & Tschann, J. M. (2001). Postabortion psychological adjustment: Are minors at increased risk? *Journal of Adolescent Health, 29*(1), 211.

Raneri, L. G., & Wiemann, C. M. (2007). Social ecological predictors of repeat adolescent pregnancy. *Perspectives on Sexual and Reproductive Health, 39*(1), 39-47.

Rector, R. E., Johnson, K. A., & Noyes, L. R. (2003). *Sexually active teenagers are more likely to be depressed and to attempt suicide* (Center for Data Analysis Report No. 03-04). Washington, DC: Heritage Foundation.

Rhein, L. M., Ginsburg, K. R., Schwartz, D. F., et al. (1997). Teen father participation in child rearing: Family perspectives. *Journal of Adolescent Health, 21*(1), 244-252.

Roye, C. F., & Balk, S. J. (1996). Evaluation of an intergenerational program for pregnant and parenting adolescents. *Maternal-Child Nursing Journal, 24*(1), 32-40.

Roye, C. F., & Balk, S. J. (1997). Caring for pregnant teens and their mothers, too. *American Journal of Maternal/Child Nursing, 22*(3), 153-157.

St. Lawrence, J. S. (1998). *Becoming a responsible teen: An HIV risk reduction program for adolescents.* Santa Cruz, CA: ETR Associates.

Santelli, J. S., Lindberg, L. D., Finer, L. B., et al. (2007). Explaining recent declines in adolescent pregnancy in the United States: The contribution of abstinence and improved contraceptive use. *American Journal of Public Health, 97*(1), 1-7.

Santelli, J. S., Morrow, B., Anderson, J. E., et al. (2006). Contraceptive use and pregnancy risk among U.S. high school students, 1991-2003. *Perspectives on Sexual and Reproductive Health, 38*(2), 106-111.

Santelli, J. S, Ott, M. A., Lyon, M., et al. (2005). Abstinence and abstinence-only education: A review of U.S. policies and programs. *Journal of Adolescent Health, 38*(1), 72-81.

Satcher, D. (2002). *Call to action to promote sexual health and responsible sexual behavior.* Report of the Surgeon General, U.S. Public Health Service, U.S. Department of Health and Human Services. Washington, DC: U.S. Government Printing Office.

Scarr, E. M. (2002). Effective prenatal care for adolescent girls. *Nursing Clinics of North America, 37*(3), 513-521.

Shearer, D. L., Mulvihill, B. A., Klermen, L. V., et al. (2002). Association of early childbearing and low cognitive ability. *Perspectives on Sexual and Reproductive Health, 34*(5), 236-243.

Sidebottom, A., Birnbaum, A. S., & Nafstad, S. S. (2003). Decreasing barriers for teens: Evaluation of a new pregnancy prevention strategy in school-based clinics. *American Journal of Public Health, 93*(11), 1890-1892.

Smith, M. A. B. (1994). Teen incentive program: Evaluation of a health promotion model for adolescent pregnancy prevention. *Journal of Health Education, 25*(1), 24-29.

Tabi, M. M. (2002). Community perspective on a model to reduce teenage pregnancy. *Journal of Advanced Nursing, 40*(3), 275-284.

Treffers, P., Olukoya, A., & Ferguson, B. (2001). Care for adolescent pregnancy and childbirth. *International Journal of Gynecology and Obstetrics, 75*(2), 111-121.

U.S. Department of Health and Human Services. (1995). *Healthy people 2000: Midcourse review.*

Washington, DC: U.S. Government Printing Office.

U.S. Department of Health and Human Services. (2000). *Healthy people 2010: Understanding and improving health (2nd ed.).* Washington, DC: U.S. Government Printing Office.

U.S. Department of Health and Human Services. (2007). *Impacts of four Title V, Section 510 abstinence education programs: Final report.* Washington, DC: U.S. Government Printing Office.

U.S. House of Representatives. (2004). *The content of federally funded abstinence-only education programs.* Washington, DC: United States House of Representatives, Committee on Government Reform.

Ventura, S. J. (1995). *Births to unmarried mothers: U.S. 1980-1992 (Vital and Health Statistics Series 21, No. 53).* Hyattsville, MD: National Center for Health Statistics.

Ventura, S. J., Matthews, T. J., Brady, E., et al. (2001). Births to teenagers in the United States, 1940-2000. *National Vital Statistics Reports, 49*(10). Hyattsville, MD: National Center for Health Statistics.

Weinstock, H., Berman, S., & Cates, W. (2004). Sexually transmitted diseases among American youth: Incidence and prevalence estimates: 2000. *Perspectives on Sexual and Reproductive Health, 36*(1), 6-10.

Whitehead, B. D., Wilcox, B., & Rostosky, S. S. (2001). *Keeping the faith: The role of religion and faith communities in preventing teen pregnancy.* Washington, DC: National Campaign to Prevent Teen Pregnancy.

Wiemann, C., & Berenson, A. (1998). Factors associated with recent and discontinued alcohol use by pregnant adolescents. *Journal of Adolescent Health, 22*(5), 417-423.

Young, T., Turner, J., Denny, G., et al. (2004). Examining external and internal poverty as antecedents of teen pregnancy. *American Journal of Health Behaviors, 28*(4), 361-373.

SUGGESTED READINGS

Abma, J. C., Martinez, G. M., Mosher, W. D., et al. (2004). *Teenagers in the United States: Sexual activity, contraceptive use, and childbearing* (Vital and Health Statistics Series 23, No. 24). Hyattsville, MD: National Center for Health Statistics.

Albert, B. (2007). *With one voice: America's adults and teens sound off about teen pregnancy.* Washington, DC: National Campaign to Prevent Teen Pregnancy.

Frost, J. J., Jones, R. K., Wong, V., et al. (2001). *Teenage sexual and reproductive behavior in developed countries: Country report for the United States* (Occasional Report No. 8). New York: Alan Guttmacher Institute.

Hoffman, S. D. (2006). *By the numbers: The public costs of teen childbearing.* Washington, DC: National Campaign to Prevent Teen Pregnancy.

Manlove, J., Papillio, A., & Ikramullah, E. (2004). *Not yet: Programs to delay first sex among teens.* Washington, DC: National Campaign to Prevent Teen Pregnancy.

Maynard, R. A. (Ed.). (2007). *Kids having kids: Economic costs and social consequences of teen pregnancy.* Washington, DC: Urban Institute.

Miller, B. C., Card, J. J., Paikoff, R. L., et al. (Eds.). (1992). *Preventing adolescent pregnancy: Model programs and evaluations.* Newbury Park, CA: Sage.

Olds, D. L., Henderson, C. R. Jr., Tatelbaum, R., et al. (1988). Improving the life course development of socially disadvantaged mothers: A randomized trial of nursing home visitations. *American Journal of Public Health, 78*, 1435-1445.

Olds, D. L., Robinson, K., Pettitt, L. M., et al. (2004). Effects of home visits by paraprofessionals and by nurses: Follow-up results of a randomized controlled trial. *Pediatrics, 114*(6), 1560-1568.

Paine-Andrews, A., Fisher, J. L., Berkley, P. J., et al. (2002). Analyzing the contributions of community change to population health outcomes in an adolescent pregnancy prevention intervention. *Health Education and Behavior, 29*(2), 183-193.

Perrin, J. M., & Dorman, K. A. (2003). Teen parents and academic success. *Journal of School Nursing, 19*(5), 288-293.

Taylor, D., & Chavez, G. (2002). Small area analysis on a large scale—The California experience in mapping teenage birth "hot spots" for resource allocation. *Journal of Public Health Management and Prevention, 8*(2), 33-45.

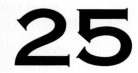

25 Substance Use Disorders

*Mary R. Haack**

FOCUS QUESTIONS

How are abuse and dependence defined?

What is the process of dependence?

What progress has been made toward reaching the *Healthy People 2010* goals related to addiction to alcohol and other drugs?

What theory of addiction is most relevant to community/public health nursing practice?

How can community/public health nurses help to prevent addictions?

How can community/public health nurses help to prevent fetal alcohol syndrome and related disorders?

What behavior patterns alert the nurse to the presence of addiction and suggest specific interventions?

How can community/public health nurses assist individuals and families recovering from addictions?

What community resources exist to help with addiction problems and how is this picture changing?

CHAPTER OUTLINE

KEY TERMS

Abstinence
Addiction
Co-dependence
Dual diagnosis

Enabler
Fetal alcohol spectrum disorders (FASDs)
Medication-assisted treatment (MAT)
Substance abuse

Substance dependence
Substance use disorders
Tolerance
Withdrawal

BACKGROUND OF ADDICTION

America's struggle with alcohol abuse, illicit drug use, and prescription drug misuse has been a significant public health problem since the inception of this country. By the year 1800, the rate of dependence on or abuse of alcohol was so high and its disruptive effects so far reaching that both Presidents George Washington

and Thomas Jefferson had suggested that people drink beer and wine rather than hard liquor. By 1900, many patent medicines, tonics, and elixirs contained liberal amounts of opium, cocaine, and alcohol, which often caused dependence on these products.

In 1914, an estimated 200,000 Americans were opiate addicts, roughly 1 of every 400 citizens. At that time, the Harrison Narcotics Act was passed requiring all narcotics

*This chapter incorporates material written for the second edition by Karen Allen and for the third edition by Katherine High. Melanie Wickham, Claudia Smith, and Frances Maurer also assisted with writing this chapter.

dealers to register with the Internal Revenue Service. The word *dealer* referred to health professionals such as physicians, dentists, and veterinarians. In 1973, President Richard Nixon declared a *War on Drugs,* and President George H. W. Bush continued with his own War on Drugs policy in 1989. As a result of the so-called crack epidemic in the mid-1980s, public policy shifted away from an illness model to a deterrence model. This shift resulted in the *Crime Bill* signed by President Bill Clinton in 1994, which called for life imprisonment for those committing three drug offenses. President George W. Bush continued the effort by the following actions:

- Reauthorizing the Drug-free Communities Act, which concentrates prevention efforts in the most severely affected communities.
- Announcing a national drug control strategy that includes efforts to limit drug supplies, reduce substance demands, and provide effective treatment to individuals with substance use disorders. However, the Office of National Drug Control Policy budget for limiting the supply side of illegal drug trafficking far outweighs the budget amount devoted to treatment.

Modern transportation, communication, and technologic growth have facilitated market penetration efforts and extended the reach of drug lords and drug dealers from international and national areas into urban, suburban, and rural U.S. communities. People at all economic levels of society are affected.

IMPACT OF SUBSTANCE ABUSE ON SOCIETY

The cost to and impact of addictions on society constitute one of the greatest health and social problems of our time, placing enormous burdens on the economy, particularly on the health care system. More than 51,000 Americans die each year in the United States as a result of alcohol and illicit drug abuse (Minino et al., 2007). Related cases of acquired immunodeficiency syndrome (AIDS) and other substance-associated health problems account for many more deaths. The cost of providing health care and associated loss of job productivity for drug abuse alone is approximately $144 billion per year (Office of National Drug Control Policy, 2004). When these costs are added to the costs of alcohol and other substances, addictions cost taxpayers between $300 and $500 billion in health care, law enforcement requirements, motor vehicle crashes, crime, and lost productivity (Fontaine, 2003; Volkow, 2003).

In addition to producing direct costs, addictions account for increased health care costs by fueling many psychiatric problems. Approximately 25% of drug abusers (5.6 million adults in 2006) have concurrent mental health diagnoses (Substance Abuse and Mental Health Services Administration [SAMHSA], 2007). In the mid-1980s through the mid-1990s, most health care provided for addicted individuals was for acute inpatient treatment. Then, mostly because of changes in health insurance compensation, many of the resources moved to community settings. The problems of addiction are of such magnitude that they have become a public health concern—one that requires the attention of all public health professionals, including community/public health nurses.

This chapter provides a clear definition of addiction, presents a broad overview of the incidence and prevalence of addiction to alcohol and illicit drugs, and describes theories of addiction relevant to community/public health nursing. The expectations in *Healthy People 2010* (U.S. Department of Health and Human Services [USDHHS], 2000), specific interventions related to the role of the community/public health nurse, and community resources for addressing the problem are discussed.

HEALTHY PEOPLE 2010 OBJECTIVES

The U.S. Department of Health and Human Services (USDHHS) developed substance abuse objectives for *Healthy People 2010* (see the *Healthy People 2010* box). The focus areas in the *Healthy People 2010* substance abuse objectives are promotion of healthy behaviors and primary prevention, areas in which community/public health nurses excel. Adolescents and children are a primary target. Efforts are aimed at discouraging the *initial* use of substances such as alcohol, tobacco, and illicit drugs. *Healthy People 2010* lacks the concentration on substance use and abuse in the elderly that was evident in the *Healthy People 2000* objectives.

DEFINITIONS

Distinguishing between the terms *abuse, dependence,* and *addiction* has been difficult, because they have been used interchangeably at times. For purposes of clarification in this chapter, definitions are provided. **Substance use disorders** is an overarching term used in the *Diagnostic and Statistical Manual of Mental Disorders (DSM-IV)* (American Psychiatric Association [APA], 2000). The term encompasses both substance abuse and substance dependence.

Substance abuse refers to a maladaptive pattern of substance use manifested by recurrent and significant adverse consequences occurring within a 12 month period (APA, 2000). Individuals may repeatedly fail to fulfill major role obligations, repeatedly use a substance in a situation in which it is physically hazardous (such as driving while intoxicated), have multiple legal problems, or have recurrent social or interpersonal problems as a result of their substance use. A diagnosis of substance abuse is preempted by the diagnosis of substance dependence if the individual has ever met dependence criteria for the given substance class.

Substance dependence refers to a cluster of cognitive, behavioral, and physiologic symptoms indicating that the individual continues to use a substance despite significant substance-related problems. Unlike substance abuse, substance dependence also includes tolerance, withdrawal, and a pattern of compulsive use. To meet dependence criteria, an individual must show three or more of the symptoms listed in *DSM-IV* in the same 12-month period (APA, 2000).

Addiction, as defined by the American Society of Addiction Medicine, encompasses the genetic, psychosocial, and environmental influences in the development of substance use, abuse, and dependence (West, 2001). This definition conceptualizes addiction as a disease similar to hypertension or diabetes. As with these diseases, addiction is a pathologic condition that has a clearly measurable, characteristic physiology and neurobiology. This definition of addiction is consistent with research that has identified genetic factors as well as environmental factors that precipitate relapse.

THE PROCESS OF ADDICTION

The *first stage* in the process of addiction is experimental and social use. The *second stage* is when problem use or abuse occurs. In this stage, alcohol and other drugs are used regularly. Use might occur during the day and while alone rather than with others. Substances are used to manipulate varying emotions.

■ HEALTHY PEOPLE 2010
Substance Abuse Objectives

Health Status Objectives

1. Reduce alcohol-related motor vehicle crash deaths to 4.8 per 100,000 population (baseline: 5.3 per 100,000 in 1998).
   - 1a. Reduce alcohol-related hospital emergency department visits (developmental, no baseline).
   - 1b. Reduce drug-related hospital emergency department visits to 349,810 (baseline: 542,250 emergency department visits by patients aged 16 to 97 years in 1998).
2. Reduce cirrhosis deaths to no more than 3.2 per 100,000 population (baseline: 9.6 cirrhosis deaths per 100,000 population in 1999; American Indians and Alaska Natives, 25.9; Hispanics 15.4; males, 13.4; in 1998).
3. Reduce drug-induced deaths to no more than 1.2 per 100,000 population (baseline: 6.8 in 1999).
4. Reduce to 0.1 cases per 1000 live births (1 per 10,000 births) the occurrence of fetal alcohol syndrome (baseline: 0.4 per 1000 live births [4 per 10,000 births] in 1995 to 1997).

Risk Reduction Objectives

5. Increase to 91% the proportion of adolescents aged 12 to 17 years who report no alcohol or illicit drug use in the past 30 days (baseline: 79% in 1998 and 2002).
6. Reduce the proportion of persons engaging in binge drinking of alcoholic beverages during the past 2 weeks.

Group	1998 Baseline	2010 Target
High school students	32%	11%
College students	39%	20%

Note: Binge drinking is defined as having five or more drinks at the same occasion.

7. Increase the percentage of 12- to 17-year-olds who perceive great risk associated with substance abuse.

Behavior Perceived as a Great Risk	2002 Baseline	2010 Target
Having five or more drinks on a single occasion once or twice per week	38%	50%
Smoking marijuana once per month	32%	36%
Using cocaine once per month	51%	57%

Service and Protection Objectives

8. Increase the proportion of persons aged 12 and older who need alcohol and/or illicit drug treatment who received specialty treatment for abuse or dependence in the past year.

Treatment	2002 Baseline	2010 Target
Illicit drug treatment	18%	24%
Alcohol and illicit drug treatment	10%	16%

9. Increase the proportion of persons who are referred for follow-up care for alcohol problems, drug problems, or suicide attempts after diagnosis or treatment for one of these conditions in a hospital emergency department (developmental, no current baseline).
10. Increase the number of communities with partnerships or coalition models to conduct comprehensive substance abuse prevention efforts (developmental, no current baseline).
11. Extend to all states and the District of Columbia administrative license revocation laws, or programs of equal effectiveness, for people determined to drive under the influence of intoxicants (current baseline: 41 states and the District of Columbia in 1998).
12. Extend to all states and the District of Columbia maximum legal blood alcohol concentration limits of 0.08% for motor vehicle drivers aged 21 years and older (current baseline: 16 States in 1998).

From U.S. Department of Health and Human Services (USDHHS). (2000). *Healthy people 2010: Understanding and improving health* (2nd ed.). Washington, DC: U.S. Government Printing Office; and USDHHS. (2006). *Healthy people 2010: Midcourse review.* Washington, DC: U.S. Government Printing Office.

Behavioral indicators in the second stage include a decline in school or work performance, mood swings, personality changes, lying and conning, change in friendships, decrease in extracurricular activities, adoption of a drug culture appearance, conflicts with family members, and preoccupation with procuring and using alcohol and other drugs. The *third stage* is dependency. Alcohol and drugs are used daily or continuously to avoid pain and depression. Use is out of control as the addict attempts to feel normal. Behavioral indicators of dependence include physical deterioration, cognitive changes, lack of concern over being caught, and absence from home, job, or other places of responsibility (SAMHSA, 1994).

EXTENT OF THE PROBLEM

In 2006, an estimated 20.4 million Americans, or 8.3% of the population 12 years of age and older, used illicit drugs (Figure 25-1). This percentage has been statistically the same since 2002. The most frequently used illicit drugs are marijuana, illicit drugs other than marijuana (most commonly psychotherapeutics), and pain relievers. Approximately 57 million or 23% of those aged 12 and older participate in binge drinking. Approximately 17 million people or 6.9% of the population engage in heavy drinking (SAMHSA, 2007). In 2006, 23.6 million people needed treatment for substance or alcohol abuse, whereas only 16% (2.5 million) actually received treatment (SAMHSA, 2007). In addition to illicit drugs, Americans are dependent on or addicted to alcohol, tobacco, and caffeine, all legal substances.

INCIDENCE AND PREVALENCE: EPIDEMIOLOGIC STUDIES

Major epidemiologic studies were conducted by the National Institute of Mental Health to estimate the prevalence (number of existing cases) and incidence (number of new cases) of psychiatric and substance abuse disorders in the U.S. population (Myers et al., 1984; Ross et al., 1988). These studies are usually referred to as the *epidemiologic catchment area* studies.

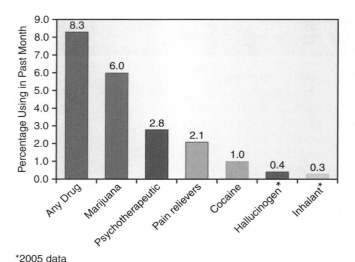

*2005 data

FIGURE 25-1 Past month's use of selected illicit drugs among persons aged 12 years or older, by type of drug, in 2006. (From Substance Abuse and Mental Health Services Administration. [2007]. Results from the 2006 National Survey on Drug Use and Health: National findings. Rockville, MD: Author.)

Study results were reported on *lifetime prevalence,* or the estimated proportion of individuals who ever have experienced particular psychiatric diagnoses (Myers et al., 1984; Robins et al., 1984). The most common diagnoses in decreasing order of prevalence were (1) alcohol abuse and dependence, (2) phobia, (3) major depressive episode, and (4) drug abuse and dependence. It is worth noting that alcoholism is by far the most common disorder, despite the tendency of many to abuse multiple drugs, and is still the most researched and written about of all substance dependencies.

The federal government conducts a biannual national survey to keep track of the incidence and prevalence of use of specific drugs. This survey, the National Survey on Drug Use and Health, is conducted by the Substance Abuse and Mental Health Services Administration (SAMHSA) of the USDHHS. Surveys were conducted in 2006 and 2008. This survey is the source of much of the epidemiologic information on substance use and abuse in the United States. Alcohol and nicotine, both legal substances, have the highest rates of addiction and costs to society. In 2006, alcohol was the most widely used and abused substance (SAMHSA, 2007).

DEMOGRAPHIC CHARACTERISTICS AND SUBSTANCE USE AND ABUSE

Demographic information is shared in an effort to describe the magnitude and scope of alcohol and illicit drug addiction in population subgroups. Because many factors influence data collection, this is a substantial, but not complete, picture of substance use and abuse in subgroups of the U.S. population. It is important to know that there are regional differences in alcohol and illicit drug use; therefore, use of a specific substance might vary across regions of the United States.

There are cultural differences in alcohol and illicit drug use, as well as socioeconomic differences *within* cultural groups. These differences should not lead community/public health nurses to stereotype a particular person's actual or potential alcohol and illicit drug use by the person's age, sex, race, socioeconomic status, geographic location, or community

setting. Nurses must recognize that alcohol and illicit drug addiction can be found in every area and social group. Community/public health nurses should also realize that one abused drug is not worse than another. They all have similar devastating effects on the individual, the family, and the community.

Some of the research on the demographic parameters related to addiction is unfortunately limited by the lack of random samples. Because addicted persons are available for study only when they appear for treatment, data for convenience samples are more frequently reported in the literature. Nevertheless, findings from these studies are interesting and have implications for further research.

Distribution by Age

Evidence from older epidemiologic studies (Myers et al., 1984; Robins et al., 1984) documents that alcohol abuse/alcohol dependence was by far the most common mental disorder in all age groups in all areas of the United States. The SAMHSA survey (2007) validates those earlier findings (Figure 25-2). In the 12- to 17-year age cohort, the use of alcohol, alone or in combination with illicit drugs, surpassed the use of illicit drugs alone. In those 18 years or older, alcohol was the substance responsible for the most dependence and abuse. Approximately 12% of current alcohol drinkers (15.6 million people) met the criteria for alcohol dependence (SAMHSA, 2007). Almost 11 million teenagers aged 12 to 20 years reported drinking alcohol in the month before the SAMHSA survey interview—approximately 28.3% of this age group. Of those teens drinking alcohol, 19% were binge drinkers and 6.2% were heavy drinkers (SAMHSA, 2007).

Addictions usually are thought to be problems of youth or adulthood, not old age. Figure 25-2 indicates that the highest dependence and abuse is among the young, especially those 18 to 25 years of age. The young also have the highest rate

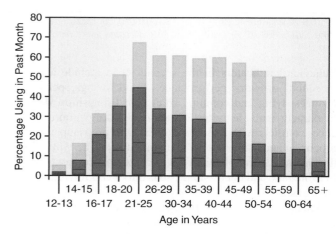

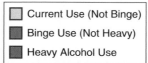

- Current Use (Not Binge)
- Binge Use (Not Heavy)
- Heavy Alcohol Use

FIGURE 25-2 Past month's alcohol use by age, 2006. (From Substance Abuse and Mental Health Services Administration. [2007]. Results from the 2006 National Survey on Drug Use and Health: National findings. Rockville, MD: Author.)

of binge drinking. Although substance dependence and abuse declines with age, the elderly are still at risk. Approximately 38% of seniors 65 years and older drink alcohol (SAMHSA, 2007). One of every 10 elders has a history of alcohol-related problems, and certain subgroups have a higher rate of alcohol problems (20% of nursing home residents and as many as 60% of elderly men admitted to acute care settings). There are also higher rates of alcohol dependence among the elderly who are widowers, single, have difficulty with the police, and live in poorer socioeconomic areas (Fontaine, 2003; Secretary of Health and Human Services, 1990).

Reports might underestimate the true rate of substance abuse among the elderly, because the signs of substance abuse are likely to be confused with the normal process of aging or degenerative brain disease (Trigoboff & Wilson, 2004). In addition, there is the potential danger of drug interactions. This population takes large amounts of prescription drugs and over-the-counter drugs for chronic problems. The rate of abuse of prescription drugs in the elderly is two to three times higher than the rate in the general population (Fontaine, 2003). Reporting does not reflect information about the use and abuse of illicit stimulants and depressants.

Distribution by Race

The epidemiologic data on lifetime prevalence rates show a varying picture of racial differences in alcohol and illicit drug use. Older prevalence studies revealed no significant differences in drug abuse and dependence in black and white populations (Robins et al., 1984). The SAMHSA survey indicates that whites have a higher rate of alcohol use and a slightly higher rate of binge drinking (24.1%) than do Hispanics (23.9%) and blacks (19.1%). Rates of alcohol use and binge drinking were lowest among the Asian cohort (SAMHSA, 2007).

Other racial minority groups, notably American Indians and Alaska Natives, have well-documented and high mortality rates that are alcohol related (National Institute on Drug Abuse [NIDA], 1990). Suicide, homicide, alcoholic cirrhosis of the liver, and unintentional injuries are among the 10 leading causes of death in these populations and are higher than in the general population. American Indians report the highest rate of binge drinking (SAMHSA, 2007; "Tobacco, alcohol, and other drug use among high school students in Bureau of Indian Affairs–funded schools—United States, 2001," 2003). However, it is impossible to generalize about drinking and drug abuse patterns for all Native American tribal groups, because there is great diversity, with some tribes being mostly abstinent. In the 1990s, tribes with alcohol-related problems started an aggressive campaign to address the issue. The sale of alcohol has been banned on some tribal lands, and alcohol and drug treatment programs have been initiated through tribal-run health centers.

Hispanics exhibit great cultural diversity in patterns of alcohol use, with some nationalities being heavier users of alcohol than others. Hispanic men exhibit a high intake mostly in their young adult years and have a higher prevalence of alcohol-related problems.

Illicit drug use is highest among American Indians and Alaska Natives (13.7%), followed by blacks (9.8%), persons who identify themselves as belonging to two or more racial/ethnic groups (8%), whites, and Hispanics. The lowest rate of reported drug use, 3.6%, is among the Asian cohort (SAMHSA, 2007).

Distribution by Gender

Men are more likely to use illicit drugs and abuse alcohol than women, but the rate of alcohol use among women is increasing. The SAMHSA survey (2007) reports the rate of illicit drug use as 10.5% in men and 6.2% in women. Men drive under the influence of alcohol at twice the rate of women. Among young persons aged 12 to 20 years, males (21.3%) are more likely than females (16.5%) to use alcohol and binge drink while underage. Still, many children of both sexes access and use alcohol before the legal drinking age.

Although the percentage of female substance users is smaller than the percentage of males, those who experience substance use and abuse are the targets of public health interventions during their childbearing years in an effort to prevent complications in their children. Approximately 12% of pregnant women use alcohol (up from 9.1% in 2002), 2.9% binge drink, and 4% use illicit drugs. Although these rates are lower than the rates of substance use among nonpregnant females, *any use of illicit drugs or alcohol during pregnancy is a health problem.*

Distribution by Socioeconomic Level

Data on the prevalence of substance dependence by socioeconomic level are not available, but data on use by educational level provide some measure of comparison. When educational level is used as an indicator of socioeconomic status, study findings show that more substance dependence is found among those at lower socioeconomic levels. The most prevalent disorder is alcohol abuse, although alcohol abuse has declined by 50% since the late 1980s. Full-time college students are more likely than other peer groups to use alcohol, binge drink, and drink heavily. In later years, however, higher educational level appears to be associated with reduced rate of continued abuse. Those who did not attend college are more likely to drink heavily than those who attended college (6.2% versus 5.4%) (SAMHSA, 2007). Illicit drug use is lower among college graduates (5.9%) than among high school graduates (8.6%) and those who did not graduate from high school (9.2%) (SAMHSA, 2007). It should be noted that those with the least financial resources and health insurance are the ones at greater risk of needing treatment (see Chapter 21).

TRENDS IN SUBSTANCE USE AND ABUSE

Trends in alcohol and drug use and dependence are monitored by several national efforts housed in the USDHHS, including the National Survey on Drug Use and Health and the National Youth Risk Survey. Alcohol abuse and dependence remain the largest substance-related problem. In 2006, approximately 15.6 million people were considered alcohol dependent or alcohol abusers. Marijuana is still the most commonly abused illicit drug. In 2006, marijuana was used by 72% of current illicit drug users. Over time, there has been some success in addressing problems associated with the use of alcohol. For example, the use of alcohol and the rate of alcohol-related motor vehicle deaths have both dropped by 50% since 1987–1988 (SAMHSA, 2006; USDHHS, 2000, 2006). Trends in the lifetime use of substances indicate a continued problem with substance use and dependence.

- Cigarette and marijuana use both declined slightly in 2001 after rising consistently from the early 1990s. The percentage of adolescents (aged 12 to 17 years) who used marijuana declined from 21.9% in 2001 to 6.7% in 2006. The number of adolescents using any tobacco product also declined. It remains to be seen if marijuana and cigarette use will continue to decline (SAMHSA, 2007).

- Cocaine use has increased since 1986 but has stabilized in recent years. The percentage of illicit drug users reporting that they had ever used cocaine was 14.4% in 2002 and 14.3% in 2006 (SAMHSA, 2007).
- Heroin use leveled off to 1.5% of illicit drug users between 2002 and 2006 (SAMHSA, 2007).
- Hallucinogen use among young adults increased until 2002, decreased in 2004, and remained stable in 2006 (SAMHSA, 2007). This was due primarily to the decrease in the use of Ecstasy (methylenedioxymethamphetamine). Use of LSD (lysergic acid diethylamide) and PCP (phencyclidine) is less common.
- The nonmedical use of pain relievers, tranquilizers, and stimulants among adolescents and young adults has increased steadily since the mid-1990s. However, illicit use of these drugs among youth 12 to 17 years of age decreased between 2002 and 2006. Illicit drug use among adults aged 50 to 54 years increased during the same period (SAMHSA, 2007).
- Steroid use among athletes has been widely publicized and is an ongoing problem.

The use of inhalants is a problem among adolescents. Some individuals combine multiple drugs for greater effect and/or combine drugs with alcohol. These practices exacerbate health consequences for the individual. Reckless use of substances in public and in private also impact the health and safety of anyone who comes in contact with a person under the influence, whether a friend, neighbor, or total stranger.

PREVALENCE OF DUAL DIAGNOSIS

Some people may exhibit mental disorders and abuse drugs, a condition called **dual diagnosis.** Approximately 10% of persons with psychiatric disorders abuse alcohol and 6% abuse drugs (Fontaine, 2003). The risk of substance use is higher for persons suffering from depression, bipolar disorder, and anxiety disorders. Frisch and Frisch (2002) reviewed several older studies and reported that participants in methadone treatment programs also used other drugs (20%) and alcohol (50%). The same reviewers indicated that almost 50% of substance abusers have a co-occurring psychiatric diagnosis.

Another type of dual diagnosis, substance dependence with a co-occurring medical condition, should be mentioned. Diseases that are strongly linked to alcohol consumption, not all of which are reversible with abstinence from alcohol, include liver disease, pancreatitis, malabsorption of nutrients, alcohol cardiomyopathy, brain damage and adult dementia, failure of reproductive function, and cancers of the mouth, larynx, and esophagus (Bauer & Hill, 2000; Fontaine, 2003; NIDA, 2007).

Individuals with dual diagnoses, that is, substance abuse and psychiatric disorders (co-occurring disorders), pose a major challenge to professionals working in the community. (See Chapter 33.) Such clients generally lack access to appropriate treatment for both disorders, have a poorer treatment outcome and a more complicated withdrawal and recovery, and are overrepresented in certain special disadvantaged populations. People with coexisting substance abuse and psychiatric disorders are at great risk for other social problems and health problems such as human immunodeficiency virus (HIV) infection and hepatitis C (Phoenix & Pelish, 2004). Social problems include homelessness, criminal activity, and relationship difficulties.

Treatment of dual diagnosis clients is problematic, because both types of treatment agencies—mental health and substance abuse—might reject the client on the basis of the other diagnosis. Research to improve the assessment and treatment of problems that coexist with substance dependence is needed, because dual diagnoses are a common and persistent health issue.

Implications for nursing services in the community are enormous. First, alcohol abuse/dependence is the most prevalent diagnosis among all *DSM-IV*–defined mental disorders in the United States, as shown by the aforementioned epidemiologic studies. The already heavy economic burden for treatment of substance abuse is increased by the coexistence of other disorders. These factors impose a high level of need for professional care by community workers, including nurses. It is likely that most clients already seen by community/public health nurses either have addictions or have family members with addictions so that their health and well-being are affected by the addictions of others.

The message is clear. In the future, community/public health nurses can be expected to assume an even greater role in the prevention and treatment of problems of substance use and dependence related to mental disorders. Nurses, for example, will be expected to identify the co-occurring problems of substance dependence and psychiatric disorder and make appropriate referrals. Community/public health nurses need to exert extra effort to advocate for appropriate treatment and resource allocations for this special, vulnerable population.

PREVALENCE OF SUBSTANCE ABUSE AMONG REGISTERED NURSES

Many researchers have attempted to estimate the prevalence of substance abuse among nurses. Research-based studies have described patterns of addiction and correlated family, personal, and professional characteristics of nurses with problems of addiction (Haack & Harford, 1984; Sullivan, 1987a, 1987b). Griffith (1999) reports that the estimate of the American Nurses Association is that 10% to 20% of nurses have substance abuse problems and that 6% to 8% of nurses are impaired due to their use or abuse of substances. Comparisons with other populations find that the rate of substance use among nurses is either similar to or lower than that in the general population (Collins et al., 1999; Fontaine, 2003).

Trinkoff and colleagues (1991) examined a large sample of nurses and reported that although alcohol abuse was low, nurses had higher rates of prescription drug use. Nurses have easy access to prescription drugs, such as tranquilizers, amphetamines, opiates, and sedatives. These drugs may be used at higher doses or more often than prescribed, or for nonapproved reasons (Trinkoff & Storr, 1998).

For nurses and for women generally, some researchers have found a strong link between psychologic symptoms that precede depression and substance abuse. Trinkoff and colleagues (2000) identified contributory conditions that increase substance abuse risk in nurses, including easy access to prescription-type drugs, job stress or role strain, and depressive symptoms.

Nurses and other health professionals who work with substance-abusing nurses must often decide how to deal with the situation. Substance use on the job represents a risk to the health and safety of patients and staff. All nurses should be aware of workplace policies that address substance use by staff. Many nurses do not report their colleagues because of punitive policies in a number of states. Beckstead's research (2002) indicates that a little more than a third of nurses working with impaired colleagues report them to supervisors. It is important to identify nurses with substance dependence to facilitate access to appropriate treatment. Nurses who are dependent on opioid-type drugs can receive buprenorphine replacement therapy in the office of a certified physician. Names of physicians who are certified to provide such therapy are available on the SAMHSA website at *http://www.SAMHSA.gov.* Each state nursing organization and state licensing agency has protocols that address the rehabilitation of nurses who abuse substances of any kind. Nurses should be aware of the Board of Nursing policies in their state and the providers that treat persons impaired by substance abuse or co-occurring psychiatric disorders (Haack & Yocom, 2002).

THEORIES OF ADDICTION

Alcohol and drug addictions appear to be part of a larger constellation of related disorders, thought to be clustered around some underlying biologic or genetic mechanism, or multifactorial cause that is yet to be discovered. A recent trend has been to create realistic models of addiction by conceptually organizing its development within a biopsychosocial framework. The biopsychosocial model has emerged to provide a broader, more holistic perspective on addiction and its prevention, treatment, and research. This model is being accepted more widely because it can more adequately explain the complex nature of addiction.

The biopsychosocial model of addiction that best fits community/public health nursing is that of the public health model (Figure 25-3). The public health model of addiction stresses that biologic, psychologic, pharmacologic, and social factors constantly interact and influence the problem of addiction in any person or group of people. As described by Mosher (1996), in the public health model, the *host* is the person who has the addiction; the *agent* is the alcohol or other drug sufficient in quantity to cause harm to the host; and the *environment* includes the social, economic, physical, political, and cultural settings in which the host and agent interact. The environment also includes the meanings, values, and norms assigned to a drug by its culture, community, and society.

It is true that alcohol and other drug addictions could not exist if the alcohol or illicit drugs were not available. Therefore, the role of addicting drugs and alcohol is that of the agent in the public health model. As shown in Figure 25-3, the addiction does not occur solely because of the agent. Some host and environmental factors also contribute to the development of addiction.

Many of the repetitive behaviors associated with addictions involve multiple brain reward regions and neurotransmitters that also regulate normal consumptive behaviors necessary to survival, such as eating and drinking (Guardia et al., 2000; NIDA, 1994). Scientists are involved in a widely publicized search for genes that predispose persons to alcoholism and

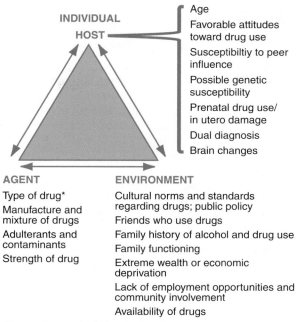

FIGURE 25-3 Public health model of addiction.

other addictions by regulating brain function. It can be stated undeniably that changes in the brain are a major cause of alcohol and other drug addictions (Trigoboff & Wilson, 2004). Prescott and colleagues (1999) and other researchers have conducted twin studies that demonstrate a genetic vulnerability to alcoholism. Identical twins of alcoholic parents have more than a 60% chance and fraternal twins a 30% chance of becoming alcoholics.

Numerous environmental conditions, such as physical and psychologic trauma, also play a part in the expression of addictions. Other environmental risk factors include economic and social deprivation, low neighborhood attachment, community norms that facilitate drug use and abuse, and availability of alcohol and other drugs (Trigoboff & Wilson, 2004).

Genetic vulnerability and environmental factors interact to produce addiction; however, addiction can apparently be induced without genetic vulnerability through the impact of the environment alone. Mosher (1996, p. 244) states, "Environmental factors—the forces that bring the agent into injurious contact with the host—are critical in the public health model of addiction. A high-risk environment creates a myriad of opportunities for public health harm." High-risk environments can be found in the family, workplace, school, and community.

EFFECTS OF ALCOHOL AND/OR DRUGS ON THE BODY

Alcohol and illicit drugs may be categorized by the effects they have on the human body (Table 25-1). Two major categories of addicting drugs are central nervous system depressants and central nervous system stimulants. Central nervous system depressants include alcohol and the drugs listed in Table 25-1. The most commonly used legal drug in this category is alcohol, and the most commonly known illegal drug is heroin. All drugs in this

TABLE 25-1   Effects of Selected Drugs and Alcohol

	Desired Effects	Health Consequences
Central Nervous System Depressants		
Alcohol, barbiturates, benzodiazepines, nonbarbiturates	Relaxation, euphoria, disinhibition, sedation, compliance with social custom, decreased tension and anxiety, decreased inhibition, mental relaxation	Death from overdose, alone or in combination with other central nervous system depressants; illnesses resulting from damage caused by chronic exposure of tissues in every organ and system of the body due to toxic effects; irreversible brain damage and resultant cognitive difficulties, fetal alcohol syndrome, trauma and accidents, respiratory depression, seizures, coma, death
Narcotics (morphine sulfate, Percodan, Dilaudid, Damerol, Dolophine, Darvon, Talwin, Stadol, heroin, codeine)	Euphoria, a thrill similar to orgasm, diminished response to pain, drowsiness, decreased anxiety, and fear	Respiratory failure, coma, death, trauma, and accidents during drug-seeking behavior; increased risk for HIV and hepatitis, and localized and systemic infections; convulsions associated with withdrawal
Central Nervous System Stimulants		
Cocaine, amphetamines, Ecstasy, MDA	Elevated mood, enhanced sexual stimulation, euphoria, releif of fatigue, increase in alertness, loss of appetite	Hypertension, increased alertness, local anesthesia, heart and respiratory rates, cardiac arrest, cerebral vascular accident, paranoia, hallucinations, seizures, death, toxic effects to fetus, increased heart and respiratory rates, irregular heartbeat, physical collapse, high fever, cardiovascular accident and cardiac arrest, psychosis
Nicotine (cigarettes, snuff, chewing tobacco, pipes, cigars)	Relaxation, relief of compliance with social custom, appetite control, increase in energy	Increased illness and absence from work, chronic obstructive lung diseases (emphysema and bronchitis associated with shortness of breath, cough, excessive phlegm), coronary heart disease, cancer of mouth and lungs, interaction of tobacco smoke with medications leading to decreased effectiveness
Caffeine (coffee, teas, colas, other soft drinks, chocolate)	Relaxation, compliance with social custom, increased wakefulness, increased alertness, diminished sense of fatigue, blocked drowsiness, facilitated mental activity	Muscle twitching, rambling thoughts and speech, heart arrhythmias, motor agitation, ringing in the ears, flashes of light, stomach complaints, breast cysts, spontaneous fetal loss
Hallucinogens		
LSD, PCP, STP, MDA, MDMA, DOM, mescaline, psilocybin, ecstasy, or MDMA	Altered perceptions, heightened awareness, sense of religious insight, increased sexual pleasure	Violence and self-inflicted injuries, memory loss and illusions, speech difficulty, convulsions, coma, ruptured blood vessels in the brain, cardiac and respiratory failure, psychotic episodes, flashbacks
Cannabis, hashish, THC	Compliance with social custom, sense of well-being, relaxation, altered perceptions, euphoria, increased appetite, relief of nausea and vomiting, heightened sensory awareness, enhanced sociability	Marijuana: dry mouth, sore throat, increased heart rate, orthostatic hypotension, bronchitis, immunosuppression, reduction in testosterone and sperm count, disruption of menstrual periods and ovulation, anxiety and extreme self-consciousness, paranoia and panic, impaired judgment, decreased REM sleep, impaired ability to carry out goal-directed tasks, apathy, social withdrawal, decreased concentration, hallucinations, and delusions
Inhalants		
Acetone, benzene, amyl and butyl nitrate, nitrous oxide, gasoline, toluene	Disorientation, increased euphoria	Mouth ulcers, gastrointestinal problems, anorexia, confusion, headache, ataxia, convulsions, death from asphyxiation, permanent brain damage, memory interference, damage to airways, lungs, kidneys and liver, nose bleeds
Anabolic Steroids	Maintenance of or improvement of athletic performance, increased muscle size and strength, increased aggressiveness	Liver damage and liver cancer, endocrine abnormalities (such as decreased plasma testosterone, decreased luteinizing hormone, atrophy of testes), decreased libido, acne, water and salt retention, stunting of bone growth in children, impotence, mood swings with paranoia, violent behavior

category have addiction potential, whether they are legal, illegal, or available by prescription. They also produce withdrawal symptoms after long-term abuse and dependent use. The most commonly used legal stimulant is nicotine. The most commonly used illegal stimulant is cocaine. Although the issue has been debated, all central nervous stimulants listed in Table 25-1 have addiction potential and produce some degree of withdrawal.

Three additional categories of drugs are hallucinogens, inhalants, and anabolic steroids. Persons using hallucinogens, including marijuana, strive for an altered perception of reality. LSD is the most potent hallucinogen. Ecstasy, popular with children and adolescents, has the properties of both a stimulant and a hallucinogen. Inhalant use is most common among children and adolescents, because inhalants are affordable and accessible. Inhalant drug use is very addicting and extremely dangerous. Inhalants include aerosols, gasoline, correction fluid, cleaning solutions, and other commonly used chemicals. Once inhaled, the solvents are rapidly absorbed and produce central nervous system effects in seconds. Consequently, the mental state is altered for 5 to 15 minutes. Although tolerance develops in long-term users, withdrawal symptoms are rare. Anabolic steroid use is most common among athletes and adolescent boys. Anabolic steroids appear to have lifelong health consequences, including increased risk of early heart disease.

> John was a 17-year-old star high school football player. He was one of the top defensive linemen in the state. His goal was to win a college scholarship and be drafted by the National Football League (NFL) after college. He knew that college and NFL linemen were large, some even weighing 300 pounds. Despite daily weight lifting and heavy caloric intake, he was unable to gain more body mass.
>
> One day he was approached by a senior classmate who suggested that he try "roids." The classmate told John that since he had started taking them he had gained 25 lb and increased his strength. The classmate told John he could get him the "roids." John knew that steroids had serious side effects, but he decided to try them. He badly wanted that scholarship.

IMPACT OF SUBSTANCE USE DISORDERS ON INDIVIDUALS AND FAMILY MEMBERS

Without question, the total effects of addiction impact all citizens, either directly or indirectly. Some of the social and human costs are outlined in the sections that follow.

INFANTS AND CHILDREN OF MOTHERS WITH PRENATAL SUBSTANCE USE DISORDERS

An estimated 1 million children per year are exposed to alcohol, tobacco, and illicit drugs during gestation (Chasnoff, 2001). Prenatal alcohol and/or drug exposure during pregnancy can have serious consequences for the infant. Different substances produce different effects, and the developing child is often exposed to multiple substances during pregnancy if the mother has a substance use disorder. Not all women who abuse alcohol or drugs give birth to babies with serious health problems. The amount of damage, which is highly variable, is related to the quantity, frequency, and timing of exposure; both maternal and fetal metabolism; individual susceptibility; and

probably differences in maternal health. Why some women manage to have healthy pregnancies despite substance abuse is not known (Haack, 1997).

Effects of Prenatal Alcohol Exposure

There is no known safe level of maternal alcohol use for the developing fetus. Each year in the United States an estimated 130,000 women drink alcohol at sufficient levels during pregnancy to put their fetuses at risk for developing alcohol-related disorders (Centers for Disease Control and Prevention, 2002). It is not just alcohol-dependent women who are at risk of having babies with these disorders. Binge drinking plays a major role by exposing the fetus to high levels of alcohol during short periods of time. Several alcohol-related developmental disorders are recognized under the umbrella term **fetal alcohol spectrum disorders (FASDs):**
- Fetal alcohol syndrome (FAS)
- Alcohol-related neurodevelopmental disorders (ARNDs)
- Alcohol-related birth defects (ARBDs)

The incidence of FAS in the United States is estimated to be 1 to 2 per 1000 births. The combined incidence of FAS, ARND, and ARBD is 10 per 1000 births (May & Gossage, 2001). The lifetime cost of care for one individual with FAS in the United States is $2 million (Lupton et al., 2004).

The Institute of Medicine has defined the diagnostic characteristics of these disorders, which are based on history of maternal alcohol use during pregnancy, facial features, small gestational age, abnormalities in the central nervous system, and failure to thrive that is not related to poor nutrition. Figure 25-4 shows an infant with FAS. A child with FASD or ARND may lack the physical features of FAS but have behavioral or cognitive abnormalities that cannot be explained by

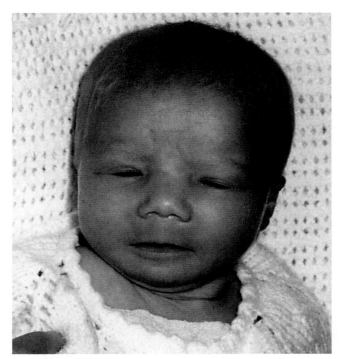

FIGURE 25-4 Infant with fetal alcohol syndrome. Note the long, smooth philtrum, thin upper lip, short nose, and flat midface. (From Hockenberry, M. J., Wilson, D., Winkelstein, M. L., et al. [2003]. *Wong's nursing care of infants and children* [7th ed.]. St. Louis: Mosby.)

environment alone. Children with apparently normal facial features can have brain damage due to fetal alcohol exposure. They may exhibit poor impulse control, inability to understand abstractions, and poor performance in school (Stratton et al., 1996). Commonly observed secondary problems include mental health problems, trouble with the law, and imprisonment. These children may be placed in foster care because their families are not able to care for them. Some children severely affected by FAS or FASD might need placement in supervised or residential care facilities.

Developmental disabilities related to maternal alcohol consumption are totally preventable. Public health nurses have a key role to play in preventing this human tragedy and economic burden to society. Nurses need to advise adolescents and women to abstain from drinking if they have the potential of becoming pregnant. Adolescents and women who drink should be advised to practice birth control until they are ready for pregnancy. Abstinence from drinking alcohol just prior to and throughout pregnancy is the wisest choice.

In any setting in which prenatal care is provided, the nurse should screen for drinking by using nonconfrontational approaches, such as questions imbedded in regular health questionnaires. Several useful instruments are available on the website of the National Institute on Alcohol Abuse and Alcoholism (NIAAA) at *http://www.niaaa.nih.gov*: TWEAK, TACE, AUDIT-C , 4P+, and the *NIAAA Clinicians' Guide*. If at-risk drinking patterns are identified, the nurse should implement a brief behavioral counseling intervention to reduce alcohol misuse.

The lives of infants and children with fetal alcohol disorders can be improved through early identification and treatment. Early intervention is important for infants whose mothers abused alcohol prenatally. Once maternal alcohol use during pregnancy is documented and a diagnosis is established, the child is eligible for early intervention services under Part C of the federal Individuals with Disabilities Education Act. These services are critical to helping the child achieve optimal functioning during his or her lifetime (Welch-Carre, 2005). (See Chapter 30.) It should be noted that it is not easy to detect FAS during the neonatal period, because the facial features associated with the syndrome are difficult to recognize and the central nervous system dysfunction might not be identified until several years after birth. Often students with FASD are misdiagnosed as having attention-deficit/hyperactivity disorder (ADHD) and are improperly medicated. Current scientific evidence suggests that although persons with FASD have attention/arousal regulation problems, their difficulties are not the same as those characterizing ADHD.

Effects of Prenatal Cocaine and Heroin Exposure

Problems that are connected with cocaine abuse include intracranial hemorrhage in the fetus and serious complications of pregnancy such as abruptio placentae. During the first 4 months of life, cocaine-exposed infants can continue to experience an abstinence syndrome and exhibit abnormal behaviors, including rapid mood changes and tremulousness. Infants exposed to cocaine in utero may have great difficulty in bonding. Although emotionally labile, they can be difficult to soothe, hold, and cuddle, which further hampers positive interactions with their mothers. If the mother does not receive guidance in parenting her baby and/or treatment for her cocaine use disorder, she may be at risk for abusing and/or neglecting her child

(see Chapter 22). Community/public health nurses can play a key role in providing or facilitating access to parenting skills training and substance abuse treatment.

Infants of mothers dependent on heroin or methadone may experience withdrawal symptoms after birth and compromised growth and development patterns. For pregnant women dependent on heroin, the policy in the United States is that it is safer for the fetus if the woman is maintained on methadone or buprenorphine. Attempts to withdraw from heroin should not be made without methadone or buprenorphine treatment.

Long-term effects of maternal substance abuse on children can include learning deficits, learning problems, attention and memory deficits, and speech and hearing impairment. Drug-exposed children are often described as *fragile*. They might be easily overstimulated and require a great deal of assistance to maintain control of their hyperexcitable nervous systems (Chasnoff, 2001). Some may require special educational environments. However, research indicates that drug-exposed children who participate in Head Start and other early interventions are able to enter mainstream kindergarten.

Community/public health nurses and other workers have performed admirably in recent years by educating pregnant and other women of childbearing age about the risks of substance use and abuse during pregnancy. However, the need for this intervention occurs anew with each generation of young women.

CHILDREN AND TEENS

The National Survey on Drug Use and Health surveys children 12 years of age and older. However, a growing number of even younger children are participating in alcohol and illicit drug use in all regions of the country. There are regional differences in degree of risk and availability of substances.

In *urban* settings, children are exposed to many facets of alcohol and drug use. Some might be involved in the drug trade that exists in the underground economy of inner cities. For example, some children younger than age 12 years are drug runners (taking drugs from dealer to buyer), drug dealers (selling drugs in schools and neighborhoods), or drug lookouts (keeping an eye out for law enforcement officers while drug dealers ply their trade). Payment for these services may actually help to support families living in poverty. Children might also be involved in picking up the drug needed by an adult and sometimes in helping to prepare the drug or give it to the adult. Children learn by example and mimic the behavior of their peer group and/or the adults in their environment. These learned behaviors contribute to the generational transmission of substance abuse in families and communities.

In *suburban* settings, substance abuse might be easier to hide, yet children are still exposed. As a reminder of this situation, a common poster and public service announcement reads, "40% of all drug use occurs in the inner city and urban areas. Where do you think the other 60% occurs?" In *rural* areas, the legal parameters are somewhat different. Legal enforcement is more difficult because there are fewer personnel or a larger geographic area to cover. There is wider use of inhalants and crystal methamphetamine among children in rural settings. In some rural communities, drinking ages might not be enforced or might be completely disregarded. Some rural communities have their own concepts about when a child can use alcohol and/or other drugs.

In all settings, children are involved in co-dependence. They might be obliged to take care of parents or siblings who are suffering from the effects of withdrawal from alcohol, marijuana, cocaine, or heroin. They might also cover for addicts in their quest to protect them from extended family members, social service workers, or law enforcement personnel.

FAMILY DYSFUNCTION AND CO-DEPENDENCE

Family dysfunction and appropriate interventions are addressed in detail in Chapters 12 and 14. Families with members who have addictions exhibit characteristic dysfunctional family patterns. Space here does not permit a full elaboration of the family dynamics associated with addiction. These dysfunctional patterns in relationships are sometimes characterized as **co-dependence.** *Co-dependence* is a term used to describe the relationship between a substance abuser and one or more persons (usually a family member) who attempt to assist and control the abuser's behavior. A co-dependent person is often an **enabler.** An enabler works to limit or eliminate the harmful consequences of the user's behavior. Therefore, the abuser is *enabled* to continue the abuse pattern because he or she does not have to face the problems brought on by his or her behavior.

One pattern identified by family theorists involves labeling or blaming (scapegoating) an individual as the sole source of the family's problems. For example, an adolescent who smokes marijuana at school is often the index case in a family with other members who have alcohol and drug problems. Nonaddicted family members are frequently "overfunctioners"; their overresponsible behaviors compensate for the irresponsible behaviors exhibited by the family member with the substance use disorder. If the overresponsible individuals are able to stop taking on responsibilities that belong to the affected family member, then that person will be more easily recruited into treatment (see Secondary Prevention later).

Sometimes, families coping with addiction reorganize and exclude the addicted person (often a parent). The parent/child or parent/spouse subsystem is left in a weaker position as a result. A strong alliance may develop between the nonaddicted partner and that partner's parent or other extended family member. Another pattern that may emerge is overcloseness between a grandparent and one or more grandchildren. This strong bond results in weakened parental authority and permits the addicted parent to underfunction in the parental role. Inner-city families with addicted members often exhibit this pattern—a strong grandparent caring for the grandchild and a weak, drug-addicted parent. Both the weak parent and the grandchild are treated as children by the grandparent. Whether or not they are addicted, parents in these families usually "triangle in" (or are overly close to) special children (see Chapters 12 and 14). If a nonaddicted parent is present, that parent is closer to the children as a general rule. Children triangled into the parental relationship, caught up in a pattern of overcloseness to one parent and distance from the other parent, cannot attend to their normal developmental tasks. They grow up either overfunctioning and overachieving, and therefore acting as parents to their parents, or significantly underfunctioning, and therefore becoming unsuccessful, inadequate adults.

Recovery from addiction is a long, painful process for both the person with the substance use disorder and family members. Recovery is likely to take years rather than months. Long recoveries underline the importance of continuing assessment, ongoing family intervention, and appropriate referrals when necessary to address emotional and physical problems. When a person's recovery is complicated by a personality disorder or psychiatric disorder, an even longer period of intervention and healing is needed. The community/public health nurse can assist such families by encouraging active participation in self-help groups, helping to establish social support systems (especially with extended family members alienated during the period of active addiction), recommending counseling, and intervening to bring dysfunctional family patterns into balance. SAMHSA has established a National Registry of Evidence-Based Programs and Practices (NREPP). The registry includes a searchable database of interventions for the prevention and treatment of mental and substance use disorders, and organizations to implement programs and practices in communities. Further information can be found at *http://www.nrepp.samhsa.gov.*

ADDICTIONS AND COMMUNICABLE DISEASES

Communicable diseases that are linked with alcohol and other drug addictions include tuberculosis (TB), sexually transmitted diseases (STDs), and serum-transmitted diseases, especially HIV infection and hepatitis B and C. These communicable diseases are discussed at length in Chapters 7 and 8.

The incidence of TB is closely related to socioeconomic status in that higher rates occur among persons in low-income groups. Crowded living arrangements increase the likelihood of exposure when someone has active TB. Poor nutrition associated with poverty, combined with addiction to alcohol and other drugs, decreases the resistance of people exposed to TB. Drug users have a two to six times greater risk of contracting TB than do nonusers (NIDA, 1999).

Homeless persons with addictions live in environmentally compromising conditions (see Chapter 21). Interactions with someone who has TB or HIV infection are highly possible, particularly if that person is under the influence of alcohol and/or other drugs. Close encounters, unprotected sex, and injection drug use contribute to the passing along of TB and HIV (see Chapter 8).

Certain groups at higher risk should be screened for TB. Among these groups are persons who inject illicit drugs and other locally identified high-risk substance users (e.g., crack cocaine users). Those with addictions are less likely to follow the medication treatment regimen for TB and therefore are more likely to have multidrug-resistant tuberculosis, which is more difficult to treat (Leshner, 2000).

The link between HIV/AIDS and addiction is well established. The ritual of needle sharing by intravenous drug users facilitates the transmission of HIV infection and other serum-borne diseases. Sex with an intravenous drug user who is infected can also play an important role (see the *Ethics in Practice* box on page 648). High-risk sexual practices are fueled by the abuse of mood-altering licit or illicit drugs, because of their effects on brain function. Higher cortical functions involving judgment, cognition, and perception are compromised, precautions are not taken, and riskier sexual behaviors occur. Individuals with substance use disorders may also engage in unsafe sexual practices, such as prostitution, to obtain money to support their addictions.

ETHICS IN PRACTICE

Conflict among Community Values

Gail A. DeLuca Havens, PhD, RN

Tom sits and listens to the rancor and divisiveness apparent in the remarks of some of the city's residents at a forum called to discuss the implementation of the syringe exchange program in the city next month. He feels a momentary twinge of regret for having brought the issue to this point. Tom is a community/public health nurse and clinical director of the municipally operated community-based health care center with the largest caseload of human immunodeficiency virus (HIV)–infected clients in the city. He understands that the critical nature of the near-epidemic proportions of the incidence of acquired immunodeficiency syndrome (AIDS) in the community requires proven interventions if the spread of HIV is to be controlled. Unfortunately, a syringe exchange program, although shown to be a very effective deterrent to the spread of the virus, comes with a large price tag: polarization of community residents because of the moral questions it raises. It is Tom's turn to speak.

"I'm pleased to see so many of our city's residents participating in the forums about the syringe exchange program. I understand that the program is very controversial. It is viewed by many as sending a message that this city condones drug addiction. It is feared that it will contribute to an increase in drug addiction. And from a practical viewpoint, it was in direct violation of one of our city ordinances, namely, the prohibition against possession of intravenous injection paraphernalia. As a point of information, the law has been amended to allow an exception such as this.

"I understand that for many of you this program represents a degradation of the prevailing moral norms that exist in this city. You are afraid that clean needles will encourage drug abuse. A well-conceived syringe exchange program, however, includes more than the exchange of contaminated equipment for clean needles and syringes. The cornerstone of such a program is the educational focus on a drug-free existence. Unfortunately, in some metropolitan areas of the United States, drug users who decide to break the habit do not have immediate access to counseling and support, but instead are placed on waiting lists for instruction and rehabilitation to help them become free of drugs. We are fortunate in our city in that we believe we have the necessary resources dedicated to the drug treatment component of the syringe exchange program to ensure that anyone wishing to enroll in the program will have immediate access.

"Syringe exchange programs have been found to be very effective interventions, with some programs 100% effective in avoiding an increase in HIV infection. Syringe exchange options have met with extraordinary success in terms of preventing or slowing HIV infection among intravenous drug users (Tempalski et al., 2007). This success has occurred without an increase in drug abuse. I believe that if we fail to initiate such a program in our city, where the incidence of AIDS is significantly higher than the national average for cities of comparable size, we will be guilty of a greater moral harm. For not only do we deny noninfected drug users in our city the means to maintain their HIV-free status, but we also reduce the likelihood that they will participate in drug abuse educational programs that have the potential to empower them to break their drug habit. I ask you to understand that by *not* initiating this program, we condemn some

fellow citizens to chronic illness and death through the uncontrolled spread of HIV. I am here this evening to respond to your questions and to ask for your cooperation and support as we prepare to begin the syringe exchange program in our city next month."

The moral issues that are present in this case exist because of differences in fundamental perspectives about what ought to be societal priorities for health care in the face of the growing numbers of HIV-positive people in the United States. The sharing of drug paraphernalia and sexual intercourse are associated with the majority of all reported cases of AIDS (Centers for Disease Control and Prevention [CDC], 2007a). The CDC estimates that between 850,000 and 950,000 people in the United States are living with HIV (CDC, 2007b).

Historically, syringe exchange programs in this country have been regarded as symbolic endorsements of illegal drug use and a perceived major threat to the integrity of our societal norms. They have been characterized as an affront to society (Shaw, 2006).

In addressing this dilemma, several fundamental questions might be posed. What obligations does society have to its individual members? Are they obligations that apply to every member of society? Do the benefits to individual members of a society to be derived from a syringe exchange program outweigh the harm to society, collectively, that is inherent in such a program? Which harm is the community willing to tolerate: the potential for harm to the community's moral norms by condoning illegal drug use and by creating a situation that might precipitate drug use or the certain harm that will befall drug users who are exposed to HIV infection through needle sharing?

When we speak about obligations, we are implying that corresponding rights exist. Certain obligations fall to a society to ensure that the rights of its individual members are met. Individual rights were not conceived as having infinite dimensions. Rather, they are defined by the rules and norms imposed on them by society. It is the existence of prevailing norms of a society and its general moral code that frequently precipitate a moral dilemma. City residents are being asked to support a program that contradicts the prevailing moral norm. Furthermore, to compound the moral tension, they are being asked to support a program for people living at the edges of society, namely, drug abusers. Do the nature of the situation and the characteristics of the people who will benefit from a syringe exchange program limit society's obligation?

One approach to the resolution of this dilemma would be for the residents of the city to refuse to condone and support a syringe exchange program, rationalizing that they have no obligation to support individuals' drug habits. An alternative approach of the city's residents, considering the positive empirical evidence, would be to support the syringe exchange program, thereby fulfilling a societal obligation to its individual members regardless of lifestyle. The city also would be protecting the public through the control of communicable disease.

Finally, where do the nurse's moral and professional obligations lie in this situation? The American Nurses Association (ANA) *Code of Ethics for Nurses* was modified substantially in 2001 so that the obligations of its members to individual members of society are clarified by the corresponding rights of clients. That is, the client has a right to nursing care that "transcends all individual differences" (ANA, 2001, p. 7). Furthermore, "An individual's lifestyle, value system and religious beliefs should be considered in planning health care with and for each patient" (ANA, 2001, p. 7). Accordingly, the nurse's practice ought to include nonjudgmental care and advocacy that respects the patient as a person and supports the patient's right to care.

Tom has chosen this approach. What would you have done?

REFERENCES

American Nurses Association. (2001). *Code of ethics for nurses with interpretive statements*. Washington, DC: Author.

Centers for Disease Control and Prevention. (2007a). *Basic information*. Retrieved May 22, 2007 from http://www.cdc.gov/hiv/topics/basic/index.htm.

Centers for Disease Control and Prevention. (2007b). *Advancing HIV prevention: New strategies for a changing epidemic*. Retrieved May 22, 2007 from http://www.cdc.gov/hiv/topics/prev_prog/AHP/default.htm.

Shaw, S. J. (2006). Public citizens, marginalized communities: The struggle for syringe exchange in Springfield, Massachusetts. *Medical Anthropology*, *25*(1), 31-63.

Tempalski, B., Flom, P. L., Friedman, S. R., et al. (2007). Social and political factors predicting the presence of syringe exchange programs in 96 US metropolitan areas. *American Journal of Public Health*, 97, 437-447.

Drug abusers and their partners often share a history of abuse as children. The resulting low self-esteem and poor ability to set interpersonal boundaries inhibit the personal assertiveness that is necessary for self-care and safe sexual practices. This combination of developmental lack in self-care and substance abuse by women or their partners often results in unsafe sexual practices. Such practices result in the spreading of STDs, including the increase in heterosexual transmission of HIV infection, chlamydia, herpes, and hepatitis B and C.

Nurses in community health settings recognize that unaddressed alcohol and/or other drug addiction have an impact on the individual, the family, and the community. Community/public health nurses should consistently screen at-risk groups to identify alcohol and other drug addictions and provide appropriate referrals for treatment.

RESPONSIBILITIES OF THE COMMUNITY/PUBLIC HEALTH NURSE

Nurses with preparation in the areas of addiction are an asset in community care settings. New and exciting opportunities have emerged for participation in a variety of community settings as the treatment emphasis has shifted from acute inpatient to community-based care. Approaches focused on at-risk, underserved populations are key. For all health professionals, emphasis should be on health promotion and primary prevention, because successful interventions have the capacity to affect the behaviors of a large segment of the population. Interventions that reduce the use of illicit drugs and increase abstinence or judicious use of alcohol save lives and ultimately reduce costs to the health care system. Whether a community/public health nurse is a novice or an expert, learning to apply the rapidly developing knowledge about addictions is facilitated by reading and having adequate reference tools at hand.

IMPORTANCE OF PRIMARY PREVENTION AND HEALTH PROMOTION

Health promotion and prevention activities should be targeted at the larger percentage of the population that is currently nonaddicted. Particular emphasis should be placed on youth, because early initiation of substance use is a precursor of long-term use, dependence, and abuse (Hawkins, 2002; Hawkins et al., 1997). Delaying the age of experimentation with substances decreases the use and abuse of substances throughout life.

One longitudinal study found that the earlier people started drinking, the more likely they were to be diagnosed as alcohol abusers. About 48% of people who began drinking at age 13 were diagnosed as alcohol dependent at some point in their lives. Only 17% of persons who started drinking at age 18 and 10% of those who started drinking at age 22 had similar diagnoses (Grant & Dawson, 1998).

TOPICS IN HEALTH PROMOTION AND PREVENTION

Areas to be addressed in health promotion include abstinence or sensible drinking limits for appropriate age groups; effects of alcohol and other drugs on the body (both immediate and long term); differences in quantity of consumption for beer, wine, and hard liquor; and appropriate use of prescribed and over-the-counter medications. Sharing specific information on intake limits is helpful. For example, recommendations on consumption limits from the NIAAA (1995) are the following:

- Men, no more than two drinks per day
- Women, no more than one drink per day
- Those 65 years of age or older, no more than one drink per day
- Although it was not addressed in the guidelines, children and adolescents up to age 18 or 21 years (depending on state law) should drink no alcohol at all

Implementing health promotion to reduce or eliminate alcohol and other drug use is consistent with *Healthy People 2010* objectives. Primary prevention involves the identification and modification of risk and protective factors that apply to alcohol and other drug use. The benefits of primary prevention include improved health, reduced medical costs and loss of time from school and work, and greatly improved quality of life for individuals, family members, and the community. Five general prevention strategies are effective in addressing alcohol and other drug addictions in the community (Center for Substance Abuse Prevention, 1994a, 1994b):

- Information dissemination: providing education or information
- Promotion of personal development: developing life coping skills

- Identification of alternatives: providing alternative experiences
- Establishment of norms and standards: advocating for a healthy environment
- Community development: mobilizing the community

These strategies can be used with individuals, families, and peer groups or with the community as a whole. As a nurse develops a planned primary prevention intervention using any of the strategies, it is important to build that program around risk and protective factors. Risk factors include attitudes, beliefs, behaviors, situations, and actions that might place a person, group, organization, or community at risk for experiencing drug addiction and its effects (Box 25-1). Risk factors predict the increased probability of future addiction. Protective factors include attitudes, beliefs, behaviors, situations, and actions that protect a person, group, organization, or community from the effects of drug addiction. For example:

- Having a healthy relationship with a caring adult role model for children and adolescents or with another caring adult for adults
- Providing a person the opportunity to contribute to and be a resource for friends, family, and community
- Experiencing success or effectiveness in school, at work, and in personal relationships
- Having self-esteem and a positive outlook

Health Education and Coping Skills

Most health education programs are aimed at children and adolescents. This is consistent with the focus of *Healthy People 2010* objectives. The most effective programs include provision of accurate information on the short-term and long-term effects of substance use, coupled with resistance training or enhancement of coping skills.

Most educational programs improve knowledge about the adverse effects of substance use. Results are mixed in terms of behavior changes (Shin, 2001). Black and colleagues (1998) analyzed drug prevention programs and found that both teacher-led and peer-led programs improved knowledge. However, peer-led programs were more effective in changing behaviors, such as in reducing cigarette smoking, alcohol use, and illicit drug use, than were teacher-led efforts. Programs that incorporate social interactions, discussion, and problem solving are more effective than straight lecture programs. Evaluation of these types of combined approaches showed that they were successful in reducing alcohol and marijuana use in middle school children, at least until they reached high school (Daugherty & Leukefeld, 1998).

There is some concern that health education programs do not have long-term effects in reducing substance use and abuse. Thombs (2000) followed students from elementary, middle, and high schools who attended Drug Abuse Resistance Education (DARE) programs. He reported that program attendance in those school years did not prevent use of substances in college.

Perhaps the best approach is one that is consistent and long term, starting early and reinforced throughout childhood, adolescence, and early adulthood. Shin (2001) recommends that programs begin early in childhood. Early childhood interventions have both short-term and more lasting effects. Early interventions are more successful in reducing the long-term use of alcohol and other substances (Corvo & Persee, 1998; USDHHS, 1997). The regularity of the message seems to have a positive effect. A program in which teens heard antidrug mes-

---

| Box 25-1 | Risk Factors for Addiction |

Individual
- Early antisocial behavior
- Alienation and rebelliousness
- Favorable attitudes toward drug use
- Susceptibility to peer influence
- Friends or siblings who use tobacco, alcohol, and drugs
- Low academic achievement
- Low self-esteem
- Delinquent behavior
- Early substance use

Family
- Child abuse and neglect
- Poor parenting skills
- Lack of clear behavioral expectations
- Lack of monitoring and supervision
- Lack of caring
- Inconsistent or excessively severe discipline
- History of alcohol and other drug abuse
- Positive parental attitudes toward alcohol and other drug abuse
- Low expectations for children's success
- Family history of alcoholism and substance abuse

Community
- Economic and social deprivation
- Low neighborhood attachment
- Community norms that facilitate drug use and abuse
- Availability of alcohol and other drugs
- Lack of employment opportunities
- Extreme wealth
- Few opportunities for youth involvement in community

Adapted from Comerci, G. D. (2002). The role of the primary care physician. In Schydlower, M. (Ed.). *Substance abuse: A guide for health professionals* (pp. 21-41). Elk Grove Village, IL: American Academy of Pediatrics; and Daugherty, R. P., & Leukefeld, C. (1998). *Reducing the risk for substance abuse: A lifespan approach.* New York: Plenum Press.

---

sages on a daily basis reduced the use of drugs among study participants ("Study: Teens who hear anti-drug ads daily less likely to use drugs," 2003).

Any health education program should have a coping skills component in which students practice how to respond in various scenarios. Even when they have no intention of participating in substance abuse, children have difficulty devising responses when offered drugs (McIntosh et al., 2003). These authors recommend that young people acquire more preparation in coping behaviors so that they can more confidently respond in situations in which drugs are encountered.

Identifying At-Risk Populations for Selected Intervention

Recognizing and targeting individuals who are at high risk for substance abuse should be part of the primary prevention strategy. Children with poor academic records are at higher risk for substance abuse (Dodgan & Shea, 2000). A multifocal program aimed at poor academic achievers and high school dropouts is more effective than a single drug education effort. Such programs aim to improve school performance, enhance interpersonal skills, provide peer support, and deliver a strong message about abstinence from illicit substances and alcohol.

Adolescents who engage in cigarette smoking are more likely to use other substances. Lenz (2003) found that freshmen college students who smoked were more likely to use marijuana and alcohol than those who did not. Other studies show a similar correlation between alcohol and tobacco use. Fifty-nine percent of heavy alcohol users smoke cigarettes (SAMHSA, 2007). A program targeted at adolescents who smoke might have the added effect of reducing other substance use.

Community-Focused Prevention

Alcohol and other drug prevention programs that are part of a broader, generic effort to promote health will be more effective. In addition, the more comprehensive the program is, the more effective it will be. A model of a comprehensive primary prevention program for a community is presented in Table 25-2. The coordinated effort facilitates a coming together of all key people and places in a community setting. Community members, employers, nurses and other health professionals, and family members need to be educated. In-school education about the effects of alcohol and other drugs on driving is an outstanding example of a prevention effort that has paid off in a decreased number of teenage fatalities in motor vehicle crashes.

Community empowerment is a strategy used in community prevention efforts. Community/public health nurses skilled in advocacy and collaboration are effective in community empowerment and mobilization. To achieve community mobilization, a community must have a sense of unity, recognize a need for action, and have the energy to act to address problems or concerns. Community mobilization efforts should focus on the enhancement of protective factors that will empower community members to make healthy choices and lead healthy lives in relation to alcohol and other drugs. The role of community/public health nursing at this level of primary prevention involves helping communities identify a shared concern regarding alcohol and other drug addiction, helping them to mobilize capacity, and helping them to become ready for focused action.

The first step for nurses in mobilizing a community is to connect with the community leadership structures. These might vary depending on ethnic group. For example, in African American communities, community leaders might be pastors or council members. The preferred point of intervention among Hispanics is the family. Among Native Americans the structures are chiefly tribal, with community action usually initiated by a small group of interested and committed people. In each community, the nurse's assessment of community systems will be a challenging process (see Chapter 15).

Community mobilization often involves coalition building. Coalitions bring different segments of a community together to solve social problems. They connect individuals and groups with current information, including success stories from other communities. Coalitions focus on systemwide changes in community environments, whereas their members address specific elements of providing services to individuals. For example, in Oroville, California, the community mobilized and created a group that worked to penalize landlords who did not try to get rid of drug activities in properties they rented. This community now has a law that fines landlords $5000 if they do not work with residents on drug issues.

The federal Center for Substance Abuse Prevention has played a major role in promoting the development of community coalitions by providing communities with millions of dollars in funding to set up partnerships for developing community programs to prevent alcohol and other drug abuse. These partnerships include community and business leaders, religious leaders, health care agencies, and law enforcement officials. Community/public health nurses need to be involved in community mobilization to empower communities in preventing alcohol and other drug addictions. One way nurses can help empower communities is helping groups to find alternatives to mood-altering drugs, smoking, and alcohol. Alternatives can be found in productive relationships, including healthy family relationships; goal-directed activities; social support for oneself and others; participation in altruistic activities; and one's lifelong adventures in growing and developing as an individual.

SECONDARY PREVENTION

Early diagnosis and treatment of addictions is important. Approximately 35% of primary care patients in community

---

TABLE 25-2   Comprehensive Model of Primary Prevention of Addiction

| Methods | Target Groups | | | | |
	Individual (across the Life Span)	Family	Peers	School/Work	Community (Culture-Specific)
Education and information	Posters	Programs	Seminars	Teacher and supervisor training	Brochure distribution
Personal development	Skill-building	Parenting training	Work teams	Supportive environment	Wellness programs
Alternatives	After-school programs	Family night	Mentors	Company teams	Park facilities
Norms and standards	Alcohol, tobacco, and other drug use principles, beliefs, and behaviors	Health care coverage for treatment	Peer support programs	SAP/EAP	Money to agencies
Community mobilization	Cleanup projects	Family support	Alcohol-free events	Coalition building	Media campaign

From Allen, K. (1996). Prevention. In K. Allen (Ed.), *Nursing care of the addicted client* (p. 94). Philadelphia: Lippincott.
EAP, Employee assistance programs; *SAP*, student assistance programs.

health centers have substance abuse or mental disorders (Olfson et al., 2003). Community/public health nurses should make every effort to identify at-risk clients and provide the appropriate brief intervention. According to SAMHSA, "brief interventions are those practices that aim to investigate a potential problem and motivate an individual to do something about his substance abuse, either by natural, client-directed means or by seeking additional substance abuse treatment." This definition, along with guidelines and best practices for brief interventions, are provided in SAMHSA's Treatment Intervention Protocol (TIP) Series No. 34, *Brief Interventions and Brief Therapies for Substance Abuse,* which can be downloaded from *http://www.kap.samhsa.gov/products/manuals/tips/index.htm.*

Early detection and treatment can mitigate the problems of addiction. Once individuals with substance use–related issues are identified, community/public health nurses can act as case managers for these individuals. They can monitor and coordinate resources and services during all stages of recovery.

It is essential that community/public health nurses take on a strong teaching and counseling role. Individuals and families need to learn about the disease concept of addictions; the predictable symptoms and relapses over the course of the illness and recovery; the management of symptoms; and possible coexisting medical and psychiatric disorders. Nurses can also lessen the effects of addiction on all family members by building on the strengths of the family. Because of their knowledge of community resources for addiction treatment, community/public health nurses can counsel family members about locating appropriate treatment resources and support groups such as 12-step self-help groups. Nursing efforts can be directed toward other family members and community resources if the member with the substance use disorder is not available.

Resources for individuals with addictions and for their family members need to be available and financially accessible. Unfortunately, that is often not the case (see Chapters 21 and 33). Community/public health nurses can advocate for insurance coverage for treatment and counseling for addictions, as well as for workplace programs addressing substance abuse.

Screening and Detection

The goal of screening for alcohol and other drug abuse or addictions is to identify persons who have or are at risk for developing alcohol or drug-related problems and to engage them in further diagnosis and treatment of their problem. There are biologic tests as well as written questionnaires for use in screening. Although many laboratory tests can detect alcohol and other drugs in urine and blood, they measure recent use rather than long-term use or dependence. Laboratory tests are best used when assessing someone to confirm a diagnosis, whereas questionnaires are best used for screening.

Various questionnaires are available for screening for alcohol and other drug abuse. If a screening result is positive, the next step for the nurse is to explore the history of an individual's alcohol and/or drug use and problems. The nurse should observe for any physical, psychologic, and social signs of dependence and dysfunction. Communication with family members can provide useful information.

Screening Tools

It is recommended that screening tools be able to detect both alcohol and drug use and be specific to the given population. For example, instruments such as CAGE-AID (Box 25-2) and the Substance Abuse Subtle Screening Inventory (SASSI) (NIAAA, 1995) are good when screening for alcohol and drug use in adults. The geriatric version of the Michigan Alcoholism Screening Test (MAST-G) (Table 25-3) is appropriate for use with seniors. The Problem Oriented Screening Instrument for Teenagers (POSIT) is the tool for use with teenagers (Table 25-4). These instruments are widely used and their validity and reliability have been established; that is, they detect alcohol and drug use as intended and can be relied upon to do so repeatedly.

Assessment and Diagnosis

According to the *DSM-IV* (APA, 2000) a dependence can be diagnosed when at least three of the following symptoms have occurred within a 12-month period:

- Tolerance to or a marked need for increased amounts of a substance to achieve the desired effect
- Withdrawal symptoms
- Unsuccessful attempts to cut down or control use
- Abandonment or reduction of important social, occupational, or recreational activities due to substance use; continuation of use despite knowledge of recurrent physical or psychologic problems

It used to be argued that to diagnose dependence the presence of two cardinal signs was mandatory. These signs are (1) tolerance and (2) withdrawal symptoms, which constitute physical dependence (or tissue dependence) on the substance. Although presence of the two signs is no longer mandatory to diagnose dependence, they indicate definite dependence if they exist. Loss of control over substance use is an indicator of dependence and can be present without tolerance or withdrawal symptoms.

Box 25-2   The CAGE and CAGE-AID (CAGE Adapted to Include Drugs) Questions

1. In the last 3 months, have you felt you should cut down or stop drinking *or using drugs?*
   ☐ Yes   ☐ No
2. In the last 3 months, has anyone annoyed you or gotten on your nerves by telling you to cut down or stop drinking *or using drugs?*
   ☐ Yes   ☐ No
3. In the last 3 months, have you felt guilty or bad about how much you drink *or use?*
   ☐ Yes   ☐ No
4. In the last 3 months, have you been waking up wanting to have an alcoholic drink *or use drugs?*
   ☐ Yes   ☐ No

Each affirmative response earns one point. One point indicates a possible problem. Two points indicates a probable problem.

The original CAGE questions appear in plain type. The CAGE Adapted to Include Drugs questions are the original CAGE questions modified by the italicized text.

From Ewing, J. (1984). Detecting alcoholism: The CAGE questionnaire. *Journal of the American Medical Association, 252,* 1905-1907, with permission (original CAGE questions); and Dube, C., Goldstein, M. G., & Lewis, D. C. (1989). *Project ADEPT volume I: Core modules.* Providence, RI: Brown University, with permission.

TABLE 25-3   Michigan Alcoholism Screening Test—Geriatric Version (MAST-G)

1. After drinking have you ever noticed an increase in your heart rate or beating in your chest?	Yes	No
2. When talking with others, do you ever underestimate how much you actually drink?	Yes	No
3. Does alcohol make you sleepy so that you often fall asleep in your chair?	Yes	No
4. After a few drinks, have you sometimes not eaten or been able to skip a meal because you did not feel hungry?	Yes	No
5. Does having a few drinks help decrease your shakiness or tremors?	Yes	No
6. Does alcohol sometimes make it hard for you to remember parts of the day or night?	Yes	No
7. Do you have rules for yourself that you will not drink before a certain time of the day?	Yes	No
8. Have you lost interest in hobbies or activities you used to enjoy?	Yes	No
9. When you wake up in morning, do you ever have trouble remembering part of the night before?	Yes	No
10. Does having a drink help you sleep?	Yes	No
11. Do you hide your alcohol bottles from family members?	Yes	No
12. After a social gathering, have you ever felt embarrassed because you drank too much?	Yes	No
13. Have you ever been concerned that drinking might be harmful to your health?	Yes	No
14. Do you like to end an evening with a nightcap?	Yes	No
15. Did you find your drinking increased after someone close to you died?	Yes	No
16. In general, would you prefer to have a few drinks at home rather than go out to social events?	Yes	No
17. Are you drinking more now than in the past?	Yes	No
18. Do you usually take a drink to relax or calm your nerves?	Yes	No
19. Do you drink to take your mind off your problems?	Yes	No
20. Have you ever increased your drinking after experiencing a loss in your life?	Yes	No
21. Do you sometimes drive when you have had too much to drink?	Yes	No
22. Has a doctor or nurse ever said they were worried or concerned about your drinking?	Yes	No
23. Have you ever made rules to manage your drinking?	Yes	No
24. When you feel lonely does having a drink help?	Yes	No

From Blow F. C., Brower, K. J., Schulenberg, J. E., Demo-Danaberg, L. M., Young, J. P., & Beresford, T. P. (1992). The Michigan Alcoholism Screening Test—Geriatric Version (MAST-G): A new elderly-specific screening instrument. *Alcoholism: Clinical and Experimental Research*, 16, 372. The Regents of the University of Michigan, 1991.
Scoring: 5 or more "yes" responses is indicative of an alcohol problem. For further information, contact Frederick Blow, Ph.D., at University of Michigan Alcohol Research Center, 400 E. Eisenhower Parkway, Suite A, Ann Arbor, MI 48104; (313) 998–7952.

Mary initially began to consume alcohol to relieve anxiety and tension. She had a family history of alcohol dependence but never thought she would become an alcoholic. At first she could control her drinking, limiting it to two or three drinks on any given occasion. As time progressed, she began to be unable to predict how much alcohol she might consume during any one episode. She would say to herself, "I'll only have one or two drinks." She would end up drinking four, five, or more drinks. Sometimes she would have blackouts with memory loss. It seemed that once she started to drink, she could no longer limit her intake or stop drinking after consuming a predetermined amount.

Tolerance, or the capacity to ingest more of the substance than other persons without showing impaired function, can be discerned in very early addiction. In our country, recognition of alcohol tolerance is blocked by the cultural myth that a man should be able to "hold his liquor." The consequence is that signs of tolerance that could lead to early intervention are often overlooked and the addiction progresses. A late-developing symptom of chronic addiction is a reduced tolerance for high blood levels of alcohol or other drugs, which develops when the diseased liver can no longer process the ingested substance as efficiently.

Withdrawal symptoms occur because the body and brain have tried to create a balance with the continual use of a drug

TABLE 25-4   Sample Question from Problem-Oriented Screening Instrument for Teenagers (POSIT)

1. Do you have so much energy you do not know what to do with it?	Yes	No
2. Do you brag?	Yes	No
3. Do you get into trouble because you use drugs or alcohol at school?	Yes	No
4. Do your friends get bored at parties when there is no alcohol served?	Yes	No
5. Is it hard for you to ask for help from others?	Yes	No
6. Has there been adult supervision at the parties you have gone to recently?	Yes	No
7. Do your parents or guardians argue a lot?	Yes	No
8. Do you usually think about how your actions will affect others?	Yes	No
9. Have you recently either lost or gained more than 10 pounds?	Yes	No
10. Have you ever had sex with someone who used intravenous drugs?	Yes	No

From National Institute of Alcohol Abuse and Alcoholism. (1995). *Assessing alcohol problems: A guide for clinicians and researchers* (pp. 431-441). USDHHS Publication No. 95–3745. Bethesda, MD: National Institutes of Health.

and when the drug is no longer taken, the systems of the body become overcompensated and unbalanced. Often, withdrawal symptoms are opposite to the direct effects of the addicting drug. For example, addiction to a central nervous system stimulant, such as cocaine or nicotine, results in withdrawal symptoms characteristic of a depressant. Conversely, addiction to a central nervous system depressant, such as alcohol, results in withdrawal symptoms characteristic of a stimulant.

After screening and assessments have been completed, the community/public health nurse or other health professional should initiate some type of intervention. A review of screening tool and other test results are a first step. Where appropriate, nurses can assist individuals with nondependent problem drinking in establishing sensible drinking goals and review positive changes that occur as a result. Persons with alcohol or other drug dependence should be referred for specialized addiction treatment. For those who are not ready to modify their behavior or seek treatment, the nurse should continue assessment, consult with the family when possible, and continue a strategy of watchful waiting for cues that the individual might be ready to address his or her addiction.

Recruitment into Treatment

Recruiting individuals into treatment usually requires some leverage and is generally most effective when the power of the family system, a partner or parent, a health care professional, an employer, the school system, the social services system, or the legal system is enlisted. Direct attempts to educate the addict might seem futile in the short run. During recovery, however, clients often mention that they did hear the information but were unable to act on it by seeking treatment. The inability of addicted people to help themselves into treatment during active addiction is characteristic. Instead, what is required is the intervention of someone (or a system) for recruitment into treatment. The beliefs that an addict has to "hit bottom" before entering treatment, has to want treatment, or has to act on his or her own to get help are false beliefs. Addicts are caught up in the powerful grip of addiction. Only later, in recovery, will they develop the capacity to help themselves.

The nurse's input can help a client at a crisis point similar to that experienced by Fred by supporting an intervention or

Fred works for a national packing and shipping company. He is divorced, lives alone, and works the evening shift at the company's local facility. Most of his socializing is done after work at his neighborhood bar, where he has a cadre of friends. He drinks seven to eight cans of beer each night, sometimes with a shot of whiskey first. He does not drink before going to work. His immediate family members live out of state and are concerned about his drinking habit, but he does not see any problem.

Fred states that his drinking does not affect his workplace performance. He has received two citations for driving while under the influence (DWI). When he received the second citation, he hired a lawyer (for $2500) and was successful in having the charges dropped. Because he already had one DWI citation, a second citation would have affected his ability to drive to work. One day he just woke up and started drinking. He did not go to work or call in sick and did not answer his phone. He stayed out for 5 days with-

out notifying his supervisor. He was in danger of losing his job of 22 years. His supervisor discussed the problem with one of his co-workers. The co-worker contacted his relatives out of state. One of his siblings flew in and was successful in convincing him to seek treatment. He entered a 30-day outpatient daily substance abuse program, and his supervisor allowed him to resume work after he completed the program.

confrontation session with concerned relatives, friends, or co-workers. During a planned confrontation the interveners share critical information with the addict. This might include the observations of family members about the addictive symptoms, the personal impact each has experienced, the impact of symptoms on job performance and the worry this creates for family members, the future implications of the addiction for the health of all family members, the current needs for treatment of the addiction, the treatment that is available, and the treatment that has been planned.

In advance of the confrontation session, family members or significant others need to be encouraged to attend Al-Anon or Alateen meetings to help understand how they have been affected by the addict and how they can begin to mobilize needed social support from others who have lived through similar situations involving addiction (see Community Resources for Practice at the end of the chapter). Family members are also encouraged to investigate treatment facilities to evaluate appropriateness and bed availability. Published materials about addiction are often helpful to family members and are readily available in bookstores, libraries, and addiction treatment offices.

Family members require emotional support and comfort. They need to hear that the problem is neither their fault nor the addict's fault. They need to know that treatment and self-help are available to help them recover.

Treatment Programs

A variety of treatment programs are available for people attempting substance withdrawal. These include the following:

- Specialty hospitals geared toward inpatient treatment
- Residential rehabilitation programs
- Extended rehabilitation care for long-term stays for recovering alcoholics and drug addicts
- Outpatient care programs consisting of daily intensive care of limited duration (1 month), which might be followed by weekly or monthly care and support groups

In the past 20 years, the use of outpatient community-based care has escalated (Figure 25-5). The increase in community-based services has been influenced by insurance reimbursement decisions and the growth in managed care.

Detoxification

Detoxification treatment for withdrawal from alcohol and other drugs might be necessary for some substance-dependent individuals. Although medical detoxification is available in hospitals, most detoxification treatment is provided in community-based outpatient programs. A person experiencing withdrawal is isolated in a quiet room and calmed by nursing care that includes frequent checks of vital signs; appropriate reassurance; reality orientation to time, place, and person; and pharmacotherapy as prescribed. Only a small percentage of persons have more serious withdrawal

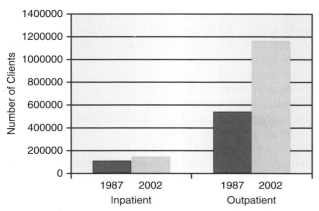

FIGURE 25-5 Census of clients in alcohol and/or drug abuse treatment by type of care, 1987 and 2002. (Data from Office of National Drug Control Policy. [2003]. *National drug control strategy update 2003.* Retrieved February 12, 2004 from *http://www.whitehousedrugpolicy.gov/publications/policy/NDCSi3/table37.htm.*)

symptoms; 1% to 3% experience seizures or delirium tremens (profound confusion, hyperactivity, and hallucinations), usually by the second or third day of withdrawal. These complications are serious, however, and require medical attention. Concurrent physical illnesses, recent and prolonged heavy alcohol intake, and previous episodes of withdrawal and/or seizure tend to produce more severe withdrawal symptoms.

Nurses and other health professionals need to focus on the goals for treatment of substance-related problems. The goals of treatment vary depending on the client: reducing alcohol and other drug use or complete abstinence from it; increasing functioning in multiple aspects of life; and preventing or reducing the frequency and severity of relapse. The following aspects of care are germane to the treatment process (SAMHSA, 1997):

- Providing education
- Establishing a therapeutic alliance
- Developing a comprehensive treatment plan
- Repeating assessments
- Monitoring progress and clinical status

TERTIARY PREVENTION

Treatment of addictions involves long periods of recovery. Tertiary prevention for alcohol and other drug addictions involves ongoing follow-up and treatment to prevent relapses and maintain recovery. Community/public health nurses should be familiar with programs for those with addictions and self-help groups for family members and significant others. Community/public health nurses can encourage continued participation in these and other community support programs and advocate for substance-free living and leisure environments. With problems of addiction, it is essential that nurses take on a strong teaching and counseling role as previously discussed. Direct nurse intervention with the addict during periods of relapse requires knowledge of relapse management, family intervention, and collaboration with members of self-help groups or referral to addiction specialists.

Twelve-Step Programs

The first recovery program was the 12-step Alcoholics Anonymous (AA) program. The AA philosophy and inspirational stories of personal recovery are found in the *Big Book*

(AA, 2001). AA is a self-help program with a spiritual base. AA provides fellowship, social support, constructive suggestions, methods that have proved effective, sponsorship of a new member by an older member, and a suggested program of hope for recovering alcoholics. Participation is strictly voluntary, and the only requirement for membership is a desire to stop drinking.

Narcotics Anonymous (NA), Gamblers Anonymous (GA), Sex and Love Addicts Anonymous (SLAA), Overeaters Anonymous (OA), and Co-dependents Anonymous (CODA) are other self-help groups that have spun off from the original 12-step AA movement. Each addresses a particular area of need.

Women for Sobriety

Women for Sobriety is a self-help group targeted specifically at women substance abusers. It does not follow the AA philosophy. The program emphasizes abstinence. The main goal is to reduce the isolation and loneliness of substance-abusing women and support their progress toward abstinence and stability.

Self-Help Groups and Programs for Spouses and Co-Dependents

Other 12-step programs modeled on AA include Al-Anon, Alateen, and Alatot. Family members of addicted individuals can educate themselves about addiction and increase their social supports. Variations of Al-Anon groups exist for other addictions, such as Gam-Anon for relatives and friends of individuals addicted to gambling.

Groups of Adult Children of Alcoholics (ACOA) are a newer development in the substance abuse field. Their growth was stimulated by the written accounts of a few pioneer authors who described the experiences of growing up in an addicted family and who suggested steps toward recovery (Wegscheider, 1981; Woititz, 1983). The ACOA groups are affiliated with Al-Anon and follow the AA model.

Family members can benefit greatly from regularly attending self-help group meetings, both as an aid to their own recovery and as a way to mobilize social support. Perhaps most importantly, they come to realize that the family, too, has developed problems living with the addiction. New members are often encouraged to seek out a sponsor, someone further along in the group process. The sponsor can be of immense assistance to a family member coping with an addicted loved one.

The co-dependence movement and CODA have created yet another type of 12-step self-help group for partners. Whereas Al-Anon groups encourage self-focus, these groups are likely to focus on relationships with others by incorporating the new language of the co-dependence movement. These include learning to establish personal boundaries in relationships, meeting one's own wants and needs in a relationship, and being able to sensitively express feelings and thoughts to one's partner. It is interesting to note that people with a history of substance dependence who are well along in their recovery often attend CODA meetings. Removal of the addiction problem helps co-dependent relationship problems to surface.

It is important for nurses who care for substance-dependent clients to become familiar with the support programs available in their communities. It is helpful for them to attend meetings to become more familiar with these resources and the services they provide.

Maintenance of Recovery

Maintaining recovery is a difficult feat. Relapse is common. More than 60% of alcoholics drink within the first 90 days after completing a treatment program (Trigoboff & Wilson, 2004). Only 1 or 2 out of 10 alcoholics remain abstinent for 1 year after treatment. Pettinati and colleagues (1982) documented that when alcoholics consistently attend AA meetings, they exhibit lower rates of relapse, a higher level of occupational and interpersonal performance, and a lower incidence of complicating psychiatric diagnoses. Positive social support, residence in a family setting, adequate socioeconomic resources, and absence of a family history of alcoholism and drug abuse have also been associated with better chances of recovery from all addictions.

Individuals with mental disorders have a more complicated recovery and are at higher risk for relapse. Today, most researchers believe that earlier and more adequate assessment of comorbid mental disorders in conjunction with appropriate treatment could decrease the incidence of relapse in these groups.

AA groups teach that relapse is the rule with addictions and that more severe alcohol dependence tends to be a key factor. By the time they enter treatment, most addicted people have experienced many unsuccessful attempts at **abstinence** from the addictive substance or process. Such episodes could be expected to continue and are, in fact, rather typical of early sobriety. Those who are newly sober should be taught that relapse is common in early recovery; they should be encouraged to quickly resume attendance at their support program after relapse occurs and to discuss the relapse with fellow members. Their social support is instrumental in avoiding further and sustained relapses. Perhaps the hardest thing for recovering addicts to understand is the need to change their social network, if that network facilitates or encourages substance use.

Severe difficulties occur in relapse prevention of drug abuse problems, particularly abuse of crack cocaine and heroin. Cravings for these drugs can be evoked when the addict is in the same environment in which the drug was abused, when talking with friends who participated in drug taking, and even when in contact with clothing worn during a period of use. Changing one's circle of friends, avoiding environments that pose dangerous temptations, and making other changes to decrease the stimulatory effect of these factors are essential to avoid further drug use. New prescription drugs to control drug craving, a major problem during recovery, are now available.

Pharmacotherapy for Substance Use Disorders

Medication-assisted treatment (MAT) is a form of pharmacotherapy and refers to any treatment for a substance use disorder that includes a pharmacologic intervention as part of a comprehensive substance abuse treatment plan. The ultimate goal of the plan is patient recovery with full social function. In the United States, MAT using Food and Drug Administration–approved drugs such as disulfiram, naltrexone, and acamprosate has been demonstrated to be effective in the treatment of alcohol dependence, and opioid dependence has been treated effectively with methadone, naltrexone, and buprenorphine (Connock, et al., 2007; Fornili & Burda-Cohee, 2006).

As part of a comprehensive treatment program, MAT has been shown to:
- Improve survival
- Increase retention in treatment
- Decrease illicit opiate use
- Decrease hepatitis and HIV seroconversion
- Decrease criminal activities
- Increase employment
- Improve birth outcomes for those with perinatal addiction

More information about MAT is available at *http://csat.samhsa.gov/publications/MedicalCommunity.aspx.*

COMMUNITY AND PROFESSIONAL RESOURCES

Community nurses have numerous community, professional, and federal resources available to assist them in addressing the problem of abuse of alcohol and other drugs with their clients. To be effective, community/public health nurses must familiarize themselves with evidence-based prevention interventions, brief interventions, effective pharmacotherapies, and the different treatment and self-help groups that are available in the communities in which their clients live and work.

It is also important to know that in some communities, none of these support groups might exist. The nurse can advocate and work to get these groups established by contacting the national headquarters of the self-help organizations. Advocacy is a major role of community/public health nursing, and this is an example of when it would be needed.

Many communities have AA but not NA or Cocaine Anonymous groups. Because many people attending AA meetings have negative feelings about persons addicted to heroin or cocaine, sending people with drug addictions to AA meetings would be a mistake. An important nursing intervention is being knowledgeable about the self-help resources in clients' communities and advocating for establishing them there if they do not exist. See Community Resources for Practice at the end of the chapter for a list of many resources for addressing substance abuse.

Many professional resources are available to nurses, including the International Nurses Society on Addictions, a professional organization of nurses who work with addicted clients in various settings. This organization provides publications and newsletters, sponsors annual conferences, and offers certification to nurses who have the responsibility of caring for addicted clients and their families and significant others.

The federal government provides free publications as well as low-cost subscriptions for materials that summarize research findings and provide guidance for developing alcohol and drug treatment and prevention programs, including the following:
- *NIDA Notes* provides drug research information and *Alcohol Alert* covers current alcohol research.
- SAMHSA's Center for Substance Abuse Treatment publishes Treatment Improvement Protocols (TIPs) for use with addicted clients and their families.
- *Prevention Pipeline* is a publication that provides information on ways to prevent alcohol and other drug addiction.

- The Center for Substance Abuse Prevention also has free publications, kits, and computer programs that can assist in providing culturally relevant prevention for communities.

FUNDING ISSUES AND ACCESS TO CARE

The Uniform Alcoholism Treatment and Prevention Act of 1974 brought treatment under the aegis of health care. A system of care eventually developed that consisted largely of 28-day inpatient programs. Very few were part of the traditional health care system, because health care practitioners had little training in treatment of addictions. Substance use disorder treatment programs have been funded primarily through federal block grants to the states, state and local taxes, and health insurance programs. Inpatient treatment centers, including those in the U.S. Department of Veterans Affairs (VA) system, have decreased drastically in size and number. Most VA treatment is now concentrated in outpatient services. Hospitals that had detoxification units have discontinued those specialty units. The burden of addiction treatment has fallen back on the more conventional outpatient system of self-help groups, jails, social service agencies, and homeless shelters and some specialty programs. A very high proportion of admissions to general hospitals are persons with substance abuse problems, although hospital personnel are not adequately trained to manage these problems.

Managed care in alcohol and other drug addiction treatment programs began in the mid-1980s. Managed care was originally designed to coordinate and mobilize health care resources to meet the needs of clients, but its effects on the addiction treatment field have been chaotic. The proliferation of managed care companies and their cost-cutting approaches have introduced as much change into treatment for addictions as they have into other sectors of the health care system (D'Ambrosio et al., 2003; Galanter et al., 2000). Providers see it as primarily a cost-saving effort that limits access and results in poor clinical decisions made by nonproviders. Many believe that the preexisting well-developed treatment system was profoundly compromised by managed care.

Multiple studies support the premise that managed care cut the costs of substance abuse treatment. Ettner, Argeriou, McCarty, and colleagues (2003) compared publicly funded programs in Iowa and found that managed care moved patients from inpatient to less costly community-based programs. McCarty and colleagues (2003) reviewed programs in four states: Arizona, Iowa, Maryland, and Nebraska. They found similar moves to community-based programs and substantial cost savings.

A major concern with managed care substance abuse programs is whether cost savings translated to poorer quality of services. An early study by the George Washington University Medical Center for Health Policy Research (1996) analyzed contracts between managed care organizations and substance abuse treatment and prevention centers on behalf of the Office of Managed Care. That study found the following with regard to managed care plans:

- The plans purchased a limited range of services, disallowing comprehensive care.
- Contracts limited providers' decision making regarding the amount or level of care required, the type of professional

most appropriate to carry out treatment, and the setting in which the services were provided.
- Communication between providers of mental health care and addiction treatment and the client's primary care providers was limited.
- Reimbursement rates were exceedingly low.

Newer studies have identified similar concerns. Rosenthal (2003) suggests that the time constraints placed on providers limit their ability to identify depression in primary care clients. Knudsen and colleagues (2003) point out that staff retention in programs is a problem because the health professionals feel that they are constrained in their decisions about treatment options. Cost-sharing fees (co-pays and coinsurance) are higher than for general medical care, which limits access for low-income individuals (Hodgkin et al., 2003).

The most important question is whether changes have impacted the long-term health and welfare of clients. In other words, do these changes provide less support and poorer outcomes in terms of the client's ability to manage his or her substance abuse problem? Alexander and colleagues (2003) reported that managed care has limited access to services and shortened treatment, jeopardizing the client's ability to succeed in treatment. Ettner, Denmead, Dilonardo, and colleagues (2003) compared services in Medicaid managed care and private programs and found that they provided equivalent services. Because almost all substance treatment programs are now under the managed care umbrella, this comparison does not address the issue of whether alternatives to managed care could produce different results.

There is a need for additional research in the area of service quality. Hutchinson and Foster (2003) point out that children's services under these programs have not been evaluated for health outcomes or quality. Levy and colleagues (2002) note that most of the evaluations performed by managed care providers look at patient satisfaction with services, not clinical outcomes. There is also a concern that the shift from inpatient to outpatient services has limited programs, because there are fewer treatment slots for patients than under the previous system (Galanter et al., 2000).

Access to treatment for addiction remains a critical problem in our health care system. Without access to effective alcohol and drug treatment, many individuals with substance use disorders engage in or exhibit behaviors that bring them into an ongoing relationship with the criminal justice system. If they are lucky enough to be diverted to a DWI court or a drug court, they will be referred and have access to treatment. The court system has now become the gateway to treatment for many individuals. However, thousands of individuals may be sent to jail or prison, or released without any assessment or referral to treatment. These individuals will continue the downward spiral associated with addiction. With the decrease in funding for prevention and treatment, it is essential that community/public health nurses know how to identify appropriate, evidence-based strategies for prevention and treatment of substance use disorders. Nurses must also facilitate referrals to resources in the community. Community/public health nurses must continue to work with other community members and leaders to ensure access to care for prevention and treatment of substance abuse dependence and addictions for all citizens.

KEY IDEAS

1. Substance abuse is a pattern of repeated, maladaptive, inappropriate use of alcohol and/or other drugs that negatively affects health. Alcohol and drug abuse and dependence are significant problems in the United States.

2. Men, the poor, and the homeless have higher prevalence rates of substance abuse and addiction than the overall population.

3. The type of substance use, abuse, and dependence varies by age group, racial/ethnic group, and geographic region.

4. Substance abuse affects all family members, not just the abuser or addict. The patterns of relationships between those addicted to substances and their loved ones are often unhealthy.

5. Community/public health nurses can help prevent FAS and related disorders.

6. Community/public health nurses are front-line health professionals who can assist those with addictions and their families. Community/public health nurses are important case finders, because they are often the first to see patterns of addiction.

7. Community/public health nurses need to recognize early signs of addiction to teach family members about addiction, teach new behaviors to family members, refer family members to treatment and self-help recovery groups, and encourage family members to confront the addict so the addict will seek care.

8. Family members of the addict often are ready to seek help before the addict is.

9. In the *Healthy People 2010* objectives, primary prevention activities are targeted toward adolescents and young adults. Interventions include school prevention programs, environmental changes (such as reduced advertising of and access to alcohol), and reductions in legal blood alcohol concentrations for motor vehicle drivers.

10. Recovery from substance addiction occurs over years and usually involves some relapses. A strong support system, including 12-step programs and self-help groups for family members, is important.

11. Access to treatment for addiction remains a critical problem in our health care system.

LEARNING BY EXPERIENCE AND REFLECTION

1. Read a daily newspaper and make note of the news reports on motor vehicle accidents, episodes of domestic quarrels or public violence, and legal problems that involve alcohol or other drugs. What major changes in society would have to occur to decrease or eliminate such incidents?

2. Have a dialogue with a friend or relative and encourage the person to share with you his or her life experiences with alcohol or other drugs. Empathize, without judgment, with positive and negative feelings as this information is shared with you. In what way do these experiences influence the kinds of choices the person makes today and his or her beliefs about the use of alcohol or other drugs?

3. Attend an open meeting of AA or NA after telephoning the local office to locate a meeting convenient for you. Note members' positive and negative feelings as they share their stories of substance abuse and recovery. Note how their experiences influence what kinds of choices they make today, what they believe about the use of alcohol and drugs, and how they value life today. How has this experience changed your previous perceptions, beliefs, and values concerning addictions?

4. Reflect in writing on your personal experiences with alcohol and other drugs. When you first used these substances, what were your initial physiologic reactions? What were your feelings and thoughts about the experience? If you abstained from using substances, reflect on that experience. Reflect on changes in the pattern of your personal experiences with alcohol and other drugs over the years. Have your subjective, physiologic, cognitive, and emotional perceptions changed from those on your very first experience? Would you like to change any patterns in the future?

5. Look at your collection of family photographs. Recall and record experiences with alcohol and other drugs that you either observed or heard about for various relatives. Compare your experiences with theirs and note similarities and differences. Share your thoughts and feelings with an understanding family member, friend, or significant other.

6. Think about your personal knowledge of and experience with colleagues who abuse alcohol or other drugs. Contact the State Board of Nursing to identify policies and procedures related to impaired professionals. Reflect on the information you obtain. Is there anything you would like to change based on your experiences and observations? Share your thoughts and feelings with a nurse colleague.

7. Record your understanding of symptoms of co-dependence before attending a meeting of CODA. After the meeting, give some thought to the belief of some that many nurses exhibit co-dependent behaviors. Compare your experiences with the experiences of those attending the CODA meeting. Do any similarities or differences exist? Share your thoughts with a trusted nurse colleague.

Dan is a successful 45-year-old salesman who owns his own business. He lives with his wife and his 18-year-old son. His problems with alcoholism have been developing insidiously since he began to drink at the age of 21 years. Heavy drinking ensued a few years later. Although his family members complain about his drinking, he denies he has a problem with alcohol. Dan has experienced some impairment of his ability to perceive distance from objects; a few days ago, his car collided with another car while he was driving, and Dan was arrested for driving under the influence. He has also had episodes of memory loss associated with drinking more heavily than usual. His beverage preference is beer, and he can easily consume two six-packs of beer in an average evening of drinking.

Dan's wife, Jan, has tried everything to get Dan to quit drinking and is embittered over his lack of cooperation, absences from home to drink, deteriorting work performance, failure to help around the house, and constant conflicts with their teenage son. Jan presents as a martyr who over functions and tries her best to selflessly care for her family but obviously neglects her own needs. She appears sad and dejected.

The community health nurse became involved in this family through a physician referral that was associated with Dan's discharge from the local hospital; he had a second serious episode of gastric bleeding secondary to long-standing gastrointestinal problems and heavy alcohol intake.

ASSESSMENT

- Assess the extent to which Dan uses alcohol and other drugs.
- Complete a biopsychosocial assessment of Dan and his family. Assess the adequacy of self-care activities.

- Assess Dan and his family members for signs and symptoms of emotional problems and addictive patterns.
- Complete a family genogram of at least three generations and identity dysfunctional patterns.
- Assess the extent of the family's resources and social support to sustain Dan and the family through an acute episode of Dan's illness.
- Assess the community resources available to Dan and the family.

NURSING DIAGNOSES

- Ineffective denial related to family history of alcoholism as manifested by repetitive refusal to admit that alcohol abuse is a problem.
- Dysfunctional family processes: alcoholism related to abuse of alcohol as evidenced by loss of control of drinking, broken promises, inability to meet emotional needs of family members and subsequent deterioration in family relationship, disruption of family roles.
- Situational low self-esteem (of wife) related to unsatisfactory spousal relationship as evidenced by declined ability to care for his or her own needs.

Following discharge from the hospital, Dan is admitted to a detoxification center, then referred to the community health clinic for further care.

Nursing Diagnosis	Nursing Goals	Nursing Interventions	Outcomes and Evaluation
Ineffective denial related to family history of alcoholism as manifested by repetitive refusal to admit that alcohol abuse is a problem.	Dan will acknowledge and accept that he abuses alcohol.	Dan will perform week long alcohol intake recall.	Dan recalls that prior to his hospitalization for gastric bleeding he consumed approximately 12 beers or more per day. On two days he also consumed 3 to 4 liquor drinks in addition to beer. "That was on Friday and Saturday though, and it's not like I'm shooting heroin or some illegal drug like that." Dan denies using other illegal drugs, but states, "I do smoke pot from time to time."
		Dan will also recall long-term alcohol recall of the last 24 years and evaluate drinking patterns.	With the nurse, Dan relates, "I didn't use to drink as much, but what's the difference? It doesn't affect me as much." Dan also reports, "the men in my family always drink. It's really not a big deal." Historically, Dan states he began drinking only on the weekends, but in his late twenties he started to drink occasionally during the week, and currently "drinks several beers a day." Dan does not associate drinking with any emotional or life changes, "I just like beer."
		Dan will list recent physical changes that are a result of long-term excessive alcohol consumption.	"The doctors tell me my stomach episode was because I drank too much, but I don't know." He attributes visual changes and memory loss to "getting older mostly." Also, he denies his recent car accident was the result of intoxication. "Well sure I got a DUI because those breathalyzers don't account for tolerance. Besides, I really do need new glasses."

Nursing Diagnosis	Nursing Goals	Nursing Interventions	Outcomes and Evaluation
	Dan will enroll in addictions counseling and adhere to agreed upon actions and goals created through counseling.	Dan will enroll in addictions counseling as mandated by the DUI court settlement.	Dan is forced to enroll in addictions counseling by the courts. His attendance at Alcoholic Anonymous meetings have been scarce at best. Dan's lawyer intervenes and insists he enroll in private addictions counseling. Dan's DUI settlement cites addictions counseling as a requirement, otherwise he may face a jail sentence. Dan has successfully attended addiction counseling for one month and states, "only two more months to go!"
		Together with an addictions counselor, Dan will create three goals for himself related to keeping sober.	Dan's three goals are, "I won't drink a lot, I won't drink a lot, and I won't drink a lot. What a bunch of baloney." While counseling attendance has improved, his reluctance to actively participate exemplifies further Dan's inability to admit to alcohol dependence.
	Dan will acknowledge the impact his alcoholism has had on his family members and their relationship.	Both Dan's wife and son have created a list that details missed family events, disappointment and/or embarrassment they have felt, and husband/father role disruption as a direct result of Dan's alcohol consumption. They will read the list to Dan.	After listening to the lists read by both his son and wife, Dan says, "I didn't know you felt this way." He apologizes and states he will try to "do better by you." However, his wife Jan reports that Dan has said this before, that both her son and herself have told him many of these same examples before, and "nothing ever changes."
		Dan will acknowledge past and present statements his family members have made about how his alcohol consumption has affected them.	After this confrontation, Dan said some things seemed familiar to him. He also stated he "felt pressured," by this "united front." "How can I work to make this better when you have already made up your minds and are conspiring against me?"

 Find additional **Care Plans** for this client on the book's website.

COMMUNITY RESOURCES FOR PRACTICE

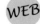 Information about each of the following organizations is found on its website, which can be accessed through the **WebLinks** section of this book's website at *http://evolve.elsevier.com/Maurer/community/*.

Alcoholics Anonymous

American Council for Drug Education

American Society of Addiction Medicine

Association for Medical Education and Research in Substance Abuse (AMERSA) (provides educational materials, including lectures slides, seminars and conference presentations, syllabi, curricula, workshop handouts, screening tools, case studies, and much more)

Fetal Alcohol Syndrome Diagnostic and Prevention Network, University of Washington, Seattle

International Nurses Society on Addictions

National Center on Addiction and Substance Abuse at Columbia University

National Center on Birth Defects and Developmental Disabilities, Centers for Disease Control and Prevention (CDC) (information on fetal alcohol syndrome)

National Clearinghouse for Alcohol and Drug Information

National Council on Alcoholism and Drug Dependence

National Inhalant Prevention Coalition

National Institute on Alcohol Abuse and Alcoholism

National Institute on Drug Abuse

Partnership for a Drug-Free America

Substance Abuse and Mental Health Services Administration (SAMHSA) (information on fetal alcohol syndrome, treatment improvement protocols, and best-practice guidelines for the treatment of substance use disorders)

U.S. Drug Enforcement Administration

STUDY AIDS   http://evolve.elsevier.com/Maurer/community/

Visit the Evolve website for this book to find the following study and assessment materials:

- Quiz
- Web Scenario
- Critical Thinking Questions and Answers for Case Studies
- Care Plans
- *Healthy People* Updates
- Glossary

REFERENCES

Alcoholics Anonymous. (2001). *The big book* (4th ed.). New York: Author.

Allen, K. (1996). *Nursing care of the addicted client.* Philadelphia: Lippincott.

Alexander, J. A., Nahra, T. A., & Wheeler, J. R. (2003). Managed care and access to substance abuse treatment services. *Journal of Behavioral Health Services and Research, 30*(2), 161-175.

American Psychiatric Association. (2000). *Diagnostic and statistical manual of mental disorders, text revision* (4th ed.). Washington, DC: Author.

Bauer, B. B., & Hill, S. S. (2000). *Mental health nursing: An introductory text.* Philadelphia: Saunders.

Beckstead, J. W. (2002). Modeling attitudinal antecedents of nurses' decisions to report impaired colleagues. *Western Journal of Nursing Research, 24*(5), 537-551.

Black, D. R., Tobler, N. S., & Sciacca, J. P. (1998). Peer helping/involvement: An efficacious way to meet the challenge of reducing alcohol, tobacco, and other drug use among youth? *Journal of School Health, 68*(3), 87-93.

Blow, F. C., Brower, K. J., Schulenberg, J. E., et al. (1992). The Michigan Alcoholism Screening Test—Geriatric Version (MAST-G): A new elderly-specific screening instrument. *Alcoholism: Clinical and Experimental Research, 16*, 372. The Regents of the University of Michigan, 1991.

Centers for Disease Control and Prevention. (2002). Alcohol consumption among women who are pregnant or might become pregnant—United States, 2002. *Morbidity and Mortality Weekly Report, 53*(50), 1178-1181.

Center for Substance Abuse Prevention. (1994a). *Invest in prevention: Prevention works in health care delivery systems [Presession materials].* Rockville, MD: U.S. Department of Health and Human Services, Substance Abuse and Mental Health Services Administration.

Center for Substance Abuse Prevention. (1994b). *Nurse training course: Prevention of alcohol, tobacco and other drug problems.* Rockville, MD: U.S. Department of Health and Human Services, Substance Abuse and Mental Health Services Administration.

Chasnoff, I. J. (2001). Perinatal exposure to maternal substances of abuse: Effects in the developing child. In Schydlower, M. (Ed.), *Substance abuse: A guide for health professionals* (pp. 293-306). Elk Grove Village, IL: American Academy of Pediatrics.

Collins, R. L., Gollnisch, G., & Morsheimer, E. T. (1999). Substance use among a regional sample of female nurses. *Drug and Alcohol Dependence, 55*(1/2), 145-155.

Comerci, G. D. (2002). The role of the primary care physician. In Schydlower, M. (Ed.). *Substance abuse: A guide for health professionals* (pp. 21-41).

Elk Grove Village, IL: American Academy of Pediatrics.

Connock, M., Juarez-Garcia, A., Jowett, S., et al. (2007). Methadone and buprenorphine for the management of opioid dependence: A systematic review and economic evaluation. *Health Technology Assessment, 11*(9), 1-171, iii-iv.

Corvo, K., & Persee, L. (1998). An evaluation of a pre-school based prevention program: Effects on children's alcohol related expectancies. *Journal of Alcohol and Drug Education, 43*(2), 36-47.

D'Ambrosio, R., Mondeaus, F., Gabriel, R. M., et al. (2003). Oregon's transition to a managed care model for Medicaid-funded substance abuse treatment: Streamrolling the glass menagerie. *Health and Social Work, 28*(2), 126-136.

Daugherty, R. P., & Leukefeld, C. (1998). *Reducing the risk of substance abuse: A lifespan approach.* New York: Plenum Press.

Dodgan, C. E., & Shea, W. M. (2000). *Substance abuse disorders: Access and treatment.* San Diego: Academic Press.

Dube, C., Goldstein, M. G., & Lewis, D. C. (1989). *Project ADEPT volume I: Core modules.* Providence, RI: Brown University.

Ettner, S. L., Argeriou, M., McCarty, D., et al. (2003). How did the introduction of managed care for the uninsured in Iowa affect the use of substance abuse services? *Journal of Behavioral Health Services and Research, 30*(1), 26-40.

Ettner, S. L., Denmead, G., Dilonardo, J., et al. (2003). The impact of managed care on the substance abuse treatment patterns and outcomes of Medicaid beneficiaries: Maryland HealthChoice program. *Journal of Behavioral Health Services and Research, 30*(10), 41-63.

Ewing, J. (1984). Detecting alcoholism: The CAGE questionnaire. *Journal of the American Medical Association, 252*, 1905-1907.

Fontaine, K. L. (2003). *Fontaine and Fletcher: Mental health nursing* (5th ed.). Upper Saddle River, NJ: Prentice Hall.

Fornili, K., & Burda-Cohee, C. (2006). Buprenorphine products for the pharmacologic management of opioid addiction: Why shouldn't advanced practice nurses prescribe? *Journal of Addictions Nursing, 17*, 139-145.

Frisch, N. C., & Frisch, L. E. (2002). *Psychiatric mental health nursing* (2nd ed.). Albany, NY: Delmar.

Galanter, M., Keller, D. S., Dermatis, H., et al. (2000). The impact of managed care on substance abuse treatment: A report of the American Society of Addiction Medicine. *Journal of Addictive Diseases, 19*(3), 13-34.

George Washington University Medical Center for Health Policy Research. (1996, June). *Principal findings from an analysis of contracts between managed care organizations and community mental health and substance abuse treatment and prevention centers.* Washington, DC: Author.

Grant, B. F., & Dawson, D. A. (1998). Age at onset of alcohol use and its association with DSM-IV alcohol abuse and dependence: Results from the National Longitudinal Epidemiologic Survey. *Journal of Substance Abuse, 10*(2), 163-173.

Griffith, J. (1999). Substance abuse disorders in nurses. *Nursing Forum, 34*(4), 19-28.

Guardia, J., Catafau, A. M., Battle, F., et al. (2000). Striatal dopaminergic D_2 receptor density measured by [^{123}I] iodobenzamide SPECT in the prediction of treatment outcomes of alcohol dependent patients. *American Journal of Psychiatry, 157*(1), 127-129.

Haack, M. R. (Ed.). (1997). *Drug-dependent mothers and their children: Issues in public policy and public health.* New York: Springer.

Haack, M., & Harford, T. (1984). Drinking patterns among student nurses. *International Journal of the Addictions, 19*, 577-583.

Haack, M. R., & Yocom, C. (2002). State policies and nurses with substance use disorders. *Journal of Nursing Scholarship, 34*(1), 89-94.

Hawkins, J. D. (2002). Risk and protective factors and their implication for the health care professions. In Schydlower, M. (Ed.), *Substance abuse: A guide for the health professional* (pp. 1-19). Elk Grove Village, IL: American Academy of Pediatrics.

Hawkins, J. D., Graham, J. W., Maguin, E., et al. (1997). Exploring the effects of age of alcohol use initiation and psychosocial risk factors on subsequent alcohol misuse. *Journal of Studies of Alcohol, 58*(3), 280-290.

Hockenberry, M. J., Wilson, D., Winkelstein, M. L., et al. (2003). *Wong's nursing care of infants and children* (7th ed.). St. Louis: Mosby.

Hodgkin, D., Horgan, C. M., Garnick, D. W., et al. (2003). Cost sharing for substance abuse and mental health services in managed care plans. *Medical Care Research and Review, 60*(1), 101-116.

Hutchinson, A. B., & Foster, E. M. (2003). The effect of Medicaid managed care on mental health care for children: A review of the literature. *Mental Health Services Research, 5*(1), 39-54.

Knudsen, H. K., Johnson, J. A., & Roman, P. M. (2003). Retaining counseling staff at substance abuse treatment centers: Effects of management practices. *Journal of Substance Abuse Treatment, 24*(2), 129-135.

Lenz, B. K. (2003). Correlates of young adult tobacco use: Application of a transition framework. *Journal of School Nursing, 19*(4), 232-237.

Leshner, A. L. (2000). Addressing the medical consequences of drug abuse. *NIDA Notes, 15*(1), 1-2.

Levy, M. E., Garnick, D. W., Horgan, C. M., et al. (2002). Quality measurement and accountability for substance abuse and mental health services in managed care organizations. *Medical Care, 40*(12), 1238-1248.

Lupton, C., Burd, L., & Harwood, R. (2004). Cost of fetal alcohol spectrum disorders. *American Journal of Medical Genetics, Part C: Seminars in Medical Genetics, 127C*(1), 42-50.

May, P. A, & Gossage, J. P. (2001). Estimating the prevalence of fetal alcohol syndrome: A summary. *Alcohol Research and Health, 25,* 159-167.

McCarty, D., Dilonardo, J., & Argeriou, M. (2003). State substance abuse and mental health managed care evaluation program. *Journal of Behavioral Health Services and Research, 30*(1), 7-17.

McIntosh, J., MacDonald, F., & McKeganey, N. (2003). Dealing with the offer of drugs: The experience of a sample of pre-teenage schoolchildren. *Addictions, 98*(7), 977-986.

Minino, A. M., Heron, M. P., Murphy, S. L., et al. (2007). Deaths: Final data for 2004. *National Vital Statistics Reports, 55*(19). Hyattsville, MD: National Center for Health Statistics.

Mosher, J. (1996). A public health approach to alcohol and other drug problems: Theory and practice. In F. D. Scutchfield & C. W. Keck (Eds.), *Principles of public health practice.* Albany, NY: Delmar Publishers.

Myers, J. K., Weissman, M. M., Tischler, G. L., et al. (1984). Six-month prevalence of psychiatric disorders in three communities: 1980 to 1982. *Archives of General Psychiatry, 41,* 959-967.

National Institute on Alcohol Abuse and Alcoholism. (1995). *Assessing alcohol problems: A guide for clinicians and researchers (USDHHS Publication No. 95–3745).* Bethesda, MD: National Institutes of Health.

National Institute on Drug Abuse. (1990). *National Drug and Alcoholism Treatment Unit Survey (NDATUS) 1990: Main findings report.* Rockville, MD: National Clearinghouse for Alcohol and Drug Information.

National Institute on Drug Abuse. (1994, September/October). NIDA reflects on 20 years of neuroscience research. *NIDA Notes,* special section. Rockville, MD: Author.

National Institute on Drug Abuse. (1999). Infectious diseases and drug abuse. *NIDA Notes, 14*(2), 1-2.

National Institute on Drug Abuse. (2007). *Medical consequences of drug abuse.* Retrieved November 18, 2007 from http://www.nida.nih.gov/consequences.

Office of National Drug Control Policy. (2003). *National drug control strategy update 2003.* Retrieved February 12, 2004 from http://www.whitehousedrugpolicy.gov/publications/policy/NDCSi3/table37.htm.

Office of National Drug Control Policy. (2004). *The economic costs of drug abuse in the United States: 1992–2002.* Washington, DC: Executive Office of the President, Office of National Drug Control Policy.

Olfson, M., Tobin, J. N., Cassells, A., et al. (2003). Improving the detection of drug abuse, alcohol abuse, and depression in community health centers. *Journal of Health Care for the Poor and Underserved, 14*(3), 386-402.

Pettinati, H., Sugarman, A. A., & Maurer, H. (1982). Four year MMPI changes in abstinent and drinking alcoholics. *Alcoholism: Clinical and Experimental Research, 6*(4), 487-494.

Phoenix, B. J., & Pelish, K. (2004). Co-existing psychiatric and substance use diagnoses. In C. R. Kneisl, H. S. Wilson, & E. Trigoboff (Eds.), *Contemporary psychiatric-mental health nursing* (pp. 506-523). Upper Saddle River, NJ: Prentice Hall.

Prescott, C. A., Aggen, S. H., & Kendler, K. S. (1999). Sex differences in the sources of genetic liability to alcohol abuse and dependence in a population-based sample of U.S. twins. *Alcoholism: Clinical and Experimental Research, 23*(7), 1136-1144.

Robins, L. N., Helzer, J. E., Weissman, M. M., et al. (1984). Lifetime prevalence of specific psychiatric disorders in three sites. *Archives of General Psychiatry, 41,* 949-958.

Rosenthal, M. H. (2003). Barriers to diagnosis, advances in therapy. *Journal of the American Osteopathic Association, 103*(8 Supplement 4), S2-S9.

Ross, H. E., Glaser, F. B., & Germanson, T. (1988). The prevalence of psychiatric disorders in patients with alcohol and other drug problems. *Archives of General Psychiatry, 45,* 1023-1031.

Secretary of Health and Human Services. (1990). *Alcohol and health: Seventh special report to the U.S. Congress from the Secretary of Health and Human Services (USDHHS Publication No. [ADM] 91–1656).* Washington, DC: U.S. Government Printing Office.

Shin, H. S. (2001). A review of school-based drug prevention program evaluations in the 1990s. *American Journal of Health Education, 32*(3), 139-147.

Stratton, K., Howe, C., & Battaglia, F. C. (1996). *Fetal alcohol syndrome: Diagnosis and epidemiology, prevention and treatment.* Washington, DC: Institute of Medicine and National Academy Press.

Study: Teens who hear anti-drug ads daily less likely to use drugs. (2003). *Alcoholism and Drug Abuse Weekly, 15*(25), 4.

Substance Abuse and Mental Health Services Administration. (2006). *Results from the 2005 National Survey on Drug Use and Health: National findings.* Rockville, MD: National Clearinghouse for Alcohol and Drug Information.

Substance Abuse and Mental Health Services Administration. (2007). *Results from the 2006 National Survey on Drug Use and Health: National findings.* Rockville, MD: National Clearinghouse for Alcohol and Drug Information.

Substance Abuse and Mental Health Services Administration, Center for Substance Abuse Treatment. (1997). *Treatment Improvement Protocol No. 24: A guide to substance abuse services for primary care clinicians (USDHHS Publication No. [SMA] 97–3139).* Rockville, MD: Author.

Substance Abuse and Mental Health Services Administration, Center for Substance Abuse Treatment. (1994). *Treatment of alcohol and other drug abuse: Opportunities for coordination (USDHHS Publication No. [SMA] 94–2075).* Rockville, MD: Author.

Sullivan, E. (1987a). A descriptive study of nurses recovering from chemical dependency. *Archives of Psychiatric Nursing, 1,* 194-200.

Sullivan, E. (1987b). Comparison of chemically dependent and nondependent nurses on familial, personal and professional characteristics. *Journal of Studies on Alcohol, 48,* 563-568.

Thombs, D. L. (2000). DARE programs. *Journal of Alcohol and Drug Education, 46*(1), 27-40.

Tobacco, alcohol, and other drug use among high school students in Bureau of Indian Affairs–funded schools—United States, 2001. (2003). *Morbidity and Mortality Weekly Report, 52*(44), 1070-1072.

Trigoboff, E., & Wilson, H. S. (2004). Substance-related disorders. In C. R. Kneisl, H. S. Wilson, & E. Trigoboff, *Contemporary psychiatric-mental health nursing* (pp. 261–303). Upper Saddle River, NJ: Prentice Hall.

Trinkoff, A., Eaton, W., & Anthony, J. (1991). The prevalence of substance abuse among registered nurses. *Nursing Research, 40*(3), 172-175.

Trinkoff, A., & Storr, C. (1998). Substance use among nurses: Differences between specialties. *American Journal of Public Health, 88*(4), 581-585.

Trinkoff, A. M., Zhou, Q., Storr, C. L., et al. (2000). Workplace access, negative proscriptions, job strain, and substance use in registered nurses. *Nursing Research, 49*(2), 83-90.

U.S. Department of Health and Human Services. (1997). *School-based drug prevention programs: A longitudinal study in selected school districts.* Research Triangle Park, NC: Research Triangle Institute.

U.S. Department of Health and Human Services. (2000). *Healthy people 2010: Understanding and improving health* (2nd ed.). Washington, DC: U.S. Government Printing Office.

U.S. Department of Health and Human Services. (2006). *Healthy people 2010: Midcourse Review.* Washington, DC: U.S. Government Printing Office.

Volkow, N. D. (2003). Bringing research and practice together to improve drug abuse prevention. *NIDA Notes, 18*(3), 1-3.

Wegscheider, S. (1981). *Another chance: Hope and help for alcoholic families.* Palo Alto, CA: Science & Behavior Books.

Welch-Carre, E. (2005). The neurodevelopmental consequences of prenatal alcohol exposure. *Advances in Neonatal Care, 5*(4), 217-229.

West, R. (2001). Theories of addiction. *Addiction, 96,* 3-13.

Woititz, J. G. (1983). *Adult children of alcoholics.* Pompano Beach, FL: Health Communications.

SUGGESTED READINGS

Alcoholics Anonymous. (2001). *The big book* (4th ed.). New York: Author.

Goldstein, A. (2001). *Addiction: From biology to drug policy* (2nd ed.). New York: Oxford University Press.

Institute of Medicine. (2006). *Improving the quality of health care for mental and substance-use conditions*. Washington, DC: National Academies Press.

Kneisl, C. R., Wilson, H. S., & Trigoboff, E. (2004). *Contemporary psychiatric-mental health nursing*. Upper Saddle River, NJ: Prentice Hall.

Kurtz, E. (1982). Why A.A. works. *Journal of Studies on Alcohol, 43*, 38-80.

Lakhani, N. (1997). Alcohol use amongst community dwelling elderly people: A review of the literature. *Journal of Advanced Nursing, 25*(6), 1227-1232.

Ma, G. X., & Henderson, G. (2002). *Ethnicity and substance abuse: Prevention and intervention*. Springfield, IL: Charles C. Thomas.

Ott, P. J., Tarter, R. E., & Ammerman, R. T. (Eds.). (1999). *Sourcebook in substance abuse: Etiology, epidemiology, assessment, and treatment*. Boston: Allyn & Bacon.

Schydlower, M. (Ed.). (2002). *Substance abuse: A guide for health professionals*. Elk Grove Village, IL: American Academy of Pediatrics.

Somervell, A., Saylor, C., & Mao, C-L. (2005). Public health nurse interventions for women in a dependency drug court. *Public Health Nursing, 22*(1), 59-64.

Substance Abuse and Mental Health Services Administration. (2007). *Results from the 2006 National Survey on Drug Use and Health: National findings*. Rockville, MD: National Clearinghouse for Alcohol and Drug Information.

West, R. (2001). Theories of addiction. *Addiction, 96*, 3-13.

Support for Special Populations

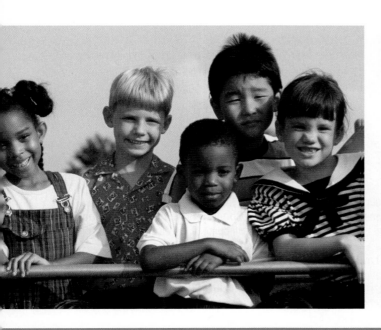

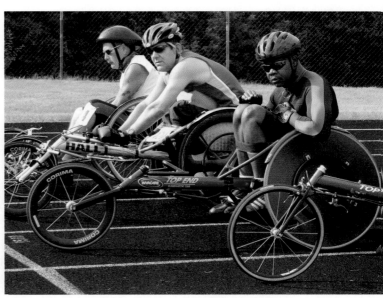

26 Rehabilitation Clients in the Community

Roslyn P. Corasaniti and Donna S. Raimondi

FOCUS QUESTIONS

What is the magnitude of disability in the United States?

What are concepts related to disability and rehabilitation?

What are some common conditions that require rehabilitation?

How does legislation affect the rehabilitation process?

What is the role of the rehabilitation nurse?

How does the rehabilitation client achieve community reintegration?

What are the responsibilities of the community/public health nurse in meeting the needs of rehabilitation clients?

What are community resources for individuals with disabilities?

CHAPTER OUTLINE

KEY TERMS

Disability

Habilitation

Handicap

Impairment

Rehabilitation

CONCEPT OF DISABILITY

The Americans with Disabilities Act (ADA) of 1990 (Public Law 101-336) defines disability as a physical or mental impairment that substantially limits one or more of the major life activities of an individual. An estimated 51.2 million Americans (18.1% of the population) live with disabilities (Centers for Disease Control and Prevention [CDC], 2006a). Of those with disabilities, approximately 77% cannot perform or have some limitation in their major life activities (play, school, work, self-care). Others are limited in their ability to perform nonmajor activities (climbing stairs, driving an automobile) (Table 26-1). The issues related to disabilities have far-reaching social and public health consequences in the United States. The national cost of disabilities totals more than $452 billion each year, including an estimated $300 billion in medical costs (Agency for Healthcare Research and Quality, 2007; U.S. Department of Health and Human Services [USDHHS], 2002). In addition, another approximately $152 billion dollars is lost in productivity each year.

Disabilities have a variety of causes and are not evenly distributed among the population. Causes of disability include congenital defects, mental retardation, traumatic injuries, and consequences of diseases (e.g., amputation in those with diabetes, altered mobility related to pain from arthritis, and altered cognition in those with schizophrenia). Although disability occurs in people of all ages, disability rates increase with age. As life expectancy and the number of aged persons in society increase, more people with disabilities will require care. We are now able to control chronic illnesses and injuries more effectively, and as a result, people with disabilities live longer.

TABLE 26-1   Disabilities among Individuals 15 Years and Older

Disability Measure	Number Disabled (in Thousands)	Percent of Population
Difficulty with specific functional activities Example: Climbing stairs Walking three city blocks	51,235	18.1
Difficulty with activities of daily living Example: Bathing/toileting	8,089	3.6
Difficulty with instrumental activities of daily living Example: Preparing meals Taking care of money/bills	13,164	5.9
Reported selected impairments Examples: Mental retardation Alzheimer's disease Learning disability	7,918	3.6
Use of assistive aid Example: Use of wheelchair or cane	11,851	5.3
Limitation in ability to work	17,385	9.4

Data from Centers for Disease Control and Prevention. (2006). *Summary health statistics for U.S. adults: National Health Interview Survey, 2005* (Vital and Health Statistics Series 10, No. 232). Hyattsville, MD: National Center for Health Statistics.

Consequently, the number of elderly people with disabilities, as well as the number of illnesses and disabilities per person, will increase (USDHHS, 2006a). Because deaths from traumatic injury have declined as a result of preventive measures and aggressive technologic treatment, the numbers of disabled individuals younger than age 65 has increased. It is estimated that two thirds of those with functional disabilities, and half of those with long-term care needs, are younger than 65 years of age (USDHHS, 2002).

Disability rates are higher among the poor (Fiscella et al., 2008; USDHHS, 2006a). Reasons for this disparity include inadequate prenatal nutrition and care, higher accident rates, less preventive care, a higher prevalence of chronic disease, and less access to treatment for health problems among poor populations. Although disability rates in the United States vary by race and ethnic group, it is important to remember that poverty is the greatest predictor of poor health and disability (see Chapter 21).

Many terms are used to describe the conditions affecting persons who live with disabilities. Several terms are defined here to establish a common frame of reference. The World Health Organization (WHO) defines an **impairment** as a dysfunction occurring at the anatomic or organ level, a **disability** as a loss in the ability to perform an activity (personal level), and a **handicap** as a disadvantage occurring at the societal level (Secrest, 2000). A handicap is any social disadvantage that exists because of a disability.

Not everyone who has an impairment is disabled, nor is every person with a disability handicapped. For example, someone may be missing a fifth finger but may be able perform all desired tasks without it. This person would not have a disability. However, if this person had been a concert pianist before the loss of the finger, such a loss would cause a disability in a major life activity (work and leisure). Community health and rehabilitation nurses seek to prevent and reduce sources of handicaps, such as stereotyping, architectural barriers, and failure to accommodate those with disabilities. Such interventions are a part of the rehabilitation process.

CONCEPT OF REHABILITATION

HISTORICAL OVERVIEW

Rehabilitation includes a wide range of activities in addition to medical care, including physical, psychosocial, and occupational therapy. It is a process aimed at enabling people with disabilities to reach and maintain their optimal levels of physical, sensory, intellectual, psychologic, and/or social functioning. Rehabilitation provides people with disabilities the tools they need to attain independence and self-determination, including means to provide and/or restore functions or compensate for the loss or absence of a function or for a functional limitation (WHO, 2007). The mission of rehabilitation is complex. Its objectives reach beyond the rehabilitation of individual clients to include educating all health care professionals, as well as the general public, to create a society in which people with disabilities have a fair chance to work, enjoy life, and live as independently as possible. Thus, a central focus of rehabilitation is the quality of life.

Historically, the problems of people with disabilities were often treated in an indifferent fashion or ignored. People had little understanding of the degree of adaptation required to successfully carry out the activities of daily living (ADLs). Indignities and isolation have long surrounded people with disabilities. Historical examples include the following (Rosen & Fox, 1972):

- Blind persons forced to beg
- Lepers shunned and ridiculed by society
- Infants with disabilities isolated and left to die in some cultures
- Crippled, malformed, and visibly ill people considered to be either cursed or possessed by the devil

Over time, attitudes moderated as the belief in the essential worth of all individuals evolved in Western thought. People with physical and mental disabilities were better tolerated. In the nineteenth century, international legislation was passed that made workplaces responsible for injuries to employees. World War II produced an interest in *functional* rehabilitation as well as care of the actual injury or injuries.

Dr. Howard Rusk, director of the Army Air Corps Convalescent and Rehabilitation Services during World War II, developed the philosophy and concept of rehabilitation medicine. He continued his work after the war at Bellevue Hospital in New York City. Other health care professionals slowly came to embrace the concept of rehabilitation (Rusk, 1972).

The World Rehabilitation Fund, founded in 1955, was an early advocate for the disabled. The fund sponsors international projects to assist people with disabilities and lobbies to create a better understanding of their problems, provide training for health care professionals in the field of rehabilitation, and increase employment opportunities for rehabilitation clients (Rusk, 1972).

Access to public spaces and transportation has been addressed by legislation and regulatory efforts. For example, in 1973 the Rehabilitation Act established the Architectural and Transportation Barriers Compliance Board. This board can hold public hearings, conduct investigations, and order the recruitment and hiring of applicants with disabilities. The act also issues regulations concerning barrier-free public facilities and educational institutions (Russel, 1973). Starting in 1983, the American National Standards Institute established standards to make buildings and facilities accessible to and usable by individuals with physical disabilities.

Modern rehabilitation nursing emerged during World War II. The contributions of rehabilitation nurses were recognized as distinct and important. Rehabilitation nursing evolved into a nursing specialty. To some extent, all nurses working with clients with impairments, chronic diseases, and acute injuries include aspects of rehabilitation in their practice.

REHABILITATION NURSING: A SPECIALTY

"Rehabilitation nursing is the diagnosis and treatment of human responses of individuals and groups to actual or potential health problems stemming from altered functional ability and [related] altered lifestyle" (American Nurses Association [ANA] & Association of Rehabilitation Nurses [ARN], 1988, p. 4). Community health nurses who provide rehabilitation must be skilled in giving comfort and performing therapy, promoting adjustment and coping, supporting adaptive capabilities, and promoting achievable independence and meaning in life (Buchanan & Neal, 2002). The community health rehabilitation nurse must possess specific knowledge and skills to provide effective nursing interventions. Expertise in the areas of psychiatric, medical, and surgical nursing is essential. Clients with mental health needs may benefit from rehabilitation services as well (see Chapter 33).

The Association of Rehabilitation Nurses (ARN) was recognized as a specialty nursing organization by the American Nurses Association in 1976. The ARN's stated purpose is "to promote and advance professional rehabilitation nursing practice through education, advocacy, collaboration, and research to enhance the quality of life for those affected by disability and chronic illness" (ARN, 2007a). The ARN publishes a journal, *Rehabilitation Nursing,* that serves as a vehicle for sharing information and rehabilitation nursing research. The organization initiated certification for specialty practice as a means of recognizing a level of rehabilitation nursing expertise. Certified nurses use the title *certified rehabilitation registered nurse (CRRN).*

In 2007, there were nearly 6000 ARN members and more than 10,000 CRRNs (ARN, 2007b). The organization continues to grow, facilitating educational, research, and professional advancement opportunities for rehabilitation nurses. Members are active in promoting the civil rights of people with disabilities and their families and in lobbying for legislation that provides an accessible environment for all citizens.

The rehabilitation nurse functions as a teacher, caregiver, case manager, counselor, consultant, client advocate, and researcher (Hoeman, 2008). Rehabilitation nurses help individuals affected by chronic illness or physical disability to adapt to their disabilities, achieve their greatest potential, and work toward productive, independent lives. They take a holistic approach to meeting patients' medical, vocational, educational, environmental, and spiritual needs (ARN, 2007c).

The goal of the rehabilitation process is to support a holistic approach to nursing care that, with the collaboration of the team, will maximize client independence (Hoeman, 2008). In the professional practice of rehabilitation nursing, the nurse must be sensitive, flexible, creative, and assertive as she or he assists clients to successfully enter or reenter a society primarily designed for able-bodied persons. Nurses must examine their beliefs and feelings about disabilities and handicaps. Not all nurses can cope with a client's lifelong consequences of devastating illnesses or injuries, such as spinal cord injury, stroke, or muscular dystrophy. A belief in the promotion of quality of life is essential. Negative attitudes toward disability create serious obstacles to the formation of a therapeutic relationship and client adaptation.

Rehabilitation nursing plays a role in, and should be a component of, all phases of recovery. For those with injuries and severe illnesses, recovery often begins with admission to the acute care facility and continues throughout community reintegration. The rehabilitation nurse is a consistent, objective resource for the client and family as they adapt to an altered self-concept, changes in roles, and different means of accomplishing ADLs. The rehabilitation nurse must work together with the client, family, and rehabilitation team, as well as the community and the environment, to achieve realistic and favorable outcomes.

For those whose impairment is discovered at birth or in childhood, the habilitative process begins with acknowledgment of the problem. Rehabilitation is the recovery of an ability that once existed, whereas **habilitation** is the development of abilities that never existed before in the child.

THE ENVIRONMENT AND THE REHABILITATION CLIENT

The environment is the critical factor in determining the extent of an individual's handicap. Disabilities can be handicapping in one situation but not in another, depending on the environment. For example, consider the person with chronic obstructive pulmonary disease whose symptoms are aggravated by walking to an office on the fifth floor in a building without elevators. When he arrives at work, his altered oxygenation affects his ability to concentrate. Such a person would be disabled in the major life activity of work. Furthermore, if the employer insisted that the employee must perform his job at that site, the individual would be handicapped. (Although the ADA, discussed later in the chapter, could make this employer's action illegal, such practices continue to occur.)

Community health nurses assist people with disabilities and their families in schools, workplaces, clinics, and homes. Nurses need to be alert to the environmental conditions encountered by disabled people in various settings. Atmospheric conditions, such as temperature, humidity, rain, wind, and snow, can affect the signs and symptoms of medical conditions like multiple sclerosis, arthritis, and chronic pain. Nurses can help clients learn to cope with such influences as they begin to reintegrate into the community. In addition, physical barriers, such as steps, curbs, features of public transportation vehicles, and doorways, can significantly hamper independent functioning. In one study, the majority of disabled persons (84.7%) reported that they had trouble with environmental barriers because of their disability. In that same study, one quarter of the disabled indicated that they were in need of home modifications but were unable to get them, and about the same number reported that they had difficulty accessing their health provider's office (CDC, 2006a).

Psychosocial Aspects of the Environment

The environment also has a psychosocial component. Attitudes of so-called able-bodied people have a profound effect on successful community reintegration. Incorrect beliefs about disabled individuals, such as that they cannot maintain jobs, attend school, or function as sexual human beings, may severely inhibit or even halt the rehabilitation process. Excessive sympathy, however, such as providing extra privileges, failing to hold the disabled person responsible for his or her actions, or attributing "good" qualities to someone because he or she is disabled, can be just as inhibiting. Both the physical and psychosocial components of the environment may require restructuring so that people with disabilities have a fair chance to work, attend school, play, and live satisfying lives (see the *Ethics in Practice* box).

ETHICS IN PRACTICE

Fear in the Community

Gail A. DeLuca Havens, PhD, APRN, BC

Rose, a community health nurse, was delighted to learn that Mr. Wilfred had bequeathed his house to be used as a community-based mental health center. It is a lovely property, but more importantly, it is situated in an attractive residential neighborhood that more closely approximates the kind of environment in which most clients of the Waveview Village Community Mental Health Center are accustomed to living. The Waveview Village clients are currently receiving day treatment in a ramshackle house on the perimeter of the commercial district. It is a noisy and dirty area where the prevalence of drug and alcohol abusers makes it unsafe to walk the streets. Clients of Waveview Village have been teased, ridiculed, and spat on over the years by people living in the neighborhood who do not comprehend the implications of mental illness and consequently are fearful of those with mental illness.

Now, a week before the ownership of Mr. Wilfred's house is to pass to the Waveview Village Corporation, Rose is attending a special session of the zoning board called in response to a petition by people living in the neighborhood of Mr. Wilfred's house. The petition requests that the board modify the existing property-use statutes to explicitly exclude community-based mental health centers from residential areas. Neighborhood residents are very agitated and fearful of having "unstable" people roaming their neighborhood. They voice concerns about personal safety, the security of personal property, and the introduction of an "undesirable element who often associate with the mentally ill" into the neighborhood.

Rose is a member of Waveview Village's board of directors. She has been asked to provide information to the zoning board about how "dangerous" clients of Waveview Village are and whether the concerns expressed by neighborhood residents are justified. Rose explains, "The clients of Waveview Village are ill. As with all illnesses, whether physical or mental, a range of diagnoses will be present in the ill population. So, too, will illnesses exacerbate, or flare up. The clients who receive care at Waveview are no exception. They are well enough to stay at home at night and benefit from social connections. They come to day treatment for counseling and supervision of their medication administration.

"Their care providers are committed to helping them remain in the community, provided they can clothe, feed, and shelter themselves and that there is no evident risk of harm to themselves or to others by their doing so. It is the opportunity to avoid potential harm to our clients that makes Mr. Wilfred's house such an attractive setting for the Waveview Village Day Treatment Program. For those of you who are not familiar with it, the present site for the day treatment program is located in an area that is not well maintained, and clients are harassed coming and going from Waveview. Relocating the day treatment program to Mr. Wilfred's house will eliminate this potential for harm to Waveview clients and will place them in an environment that is more comfortable and familiar to them. I hope that the board's decision is a favorable one for Waveview's clients."

Several days later, Rose receives a letter from the zoning board stating that the board is postponing its decision to allow its members time to become personally acquainted with some of the clients of Waveview Village. The letter asks her to arrange whatever kind of individual or group meetings she thinks would be most comfortable for the clients, while still affording the members of the zoning board the opportunity to get to know them. Usually this type of request would be rejected, because it breaches client confidentiality and discriminates on the basis of their medical diagnoses. However, a number of Waveview clients, knowing that Rose had been advocating for the program to relocate to Mr. Wilfred's house, have approached her, volunteering to provide statements to the board in person. What should Rose do in this situation? Should she follow up on the clients' offers and ask them to meet with members of the zoning board, knowing that such a request will breach their confidentiality? Or should she refuse to comply with the board's request?

Community health nurses develop direct contacts with clients and their social networks, as well as relationships with mental health providers. These interfaces allow nurses to serve as natural intermediaries between the client and the larger systems of social and mental health services. Evidence of this intermediary relationship is observed in the fact that Waveview clients have approached Rose to volunteer to talk with members of the zoning board, as well as that fact that the zoning board has asked Rose to arrange opportunities for them to come to know some of Waveview's clients. If Rose accepts the offers of the clients who have volunteered to meet with members of the zoning board, she will do so only after first ensuring that the clients understand that their actions will breach the confidentiality regarding their illness. She is also aware that she is contributing to that infringement. However, from a utilitarian perspective, she perceives her action to be doing the greatest possible good (Beauchamp & Childress, 2001). Furthermore, the *Code of Ethics for Nurses* explicitly indicates, "Nurses should actively promote the collaborative multi-disciplinary planning required to ensure the availability and accessibility of quality health services to all persons who have needs for health care" (American Nurses Association, 2001, p. 11).

Continued

Given that context, presuming that the zoning board decides in favor of the day treatment center, sacrificing the confidentiality of a few clients to gain access to a treatment environment that is safe and therapeutic for all may be justified.

The American Nurses Association *Code* also clearly states, however, that "the nurse safeguards the patient's right to privacy" and "advocates for an environment that provides for sufficient physical privacy … and policies and practices that protect the confidentiality of information. … The rights, well-being, and safety of the individual patient should be the primary factors in arriving at any professional judgment concerning the disposition of confidential information received from or about the patient. … The standard of nursing practice and the nurse's responsibility to provide quality care require that relevant data be shared with those members of the health care team who have a need to know … only those directly involved with the patient's care" (American Nurses Association, 2001, p. 12).

On the other hand, if Rose refuses to arrange the meetings between the client volunteers and the members of the zoning board, she will be doing so to protect the confidentiality of the client volunteers. In this regard, Rose will be acting from a deontologic perspective, the essence of which is that some actions are right (or wrong) for reasons other than their consequences (Beauchamp & Childress, 2001). However, Rose's refusal of the board's request does not actively encourage the board to rule in favor of the day

treatment program. In fact, it most likely compromises any opportunity to use Mr. Wilfred's house for the Waveview Village Day Treatment Program.

An alternative that Rose might consider is to suggest to Waveview's management staff that she work with them in arranging an open house event, inviting the residents of the neighborhood in which Mr. Wilfred's house is located to visit the present day treatment facility to see firsthand what it contains, how it is organized, and where it is located. Waveview staff, management personnel, and members of the board of directors would be available to discuss the philosophy, mission, and treatment goals of the Waveview Village Day Treatment Program with visitors and to answer their questions. As people become informed about a topic, they often change their opinions related to it. This strategy has the potential to diffuse the objections and resistance to relocating Waveview to Mr. Wilfred's house and to preserve the privacy of its clients.

Which course of action would you choose?

REFERENCES

American Nurses Association. (2001). *Code of ethics for nurses with interpretive statements*. Washington, DC: Author.

Beauchamp, T. L., & Childress, J. F. (2001). *Principles of biomedical ethics* (5th ed.). New York: Oxford University Press.

Cost and Access Issues

Clients and families frequently have concerns about the availability and cost of health care. These concerns bring additional stress to an already stressful environment. Medicare pays for inpatient rehabilitation and selected home health care services for the elderly and other disabled individuals who receive Social Security disability payments, regardless of age. Medicare requires a 2-year wait for eligibility for young disabled persons who do not already qualify for Medicare because of age (USDHHS, 2007). Rehabilitation services under Medicaid vary by state. Private health insurance programs vary widely in the type of coverage provided to disabled and chronically ill people.

In an effort to curb the cost of care, government health plans (Medicare and Medicaid) and private insurers have turned to health maintenance organizations and other forms of managed care. One strategy, initiated in managed care programs and expanded into private insurers, has been the institution of strict case management programs for people with chronic illnesses and other types of high-cost conditions (Cohen & Cesta, 2005; Wallace et al., 2001). Rehabilitation nurse specialists and community health nurses are often the case managers for these individuals.

The change to managed care and case management arrangements has been anxiety provoking for some disabled individuals, particularly in light of publicity about poor quality in some managed care arrangements (see Chapters 3 and 4). Although there has been widespread public concern about the quality of care provided in managed care, there are no substantial data at this time to indicate that managed care provides less or lower-quality care. Some studies of chronically ill clients show that

managed care clients receive worse care for physical conditions, whereas others show the opposite (Lee-Feldstein et al., 2002; Sultz & Young, 2004). Because many disabled and chronically ill clients are new to the constraints of managed care, the ambiguous information about quality issues further increases their stress level.

MYTHS ABOUT DISABILITY

IMPACT ON EMPLOYMENT

Myths abound regarding the interest, motivation, and capability of people with disabilities with regard to work. For example, some people believe that those with disabilities need someone to take care of them because they do not fit into the workplace and making the workplace fit them would be too costly. Others believe that disabled persons do not want to work because they receive enough income from the government. Still others believe that people with disabilities do not make good employees because they are unreliable, dependent, frequently absent from the job because of illness, and too expensive to employ because of their health care costs. All of these myths and stereotypic notions are inaccurate.

Nurses must remember that those with disabilities are people first. Abrasive personalities and behavioral characteristics can be found in any group of individuals. There are competent employees and those who demonstrate poor work habits and attitudes, regardless of the presence or absence of disability. Studies conducted by disability organizations, the Rehabilitation Services Administration, the President's Committee on Employment of People with Disabilities, and others clearly indicate that the attendance rates of workers with disabilities are equal to or better than those of their nondisabled counterparts. The employment of the disabled worker might involve some accommodations. Employers who had made accommodations for employees with disabilities reported multiple benefits as a result. The most frequently mentioned direct benefits were that (1) the accommodation allowed the company to retain a qualified employee, (2) the accommodation eliminated the costs of training a new employee, and (3) the accommodation increased the worker's productivity (Job Accommodations Network [JAN], 2005).

The most widely mentioned indirect benefits employers received were that (1) the accommodation increased over-all company productivity, (2) the accommodation increased overall company morale, and (3) providing the accommo-dation ultimately improved interactions with co-workers and customers. In addition, a significant number of employ-ers said that the accommodation helped improve workplace safety (JAN, 2005). In addition, 49% of employers believed that they received more than $10,000 in business value for the accommodations they made for employees with disabilities (JAN, 2003). Some of the barriers people with disabilities encoun-ter when securing and maintaining employment are listed in Box 26-1.

Potential employers have expressed concern about hiring people with disabilities. Their fears have been based in part on the anticipation that providing work site accommodations for these employees might be costly. The Job Accommodations Network (JAN), a consultative service of the President's Committee on Employment of People with Disabilities, is an international information network and consulting resource for accommodating persons with disabilities in the workplace (JAN, 2005). This is a free service with a data bank of more than 20,000 possible accommodations. The JAN reports that the cost of reasonable accommodations varies, but most are inexpensive (Figure 26-1).

Job accommodation is usually not expensive. It is often as simple as a rearrangement of equipment. It can reduce work-ers' compensation and other insurance costs, increase the pool of qualified employees, and create opportunities for persons with functional limitations. The following are examples of job accommodations:

- A mail carrier with a back injury could no longer carry his mail bag. A cart was purchased for $150, which allowed him to keep his route.
- A woman who used a wheelchair could not sit at her desk because her knees would not fit under it. The center desk drawer was removed, which allowed the employee to sit and work comfortably at the desk. This simple modification cost the company and the worker nothing.
- A medical technician who was deaf could not hear the buzz of a timer, which was necessary for specific laboratory tests. A $26.95 indicator light was attached.

Individuals with disabilities should be well informed regarding their rights under the ADA. Excellent informa-tion, including a *Guide for People with Disabilities Seeking Employment*, is available at the JAN website (see Community Resources for Practice at the end of the chapter).

Box 26-1   Barriers Encountered by People with Disabilities Seeking Employment

- **Lack of educational preparation.** Students with disabilities who do not attend college might have little vocational prepara-tion. These students will face unemployment, social isolation, and greater difficulties achieving integration into their communities. The U.S. Department of Education's National Institute of Disability and Rehabilitation Research declared effecting the transition of disabled students from high school to the workforce to be a priority initiative (LaPlante et al., 1992).
- **Inadequate preparation in independent living skills.** Limited social, self-care, economic, or job skills may make it difficult for persons with disabilities to live independently in the community. Social and vocational supports and assistive technologies can reduce disabled persons' dependence on caregivers.
- **Feelings of the person with a disability and an employer that the person does not fit into the work environment.** Discrimination in the workplace continues. Individuals who sus-tain work-related injuries continue to quit and/or be fired from their jobs. Neither the employer nor the employee has information about job restructuring or work site accommodations. The passage of the Americans with Disabilities Act in 1990 and other legislation has facilitated discussions of workers' and employers' fears and attitudes regarding the disabled and workplace accommodation.
- **A belief that provision of income supplements discourage employment.** When employers and others believe that people with disabilities who receive welfare benefits or Social Security disability subsidies have sufficient income and are satisfied, they are not inclined to consider employment for them. Although mini-mum-wage jobs still leave people near poverty, some people with disabilities may be reluctant to give up a government subsidy for a paycheck, particularly if health benefits are not included with the job. Supplements to the Americans with Disabilities Act have reduced this problem, but it still exists.
- **A belief that people with disabilities are more unreliable in job attendance because of frequent illness.** Some people with dis-abilities may be more susceptible to disability-related illnesses (e.g., urinary tract infections and skin breakdown in persons with paraple-gia), but this possibility does not permit discrimination in hiring.

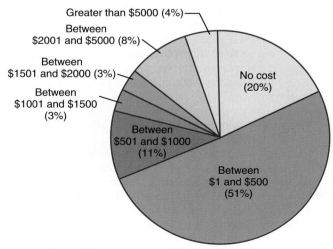

FIGURE 26-1 Percentages of workplace accommodations by cost. (Data from Job Accommodations Network. [2003]. *Accommodations benefit/cost data.* Retrieved November 25, 2003 from *http://www.jan.wvu.edu/medou/Stats/BenCosts0799.html*).

COMMUNITY LIVING ARRANGEMENTS

Society has fostered the myth that people with disabilities must be taken care of and cannot live independently. Much of the public perception has focused on those with developmental disabilities or mental illnesses living in group homes and older adults in nursing homes. Efforts are needed to assess the needs of people with disabilities and to project the future housing needs of all citizens.

The 1988 Fair Housing Amendments were designed to increase the access to housing opportunities for people with disabilities (U.S. Department of Education, 1988). Although these amendments do not cover all dwellings, multifamily housing units built after May 1991 are required to consider the needs of people with disabilities in accessing common building areas, kitchens, bathrooms, and environmental controls (e.g., light switches and thermostats).

A variety of living arrangements are available for people with disabilities, based on their income, functional status, and existing support systems. Some of these are described in Box 26-2.

BOX 26-2 Alternative Living Arrangements Available for People with Disabilities

- **Nursing homes**—Most nursing homes are privately run facilities for chronically ill clients. Available services range from fully accredited rehabilitation programs to total nursing care. For Medicaid to pay for nursing home care, a person's assets must be almost depleted (see Chapters 3 and 4). Older adults are typically the long-term residents in these facilities. Young people in their twenties or thirties who have spinal cord injuries, severe multiple sclerosis, acquired immunodeficiency syndrome, or amyotrophic lateral sclerosis become residents of nursing homes because there are no other alternatives available to them in the community.
- **Group homes**—Group homes and supervised living quarters provide people with disabilities the structure and support to live outside of institutions. These living situations typically provide housing for two to four adults who may be developmentally disabled or have a head injury or a chronic mental illness.
- **Transitional living**—In transitional living, people recovering from a head injury or other conditions may try out their independent living skills in a supportive environment. These are short-term, post-hospital facilities. Clients are generally expected to participate in a structured program (work, prevocational, or therapeutic activity) during the day and organize their meals and leisure activities in the evenings and on weekends. Staff are available to assist in problem solving, facilitation, socialization, and conflict negotiation.
- **Senior and disabled citizen housing**—Senior and disabled citizen housing offers living units designed to accommodate the needs of older adults and those with disabilities, regardless of age. These housing programs offer security, social activities, and transportation to community activities and shopping.
- **Independent living apartments**—Those with financial assets can purchase lifetime residence and care in independent living apartments. Medical, rehabilitation, and other support services are offered to address specific needs. Those who ultimately require 24-hour nursing care will find it accessible in life care communities.
- **In-home residences with support services**—Individuals with disabilities and their caregivers may take advantage of a variety of community support services. The following programs are usually available for children and adults (eligibility requirements may vary): home health, in-home aid and personal care, respite care, Meals on Wheels, daycare, information and referral, and support groups (see Chapters 30 and 31).

Additional information about housing resources can be obtained by contacting a state's office on aging, department of housing and community development, health department, or developmental disability administration. Mental health associations, independent living centers, the federal Division of Vocational Rehabilitation (Rehabilitation Service Administration), and head injury foundations may also have information about the location of specialized housing and community programs for people with specific disabilities.

MAGNITUDE OF DISABILITY IN THE UNITED STATES

TYPES OF DISABILITIES

Disability is a result of impairments that often occur because of injury or chronic disease. The National Health Interview Survey (NHIS), a continuous, nationwide household survey conducted by the U.S. Bureau of the Census, includes questions about disability and health. According to NHIS data, the six most prevalent chronic conditions causing disability are arthritis and orthopedic deformities or impairments, heart disease and other circulatory problems, diabetes, asthma and other respiratory problems, and mental health problems (U.S. Bureau of the Census, 2006). However, more people report having these chronic impairments and diseases than report being disabled by them. Consequently, community health nursing efforts to prevent disability must address prevention and adequate treatment of these chronic conditions. Many of the *Healthy People 2010* objectives (USDHHS, 2006b) specify targets for reducing the prevalence of chronic diseases and impairments as well as improving access to treatment and accommodation for people with disabilities. (See the *Healthy People 2010* box on page 673.)

Chronic Illness and Disability

Many people with chronic illness have one or more disabilities as a result of that illness. It is estimated that 79 million Americans have one or more types of coronary artery heart disease, and 700,000 have strokes each year. Stroke is a leading cause of serious long-term disability in the United States (CDC, 2003). Half of all stroke clients will have residual physical and/or social disabilities (American Heart Association [AHA], 2007). Those clients need rehabilitative therapies. The estimated direct and indirect cost of stroke in the United States for 2007 was $62 billion (AHA, 2007). In addition, there are approximately 3 million new clients with cardiac disease each year who would benefit from cardiac rehabilitation programs (Brewer et al., 2002).

People with orthopedic disabilities represent 38% of the total number of Americans with disabilities (CDC, 2001). Included in this category are two of the leading causes of disabilities, arthritis and orthopedic impairments, which inhibit a person's ability to work and function independently.

Mental illness is a source of *functional* disability. More than 22% of adults in the United States have experienced serious mental illness in the past 12 months (Kessler et al., 2005). The mentally ill are not often thought of as candidates for rehabilitation services. There are many mentally ill people living in community placements as a result of the push toward deinstitutionalization (see Chapter 33). Research indicates that these individuals benefit from comprehensive programs of

■ HEALTHY PEOPLE 2010 ■
Objectives for Persons with Disabilities

1. Include in the core of all *Healthy People 2010* surveillance instruments a standardized set of questions that identify "people with disabilities" (baseline: no instruments contain a standardized set in 1999).

2. Reduce to 17% the proportion of children and adolescents with disabilities who are reported to be sad, unhappy, or depressed (baseline: 31% of children and adolescents aged 4 to 11 years in 1997).

3. Reduce to 7% the proportion of adults with disabilities who report feelings such as sadness, unhappiness, or depression that prevent them from being active (baseline: 28% of adults 18 years and older in 1997).

4. Increase to 79% the proportion of adults who participate in social activities (baseline: 61% of adults aged 18 years and older in 2001).

5. Increase to 84% the proportion of adults with disabilities reporting sufficient emotional support (baseline: 71% of adults aged 18 years or older in 2001).

6. Increase to 96% the proportion of adults with disabilities reporting satisfaction with life (baseline: 80% of adults aged 18 years or older in 2001).

7a. Decrease to 46,681 the number of people aged 22 years or older with disabilities in congregate care facilities consistent with permanency planning principles (baseline: 93,362 persons in 1997).

7b. Reduce to zero the number of persons aged 21 years and under in congregate care facilities (baseline: 24,300 persons in 1997).

8. Eliminate disparities in employment rates between working-age adults with and without disabilities (*Healthy People 2010* target is 80% of disabled employed) (baseline: 43% of adults aged 18 through 64 years with disabilities were employed in 1997).

9. Increase to 60% the proportion of children and youth with disabilities who spend at least 80% of their time in regular educational programs (baseline: 45% of children and youth aged 6 to 21 years with disabilities in the 1995-1996 school year).

10. Increase to 63% the proportion of people with disabilities who report having access to health and wellness and treatment programs and facilities (baseline: 48% of persons over age 18 in 2002).

11. Reduce to 7% the proportion of people with disabilities who report not having the assistive devices and technology needed (baseline: 10% of people aged 18 years and older in 2002).

12. Reduce the proportion of people with disabilities reporting environmental barriers to participation in home to 9%, in school to 5.7%, at work to 7%, and in the community to 7% (baseline: 10% at home, 6.1% in school, 7.7% at work, and 11% in the community in 2002).

13a. Increase the number of states and the District of Columbia that have public health surveillance and health promotion programs for people with disabilities and caregivers (baseline: 14 states and the District of Columbia in 1999).

13b. Increase the number of tribes that have public health surveillance and health promotion programs for people with disabilities and caregivers (developmental—no baseline).

Specific Chronic Disease Objectives Related to Rehabilitation

Arthritis

2.2 Reduce to 33% the proportion of adults with doctor-diagnosed arthritis or joint symptoms chronic joint symptoms who experience a limitation in activity due to arthritis (baseline: 36% of adults in 2000).

Diabetes

5.10 Reduce the rate of persons with diabetes who experience lower-extremity amputations to 2.9 per 1000 persons (baseline: 6.6 per 1000 persons with diabetes in 1997 to 1999).

Hypertension (for stroke control)

12.11 Increase to 98% the proportion of adults with high blood pressure who are taking action (losing weight, increasing physical activity, reducing sodium intake) to help control their blood pressure (baseline: 84% of adults with high blood pressure in 1998).

Injury Prevention

15.17 Reduce the rate of nonfatal injuries caused by motor vehicle crashes to 933 per 100,000 population (baseline: 1181 per 100,000 population in 1998).

Mental Health

18.4 Increase to 54% the proportion of persons with serious mental illness who are employed (baseline: 52% in 2002).

Respiratory Disease

24.9 Reduce to 1.9% the proportion of adults whose activity is limited due to chronic lung and breathing problems (baseline: 2.5% of adults aged 45 years and older in 1997).

From U.S. Department of Health and Human Services. (2000). *Healthy people 2010: Understanding and improving health* (2nd ed.). Washington, DC: U.S. Government Printing Office; and U.S. Department of Health and Human Services. (2006). *Healthy people 2010: Midcourse Review.* Washington, DC: U.S. Government Printing Office.

community care that include rehabilitation services (Wadhwa & Lavizzo-Mourey, 1999).

Some impairments and chronic diseases are associated with greater disability than others. Table 26-2 identifies common chronic conditions that cause limitation in a major activity. More than 85% of persons with mental retardation have a limitation of 30% or more, and 60% of those who are blind in both eyes have a similar degree of disability. Arthritis is the leading cause of disability; approximately 17.4 million people have activity limitations because of their arthritis (CDC, 2006b).

Personal Care Needs

Approximately 10.2 million people have difficulty carrying out one or more of six ADLs (U.S. Bureau of the Census, 2006). Most rely on a child or spouse to assist with care. Only 11% paid for care attendants, which can be costly. Because the disabled are at greater risk of poverty and lack of health insurance, they are often unable to pay for personal care. Many insurance programs do not pay or pay for a limited amount of care. Approximately 23% to 27.8% of the disabled live alone (U.S. Bureau of the Census, 2006), which means that they often cannot rely on friends or family members to assist

TABLE 26-2 Selected Conditions as Main Cause of Disability in Adults 21 to 64 Years, United States, 2002

Chronic Condition	Number of Persons (in Thousands)	Percentage of Disabled with Specific Condition
Arthritis	17,400	8.3
Back or spine problem	8,094	22.9
Heart trouble/hardening of the arteries	2,094	5.9
Lung or respiratory problem	1,738	4.9
Deafness or hearing problem	1,566	4.4
Limb/extremity stiffness	1,522	4.3
Mental or emotional problem	1,654	4.7
Diabetes	2,256	6.4
Blindness or vision problem	1,029	2.4
Stroke	462	1.3
Broken bone/fracture	899	2.5
Mental retardation	462	1.3
Cancer	889	2.5
High blood pressure	1,954	5.5
Head or spinal cord injury	494	1.4
Learning disability	341	1.0
Alzheimer's disease/ senility/dementia	61	0.17
Kidney problems	400	1.1
Paralysis	212	0.6
Missing limbs	215	0.6
Other	6,983	19.8

Data from U.S. Bureau of the Census. (2006). *Americans with disabilities: 2002* (Current Population Reports, P70-107). Washington, DC: U.S. Department of Commerce; and Centers for Disease Control and Prevention. (2006). Prevalence of doctor-diagnosed arthritis and arthritis-attributable activity limitation—United States, 2003-2005. *Morbidity and Mortality Weekly Report, 55*(40), 1089-1092.

with personal care needs. The federal government has been considering changes to insurance programs that would help the disabled with personal care expenses. These efforts are discussed later in the chapter.

Spinal Cord and Traumatic Brain Injury and Disability

Approximately 1.4 million people experience traumatic brain injury (TBI) and 7800 persons sustain a spinal cord injury each year in the United States (CDC, 2006c; Spinal Cord Injury Information Network, 2006). Spinal cord and head injuries are most common in young men between 17 and 34 years of age. Approximately one in four of those injured have residual deficits that affect their cognition and ability to live and function independently (Dufour et al., 2000). Their lifelong disabilities have an impact on their lives and the lives of their family members. Both spinal cord injuries and TBIs require intensive, long-term health care. Most family members still experienced a sense of crisis 4 to 5 years after the injury. There

are an estimated 5.7 million persons who require long-term care or lifelong help in performing ADLs as a result of TBIs and spinal cord injuries (CDC, 2006c; National Spinal Cord Injury Association, 2007).

Although the numbers are difficult to estimate, it is apparent that many children are surviving congenital and traumatic illness or injury. Many of these children have physical and developmental disabilities. An estimated 17% of U.S. children are born with disabilities that result in developmental delays (CDC, 2006d). Chapters 27 and 30 discuss programs that identify these children, prevent further disability, promote development and learning, and foster integration into the community.

DISABILITY BY AGE GROUP

Disability rates increase with age (Figure 26-2). However, higher percentages of children, adolescents, and those older than 85 years of age receive assistance because of limitations in carrying out basic life activities. Children are more likely to have mental or developmental impairments than are adults. Almost 25% of those with limitations in performing basic life activities, such as dressing and food preparation, do not receive help from others. The percentage of persons who are in need but do not have assistance increases with age (U.S. Bureau of the Census, 2006). These data substantiate the need for and importance of community health nurses as direct interventionists and case managers. Professionals who assist people with disabilities in community settings collaborate with clients to establish realistic goals that will foster the maintenance of independent functioning.

DISABILITY BY EMPLOYMENT STATUS AND GENDER

People with disabilities who are able to work have seen some improvement in employment rates during the past 10 years. For the disabled, however, acquiring and keeping a job is still more difficult than it is for those without disabilities. In 2000, the employment rate was 81.7% for the nondisabled but only 27% for the disabled (Kaye, 2003). The severity of disability influences employability. Those with a nonsevere disability are three times more likely to be employed than those with a severe disability (Stoddard et al., 1998). Gender differences exist in disability and work. Women with both severe and less severe disabilities are less likely to be employed than men with disabilities (Kaye, 2003; USDHHS, 2006a). Employment is lowest for people with a mental disability and low for those with a physical or sensory disability (Figure 26-3).

Injury and chronic disease patterns also vary by gender. Among adolescents and young adults who sustain traumatic injuries, males are twice as likely as females to sustain severe injuries (CDC, 2006e). Such injuries most often result from vehicular accidents, unintentional falls, and assaults. When examining the causes of disability among older adults, one must be cognizant of the fact that women continue to live longer than men. Therefore, it is no surprise that women experience more strokes than men. Men and women are at equal risk for heart attacks, which was not the case in the past. Perhaps the increase in women's risk is the result of an increased participation in the workforce, an increase in smoking, and stresses equal to or greater than those encountered by their male counterparts.

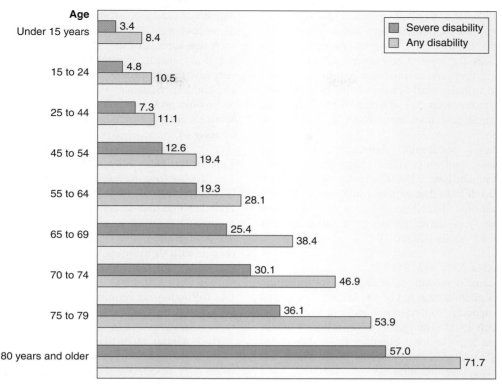

FIGURE 26-2 Disability prevalence and the need for assistance by age, 2000 (in percent). (From U.S. Bureau of the Census. [2006]. *Americans with disabilities: 2002* [Current Population Reports, P70-107]. Washington, DC: U.S. Department of Commerce.)

LEGISLATION

Legislation to protect and promote the rights of people with disabilities is a critical component of rehabilitation. Nurses should have basic knowledge about legislation affecting the civil rights of people with disabilities. The following sections discuss major legislative initiatives that have helped to expand the employability and integration of people with disabilities in the community.

EMPLOYERS' LIABILITY LAWS

In 1911, the first workmen's compensation laws were enacted in this country to provide financial support for workers unemployed because of work-related injuries. In 1920, the first civilian rehabilitation program was established by means of the Smith-Fess Act (Civilian Rehabilitation Act). This program provided vocational rehabilitation services through state boards of vocational rehabilitation to people disabled in industry (Van de Bittner, 1987).

VOCATIONAL REHABILITATION ACTS

The Social Security Act of 1935 established permanent authorization for vocational rehabilitation. It also established old-age insurance, aid to the blind, and services for crippled children. Amendments to the Vocational Rehabilitation Act have been enacted periodically. In 1943, the Vocational Rehabilitation Program was broadened to include emotionally disturbed and mentally retarded persons and to provide maintenance money for living expenses and occupational tools. Training grants were authorized for the preparation of professional rehabilitation personnel in 1954. These amendments also authorized federal support for research.

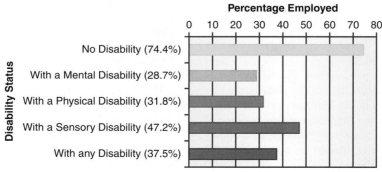

FIGURE 26-3 Employment percentages by disability status. (From U.S. Bureau of the Census. [2005]. *American community survey*. Retrieved March 5, 2007 from *http://factfinder.census.gov/servlet/STTable*.)

During the 1960s, the Council of State Governments published the Workmen's Compensation and Rehabilitation Law, which contained detailed provisions governing vocational rehabilitation services for injured employees. Other amendments passed during that decade provided federal assistance to plan, equip, and initially staff rehabilitation facilities and workshops, authorized funds for evaluation to determine rehabilitation potential, and mandated follow-up services to clients and families.

In 1975, mandatory vocational rehabilitation laws were enacted in California, and most states followed with some form of vocational rehabilitation law. Currently all states have workers' compensation laws that require employers to assume the cost of occupational disabilities without regard to any fault involved. Employers, therefore, are spared civil lawsuits involving negligence (Van de Bittner, 1987).

REHABILITATION ACT OF 1973
One of the most critical reforms affecting the rehabilitation movement was the Rehabilitation Act of 1973. This act required state rehabilitation agencies to develop an individualized, written care plan for each client. The plan is to be designed jointly by the rehabilitation team and the client; it must state long- and short-term goals and spell out the terms under which services are offered. The Rehabilitation Services Administration under the U.S. Department of Education administers rehabilitation programs authorized by the act. The provisions of the Rehabilitation Act include the following (Van de Bittner, 1987):

- Requires the development of affirmative action programs for employment of disabled people in departments and agencies of the executive branch of the federal government
- Establishes the Architectural and Transportation Barriers Compliance Board to develop standards for compliance with regulations to overcome architectural, transportation, and communication barriers in public facilities
- Forbids discrimination against otherwise qualified disabled persons in any federally assisted program or activity
- Entitles children with disabilities to a free, appropriate public education in the least restrictive setting
- Ensures that qualified people with disabilities may not be denied entrance to postsecondary educational and vocational programs or discriminated against in recruitment or admission to these programs
- Prohibits employers from refusing to hire disabled people if they meet the job requirements
- Prohibits preemployment inquiries about disabilities
- Requires all federally assisted programs to provide facilities that are accessible and usable
- Requires all new facilities built with federal funds be barrier free

CATASTROPHIC CARE ACT
When the Medicare Catastrophic Coverage Act of 1988 was enacted, it was described as historic health care legislation that provided the largest expansion in the Medicare program since its inception in 1966. Most of the act was repealed because of opposition to the funding mechanism by middle- and upper-income retirees. The law never addressed insurance needs for the cost of long-term nursing home care. Eliminated as part of the repeal were unlimited coverage of hospital and physician costs once out-of-pocket expenses reached preset limits,

outpatient prescription drug coverage, and extended nursing home coverage.

A few aspects of the act were retained, including the mandate for states to expand Medicaid coverage to include not only low-income elderly but also low-income pregnant women and children. States also were required to increase the amount of income and assets that may be kept by a person whose spouse's nursing home costs are being paid by Medicaid (see Chapter 4).

TECHNOLOGY-RELATED ASSISTANCE ACT
The Technology-Related Assistance for Individuals with Disabilities Act of 1988 (Public Law 100-407), known as the *Tech Act,* and amendments passed in 1994 offer grant money to states interested in establishing programs for informing the public about the benefits of assistive technologies for people with disabilities. These programs are required to be statewide, and the activities initiated with the federal funding are to be eventually funded by state and local resources. The following six requirements are to be addressed in each program:

- *Conduct a needs assessment.* Each state is required to survey the potential needs that people with disabilities might have for assistive technologies.
- *Identify resources.* The delivery of assistive technology services must be coordinated between public and private agencies.
- *Provide assistive technology devices and services.* Each state must provide assistive devices and related services directly to consumers; provide funding to consumers, enabling them to purchase the product or service they desire; and establish facilities to loan equipment or provide funding to people who make assistive devices for those with disabilities, including wheelchairs, computers, and modified eating utensils.
- *Disseminate information.* Strategies are required to inform the public about the benefits and availability of assistive technologies. Computer databases and print and electronic media should be used.
- *Provide training and technical assistance.* States must teach consumers and professionals how to use assistive technologies.
- *Support public and private partnerships.* States must encourage the public and private sectors to work more closely together to meet the assistive technology needs of the community.

AMERICANS WITH DISABILITIES ACT
The ADA was enacted in 1990. It provides protection from discrimination to the 49 million Americans with disabilities. This act extends the protection of civil rights to people with physical and mental handicaps and chronic illnesses (ADA Consultants, 1992; Craven & Gleason, 2002; Spears, 1990).

The ADA deals with access to employment, government services, public accommodations, public transportation, and telecommunications. Five key provisions are as follows:

- All state and local government agencies and businesses open to the public must make their services available to people with disabilities unless the cost to do so is excessive.
- Interstate and commuter rail systems, and local and intercity bus lines must accommodate passengers in wheelchairs.

- All businesses with 15 or more employees are required to disregard handicaps in hiring decisions.
- All telephone companies are required to provide special services for people with speech or hearing impairments.
- Food industry employers can reassign workers with diseases that are transmitted through contact with food (e.g., salmonellosis, hepatitis A).

Amendments to the ADA in 1999 refined the law to encourage the disabled to continue employment. Vocational rehabilitation, employment assistance, and other social support services can now be provided without a disabled person's risking loss of Medicaid or disability insurance support. Prior to the 1999 amendments, many disabled were in a catch-22 situation: work and lose medical and assistance benefits, or remain unemployed and limit their social, emotional, and physiologic well-being (Craven & Gleason, 2002).

The ADA intended to integrate the disabled, whenever possible, into the community. In 1999 the Supreme Court upheld the right of such integration when it ruled in *Olmstead v L.C. and E.W.* that the states could not require institutional care for mentally ill patients when their care providers determined that the patients were able to be placed in community settings (Center for an Accessible Society, 2007). Community rather than institutional care is the goal for many disabled persons.

FAMILY AND MEDICAL LEAVE ACT

The Family and Medical Leave Act of 1993 provides employees with up to 12 weeks of unpaid leave per year to care for a newborn or recently adopted child; a foster child; a spouse, parent, or child with a serious health condition; or the employee's own serious health condition. This law applies to all public and private employers with 50 or more employees and is enforced by the Department of Labor.

Although not everyone can afford unpaid leave, the act allows family members to care for each other during times of serious health problems, such as recuperation from surgery for correction of congenital defects or recovery from a spinal cord injury. Health care insurance continues during the worker's absence, and the worker is guaranteed his or her job or an equivalent job on return to work.

BALANCED BUDGET ACT OF 1997

The Balanced Budget Act of 1997 imposed stricter limits on Medicare reimbursement for home care services. The act narrowed the definition of *home-bound.* Persons were no longer eligible for home care benefits if they were able to leave home for any reason other than to obtain medical services. As a result, the number of persons 65 years or older eligible for Medicare home care funding declined by 50% between 1997 and 2000 (USDHHS, 2002). This restriction runs counter to accepted rehabilitative and custodial care practices in which people are encouraged to remain as active as possible within their physical limitations.

COMMUNITY LIVING LEGISLATION

Most disabled individuals who qualify for long-term care support services must use the Medicaid program. This program is heavily weighted toward institutional care. Home and community-based support services represent just 12.5% of Medicaid's annual expenses (U.S. Congress, House, 2007).

Two new federal legislative efforts are an attempt to help the disabled stay in the community and access support services as needed. The Community Living Assistance Services and Support Act would provide for an insurance program administered by the U.S. Department of Health and Human Services, much like the optional Medicare part B and D programs. It would be a voluntary program in which premiums would be pooled. If a person used the program and became disabled, he or she would receive cash benefits to pay for assistance services (Disability Policy Seminar, 2007). This legislation has been considered by Congress in the past several years, but has not been passed.

The second bill is entitled the Community Choice Act of 2007 (House Resolution 1621) (U.S. Congress, House, 2007). It would required Medicaid to pay for community-based attendants and support services and increase federal funding for the Medicaid program. There has been no action on this bill.

CONDITIONS NECESSITATING REHABILITATION

IMPACT OF INCREASING LIFE SPAN

Approximately 36.3 million Americans, or 12.4% of the population, are 65 years of age or older. The elderly population is the fastest growing segment of the population in the country (USDHHS, 2006a). By the year 2050, one American in five will be older than 65 years of age. Because of advancing age, lengthening life span, and prevalence of chronic illness, this heterogeneous group is one of the largest consumers of health care services, regardless of the setting. The elderly make up the largest population of community-based rehabilitation clients (Gender, 2008). Thirty-four percent of elderly Americans cannot independently perform at least one basic ADL (USDHHS, 2006a). Arthritis, atherosclerosis, and osteoporosis are some of the conditions that influence an older person's ability to perform ADLs.

The incidence of sudden, critical illnesses, such as heart attacks and strokes, also increases as individuals age. In addition, the survivors of heart attacks and strokes are often left with residual effects. After a heart attack, diet and mobility may require alteration. Fear of another heart attack might inhibit a person's ability to work, enjoy leisure activities, or have a satisfying sexual relationship. After a stroke, mobility, manual dexterity, speech, elimination functions, and safety awareness can all be affected. After rehabilitation in a rehabilitation facility, additional community follow-up involving various therapy modalities is often recommended. Home health care, clinic services, or nursing home care might be required. Respite care might be helpful for family members who are caregivers.

These critical illnesses influence nearly all aspects of clients' and their families' ADLs. Role changes, fear, anxiety, and the ability to provide adequate care must be assessed in the community environment. Safety issues, such as the ability to summon help if left alone at home, crime prevention, and cognitive abilities (e.g., judging whether water is too hot to bathe in or remembering how to transfer from a wheelchair to a toilet without falling), are of critical importance. If there are steps in the home, is the cardiac client able to climb them without compromising cardiorespiratory status? Is there an adequate family or social support system for these clients?

These issues indicate that the integration of these clients into the community environment is an ongoing process.

Following through with medical treatment regimens is of critical importance to those with chronic diseases. People who experience a sudden onset of illness might have to learn a regular regimen of medications. Compliance with diets and medication schedules and the reestablishment of sexual and social relationships take time. The community health nurse may be notified of problems only after complications develop from a chronic condition. Difficulties may result from a failure to understand the treatment regimen (e.g., medication administration or nutritional needs). Cost factors can also influence a person's ability to adhere to recommended health care practices.

TRAUMATIC INJURIES

There are many types of traumatic injury. TBI is the most common condition requiring extensive rehabilitation efforts. An estimated 5.3 million Americans live with disabilities resulting from TBI. Annually, more than 1.4 million people sustain a brain injury (CDC, 2006c). Approximately 80,000 each year are left with lifelong disabilities as a result of TBI (Brain Injury Association of America, 2007). The average survivor of TBI requires 5 to 10 years of rehabilitation. TBI costs the country an estimated $60 billion per year in medical costs and lost wages (CDC, 2006f). The severity of the injury influences the degree of residual deficit and the person's subsequent need for medical and social support services in the community. People who sustain head injuries might have permanent functional deficits in one or more of the following areas: cognition, performance of ADLs, manipulation, bowel and bladder function, mobility, speech, vision, educational performance, memory, concentration, attention, and behavior.

It is estimated that the incidence of spinal cord injury, not including those who die at the scene of the accident, is approximately 11,000 new cases per year (Spinal Cord Injury Information Network, 2006). The number of people in the United States who live with a spinal cord injury is estimated to be between 250,000 and 400,000 (National Spinal Cord Injury Association, 2007).

Those with spinal cord injuries are another significant group requiring extensive rehabilitation. Approximately 85% of persons who sustain a spinal cord injury and survive past the first 24 hours live for at least 10 years after the injury (National Spinal Cord Injury Association, 2007). Client needs in this population are extensive and vary with the level and type of injury (i.e., complete or incomplete nerve damage). Important issues to consider include:
- Does the client have use of his or her hands?
- How has fine motor control been affected?
- To what extent is the client capable of performing ADLs, such as bathing, dressing, and toileting, and managing emergency situations?

Because of significant advances in health care technology and practice, more persons are surviving severe traumatic injuries. For example, approximately 87% of patients hospitalized for TBI recover sufficiently to be discharged from the hospital (CDC, 2006f). The residual effects of traumatic injuries often require many lifestyle adaptations. A polytrauma client—for example, one who has experienced multiple fractures, contusions, and lacerations—might have to deal with chronic pain for the rest of his or her life. Traumatic amputation, or amputation because of an inability to maintain or restore adequate circulation, may result from these injuries. Mobility, ability to work, sexual identity, and self-concept are affected. Wound healing and the threat of infection may continue for an indefinite period of time, depending on the complexity of the injuries. Financial hardship may result if the client is unable to work or health insurance coverage is inadequate.

Many areas must be assessed to facilitate community reintegration of persons who sustain catastrophic injuries. These include:
- Extent and type of community services required
- Degree of supervision or care needed
- Sources of provided care

Family, friends, and paid caretakers are potential sources of supervision and care. Community-based rehabilitation nurses are often responsible for teaching and initial supervising of caregivers in providing appropriate, safe physical care. They are also a primary source of referrals to community-based assistance services, such as caregivers, home maintenance services, and companion, transportation, and financial resources.

Psychosocial needs are critical. The client's educational and vocational interests should be explored. A person with a head or spinal cord injury might be unable to return to a former occupation or academic course of study. Family roles may have to be altered to accommodate the individual's disability. Spouses of those with a spinal cord injury experience more role change than do parents of the injured person; new ways to express sexuality may have to be learned (Duchene, 2008). The issue of substance abuse should also be explored, because alcohol or other drug abuse is often a contributing factor in accidents resulting in traumatic injury.

Traumatic injuries influence all physical and psychosocial aspects of the lives of clients, their families, and their friends. The same can be said of persons and families affected by chronic illnesses. After returning to the community, rehabilitation clients might be in danger of being "lost" by the health care system. Follow-up health care appointments may be infrequent, and problems may develop between visits and worsen. Clients may choose not to seek or maintain health care contacts because of depression or anger, or they might fail to recognize (or refuse to acknowledge) a problem's existence. To be effective, the rehabilitation community health nurse must be available over a period of time to reassess the client's readiness to accept rehabilitative care. Instead of waiting for the client to seek care, providers must offer care where the client lives, works, or plays.

RESPONSIBILITIES OF THE REHABILITATION NURSE

The responsibilities of the community-based rehabilitation nurse are varied and challenging. Box 26-3 lists several practice environments and describes the focus of nursing care for the disabled person in each environment. As in any nursing specialty, the role of caregiver is important. The nurse must develop flexible and creative interventions and an acceptance of the clients' rights to determine their care when dealing with clients who must adapt the ways in which they carry out *every* aspect of their lives.

Box 26-3 **Practice Environments for Community-Based Rehabilitation Nurses and Focus of Nursing Care**

- **Outpatient rehabilitation clinics**—Focus is on reintegration of client into his or her community.
- **Assisted living facilities**—Focus is on maintaining optimal level of health for the client within the constraints of the client's disabilities and health.
- **Home health care**—Focus is on providing nursing care in the client's home.
- **Schools**—Focus is on providing hands-on nursing care to disabled children and education, counseling, and referral services for parents, teachers, and children.
- **Case management**—Focus is on acting as a liaison and planning for the ongoing health care needs of a disabled person. The nurse may provide health education, health promotion, and referral services as well.

Adapted from Parker, B. J. (2002). Community and family-centered rehabilitation nursing. In P. A. Edwards (Ed.), *The specialty practice of rehabilitation nursing: A core curriculum* (4th ed.; pp. 17-41). Glenview, IL: Association of Rehabilitation Nurses.

TEAM MEMBER AND CASE MANAGER

The first step in assisting a client in adjusting to physical limitations is an assessment of the client's physical, mental, and emotional status. The nurse case manager needs to assess a client's health status, functional skills, psychosocial status, environment, and financial status (McCollum, 2008). Box 26-4 provides examples of assessment measures helpful in determining the needs and issues of concern for each person.

Primarily, the nurse and other members of the health care team need to remember that the client is the captain of his or her care team. The nurse or another team member might disapprove of a treatment option chosen by the client, but the team must respect the client's wish. For instance, a client

---

Box 26-4 **Selected Assessment Measures for Use with Persons with Disabilities**

- **Activities of daily living (ADLs) tools**—Measure ability to feed, bathe, groom, dress self. Assesses mobility, such as chair to bed transfer, stair climbing, and ability to handle a wheelchair. Measure bowel and bladder control and ability to toilet alone or with assistance.
  Sample tool: Barthel Index
- **Instrumental ADLs scales**—Assess areas of social and economic capabilities. Look at mental health, physical health, and ADLs. For example, can a person pay bills by themselves, handle bank accounts, make and keep doctors appointments?
  Sample tool: OARS (Older American Resources and Service): 1-ADL
- **Cognitive status tools**—Assess ability to reason; orientation to time, person, and place; and mood level.
  Sample tools: Mini-Mental State Examination, Depression Scale
- **Quality-of-life tools**—Assess a person's feelings and emotions as well as physical and social activities.
  Sample questions: Does the person have a social life outside the home? How is the person adjusting to physical or mental limitations? Does the person have an active support system?
  Sample tool: MOS (Medical Outcome Survey) three-item survey

---

might elect to use a wheelchair for mobility rather than an artificial limb. Every team member should strive to incorporate the client's cultural and spiritual beliefs into all aspects of care and must avoid imposing her or his own attitudes and values on the client.

An important characteristic of a community-based rehabilitation nurse is the ability to work collaboratively with other health care professionals (Figure 26-4). This becomes essential as more persons with disabilities are covered by managed care arrangements (Boylan & Buchanan, 2008). Occupational, physical, speech, and recreational therapists and vocational counselors are some of the specialists working to enhance the rehabilitation process. If a community health nurse is assessing a client's ability to self-administer medications in the home and notices that the client is not using the dressing techniques taught by the occupational therapist, the nurse should reinforce the proper method. The occupational therapist may need to be notified, and additional home visits may be necessary. Thus, the nurse needs to be aware of all treatment interventions advocated by the team and support continuity of interdisciplinary care.

The nurse case manager's efforts are geared toward helping clients reintegrate into community and independent living. It is crucial that community-based rehabilitation nurses have a very good knowledge base about what community resources are available and how they fit the client and family. A list of potential resources is provided in Community Resources for Practice at the end of the chapter. As case managers and client advocates, community health and rehabilitation nurses can ensure that clients smoothly transition between inpatient,

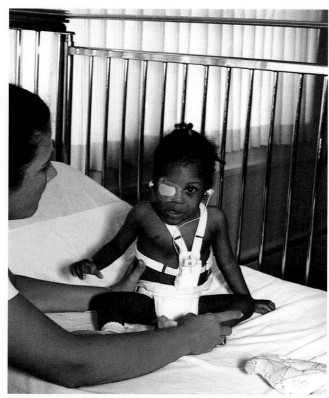

FIGURE 26-4 Many people are involved in the rehabilitation of this young child. Members of the interdisciplinary team, including the parent or caregiver, collaborate to assess, plan, implement, and evaluate the child's care.

custodial, and home care as their physical and financial needs change. For example, a client who no longer requires acute care will need to find an appropriate rehabilitation placement; a client whose private health insurance benefits are depleted needs to find alternate funding to continue the rehabilitation process. There are many stumbling blocks to successful community interventions. As the number of persons who survive traumatic illnesses and injuries grows, community health practitioners will become more and more critical to successful community reintegration.

EDUCATOR

The primary role of the rehabilitation nurse, whether in the inpatient, outpatient, or home setting, is that of client-family educator. The rehabilitation nurse helps the client and family learn new skills that must be applied continuously in all components of daily living. Common nursing diagnoses used by rehabilitation nurses in the care of clients appear in Box 26-5. Functions such as walking or speaking might be taken for granted, but when a person is forced by illness or injury to relearn these skills, the emotional stress is great.

Education should include how to prevent complications or further disability and how to promote healthy lifestyles and behaviors to minimize further problems. For example, paraplegics are prone to lower limb atrophy. The benefits of regular passive exercise in reducing or minimizing limb atrophy should be part of any education program for new paraplegics and their families.

Cindy Barson is a community-based rehabilitation nurse and a volunteer with the Multiple Sclerosis (MS) Society. She is asked by the director of the society to present an educational program to women with MS. Cindy knows that clients with MS develop physical limitations. She also knows that women with MS are at greater risk for osteoporosis and fracture than are women in the general population (Sharts-Hopki & Sullivan, 2002). Based on this knowledge, she develops an educational program for a group of women with MS that includes the following goals:

- Increasing their knowledge about osteoporosis
- Increasing their knowledge about the increased risk of osteoporosis associated with MS
- Helping them identify preventive measures to reduce the risk of osteoporosis
- Assisting them with a plan to consult their physicians to assess their own individual risk and develop appropriate preventive measures.

COUNSELOR

Often the diagnoses used with newly disabled people focus on their physical limitations and difficulties. Community-based rehabilitation nurses use additional diagnoses to focus on issues of community reintegration, including ineffective individual and/or family coping, noncompliance, health management deficit, and impaired thought processes. One of the most important areas to address is the emotional concerns of the disabled individual and family members who are the caregivers. Pryor (2008) advises nurses to understand that newly disabled people usually experience a period of grieving as they learn to deal with their physical limitations. One way to assist clients in that process is to emphasize the clients' positive areas of strength rather than just their limitations. Box 26-6 provides a list of areas helpful to nurses who employ this strategy.

For those family members who must adjust to caring for a person with a disability, emotional support and education are crucial. Hertzberg (2008) reports that family members perceive their task as daunting, and both physically and emotionally draining. A broad range of concerns have been expressed by relatives of persons with new disabilities (Smith & Testani-Dufour 2002; Verhaeghe et al., 2005). Their concerns include educational needs related to physical care assistance, disease or condition progression, availability of community resources, and future needs of the family member. Family members also express a need for information related to financial reimbursement and limitations imposed by insurance providers. They also desire emotional support and understanding in adjusting to their newly acquired responsibilities. All these areas should be part of counseling efforts for clients with chronic illnesses or disabilities and their families.

CASE FINDER

The role of the case finder is useful in locating clients who need help but are outside the health care system. Financial concerns may keep clients from receiving health care services and adhering to good health practices. Holding free health

---

BOX 26-5   Frequent Nursing Diagnoses for Rehabilitation

- Impaired physical mobility
- Self-care deficit
- Alteration in urinary elimination pattern
- Impaired skin integrity
- Alteration in bowel elimination pattern
- Potential for injury
- Knowledge deficit
- Impaired verbal communication
- Decreased activity tolerance
- Alteration in nutrition
- Alteration in thought process, memory
- Altered family process
- Social isolation
- Sleep pattern disturbance
- Independence/dependence conflict
- Diversional activity deficit
- Powerlessness/hopelessness

BOX 26-6   Strategies to Assist Coping with Disability

- Allow the client to talk about his or her disability.
- Maximize the wellness aspect.
- Build on the client's assets.
- Help the client compensate for limitations.
- Help the client cope with or modify negative environmental factors.
- Mobilize resources.
- Help identify social supports.
- Maximize the client's available energy.
- Promote healthy ego integrity.
- Encourage hope.

screening clinics is often helpful in locating persons with disabilities who are not receiving health care services. For example, a blood pressure screening clinic gives the nurse an opportunity to assess blood pressure *and* case-find clients with other physical, financial, and education needs. Community health nurses can speak about topics of rehabilitation and community reintegration to senior citizen centers, parent-teacher organizations, and support groups for survivors of devastating illnesses and injuries. The nurse should make a point of asking those present if they know of potential clients or families who are in need of rehabilitation services and should come prepared to follow up on any concerns.

CLIENT ADVOCATE

Often client frustration and difficulties stem from inadequate community resources, such as financially unattainable health care, lack of public transportation, or discriminatory attitudes. The nurse can advocate for accessible health care for all citizens.

> Jay Albert is a community-based rehabilitation nurse working as a case manager for a private social service agency. One of his clients, Alice Sumers, has muscular dystrophy. She wanted to visit her family in California, but discovered that the airlines were reluctant to transport her because of her physical limitations and need for assistive devices (Klemme, 2003). Ms. Sumers voiced her disappointment to Jay on one of his visits. Jay determined that Ms. Sumers was able to travel if the airlines would assist with her transfer to and from the airline seat, and provide additional storage for her power wheelchair. He contacted three airlines on behalf of Ms. Sumers and was able to convince one to allow her to travel. The airline agreed to transport Ms. Sumers if she had a medical clearance from her physician, booked a first-class ticket on a nonstop flight each way, and provided an able-bodied traveling companion. At the end of her 2-week trip, Ms. Sumers reported back to Jay that she had an enjoyable time.

There are no common denominators for the disabled population as a whole. Problems range from obvious physical limitations (loss of a limb or use of a wheelchair for mobility) to no visible sign of disability (such as cognitive deficits following a head injury). The nurse as advocate must have knowledge of current laws, especially those regarding financial entitlement, and existing support services. Nurses must also know what services are needed but unavailable. For example, a community health nurse may assist several persons with disabilities to form their own support group.

Formal mechanisms for advocacy, such as legislative lobbying and work through professional health care organizations, are excellent means for advocating for the rights of people with disabilities. Other sources of help for advocacy activities are government, voluntary, and professional organizations such as the Association of Rehabilitation Nurses (see Community Resources for Practice at the end of the chapter).

Day-to-day experiences also have the potential to suggest civil rights issues. For example, during a routine shopping trip a nurse may notice many barriers that restrict or prohibit the activities of disabled persons. Are there adequate parking facilities for the disabled at local shopping malls, grocery stores, churches, and schools? If so, are these parking spaces occupied by cars that do not have handicapped license tags?

Such vehicles should be reported to the facility's management immediately. Do public buildings advertise themselves as being accessible to people with disabilities but have heavy doors that are difficult to open, even by able-bodied persons? A wheelchair ramp to a doorway is useless if the doors cannot be opened by someone with limited upper body strength or coordination.

In their daily lives, health professionals should make it a practice to review the environment for barriers to persons with disabilities. A letter to management identifying such barriers will carry more influence if it contains not only a complaint but also a reference to applicable legislation and a statement that the writer is a health care professional.

COMMUNITY REINTEGRATION ISSUES

Wellness can be defined as being sound in body, mind, and spirit. It is an ongoing, dynamic process. Ultimate responsibility for wellness rests with the client. As the rehabilitation client adapts in and modifies the environment, the nurse must be aware of factors in the community that facilitate or inhibit successful community reintegration. Box 26-7 presents a guide for assessing health problems and barriers for persons with disabilities in the community. Access to health care, availability of physical and interpersonal resources, safety, attention to psychosocial concerns, and promotion of a barrier-free environment are essential for well-being.

Promotion of health among those with disabilities fosters optimal use of personal strengths and resources, and prevents further disability. New or existing resources must be evaluated for availability, accessibility, and acceptability. Community health nurses in rehabilitation can propose new services and modifications to existing ones.

> Bill, a 30-year-old construction worker, fell and sustained an injury resulting in an L4-L5 complete spinal cord injury. Following the acute care phase of hospitalization, Bill was transferred to the rehabilitation hospital in his community, where he worked with nursing, physical therapy, occupational therapy, and recreation therapy personnel. He and his family attended classes on spinal cord injury, learned to care for his physical needs, and participated in discharge planning to help with the transition to his home environment.
>
> As part of Bill's discharge plan (1) an assessment of his home was conducted by physical and occupational therapists to identify accessibility issues and plan renovations necessary for him to be independent at home, (2) a home health agency was contracted to provide nursing care as needed, and (3) an outpatient therapy center was scheduled to continue his physical rehabilitation. An employment assessment indicated that he would no longer be able to work at the same job. A workmen's compensation case manager was assigned to assist him. His case manager made a referral to the local vocational rehabilitation agency. Bill participated in vocational assessment and counseling and explored possible career choices. Bill wished to remain in the construction business. He received vocational training in drafting and attended the local community college for business classes. His vocational training included adaptive driving with hand controls so that he could drive himself to school and work.

| Box 26-7 | **Guidelines for Assessing Community Reintegration Needs of Persons with Disabilities** |

Access to Health Care

- Are health care facilities (inpatient and outpatient) and practitioners' offices architecturally accessible?
- Does the client have access to either private or public transportation that may be used by a person with his or her specific disability?
- Is telemedicine available?
- Are needed health care programs available? (Substance abuse treatment programs may not be accessible or available.)
- Are needed health care programs financially accessible?
- Are negative attitudes on the part of the client, family, or health care professionals prohibiting adequate health care? (Feelings regarding sexuality counseling or employment capability may have a major impact on community reintegration.)
- Does the client want to promote his or her own wellness?

Community Resources

- Are community resources financially, attitudinally, and architecturally accessible?
- Are the sources used credible?
- Does the client/family know how to locate and access resources? This may be a particular problem in a rural area in which resources and transportation may be limited.
- The telephone book may be a valuable resource for locating community resources. Does the client/family have the necessary reading and verbal skills to use this method?
- The Internet is a valuable resource for locating community and national resources. Does the client have access to the Internet? Does the client have the computer skills necessary to use the Internet? The public library often offers free Internet access and training.
- Is there a mayor's/governor's office on disability in the client's city/state?
- Has the rehabilitation team investigated community resources available in the client's environment and have they notified both the client and the resource agencies?
- Does the health care professional make it a point to network with key community resource personnel?

Safety

- Has the home been assessed for potential safety problems? The local fire department will often provide a free checklist and/or walkthrough.
- Do the client and family know how to assess workplaces, schools, and recreational areas for potential problems?
- Does the client have a plan in the event that he or she must summon help? (For example, how will a person with a communication disorder report an emergency situation over the telephone?)

- Has crime prevention been addressed? An individual using a wheelchair may be especially vulnerable to street crime.

Psychosocial Issues

- What role changes have taken place as a result of the client's disability?
- What are the financial resources and what effects do they have on wellness?
- If the person with a disability requires assistance with activities of daily living, are other members of the family unit feeling neglected by the caregiver?
- Is the caregiver given a chance to grieve? Is he or she devoting all energy to the person with the disability and in danger of compromising his or her own wellness?
- Has the family been assessed for adequate coping skills?
- Does the client have emotional as well as physical support systems?
- Are the developmental tasks of the client and family being addressed?

Promotion of a Barrier-Free Environment

- What attitudinal barriers exist in the client's environment? Are there feelings that individuals with disabilities cannot adequately work, attend school, or enjoy leisure activities?
- How is the client's sexuality viewed by himself or herself and others?
- Does the client have a negative outlook? Does he or she avoid interpersonal relationships or refuse to maintain wellness, look for a job, attend school, or interact with the health care system?
- Is there adequate housing for individuals with disabilities?
- Is there barrier-free public and/or private transportation?
- If the client requires 24-hour care, how are these caregivers located, evaluated, and trained?
- Are the client's place of worship, school, work setting, and shopping facilities accessible?
- What advocacy groups exist in the community? What barriers exist to these groups?
- Do health care providers have feelings that negatively influence their ability to provide adequate care for the disabled?
- Has the client/family been taught to plan ahead when going to a new setting for the first time? Are schools, restaurants, and stores assessed before using?
- What provisions are available for travel and vacations? Resources for traveling with a disability can be located on the Internet.

He received regular psychologic counseling to assist him with the transitions related to returning to work and school.

Over the next few years, Bill completed his business degree and training in computer-aided drafting. He returned to work full time for his previous employer. The company provided him with the reasonable accommodations he required to function independently in his wheelchair, for example, an extra handrail in the handicapped toilet stall and a lower-pile carpet in common traffic areas of the office. With the support of his family, community resources, rehabilitation team, and a cooperative employer, Bill was successfully reintegrated and adjusted well to his new disability.

Rehabilitation clients experience the loss of a variety of skills. Adults with disabilities, as well as the parents of an infant or child recently diagnosed with an impairment or disability, mourn the loss of full functioning. It is important that both the client and the family be given the opportunity to grieve. The nurse assists the client in acknowledging the loss, allows expression of grief, and provides information about the disabling condition. This support will foster realistic expectations and hope for the future. Throughout this chapter, barriers to community reintegration of the rehabilitation client have been identified. The community health nurse and the entire rehabilitation team should make every effort to accurately identify and reduce or eliminate barriers to the successful community reintegration of their disabled clients.

KEY IDEAS

1. Rehabilitation is a dynamic process that aids a person with disabilities in successfully achieving well-being and the highest level of function possible. This process must also involve successful community integration.

2. Society in general and health care professionals in particular have a long history of treating citizens with disabilities as second-class people. A key characteristic of any rehabilitation specialist is the belief in quality of life and the right of all persons to live satisfying, productive lives.

3. As the U.S. population continues to age, the demand for rehabilitation services in the community will continue to grow.

4. As a member of an interdisciplinary team, the community/public health nurse must have the ability to collaborate with a variety of health care professionals.

5. The nurse must be a client advocate, aware of legislation and community factors that affect the disabled person's ability to integrate successfully into the community.

6. A component of this advocacy role includes being able to assess barriers to wellness that affect both clients and their families.

7. Managed care affects the financial accessibility of services and the choice of providers for persons with disabilities.

8. One of the biggest barriers to successful rehabilitation is the possibility of a client's getting "lost" in the health care system. The rehabilitation client must be able to access the health care system, especially after returning home from an inpatient setting. The rehabilitation community/public health nurse must be aware of ways to keep the door to wellness open.

CASE STUDY Advocating for Rehabilitation Clients

A community health nurse is attending a small state university part time. She is working on a master's degree and has a particular interest in people with disabilities. On the first evening of class, she is surprised to find that the class has been moved from one building to another. The first location was close to the parking lot, next to the library, and a popular classroom setting for students and professors. The new location is a considerable distance from the parking lot and is referred to in a negative manner by most students and faculty. It is "too far from everything," parts of the building are still under construction, and the heating system is not working properly.

The nurse listens to her classmates grumble as they walk to the new building. It seems that one of the students uses a wheelchair, and the class had to be relocated to the newer, wheelchair-accessible building. She tries to point out that communities have an obligation to provide barrier-free academic settings, but no one really wants to listen. Most of the students in this business class are not health care professionals and are not happy about being inconvenienced. This class is an elective for the nurse, who hopes to enhance her budgetary skills. The nurse believes she will also have an opportunity to be a client advocate.

The disabled student is approximately half an hour late for class. She seems nervous and uncomfortable when she arrives. The professor comments that the class has undergone considerable inconvenience on her behalf, and she should plan to arrive on time in the future. The student is a paraplegic who must do wheelchair pushups several times an hour to relieve pressure on her sacrum. This causes several giggles from watching classmates and another comment from the professor about distracting the class. At break time, the disabled student wheels herself from the room in tears.

The nurse attempts to follow the student, but finds that there is no wheelchair-accessible bathroom on this floor. It is still being constructed. The only accessible bathroom is two floors down. The nurse finds the student, introduces herself as a nurse, and offers to assist her. She is surprised when the student angrily refuses her help with the comment, "You nurses don't understand what it's like to be this way!" The student does not return to class after the break.

The nurse approaches the professor privately and discusses the need for successful community reintegration. She points out the need for the wheelchair pushups and the importance of wheelchair-accessible bathrooms. The nurse may also share this information with her classmates. She should probably examine her own feelings in this situation, because she did not intervene until after the disabled student left the class in tears. For example, the nurse may also be feeling resentful at being inconvenienced.

The nurse has several options for action. He or she could contact the campus office responsible for implementing the ADA to report her observations and make suggestions. She might also involve some of her classmates in touring the campus and classroom building to identify barriers to wheelchair mobility. It is likely that some of them will continue to hold negative attitudes, but a practical, concrete illustration of barriers may be more effective than verbal arguments. She could also find out about the existence of advocacy groups for disabled persons on campus.

The nurse may help the disabled student gain access to appropriate assistance for community reintegration. This is a particularly difficult issue. The student has already refused assistance. If she does not return to class, the nurse may contact student health services and request that they attempt to contact the student. The student with the disability may benefit from help in planning her ADLs. She may need help in assessing new situations for potential barriers. If the student with the disability is not found, or if she continues to refuse assistance, the nurse cannot ethically pursue the matter. However, she can continue to work to promote a barrier-free environment in her academic setting.

The success of the plan does not depend totally on the ability of students and professors to acknowledge the barriers that are present and eliminate them. Realistically, the nurse must evaluate her impact on the academic setting by both long-term and short-term changes. If, as a result of this nurse's efforts on campus, awareness of the rights of persons with disabilities has been increased and acknowledged, then the nurse has been an effective client advocate. An important factor is the realization that nursing takes place in all settings and at all times with a variety of roles, not merely within the professional work setting.

See **Critical Thinking Questions** for this Case Study on the book's website.

LEARNING BY EXPERIENCE AND REFLECTION

1. As you go about your day, take time to imagine what life would be like if you used a wheelchair for mobility. Attend class, go shopping, and see a movie, all from the viewpoint of a person with a disability. What barriers did you encounter? How would you attempt to eliminate these barriers? How do you feel about living with a disability?

2. Visit a supervised living arrangement, such as senior housing or a group home. Identify the criteria for residency, the services available, and the home's ambiance. What nursing care is available and from whom?

3. Explore a supply store or catalogue that sells equipment for environmental adaptation and assistive devices for the disabled. Notice what equipment and devices are available, and their cost.

4. Participate with a rehabilitation nurse, physical therapist, occupational therapist, or vocational rehabilitation counselor as he or she makes an assessment and plans care.

5. Recall a time you felt uncomfortable in the presence of someone with a disability. Role-play alternative ways of relating to the person that emerge from different attitudes.

COMMUNITY RESOURCES FOR PRACTICE

Information about each of the following organizations can be found on its website, which can be accessed through this book's website at http://evolve.elsevier.com/Maurer/community/.

Access Abroad
ADA Information Line
Alliance for Technology Access
American Association for Health and Disability (AAHD)
American Heart Association
American Stroke Association
Association of Rehabilitation Nurses
Brain Injury Association of America
Christopher and Dana Reeve Resource Center
Commission on Accreditation of Rehabilitation Facilities
Consortium for Citizens with Disabilities
Developmental Disabilities Nurses Association
Disability Information and Resources
Disability Travel
Job Accommodation Network
Library of Congress National Library Service for the Blind and Physically Handicapped
Mobility International USA (MIUSA)
National Clearinghouse on Disability and Exchange (NCDE)
National Clearinghouse of Rehabilitation Training Materials
Disabled Sports, USA
National Institute of Arthritis and Musculoskeletal and Skin Diseases Information Clearinghouse
National Multiple Sclerosis Society
National Rehabilitation Information Center
National Stroke Association
Paralyzed Veterans of America
Spina Bifida Association of America
Special Olympics

STUDY AIDS   http://evolve.elsevier.com/Maurer/community/

Visit the Evolve website for this book to find the following study and assessment materials:

- Quiz
- Web Scenario
- Critical Thinking Questions and Answers for Case Studies
- Care Plans
- *Healthy People* Updates
- Glossary

REFERENCES

ADA Consultants. (1992). *What every rehab professional in the USA should know about the ADA*. South Miami, FL: Author.

Agency for Healthcare Research and Quality (2007). *Improving health care for Americans with disabilities*. U.S. Department of Health and Human Services. Retrieved July 11, 2007 from *http://www.ahrq.gov/news/focus/focdisab.htm*.

American Heart Association (2007). American Heart Association: Heart disease and stroke statistics. *Circulation, 115*, e69-e171. Retrieved May 4, 2007 from *http://www. Americanheart.org/*.

American Nurses Association & Association of Rehabilitation Nurses. (1988). *Rehabilitation nursing: Scope of practice, process and outcome criteria for selected diagnoses*. Washington, DC: American Nurses Association.

Association of Rehabilitation Nurses (2007a). *ARN facts*. Retrieved May 1, 2007 from *http://www. rehabnurse.org/about.index.html*.

Association of Rehabilitation Nurses (2007b). *ARN membership*. Retrieved May 1, 2007 from *http:// www.rehabnurse.org/membership/index.htm*.

Association of Rehabilitation Nurses (2007c). *ARN: What do rehabilitation nurses do?* Retrieved

May 1, 2007 from *http://www.rehabnurse. org/about/definition*.

Boylan, L. N., & Buchanan, L. C. (2008). Community-based rehabilitation. In S. P. Hoeman (Ed.), *Rehabilitation nursing: Prevention, intervention, and outcomes* (4th ed.; pp. 178-191). St. Louis: Mosby.

Brain Injury Association of America (2007). *A comparison of traumatic brain injury and leading injuries or diseases*. McLean, VA: Author. Retrieved July 7, 2007 from *http:// www.biausa.org/elements/aboutbi/factsheets/ TBIincidence.pdf*.

Brewer. L., Phillips, B. R., & Boss, B. J. (2002). Cardiac and cardiovascular rehabilitation. In S. P. Hoeman (Ed.), *Rehabilitation nursing: Process, application, and outcomes* (3rd ed.; pp. 723-748). St. Louis: Mosby.

Buchanan, L. C., & Neal, L. J. (2002). Community-based rehabilitation. In S. P. Hoeman (Ed.), *Rehabilitation nursing: Process, application, and outcomes* (3rd ed.; pp. 114-134). St. Louis: Mosby.

Center for an Accessible Society, (2007). *Supreme Court upholds ADA "integration mandate" in Olmstead decision.* Retrieved July 10, 2007 from *http://www.accessiblesociety.org/topics/asa/olmsteadoverview.htm.*

Centers for Disease Control and Prevention. (2001). Prevalence of disabilities and associated health conditions among adults—United States, 1999. *MMWR, 50*(7), 120-125.

Centers for Disease Control and Prevention. (2003). Public health and aging: Hospitalization for stroke among adults aged >65 years—United States, 2000. *Morbidity and Mortality Weekly Report, 52*(25), 586-589.

Centers for Disease Control and Prevention. (2006a). Environmental barriers to health care among persons with disabilities—Los Angeles County, California, 2002-2003. *Morbidity and Mortality Weekly Report, 55*(48), 1300-1303.

Centers for Disease Control and Prevention. (2006b). Prevalence of doctor-diagnosed arthritis and arthritis–attributable activity limitations—United States, 2003-2005. *Morbidity and Mortality Weekly Report, 55*(40), 1089-1092.

Centers for Disease Control and Prevention. (2006c). Brain injury awareness month—March 2006. *Morbidity and Mortality Weekly Report, 55*(8), 201.

Centers for Disease Control and Prevention (2006d). *Monitoring developmental disabilities.* Retrieved July 11, 2007 from *http://www.cdc.gov/ncbddd/dd/ddsurv.htm.*

Centers for Disease Control and Prevention. (2006e). *Facts about traumatic brain injury.* Atlanta: Author.

Centers for Disease Control and Prevention. (2006f). Incidence rates of hospitalization related to traumatic brain injury—12 states, 2002. *Morbidity and Mortality Weekly Report, 55*(8), 201-204.

Centers for Disease Control and Prevention. (2006g). *Summary health statistics for U.S. adults: National Health Interview Survey, 2005* (Vital and Health Statistics Series 10, No. 232). Hyattsville, MD: National Center for Health Statistics.

Centers for Disease Control and Prevention. (2006h). Prevalence of doctor-diagnosed arthritis and arthritis-attributable activity limitation—United States, 2003-2005. *Morbidity and Mortality Weekly Report, 55*(40), 1089-1092.

Cohen, E., & Cesta, T. (2005). *Nursing case management from essentials to advanced practice application* (4th ed.). St. Louis: Mosby.

Craven, G. T., & Gleason, C. A. (2002). Legislation and policy. In S. P. Hoeman (Ed.), *Rehabilitation nursing: Process, application, and outcomes* (3rd ed.; pp. 37-44). St. Louis: Mosby.

Disability Policy Seminar. (2007). Fact sheet: Community Living Assistance Services and Supports Act (CLASS Act). Presented at the 2007 Disability Policy Seminar: New Congress, New Opportunities, Washington, March 4-6, 2007, hosted by ARC of the United States, American Association on Intellectual and Developmental Disabilities, Association of University Centers on Disabilities, United Cerebral Palsy, and National Association of Councils on Developmental Disabilities.

Duchene, P. M. (2008). Sexuality education and counseling. In S. P. Hoeman (Ed.), *Rehabilitation nursing: Prevention, intervention, and outcomes* (4th ed.; pp. 560-585). St. Louis: Mosby.

Dufour, L., Williams, J., & Coleman, K. (2000). Traumatic injuries: Traumatic brain and spinal cord injury. In P. A. Edwards (Ed.), *The specialty practice of rehabilitation nursing: A core curriculum* (4th ed.; pp. 189-210). Glenview, IL: Association of Rehabilitation Nurses.

Fiscella, K., & Williams, D. R. (2008). Health disparities based on socioeconomic inequities: Implications for urban health care. In C. Harrington & C. L. Estes (Eds.), *Health policy: Crisis and reform in the U.S. health care delivery system* (5th ed.; pp. 49-60). Sudbury, MA: Jones & Bartlett.

Gender, A. R. (2008). Administration and leadership. In S. P. Hoeman (Ed.), *Rehabilitation nursing: Prevention, intervention, and outcomes* (4th ed.; pp. 124-145). St. Louis: Mosby.

Hertzberg, D. L. (2008). Rehabilitation nursing care of people with intellectual/developmental disabilities. In S. P. Hoeman (Ed.), *Rehabilitation nursing: Prevention, intervention, and outcomes* (4th ed.; pp. 610-631). St. Louis: Mosby.

Hoeman, S. P. (2008). History, issues, and trends. In S. P. Hoeman (Ed.), *Rehabilitation nursing: Prevention, intervention, and outcomes* (4th ed.; pp. 1-13). St. Louis: Mosby.

Job Accommodations Network (2003). *JAN Accommodation benefit/cost data.* Retrieved November 25, 2003 from *http://www.jan.wvu.edu/medou/stats/bencosts0799.html.*

Job Accommodations Network (2005). *JAN workplace accommodations: Low cost, high impact* (Fact Sheet Series). Retrieved May 4, 2007 from *http://www.jan.wvu.edu/media/LowCostHighImpact.doc.*

Kaye, H. S. (2003). *Improved employment opportunities for people with disabilities.* San Francisco: University of California, Institute for Health and Aging, Disability Statistics Center.

Kessler, R. C., Chiu, W. T., Demler, O., et al. (2005). Prevalence, severity, and comorbidity of 12-month DSM-IV disorders in the national comorbidity survey replication. *Archives of General Psychiatry, 62*(6), 617-627.

Klemme, K. L. (2003). Transportation of a client with muscular dystrophy on commercial air: A unique setting for a rehabilitation nurse. *Rehabilitation Nursing, 28*(2), 40-41.

LaPlante, M. P., Miller, S., & Miller, K. (1992, May). People with work disability in the U.S. *Disability Statistics Abstract,* No. 4. Washington, DC: U.S. Department of Education, National Institute on Disability and Rehabilitation Research.

Lee-Feldstein, A., Feldstein, P. J., & Buchmueller T. (2002). Health care factors related to stage at diagnosis and survival among Medicare patients with colorectal cancer. *Medical Care, 40*(5), 359-361.

McCollum, P. L. (2008). Case management. In S. P. Hoeman (Ed.), *Rehabilitation nursing: Prevention, intervention, and outcomes* (4th ed.; pp. 192-199). St. Louis: Mosby.

National Spinal Cord Injury Association (2007). *More about spinal cord injury.* Accessed July 7, 2007 from *http://www.spinalcord.org/html/factsheets/spinstat.php.*

Parker, B. J. (2000). Community and family-centered rehabilitation nursing. In P. A. Edwards (Ed.), *The specialty practice of rehabilitation nursing: A core curriculum* (4th ed.; pp. 17-41). Glenview, IL: Association of Rehabilitation Nurses.

Pryor, J. (2008). Patient and family coping. In S. P. Hoeman (Ed.), *Rehabilitation nursing: Prevention, intervention, and outcomes* (4th ed.; pp. 448-474). St. Louis: Mosby.

Rosen, E., & Fox, I. G. (1972). *Abnormal psychology.* Philadelphia: W. B. Saunders.

Rusk, H. (1972). *A world to care for.* New York: Random House.

Russel, H. (1973). *Affirmative action for disabled people.* Washington, DC: U.S. Government Printing Office.

Secrest, J. A. (2000). Rehabilitation and rehabilitation nursing. In P. A. Edwards (Ed.), *The specialty practice of rehabilitation nursing: A core curriculum* (4th ed.; pp. 2-15). Glenview, IL: Association of Rehabilitation Nurses.

Sharts-Hopki, N. C., & Sullivan, M. P. (2002). Beliefs, perceptions, and practices related to osteoporosis risk reduction among women with multiple sclerosis. *Rehabilitation Nursing, 27*(6), 232-236.

Smith, M. S., & Testani-Dufour, L. (2002). Who's teaching whom? A study of family education in brain injury. *Rehabilitation Nursing, 27*(6), 209-214.

Spears, J. (1990). Legislative department. *Rehabilitation Nursing, 15*(2), 98.

Spinal Cord Injury Information Network (2006) *Facts and figures at a glance—June 2006.* Retrieved July 12, 2007 from *http://www.spinalcord.uab.edu/show.asp?durki=21446.*

Stoddard, S., Jans, L., Ripple, J. M., et al. (1998). *Chartbook on work and disability in the United States, 1998*. Washington, DC: U.S. National Institute on Disability and Rehabilitation Research.

Sultz, H. A., & Young, K. M. (2004). *Health care USA: Understanding its organization and delivery* (4th ed.). Sudbury, MA: Jones & Bartlett.

U.S. Bureau of the Census. (2005). *American Community Survey*. Retrieved March 5, 2007 from *http://factfinder.census.gov/servlet/STTable*.

U.S. Bureau of the Census. (2006). *Americans with disabilities: 2002* (Current Population Reports, P70-107). Washington, DC: U.S. Department of Commerce.

U.S. Congress, House (2007). *Community Choice Act of 2007*. House Resolution 1621. 110th Congress, 1st session. Published in the Congressional Record, House of Representatives, March 21, 2007. Retrieved April 24, 2008 from *http://www.thomas.gov/cgi-bin/query/D?r110:12:.temp/~110N8sWrS*.

U.S. Department of Education. (1988). *Summary of existing legislation affecting persons with disabilities*. Washington, DC: U.S. Government Printing Office.

U.S. Department of Health and Human Services. (2002). *Health, United States 2002*. Washington, DC: U.S. Government Printing Office.

U.S. Department of Health and Human Services. (2006a). *Health USA 2006*. Washington, DC: U.S. Government Printing Office.

U.S. Department of Health and Human Services. (2006b). *Healthy people 2010: Midcourse review*. Washington, DC: U.S. Government Printing Office.

U.S. Department of Health and Human Services (2007). *Health highlights: April 11 2007: Groups demand end to two-year Medicare wait for disabled people*. Office of Minority Health. Retrieved July 11, 2007 from *http://www.omhrc.gov/templates/news.aspx?ID=603614*.

Van de Bittner, S. (1987). Reintegration of the client into the community. In C. Mumma (Ed.), *Rehabilitation nursing: Concepts and practice, a core curriculum* (2nd ed.; pp. 1-25). Evanston, IL: Rehabilitation Nursing Foundation.

Verhaeghe, S., Defloor, T., & Grypdonck, M. (2005). Stress and coping among families of patients with traumatic brain injury. *Journal of Clinical Nursing, 14*(8), 1004-1012.

Wadhwa, S., & Lavizzo-Mourey, R. (1999). Do innovative models of health care delivery impact quality of care for selected vulnerable populations? A systematic review. *Journal of Quality Improvement, 25*(8), 408-421.

Wallace, S. P., Avel, E. K., Stefanowicz, P., et al. (2001). Long term care and the elderly population. In R. M. Anderson, T. H. Rice, & G. F. Kominski (Ed.), *Changing the U.S. health care system: Key issues in health services, policy, and management* (pp. 205-223). San Francisco: Jossey-Bass.

World Health Organization (2007). *Concept paper: World report on disability and rehabilitation*. Retrieved May 4, 2007 from *http://www.who.int/disabilities/care/en/*.

SUGGESTED READINGS

Alexander, T. T., Hiduke, R. J., & Stevens, K. A. (Eds.). (1999). *Rehabilitation nursing procedure manual* (2nd ed.). New York: McGraw-Hill.

Association of Rehabilitation Nurses. (2000). *Standards and scope of rehabilitation nursing practice*. Glenview, IL: Author.

Center for Functional Assessment Research, Department of Rehabilitation Medicine. (1990). *Guide for use of the uniform data set for medical rehabilitation including the Functional Independence Measure (FIM)*. Buffalo: State University of New York.

Edwards, P. (Ed.). (2000). *The specialty practice of rehabilitation nursing: A core curriculum* (4th ed.). Glenview, IL: Association of Rehabilitation Nurses.

Hoeman, S. (Ed.). (2008). *Rehabilitation nursing practice: Prevention, intervention, and outcomes* (4th ed.). St. Louis: Mosby.

Modrein-McCarthy, M. A., & McGuire, S. L. (1997). Keeping current: Ten important information resources to help rehabilitation nurses. *Rehabilitation Nursing, 22*(2), 88-92.

Watson, P. (1990). The Americans with Disabilities Act: More rights for people with disabilities. *Rehabilitation Nursing, 15*(6), 325-328.

27 Children in the Community

Anne Rath Rentfro

FOCUS QUESTIONS

What are common health care needs of children from birth through adolescence?

Who are the children "at risk" who require community/public health nursing interventions?

What is the impact of poverty on child health?

What is the role of the community/public health nurse in caring for a child with special health care needs?

What community resources are available to promote the health of children?

How do the various health care funding programs affect the community/public health nurse's role with children?

CHAPTER OUTLINE

Children in the United States
 Demographics
 Impact of Poverty on Child Health
 Legal Parameters Guiding the Care of Children
 History of Community Health Care for Children
 Financing Health Care for Children
Families and Communities with Children
 Children and Their Family Constellations

Developmental Tasks of Families
Cultural/Ethnic Influences on Health Care
Common Health Needs of Children
 Health Promotion/Disease Prevention
 Environmental Safety
 Psychosocial Wellness
Children at Risk
 Biophysical Risk Factors

Environmental Risk Factors
Support Services
Community Health Care for Children with Special Needs
 Specific Conditions Requiring Home Care
 The Child Requiring Use of a Ventilator
Community/Public Health Nursing Responsibilities
Trends in Child Health Services

KEY TERMS

CHILDREN IN THE UNITED STATES

Children have unique needs and health concerns. Community/public health nurses whose practice includes families and children need to be aware of the special needs and health risks of children in the United States.

DEMOGRAPHICS

In 2005 there were more than 73 million children under the age of 18 in the United States, representing approximately 25% of the population. Approximately 58% of American children are non-Hispanic white, 20% are Hispanic, 15% are black, 4% are Asian/Pacific Islander, and 1% are American Indian/Alaska Native (U.S. Census Bureau, 2004).

More than 17% of children (12.3 million) less than 18 years of age live in poverty in the United States (Nilsen, 2007). More than 34.2% of African American children and 27.7% of Hispanic children live in poverty, compared to 9.5% of white children (Nilsen, 2007). Forty-three percent of children from single-parent households live in poverty (*Child Trends DataBank—Children in Poverty,* 2006). Children living in homes with female householders and no spouse present are particularly vulnerable to poverty because women earn less than men, and because there is only one adult wage earner in the family.

IMPACT OF POVERTY ON CHILD HEALTH

Low household income is consistently associated with poor health (see Chapter 21). **Poverty** (that is, inadequate food, clothing, and shelter) negatively affects children's health and well-being in a number of ways. Death rates are higher for poor children, who are more likely to be born prematurely or at low birth weight. Depression and conduct disorders occur more often, and violence is commonly encountered. Chronic health problems, injuries, adolescent pregnancy, substance abuse, school failure, and school dropout are all more common in children who live below the poverty level (Bauman et al., 2006; Borders et al., 2007). Obesity and sedentary behavior are more likely to occur in poor children, with associations also noted among poverty, stress, and adverse health outcomes such as compromised immune systems (Nilsen, 2007).

Poor families focus on basic survival with crisis-oriented rather than preventive approaches to health. Barriers to health care services—such as unavailable transportation, high costs, geographic inaccessibility, cultural differences, inaccessible hours of operation, or lengthy eligibility processes—complicate health care delivery (Bauman et al., 2006; Shi et al., 2007). Eligible families often receive services from several sources such as Temporary Assistance to Needy Families (TANF) and Medicaid. Fragmentation of services, however, occurs with multiple agency involvement. Nurses play an important role in coordinating programs and ensuring services for families in need. Eight million children lack health insurance and most of them live in employed families (Kaiser Commission, 2007). Three out of every four of these children who are eligible for assistance are not enrolled (Hoffman, 2007; Kaiser Commission, 2007).

LEGAL PARAMETERS GUIDING THE CARE OF CHILDREN

Because children are minors, parents or guardians make legal decisions for them. Guardians act as protectors and should advocate for the child's best interests. Faced with multiple family constellations and potential health care situations, the legal system in most states clarifies who makes decisions for the child (see Chapter 6). State laws determine legal age, which is closely related to chronological age rather than maturational or mental age (see Chapter 6).

General policies, often set by state legislation, categorize and label children based on preset criteria, which are often based solely on age (Tillett, 2005). For example, the age that children enter public school is legislated on the basis of age rather than developmental readiness for school. An example of a situation where policy is not strictly aligned with age alone is that of the emancipated minor. An **emancipated minor** is an adolescent who is legally under-age, but recognized legally as an adult under circumstances prescribed by state law. Situations resulting in emancipation vary from state to state, but usually include pregnant female adolescents, high school graduates, married adolescents, military personnel, or adolescents living independently from their parents or guardians (Tillett, 2005). Some minors may consent to certain medical and surgical procedures without notifying their parents or guardians. The types of services vary but generally include treatment for sexually transmitted diseases (STDs), human immunodeficiency virus (HIV) counseling, contraceptives, pregnancy, drug and alcohol problems, outpatient mental health counseling, and emergency situations (Tillett, 2005).

Regardless of emancipation status, nurses can act as advocates to encourage their participation in decision making for children in health care. Health care providers and parents frequently make decisions for younger children. Community health nurses should, when possible, give children opportunities to express opinions about decisions that affect them. In addition, a child whose parents refuse lifesaving measures for that child based on religious practices has the legal right to petition the court. Nurses often present information about options to families; therefore knowledge about broadened options available to these families for adequate decision making is essential. For example, even the family may be unaware that some isolated protein preparations may be acceptable alternatives for people who have religious restrictions to transfusion (Sniecinski & Levy, 2007).

Community health nurses participate in the legal aspects of children's health in cases of child abuse or neglect (see Chapter 23). Some situations in which nurses encounter these issues are obtaining consent from minors for sensitive services, such as sexually transmitted disease (STD) treatment, family planning, or abortion services, or obtaining consent when parents or guardians refuse needed care for their child (see Chapter 6). Nurses who know local laws and maintain a relationship with child protective services become advocates for children in the community.

HISTORY OF COMMUNITY HEALTH CARE FOR CHILDREN

Since the 1880s, community health nurses assisted new mothers to care for their newborn children. This important role decreases high infant death rates and child neglect (Izzo et al., 2005; Kitzman et al., 2000; Olds et al., 2004). Postpartum home visits provide healthy childcare measures, including information about sanitation and nutrition, to new mothers to foster and maintain health. Outcome indicators using automated informatics such as the Omaha System indicate that public health nursing continues to provide positive outcomes (Monsen et al., 2006).

At the beginning of the 20th century, infection continued to kill many children. Sick children remained at home for care. Community health nurses played a vital role in infection control through home risk assessment, family education about infection control, and care of the sick. Nurses monitored quarantined families; however, lack of sophisticated medical technology led to death for many ill children. By the middle of the century, the focus of community health nurses expanded to include education about the growth and development of children. In 1932 the National Organization of Public Health Nursing identified family health as the primary focus for public health nursing practice (Edgecomb, 2001).

Before World War II, support services for children with significant disabilities were minimal. Some families institutionalized disabled children, while others cared for them at home without external resources to facilitate coping. In 1935 Title V of the Social Security Act authorized the Crippled Children's

Services (CCS) programs, later renamed the Title V Children with Special Health Care Needs (CSHCN) programs. This federal and state partnership provides funds for infrastructure development and direct care for children with special health care needs (Social Security Administration, 2006). In 1989 program enhancements included a focus on development of family-centered, community-based, and coordinated systems of care for special needs children.

By the late 1950s, immunization programs prevented many communicable diseases, resulting in a shift in emphasis to students with special needs. When possible, special needs children were placed in special classes in schools. Educational rights and services for children with disabilities changed dramatically with the 1975 enactment of Public Law (PL) 94-142, Education for All Handicapped Children Act. This law guaranteed *free* and *appropriate* education for all children with disabilities ages 6 through 21 years in the least restrictive environment. Subsequent amendments (PL 99-457 and PL 102-119) expanded eligibility to all children with disabilities from birth through age 21 (U.S. Department of Education, 2007).

Currently, the development and implementation of high-technology care have resulted in an entirely new population for community health nurses (Remke & Chrastek, 2007). The number of children surviving the perinatal period with significant impairment has grown rapidly with a corresponding rise in the need for programs to maximize human potential and minimize economic costs associated with such disability (Nolan et al., 2005). The **technology-dependent** or medically fragile child now challenges health care. Providing optimal care in the home, while promoting normal growth and development for these children in schools and communities, introduces new issues for nurses in the community (for example, community care for ventilator-dependent children [Carnevale et al., 2006; *Pediatrics,* 2005]).

In general, nurses' goals for community health today have changed minimally from those of 100 years ago. Goals continue to emphasize health promotion, disease prevention, and risk reduction for the child, the family, and the community. Techniques used and resources available to reach contemporary goals, however, are diverse and vary from one state to another. Nursing responsibilities in the community continue to be assessing the child and the family and planning interventions using appropriate resources.

FINANCING HEALTH CARE FOR CHILDREN

Access to health care is directly related to a family's ability to pay for that care (see Chapters 3 and 4). Children's health care may be financed by private insurance, Medicaid, the **State Children's Health Insurance Program (SCHIP),** state Title V CSHCN programs, or other sources, such as nonprofit organizations providing care to low-income families. Offering clear access to programs provides the basic foundation to reduce the number of uninsured children. It is estimated that three of four children who are eligible for SCHIP or Medicare do not access these funds (Kaiser Commission, 2001). Effective access measures include expanding eligibility requirements, developing outreach mechanisms, and reducing administrative barriers. Data indicate that when such measures are used, significant reductions (from 23% to 15%) in the number of uninsured children occur (Kaiser Commission, 2001; Pulcini, 2007).

Many children receive care through employer-based health insurance plans of their parent. Employers continue to increase employees' share of premium costs. Some employers limit health coverage solely to their employees, excluding families. For many families, cost of health insurance coverage becomes prohibitive (see Chapters 4 and 21). Coverage for needed services such as well-childcare and family planning, or specialized services such as long-term speech therapy for a child with cognitive or developmental delays, may be limited. **Managed care programs,** with limitations on choices and providers, is the form of employer-provided health insurance for most families. Managed care provides opportunities for better coordination of care, but concern develops about provider-client relationships and access to specialty care providers.

For those who cannot afford health care, federal service falls into two categories. One method uses grants to encourage the availability of specific health care services to specific populations, such as maternal and child health care services, immunization programs, community and migrant farm worker health centers, and physician services in underserved locations (Hoffman, 2007). The second method is the Medicaid program, which provides health care for the poor.

Many poor children receive care funded through the Medicaid program (Title XIX of the Social Security Act) (see Chapter 4). Medicaid, a form of health insurance for low-income and disabled individuals, is financed by federal and state funds. States administer the program, choosing to pay for services in various ways, most frequently through managed care plans or on a fee-for-service basis. Medicare enrollments experienced a sevenfold increase in the 1990s, which was attributed to the managed care movement. This improvement in access to care and cost control has stabilized in the past few years (Kaiser Commission, 2001).

An important component of the Medicaid program for children is the **Early and Periodic Screening, Diagnosis, and Treatment (EPSDT) program.** It is a separately mandated program serving children from birth to age 21. As with Medicaid, it funds but does not provide direct services. The goal of EPSDT is to ensure that all children enrolled in Medicaid receive a basic set of comprehensive services to promote health and identify and treat problems at early stages. EPSDT services follow a prescribed schedule and include well-childcare; immunizations; laboratory studies; **anticipatory guidance;** mental health, vision, dental, and hearing screenings; tobacco avoidance information; and treatment for any identified conditions. The EPSDT program is an excellent resource for serving low-income adolescents, who often are without health care.

In 1997 Congress passed legislation authorizing Title XXI of the Social Security Act, SCHIP. This program allows states to provide health insurance to children whose families are above the financial eligibility for Medicaid, either through expansion of the Medicaid program or development of a new children's health insurance program (Pulcini, 2007). States retain significant flexibility in establishing eligibility, subsidies, payment rates, and use of health plans, although the federal Health Care Financing Administration (HCFA) must approve each state's plan. The benefit package offered by the state must be at least equal to the level of typical commercial health insurance and includes preventive, primary, specialty, dental, and vision care. Although the SCHIP program has experienced successes, the state to state flexibility results in wide variations of uninsured children from the highest in Texas (20.4%) to the lowest in Massachusetts (5.6%) (Kaiser Commission, 2001). After protracted negotiations and several Presidential vetoes, SCHIP funding was continued through March of 2009.

Title V of the Social Security Act authorizes the state CSHCN programs (formerly called Crippled Children's Services) to provide care to eligible children with severe or chronic illnesses. States may set up specialty care networks and clinics or contract with providers to pay for care on a fee-for-service basis. Program names, eligibility requirements, and benefit packages may vary by state but often include specialty health care therapies, medications, equipment, and home health care.

In addition to public and private sources of health insurance, community-based, nonprofit agencies and clinics may provide care to children and families who have no other source of payment. These include community and migrant health care centers, charitable care programs, the Indian Health Service, and others. The community health nurse must become familiar with all potential sources of low-cost health care within the community.

FAMILIES AND COMMUNITIES WITH CHILDREN

CHILDREN AND THEIR FAMILY CONSTELLATIONS

Children live in almost every conceivable form of family constellation (see Chapter 12). Although most children's families consist of what would be considered the *nuclear family* that consists of husband, wife, and their children (adopted or natural), many experience an alternative family environment at some point during their childhood with fewer children living with married parents than in years past. Grandparents play a vital role in many homes. As divorces and remarriages increase, the number of children in *blended families* with stepparents, stepsiblings, and extra sets of grandparents also increases. These children must make adjustments when remarriage occurs. Blended or *reconstituted families* are the fastest growing family constellation (London & Fairlie, 2005).

In 2005, 68% of children younger than 18 years of age usually lived with both parents; however, 25% lived with only their mothers, and 6% lived with only their fathers. Marked differences exist across racial lines, with more white children living in two-parent homes than black or Hispanic children (American Community Survey, 2005).

Extended families, which include the nuclear family along with blood relatives or those related by marriage, play an important role in community health nursing (Musick & Mare, 2004). Today, children are often raised within an extended family with grandparents, aunts, uncles, and cousins. Extended families change the dynamics of nurses' interactions with children. For example, the teenage mother frequently lives with her mother, who may help care for the baby. Both caregivers should be included in well-baby care counseling. New teen mothers and more experienced grandmothers may differ in their learning needs. Some children live in multiple "families" that share common ownership of property and goods (communal families), and others are raised by same-gender couples (nontraditional families) (Perlesz et al., 2006).

Additionally, families with foster-care and homeless children require extensive community resources and support. Community health nurses locate, facilitate access, and coordinate care for these children and their families. Homeless and foster-care children typically have significant health care needs and are likely to be eligible for Medicaid and other community services. Nurses act as advocates, seek appropriate community sources, and coordinate care among multiple agencies (Musick & Mare, 2004).

DEVELOPMENTAL TASKS OF FAMILIES

Developmental tasks contribute to overall health in childhood. Children must accomplish physical, cognitive, and psychosocial tasks to progress toward maturity (Table 27-1). For example, sitting alone, walking, learning concepts of time and numbers, and development of trust and sense of self are tasks required for this progression. Families work to master a set of developmental tasks, as well. Developmental tasks of families involve interaction among family members rather than developmental tasks of the individual child. Family developmental tasks aim toward strengthening the family unit (Hockenberry & Wilson, 2006). Family developmental stages include aspects of physical requirements, cultural practices, and development of the family's values and aspirations (see Unit Three, Family as Client).

Duvall's eight stages for families based on age and school placement of the oldest child are generally accepted as the foundation for family development theory. Four stages affect families with children younger than 18 years of age: stages II through V. These stages include families with infants and toddlers (II), preschoolers (III), school-age children (IV), and adolescents (V). Critics of this model note that these stages were developed for two-parent families and are neither appropriate nor accurate for other family constellations, for families who have a child with a chronic condition, or for some cultural groups (see Chapter 10). Contemporary family structures extend well beyond the nuclear family. More than 25% of children live within a blended family structure. Single-parent, grandparent, and gay parent arrangements occur more commonly now than ever before. Values of affection and moral responsibility rather than biology alone bond contemporary families (Musick & Mare, 2004; Perlesz et al., 2006).

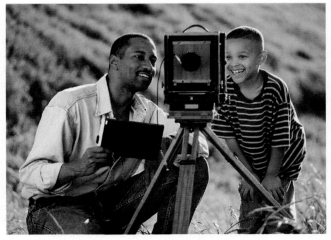

Son enjoys receiving a photography lesson from his father.

TABLE 27-1   Developmental Tasks for Infants and Children (Includes Physical, Psychosocial, and Cognitive)

	Age	Task
Infancy	3 months	Decrease in primitive reflexes except protective and postural reflexes
		Social smile (indicates development of memory traces)
	4 months	Laugh
	5 months	Birth weight doubles
		When prone, can push up on arms
		Rolls over
	6 months	Teething begins
		Sits with support
		Exhibits "stranger anxiety" (is wary of strangers and clings to mother)
	8 months	Sits alone
		Crawls
	9 months	Pincer grasp
		Holds own bottle
	10 months	Stands with support
	12 months	Birth weight triples
		Takes first steps alone
		Develops trust
		Speaks five words
		Claps hands, waves bye-bye
Toddlerhood	13 months-2.5 years	Masters walking
		Climbs stairs
		Feeds self (autonomy)
		Language (increases to 400 words and 2- to 3-word phrases)
		Toilet training and bowel and bladder control
		Separation anxiety (screams when the mother leaves)
School age	2.5-4 years	Increased vocabulary, uses sentences
		Alternates feet on steps
		Copies circles and lines
		Builds a tower of blocks
		Concepts of causality, time, and numbers begin
		Body image develops
		Role plays
		Enculturation begins
		Development of conscience begins
		Fears loss of body integrity
	5-12 years	Vision matures by age 6 years
		First baby tooth is lost at age 6 years; all permanent teeth except final molars are in by age 12 years
		Develops peer relationships
		Enjoy activities, groups, and teams
		Morality develops
		Cognitive development: concepts of time and space, reversibility, conservation, parts and whole
		Can classify objects in more than one way
		Reading and spelling and math concepts develop
		Puberty begins: age 9 years for girls; age 11 years for boys
		Sense of industry
Adolescence	13-19 years	Secondary sex characteristics develop
		Attains adult growth
		Adjusts to body changes
		Menses begin
		Abstract thought develops
		Develops an identity
		Fantasizes role in different situations
		Increased heterosexual interests
		Increased peer influences

Compiled from Selekman, J. (1996). *Pediatric nursing.* Springhouse, PA: Springhouse; Ball, J., & Bindler, R. (2002). *Pediatric nursing: Caring for children* (2nd ed.). Nowwalk, CT: Appleton and Lange; Wong, D. (2003). *Whaley and Wong's nursing care of infants and children* (7th ed.). St. Louis: Mosby.

Developmental tasks for the early childbearing family (stage II) include the development of parenting skills, new communication patterns, and tasks related to time and energy management. Parents and grandparents adjust to their new roles, and the infant is integrated into the family unit. Throughout this process, parents attempt to maintain and strengthen their marital bond (Hockenberry & Wilson, 2006).

Families often decide about the size of their family while their first child is at the preschool age. When 3- and 4-year-old children begin preschool, issues related to separation for both parent and child are manifested. Children commonly experience illnesses and illness often requires alternative care arrangements for working parents. Family stresses may stem from dealing with these issues. Children become socialized to their home values and cultural practices, whereas adult members of the family attempt to meet their own needs for privacy and make employment decisions. At this stage, children identify with the same-gender parent; therefore availability of an adult of the child's same gender is important.

Parents of school-age children adjust to influences of a third party (the school) on their child's life and must adapt to the impact of the child's peers and teachers. During this stage child's tasks center on school achievement, while parents continue to develop a satisfying marital relationship. Adolescents deal with increasing autonomy and independence, while parents return to their own marital and career issues along with concern for the older generation (Hockenberry & Wilson, 2006).

Because of the multiple variables that may interfere with these tasks, making generalizations are invalid. Adolescent's psychosocial developmental tasks may conflict with family developmental tasks. For example, the adolescent's psychosocial task to seek role identity may conflict with the family task to take responsibility for the needs of another human being.

Community health nursing is family health nursing. Nurses facilitate communication among family members and support families' endeavors to meet family and individual needs. Parenting is a learned skill rather than an innate one. Each developmental stage raises new issues and concerns for parents. As parents learn to address these issues, they grow along with their children.

CULTURAL/ETHNIC INFLUENCES ON HEALTH CARE

Community health care is culturally sensitive. The increasing diversity of our population challenges community health nurses to become or remain culturally competent (see Chapter 10). Home and community care must be appropriate and acceptable to the culture to be successful (see the *Ethics in Practice* box).

ETHICS IN PRACTICE

Cultural Differences

Gail A. DeLuca Havens, PhD, APRN, BC

The monthly immunization clinic is always busy. Since it opened 4 months ago, the number of new enrollees at this site in the eastern part of the city has continued to rise each month. It pays to advertise, thinks Martin, a pediatric nurse who practices at the Eastside Primary Care Center. No doubt providing immunizations at no cost, or for a nominal fee, is an influential factor too.

Martin enters an examination room to begin a visit with his next clients, 9-month-old twin infants and their preschool siblings, ages 3 and 4. Their mother, Mrs. Flores, converses in Spanish. Because all employees of the primary care center speak both English and Spanish, Martin is able to talk directly with Mrs. Flores. He learns that her native tongue is the language of the Ojibwes but that she has learned Spanish since her marriage.

Mrs. Flores has brought her preschoolers to the clinic to begin their routine immunizations. However, when asked about the twins, she refuses to give permission for their routine immunization series. When talking with Mrs. Flores, Martin learns that the mother's tribal beliefs include not "poisoning" babies with man-made medicines. She relates, also, that her neighbor's baby became very ill 2 months ago after receiving his first set of routine immunizations and that he is still "not right." Martin attempts to explain to Mrs. Flores that her twins are at greater risk without their routine immunizations. Without alarming her, he tries to impress upon Mrs. Flores that now is a particularly bad time to leave her twins unprotected because of the increase in confirmed cases of "whooping cough" in this section of the city during the past 3 months. He explains that the disease is very contagious and severe. Martin acknowledges that there are risks with immunizations as well but that the risks related to whooping cough far outweigh those associated with immunization (American Academy of Pediatrics, 2007).

Mrs. Flores disagrees that her babies are unprotected because she is breast-feeding them. She recounts the beliefs of her tribe about the physical and social misfortunes that befall members later in life who do not acknowledge, by their actions at the beginning of life, their belief in the protective power of the natural, traditional ways of nurturing the well and treating the sick. Because these actions fall to parents on behalf of their children, she is frightened for her babies' future well-being if she allows them to be immunized with "bad medicine" before they are 2 years old (Dodgson & Struthers, 2003). Martin acknowledges Mrs. Flores' confidence in traditional ways as being necessary and sound but tells her that her breast milk will not prevent her twins from getting "whooping cough" (Ahmann, 2005). Mrs. Flores is adamant, and after having her preschoolers immunized with the first series of vaccines, she leaves the clinic without the twins having been immunized.

What should Martin do? Should he simply document Mrs. Flores' refusal and file the twins' records, forgetting about the conversation? What, if any, obligation does Martin have to the twins? Should he continue to try to convince Mrs. Flores to have them immunized? If Martin chooses to follow up, how can he be most effective in working with Mrs. Flores to find a culturally acceptable approach to immunizing her babies?

If Martin decides not to follow up with Mrs. Flores and her twins, he would be practicing within the parameters of his position at the primary care center. His responsibilities do not include community outreach, only the provision of primary care to those who come to the center seeking it. Attempting, although unsuccessfully, to convince Mrs. Flores to accept immunizations for her twins has fulfilled his job-related obligation. In this situation, Mrs. Flores is acting on behalf of her children, the clients, when deciding against immunizations. In fact, the *Code of Ethics for Nurses* (American Nurses Association, 2001, p. 8) indicates that:

> Patients have the moral and legal right to determine what will be done with their own person; to be given accurate, complete, and understandable information in a manner that facilitates an informed judgment; to be assisted with weighing the benefits, burdens, and available options in their treatment, including the choice of no treatment; to accept, refuse, or terminate treatment without deceit, undue influence, duress, coercion, or penalty; and to be given necessary support throughout the decision-making and treatment process.

An alternative course of action is for Martin to follow up with Mrs. Flores and her twins. Although Martin respects the autonomy of the twins, as expressed by their mother, he is motivated to continue dialogue with Mrs. Flores. The Code describes the nurse's respect for the worth, dignity, and human rights of every individual (American Nurses Association, 2001). It does not qualify the nurse's respect by indicating that it applies only when the client is in the nurse's practice setting. Perhaps the twins will not contract pertussis before it is culturally acceptable for them to be immunized; however, given the growing incidence of pertussis in this part of the city, they could contract the disease and even be left with extreme and irreversible brain damage because of the hypoxia associated with prolonged coughing spasms (American Academy of Pediatrics,

2007). He believes that cross-cultural differences have resulted in conflicting views about how to prevent harm to the twins.

The American Nurses Association's *Code of Ethics for Nurses* (2001, p. 7) describes the need for health care as "universal, transcending all individual differences," which is Martin's specific interest in this situation. Recognizing the complex factors that influence behaviors surrounding states of health and illness within cultures is fundamental to competent nursing practice (Andrews & Boyle, 2003). Martin perceives it to be his personal responsibility to maintain competency in his practice. A consultation with colleagues practicing in the community should give Martin some insight into how best to approach Mrs. Flores. Perhaps they could identify people in the community who are culturally sensitive to Native American value systems and who might be willing to collaborate with him in approaching Mrs. Flores about the immunization of the twins or help him better understand her perspective. Enlisting the assistance of a respected member of a specific cultural community is often an effective strategy in negotiating over health beliefs with a client from that culture. In this situation, such action could be helpful to the twins, Martin, and Mrs. Flores.

REFERENCES

Ahmann, E. (2005). Tiger Woods is not the only "Cablinasian:" Multi-ethnicity and health care. *Pediatric Nursing, 31*(2), 125-129.

American Academy of Pediatrics, (2007). *2007 Immunization schedule released!* Retrieved May 22, 2007, from http//www.cispimmunize.org.

American Nurses Association. (2001). *Code of ethics for nurses with interpretive statements.* Washington, DC: American Nurses Publishing.

Andrews, M. M., & Boyle, J. S. (2003). *Transcultural concepts in nursing care.* Philadelphia: Lippincott Williams & Wilkins.

Dodgson, J. E., & Struthers, R. (2003). Traditional breastfeeding practices of the Ojibwe of northern Minnesota. *Healthcare for Women International, 24,* 49-61.

Child-rearing traditions vary. Breast-feeding, introducing solids, and toileting customs might have cultural influences (Hockenberry & Wilson, 2006). Family decisions about health and childcare differ from culture to culture. Knowing child care practices and identifying key family decision makers help nurses plan interventions that incorporate all persons responsible for childcare. Chapter 10 includes a broader discussion of the influences of culture. Expected behavior of children varies from one culture to another, as well (Leininger & McFarland, 2006). It is important for the community health nurse to determine how children are viewed in the community and what the expected age-related behaviors are for that culture.

COMMON HEALTH NEEDS OF CHILDREN

HEALTH PROMOTION/DISEASE PREVENTION

Private health insurance and governmental funding agencies are more frequently oriented toward the individual and treatment of preexisting conditions. They are not family oriented, nor do they focus on health promotion and disease prevention, except for selected health maintenance organizations (HMOs). Core functions for community health nursing include promoting health and preventing disease. In many communities, public health agencies provide these services. As health care reform initiatives continue, greater emphasis on health promotion and disease prevention may evolve. Community health nurses and the nursing

profession could provide the leadership necessary to promote health and disease prevention for families. Nurses can contribute to empiric research to evaluate cost savings evidenced by prevention measures and early interventions that decrease morbidity and mortality. When these efforts produce cost savings, health care insurers and managed care organizations are more likely to permit these preventive measures as standard protocol.

Screening, education, counseling, and anticipatory guidance facilitate health maintenance, health promotion, and wellness. Families with newborn infants have numerous health-promotion and primary prevention needs. Well-child care (e.g., bathing, feeding, holding, and diapering) and interpreting the communication cues of the infant are important for all new parents to know. In addition, parents are learning and adjusting to their new roles (Edelman & Mandle, 2006; Hockenberry & Wilson, 2006). Parents usually welcome community health nurses and eagerly solicit support and advice.

Parents need information about normal growth and development and how to promote physical, psychosocial, and cognitive development throughout childhood. Knowing what age-appropriate developmental tasks to expect, how to implement age-appropriate stimulation (Table 27-2), and how to handle the physical health problems common to young children (Table 27-3) help parents cope with the changes that occur. Community health nurses also help families recognize the importance of preventive health care (immunizations and

TABLE 27-2   Age-Appropriate Play Activities

Infancy—Interaction primarily between caregiver and baby	
Birth to 3 months	Rocking, cuddling, touching, massaging, singing, talking to infant: hanging brightly colored objects; looking in mirror; "people watching" Music, floor time with toys in reach
4 months	"Busy box" on the side of the crib or a "cradle gym" across the top to encourage reaching out
6 months	Toys, plastic cups, pot lids, spoons, clutch ball, squeaky toys, water and water play (always supervised)
9 months	Teething toys, toys that make noise when moved, boxes, large books, toys that can be pushed when crawling
12 months	Blocks, stacking cups, baby safe cars, dolls, books, singing, cuddling, reading
Toddler—Observes others at play but little cooperative play yet	Filling and dumping containers, stacking blocks, reading, singing, toys that can be carried, pushed, thrown, or dropped or can aid in walking
Preschool—Play becomes more interactive	Gross motor activities like riding a tricycle, playing ball, painting, stringing beads, arts and crafts, guessing games, puzzles, reading, fantasy play
School age— Play is a social experience	Collections, games, group activities, bikes, skates, sports, reading

Data from Bowden, V., Dickey, S., & Greenberg, C. (1998). *Children and their families: The continuum of care.* Philadelphia: W. B. Saunders.

well-child care checkups) to maintain their child's health and identification of problems at an early stage.

Community health nurses provide explanations of recommended immunization schedules and the diseases they prevent (see Chapter 8). Encouraging immunization of children not only prevents disease in the child but also protects communities. Community health nurses assess children's immunization status, and encourage parents to maintain current immunizations for their children. Immunization information changes regularly, requiring continuous updates for nurses.

Adjusting to parenting and the needs of children is not limited to families with newborns. As families deal with toddlers, school-age children, and teens, they need information about the physical, psychosocial, emotional, cognitive, safety, and nutritional needs of their children. By attending to the changes in their children as they develop, parents will be better prepared to prevent illness and accidents. Table 27-4 provides a list of health needs and other issues common to different age groups. Because risks and needs change with a child's age, continued education and support for parents is part of the community nursing role.

ENVIRONMENTAL SAFETY

A safe environment is a priority for young children. Nurses have the unique opportunity to directly assess homes for safety and

make prevention-focused recommendations to the family during home visits (Ehiri et al., 2006). Safety needs change as children grow and their mobility, dexterity, and curiosity mature. The nurse can help parents identify and alleviate risks in the home environment and community (McDonald et al., 2005). A list of suggested measures for home safety is provided in Box 27-1.

Entering a home to visit the family of a 6-year-old child who is ventilator dependent, the nurse notices the mother cleaning the floor. The family consists of a single mother, the 6-year-old child, and a 2-year-old. The nurse dialogues with the mother about how numerous household items, such as detergents for cleaning, can be dangerous to toddlers. The conversation centers on toddlers' inquisitiveness and the need for constant supervision. While reinforcing positive attributes of toddlerhood, the nurse gears the discussion toward accident potential based on developmental tasks that a toddler encounters. Toddlers explore their world with newfound mobility, challenging the family members' ability to keep them safe and provide constant supervision. Rather than restraining curiosity, mothers are encouraged to observe the toddler's novel approach to the world. Removing hazardous substances with emphasis on constant supervision is one strategy. Toddlers' creativity far surpasses the adults' capacity to anticipate hazards.

Accidents, particularly motor vehicle accidents, are the primary cause of death for children from 1 to 18 years of age (see Chapter 26). Most accidents occur in or near the home and can be prevented. Safety-proofing homes, as well as increasing supervision for infants, toddlers, and preschoolers, will decrease injury incidence. Assessing the environment for lead-based paint on windows, toys, old baby furniture; installation of gates across high-risk areas such as stairs; and keeping medications and toxic substances in their original containers out of children's reach in locked cabinets provide a safer environment. In addition to these interventions, using car seats and bicycle helmets significantly decreases vehicular mortality and morbidity.

For older children and adolescents, substance abuse and other high-risk behaviors influence the incidence of accidents and injuries. Effective risk-reduction interventions for school and the community provide straightforward information that incorporates peers whenever possible (Messias et al., 2006). High school students in groups (e.g., Students Against Drunk Driving) use peer pressure and peer education to reinforce the dangers of drinking and driving, as well as the need for seat belts (Delp et al., 2005; Emmons et al., 2005). Parents should be aware that they serve as role models with either positive or negative behaviors for these actions as well.

Homicide and suicide rates increase in the adolescent population and are correlated with the use of alcohol and illegal drugs. Teaching nonviolent conflict resolution along with increasing awareness of the association between weapons and risk of injury are strategies to address the issue of increased violence among adolescents (May et al., 2005; Piper et al., 2006) (see Chapter 23).

PSYCHOSOCIAL WELLNESS

Psychosocial wellness depends on emotional well-being, as well as physical health and safety precautions. Consistency in care promotes trust and a sense of control for young children. As children grow, their need to share their feelings with others

TABLE 27-3 Common Health Problems in Young Children

Problem	Comments	Interventions
Teething	Begins around age 6 months when lower central incisors arrive Molars arrive during toddlerhood Caries develop mostly during preschool and school age	Teething biscuits Hard teething toys Acetaminophen for irritability Use fluoride until age 12 Brush teeth from age 3 Prevention: annual dental checkups from age 5 Encourage brushing after meals
Bottle mouth syndrome	Results from sleeping with juice- or milk-filled bottle and having long-term contact between the nipple and the teeth	Give a bottle of water or have the child finish the bottle and take an empty or clean bottle to bed
Toddler does not begin to speak		Assess hearing Assess the amount that the child is spoken to at home
Iron deficiency anemia	Child's iron supply from birth is depleted by age 4 to 6 months	1. Begin iron supplements or iron-enriched foods at 4 to 6 months of age 2. Limit milk or formula intake to no more than 30 oz/day
Temper tantrums	Common and normal during toddlerhood Prevent by keeping routines simple and consistent; set reasonable limits; provide choices	1. Provide a safe environment during a tantrum 2. Help the child regain control; attempt distraction; remove the child to a neutral area until control is achieved 3. Do not reason, threaten, promise, or hit 4. Respond consistently
Streptococcal pharyngitis		Throat culture is needed to confirm Antibiotics are essential to prevent development of rheumatic fever or glomerulonephritis Treatment of a sore throat is dependent on age
Urinary tract infections	May be related to poor hygiene, fecal contamination, or sexual abuse	Assess for frequency, burning, foul-smelling urine, fever, irritability Refer for treatment with antibiotics Teach the child to wipe from front to back Avoid bubble baths Promote use of cotton underwear
Diaper rash		Change diaper frequently; clean skin with water at each changing and then dry skin well; avoid plastic coverings; use a thin layer of A&D ointment or zinc oxide; wash diapers thoroughly with mild soap and rinse well; expose diaper area to air if possible during the day
Constipation	Defined as hard consistency to the stools; not related to straining or grunting during defecation	1. Increase liquids in the diet 2. Add karo syrup (1 tsp to 3 oz of formula or milk) Increase fluid intake; use cool mist vaporizers; use a bulb syringe to remove nasal mucus; give acetaminophen
Upper respiratory infection	6 to 9 per year is normal	Refer for treatment with antibiotics and decongestants
Otitis media	The child may exhibit irritability, fever, and pulling on the ear lobe	

increases. Open lines of communication become most important to establish and maintain trust. Infants need warm, caring environments to develop trust. Hostile environments in which children receive little nurturing from consistent caregivers may lead to withdrawal (Vig et al., 2005). Toddlers begin to develop autonomy as they acquire and practice new skills. Safe and supportive environments that allow for growth promote positive self-esteem and self-confidence in children. Preschoolers begin to initiate activities, which leads to a sense of purpose and satisfaction. School-age children acquire reading, writing, math, and social skills, resulting in feelings of competence and enjoyment of learning (Hockenberry & Wilson, 2006). As adolescents move into their healthy adulthood they separate from family while maintaining emotional ties (Christie & Viner, 2005; Jenkins et al., 2005).

Community health nurses who teach parenting skills should emphasize the important roles that emotional support, encouragement, and listening have in child development, as well as the stages of appropriate development. Parents should initiate and encourage discussion of sensitive topics. Nurses can help parents and children role play sensitive conversations, such as those regarding sex education and clarification of values. Some

TABLE 27-4	**Selected Examples of Health Needs and Issues for Children and Adolescents**
Ages 1-5 years	Sleeping concerns (resistance to going to bed, night awakening, sleeping with bottle, nightmares and terrors)
	Eating concerns (decreased appetite, "picky" eating, food jags, pica)
	Behavioral concerns (distractibility, lack of control, demanding or aggressive behavior, biting, hitting, temper tantrums, breath-holding spells, impulsiveness)
	Emotional concerns (shyness, fears, separation problems, and anxiety)
	Speech or language concerns (shyness, fears, separation problems, and anxiety)
	Autism
	Undersocialization, few or poor peer relationships
	Infections, illnesses
	Baby bottle tooth decay
	Lead poisoning
Ages 5-11 years	School concerns (learning disabilities, underachievement, failure to do homework, frequent school absence or tardiness and school avoidance, lack of motivation)
	Behavioral concerns (hyperactivity, distractibility, disobedience, temper outbursts, lying, aggression, fighting, stealing, vandalism, fire setting, violence)
	Peer concerns (inability to get along with other children, shyness, lack of friends)
	Emotional concerns (separation problems, depression, anxiety, low self-esteem, threat of suicide)
	Risk-taking behavior (smoking, sexual activity, use of alcohol, drugs, or tobacco)
	Weight and height concerns (short stature, obesity, eating disorders)
Ages 11-21 years	School concerns (poor grades, underachievement, disinterest, truancy)
	Vocational concerns
	Behavioral concerns (disobedience, aggression, violence, homicide)
	Social concerns (lack of friends, negative peer influence, withdrawal from family)
	Emotional concerns (depression, anxiety, schizophrenia, confusion about sexual orientation, low self-esteem, threat of suicide, suicide)
	Early sexual activity, inappropriate sexual behavior, pregnancy, sexually transmitted diseases, infection with HIV
	Substance abuse (alcohol, drugs, tobacco, steroids)
	Poor safety behaviors (drunk driving, failure to use seat belts or helmets)
	Medical concerns (acne, myopia, scoliosis, problems with menstruation)

From Green, M., & Palfrey J. S. (Eds.). (2002). *Bright futures: Guidelines for health supervision of infants, children, and adolescents.* Arlington, VA: National Center for Education in Maternal and Child Health. Available online at www.brightfutures.org/.

BOX 27-1	**Safety Measures for Infants and Young Children**

Safety Measures for Infants
- Support the infant's head.
- Keep the crib rails up.
- Do not place pillows in the crib.
- Never leave an infant unattended on the dressing table.
- Do not prop bottles.
- Use bumper pads in the crib.
- Use approved car seats.
- Never leave an infant unattended in the bathtub.
- No pins, plastic, or small objects should be present in a child's environment.
- No hanging electrical cords should be present in a child's environment.
- No bean bag toys should be present in a child's environment.

Safety Measures for Toddlers
- Put safety plugs in all electrical outlets.
- Place gates across stairways.
- Lock cabinets for medication and cleaning agents and poisons; keep poisons in original containers.
- Do not keep any dangerous plants in the child's environment.
- When the child begins to climb over the crib rails, it is time for the child to have a bed.

- Pot and cup handles should be positioned away from the edges of the table or the stove.
- Keep medication in child-proof containers and out of reach.
- No toys with sharp edges or small parts should be present in a child's environment.
- Reinforce that pills are not candy.
- No peanuts or popcorn should be present in a child's environment.

General Environmental Safety
- Decrease cigarette smoke in the child's environment.
- Remove lead paint on windows, toys, or furniture.
- Decrease use of powder or aerosols in the child's environment.
- Install screens in the windows.
- Clear play areas of debris.
- Ensure food storage is appropriate for the foodstuffs.
- Damp dust the child's environment.
- Keep insect and rodent traps and poisons out of the reach of children.
- Install smoke detectors.
- Keep matches out of the reach of children.
- Keep guns out of the reach of children.

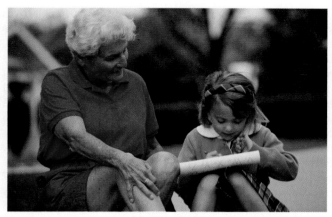

Granddaughter practices writing the alphabet under the watchful eye of her grandmother. Grandparents are increasingly playing a more important role in the lives of their grandchildren, often providing after-school or full-time baby-sitting or permanent custodial care.

nurses may be uncomfortable with these topics and may need to practice with their colleagues before attempting parental interventions (Christie & Viner, 2005).

Adolescence is a time of growing independence, with less reliance on parents, greater influence of peers, and exposure to a variety of hazards. As such, this is often a time of significant anxiety for parents. Communication is the key to enhancing a strong family system for the family with adolescents. Community health nurses should encourage parental/adolescent communication that includes promoting communication, providing information about sexuality, explaining risks involved with substance use, and promoting automobile safety. Quality mental health for teenagers is an essential, but frequently unavailable resource. Freedom within age-appropriate limits, support, and authoritative rather than punitive relationships cultivate higher self-esteem in children and adolescents (Christie & Viner, 2005).

Adolescents benefit from a family that stays available to them in times of crisis and for problem solving. Parents benefit from suggestions about how to help children develop a positive self-image. Empowering parents to set limits for their children and to check whether responsible adults are present when their children visit others is appropriate. Encouraging parents to share their concerns empowers families to work through their frustrations in a positive way. With the increased number of working parents, time to discuss their child-rearing issues with others may be limited. Attending school, clubs, or other group meetings where adolescents and their parents gather facilitates communication with other parents.

Adolescents frequently share information with nurses that they will not want to share with their parents; therefore separate interview time should be arranged. Adolescents may seek information and counseling about birth control, HIV, other sexually transmitted diseases, and abortion, or they may share concerns regarding school, peer relationships, or other difficult issues. Nurses should provide information to promote healthy behaviors with a nonjudgmental approach that is appropriate for both age and culture. Whenever possible, nurses should encourage adolescents to share health concerns with their parents. Community health nurses frequently act as a bridge for communication between the parents and the child (Hockenberry & Wilson, 2006).

Dolores Coronado, a family nurse practitioner, has worked at an urban clinic serving a predominantly Mexican American population. Many adolescents who visit the clinic for gynecologic problems are first-generation children of Mexican parents. The parents hold traditional values of their heritage. The adolescents often share concerns with Dolores about conflicts with their parents about their sexuality. Recently, a 15-year-old client confided in Dolores that she and her boyfriend have been sexually active and that she thought she was pregnant. After the pregnancy was confirmed, the adolescent shared her concern about what her parents would think if they found out that she had been to the clinic for an appointment. Dolores took the opportunity to allow the adolescent to express her fears about talking to her parents. Using the strategy of role playing, Dolores guided her through a simulated interaction that mimicked a potential interchange with her parents. During this role playing, Dolores and the young woman were able to pursue issues related to sexuality and health promotion for adolescents. By the end of the appointment, the young woman verbalized that she was more confident about approaching a conversation with her parents.

One important concern for children of all ages is exposure to violence. Some children may be directly exposed to family, school, or neighborhood violence. Furthermore, entertainment media (e.g., movies, television) and news venues (e.g., school shootings, acts of terrorism) expose children to violence. Health care personnel who care for children should be alert to children's violence-related concerns (*Pediatrics*, 2006). For additional discussion of children and violence, see Chapters 23 and 30.

CHILDREN AT RISK

Biophysical situations, psychologic conditions, or environmental situations place children at risk for alterations in physical, cognitive, or psychosocial development. Many factors might place a child at risk, but even a single factor could produce developmental problems. Assessment and early intervention are important elements in the quest to limit a child's risk.

BIOPHYSICAL RISK FACTORS
Infants and Young Children

Risks from biophysical situations can occur before, during, or after the birth of the infant. These risks include tobacco, drug, and alcohol use by the mother before and during the pregnancy, congenital and chromosomal anomalies, central nervous system deficits, prematurity, and serious illness during early infancy. Approximately 12,000 infants (1 to 2 per 1000 live births) are born annually with fetal alcohol syndrome spectrum disorders (Centers for Disease Control and Prevention [CDC], 2005). See Figure 24-4 for a photograph of a child born with fetal alcohol syndrome. Approximately 4% of pregnant woman ages 15 to 44 years report using illicit drugs (Substance Abuse and Mental Health Services Administration, 2006).

In 2005 the Centers for Disease Control and Prevention (CDC) identified approximately 600 new cases of HIV/AIDS in individuals younger than 20 years of age, three fourths of whom are between the ages of 15 and 19 (CDC, 2007d). More than 10,000 children under age 14 are infected with HIV with 90% of the cases acquired perinatally (CDC, 2007d).

The number of children who survive neonatal drug withdrawal, serious conditions related to prematurity, chronic childhood illnesses, and many childhood concerns has increased. In addition, more children are diagnosed with learning disabilities, autism, and attention-deficit hyperactivity disorder than ever before (Hack et al., 2005). Advances in medical science save some children who would have died from their conditions only a few years ago. The result is an increased prevalence of chronic conditions, such as premature infants who develop bronchopulmonary dysplasia (Donn & Sinha, 2006). These children risk dependence on oxygen or assisted ventilation in childhood, increasing the possibility of chronic respiratory problems for life.

Infant Mortality Rate and Causes of Death. Infant mortality rates provide an indicator of the health status of a community, a state, or the nation. Infant mortality is defined as death that occurs during the first year of life. The *Healthy People 2010* objectives set a goal to reduce mortality rates to 4.5 per 1000 live births (U.S. Department of Health and Human Services, 2006). The U.S. infant mortality rate in 2004 was 6.78 per 1000 live births, compared to 6.84 in 2003 (Mathews & MacDorman, 2007). Infant mortality rates continue to drop for all racial/ethnic groups, yet health disparities remain. The mortality rate is highest for babies born to non-Hispanic black mothers (13.6 per 1000 births). In other groups, mortality rates are lower, but vary by race or ethnic background. For example, the mortality rate for infants of Puerto Rican mothers is 7.8 per 1000; for Cuban mothers the rate is 4.6; and for Asian and Pacific Islander mothers, 4.7 (Mathews & MacDorman, 2007). Although neonatal mortality rates are declining, infants with very low gestational ages and birth weights continue to influence U.S. infant mortality more than any other group (Mathews & MacDorman, 2007).

■ HEALTHY PEOPLE 2010 ■
Objectives for Children

1. Reduce the infant mortality rate to no more than 4.5 per 1000 live births. (Baseline: 7.2 in 1998.)
2. Reduce low birth weight to no more than 5% of live births and very low birth weight to no more than 0.9% of live births. (Baseline: 7.6% and 1.4%, respectively, in 1998.)
3. Reduce the fetal death rate (20 weeks or more of gestation) to no more than 4.1 per 1000 live births plus fetal deaths. (Baseline: 6.8 per 1000 live births plus fetal deaths in 1997.)
4. Increase to at least 90% the proportion of all pregnant women who begin prenatal care in the first trimester of pregnancy. (Baseline: 83% of live births in 1998.)
5. Reduce the rate of child deaths.

	Target Goal	1998 Rate per 100,000
Children ages 1 to 4 years	20	34.1
Children ages 5 to 9 years	13	17.2

6. Reduce the occurrence of developmental disabilities arising from events in the prenatal and infant periods.

Developmental Disability	Target Goal	1991-1994 Rate per 10,000
Mental retardation	124.5	131
Cerebral palsy	31.6	33.3

7. Ensure appropriate newborn bloodspot screening and follow-up. (Developmental: no current baseline.)

Specific Health Risks or Prevention Areas
Iron Deficiency

8. Reduce iron deficiency to 5% or less among children ages 1 and 2 years, and to less than 1% among children ages 3 and 4 years. (Baseline: 9% of children ages 1 and 2 years; 4% of children ages 3 and 4 years from 1988 to 1994.)

Blood Lead Levels

9. Eliminate elevated blood lead levels in children. (Baseline: 4.4% of children ages 1 to 5 years had blood lead levels exceeding 10 mcg/dl during 1991 to 1994.)

Asthma

10. Reduce asthma death rate to no more than 0.9 per million children ages 5 to 14 years. (Baseline: 3.1 per million for children ages 5 to 14 years in 1999.)
11. Reduce emergency department visits for asthma to no more than 80 per 10,000 children under 5 years of age and to no more than 50 per 10,000 children and adults ages 5 to 64 years. (Baseline: 150 per 10,000 for children under 5 years; 71.1 per 10,000 for children and adults ages 5 to 64 years in 1995 to 1997.)

Fire Deaths

12. Reduce residential fire deaths to no more than 0.2 per 100,000 people. (Baseline: 1.2 per 100,000 for all ages in 1999.)

Poisoning

13. Reduce nonfatal poisoning to no more than 292 emergency room visits per 100,000 people. (Baseline: 348.3 per 100,000 for all ages in 1997.)

Neural Tube Defects

14. Reduce the incidence of spina bifida and other neural tube defects to 3 per 10,000 live births. (Baseline: 6 per 10,000 in 1996.)
15. Increase to at least 80% the proportion of women of childbearing age who take a vitamin with the recommended 0.4 mg (or 400 mcg) of folic acid daily. (Baseline: 21% in 1991 to 1994.)

Injury Prevention

16. Increase the use of child restraints to 100% of motor vehicle occupants. (Baseline: 92.9% of all children 4 years and younger in 1998.)
17. Increase the number of states requiring helmets for bicycle riders. (Baseline: 10 states required helmets for bicycle riders under 15 years in 1999.)
18. Reduce to 4.9% the proportion of adolescent students carrying weapons on school property. (Baseline: 6.9% of students in grades 9 to 12 in 1999.)

From U.S. Department of Health and Human Services (USDHHS). (2000). *Healthy People 2010: Understanding and improving health* (2nd ed.). Washington, DC: U.S. Government Printing Office; and U.S. Department of Health and Human Services (USDHHS). (2006). *Healthy People 2010: Midcourse review.* Washington, DC: U.S. Government Printing Office.

The primary causes of mortality from birth to 1 year of age are listed in Chapter 7. Congenital anomalies, prematurity/low birth weight, sudden infant death syndrome, and unintentional injury account for most of all deaths (Mathews & MacDorman, 2007). Community health nurses participate in prevention efforts to reduce infant mortality rates, including anticipatory health teaching and supportive measures for pregnant women and their families.

Low-Birth-Weight Infants. Low birth weight contributes to infant mortality, birth injuries, neurologic defects, and mental retardation. As more low-birth-weight infants survive, the number of associated health problems increase. Low birth weight is associated with cerebral palsy, seizure disorders, developmental delay, decreased school achievement, learning disabilities, attention-deficit hyperactivity disorder, visual and hearing deficits, and autism (Hack et al., 2005). Early prenatal care produces lower numbers of infants with low birth weights. However, many pregnant women do not receive adequate prenatal care. Certain racial groups receive inadequate or late prenatal care. Pregnant adolescents also tend to delay prenatal care (see Chapter 24). Other factors contributing to low birth weight include inadequate nutrition and maternal tobacco use during pregnancy.

Toddlers and Preschoolers and School-Age Children

Accidents lead the causes of death among children and young adults (Mathews & MacDorman, 2007). Toddlers and preschoolers need active protection from accidents and injuries. Increased mobility and exploration in young children contribute to the risk. Home safety, including removing matches, medicines, poisons, and other hazardous items, helps to limit danger. Families who secure play areas and reduce exposure to traffic and water avoid the dangers associated with this age group. School-age children should be taught general safety considerations, use of helmets and seat belts, safety with others, and safe bicycle use (see Table 27-3).

Adolescents

Three main causes of injury and death among teenagers are accidents, especially motor vehicle accidents, suicide, and homicide (CDC, 2007a). Adolescents generally dismiss dangers associated with high-risk behaviors. Alcohol and drug use contributes to this tendency. Unprotected sex results in births and sexually transmitted diseases in adolescents. Even with recent declines, the United States continues to have one of the highest adolescent pregnancy rates of the industrialized nations (Santelli et al., 2007) (see Chapter 24).

ENVIRONMENTAL RISK FACTORS

Environmental risks for children include poor quality care, inadequate amounts of physical or environmental stimulation, or an unsafe environment. Additional environmental risks include maternal deprivation, poverty, inadequate nutrition, and inadequate social supports for the family.

Although morbidity is usually considered in its physical context, the emotional effects of living in poverty, living with chronic illness, or increased risk of abusive homes must also be considered (Bauman et al., 2006). Conditions such as failure to thrive, associated with poor quality parenting, as well as maladaptive coping mechanisms and delinquency have become more prevalent among school-age children and adolescents.

In the United States the leading causes of death for children are unintentional injury, homicide, and suicide. Disparities in injury rates continue to exist between white and minority children. Firearms are used over 80% of the time in homicide and suicides in black and Hispanic adolescents (CDC, 2007b). Public health prevention strategies that target mechanisms most hazardous to minorities of each age group are needed to close these gaps.

Child Abuse and Neglect

Maltreatment often goes unreported; therefore child abuse and neglect most likely exceeds 1 million cases annually (CDC, 2007c) (see Chapter 23). Perpetrators of abuse or neglect may be parent(s), baby-sitters, or teachers, that is, anyone with access to the child. Community health nurses remain in a prime position to observe abusive behavior because of their contact with caregivers. Observing caretaker interaction, assessing children for signs of abuse or neglect, and also assessing environmental safety and hygienic conditions include initial actions for the nurse. Reporting suspected child abuse and neglect to the police or the child protective service agency is mandatory in all states for all health professionals, including nurses. Local laws and procedures guide appropriate reporting for community health nurses. Moreover, nurses who care for children hold responsibility for staying informed about child protective laws and procedures. Families in abusive situations need parenting role models and support systems during stressful periods. Hotline or crisis telephone numbers, such as CHILDHELP (copyright National Child Abuse Hotline), The National Domestic Violence Hotline, and Parents Anonymous, provide help for people in traumatic situations. Furthermore, parents benefit from early intervention or family preservation services aimed at changing behavior at its earliest point (CDC, 2007c). Community health nurses may use **role modeling** strategies to shape appropriate parenting behaviors.

SUPPORT SERVICES
Home Health Visiting for the Child/Family Unit

Successful maternal-child home visiting programs aim to promote health promotion and provide **primary prevention** (Keefe et al., 2006; Olds, 2006). Specific populations served include women reluctant to use the health care system, and families considered at high risk to develop future problems. Pregnant adolescents, those living in poverty, and women with a premature infant being discharged to the home receive care (see Chapters 21 and 24) (Olds, 2006). Visits with these families focus on the whole family, incorporating family dynamics into planning.

Studies demonstrate reduction in anxiety with increased infant health when regular nurse visits occur. Fewer accidents and emergency department visits result. With home visits by community health nurses, families with identified child abuse incidents show improvements in home safety and maternal-infant interactions and use of positive discipline techniques as a substitute for physical discipline (Barlow et al., 2007). Despite research that repeatedly demonstrates decreases in mortality and morbidity in infants with early intervention measures, third-party reimbursement for home visits rarely occurs. Public health clinics operate successfully in many communities but often require families to travel to the centers, rather than using home visits. Case management for low-income pregnant women in many states reimburses for home visits by nurses employed by local health departments or health centers.

Home health visits by community health nurses also aim for early identification and treatment of illness and disabling conditions. Using developmental and family assessments helps to identify children at high risk for future problems. Interventions appropriate for community health nurse home visits include teaching parents to implement measures to promote growth, development, and safety; ensuring that children receive proper nutrition; and addressing adequacy and accessibility of family health care.

Resources

In the United States, families at risk may receive multiple services. Customary health services include screening and well-child care at public clinics or private medical practices. Agencies provide immunizations, developmental screening, and parent education (e.g., parenting skills, safety practices, and nutritional and developmental needs). Pediatric nurse practitioners, employed by many community agencies, provide expert primary care services. Community health nurses provide child health screening and anticipatory guidance to parents. Referral occurs for children with developmental delays or unmet health care needs.

Preschools and schools use EPSDT examinations to identify health problems and initiate referrals for appropriate services (Meurer, 2005). Nurses working in well-child clinics and making home health visits also perform screenings. Screening includes vision and hearing, lead detection, developmental assessments, and routine physical examinations.

Growth and development along with school functioning rely on promotion of adequate nutrition for poor families. The Special Supplemental Food Program for Women, Infants, and Children (WIC) provides food vouchers for high-protein, vitamin-rich food for pregnant women, new mothers, infants, and young children. Provision of healthy food to pregnant women increases the chance that their children will be healthy and of a normal weight. Financial savings from decreased hospital care for newborns and from improved health of high-risk infants and children have been attributed to WIC (Lee et al., 2006). Food Stamps and federally funded school breakfast and lunch programs help to ensure adequate food for children attending school.

Other health-promotion services include foster grandparents' programs (intergenerational support) or big brother and sister programs to provide someone who cares and is a role model; preschool education; Special Olympics; and creative programs for adolescents. Adolescent pregnancy prevention programs have included the use of incentives to stay in school; job training programs; and access to information about sexuality, sexually transmitted diseases, acquired immunodeficiency syndrome, and birth control. One nonprofit organization of families, health professionals, and educators that strives to support and facilitate home care for technology-dependent children is Sick Kids Need Involved People (SKIP).

Children with disabilities and those with chronic conditions need additional medical and support services. These special children require regular health care as well as special care for their chronic illness. Health care services are available from children's hospitals and through the state Title V Community Health Center Network (CHCN) programs. Family support services are available from a variety of disease-specific organizations. Numerous organizations (listed at the end of the chapter under Community Resources for Practice) serve children with special needs and their families. In addition to disease-specific services, the Indian Health Service and other organizations such as the National Easter Seal Society, March of Dimes Birth Defects Foundation, and Muscular Dystrophy Association provide financing for health services, support services, and educational information for children and parents.

Parents who provide continuous care for a child with special needs benefit from frequent breaks in their routines to maintain their own mental health. Respite care offers parents a break from the routine, continuous care of the child, either for a short period each day or for a more prolonged time. This care may be offered in the home or in another facility but can be difficult to find and even harder to finance. Respite allows parents time to be together and to do activities with their other children. Some health insurance plans pay for respite care, and the developmental disabilities system will often fund respite for its clients.

Numerous other programs offer support for children with disabilities or special needs and their families. The developmental disabilities system provides help to families for children with developmental disabilities. Services include case management, direct services, or specialized funding in addition to parent support programs. The Social Security Administration's Supplemental Security Income (SSI) program provides monthly funds and access to Medicaid for disabled or blind children and youth. Funds provide additional care, home modification, and respite care. Medicaid provides access to health care services. Special education, including school-based health, education, and support services, occurs for children with learning needs as well as physical disabilities. Parents attend support and education programs, including parent to parent support, parent support groups, and parent training programs.

Children's Defense Fund (CDF), a private organization and the premier advocacy group for children, serves as an advocate for children, especially poor, minority, and handicapped children. This organization's goal is to educate the nation about children's needs and encourage preventive investment for children before they get sick, drop out of school, or get into trouble. The CDF initiative focuses on programs and policies that affect large numbers of children. Furthermore, the organization monitors development and implementation of federal and state policies.

Early Intervention for Children at Risk

In 1975 the federal government recognized that handicapped children had a constitutional right to a free public education in the least restrictive environment (PL 94-142, Education for All Handicapped Children Act). This law includes children with physical impairments, learning disabilities, and mental and emotional disabilities.

Before this act, children with chronic conditions and disabilities learned at home without peer contact; learned in separate classrooms or schools with only special needs children; or received inadequate education or no education at all. Public Law 94-142 was amended in 1986 through PL 99-457 and expanded coverage for high-risk children from birth. PL 99-457 (Education for All Handicapped Children

Act Amendments of 1986) authorizes a discretionary state grant program focusing on comprehensive early intervention for high-risk children from birth through school age, with the intent of providing financial incentives to states to develop and implement comprehensive, coordinated, multidisciplinary, and interagency programs. This law was among the first proactive measures adopted by Congress.

The federal government enacted the law but provided no funding. Each state's legislature determines whether the state will develop and fund an early intervention program. The state decides who the special at-risk or handicapped population will be. Eligibility criteria and the definition of developmental delay differ from one state to another. However, the law does specify services for children who are or may be, as a result of a current condition, developmentally delayed.

In 1991, PL 94-142 and PL 99-457 were renamed the Individuals with Disabilities Education Act (IDEA). Implementation of IDEA requires a great deal of leadership to enhance communication among service providers and organizations to prevent replication of services and provide comprehensive care. The community health nurse is in an ideal position to participate in this case management process. Chapter 30 provides a more detailed discussion of federal laws and school programs affecting children at risk. Over the past 30 years, IDEA has been amended regularly. Most recently the law was amended to restructure the regulations and included issues related to special education teachers' certification, workloads, and evaluations; Individual Education Plan (IEP) team attendance as well as IEP procedural changes; learning disability assessment; due process issues; and transition services for older children (Office of Special Education and Rehabilitation Services, 2005).

Daycare and Nursery School

Nursery school programs initially intended to enhance learning ability, promote social skills, and provide necessary remedial learning time. Typically, nursery schools served children 3 and 4 years old and met a few mornings a week or full days, 5 days a week. **Head Start** provides educational, nutrition, health services, and parent involvement opportunities to low-income children. Health services include nutrition, dental, medical, and mental health services. Home Start provides parents with guidance, suggested learning activities, and positive reinforcement to encourage stimulation of the child's learning in the home environment.

Daycare programs developed as an alternative to home baby-sitting for parents who were not at home during the day. Initially daycare programs intended to provide alternative childcare service, not education. Terms such as "nursery school," "preschool," and "daycare" hold blurred meanings. Some parents seek daycare for their children as young as a few weeks of age. Finding quality childcare, particularly in licensed facilities with high standards of care and small staff-to-children ratios, may be difficult. Adequate childcare is expensive and many families must make due with substandard arrangements. Childcare for one child costs approximately half of the wages for a full-time worker earning minimum wage. Some families opt to leave children at home alone because of the cost of daycare. The effect of daycare on children's growth and development has been studied for a long time. There has been no definitive conclusion as to whether daycare arrangements are good or bad for children (Shpancer, 2006).

Demands for specialized daycare have emerged, such as the need for "sick" daycare, that is, a daycare facility that accepts sick children in order to prevent missed workdays for parents. With increases in the number of working parents, additional needs exist for after-school care. Care should be taken to ensure children are in safe arrangements. Programs that stress health practices are important. Health issues to address would include hand-washing, brushing teeth after meals, proper disposal of soiled clothes and diapers, role modeling, implementing environmental safety measures, and enhancing social interaction and language skills, especially for children from non–English-speaking homes. Care environments that use a variety of play materials promote social skills. Supervision by a supportive and nurturing adult encourages mastery of developmental tasks with small groups of same-age children. Discipline includes redirection to positive behaviors, encouragement of children to use their words to resolve conflicts, and brief separation from the group if necessary. Above all, the environment should be one of caring and acceptance.

Nurses act as consultants to on-site care providers in daycare and preschool settings. They can teach the aforementioned content to daycare staff, facilitate parent group sessions, and have sessions with older children. In some areas, nurses play a role in daycare licensure by monitoring the implementation of standards and regulations.

Infection control in daycare is critical. One of the prime concerns for children in daycare is the easy spread of pathogens, which is, in part, due to children's lack of hygienic experience and higher risk for developing contagious diseases, the numerous instances of bodily contact, and the likelihood that some young children are not able to control their bodily functions. Implementation of precautions, including using gloves to change diapers, cleaning between children, and developing policies about how to treat sick children, must be accomplished consistently. Teaching and promoting adequate hand-washing for caregivers and children is the single most important infection control measure.

COMMUNITY HEALTH CARE FOR CHILDREN WITH SPECIAL NEEDS

Children with chronic conditions, especially children requiring technological care at home, frequently require services of the community health nurse. **High-technology home care** includes ventilator care, gastrostomy and nasogastric tube care, total parenteral nutrition, ostomy and dressing care, and apnea monitoring. Home routines with family interactions benefit the child and eliminate the stress of the hospital setting for both children and parents. Since the early 1980s, care has shifted from the hospital to the home setting. Hospital settings increase risk for contracting nosocomial infections because of an increased number of invasive procedures, multiple caretakers, and risk of contact with organisms from other children and staff. Altered environments from increased noise level, constant lighting, and large numbers of people result in sensory overload, sleep deprivation, and decreased learning opportunities. For these reasons, hospital environments limit growth and development.

Children with chronic conditions deserve the same home and family experiences as any child. Home care provides access to these experiences. Home care promotes **normalization** and self-care. Home care requires intensive discharge planning, with the collaboration of acute care and community health nurses. In the home, the parents resume the role of the primary caregiver, a role they otherwise may not have assumed. The child adapts to parents as caregivers. The parent who has been a visitor and bystander will replace multiple hospital caregivers when the child is discharged. Family goals aim to successfully bond with the child, provide appropriate care, and promote development. Parents often feel incompetent about the caregiver role or angry with others for having better understanding of their child. Nurses facilitate attachment and improved parental confidence by treating parents as equal partners and by acting as mentors while parents learn technical skills.

Although home care for some children with chronic conditions has many positive assets, there may be drawbacks. Home environments become disrupted with high-technology home care. Special equipment and structural adjustments limit living space. Siblings feel displaced or frightened by equipment or procedures, and by disrupted routines. Brother and sisters often serve as caregivers. Families generally feel isolated, but finding alternative caregivers is difficult. Demands of caregiving, careers, household duties, and other children in the household limit leisure time and cause stress.

Perhaps funding presents the greatest impediment to providing high-technology care in the home. Funding processes involve long waiting periods, negotiations, and evidence of discharge planning. Although third-party payers generally pay completely for inpatient care, similar care in the home may not receive funding. Numerous studies provide evidence for the cost-effectiveness of home care, yet third-party payers, including governmental agencies, often fail to acknowledge these data. Insurance companies now realize that working with parents, hospitals, and home care agencies provides quality home care at the best cost (Berman et al., 2005). Nurses, frequently employed as case managers, assess needs, coordinate efforts, and reduce duplication of services. Even in the wake of insurance coverage, there are **hidden costs** to families that are not immediately obvious. Families may lose job advancement opportunities, and they may make choices to accommodate the need of the disabled child at the expense of other family members.

The availability of improved, smaller, more portable equipment reduces risks for children confined to home. Portable ventilators, backpacks to carry continuous infusion pumps for toddlers, and motorized wheelchairs for children improve access to community participation for the child and family. Equipment rental or purchase, supplies, cleaning agents, electricity, vender service contracts, and innumerable other issues factor into the cost of home care.

Chronically ill children need well-child or regular preventive care just as any other child. Care plans, services, and equipment needs should be reviewed annually. For example, when an infant becomes a toddler with increased mobility needs, the child's assistive-device needs will also change. Parental knowledge and expectations are other areas for regular review. Nurses intervene with clarification, discussion, and education when unrealistic parental expectations surface. As children mature, their sense of independence and their role in their own care change. The nurse and family members who stay attuned to the child's needs better accommodate developmental changes.

Many technology-dependent children attend school. Community health nurses facilitate school attendance when medically feasible and desirable. Children in school engage in developmentally appropriate activities with peers, and participate in classroom learning. School also provides an important source of respite care for parents of these children, so that parents can work, attend to other children, or carry out household activities. Treatments may occur at the school or in the home before or after school.

SPECIFIC CONDITIONS REQUIRING HOME CARE

Technology-dependent and **medically fragile children** are a growing target population for community health nursing services. Their chronic conditions and needs are multiple and varied. The nursing literature addresses the special needs of the following groups:

- Terminal hospice care for children with cancer, including family support before, during, and after the death
- Infants born with spina bifida or other congenital anomalies for whom no surgical correction will be performed
- Younger siblings of children who died of sudden infant death syndrome who require an apnea monitor
- Children requiring peritoneal dialysis
- Children with hemophilia who are receiving clotting factor replacements
- Children requiring assistance with diabetes control, especially children who are ready to learn self-injections and self–blood glucose monitoring
- Children requiring pain control at home, for whom frequent pain assessments and medication adjustments are needed
- Children receiving parenteral nutrition, nasogastric or gastrostomy feedings, or intravenous antibiotics

THE CHILD REQUIRING USE OF A VENTILATOR

Ventilator-dependent children require more community and home health services than almost any other children. Medically stable children with families who have the desire, time, and resources to meet the child's needs make candidates for care at home. Some areas of the United States do not have licensed home care agencies or qualified nursing personnel who can support ventilator care in the home.

Numerous benefits exist for home care of ventilator-dependent children, including the following advantages: fewer infections, improved nutrition, increased socialization, and improved motor skills compared with institutionalized children (Carnevale et al., 2006). Although there is a risk of accidental death related to complex care provided in the home, studies provide some evidence that ventilator-dependent children can receive care safely outside of the critical care setting (Ambrosio et al., 1998; Hockenberry & Wilson, 2006). Electrical equipment requires an adequate number of grounded outlets. A second ventilator needs to be available as a backup for ventilator failure and to facilitate movement from one area of the home to another. Family must keep a suction machine, suction catheters, tracheotomy tubes, ties, dressings, and ventilator tubing available in the home for daily care and maintenance. Community health nurses assist families with their plan to maintain the homelike, safe, accessible, and normalized environment. For safety, community health nurses coordinate the notification of local fire and rescue units; gas, electric, and telephone companies; the emergency departments of the hospitals; city or township services for street clearing in inclement weather; and the child's school.

Home care reduces health care costs as much as 80% to 90% for some children who are dependent on technology (Hawkins et al., 2006). Cost studies include the costs of equipment, supplies, oxygen, nursing care, special diets, and therapies. Many cost-related studies, however, fail to address a family's out-of-pocket expenses. These expenses include structural changes to the home, intercom systems, and higher utility bills. Parents may need to adjust work schedules or eliminate working outside the home altogether in order to care for the child.

With the accountability of hidden costs, the question remains whether significant cost savings exist. Hawkins and colleagues (2006) estimate that home care, factoring in caregiver time value or forfeited wages, remains less costly in 70% of situations. These authors claim that most caregivers are women who were not in the labor market or held low-paying jobs. One important benefit to home care is the degree of family interaction (Carnevale et al., 2006). Medically fragile children benefit by being in familiar surroundings with family, friends, and pets, enabling them to participate more fully in the activities of daily living.

Marital and family distress may develop in families involved in home care. Some problems parents have identified include lack of parental support groups, lack of privacy related to home nursing care, restrictions on the parents' travel or social activities, stressful time schedules, disrupted sleeping patterns, insufficient financial assistance, physical and mental exhaustion, and stress involved in dealing with these conditions (Carnevale et al., 2006).

Parents may feel overwhelmed and inadequate, resulting in dependence on the nurses who assist or manage care. They may feel great relief when care is provided. Families who develop dependency issues need support and encouragement to resume their role in the care. Respectful communication encourages parents to share their needs as caregivers. Current funding and insurance restrictions may be barriers to care for families with technology-dependent members. Community health nurses should assess families for signs of stress and burnout. Acknowledging parents' heavy responsibilities sometimes reenergizes primary caregivers. Respite opportunities available in the community can help to alleviate stress and burnout.

COMMUNITY/PUBLIC HEALTH NURSING RESPONSIBILITIES

A primary goal of nursing is to attain, regain, or maintain health for children and their families. This goal involves the nursing roles of care provider, educator, coordinator, advocate, and systems' change agent. Provision of direct care requires a knowledge base in child and family development, as well as preventive, acute, and chronic care needs of children. Nurses assess growth and developmental level; family dynamics; priorities, strengths, and needs; cultural determinants of care; and environment. This expertise allows nurses to plan family-centered, community-based, culturally-competent, comprehensive care. Community health nurses focus on the following:

- Promoting normal growth and development and general wellness
- Enhancing the nutritional, dental, and immunologic status of the child
- Providing a safe environment
- Promoting healthy family interactions

As direct-care providers, community health nurses act as case finders to locate children and families who need community resources and to facilitate access to appropriate services. A particular challenge for the community health nurse is reaching families who are reluctant to use existing health care services.

A home health nurse, Lori, visits a family with five children under the age of 8 years old. She is making a home visit to a new client who is the grandfather of the children. The grandfather, Lawrence, has come to live with his daughter because he suffered a cerebral vascular accident with severe paralysis to the right side. When completing the admission assessment, Lori discovers that the children have not received regular health care. The mother, Kacy, cannot afford the insurance that her employer provides. Her own health insurance is subsidized by her employer, but the family coverage is not. The cost of insuring the children is prohibitive. She is reluctant to obtain information about Medicaid, because she is embarrassed about what people might think. She is sure that her income will place her slightly above the poverty level. Lori informs Kacy about a state program that was developed for families. She explains to Kacy that the program has a toll-free number. With one telephone call, she is able to begin the enrollment process. The state program streamlines the three programs for children's health insurance. With one enrollment, the family would be evaluated for Medicaid, the state Children's Health Insurance Program (CHIP), and another group insurance program for people in a higher income bracket. Having this telephone number available as a resource, Lori was able to reach this family and help them to take action to promote the health of the children.

Nurses educate families through teaching and role modeling. Families require information about development, health promotion, parenting skills, and community resources. Families with medically fragile children need education about the child's condition, care needs, and specialized resources, as well as supervision and training in specialized care procedures.

As families choose and access needed services, they often need assistance to coordinate care among providers and service systems. Coordinating care remains a core function for community health nurses. Nurses evaluate and modify plans regularly in order to coordinate and refer families to the appropriate resources.

Community health nurses assume the **advocacy** role to reduce obstacles for individual families. Advocacy for families takes the form of clarifying information for providers, providing additional information to families to increase their understanding of the service system, or providing ongoing support and assistance as families work to access care. Nurses also function as change agents in unresponsive systems. System-level change occurs through participation on community-based boards and educating and informing policymakers.

After more than 15 years as a public health nurse, Maureen had become quite active in her community. In particular, she became involved in a new organization called Healthy Communities. This organization brought people together from all areas of the community. The overall mission of the organization was to develop ways to strengthen the community in vital areas. Although the organization focused on environmental and educational issues, Maureen, from the nursing perspective, was most interested in the traditional health issues. One issue of particular interest to her was the issue of childhood obesity. Maureen assumed the role of facilitator of the group interested in this issue. As facilitator, Maureen was able to promote a search for programs that were most effective in addressing childhood obesity. Several members of Healthy Communities were involved with the local school district. The Healthy Communities organization financed a team from the school district to visit schools that had already implemented one of the researched programs. Board members of Healthy Communities visited the school district administrators and described the program. The team that made the site visit prepared a budget for program implementation. Implementation of the program commenced the following school year. Because of Maureen's advocacy and community involvement, Healthy Communities was able to act as a catalyst in this process.

TRENDS IN CHILD HEALTH SERVICES

Economic trends continue to influence the availability and quality of health care provided to children. Health care services for both wellness and illness need to be available and accessible. Early screening and developmental assessments prevent further disabilities. Governmental trends must focus on finding sufficient funding for federal and state programs for home care and childcare as part of the continuum of health care services for children. Refunding for the SCHIP program is currently under federal review. Many states are dissatisfied with the federal funding formula, which has put greater stress on state health budgets (see Chapter 4).

One of the primary needs of families is the availability of quality childcare. This will be especially true as welfare reform moves many mothers into employment at potentially low wages. This need for childcare must be addressed with solutions that include care for mildly ill children, technology-dependent children, and those with other special needs, as well as infants and older children needing after-school care.

Improved treatment modalities and survival rates will continue to increase the number of children requiring home health care services. Community health care agencies must respond to this expanding population. This requires nurses who are knowledgeable in growth and development, family dynamics, and public policies affecting children, and competent in nursing care for acute and chronic illnesses and disabling conditions.

Nursing must be involved as states continue to implement and modify their programs that serve children, such as early intervention, Medicaid (including the transition to managed care), SCHIP, and others. Nursing has a long history of working with children with disabilities and children at risk and is the ideal profession to coordinate care for these children.

Community health care services cannot just focus on the child with chronic conditions. A refocusing on provision of preventive and primary care to all children is mandatory, especially in light of resurgent measles and mumps epidemics, the increase in tuberculosis, outbreaks of infectious agents such as *Escherichia coli,* the increasing rate of childhood obesity, and other child health problems in the United States. Public health initiatives and creative community health approaches to decrease the risk factors that result in mortality and morbidity for children are needed.

The increased emphasis on normalization of children with chronic conditions will enhance the role of school nurses. It will also promote home care services for the medically fragile or technology-dependent child (see Chapter 30). The effectiveness of home care must continue to be empirically supported, and the information used to change public policy related to third-party funding for home care. The United States must focus on providing sufficient services for childcare, home care, and health care for children and adolescents.

Finally, the needs of special groups of children must be addressed. Improving the quality of foster care and removing obstacles to adoptions, especially for technology-dependent children, are essential. Affordable and available group homes and respite facilities must be available to support families and provide continuing quality care for their children. The community health nurse can help assure the quality of health care services for these vulnerable children, advocate on behalf of these children, and support families in decision making and providing care.

KEY IDEAS

1. The responsibilities of community/public health nurses in child health include health promotion, disease prevention, risk reduction efforts, and case management, as well as home health care.
2. Community/public health nursing care is culturally sensitive and recognizes and supports the physical, cognitive, psychosocial, and environmental priorities and needs of children and their families.
3. Children in the community may have many health problems, both chronic and acute. Some of these problems include infectious diseases, chronic illnesses such as asthma, and environmental risks such as lead exposure and injury. Accidents are the main cause of death of children from 1 to 18 years of age.
4. Children in poverty are at greater risk for health problems (e.g., low birth weight, increased infant mortality, and increased incidence of chronic illnesses) and exposure to environmental and safety hazards than are children of other income groups. They may also have less access to health care services.
5. Primary prevention and early identification and intervention services are targeted to groups of children and adolescents who are especially at risk of poorer health: children living in poverty, those with chronic illnesses and disabilities, and teenage parents.
6. Public funding for child health services is variable. Eligibility criteria may vary by state; thus children with similar needs may receive funding in one state but not in another.
7. Children with special needs require multiple resources and services from a variety of agencies and providers. For those needing long-term care, home is the most desirable place to receive care. Community resources are not always available to support home care.

8. Community/public health nurses need to be knowledgeable about resources available within the community to support children and their parents.

9. Federal law established human rights regarding educational and school health care services for children with disabilities. These laws provide for public education, school support services, and early screening and interventions to reduce developmental delays and encourage the mental, physical, and emotional development of children with special needs.

10. At present, there are few high-quality daycare facilities for children of working parents; the shortage is most pronounced for those children with special needs. This shortage is expected to continue to increase and affects after-school care for school-age children of working parents as well.

11. Community/public health nurses involved with children's services need to advocate for improved funding, expansion of existing services, and creation of policies and additional support services to help families maximize the health and well-being of their children. In addition, services should be family friendly, easy to access, and coordinated with other services in the community.

12. Above all, the community/public health nurse must remember that regardless of their age, environmental situation, or physical and mental ability, children are children first. Caregivers should take care to allow them as many of the delights of childhood as possible.

THE NURSING PROCESS IN PRACTICE | **A Child with Special Health Care Needs (by Jennifer Maurer Kliphouse)**

Daniel is 6 years old. He lives with his mother and two younger sisters. His parents are divorced, and his mother wants to return to her job as a waitress if she can find affordable childcare. Daniel was born with a large myelomeningocele (spina bifida) that was repaired shortly after birth, leaving him paralyzed from the waist down. At 3 months of age, he received a ventriculoperitoneal shunt for hydrocephalus. He has just received his first wheelchair. Home care visits are requested because he has been having frequent urinary tract infections, most likely related to his need for catheterization every 4 hours. His mental development is slightly delayed (mental age of 5 years), but he is continuing to progress. Daniel is about to start regular school.

ASSESSMENT

- Assess the mother's technique for catheterization as well as the technique of significant others who perform this task on Daniel.
- Assess the physical, psychologic, and social needs of the child and family.
- Explore the readiness of Daniel to learn to assist with clean intermittent catheterization.
- Assess the home environment for wheelchair accessibility and safety.
- Assess the school environment for readiness to accommodate Daniel's special needs, and assess the mother's knowledge of special services available at the school.

- Assess the mother's childcare options and the ability of caregivers to provide needed care.
- Assess the specific health-promotion and maintenance activities of the mother and two siblings.

NURSING DIAGNOSES

- Knowledge deficit related to information misinterpretation regarding catheterization by the mother and caregivers as evidenced by (AEB) increased urinary tract infections in Daniel
- Impaired wheelchair mobility related to cognitive unfamiliarity with use of wheelchair AEB lack of independent ambulation via wheelchair
- Impaired home maintenance management related to insufficient finances AEB an environment that is not wheelchair accessible
- Ineffective role performance related to inadequate support systems AEB the inability of the mother to find adequate childcare that would allow her to return to work
- Knowledge deficit of school system related to lack of exposure AEB limited knowledge of role in educating a child with a chronic condition
- Health-seeking behaviors related to active participation in immunization maintenance and active involvement in appropriate health care maintenance of child with myelodysplasia

Nursing Diagnosis	Nursing Goals	Nursing Interventions	Outcomes and Evaluation
Knowledge deficit related to information misinterpretation regarding catheterization by the mother and caregivers AEB increased urinary tract infections in Daniel	Daniel's mother and other caregivers will demonstrate appropriate clean technique when performing a catheterization.	Observe the mother's and caregivers' catheterization technique. Provide simple step-by-step instruction brochure and corrective information as needed.	Daniel's mother consistently demonstrated appropriate catheterization technique and care of equipment. However, Daniel's father did not demonstrate appropriate clean technique. After speaking with the nurse, Daniel's father stated that he felt "intimidated" by the catheterization process. About 1 month after instruction by the nurse on the catheterization process and clean technique, Daniel had yet to have a recurrent urinary tract infection. Although some children younger than 6 are able to demonstrate clean intermittent catheterization, Daniel does not have the physical coordination or ability to understand the importance of clean technique. Therefore he is not a candidate for self-catheterization at this time. Both the nurse and Daniel's parents expect he will be ready to begin learning within the year.

Continued

Nursing Diagnosis	Nursing Goals	Nursing Interventions	Outcomes and Evaluation
Impaired wheel-chair immobility related to unfamiliarity with the use of a wheelchair AEB lack of independent ambulation via wheelchair	Daniel will adapt to and appropriately use his wheelchair.	Provide anticipatory guidance related to the growth and developmental needs of the child entering school, as well as his physical, psychologic, and cognitive needs. 1. Collaborate with a physical and/or occupational therapist. 2. Practice transfer maneuvers around barriers. 3. Review and demonstrate proper seating alignment as well as motoring of wheelchair.	Daniel stated he was excited to have a wheelchair and expressed hope that it would provide increased independence. Daniel received several occupational and physical therapy consults. He adapted quickly to the use of a wheelchair and was able to demonstrate safe wheelchair use and transfer technique independently. About 1 month later, Daniel appeared proficient in wheelchair use and even showed the nurse several "cool tricks."
Impaired home maintenance management related to insufficient finances AEB an environment that is not wheelchair accessible	Daniel's mother will secure resources and make the necessary modifications in the home.	Coordinate access to community resources for home modifications.	As Daniel's mother was his full-time care provider, she had limited financial resources. A social worker contacted several volunteer agencies to help the family make the necessary home modifications. A local hardware store provided raw materials necessary for a ramp entrance and minor doorway expansions in the house, while another community agency provided free skilled labor.

 Find additional **Care Plans** for this client on the book's website.

LEARNING BY EXPERIENCE AND REFLECTION

1. When you were a child, whom did you know who had special health care needs? How were their needs addressed in your school? How were their needs addressed in the community? What supports were available to their families? How did you and your peers respond to the child with a special need?
2. Interact with and assess a child with a chronic condition or special need. Does the child appear to focus more on the illness and disability or on the common concerns of childhood?
3. How would you feel if your own child was born prematurely, developed bronchopulmonary dysplasia, and was now ready to be discharged to your home on a ventilator?
4. How would you counsel an unmarried, poor, 16-year-old female who is now pregnant with her second child and who is using cocaine? What anticipatory guidance would you provide, and what community resources would be appropriate for her use?
5. Consider how you might resolve the conflict of promoting health care and preventive measures with poor homeless families who share one room for two families and have no physical resources or utilities. Explore your community's resources and identify any that might meet the needs of this family.

COMMUNITY RESOURCES FOR PRACTICE

Information about each organization listed below can be found on its website, which can be accessed through the book's website at *http:// evolve.elsevier.com/Maurer/community/.*

Alliance of Genetic Support Groups
American Cancer Society
American Heart Association National Center
American Juvenile Arthritis Organization
Association of Birth Defect Children
Association of Retarded Citizens
Asthma and Allergy Foundation of America
Candlelighters Childhood Cancer Foundation, Inc.
Child Help USA
Children's Defense Fund
Children's Hospice International
Cystic Fibrosis Foundation
Elizabeth Glaser Foundation (Pediatric AIDS)
Epilepsy Foundation of America
Families USA: Policy Action Network
Family Voices
Housing and Urban Development (HUD)—People with Disabilities
HRSA Maternal and Child Health Bureau
Juvenile Diabetes Research Foundation
Learning Disabilities Association of America
March of Dimes Birth Defects Foundation
Muscular Dystrophy Association
National Association for Down Syndrome
National Dissemination Center for Children and Youth with Disabilities
National Easter Seal Society
National Hemophilia Foundation
United Cerebral Palsy Association, Inc.

Visit the Evolve website for this book to find the following study and assessment materials:

- Quiz
- Web Scenario
- Critical Thinking Questions and Answers for Case Studies
- Care Plans
- *Healthy People* Updates
- Glossary

REFERENCES

Ambrosio, I. U., Woo, M. S., Jansen, M. T., et al. (1998). Safety of hospitalized ventilator-dependent children. *Pediatrics, 101*(2), 257-259.

American Community Survey (2005). *United States—Children characteristics.* Retrieved May 31, 2007, from *http://factfinder.census.gov/servlet/STTable?_bm=y&-qr_name=ACS_2005_EST_G00_S0901&-geo_id=01000US&-ds_name=ACS_2005_EST_G00_&-_lang=en&-format=&-CONTEXT=st.*

Ball, J. & Bindler, R. (2002). *Pediatric nursing: Caring for children* (2nd ed.). Norwalk, CT: Appleton & Lange.

Barlow, J., Davis, H., McIntosh, E., et al. (2007). Role of home visiting in improving parenting and health in families at risk of abuse and neglect: Results of a multicentre randomized controlled trial and economic evaluation. *Archives of Disease in Childhood, 92*(3), 229-233.

Bauman, L. J., Silver, E. J., & Stein, R. E. K. (2006). Cumulative social disadvantage and child health. *Pediatrics, 117*(4), 1321-1328.

Berman, S., Rannie, M., Moore, L., et al. (2005). Utilization and costs for children who have special health care needs and are enrolled in a hospital-based comprehensive primary care clinic. *Pediatrics, 115*(6, Suppl), e637-642.

Borders, A. E., Grobman, W. A., Amsden, L. B., et al. (2007). Chronic stress and low birth weight neonates in a low-income population of women. *Obstetrics & Gynecology, 109*(2, Pt 1), 331-338.

Bowden, V., Dickey, S., & Greenberg, C. (1998). *Children and their families: The continuum of care.* Philadelphia: W.B. Saunders.

Carnevale, F. A., Alexander, E., Davis, M., et al. (2006). Daily living with distress and enrichment: The moral experience of families with ventilator-assisted children at home. *Pediatrics, 117*(1, Suppl), e48-60.

Centers for Disease Control and Prevention (2007a). *Scientific data, surveillance, & injury statistics—NCIPC.* Retrieved June 6, 2007, from *http://www.cdc.gov/ncipc/osp/charts.htm.*

Centers for Disease Control and Prevention (2007b). Surveillance summaries: Fatal injuries among children by race and ethnicity—United States, 1999-2002 (electronic version). *Morbidity and Mortality Weekly Report, 56*(SS-5), 1-20. Retrieved June 15, 2007 from *http://www.cdc.gov/MMWR/preview/mmwrhtml/ss5605a1.htm.*

Centers for Disease Control and Prevention (2007c). Notice to readers: National child abuse prevention month—April 2006 (electronic version). *Morbidity and Mortality Weekly Report, 55*(13), 370-371. Retrieved June 15, 2007 from *http://www.cdc.gov/MMWR/preview/mmwrhtml/MM5513a6.htm.*

Centers for Disease Control and Prevention (2007d). *Cases of HIV infection amd AIDS in the United States and dependent areas, 2006* (vol. 17). Atlanta, GA: United States Government. Retrieved June 1, 2007, from *http://www.cdc.gov/hiv/topics/surveillance/resources/reports/.*

Centers for Disease Control and Prevention (2005). *Fact sheets, fetal alcohol syndrome, NCBDDD, CDC.* Retrieved June 1, 2007, from *http://www.cdc.gov/ncbddd/factsheets/FAS.pdf.*

Child Trends DataBank—Children in poverty (2006). Retrieved June 17, 2007, from *http://www.childtrendsdatabank.org/indicators/4Poverty.cfm.*

Christie, D., & Viner, R. (2005). ABC of adolescence: Adolescent development…first in a series of 12 articles. *BMJ, 330*(7486), 301-304.

Delp, L., Brown, B., & Domenzain, A. (2005). Fostering youth leadership to address workplace and community environmental health issues: A university-school-community partnership. *Health Promotion Practice, 6*(3), 270-285.

Donn, S. M., & Sinha, S. K. (2006). Minimizing ventilator induced lung injury in preterm infants. *Archives of Disease in Childhood—Fetal and Neonatal Edition, 91*(3), F226-230.

Edelman, C. L., & Mandle, C. L. (2006). In C. L. Edelman & C. L. Mandle (Eds.), *Health promotion throughout the life span* (6th ed.). St. Louis, MO: Elsevier Mosby.

Edgecomb, G. (2001). *Public health nursing: Past and future: A review of the literature.* Denmark: World Health Organization (Public Health Nursing Europe). Retrieved May 31, 2007, from *http://www.rcm.org.uk/info/docs/060105163054-331-1.pdf.*

Ehiri, J. E., Ejere, H. O. D., Magnussen, L., et al. (2006). Interventions for promoting booster seat use in four to eight year olds traveling in motor vehicles. *Cochrane Database of Systematic Reviews, 2.*

Emmons, K. M., Puleo, E., Park, E., et al. (2005). Peer-delivered smoking counseling for childhood cancer survivors increases rate of cessation: The partnership for health study. *Journal of Clinical Oncology, 23*(27), 6516-6523.

Green, M., & Palfrey, J. S. (Eds.). (2002). *Bright futures: Guidelines for health supervision of infants, children, and adolescents.* Arlington, VA: National Center for Education in Maternal and Child Health.

Hack, M., Taylor, H. G., Drotar, D., et al. (2005). Chronic conditions, functional limitations, and special health care needs of school-aged children born with extremely low-birth-weight in the 1990s. *JAMA: Journal of the American Medical Association, 294*(3), 318-325.

Hawkins, M. R., DiehlSvrjcek, B., & Dunbar, L. J. (2006). Caring for children with special healthcare needs in the managed care environment. *Lippincott's Case Management, 11*(4), 216-223.

Hockenberry, M. J., & Wilson, D. (2006). *Wong's nursing care of infants and children* (8th ed.). St. Louis, MO: Mosby.

Hoffman, C. B. (2007). Simple truths about America's uninsured. *American Journal of Nursing, 107*(1), 40-43.

Izzo, C. V., Eckenrode, J. J., Smith, E. G., et al. (2005). Reducing the impact of uncontrollable stressful life events through a program of nurse home visitation for new parents. *Prevention Science, 6*(4), 269-274.

Jenkins, S. M., Buboltz, W. C., Jr., Schwartz, J. P., et al. (2005). Differentiation of self and psychosocial development. *Contemporary Family Therapy: An International Journal, 27*(2), 251-261.

Kaiser Commission (2007). *The Kaiser Commission on Medicaid and the Uninsured: A decade of SCHIP experience and issues for reauthorization* (Foundation Report No. 7574). Washington, DC: The Henry K. Kaiser Family Foundation. Retrieved May 3, 2007 from *http://www.kff.org/medicaid/206803-index.cfm.*

Kaiser Commission (2001). *Medicaid and managed care* (Foundation Report No. 2068-03). Washington, DC: The Henry K. Kaiser Family Foundation. Retrieved May 3, 2007 from *http://www.kff.org/medicaid/7574.cfm.*

Keefe, M. R., Karlsen, K. A., Lobo, M. L., et al. (2006). Reducing parenting stress in families with irritable infants. *Nursing Research, 55*(3), 198-205.

Kitzman, H., Olds, D. L., Sidora, K., et al. (2000). Enduring effects of nurse home visitation on maternal life course: A 3-year follow-up of a randomized trial. *JAMA, 283*(15), 1983-1989.

Lee, B. J., Mackey-Bilaver, L. M., & Chin, M. (2006). *Effects of WIC and food stamp program participation on child outcomes (Electronic Government Report No. 27)*. Washington, DC: United States Department of Agriculture (WIC).

Leininger, M., & McFarland, M. R. (2006). *Culture care diversity and universality* (2nd ed.). Sudbury, MA: Jones & Bartlett.

London, R. A., & Fairlie, R. W. (2005). *Economic conditions and children's living arrangements* (Working Paper No. 05-27). University of Michigan: National Poverty Center. Retrieved May 31, 2007 from *http://www.ncp.umich.edu/publications/working_papers/index.php?publication_id=53*.

Mathews, T. J., & MacDorman, M. F. (2007). Infant mortality statistics from the 2004 period linked birth/infant death data set. *National vital statistics reports, 55*(15). Retrieved June 5, 2007, from *http://www.cdc.gov/nchs/data/nvsr/nvsr55/nvsr55_14.pdf*.

May, P. A., Serna, P., Hurt, L., et al. (2005). Outcome evaluation of a public health approach to suicide prevention in an American Indian tribal nation. *American Journal of Public Health, 95*(7), 1238-1244.

McDonald, E. M., Solomon, B., Shields, W., et al. (2005). Evaluation of kiosk-based tailoring to promote household safety behaviors in an urban pediatric primary care practice. *Patient Education and Counseling, 58*(2), 168-181.

Messias, D. K. H., Moneyham, L., Murdaugh, C., et al. (2006). HIV/AIDS peer counselors' perspectives on intervention delivery formats. *Clinical Nursing Research, 15*(3), 177-196.

Meurer, J. R. (2005). Medicaid Policy Statement. *Pediatrics, 116*(1), 274-280.

Monsen, K. A., Fitzsimmons, L. L. M., Lescenski, B. A. C., et al. (2006). A public health nursing informatics data-and-practice quality project article. *CIN: Computers, Informatics, Nursing, 24*(3), 152-158.

Musick, K., & Mare, R. D. (2004). *California Center for Population Research: Recent trends in the inheritance of poverty and family structure*. Los Angeles, CA: University of California.

Nilsen, S. (2007). *Poverty in America: Economic research shows impacts on health status and other social conditions as well as the growth rate* (Government No. GAO-07-353T). Washington,

DC: United States Government Accountability Office (poverty). Retrieved June 15, 2007, from *http://www.gao.gov/new.items/d07344.pdf*.

Nolan, K. W., Young, E. C., Hebert, E. B., et al. (2005). Service coordination for children with complex healthcare needs in an early intervention program. *Infants and Young Children, 18*(2), 161-170.

Office of Special Education and Rehabilitation Services. (2005). Proposed rules for the assistance to states for the education of children with disabilities. *Federal Register, 70*(118), 35782-35792.

Olds, D. (2006). Progress in improving the development of low birth weight newborns. *Pediatrics, 117*(3), 940-941.

Olds, D. L., Kitzman, H., Cole, R., et al. (2004). Effects of nurse home-visiting on maternal life course and child development: Age 6 follow-up results of a randomized trial. *Pediatrics, 114*(6), 1550-1559.

Pediatrics. (2006). The pediatrician and disaster preparedness. Policy statement. *Pediatrics, 117*(2), 560-565.

Pediatrics. (2005). Care coordination in the medical home: Integrating health and related systems of care for children with special health care needs. Policy statement. *Pediatrics, 116*(5), 1238-1244.

Perlesz, A., Brown, R., Lindsay, J., et al. (2006). Family in transition: Parents, children and grandparents in lesbian families give meaning to 'doing family'. *Journal of Family Therapy, 28,* 175-199.

Piper, T. M., Tracy, M., Bucciarelli, A., et al. (2006). Firearm suicide in New York City in the 1990s. *Injury Prevention, 12*(1), 41-45.

Pulcini, J. (2007). The State Children's Health Insurance program. *American Journal of Nursing, 107*(3), 29-30.

Remke, S. S., & Chrastek, J. R. (2007). Hospice & palliative care. Improving care in the home for children with palliative care needs. *Home Healthcare Nurse, 25*(1), 45-53.

Santelli, J. S., Lindberg, L. D., Finer, L. B., et al. (2007). Explaining recent declines in adolescent pregnancy in the United States: The contribution of abstinence and improved contraceptive use. *American Journal of Public Health, 97*(1), 150-156.

Selekman, J. (1996). *Pediatric nursing*. Springhouse, PA: Springhouse.

Shi, L., Stevens, G. D., & Politzer, R. M. (2007). Access to care for U.S. health center patients and patients nationally: How do the most vulnerable populations fare? *Medical Care, 45*(3), 206-213.

Shpancer, N. (2006). The effects of daycare: Persistent questions, elusive answers. *Early Childhood Research Quarterly, 21*(2), 227-237.

Sniecinski, R., & Levy, J. H. (2007). What is blood and what is not? Caring for the Jehovah's Witness patient undergoing cardiac surgery. *Anesthesia & Analgesia, 104*(4), 753-754.

Social Security Administration (2006). *Social Security online—history*. Retrieved May 31, 2007, from *http://www.ssa.gov/history/35actv.html*.

Substance Abuse and Mental Health Services Administration (2006). *Results from the 2005 National Survey on Drug Use and Health: National findings, SAMHSA,* (Office of Applied Studies, NSDUH Series H-30, DHHS Pub No. SMA 06-4194). Rockville, MD: Author. Retrieved June 1, 2007 from *http://www.oas.samhsa.gov/nsduh/2k5nsduh/2k5results.pdf*.

Tillett, J. (2005). Adolescents and informed consent: Ethical and legal issues. *Journal of Perinatal & Neonatal Nursing, 19*(2), 112-121.

U.S. Census Bureau (2004). *2005 American Community Survey*. Retrieved August 22, 2006, from *http://factfinder.census.gov/servlet/ACSSAFFFacts?_event=Search&geo_id=&_geoContext=&_street=&_county=cameron+county&_cityTown=cameron+county&_state=04000US48&_zip=&_lang=en&_sse=on&pctxt=fph&pgsl=010*.

U.S. Department of Education. (2007). *Archived: 25 year history of the IDEA*. Washington, DC: U.S. Government Printing Office.

U.S. Department of Health and Human Services. (2006). *Healthy People 2010: Midcourse review*. Washington, DC: U.S. Government Printing Office.

Vig, S., Chinitz, S., & Shulman, L. (2005). Young children in foster care: Multiple vulnerabilities and complex service needs. *Infants and Young Children, 18*(2), 147-160.

Wong, D. (2003). *Whaley and Wong's nursing care of infants and children* (7th ed.). St. Louis: Mosby.

SUGGESTED READINGS

Annie E. Casey Foundation. (2008). *Kids count 2008 data book online*. Baltimore, MD: Author. Retrieved August 20, 2008, from *http://www.kidscount.org/datacenter/databook.jsp*.

Centers for Disease Control and Prevention. (2008). *Life stages and specific populations: Children*. Retrieved August 18, 2008, from *http://www.cdc.gov/LifeStages/Children.html*.

Children's Defense Fund. (2005). *The state of American's children, 2005*. Retrieved August 18, 2008, from *http://www.childrensdefense.org/site/PageServer?pagename=publications*.

Children's Defense Fund. (2007). *The America's Cradle to Prison Pipeline report*. Retrieved August 18, 2008 from *http://childrensdefense.org/site/PageServe?pagename=publications*.

Edelman, M. (2008). *The sea is so wide and my boat is so small: Charting a course for the next generation*. New York: Hyperion.

28 Older Adults in the Community

*Meredith Wallace**

FOCUS QUESTIONS

What does it mean to be old?

What crises do aging families experience?

What are the common health care needs of older adults?

What support systems are available to meet the needs of an aging society?

How have community resources been organized and developed to promote a coordinated and comprehensive system of care for older adults?

What are the responsibilities of the community/public health nurse in meeting the needs of an aging population?

CHAPTER OUTLINE

KEY TERMS

Aging
Case management
Congregate housing
Durable power of attorney
Foster care
Geriatric Evaluation Service (GES)

Gerontology
Group homes
Home care
Life-care (continuous-care) community
Living wills
Long-term care

Medical daycare
Multipurpose senior centers
Retirement communities
Respite care
Social daycare

With the growing population of people 65 years of age and older, complex and unique health care needs have emerged that call for knowledge and expertise in the field of gerontology. **Gerontology** has been defined as the study of aging persons and of the process of aging (Miller, 2004). The term gerontology is derived from the root word *gera* or *geron,* meaning "great age" or "privilege of age."

At the onset of the 20th century, older adults made up only 4% of the U.S. population (3.1 million individuals). By mid-century, this number had grown to 12.3 million older adults or

approximately 8% of the population (Rice & Fineman, 2004). Growth in the older adult population will continue to increase as the "baby boomers" turn 65 years of age beginning in 2011. By 2050 it is projected that 20% of Americans will be older than age 65 (U.S. Department of Health and Human Services [USDHHS], 2003).

Regardless of which clinical setting nurses choose to work, the majority of nurses will care for older adults in their careers. In fact, the American Association of Colleges of Nursing (American Association of Colleges of Nursing [AACN], 2007)

*The author would like to acknowledge Erin Comstock, Sarah Brett Hartmann, and Theresa Petrone for their contributions to this chapter. This chapter incorporates material written for the third edition by Teri A. Murray states that nurses are the largest members of hospital staffs and are the primary providers of older adult care in both hospitals and nursing homes. Consequently, nurses must be knowledgeable about the unique health care needs of an increasingly aging population. It is particularly important for community health nurses to understand the needs of older adults, because only about 5% of the Medicare population resides in long-term care facilities, leaving the remaining 95% of older adults living in the community. Approximately 2% of older adults living in the community require assistance to remain living independently (Federal Interagency Forum on Aging-Related Statistics, 2004).

This chapter explores the role of older adults in the family and community in light of developmental and sociocultural influences, unique crises experienced by aging families, and the need for support systems to assist families coping with the crises of aging. Common health care needs of older adults in the areas of nutrition, medication, mobility, and social isolation are reviewed. The influence of poverty is examined in view of its impact on the health of older Americans and their ability to secure needed health care services.

Legislative trends in health care and social services for older adults arising in response to the changing demography of the U.S. population are identified. These political actions have had great influence on the development and organization of community resources for older adults. The federal, state, and local governments and social concern for the welfare of older adults have resulted in the development and organization of nationwide services for older adults. Finally, the responsibilities of the community health nurse as facilitator-collaborator, advocate, teacher, and case manager in working with the older adult client in the community are explored.

AGING

MEANING

Aging can be viewed in both objective and subjective terms. What does it mean to be old in contemporary Western society? Is one "old" when he or she reaches the age of 65 years? In 1935 the federal government adopted 65 years as the official threshold of "elderliness."

Aging is a universal human experience that culminates in an end. It is a dynamic state of existence that changes with one's perspective. Meanings of old age are based on societal views of aging, cultural beliefs about the meaning of being old, and values associated with old age.

MYTHS

Common myths about older adults are that they are frail, senile, unhealthy, unhappy, set in their ways, irritable, lacking in interest in matters of sexuality, and ineffective and undependable as workers (Cruikshank, 2003). In fact, 80% of older persons are healthy enough to engage in normal activities. Although reaction time slows with age, older persons are not senile and do not have serious memory deficits. Older people are not set in their ways. Most have had to adapt to such major life events as retirement, having children leave home, and declining health.

Studies also show that older working Americans work as effectively as their younger counterparts. They change jobs less frequently, have fewer job-related accidents, and have lower rates of absenteeism. Most older adults also report that they feel relatively satisfied most of the time. Most do not feel any significant restriction on their daily life (Rice & Fineman, 2004). Overall, older adults experience frequent social contacts with friends or relatives, participate in church-related activities or voluntary organizations, and continue to have interest in and a capacity for sexual relations (Miller, 2004). Some facts about older adults are listed below (Federal Interagency Forum on Aging-Related Statistics, 2004; USDHHS, 2003):

- The majority of older adults live independently in the community; 2% live in community-housing; only 5% live in nursing homes.
- Persons 65 years of age can expect to live for more than 18 additional years.
- Two of three older workers retire before age 65 years.
- Half of older adult women are widows, many of whom live alone.
- Older adults consume 30% of all prescription medications, and 25% of all over-the-counter medications.
- Approximately 10% of noninstitutionalized older adults receive help with at least one activity of daily living (e.g., bathing or showering, dressing, eating, getting in or out of bed or a chair, walking, and using the toilet) compared with 91% of institutionalized older adults, who comprise 5% of all Medicare beneficiaries 65 years of age and older.
- Informal networks of family, friends, and neighbors provide most health and social services to older adults.

CHRONOLOGY

Chronology is a poor measure of aging, as persons 65 years and older may span an age range of 40 or more years and may experience diverse and unique needs during this time. For this reason, some theorists make a distinction between the *young-old* and the *old-old*. The old-old have been defined as persons 85 years and older, and the young-old are persons between the ages of 65 and 74 years (Leppik, 2006). Other theorists argue that aging should be defined not in terms of chronology but in terms of biopsychosocial functioning (Ebersole et al., 2004). However aging is defined, a growing aging population is a demographic reality with definite health care implications. An increase in the prevalence of chronic diseases and functional impairments (i.e., the ability to perform activities of daily living) can be expected. The need for health care services for chronically ill persons will increase. An increase in chronic illness and residual disability will necessitate more long-term care. Medical care expenditures will increase in proportion to the greater number of older adults in need of health care services. These trends will require that health care providers have a thorough understanding of the unique health care needs of a growing aging population (Goulding et al., 2003).

ROLE OF OLDER ADULTS IN THE FAMILY AND THE COMMUNITY

Less than half of all children born at the turn of the 20th century could expect to live to age 65. Today, approximately 80% can expect to live to age 65 and one third to age 85. Americans now live longer than ever before. Currently, 12.4% or more than 35 million people in the United States are older than age 65 (Rice & Fineman, 2004).

DEVELOPMENTAL TASKS AND CRISES OF AGING FAMILIES

As people age, they face new challenges, new life experiences, and new life crises. Erikson and colleagues (1986) conceived the primary developmental task of old age as the achievement of integrity over despair. *Integrity* refers to a sense of wholeness and meaning in one's past and present experiences. *Despair* involves a sense of dread and hopelessness and the feeling that life lacks meaning and purpose. The developmental task of old age includes the reaffirmation of meaning in life and the acceptance of the inevitability of death (Erikson et al., 1986).

Maintaining a sense of wholeness and purpose may represent a challenge in the midst of declining health and significant alterations in major life roles and relationships. Such major developmental life events as retirement, loss of significant others, and the dependency incurred by declining health produce multiple role changes and may precipitate a major life crisis, or may be viewed as an opportunity for growth (Newman & Newman, 2005).

Retirement as a Developmental Task

Role changes that accompany the aging process are often abrupt and undesired (Ebersole et al., 2004). A person's occupation represents a significant societal role that may be interrupted by illness or retirement, both of which may be viewed as undesirable. *Retirement* is a withdrawal from a given service in society; operationally, retirement is measured by counting those who are no longer employed full-time. Most people older than 65 years are retired; however, some continue to work out of necessity or desire. There were 20% of men and 11.3% of women older than age 65 in the civilian labor force in 2002 (U.S. Bureau of the Census, 2006a).

Advantages of retirement include freedom from work, more leisure time, and the eligibility to collect retirement benefits or pensions. Despite these advantages, some may feel useless, unproductive, or worthless after losing this significant role. Men, in particular, who retire unwillingly, are at a significant risk for alcoholism, depression, and suicide. For this reason, it is important that persons receive adequate support and counselling in preparation for retirement. The community health nurse working in home settings and skilled in working with families is uniquely prepared to provide this service. The occupational health nurse can engage in preretirement planning with clients in the middle years, long before retirement becomes a reality.

Although federal legislation prohibits mandatory retirement based on age, most workers in private or government sectors may still be encouraged to leave work through early retirement incentive programs (Ebersole et al., 2004). The community health nurse may be responsible for coordinating preretirement planning programs. These programs should include information on attitudes toward retirement, retirement benefits, legal aspects of retirement, the effects of retirement on family relationships, and possible uses of leisure time. The American Association of Retired Persons (AARP), a national organization devoted to the needs of older Americans, publishes a package of training materials for coordinators of preretirement programs.

Loss and the Older Adult Population

Women are more likely to experience the loss of a spouse. With increasing age, the proportions of women who are widowed rose rapidly: 26.2% of women ages 65 to 74 and 75.5% of women 85 and older are widowed compared with 7.3% and 32.5% of men, respectively (U.S. Bureau of the Census, 2006a). The death of a spouse or loss of another significant person through death or relocation (e.g., children leaving home) represents a major life crisis that requires support and intervention. The loss of a loved one is an important predictor of physical and emotional decline in the older adult client. Clients who experience the loss of a spouse or significant other may grieve not only for the lost person but also for the loss of multiple roles provided by that person (e.g., loss of a lover, a homemaker, a comforter, a provider). Widows are less likely to remarry than widowers, because older adult women significantly outnumber older adult men. In addition, the loss of a spouse may necessitate relocation, which further contributes to the sense of loss and the disruption of integrity in one's life.

As people age, they are likely to experience the death of significant others of their own age and cohort. The loss of a significant other represents the loss of a part of one's past and of life history. The experiences shared with the lost person and the ability to fondly recall memories together are partially lost when the co-creator of these memories is no longer present. Anger, guilt, loneliness, and depression are common outcomes.

The community health nurse can provide support by encouraging reminiscence (i.e., by acknowledging meaningful past experiences and times of distress and by assisting the client to identify past coping mechanisms), assessing for signs of depression and suicidal intention, and assisting clients to grieve. Clients may be referred to support groups in the community that provide an opportunity to share experiences, to draw on others for support, and to establish new relationships.

Declining Health. The multiple losses experienced with aging are represented not only through the loss of significant others but also through the experience of declining health. Seventy-three percent of older adults rate their health as good or better (Federal Interagency Forum on Aging-Related Statistics, 2004). The chance of experiencing health impairment increases with age, and those with more than one chronic condition report greater limitations. In 2006, 36% of persons 75 or older reported having three or more chronic conditions (USDHHS, 2006).

Dependency. The likelihood of increased disability with age also increases the likelihood of dependency on others (Figure 28-1). This increased dependency may produce feelings of guilt, anger, frustration, and depression in clients and their families.

Research indicates that approximately 79% of older adults who need long-term care reside at home and receive care from informal caregiving systems (e.g., family, friends, or neighbors) and 59% of the U.S. adult population either is or expects to be a caregiver (Centers for Disease Control and Prevention and Merck Institute for Aging and Health, 2004). Most of the burden for family caregiving falls to middle-age and young-old adults. The term "sandwich generation" refers to middle-age persons who are juggling the support for adolescent and college-bound children and the care of parents. In fact, with the increase in life expectancy, middle-age persons may find that four generations are ultimately dependent on them (i.e., children, grandchildren, parents, and grandparents), and older adults (65 years and older) may be expected to care for old-old parents.

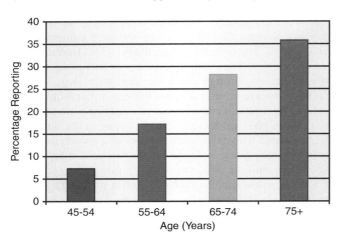

FIGURE 28-1 Risk of disability increases with age. Percentage of adults who report three or more chronic conditions. (From U.S. Department of Health and Human Services. [2006]. *Health, United States, 2006.* Washington, DC: U.S. Government Printing Office.)

Many women and men balance multiple and competing demands to care for an older adult family member (National Family Caregiver's Association, 2007a). The pool of family caregivers is dwindling. In 1990 there were 11 potential caregivers for each person needing care, compared with the projected ratio of 4:1 in the year 2050 (Mid-East Area Agency on Aging, 2003). Caregivers report increased stress and are often placed in economic jeopardy because of care needs. One study found that American businesses lose between 11 and 29 billion dollars yearly because of employees' needs to care for loved ones, and that the value of unpaid caregiving for older adult family members is near 200 billion dollars (Mid-East Area Agency on Aging, 2003). The level of caregiving required often demands significant readjustment in employment or job resignation, which may lead to financial burden and a significant alteration in family relationships. This problem is compounded by the scarcity of services available to support family caregivers.

Older age brings adjustments for the entire family, with changing roles and relationships. Intergenerational dependency and support of the aging family are greatly influenced by marital and health status, culture and ethnicity, and quality of family relationships. Family members must be recognized as highly significant in promoting the health of older clients. The community health nurse should assess the family support system, anticipate future needs and crises, and help families to plan ahead for potential crises. Family members should be encouraged to discuss their concerns and their past and present coping behaviors. The dependent older adult client should be incorporated into the family's plans as much as possible. The community health nurse can also explore with the family the available resources in the community to meet client and family needs. Common problems encountered in working with an older adult dependent family member include a lack of awareness of services in the community, the need for respite care for families assuming caregiving responsibilities, and the guilt, resentment, and frustration that arise in attempting to provide care and support to the older adult client (see the *Ethics in Practice* box).

ETHICS IN PRACTICE

When Roles Reverse: Caring for a Parent

Gail A. DeLuca Havens, PhD, APRN, BC

Nancy waves to Mrs. Costello, as she does each day when she passes the older woman sitting on the porch of her daughter's home. Today, though, Mrs. Costello does not respond. Puzzled, Nancy finishes her walk. Nancy, a community health nurse clinical specialist and a certified gerontologic nurse, practices in the state agency for the aging. Mrs. Costello is the mother of one of her best friends and long-time neighbor, Peggy. After dinner, Nancy telephones Peggy and asks if she may come visit for a few minutes. Peggy sounds welcoming, but her voice is somewhat hesitant.

Nancy is shocked to see the change in Mrs. Costello since she last saw her 2 weeks ago. She is disheveled and smells of urine. Her clothing is stained with food and she appears to have lost weight. Both of her arms are wrapped in elastic bandages and suspended in slings, which explains why she could not wave to Nancy this afternoon. Peggy explains that her mother fell this morning and, according to their family doctor, sprained both of her arms. Mrs. Costello looks downward, seemingly to avoid even nonverbal communication with Nancy. Nancy recalls that any unusual trace of what one might consider fear exhibited by an elder in the presumed safe atmosphere of his or her home, or in the presence of a caregiver, is a cue for further assessment (Turkoski, 2003). Peggy shows little interest in talking further, so Nancy leaves.

The next day Nancy keeps remembering Mrs. Costello's appearance and affect. She is unnerved as she begins to recall other incidents of "accidents" that Mrs. Costello has had over the past few months. Nancy realizes that it is possible that Mrs. Costello is being abused by her family. Before Nancy starts out on her walk that evening, she calls Peggy to see whether she would like to join her. Peggy agrees.

During their walk Nancy raises the subject of Mrs. Costello's accidents. Initially Peggy denies any recollection of Mrs. Costello having multiple accidents. She is evasive and becomes somewhat hostile. Then as their walk draws to a close, Peggy begins to cry. She is overwhelmed by the multiple responsibilities in her life. Her mother is requiring increasingly more care and supervision. Peggy's husband is not as understanding of the constraints placed on their spousal relationship by Peggy's responsibility to care for her mother as he was when Mrs. Costello first moved in with them 2 years ago.

Peggy tells Nancy that she has far less patience with her mother than she used to have. "It is so frustrating to have to care for a parent as if she were your child. It makes me resentful and angry. And now that my mother's memory is really beginning to fail, I find that I have much less tolerance for her behavior than I ever did. Nancy, I realize that I am not treating my mother well. You are an expert in caring for the elderly. Would you please help me?"

"Peggy, have you been the cause of the accidents that your mother has had?"

"Yes, but I realize that I have been very wrong in treating her in the way that I have. That's behind me now. I just need help coping."

How should Nancy respond to her friend's call for help? Should she try to work with Peggy and introduce her to strategies for coping with her mother, give her ongoing support and encouragement, and hope that a positive relationship will be reestablished between Mrs. Costello and her family in the process? Or should Nancy talk to Mrs. Costello to determine her wishes in this matter? Should Nancy, even though the problem is unrelated to her work responsibilities, report her findings to the elder ombudsman at the Council on Aging, advocating as she would for any elderly client in the context of her work?

Because family dysfunction can occur gradually over a long period of chronic stress, it is important in a situation of this nature that deliberation be thoughtful and not precipitous (Fulmer, 2003). Nancy could talk with Mrs. Costello. It is Mrs. Costello's right to choose what will happen to her (American Nurses Association, 2001).

There would be several advantages in a decision that would include Nancy helping her friend learn how to cope with her mother. Most importantly, it would allow Mrs. Costello to continue to live with her family. When the suspicion of elder abuse is reported, removal of the elder to a nursing home often occurs. If Mrs. Costello agreed, having her remain at home, supported emotionally and cared for by her family, would be to her benefit (Congdon, 2001). Helping Peggy would develop skills Peggy needed to cope constructively with the ongoing care of an elder. This expertise would have long-term benefits for Mrs. Costello, as it would enable Peggy, her primary caregiver, to become more skilled in caring for her. This strategy would serve as well to bolster Peggy's self-confidence and belief that she can care for her mother appropriately. Finally, such a decision would avoid having to expose Peggy to legal penalties resulting from reported abuse, which would help to maintain the psychologic equilibrium of the family unit. A disadvantage of such a strategy would be the need for Nancy to maintain objectivity in such a situation. Is the successful separation of professional and personal roles a realistic expectation?

Mrs. Costello, however, needs an advocate. She is being physically harmed by her daughter. Given her physical appearance and affect, it is also likely that she is a victim of active neglect, that is, the intentional omission of caregiving activities (Westley, 2005). Reporting of Mrs. Costello's situation to Adult Protective Services would trigger an investigation and eventual protection of Mrs. Costello from further physical and psychologic harm. However, would it be in Mrs. Costello's best interest, considering that such protection would likely be accomplished by removing her from the family unit? Nancy recalls how delighted Mrs. Costello was 2 years ago when she moved into her daughter's house. Nancy must decide what is the greater harm. Another consideration in choosing to report the abuse is the enduring psychologic trauma Mrs. Costello and Peggy will experience, knowing that mother and daughter must be separated to avoid repeated episodes of abuse. Finally, there is the matter of Peggy confiding in Nancy and asking her for help. Is the nature of Peggy's communication with Nancy confidential? If so, given this situation, what obligation does Nancy have to maintain confidentiality?

Another alternative to be considered is respite care for Mrs. Costello combined with counseling for Peggy or for Peggy and her husband. This approach contains the advantages of removing Mrs. Costello, temporarily, from Peggy's home and focusing on the family as a unit (Congdon, 2001). Counseling with an expert, other than Nancy, who is not personally involved in the situation could then begin.

Because Nancy is familiar with respite and counseling services in the area, she could make recommendations to Peggy from a professional perspective. This strategy has several advantages. It removes Mrs. Costello from harm, but on a temporary basis. All things being equal, this is a positive intervention, as the plan includes Mrs. Costello eventually returning to her daughter's home. It gives the family the opportunity to receive counseling without the pressure of caring for Peggy's mother. This ought to be a therapeutic arrangement as well as a constructive one, because Mrs. Costello likely will return to her family's care when they become better prepared to deal with the demands and the stress of caring for an elder. Finally, such a strategy clarifies Nancy's role in the situation and avoids the difficulties that often occur when one attempts to blend professional and personal roles. Nancy decides that if Peggy does not seek respite care and counseling, Nancy can then report the situation to Adult Protective Services.

REFERENCES

American Nurses Association. (2001). *Code of ethics for nurses with interpretive statements.* Washington, DC: American Nurses Publishing.

Congdon, J. G. (2001). *Scope and standards of gerontological nursing practice* (2nd ed.). Washington, DC: American Nurses Publishing.

Fulmer, T. (2003). Try this: Best practices in nursing care to older adults. Elder abuse and neglect assessment. *Journal of Gerontological Nursing, 29*(6), 4-5.

Turkoski, B. B. (2003). Ethical dilemma: Is this elder abuse? *Home Healthcare Nurse, 8,* 518-551.

Westley, C. (2005). Elder mistreatment: Self-learning module. *MEDSURG Nursing, 14*(2), 133-137.

SUPPORT SYSTEMS FOR AGING FAMILIES IN THE COMMUNITY

Because families provide most of the caregiving to older adults, programs for respite and support are needed to improve caregiver coping and to encourage a continued willingness to care for older adults (Stoltz et al., 2004). A variety of support systems are available in the community that might assist in meeting the diverse needs of dependent older adults and their families. The U.S. Administration on Aging (AOA), along with the National Family Caregivers Support Project Program, has developed resource guides to assist families who are involved in caregiving. Some national resources specific to the needs of the older adult population are listed under Community Resources for Practice at the end of the chapter. Older adults who receive social support can function independently for much longer than those who lack these needed services.

Most older adults want to remain in their own home whenever possible, and if this is not possible, most prefer some sort of community-based living arrangement rather than a nursing home. Most (95%) older adults live in the community or in community-based assisted living care. Support services that help to maintain their independence or assist family members to provide care are essential needs in every community.

Long-Term Care

Long-term care refers to a comprehensive range of health, personal, and social services that are coordinated and delivered over a period of time to meet the changing physical, social, and emotional needs of chronically ill and disabled persons. Long-term care may be delivered in the home, in the community, or in an institutional setting (Feldman & Kane, 2003). Long-term care services may be provided to clients who exhibit a degree of functional impairment that necessitates assistance with activities of daily living (e.g., bathing, dressing, toileting, eating) or instrumental activities (e.g., meal preparation, housework, shopping). Twenty-five percent of older adults possess at least a mild degree of functional disability or difficulty carrying out personal care and home management activities. A total of 52% of adults 65 or older reported a disability in 2002 (U.S. Bureau of the Census, 2006b). Long-term care services focus on assisting the client to maintain independent functioning to the fullest extent possible.

Home Care

Because support systems in the community may be confusing, fragmented, or unknown to the family, the community health nurse must coordinate in-home and community services to meet family health care needs (Robinson & Street, 2004). **Home care** refers to a range of health and supportive services provided in the home to persons who need assistance in meeting health care needs. These services, provided through home health agencies, hospitals, or public health departments, include skilled nursing care, occupational therapy, physical therapy, speech therapy, personal care (e.g., bathing, dressing, and toileting), assistance with meals, meal preparation, and housekeeping. The National Association for Home Care

represents the facilities and organizations that provide home care services. Various types of home care services are summarized in Box 28-1. Chapter 31 provides a detailed discussion of home care.

Respite Care

Respite care refers to the provision of temporary, short-term relief to family caregivers (National Family Caregiver's Association, 2007b). Trained personnel care for the older adult client while the caregiver is away for a period of hours, days, or even weeks. Respite care services may be sponsored by churches, synagogues, nursing homes, home health agencies, volunteer agencies, or for-profit agencies. Care may be provided at home, in institutions (nursing homes, hospitals), or in community-based (adult daycare) centers. One of the most important problems with respite care is cost. Few respite services are reimbursed by private or public health insurance. Paying for respite services out of pocket is often beyond the reach of many families.

Adult Daycare

Adult daycare can serve as an out-of-home form of respite care for family caregivers. Adult daycare centers offer a variety of services for persons who require some assistance but not 24-hour care. The centers may provide health and physical care and recreational, legal, and financial services. Transportation is usually provided to the program. Adult daycare provides a structured program for dependent, community-based elders who have difficulty performing activities of daily living or who require attention or support during work hours when significant others are not available. Adult daycare programs may provide hot meals, assistance with medications and personal care, counselling, therapy, and recreational activities. The National Institute of Adult Day Care is the national organization representing adult daycare programs. Daycare may be offered through community centers, including local senior citizen centers, religious organizations, retirement homes, nursing homes, or hospitals.

Adult daycare may be classified according to its primary objective. **Medical daycare** programs are closely affiliated with hospitals or nursing homes and are aimed at providing

---

Box 28-1 Types of in-Home Services

Home-delivered meals. Provides hot meals to senior citizens who are housebound or unable to cook.

Friendly visiting services. Provides routine home visits to older adult clients who need companionship.

Emergency response systems. Provides an immediate and accessible way of notifying appropriate authorities in case of medical emergency.

Telephone reassurance programs. A program in which volunteers make daily calls to older adults living alone.

Personal care services. Provision of household and personal care (such as homemaker and home health aide services) under the direction of a health professional.

Chore services. Provides help in home maintenance, minor repairs, house cleaning, and yard work.

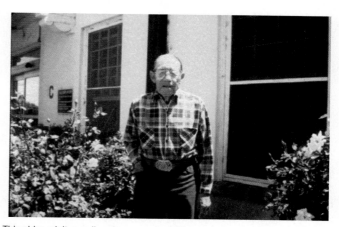

This older adult man lives in an apartment in a retirement community. He helps maintain the gardens in the community, which gives him a purpose and makes him feel useful.

comprehensive rehabilitation and support services, frequently to clients who have recently been discharged from a hospital. The objective of medical daycare is to restore or maximize physical and mental functioning to the fullest extent possible. **Social daycare** programs are designed to meet the needs of chronically disabled clients and to provide an opportunity for socialization, recreation, monitoring, and other social services. The goal of these types of programs is to maximize physical and social well-being and to prevent or delay hospitalization (Miller, 2004).

Multipurpose senior centers are community centers that provide lunch programs, home-delivered or congregate meals, socialization, recreational activities, health counselling and screening, information and referral services, and legal and financial counselling services to older adults and their families (Miller, 2004). Senior centers attempt to meet the needs of both well and frail older adults in the community. A senior center may also offer adult daycare programs to frail older adult clients. In a senior center, one important nursing role is health education aimed at encouraging health promotion and disease prevention activities.

Community-Based Living Arrangements

Other forms of community-based support systems include **foster care,** in which the older adult client is cared for in a personal residence by a family licensed through a social service agency to provide meals, housekeeping, and personal care services. **Group homes** provide shared living arrangements for a group of older adults who are jointly responsible for food preparation, housekeeping, and recreation. **Congregate housing** describes a variety of group housing options for the older adult in which housing is supplemented by services such as 24-hour security, transportation, recreation, and meals (Miller, 2004). Congregate housing can be an apartment, a single room, or a single room with shared group space. **Retirement communities** are residential developments designed for older people who may own or rent the units. Recreational and some support services are available. In most retirement communities, residents must contract for health care services on their own.

A **life-care (continuous-care) community** is a form of retirement housing that provides comprehensive health and social services to the older adult. Residents move from one level (independent living) to others within the community as their health care needs change (Pratt, 2004). For example, an older person might first purchase or rent a home or apartment and then move to congregate living, assisted living, or a nursing home as the need arises. Life-care communities usually require that clients have financial assets to pay for entry into the community.

Nursing Homes

Most elderly do not use nursing home care. Approximately 5% of people will require nursing home care at some time in their lives (Federal Interagency Forum on Aging-Related Statistics, 2004). The percentage of people 65 years and older living in nursing homes declined from 5.1% in 1990 to 3.6% in 2004 (Alecxih, 2006). The decline in nursing home use by the elderly is attributed to the growth of alternative community caregiving arrangements. Still most nursing home residents are elderly. About 94% of the nursing home population was 65 years and older in 2004 (Alecxih, 2006). Nursing homes provide continuous nursing care, rehabilitation, social activities, supervision, and room and board in state-licensed facilities. Considering nursing home placement is often a painful and traumatic experience for both the client and the family. Families may feel guilt and despair at being unable to maintain their older adult loved one at home. It is important that the older person be involved as much as possible in the decision-making process. The AARP and the Center for Medicare and Medicaid Services (CMS) publish valuable consumer information to assist families in choosing a nursing home that will best meet their needs. **Website Resource 28A** contains a sample assessment tool for evaluating nursing homes.

There are many resources currently available to help with making nursing home choices. Many organizations, such as the AARP, Center for Medicare and Medicaid Services, and state health departments, are working together to develop clear, concise, comprehensive, and consumer-friendly information profiling nursing homes to inform the public about the quality of care. Using specific checklists or tools along with information gathered during a visit to the nursing home would be most helpful in allowing one to make a good choice.

SOCIOCULTURAL INFLUENCES

As a group, the older adult population represents a diversity of beliefs, values, and cultural practices. Differences in beliefs and values may be attributed to ethnic, cultural, and generational influences. Culture is a learned way of thinking and acting. The behavioral, intellectual, and emotional forms of life expression represent a cultural heritage that is passed on from generation to generation.

A cohort refers to a group of people who share similar characteristics. People born in the same time period (i.e., within approximately 10 years) represent an age cohort. People growing up in different historical eras have lived through similar major life events (e.g., World War II, the Great Depression). These events, however, may affect persons differently depending on their age at the time the events were experienced. Differences in age ranges among older adults may span as much as 40 years, indicating that the older adult population is a heterogeneous group of people who have lived through a diversity of life experiences that have helped to shape them in unique and unpredictable ways. Therefore when working with older adult clients and their families, the community health nurse should approach each person as a unique individual.

The community health nurse can assess the influence of the client's ethnic and cultural heritage on beliefs, values, and health care practices (refer to Chapter 10 for assessment tools). Specific areas affected by ethnic and cultural orientation include perception of women's roles, social responses to a growing aging population (changes in legislation, creation of federal programs, emergence of special interest groups), and changes in role performance and opportunities (Betancourt et al., 2003). Other significant sociocultural influences include family relationships, customs, and habits; religious practices; diet; work and leisure activities; beliefs about pain, illness, and death; forms of verbal and nonverbal expression; and the ethnic and cultural orientation of the surrounding community. Family rituals and practices that are meaningful to the client and do not pose a threat to health or safety should be respected (Ebersole et al., 2004).

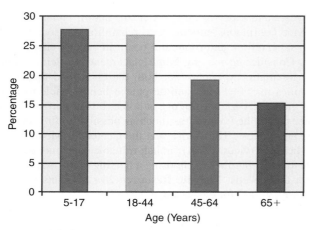

FIGURE 28-2 Percentage of people in the United States who speak a language other than English at home. (Data from U.S. Bureau of the Census. [2000]. *Census 2000 Summary File 3 [SF3], PCT14. Language density by linguistic isolation by age for the population 5 years and over in households [28]. Washington, DC: Author.)*

A community with similar cultural practices, beliefs, and values tends to reinforce the client's and family's cultural heritage. Foreign-born older adults who recently immigrated to the United States may have difficulty communicating in English and may live in a community that is foreign to their cultural orientation. Approximately 15% of all older adults speak a language other than English at home (Figure 28-2) and may live with family members who have difficulty with the English language.

Foreign-born residents may require assistance in locating and using needed community resources, including a support network of persons who share their ethnic heritage and reinforce their cultural practices. The community health nurse may also advocate for the needs of these non–English-speaking persons by increasing community awareness of the need for bilingual service providers, publications, and community announcements. Services most acceptable to older adult members of ethnic groups are usually those provided in their community by persons who are conversant in their native language and are sensitive to their cultural practices and beliefs. (See Chapter 10 for a detailed discussion of cultural influences.)

In general, when examining social and cultural influences, the community health nurse requires knowledge of the historical and cultural traditions that have shaped and influenced the personal life experiences of older adult clients and families. These experiences will exert a significant impact on the client's physical, psychologic, social, and economic well-being.

COMMON HEALTH NEEDS OF OLDER ADULTS

Four of five older adults experience at least one chronic condition, and many suffer from multiple chronic diseases. Common chronic conditions seen in older adults are the following:

- Arthritis
- Cancer
- Cataracts
- Diabetes
- Hearing loss
- Heart disease
- Hypertension

- Osteoporosis/hip fractures
- Stroke
- Varicose veins

According to the Centers for Disease Control and Prevention (CDC, 2004), some of the most common complaints of the older adult are arthritis (37%), hypertension (47%), and heart conditions (32%). The likelihood of disability increases with age. Disability rates rose with age for both males and females. Disability rates were higher for women (55.9%) than men (47.4%) ages 65 and older (U.S. Bureau of the Census, 2006b). Persons 65 years or older average 34.6 disability days per year compared with 13.4 days for persons younger than 65 years. Disability days represent days when persons have to reduce their normal activities because of illness or injury, days of confinement to bed, and days lost from work or school.

The prevalence of chronic disease and disability in older adults produces a number of health care needs. Preventive care is also needed for older adults who are healthy to maintain wellness and prevent the onset of illness or disability. The community health nurse should encourage such health promotion behaviors as a balanced diet, regular exercise, stress management, routine medical and dental evaluations, monthly breast or testicular self-examination, annual mammography, and influenza (annually) and pneumonia (one time only) immunizations. Chapters 18 and 19 provide an in-depth discussion of health promotion and screening.

NUTRITIONAL NEEDS

Nutritional needs in older adults may be affected by normal physiologic changes associated with aging and psychosocial and environmental factors that affect nutrition (Box 28-2). Dietary planning should take into consideration cultural preferences, religious observances, behavioral patterns (e.g., timing of meals), and special dietary needs (e.g., low-fat, cholesterol, diabetic, low-salt). Eliciting a diet history may help the com-

---

Box 28-2   **Factors Influencing Nutrition in Older Adults**

Physiologic Factors
Decrease in digestive enzymes and in intestinal motility
Activity reduction—unable to prepare or feed self
Dental problems (e.g., poorly fitting dentures may limit intake and predispose to nutritional deficiencies)
Sensory losses (e.g., decreased taste, vision, hearing)
Physical illness

Psychosocial Factors
Inadequate income to purchase nutritional foods
Lack of motivation to prepare balanced meals (e.g., client lives alone)
Inadequate knowledge of basic nutrition
Poor life-long eating habits
Depression
Grief/bereavement
Substance abuse or polypharmacy
Culturally inappropriate meals

Environmental Factors
Accessibility of shopping areas
Adequacy of space and equipment to store and prepare food

munity health nurse to identify dietary patterns and habits. General nutrition education should stress adherence to a balanced diet; maintenance of ideal body weight; limited intake of alcohol, fats, and sugars; increased intake of dietary fiber; and avoidance of excessive salt intake. Most older adults are deficient in vitamin D intake, and therefore a calcium supplement would be helpful (Mahan & Escott-Stump, 2004).

Decreases in hearing, vision, and taste may diminish food appeal. In addition, clients may be unwilling to eat in noisy, public places. When eating out, quiet, well-lit dining areas should be sought to enhance the dining experience.

Decreases in intestinal motility may predispose clients to constipation and overuse of laxatives. Fluid and fiber should be incorporated into the diet to compensate for decreases in intestinal motility. Thirst sensation may be diminished, so adequate water intake (2200 to 2900 ml/day) should be encouraged and monitored (Davidhizar et al., 2004). For clients who prefer not to cook for themselves or who have difficulty getting to the store, the community health nurse may wish to investigate home delivery services provided through neighborhood groceries, home-delivered meal services (e.g., Meals on Wheels), or congregate eating programs. The local senior center may provide transportation for shopping or "eating together" programs in which seniors gather for a hot meal in a group setting. Clients experiencing financial difficulties may be eligible for the federal food stamp program. Nutritional information for seniors is available through the National Institute on Aging and the AARP.

MEDICATION USE

Older adults consume approximately 34% of all prescription medication and 30% of over-the-counter medication (American Public Health Association, 2005). Prescription drug costs increased by 10% each year from 1991 to 2001 and increased 8.6% in 2005 (PriceWaterhouseCoopers, 2006; Stunk & Ginsburg, 2003). The rising cost of prescription drugs is a hardship for many older adults, especially those who have limited income sources. This concern has led to passage of a prescription drug plan for Medicare (see Box 28-4 later in this chapter, as well as Chapters 3 and 4).

The following conditions place older clients at a higher risk for adverse drug reactions:

- Normal aging changes that affect the absorption, distribution, metabolism, and excretion of drugs in the body
- Conditions, such as bed rest, dehydration, congestive heart failure, and stress, that affect the body's response to drugs
- The use of multiple drug regimens to treat concurrent health problems (Ebersole et al., 2004)

Older adults usually take drugs over long periods for chronic conditions. Approximately 25% to 50% of older adults who take prescription medications are noncompliant (Miller, 2004). In one study of 17,000 older Medicare beneficiaries, 52.1% reported medication nonadherence, with 26.3% reporting that nonadherence was related to cost (Wilson et al., 2007). The reasons for noncompliance are numerous and include the following:

- Lack of finances
- Lack of knowledge of the reason for taking medications or the nature of the illness
- Conflicts with cultural or religious beliefs
- Sense of hopelessness about getting better
- Inaccessibility of pharmacy services
- Complexity of drug regimens
- Inadequate supervision
- Inability to open drug container because of sensory-motor impairments
- Desire to avoid unpleasant side effects
- Fear of drug dependency

In addition to failing to take medication, the older adult often uses medication inappropriately. They may continue to use outdated or discontinued medication or share pills with others. Many fail to report the use of over-the-counter drugs to their physician, a failure that could result in adverse drug reactions with prescribed medications. Approximately 82% of older adults use over-the-counter medication (Miller, 2004). Among persons misusing over-the-counter drugs, the American College of Emergency Physicians (2004) report that one of two Americans misuse common pain relievers.

Drug misuse may occur through errors in prescription, the use of prescription drugs without physician supervision, or physician over-prescription. In addition, lack of knowledge of how to take medications properly, self-medication without physician consultation, or receiving medications from multiple physicians without each provider's knowledge may contribute to drug misuse. Age- and disease-related conditions and multiple drug regimens also compound the problem and may lead to adverse drug reactions or drug overdose (Weingart et al., 2005).

To improve client compliance, the community health nurse working with the older adult client should assess all prescription and over-the-counter drugs in use, including vitamin and mineral supplements, by obtaining a thorough drug history. Older adult clients should be monitored for adverse drug reactions, potential interactions between drugs, and compliance with prescribed regimens. The community health nurse should teach the client and family about the purpose, use, appropriate dosage, and side effects of all drugs. Instructions should be given verbally and in writing to facilitate retention of information. For clients with memory impairment, a calendar or schedule may be developed for taking medications; times for taking medications may be associated with daily activities, such as meals or bedtime (Ebersole et al., 2004).

The client may be advised to select pharmacies that are able to monitor the client's complete medication profile and alert the client and health care provider to potential adverse drug interactions. Providers are also responsible for explaining drug use and seeking validation of client understanding. Clients may request large-print medicine labels to facilitate readability and flip-off (versus child-proof) caps to allow for ease of opening. The community health nurse may also investigate pharmacies that offer discounts to senior citizens and generic drugs to decrease the cost of medications.

In addition to medication misuse because of lack of knowledge or physical or cognitive impairment, the older adult client may abuse drugs in an attempt to cope with depression and loss. Substance abuse is difficult to identify in the older adult client, because family members may attempt to protect the client by covering up the problem. The problem may become visible only when the behavior of a person living alone begins to draw the attention of others. For example, neighbors may become concerned when basic home repairs are not made, or family members, on visiting the client, may find their loved one unkempt or poorly nourished. The community health nurse can develop outreach programs to reach older persons who are drug-dependent and to educate the public and health professionals about the unique causes and manifestations of substance misuse and abuse in the older adult population. (See Chapter 25 for a detailed discussion of substance abuse in the community.)

MOBILITY

Deaths related to falls increase with age (see the *Healthy People 2010* box). Adults 65 years and older are more likely to experience a fall-related mortality than are younger age groups (Gleberzon & Hyde, 2006). Falls are the most frequent injury and cause of hospital admissions for trauma among older adults (Gleberzon & Hyde, 2006). Falls account for 40% of the admissions to long-term care facilities (Marshall, 2006). The risk for falling is increased in older adults because of confusion, disturbances in gait, alterations in musculoskeletal functioning, medication side effects, unfamiliarity with new surroundings, poor eyesight, and orthostatic hypotension, which may produce dizziness and syncope (Gleberzon & Hyde, 2006).

■ HEALTHY PEOPLE 2010 ■
Selected Health Objectives for Older Adults

Physical Activity

1. Increase to 50% the proportion of adults who engage in moderate physical activity for at least 30 minutes per day, 5 or more days per week. (Baseline: 32% of adults in 1997.)
2. Increase to at least 30% the proportion of adults who perform physical activities that enhance and maintain muscular strength and endurance 2 or more days per week. (Baseline: 18% of adults in 1998.)

Safety

3. Reduce suicides to no more than 9.6 per 100,000 people. (Baseline: age-adjusted 11.2 per 100,000; 38.7 per 100,000 for white males ages 65 and older in 1995.)
4. Reduce deaths from falls to no more than 3.3 per 100,000 people. (Baseline: 17.2 per 100,000 for persons 65 to 84 years and 107.9 per 100,000 for persons age 85 or older in 1998.)
5. Reduce residential fire deaths to no more than 0.2 per 100,000 people. (Baseline: 3.2 per 100,000 for persons 65 years and older in 1998.)

Chronic Disabling Conditions

6. Reduce to 33% the proportion of adults with doctor-diagnosed arthritis who experience a limitation in activity because of arthritis or joint symptoms. (Baseline: 36% in 2002.)
7. Decrease to 8% the proportion of adults with osteoporosis. (Baseline: 10% of adults 50 or older from 1988 to 1994.)
8. Increase to 79% the proportion of adults with disabilities who participate in social activities. (Baseline: 61% in 2001.)
9. Reduce to 14.0 per 10,000 the proportion of adults age 65 and older who are hospitalized for vertebral fractures associated with osteoporosis. (Baseline: 17.5 per 10,000 in 1998.)

Health Promotion and Screening

10. Increase the rate of immunization coverage among adults 65 years and older.

Recommended Immunization	1998 Baseline	2010 Target
Noninstitutionalized adults 65 years of age or older		
Influenza vaccine	64%	90%
Pneumococcal vaccine	46%	90%
Noninstitutionalized high-risk adults 18 to 64 years of age		
Influenza vaccine	26%	60%
Pneumococcal vaccine	13%	60%
Institutionalized adults (long-term care or nursing homes)		
Influenza vaccine	59% (baseline 1997)	90%
Pneumococcal vaccine	25% (baseline 1997)	90%

11. Decrease the incidence of invasive pneumococcal infections to 42 per 100,000 persons ages 65 and older. (Baseline: 62 per 100,000 ages 65 or older in 1997.)
12. Increase to at least 90% the proportion of people ages 65 and older who have participated during the proceeding year in at least one organized health promotion program. (Baseline: 12% in 1998.)
13. Increase to 60% the proportion of adults who are at a healthy weight. (Baseline: 36% of adults 60 or older from 1984 to 1994.)
14. Increase the proportion of persons 18 years and older counseled about health behaviors.

Health Behavior	2001 Baseline	2010 Target
Physical activity or exercise	45%	54%
Diet and nutrition	43%	56%
Smoking cessation	66%	72%
Risks associated with drinking	11%	17%

Access

15. Reduce the proportion of persons 65 and older with long-term care needs who do not have access to the continuum of long-term care service.

Care Need	2001 Baseline	2010 Target
Home health care	9.6%	7.7%
Adult daycare	2.9%	2.3%
Assisted living	3.3%	1.8%
Nursing home care	1.1%	0.8%

16. Increase to 96% the proportion of adults who have a specific source of ongoing care. (Baseline: 87% in 1998.)

From U.S. Department of Health and Human Services. (2000). *Healthy People 2010: Understanding and improving health* (2nd ed.). Washington, DC: U.S. Government Printing Office; and U.S. Department of Health and Human Services. (2006). *Healthy People 2010: Midcourse review.* Washington, DC: U.S. Government Printing Office.

Arthritis is a leading cause of morbidity in persons 65 years of age and older (U.S. Bureau of the Census, 2005). Approximately 19.3% of persons older than 75 years of age and 11.8% of persons between the ages of 65 and 74 reported activity limitations from arthritis (U.S. Bureau of the Census, 2005). The loss of muscle strength, painful joints, and stiffness affect gait and limit range of motion (Ebersole et al., 2004).

Osteoporosis is prevalent in postmenopausal women and in men older than 80 years. Estrogen deficiency accelerates the loss of bone mass associated with aging and may lead to back pain, deformity, or loss of height because of osteoporotic bone changes. Clients with osteoporosis are at a greater risk for sustaining fractures with little or no trauma.

Activity limitations imposed by chronic illness further compromise mobility in the older adult client. Approximately 42% of adults 65 years and older have a low level of overall physical activity and did not engage in recommended amounts of physical activity (USDHHS, 2003). The U.S. Bureau of the Census (2005) reports that over 20% of the 65 and older population have difficulty leaving their homes.

The community health nurse may assist the older adult client to maintain flexibility, muscle strength, and bone mass through counselling about sound nutritional practices and through encouraging adoption of exercise programs that strengthen muscle and improve cardiovascular function. Exercise becomes especially important in later life because it can slow, stop, or reverse physical decline (Melov et al., 2007). Walking, calisthenics, water aerobics (calisthenics performed in a swimming pool), and cycling on a stationary bicycle are examples of activities that provide an excellent form of exercise with a minimum degree of stress on joints (Warshaw, 2005). Exercise groups can improve social interaction. Walking is the most popular form of physical activity for older adults (U.S. Bureau of the Census, 2005) and provides increased social interaction and an increased sense of well-being (Ebersole et al., 2004).

All five senses become less acute with age. Sensory impairment affects both perception and the ability to move around in the environment. Approximately 15.6% of older men and 13.2% of older women have one or more sensory disabilities (U.S. Bureau of the Census, 2005). One of every 20 Americans 85 years of age or older is legally blind. Many more older adults need glasses and have difficulty with night vision.

The leading causes of blindness in persons 65 years of age and older include glaucoma (increased intraocular pressure), macular degeneration (which leads to loss of central vision), cataracts (a clouding or opacity of the lens of the eye), and diabetic retinopathy. These conditions may lead to a decrease in visual acuity, a decrease in depth perception, a decrease in peripheral vision, a decreased tolerance to glare, and a decreased ability of the lens of the eye to focus on objects. Visual and hearing impairments may mask warning signs in the environment, predisposing older adults to accidental injury. When caring for clients who have sensory impairments that may compromise mobility, the community health nurse should identify hazards in the environment, teach the client and the family about home safety, and promote an environment that encourages both independence and safety (Ebersole et al., 2004). Many environmental hazards are associated with falls or near falls, including attempting to negotiate in the dark and walking on slippery floor coverings and uneven walking surfaces. Herwaldt and Pottinger (2003) report that falls could be reduced by improving positional stability, alertness, and attention in older adults.

Information about transportation services for older adult clients may be obtained by contacting the local office on aging or the local senior center. The area agency on aging may contract with a local taxi company to provide transportation to seniors at a discounted rate. In some localities, mass transit buses and subways receive federal funding from the Department of Transportation and provide discounted rates for senior citizens. These discounts may be available on a 24-hour basis or restricted to non–rush hour times. Medicare cards may enable the older adult client to ride at half fare, or reduced fare cards may be obtained from the local office on aging. The American Red Cross may provide emergency transportation when an older adult client is discharged from a hospital or emergency department. Local governments or community agencies may also sponsor "senioride" programs, which provide door-to-door transportation to older adults at a minimal cost.

SOCIAL ISOLATION

Twenty-eight percent of people 65 or older live alone (U.S. Bureau of the Census, 2004). Older women are more likely to live alone than are men. In 2006, 75.1% of men 65 to 74 years were married and living with their spouse, whereas only 54.3% of women in the same age group did so (U.S. Bureau of the Census, 2006a). Living alone, coupled with the prevalence of sensory-perceptual and mobility impairments, cognitive impairment, and chronic illness, places the older adult client at a higher risk for social isolation. It is imperative that community health nurses assess the older adult's social support network, including family, peers, church-related, and other groups; professional caregivers; and other more informal caregivers. Social support through friends, relatives, and acquaintances can be of great value in giving life meaning (Yeh, 2004). Low levels of social support are associated with higher rates of health problems.

Mental Health Disorders

Social isolation may be a symptom of a mental health disorder. Depression and dementia are the two most common mental health disorders in older adults.

Depression. It is estimated that 10% to 65% of older adults may experience depression. Depression may be characterized by a persistent sad or depressed mood (i.e., at least 2 weeks), loss of pleasure in previously enjoyable activities, impaired thinking and concentration, or recurrent thoughts of death or suicide. Depressed clients may also experience insomnia or hypersomnia (increase in sleep), early morning awakening, loss of interest in activities, feelings of guilt, fatigue, loss of appetite, weight gain or loss, agitation, and feelings of helplessness or hopelessness (Miller, 2004).

Geriatric depression may develop as a result of actual or perceived losses, environmental stresses, neurologic or endocrine disorders, adverse effects of medication, infection, or alcohol consumption (Hutman et al., 2005). Treatment of depression in older adults may be delayed or never pursued, because sadness and loss are often thought to be normal consequences of aging. Depression may also be inappropriately regarded as a normal consequence of senility. Depression may not be identified early in clients who live alone and have few social contacts. Older adult depressed clients may report anxiety, physical symptoms such as chronic pain or worries about the body, or a loss of concentration and difficulties with memory.

Older adults account for nearly 13% of the population but commit 16% of the suicides (National Institute of Mental Health, 2007). Men accounted for 85% of suicides among persons ages 65 years and older in 2001 and actually have higher suicide rates than men in all age groups except males 40 to 44 years old (U.S. Bureau of the Census, 2005). Older adults who live alone, perceive themselves as friendless, have few meaningful attachments to the community, and have little social support are more vulnerable to psychiatric illness, depression, and suicide (Yeh, 2004). Warning signs of suicidal intent include verbal clues indicating a desire to commit suicide (e.g., "others would be better off without me"), behavioral clues (such as getting personal affairs in order or changing one's will), and situational clues (e.g., significant loss, death of spouse, diagnosis of illness, recent undesired move, family conflict) (Smith & Jaffe, 2007). Detecting suicide ideation in older adults may be more difficult because they do not provide as many verbal cues as younger adults (Miller, 2004).

It is important for the community health nurse to monitor for signs and symptoms of depression, to be alert to subtle differences in behavior, and to refer clients to the appropriate resources for medical evaluation, counselling, and support. Social interactions seem to alleviate or reduce the risk for depression (Yeh, 2004).

Clients who are struggling with feelings of worthlessness and low self-esteem may also benefit from therapeutic reminiscence. The notion of reminiscence or life review involves a reflection on past life experiences with the goal of building self-esteem and understanding, stimulating thinking, transmitting a cultural heritage, and finding meaning, worth, and acceptance in life. The use of group reminiscence in nursing homes has reduced the level of depression in participating residents (Ebersole et al., 2004).

Reminiscence is, in essence, communicating comforting memories (Ebersole et al., 2004). A story recounts both the joys and struggles of human experience. Persons may be assisted in telling their stories through involvement in the following activities that invite storytelling:

• Sharing memorabilia and family pictures
• Participating in reminiscence support groups
• Constructing family trees or scrapbooks
• Writing or audio taping a personal autobiography
• Creating safe, supportive environments that permit disclosure
• Demonstrating a nonjudgmental, open, accepting attitude to the client's disclosures

The community health nurse can teach the family the value of reminiscence and techniques for facilitating reminiscence and can, thereby, assist persons in finding meaning in their memories and coming to terms with unresolved life conflicts.

Dementia. Dementia is a serious cognitive impairment involving thought, memory, or personality (Miller, 2004). Dementia may be caused by a variety of diseases. The most common type of dementia is Alzheimer's disease. Alzheimer's disease affects 8% to 15% of persons older than age 65, with the number of cases doubling every 5 years of age after the age of 60. Alzheimer's disease is prevalent in approximately 3% to 20% of persons older than 65 years and in 50% of persons who are 85 or older (National Institute on Aging, 2004).

The costs of caring for Alzheimer's clients are tremendous in both monetary and personal costs. The annual direct and indirect costs for caring for persons with Alzheimer's disease are estimated at $100 billion (National Institute on Aging, 2003). Alzheimer's disease is responsible for most cases of dementia, currently estimated at 4.5 million Americans (Smith & Buckwalter, 2005). It is the leading cause of nursing home placement. In 2004 approximately 45% of nursing home beds were occupied by clients with dementia, an increase of 8% between the years 1998 and 2004 (Harrington et al., 2005).

The exact cause of Alzheimer's disease is unknown. The diagnosis is established by ruling out all other possible causes of dementia. Ultimately, the diagnosis can only be positively confirmed at autopsy, at which time distinct changes in the brain may be evident. The disease is progressive, presenting initially with subtle changes in memory and personality (e.g., decrease in attention span, forgetfulness, losing or misplacing items). Nurses should be alert to behavior and cognitive changes associated with Alzheimer's disease. There are a number of quick assessment tools to help evaluate cognitive abilities, including the Mini Mental States Exam. Even without a formal tool, it is suggested that nurses test a number of functions for cognitive impairment (Box 28-3). The disease progresses over a period of years to complete disorientation, extreme agitation or apathy, incontinence, complete loss of self-care ability, and loss of language (Ebersole et al., 2004; Miller, 2004).

Respite care and eventual nursing home placement may need to be considered for the client with Alzheimer's disease. Unfortunately, not all nursing homes can accommodate clients with Alzheimer's disease. The Alzheimer's Association is a family-established, volunteer-operated, national organization that provides family support, education, advocacy, referral services, and research funding. Local chapters within the community sponsor family support groups.

Families caring for clients with Alzheimer's disease will also likely require legal and financial consultation. Legal consultation is needed to assist the family in getting the client's legal affairs in order before he or she is no longer competent to make legal decisions about medical care and handling of property and assets (see Chapter 6). Financial consultation is needed to assist the family in preparing for the financial burden

---

BOX 28-3 Suggested Cognitive Assessment Areas

1. Orientation: Determine if the client is oriented to time, person, and place.
2. Memory and retention: Name several items and later ask the client to recall them.
3. Remote memory: Ask about events in early life such as childhood or school.
4. Three-stage command: Ask the client to perform three simple acts in succession.
5. Judgment: Supply a proverb and ask for an interpretation, for example, "The early bird catches the worm"; or provide a situation and ask the client what to do, for example, "You see a house on fire; what would you do?"
6. Calculation: Provide simple arithmetic problems or ask the client to count backward from 100 or 50 by 5 or 3.

likely to be incurred as the client's condition deteriorates and he or she requires greater assistance in meeting personal and health needs. The Alzheimer's Association may supply families with referrals for these important services. Referrals for legal services may also be obtained through the local department on aging, legal aid society, bar association, or legal clinics in law schools.

The term pseudodementia describes cognitive deficits that mimic organic mental disorders but that are reversible when the underlying condition is treated. Approximately 15% of cognitively impaired older adults have a medical condition that, if treated, will alleviate symptoms of dementia (Miller, 2004). Pseudodementia may be caused by depression, social and environmental stresses, sensory-perceptual impairment, or side effects of medications. Often, clients with depression are inappropriately diagnosed as having dementia because of the memory impairments that may accompany the depressed state.

Hearing Loss

Hearing loss may contribute to social isolation because of the embarrassment or frustration that sensory-impaired persons experience when they are unable to hear and respond appropriately in social settings or because of the stigma associated with hearing loss. Approximately 30% to 50% of persons 65 years of age and older experience hearing loss significant enough to interfere with their ability to communicate (Ebersole et al., 2004). The community health nurse may assess for the presence of a hearing impairment and refer the client for audiologic evaluation and treatment. The nurse provides support, counselling, and advice on locating affordable resources (e.g., funding for a hearing aid that is not covered by Medicare) and securing appropriate intervention. One of the most common problems seniors find in adjusting to a hearing aid is background noise. Most hearing aids amplify all sounds and do not distinguish between distant and near sounds. As a result, many seniors do not use their hearing aids. Sometimes the hearing aid technician can reduce the level of distracting noise. Helping friends and family to understand the problem and reducing the intensity of background sounds such as loud conversations and music will help. There is new technology that uses computer chips to distinguish the distance of the sound source and modifies intensity as needed. These hearing aids are very expensive but should become more affordable as the technology evolves.

Incontinence

Incontinence, or the involuntary loss of control of urination or defecation, is a significant cause of disability and dependency in the older adult population. Incontinence is a leading cause of institutionalization of persons older than age 65 (Ebersole et al., 2004). Incontinence may contribute to social isolation through embarrassment, feelings of loss of control, low self-esteem, and infantilization. Gray (2003) reports that between 10% and 58% of women and between 6% and 28% of men experience daily incontinence.

Even if not incontinent, older adults have a higher frequency of nocturnal urination. Two thirds of persons 65 and older report it necessary to go to the bathroom during the night. Night bathroom visits place older adults at risk for accidents and injuries because many have difficulty with visibility, mobility, or initial positional orientation. The community

health nurse works with the older client and family to assist in coping with this serious problem. Interventions may include encouraging regular toileting, reducing liquid intake at night, teaching Kegel exercises (a series of exercises that strengthen the pelvic floor), or investigating pharmacologic options with the client. If older clients are taking long-acting diuretics, the medication should be taken in the morning to reduce the risk of late-night voiding.

VICTIMIZATION

Older adults are vulnerable to being victimized. Because of increased dependency and the potential for chronic health impairment, older adults may be placed in situations in which they are less able to advocate for their own needs. Older adults may be abused or neglected by caregivers or be victims of criminal practices.

Elder Abuse and Neglect

Elders are at risk for abuse and neglect from family members and other caregivers. Families experiencing the stress of caring for a chronically ill member are at a high risk for elder abuse or neglect. More than half a million older adults are victims of abuse each year (Administration on Aging, 2004). Older adults rarely report acts of abuse. This failure to report abuse or neglect may be due to physical or mental impairment; fear of injury, retaliation, or abandonment; or fear of not being believed or taken seriously (Miller, 2004). Financial abuse is a common, but usually difficult, problem to detect. Nurses who provide care to older adult clients in all settings should be sensitive to signs of financial abuse and know what to do in such situations. (See Chapter 23 for a detailed discussion of family violence and interventions.)

Self-Neglect. One of the most common forms of elder abuse is self-neglect. Social isolation places older adults, especially those who are depressed and live alone, at risk for neglecting themselves and their living space. Community nurses should be especially vigilant to early signs of depression and neglect, such as poor hygiene, untidy or unkempt living arrangements, or failure to seek medical care. Suicide potential must be assessed. Quick intervention coupled with closer supervision and increased social interaction can reduce the risk for self-neglect. Some elders resist interventions, however well-meaning. One of the most difficult things for nurses to accept is that these older adults, if mentally competent, have the right to continue living in hazardous states (see Chapter 6).

Criminal Victimization. Concerns about criminal victimization may contribute to social isolation in the older adult by breeding suspicion, mistrust, and fear of leaving home. Although the incidence of crime is no higher in the older adult population than in the general population, the consequences of criminal victimization may be greater (Ebersole et al., 2004). For example, a client who has been physically assaulted may sustain a hip fracture during a fall. Recovery may involve bed rest or other mobility limitations that may increase the client's risk for developing pneumonia.

Crime is a major concern of older adults because of their heightened sense of vulnerability. Older adult clients who are frail and live in inner-city neighborhoods where the incidence of crime is high are often prime targets for criminal victimization, such as robbery and assault. Frequently performed crimes against older adults include purse-snatching, fraud, theft of checks from the mail, vandalism, and harassment. The community health nurse works with older clients in the community to educate them about crime prevention, protection from fraud and harassment, and sources of emotional, financial, and legal assistance should they experience criminal victimization.

Mr. Tillman Arnold is a 78-year-old man living alone in a row house in a mid-sized city. Tom Fisher, a community health nurse, is assigned to do home visits after Mr. Arnold's discharge from the hospital, where he had a broken arm repaired. On Tom's first visit, he finds four teenage boys sitting on Mr. Arnold's porch. Tom asks Mr. Arnold if they are family members, and Mr. Arnold responds "These boys just hang around my house. I tell them to go away and they just laugh at me. I'm afraid to go out to get my mail; they try to trip me." Tom suspects the boys may be involved in the "accident" that caused Mr. Arnold to break his arm.

IMPACT OF POVERTY ON OLDER ADULTS

In the past decade, the income status of the older adult population has improved because of an increase in Social Security benefits (i.e., the National Retirement Income Supplement Program) and improvements in private pension plans. Nevertheless, on retirement, the older adult may experience a 40% to 60% drop in income.

Approximately 9.4% of older adults live below the poverty line (DeNavas-Walt & Smith, 2007). Poverty levels are higher for minorities, women, and persons 75 years and older. Older adult widows are primary victims of poverty. Three of four older adult poor persons are women. Both older adult men and older adult women may have inadequate pension income because of previous limited employment opportunities, frequent job changes, or low-wage jobs with no employer-sponsored pension plans. In addition, women may experience lower pension income because of interruption in work history for child rearing or the cessation/reduction of a pension related to the death of a spouse.

Because older adults often have inadequate income for immediate expenses, they may deprive themselves of needed goods and services to avoid selling their homes (Ebersole et al., 2004). The Federal Interagency Forum on Aging-Related Statistics (2004) reported that 39% of older adult income comes from Social Security, 25% from earnings, and only 19% from pensions, an economic reality that can significantly affect the adequacy of income over time. Although more current information is not presently available, the changes in pension composition and the losses in guaranteed pensions probably indicate that inflation-protected pensions are becoming less common. Fortunately, Social Security benefits are indexed for cost of living. However, benefits are reduced if the recipient earns more than a certain amount of money. Critics have labelled this practice as an unfair penalty for older workers. For 51% of persons 65 years and older, Social Security payments are the source of 90% to 100% of their income (Social Security Administration, 2006). The number of elders dependent on Social Security income has increased 13% since 1995. This is troubling, because it indicates that older adults have less supplemental income at a time when the stability of the Social Security system is under question.

Older adults are the heaviest users of health services. Health care spending in this group accounts for one third of the personal health care expenditures in the nation. Despite the benefits of Medicare, older adults spend approximately 21% of their income on medical care (National Clearinghouse for Long-Term Care Information, 2007). As discussed in Chapter 4, Medicare does not cover costs and services such as deductibles, co-insurance premiums, additional charges when Medicare rates are not accepted as full payment, and charges for long-term care, dental care, eyeglasses, hearing aids, and preventive care. Often, older persons must purchase additional supplemental insurance (referred to as "Medigap" policies) to cover the gaps in Medicare coverage. Consequently, older adults who cannot afford to pay for services not covered by Medicare or for Medigap policies may be denied access to needed services.

Because some states set Medicaid eligibility requirements below the federal poverty line, many poor older adults do not qualify for Medicaid. Although new legislation in recent years has allowed older adults to maintain a portion of their assets and remain eligible for Medicaid, many nursing home residents still must deplete their financial assets and become financially destitute before receiving federal aid. Costly long-term nursing home stays often leave both the client and his or her spouse impoverished. The average cost of nursing home care is now $74,500 per year (New York Life, 2007). Persons at greatest risk for "spending down" their economic assets to reach Medicaid eligibility levels include those suffering from chronic debilitating illnesses who have limited incomes.

Poor older adults may lack available, affordable health care services, the transportation needed to reach these services, or the knowledge of where to look for services. Services that are fragmented, inadequately covered, and inaccessible leave significant gaps in health care. Because older adults often demonstrate multiple health care needs, they require a comprehensive continuum of services that are integrated and coordinated.

DEVELOPMENT AND ORGANIZATION OF COMMUNITY RESOURCES

Community resources have been established historically through federal, state, and local initiatives that have effected needed social action for the welfare of older adults. Several pieces of important legislation have been passed to assist in meeting the needs of older Americans. Some legislation has had an adverse effect on the older adult. In Box 28-4, some of the pertinent pieces of legislation affecting services and access to care in the community are reviewed.

IMPACT OF LEGISLATION ON SERVICES

From the 1930s through the 1970s, most legislation was aimed at improving the economic situation, enhancing access to medical care, and encouraging the emergence of support services for older Americans. For younger people, it is difficult to understand there was a time when most older people were poor, few qualified for pensions, most could not retire because no job meant no income, and many could not afford to pay for health care or health insurance. Social Security and Supplemental Security Income provided a modest income for those too old or too sick to work. Medicare and Medicaid increased accessibility to health care. By 2005, 95% of persons 65 years and older had Medicare coverage (DeNavas-Walt & Smith, 2007). The

Box 28-4   Selected Legislation Affecting Support and Services for Older Adults

The websites related to these legislative acts can be accessed through this book's website. See the Community Resources for Practice box at the end of the chapter for more details.

Social Security Act

Passed in 1935, this act provided for a national retirement income system and a system of federal grants to assist states in providing support to aged, disabled, and blind persons and to dependent children.

In 1965 *Title 18* of the Social Security Act established *Medicare,* a federal program providing hospital and medical insurance to persons entitled to Social Security.

Title 19 of the Social Security Act was enacted to provide health care coverage for low-income persons, *Medicaid.*

Supplemental Security Income is a federally funded program that ensures a minimum monthly income to aged, blind, and disabled persons who are not covered by Social Security or for whom Social Security is insufficient.

Older Americans Act

Enacted in 1965 to promote the welfare of older adults, the Older Americans Act (OAA) developed congressional policies related to aging, defined responsibilities of state and local governments, and provided for demonstration projects, research, and training programs. The OAA called for better coordination of resources and state assistance in developing new programs for older adults. It established a network of state and *local area agencies on aging* (AAAs), which are responsible for planning, coordinating, and funding local services and programs for persons 60 years of age and older.

In 1981 an amendment to the OAA mandated the development of a *State Ombudsman Program* to provide liaison services between nursing home residents and their families and nursing home administration. The state-appointed ombudsman investigates problems and complaints in skilled nursing, residential care, and other health-related facilities and works with the health care administration to resolve grievances.

Title 2 of the OAA established the *Administration on Aging* (AOA) as a division of the U.S. Department of Health and Human Services. The focus of the AOA is the development and coordination of federal programs for older adults.

Title 3 of the OAA provided for programs for older adults to be established at a state level. The *State Unit on Aging* (SUA), an office within each state government, was established to develop a statewide plan for providing services to older adults.

The OAA then laid the foundation for the development of a *National Network on Aging* (NNOA). The NNOA is a program for establishing and maintaining a coordinated, nationwide system of services for older adults. It is nationally coordinated and funded.

Omnibus Reconciliation Act 1981

This act shortened acute inpatient hospital stays in the Medicare program. It forced patients out of acute care institutions and into community-based institutional care, long-term care, and other community-based supportive services. Most of the patients affected were older adults.

For the Medicaid program, the act allowed states greater flexibility in determining the scope of services, eligibility requirements, and types of populations served by the program. The impact of this action included curtailment of "optional services" and elimination of some previously served populations, including some low-income older adults. Most mental health care was termed "optional," and some states drastically curtailed these services.

Omnibus Reconciliation Act 1987

This act aimed to improve the standards of nursing home care, expand coverage by registered and licensed practical nurses in nursing homes, and require formal training, in-service education, and competency-based evaluation of nurses aides working in nursing homes. Standards were to be implemented by 1990.

Medicare Catastrophic Coverage Act 1988/1989

This act protected against financial ruin for the spouse of a Medicare client who needed nursing home care. The spouse was allowed to keep the house and designated financial assets. Before this act, the spouse living in the community could be compelled to sell the house and deplete all assets before Medicaid would pick up coverage for nursing home care.

Omnibus Reconciliation Act 1990

This act provided some health promotion and screening for Medicare clients who use federally qualified health centers (FQHCs) in medically underserved, low-income areas. Preventive services included physical examinations, immunizations, cholesterol checks, limited blood work, and counseling related to diet, exercise, substance abuse, and injury prevention. This act does not provide such services for other Medicare recipients.

Section 1115 Waivers for Medicaid, Expanded 1993

This legislation allowed states flexibility in the provision of health care services. All the waivers permit enrolling Medicaid beneficiaries in managed care organizations and expanding coverage to working poor families not previously covered by Medicaid.

Balanced Budget Act 1997

Medicare recipients and their physicians may privately contract to pay for services, even if those services are qualified reimbursable by Medicare. The following are conditions of these contracts:

- Services provided must be specified in the contracts and signed in advance of treatment. Both the physician and the recipient must agree not to bill Medicare.
- Clients must be informed that there is no limit on the amount the physician can charge.
- A private contract is not permitted in an emergency situation.
- Clients must be informed that the services could be covered by Medicare if performed by another physician.
- Authorized the National Family Caregiver Support Program, which funds programs administered through state agencies to provide support services to caregivers. Services include information, caregiver assistance, counseling, support groups, respite care, and other home-based and community-based services to families caring for frail older members.

Medicare Prescription Drug and Modernization Act 2003

- Adds a prescription drug plan for seniors to the Medicare program, starting in 2005.
- Plan will make seniors choose between Medicare Advantage (replaces Medicare+Choice, the managed care plan option); Medicare-enhanced fee-for-service (EFFS), or a prescription drug plan (PDP) if staying in the current Medicare program.
- Provides new enrollees in Medicare with an initial physical examination and other primary prevention services. Current enrollees are not eligible for these services.
- Plans to improve the health promotion and disease prevention areas in Medicare.

Older Americans Act established community support services and legal safeguards against mistreatment in nursing homes.

During the 1980s a series of federal actions designed to cut costs in service programs affected some older adults. In 1981 the first of a series of Omnibus Reconciliation Acts (OMBAs) allowed states more latitude in determining eligibility and services for Medicaid clients. Consequently, some low-income older adults were cut from the program, and there was wider variation in services provided among the states. The same bill increased the hospital discharge rate of Medicare clients, increasing the demand for community support services. Because of this Medicare change, there was a proliferation of for-profit community-based home care services that were significantly impacted by the 1997 Balanced Budget Act that reduced the length of stay in home care (Murkofsky et al., 2003). Expanded oversight of these organizations is needed to ensure proper services are provided to Medicare recipients. For additional information on the impact of budget efforts, refer to Chapters 3 and 4.

Although many OMBAs had adverse effects on older adults, the OMBA of 1987 enhanced safety factors for nursing home residents. It also expanded nursing's role in skilled nursing and intermediate care facilities because of the requirement for additional quality oversight (see Box 28-4).

In 1993 President Clinton directed the Health Care Financing Administration to streamline Section 1115 waivers for the Medicaid program. The most significant impact was an increase in enrollment in Medicaid managed care, which affected Medicaid-eligible older adults. Medicare clients have also been offered managed care coverage, but it is a voluntary choice and not mandated (see Chapter 4).

Most of the actions in the 1980s and early 1990s were designed to reduce the costs of health care services. Rising public concern about the quality of services has led to new legislative and regulatory efforts to ensure quality of care. These efforts include designing quality measures to evaluate managed care organizations; consideration by Congress of a "patient's bill of rights"; state legislation requiring specific services of managed care organizations; and attempts to eliminate the "gag order" from physician contracts with managed care organizations. Refer to Chapters 3 and 4 for additional details on these measures.

In 2003 Congress passed the Medicare Reform Act (see Box 28-4), known as the Medicare Prescription Drug and Modernization Act (Part D). The intent of this act was to make prescription drug coverage available for seniors on Medicare. Starting in 2005 Part D has made some progress in helping seniors with medication access. In 2006 The Kaiser Family Foundation study found that the percentage of seniors without prescription drug coverage fell to 8% compared with 33% in the year before Part D took effect (Hoadley et al., 2006). That same report found that prescription co-pays for seniors was more costly in Part D than for seniors who had coverage from their employer plan or the Veterans Administration. Other issues with Part D coverage are under investigation (see Chapter 4).

The remainder of the act includes funding for managed care competition against the standard Medicare program, reorganizes the cost of care for services under the Medicare program, adds additional incentives to reduce hospital days, provides for several models of drug coverage plans from which seniors must choose, bans the Medicare program from negotiating price discounts for medication, and discourages the importation of drugs from other countries. Chapter 4 addresses some of these issues in more detail. The effects of these changes are impossible to determine at this time, because most of the act did not take effect until 2006. It will be several more years for the actual results, impact on seniors, benefits or problems, and costs to become evident.

Nursing organizations have been at the forefront of support for oversight measures to ensure both quality of and access to health care services. The American Nurses Association (ANA) has supported universal access to health care and has developed *Nursing Blueprint for Managed Care,* a companion policy statement to *Nursing Agenda for Health Care Reform* (ANA, 1997). Nurses are also becoming involved in the evaluation of health care services. In 2003 the ANA adopted principles to guide evaluation of the Medicare prescription drug plan and remain committed to a reliable and affordable prescription benefit for older Americans (ANA, 2007; McKeon, 2003).

It is especially important for nurses to act as advocates and to monitor the caliber of health services provided to older adults. Many older adults are not accustomed to navigating a complicated health system and are often unaware of their rights with reference to access to second opinions, appeals of denied services, and questions of billing errors. In the community, it is often the nurse who sees older adults on a regular basis and must assist them in obtaining relief. In the wake of the Medicare Reform act, nurses should be alert to how these changes benefit or compromise the care provided to the country's senior citizens.

ROLE OF SPECIAL INTEREST GROUPS

In addition to federal, state, and local government initiatives, special interest groups and organizations may serve as advocates in effecting needed social action for the welfare of older Americans. The most notable group is the American Association of Retired Persons (AARP), the nation's largest nonprofit, nonpartisan organization of people 50 years and older, with approximately 38 million members (AARP, 2006). The AARP offers a variety of membership benefits and educational and community service programs that are provided through a national network of volunteers and local chapters. In addition, the AARP sponsors policy research and analysis and is an effective lobbying group at both the federal and the state levels.

Other senior advocacy and political action groups, such as the Gray Panthers, the National Council of Senior Citizens, the National Retired Teachers' Association, and the National Caucus on the Black Aged, work independently or in cooperation with other organizations to advocate for the needs of the older adult population and to promote legislation that preserves and protects the rights of older Americans. Because a higher percentage of older adults vote than do their younger counterparts, the older adult population is recognized as a powerful political force.

TRENDS IN HEALTH CARE SERVICES FOR OLDER ADULTS

America has witnessed tremendous changes in health care policies and priorities as the number of older Americans has continued to grow. Major social policy issues and concerns, centering on the aging of the "baby boom" population (i.e., those born from 1945 to 1964) and the reduced birth rate of succeeding cohorts, necessitate that younger people bear a heavier burden in paying for retirement, Social Security, and health benefits for aged persons in the future. The condition of the economy is also likely to affect the ability of older Americans to care for themselves and the ability of the government to provide needed support. The need for long-term care will continue to escalate as the population ages. Currently, many community support services and other types of long-term care arrangements are limited and too costly for many older adults. At the same time, there is a national push to place greater emphasis on health promotion and disease prevention. For older adults, good health habits can improve health status and reduce the length of infirmity before death.

HEALTHY PEOPLE 2010

Healthy People 2010 identifies national health-promotion and disease prevention objectives and sets forth a national agenda for promoting and protecting the health of the American people. *Healthy People 2010* has less emphasis on the specific health needs of older adults than did *Healthy People 2000*. Although *Healthy People 2010* does selective age aggregate targeting, many of its objectives are targeted at the entire adult population. The *Healthy People 2010* box earlier in this chapter identifies some of the initiatives that address older adults. Many of these are related to reducing risks and encouraging a healthy lifestyle.

PATIENT'S SELF-DETERMINATION ACT

Because of concern that medical care wishes of older adults were not being followed, Congress enacted the Patient's Self-Determination Act as part of the Omnibus Reconciliation Act of 1990 and amended it in 1992. This act applies to all Medicare and Medicaid provider organizations, including community-based health services. It requires that each health care facility maintains written policies and procedures for advance directives (i.e., directions given in advance to a health care provider articulating a client's wishes regarding health care decisions).

Under this law, clients have the right to make their own health care decisions, refuse medical treatment, and establish advance directives. Advance directives may take the form of living wills or durable powers of attorney. **Living wills** enable persons to document in advance their decisions regarding medical care should the time come when they are incapable of expressing their wishes. The living will defines under what conditions, if any, life-sustaining measures may be instituted. A **durable power of attorney** is a written document giving another adult the right to make health care decisions on one's behalf, in the case of incompetence or inability to render these decisions independently. For additional information, refer to Chapter 6. The Patient's Self-Determination Act is an important document. It allows older adults, who are more vulnerable to chronic and long-term illness and are more likely to face difficult health care decisions, some assurance that their wishes will be followed.

NATIONAL CONFERENCES ON AGING

In the wake of elder concerns and in response to the changing demography of the population, the White House has sponsored

four National Conferences on Aging, one each decade since 1961. The most recent National Conference on Aging was held in 2005. Each conference has outlined major concerns of the older adult population and made specific recommendations to address these concerns. The latest White House Conference on Aging made extensive recommendations with a goal of developing a coordinated comprehensive long-term care strategy addressing issues of finance, choice, quality, service delivery, and the long-term care workforce, both paid and unpaid (White House Conference on Aging, 2005). Recommendations from this conference are summarized in Box 28-5.

PROBLEMS IN LONG-TERM CARE

Long-term care encompasses both health and social support services. Current problems in long-term care include fragmentation of services, high cost of services, difficulty locating and using appropriate resources, limited funding for long-term care, insufficient community-based alternatives to nursing home care, and inadequate support to family and informal support networks that provide the greatest amount of long-term care to older adults.

As discussed in Chapters 3 and 4, Medicare offers only limited coverage for long-term care and Medicaid covers only select impoverished elders in nursing homes and other limited living arrangements. Policymakers have been reluctant to expand long-term care services in public insurance programs, and long-term care services are not included in the standard policies for most private insurance. Medicare pays only a small amount of nursing home costs directly related to skilled nursing and rehabilitative services, while over half of nursing home residents assume the cost of their nursing home stays from personal resources that are quickly exhausted (Marshall, 2006). Medicaid pays for most nursing home stays for older adults with limited assets and financial resources (Marshall, 2006). Specific long-term care insurance policies are on the market, but premiums are costly, ranging from $630 to $700 per month or higher for persons age 70 (Consumer Reports, 2003; Office of Personnel Management, 2002). The cost makes these plans unavailable for many seniors, especially for the 51% of seniors whose only income is Social Security.

With an ever-expanding older population, the issues of cost will continue to affect policy decisions. Many are concerned that cost-cutting efforts in health care have peaked, and that any money saved in hospitalization costs is being used to provide community-based services. Easing the restrictions on coverage of long-term care would dramatically escalate those community-based health care costs. As it is, Medicare has moved to reduce costs and increase oversight of home health care, one of the fastest rising cost areas in that program.

Physicians for a National Health Plan advocate universal coverage for preventive, acute, and long-term care. Such a policy, they contend, would eliminate the substitution of acute care services for long-term care and prevent unnecessary nursing home placements. The ANA (2007) remains committed to universal access to health care. Many solutions have been proposed and are summarized as follows:

1. Expand Medicaid to cover long-term care for all, similar to the recommendation of Physicians for a National Health Care Program.

| Box 28-5 | Summary of White House Conference on Aging 2005 Resolutions |

1. Reauthorize the Older Americans Act within the first 6 months following the 2005 White House Conference on Aging.
2. Develop a coordinated, comprehensive long-term care strategy by supporting public- and private-sector initiatives that address financing, choice, quality, service delivery, and the paid and unpaid workforce.
3. Ensure that older Americans have transportation options to retain their mobility and independence.
4. Strengthen and improve the Medicaid program for seniors.
5. Strengthen and improve the Medicare program.
6. Support geriatric education and training for all health care professionals, paraprofessionals, health profession students, and direct care workers.
7. Promote innovative models of noninstitutional long-term care.
8. Improve recognition, assessment, and treatment of mental illness and depression among older Americans.
9. Attain adequate numbers of health care personnel in all professions who are skilled, culturally competent, and specialized in geriatrics.
10. Improve state- and local-based integrated delivery systems to meet 21st century needs of seniors.
11. Establish principles to strengthen Social Security.
12. Promote incentives for older workers to continue working and improve employment training and retraining programs to better serve older workers.
13. Develop a national strategy for supporting informal caregivers of seniors to enable adequate quality and supply of services.
14. Remove barriers to the retention and hiring of older workers, including age discrimination.
15. Create a national strategy for promoting elder justice through the prevention and prosecution of elder abuse.
16. Enhance the affordability of housing for older Americans.
17. Implement a strategy and plan for accountability to sustain the momentum, public visibility, and oversight of the implementation of 2005 WHCOA Resolutions.
18. Foster innovations in financing long-term care to increase options available to consumers.
19. Promote the integration of health and aging services to improve access and quality of care for older Americans.
20. Encourage community designs to promote livable communities that enable aging in the home.
21. Improve the health and quality of life of older Americans through disease management and chronic care coordination.
22. Promote the importance of nutrition in health promotion and disease prevention and management.
23. Improve access to care for older adults living in rural areas.
24. Provide financial and other economic incentives and policy changes to encourage and facilitate increased retirement savings.
25. Develop a national strategy for promoting new and meaningful volunteer activities and civic engagements for current and future seniors.
26. Encourage the development of a coordinated federal, state, and local emergency response plan for seniors in the event of public health emergencies or disasters.
27. Enhance the availability of housing for older Americans.
28. Reauthorize the National and Community Service Act to expand opportunities for volunteer and civic engagement activities.
29. Promote innovative evidence-based and practice-based medical and aging research.
30. Modernize the Supplemental Security Income (SSI) Program.
31. Support older adult caregivers raising their relatives' children.
32. Ensure appropriate recognition and care for veterans across all health care settings.
33. Encourage redesign of senior centers for broad appeal and community participation.
34. Reduce health care disparities among minorities by developing strategies to prevent disease, promote health, and deliver appropriate care and wellness.
35. Educate Americans on end-of-life issues.
36. Develop incentives to encourage the expansion of appropriate use of health information technology.
37. Prevent disease and promote healthier lifestyles through educating providers and consumers on consumer health care.
38. Promote economic development policies that respond to the unique needs of rural seniors.
39. Apply evidence-based research to the delivery of health and social services where appropriate.
40. Improve health decision making through promotion of health education, health literacy, and cultural competency.
41. Strengthen the Social Security Disability Insurance Program.
42. Evaluate payment and coordination policies in the geriatric health care continuum to ensure continuity of care.
43. Encourage appropriate sharing of health care information across multiple systems.
44. Ensure appropriate care for seniors with disabilities.
45. Strengthen law enforcement efforts at the federal, state, and local levels to investigate and prosecute cases of elder financial crime.
46. Review alignment of government programs that deliver services to older Americans.
47. Support older drivers to retain mobility and independence through strategies to continue safe driving.
48. Expand opportunities for developing innovative housing designs for seniors' needs.
49. Improve patient advocacy to assist patients in and across all care settings.
50. Promote enrollment of seniors into the Medicare Prescription Drug Program with particular emphasis on the limited-income subsidy.

Data from White House Conference on Aging. (2005). *Final report of the 2005 White House Conference on Aging.* Washington, DC: Author.

2. Expand private health insurance to all.
3. Expand Medicare to include universal public long-term care insurance.
4. Provide a combination of public and private partnerships in which people who can afford private insurance do so, but Medicaid would ensure care under catastrophic circumstances.

All these alternatives and others will be hotly debated in the near future, as the nation tries to resolve the problems of long-term care. Nurses, especially community health nurses, have a unique perspective of the problems and needs of older adults who require long-term care. They should articulate these issues in the policy arena to expand and improve the quality of services available to older adults and others with long-term care needs.

RESPONSIBILITIES OF THE NURSE WORKING WITH OLDER ADULTS IN THE COMMUNITY

The community health nurse may function as a *facilitator-collaborator, advocate, teacher,* or *case manager* in assisting older adult clients and their families in the community to maintain and improve health and well-being. The responsibilities of the community health nurse are carried out using the nursing process. The community health nurse assesses the client, family, and community to determine actual or potential health care needs and resources. A comprehensive assessment should include physical, psychosocial, spiritual, functional, developmental, and environmental factors. Data from the comprehensive assessment are used to develop nursing diagnoses that are individual-, family-, and community-focused.

CASE MANAGEMENT

Based on a comprehensive assessment of needs, the community health nurse collaborates with the client and family in jointly setting mutually acceptable goals. A nursing care plan is developed and implemented to meet family health promotion goals. In implementing the plan of care, the nurse needs to function as a *case manager,* referring the client and family to appropriate resources and monitoring and coordinating the extent and adequacy of services to meet family health care needs. Today, the community nurse as case manager is needed to manage the wide variety of fragmented community-based services available for at-risk elders (Schein et al., 2005).

Case management is the process by which services are organized and coordinated to meet client needs. In working with frail older adult clients with multiple health problems, case management is an essential service that is frequently required over a long period. Nurses should be aware that an important goal for older adults is to maintain as much independence as possible for as long as possible. The need for case management may increase in intensity and complexity as individual and family needs change. For example, an older adult client returning home from the hospital after experiencing a stroke may require a variety of services. The community health nurse functions as a case manager by locating and coordinating resources in the community to meet client needs. Services may include in-home personal care, transportation, assistance in restructuring the home environment to facilitate mobility and wheelchair accessibility, physical therapy, or speech therapy. In this example, evaluation of case management is based on the client's adjustment to the home environment once resources are in place, improved access to needed services such as physical and speech therapy, and avoidance of repeated hospitalization or the need for nursing home care.

> Jennifer Johnson returned home from the hospital after suffering from a cerebrovascular accident (CVA). The residual effects of Mrs. Johnson's CVA were left-sided weakness with hemiparesis and difficulty speaking. Mrs. Johnson lived alone and needed assistance in understanding her medication regimen. Mary Jenkins, the nurse, was able to coordinate the needed services for Mrs. Johnson. Nurse Jenkins arranged for Mrs. Johnson to receive home health rehabilitative services. A physical therapist was scheduled to visit Mrs. Johnson twice weekly to instruct her on therapeutic exercises and a home exercise program to increase strength in her left extremities; a speech/language pathologist was scheduled to evaluate her speaking difficulties and develop a plan of care to improve functioning; and an occupational therapist was scheduled to assess her ability to perform activities of daily living and to order appropriate adaptive equipment, if needed. The home care nurse was scheduled to instruct Mrs. Johnson on the medication regimen, signs and symptoms to report, and safety measures, as well as to continually assess Mrs. Johnson's ability to manage in the home independently. Additionally, Nurse Jenkins arranged transportation services to and from the physician's office as needed as well as ensuring that Mrs. Johnson received daily "Meals On Wheels."

Case management programs for older adults are offered in many states through the local health department or office on aging. **Geriatric Evaluation Service (GES)** is an example of a program that provides assistance to older adults and functionally disabled adults who are at risk of institutionalization. The goal of GES is to maintain the individual in the community or in the least restrictive environment and to promote the highest possible level of independence and personal well-being. GES teams, located in local health departments, assess the health status and psychosocial needs of the client and develop a plan of care to address these needs. The GES team is usually composed of a nurse, a social worker, and, as needed, a psychiatrist and a psychologist. Following this comprehensive assessment, case management services are provided to assist the client in obtaining needed community resources.

Under the Nursing Home Reform Act of 1987, GES personnel are also federally mandated to conduct preadmission screening and annual resident reviews of persons seeking nursing home placement or persons currently residing in a nursing home who are suspected of having a diagnosis of mental illness or mental retardation. GES evaluates these clients annually to determine whether nursing home placement is the most appropriate health care setting to meet their needs. Finally, GES evaluates persons 65 years and older who are referred for admission to a state psychiatric facility to determine the least restrictive environment appropriate for the client.

Carr (2005) asserts that case management is a cost-effective solution to providing comprehensive care to older adults, especially in attempts to improve health outcomes and rehabilitation. Nurses are in a position to visit more frequently and to closely monitor services to meet a client's changing health care needs over time. The nurse should ensure that services are not overutilized or underutilized. To that end, the nursing care plan may require modification of services as needs and the situation change.

ADVOCACY

Effective case management requires a broad knowledge base of the diversity of health, social, and supportive community resources. By having a case manager, the confusion that may come from contact with multiple persons in the health care team is eliminated (Schein et al., 2005). To function effectively as a case manager, the community health nurse must assume a strong *advocacy* role.

Key elements of the advocacy role include a sensitivity to the needs of the client and family, a broad knowledge base of available community resources and supports, and the ability to communicate a professional assessment of client and family needs to the appropriate service providers. Persistence is also needed when acting on behalf of the family, because much time and patience are often required to locate and channel the client into the appropriate resource or support service. For example, home care services are often fragmented and decentralized, preventing older adults from easily making arrangements to safely remain at home. Frail older adult clients who require multiple home care services often find that coordinating needed services is complex and overwhelming. Families may consider nursing home placement simply because it is easier to arrange than it is to unravel the complex and fragmented mix of community support services. By assisting frail older adults to locate and receive services that enable them to carry out activities of daily living and remain independent in the community, nursing home placement may be delayed or avoided.

TEACHING AND COUNSELLING

Teaching and counselling are also essential responsibilities of the community health nurse in working with aging families. Clients and families often require teaching related to the disease processes being experienced, management of symptoms, mobility, medications, diet, bowel and bladder function, normal health promotion activities, and recommendations for health screening. Health promotion activities are an important element of nursing care, even when older adults have one or more chronic illnesses. They and their family members should be taught the value of behavior modification in improving the quality of health in chronic conditions.

A 72-year-old female, Mrs. Mary Hart, was recently diagnosed with osteoporosis. The home care nurse, Judy Ellis, was assigned to visit. She found Mrs. Hart lived alone, but her daughter checked on her daily. The nurse provided instructions on management of Mrs. Hart's back pain. She reviewed with Mrs. Hart the need for her to increase her dietary intake of calcium and vitamin D, the medication regimen for calcitonin (which slows bone loss), and self-care measures, such as diet, exercise, and safety (fall prevention activities), to assist her in the management of her disease process. On her next visit, the nurse plans to perform a home assessment to check for fall risks. She hopes to have Mrs. Hart's daughter present at that time to facilitate any changes to the home that she might recommend.

Counselling includes the provision of family and caregiver support, assistance in coping with and adjusting to the normal consequences of aging, assistance with the grieving process and coping with loss, and improvement of interpersonal communication between family members. Clients should also be counselled on how to locate appropriate community resources and what questions to ask in investigating agencies. The AARP publishes valuable consumer information to assist clients and caregivers who are investigating community resources.

Many of the nurse's interventions are directed at the caregiver. Teaching and counseling of caregivers focuses on accepting respite care and in-home services, planning and anticipating future health care needs and services, and teaching caregiving and assessment skills. It is estimated that 53.6% (13.7 million) of older noninstitutionalized persons live with their older adult spouses and that family members provide approximately 80% of the care for older adults (AARP, 2005). The experience of caregiving may be stressful as the caregiver seeks to help others while coping with their own health problems. Sullivan (2007) reports that the experience of caregiving has been shown to result in the onset of depression, grief, fatigue, decreased socialization, and health problems for the caregiver. Schumacher and colleagues (2006) recommend that the nurse form a partnership with the caregiver, providing guidance and support and encouraging respite care when appropriate.

Community health nurses are uniquely qualified to conduct comprehensive assessments and to help the family bridge the gap between social and health care needs and services in the population. In addition, the community health nurse as case manager is uniquely qualified to decrease fragmentation of services and to refocus services from an acute illness model to a preventive model of care.

COLLABORATION

The community health nurse may collaborate with the family and other providers to facilitate improved health and well-being. Collaboration involves working together with others to meet a common goal. On a broader scale, the community health nurse may collaborate with local and state governments to provide more comprehensive services for older adults by acting as a representative of consumer interest groups before state regulatory bodies and local health planning commissions and by lobbying for legislation that promotes expanded services for the older adult person. The community health nurse may work with a coalition of providers and citizen groups to advocate for the needs of the older adult population or may participate in hearings of area agencies on aging to advocate for greater community-based long-term care services.

The community health nurse may also engage in valuable community services such as the following:

- Coordinating the preparation of a directory of community resources for older adults
- Developing telephone hotlines to provide information on long-term care
- Holding public education forums and seminars on the needs of the older adult population in the community
- Educating the community about long-term health care coverage
- Conducting surveys and publicizing price information on long-term care in the community
- Meeting with corporations to explore long-term care and retirement options for employees
- Organizing, coordinating, or supervising paid or volunteer programs (such as Friendly Visitors), family respite care, or self-help and support groups

The community health nurse may also be involved in supporting federal policies that provide and finance care for older adults, such as legislation that provides greater financial protection against catastrophic costs not covered by Medicare. Finally, through mass screening efforts, the community health nurse can promote preventive health education, screening, and referral services to older adults.

KEY IDEAS

1. As the number of older Americans continues to grow, the need for health care services for the older adult population will escalate.
2. Because most older adult Americans live independently in the community, community/public health nurses are responsible for delivering health care services to a large segment of the older adult population.
3. As society continues to age, the amount of chronic disease and functional impairments in the population will increase.
4. The community/public health nurse is responsible for facilitating utilization of needed resources by collaborating with service agencies; coordinating care to ensure systematic, comprehensive delivery of needed services; and advocating for the needs of older Americans. Advocacy is accomplished through community education and support of legislation that promotes a healthy, vital, and meaningful aging experience for older adults.
5. Through concerted efforts at the local, state, and federal levels to address the needs of older Americans, the nation's health care system may move to a more comprehensive and holistic vision for improving quality of care throughout the life span.
6. Through teaching, counselling, case management, advocacy, and collaboration with the client, family, and other providers, the community health nurse can effect needed social change for the welfare of older adults.

THE NURSING PROCESS IN PRACTICE ▶ An Older Adult Couple at Home (by Jennifer Maurer Kliphouse)

Mr. Walter, an 80-year-old white male, lives with his 76-year-old wife in their home. Mrs. Walter, diagnosed with Alzheimer's disease 5 years ago, has been experiencing progressive memory impairment. Though she continues to dress and feed herself, she requires minimal assistance. In the last 6 months, she has had difficulty naming objects and is unable to recall recent events. In the afternoon, she begins looking for the children and does not respond to redirection. At night she wanders through the house, and last winter she went into the yard in her nightgown. Furthermore, Mrs. Walter becomes anxious when she is unable to perform a task and requires a great deal of assurance and encouragement. She denies awareness of a decline in cognitive functioning.

Mr. Walter, increasingly frustrated and overwhelmed with caregiving activities, states, "You work all your life and for what? It doesn't make sense. I don't understand why these doctors just can't fix her. These young guys don't know what they are doing." Although they have two adult children and six grandchildren living in a 5-mile radius, Mr. Walter notes, "My children do not visit because they do not want to see their mother acting this way. It is just the two of us."

On the initial home visit, the community health nurse noted that both Mr. and Mrs. Walter appeared disheveled and unkempt. Their clothes had dried food stains, and Mrs. Walter's hair was not combed. Unwashed dishes remained piled in the sink. Mr. Walter complained he "feels tired all the time," and repeatedly stated, "We would both be better off dead."

ASSESSMENT

Based on a thorough assessment of individual and family needs, the community health nurse developed a mutually acceptable plan of care with the family. The nursing assessment addressed the physical, psychologic, social, spiritual, and environmental needs of the client and the family.

- Assess for the presence of depression, suicidal intentions, social isolation, ability to meet nutritional needs, compliance with medication, and self-care behavior.
- Assess the degree of family and social supports available to assist the client and the family through a crisis of coping with chronic illness (e.g., transportation, financial assistance, legal assistance, caretaking, respite care).
- Assess for the presence of abuse or neglect because of ineffective family coping (see Chapter 23).
- Assess the potential for injury as a result of Mrs. Walter's declining cognitive function and night wandering.

The community health nurse formulated the following list of nursing diagnoses, which will be used to create, implement, and evaluate the effectiveness of the nursing care plan for this family.

NURSING DIAGNOSES

- Caregiver role strain related to unrelenting and complex requirements secondary to progressive dementia as evidenced by (AEB) Mr. Walter's complaint of chronic fatigue and statement, "We would both be better off dead."
- Compromised family coping related to chronic illness of a family member AEB Mr. Walter's statement, "My children do not…want to see their mother acting this way."
- Powerlessness related to the chronic disease process of Alzheimer's disease AEB Mr. Walter's statement, "You work your whole life, and for what?"
- Risk for injury to Mrs. Walter related to decrease in or loss of short-term memory AEB wandering at night, decreasing response to redirection and comfort.
- Impaired memory related to degenerative brain disease AEB Mrs. Walter's inability to recall names of everyday objects.
- Ineffective role performance AEB Mr. Walter feeling overwhelmed with caregiver duties and his inability to perform activities of daily living (as seen by the unkempt appearances of Mr. and Mrs. Walter and their home).
- Social isolation related to loss of usual social contacts secondary to chronic illness AEB Mr. Walter's observation, "It's just the two of us."
- Spiritual distress related to chronic dementing illness of family member as evidenced by Mr. Walter's reflection that they would both be better off dead.

Continued

Nursing Diagnosis	Nursing Goals	Nursing Interventions	Outcomes and Evaluation
Caregiver role strain related to unrelenting and complex requirements secondary to progressive dementia AEB Mr. Walter's complaint of chronic fatigue and the statement, "We would both be better of dead"	The client and family will verbalize knowledge of the disease process.	The community health nurse provides immediate education about the pathologic changes in the brain as a result of Alzheimer's disease, discussing specific changes in Mrs. Walter's cognitive and physical functioning. Knowledge of the disease process provides Mr. Walter a deeper understanding of the changes he witnesses in his wife's behavior and physical abilities.	Mr. Walter verbalized an understanding of the disease process and how its progression is reflected in his wife's behavior and abilities.
	The client and family will use services to attain additional caregiver support.	A referral to a local Alzheimer's Association chapter for further education regarding the disease will increase Mr. Walter's knowledge base and provide information for support groups, respite care, and consumer information.	Mr. Walter agrees to participate in a support group that offers open discussion about the effects on his relationship with his wife and changes in his own daily activities impacted by the progression of Alzheimer's disease.
		The community health nurse investigates local agencies, both charitable and for profit, to offer a variety of sources for assistance with daily living activities (e.g., meal preparation, housekeeping, minor house repairs).	The Walters hire a respite caregiver to afford Mr. Walter personal time for increased social interaction and/ or activities outside the home. Local charity services provide Meals on Wheels and housekeeping services three times weekly.
	The client and family will communicate to the community health nurse and each other, as appropriate, their feelings and concerns in coping with the experience of chronic illness.	The community health nurse provides the client and family a counseling and mental health evaluation referral to assess for depression, potential threat of self-harm, and potential for abuse or neglect.	The department of aging and social services offered social work consultation, which Mr. Walter denied, stating, "I don't need a shrink." Though Mr. Walter refused social work services, he reported both increased insight of the disease process and psychologic relief from respite and charitable services. The community health nurse will continue to monitor the situation.

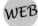 Find additional **Care Plans** for this client on the book's website.

LEARNING BY EXPERIENCE AND REFLECTION

1. Assess your home environment for the presence of safety hazards. What modifications must be made in your home if you suddenly needed to assume care for a frail, dependent, older adult family member?

2. Institute a dialogue with an older adult client or family member. Encourage him or her to share a part of his or her life story. Storytelling may be enhanced by sharing family pictures or memorabilia, asking open-ended questions that invite reminiscence, taking a family history, and supporting past recollections. Empathize with and acknowledge positive and negative feelings that the person may experience as his or her life story is shared. In what way does past experience influence who the person is today (e.g., choices, beliefs, and values)?

3. Ask an older adult parent and an adult child to recall a shared past experience. Compare the perceptions between generations. In what ways are the life stories similar? In what ways are they different? What might influence the storytellers' perceptions? In what way do you become a part of the life story by sharing in past and present experi-

ences? How is your life story changed by being with the clients?

4. Reflect in writing on your perceptions of old age. What do you think it is like to be old? Share your reflections with an older family member or significant other.

5. Take time to review old family photographs, scrapbooks, or memorabilia. Reflect on the changes you can see in yourself over the years. What patterns do you see emerging in your past? In what ways are you the same or different? What do you think you will be like as you grow older?

6. Interview an older adult client or family member regarding the most difficult choices he or she has had to make in life. What were the conditions surrounding these choices? How was a decision made? How does the person feel about the decisions he or she made?

COMMUNITY RESOURCES FOR PRACTICE

Information about each organization listed below can be found on its website, which can be accessed through this book's website at *http://evolve.elsevier.com/Maurer/community/*.

Administration on Aging

Agency for Healthcare Research and Quality

Alzheimer's Association

Alzheimer's Disease Education and Referral Center (ADEAR)

American Association for Geriatric Psychiatry

American Association of Homes and Services for the Aging

American Association of Retired Persons

American Geriatrics Society

American Public Health Association

American Society on Aging

American Speech, Language, and Hearing Association

Arthritis Foundation

Family Caregiver Alliance

Gerontological Society of America

Gray Panthers

Institute for Retired Professionals

National Alliance for Caregiving

National Association for Home Care & Hospice

National Caucus and Center for the Black Aged

National Citizen's Coalition for Nursing Home Reform

National Council of Senior Citizens

National Family Caregivers Association

National Institute on Aging

National Long Term Care Ombudsman Resource Center

National Senior Citizens Law Center

Office of Disability and Income Security Programs, Social Security Administration

Older Americans Act, Administration on Aging

Older Women's League

Social Security Administration

STUDY AIDS   http://evolve.elsevier.com/Maurer/community/

Visit the Evolve website for this book to find the following study and assessment materials:

- Quiz
- Web Scenario
- Critical Thinking Questions and Answers for Case Studies

- Care Plans
- *Healthy People* Updates
- Glossary

WEBSITE RESOURCES

These items supplement the chapter's topics and are also found on the Evolve site:

28A: Nursing Home Evaluation Checklist

28B: Guide to Choosing a Nursing Home

REFERENCES

Administration on Aging, U.S. Department of Health and Human Services, (2004). *Factsheets: Elder abuse prevention*. Retrieved June 20, 2007, from *http://www.aoa.gov/press/fact/alpha/fact_elder_abuse.asp*.

Alecxih, L. (2006). *Nursing home use by "oldest old" sharply declines*. Falls Church, VA: The Lewin Group. Presented at the National Press Club, November 21, 2006.

American Association of Colleges of Nursing. (2007). *Your nursing career: A look at the facts*. Washington, DC: Author.

American Association of Retired Persons, (2005). *Profile of older Americans*. Retrieved July 14, 2007, from *http://www.aarp.org/*.

American Association of Retired Persons. (2006). *Annual report 2006*. Washington, DC: Author.

American College of Emergency Physicians, (2004). *New research shows approximately half of Americans misuse common over-the-counter (OTC) pain relievers*. Retrieved July 25, 2007, from *http://www.acep.org/webportal/Newsroom/NR/general/2004/NewResearchShowsApproximatelyHalfofAmericansMisuseCommonOvertheCounter-OTCPainRelievers.htm*.

American Nurses Association. (1997). ANA group boldly acts to shape health care change. *The American Nurse, 29*(6), 1-12.

American Nurses Association. (2007). *Nursing legislative and regulatory initiatives for the 110th*

Congress: Patient safety/advocacy. Washington, DC: ANA Department of Government Affairs. Accessed at *http://www.anapoliticalpower.org*.

American Public Health Association, (2005). *Fact sheet: Prescription medication use by older adults*. Retrieved September 1, 2007, from *http://www.medscape.com/viewarticle/501879*.

Betancourt, J. R., Green, A. R., Carrillo, J. E., et al. (2003). Defining cultural competence: A practical framework for addressing racial/ethnic disparities in health and health care. *Public Health Reports, 118*, 293-302.

Carr, D. (2005). The case manager's role in optimizing acute rehabilitation services. *Professional Case Management, 10*(4), 190-200.

Centers for Disease Control and Prevention, (2004). *National Center for Health Statistics 2004.* Retrieved January 20, 2004, from *http://www.cdc.gov/nchs.*

Centers for Disease Control and Prevention and Merck Institute for Aging and Health, (2004). *The state of aging and health in America.* Retrieved July 13, 2007 from *http://www.cdc.gov/aging/pdf/saha_2007.pdf.*

Consumer Reports. (2003). Do you need long-term-care insurance? *Consumer Reports, 68*(11), 20-24.

Cruikshank, M. (2003). Learning To Be Old author takes hard look at myths of aging. *Aging Today, 24*(1), 3.

Davidhizar, R., Dunn, C. L., & Hart, A. N. (2004). A review of the literature on how important water is to the world's older adult population. *International Nursing Review, 51,* 159-166.

DeNavas-Walt, C., & Smith, J. (2007). *Income, poverty, and health insurance coverage in the United States: 2006. U.S. Bureau of the Census, Current Population Reports, P60-233.* Washington, DC: U.S. Government Printing Office.

Ebersole, P., Hess, P., & Luggen, A. (2004). *Toward healthy aging: Human needs and nursing responses* (6th ed.). St. Louis: Mosby.

Erikson, E., Erikson, J., & Kivnick, H. (1986). *Vital involvement in old age.* New York: W. W. Norton.

Federal Interagency Forum on Aging-Related Statistics. (Nov 2004). *Older Americans 2004: Key indicators of well-being.* Washington, DC: U.S. Government Printing Office.

Feldman, P. H., & Kane , R. L. (2003). Strengthening research to improve the practice and management of long-term care. *The Milbank Quarterly, 81*(20), 179-220.

Gleberzon, B., & Hyde, D. (2006). Hip fracture presenting as a mechanical low back pain subsequent to a fall: A case study. *Journal of Canadian Chiropractic Association, 50*(4), 255-262.

Goulding, M. R., Rogers, M. E., & Smith, S. M. (2003). Health and aging: Trends in aging United States and world wide. *MMWR, 52*(06), 101-106.

Gray, M. L. (2003). Gender, race and culture in research on urinary incontinence. *American Journal of Nursing, 103*(Suppl), 20-25.

Harrington, C., Carillo, H., & Mercado-Scott, C. (2005). *Nursing facilities, staffing, residents, and facility deficiencies, 1998 through 2004.* University of California, San Francisco. Retrieved July 17, 2007, from *http://www.pascenter.org/publicaitons/publication_home.php?id=250.*

Herwaldt, L. A., & Pottinger, J. M. (2003). Preventing falls in the older adult. *Journal of the American Geriatric Association, 51*(8), 1175-1177.

Hoadley, J., Hargrave, E., Cubanski, J., et al. (2006). *An in-depth examination of formularies and other features of Medicare drug plans.* Menlo Park, CA: The Kaiser Family Foundation.

Hutman, S., Jaffe, J., & Segal, J. (2005). *Suicide prevention: Depression in older adults and the elderly.* Retrieved July 26, 2007, from *http://www.helpguide.org/mental/depression_elderly.htm.*

Leppik, I. E. (2006). Epilepsy in the elderly. *Epilepsia, 47*(suppl 1), 65-70.

Mahan, L. K., & Escott-Stump, L. (2004). *Krause's food, nutrition, and diet therapy* (11th ed.). Philadelphia: W. B. Saunders.

Marshall, R. T. (2006). *Nursing home issues.* Retrieved July 26, 2007, from *http://www.elder-web.com.*

McKeon, E. (2003). Prescription drug access: The ANA adopts principles to evaluate congressional Medicare proposals. *American Journal of Nursing, 103*(9), 106.

Melov, S., Tarnopolsku, M. A., Beckman, K. et al. (2007). Resistance exercise reverses aging human skeletal muscle. *PLoS One, 5,* 1-9.

Mid-East Area Agency on Aging, (2003). Mid-East Area Agency on Aging. (2003). *Caregiving statistics.* Retrieved February 13, 2004, from *http://www.mecaaa.org/Caregiving%20statistics.htm.*

Miller, C. A. (2004). *Nursing for wellness in older adults: Theory and practice* (4th ed.). Philadelphia: Lippincott Williams & Wilkins.

Murkofsky, R. L., Phillips, R. S., McCarthy, E. P. et al. (2003). Length of stay in home care before and after the 1997 balanced budget act. *Journal of the American Medical Association, 289*(21) 2841-2848.

National Clearinghouse for Long-Term Care Information, (2007). National Clearinghouse for Long-Term Care Information. (2007). *Paying for long-term care.* Retrieved July 19, 2007, from *http://www.longtermcare.gov.*

National Family Caregiver's Association, (2007a). *Caregiving statistics.* Retrieved July 24, 2007, from *http://www.nfcacares.org/who_are_family_caregivers/care_giving_statstics.cfm#1.*

National Family Caregiver's Association, (2007b). *RESPITE: Time out for caregivers.* Retrieved July 24, 2007, from *http://www.thefamilycaregiver.org/caregiving_resources/v3_a4.cfm.*

National Institute on Aging, U.S. Department of Health and Human Services. (2003). *2001-2002 Alzheimer's disease progress report.* Bethesda, MD: Author.

National Institute on Aging, U.S. Department of Health and Human Services, (2004). *General information on Alzheimer's disease.* Retrieved February 13, 2004, from *http://www.alzheimers.org/generalinfo.htm#howmany.*

National Institute of Mental Health, (2007). *Older adults: Depression and suicide facts.* Retrieved July 26, 2007, from *http://www.nimh.nih.gov/publicat/elderlydepsuicide/cfm.*

Newman, B. M., & Newman, P. R. (2005). *Development through life: A psychosocial approach.* Belmont: Thomson Wadsworth.

New York Life, (2007). *Average cost of nursing home care rises 6% year over year.* Retrieved August 29, 2007, from *http://www.newyorklife.com/cda/0,3254,15833,00.html.*

Office of Personnel Management, (2002). Federal Long Term Care Insurance Program (FLTCIP). Retrieved February 15, 2004, from *http://www.pwc.com/extweb/pwcpublications.nsf/docid/e4c0fc004429297a852571090065a70b.*

Pratt, J. R. (2004). *Long-term care: Managing across the continuum.* Sudbury, MA: Jones & Bartlett.

PriceWaterhouseCoopers, (2006). *The factors fueling rising healthcare costs, 2006.* Retrieved May 11, 2007, from *http://www.ahip/redirect/PwCostofHC2006.pdf.*

Rice, D. P., & Fineman, N. (2004). Economic implications of increased longevity in the United States. *Annual Review of Public Health, 25,* 457-473.

Robinson, A., & Street, A. (2004). Improving networks between acute care nurses and an aged care assessment team. *Journal of Clinical Nursing, 13,* 486-496.

Schein, C., Gagnon, A. J., Chan, L., et al. (2005). The association between specific nurse case management interventions and elder health. *Journal of the American Geriatrics Society, 53*(4), 597-602.

Schumacher, K., Beck, C. A., & Marren, J. M. (2006). Family caregivers: Caring for older adults, working with their families. *American Journal of Nursing, 106*(8), 40-50.

Smith, M., & Buckwalter, K. (2005). Behaviors associated with dementia. *American Journal of Nursing, 105*(7), 40-53.

Smith, M., & Jaffe, J., (2007). *Suicide prevention: Understanding and helping a suicidal person.* Retrieved July 26, 2007, from *http://www.helpguide.org/mental/suicide_prevention.htm.*

Social Security Administration. (2006). *Income of the population 55 or older, 2004 (SSA Pub No. 13-11871).* Washington, DC: Author.

Stoltz, P., Uden, G., & Willman, A. (2004). Support for family carers who care for an older adult person at home—a systematic literature review. *Scandanavian Journal of Caring Science, 18,* 111-119.

Stunk, B. C., & Ginsburg, P. B. (2003). Tracking health care costs: Trends stabilize but remain high in 2002. *Health Affairs, Web Exclusives: A Supplement to Health Affairs,* W3-266-274.

Sullivan, T.M. (2007). Caregiver strain index (CSI). In *Try this: Best practices in nursing care to older adults (issue 14).* New York: The Hartford Institute for Geriatric Nursing, New York University, Division of Nursing.

U.S. Bureau of the Census. (2000). *Census 2000 Summary File 3 (SF3), PCT14. Language density by linguistic isolation by age for the population 5 years and over in households (28).* Washington, DC: Author.

U.S. Bureau of the Census, (2003). *American factfinder.* Retrieved January 20, 2004, from *http://www.factfinder.census.gov.*

U.S. Bureau of the Census. (2004, December). *We the people: Aging in the United States (Report CENSR-19).* Washington, DC: Author.

U.S. Bureau of the Census, (2005). *65+ in the United States: 2005.* Retrieved July 27, 2007, from *http://www.census.gov/prod/2006pubs/p23-209.pdf.*

U.S. Bureau of the Census, (2006a). *The older population in the United States: 2006.* Retrieved August 27, 2007, from *http://www.census.gov/ population/socdemo/age/age_2006.htm.*

U.S. Bureau of the Census. (2006b). Americans with disabilities: 2002. *Current Population Reports (P70-107).* Washington, DC: Author.

U.S. Department of Health and Human Services. (2000). *Healthy People 2010.* Washington, DC: U.S. Government Printing Office.

U.S. Department of Health and Human Services. (2003). *Health, United States, 2003.* Washington, DC: U.S. Government Printing Office.

U.S. Department of Health and Human Services. (2006). *Health, United States, 2006.* Washington, DC: U.S. Government Printing Office.

Warshaw, R. (2005). *Joint effort pays off: Exercise benefits sore knees, hips, shoulder and other joints that hurt. Healthy Women Take 10.* Retrieved July 17, 2007, from *http://www.healthywomen.org.*

Weingart, S. N., Pagovich, O., Sands, D. Z., et al. (2005). What can hospitalized patients tell us about adverse events? Leaning from patient reported incidents. *Journal of General Internal Medicine, 20,* 830-836.

White House Conference on Aging. (2005). *Report to the President and the Congress, The booming dynamics of aging: From awareness to action.* Retrieved September 1, 2007, from *http://www. whcoa.gov.*

Wilson, I. B., Schoen, C., Neuman, P., et al. (2007). Physician-patient communication about prescription medication nonadherence: A 50-state study of America's seniors. *Journal of General International Medicine, 22,* 6-12.

Yeh, S.-C. J. (2004). *Living alone, social support, and feeling lonely among the elderly.* Sydney, Australia: Institute of International Health.

SUGGESTED READINGS

American Nurses Association, (2007). *Nursing legislative and regulatory initiatives for the 110th Congress: Patient safety/advocacy.* Washington, DC: ANA Department of Government Affairs. Accessed at *http://www.anapoliticalpower.org.*

Bettleheim, A. (2001). *Aging in America.* Washington, DC: CQ Press.

Centers for Medicare and Medicaid Services, U.S. Department of Health and Human Services, (2007). *Prescription drug coverage: Basic information.* Accessed September 1, 2007, from *www. medicare.gov/pdp-basic-information.*

Kausler, D. H., & Kausler, B. C. (2001). *The graying of America: An encyclopedia of aging, health, mind, and behavior* (2nd ed.). Chicago: University of Chicago Press.

Settings for Community/ Public Health Nursing Practice

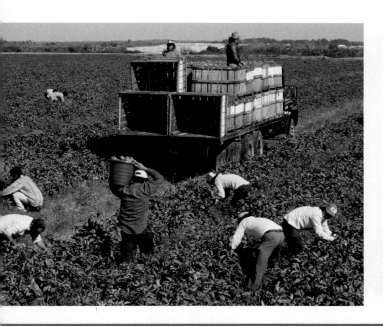

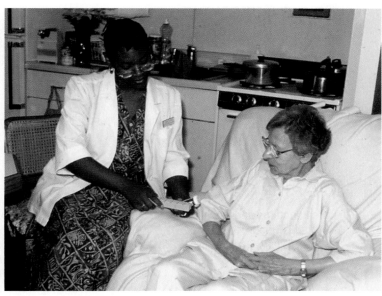

FOCUS QUESTIONS

What are the core functions and essential services of public health?

What are the responsibilities of the state health agency and local health department?

What is the impact of funding sources on public health services to communities?

What health services and populations have traditionally been a focus of public health nursing?

How is nursing in local health departments organized?

What are the various responsibilities of the public health nurse in the local health department?

How can the MAPP Model and the *Healthy People* objectives be used to plan nursing services for populations?

What are future trends for nursing in state and local health departments?

CHAPTER OUTLINE

KEY TERMS

Core functions of public health
Direct health care services
Essential public health services

Local health department (LHD)
MAPP Model
Population-based health services

Public health infrastructure
State health agency (SHA)
Superagency

CORE FUNCTIONS AND ESSENTIAL SERVICES OF PUBLIC HEALTH

Under the U.S. Constitution, states retain the power to protect the health and welfare of their residents (see Chapter 3). Consequently, states have the primary responsibility for public health functions. They address these responsibilities through the **state health agency (SHA)**. States delegate some of that responsibility to local health departments. Thus in the United States, state and local health departments perform the major portion of public health activities. The 1988 Institute of Medicine (IOM) report titled *The Future of Public Health* indicated public health functions were poorly focused and the **public health infrastructure** was inadequate. It further noted that funding for public health was sporadic and inadequate to meet the needs of the nation's health. In 2003 another IOM report noted fragmentation, inadequate funding, insufficient accountability, and lack of partnerships with other health care service providers persist (Institute of Medicine [IOM], 2003a).

*The authors acknowledge the contribution of Glenda Kelly for her work on this chapter in the previous edition.

TABLE 29-1   Public Health Core Functions and Essential Public Health Services

Core Functions	Services
Assessment of population health Policy development Assurance of high-quality public health services	Monitor health status to identify and solve community health problems Diagnose and investigate health problems and health hazards in the community Inform, educate, and empower people about health issues Mobilize community partnerships to identify and solve health problems Develop policies and plans that support individual and community health efforts Enforce laws and regulations that protect health and ensure safety Link people to needed personal health services and ensure the provision of health care when otherwise unavailable Assure a competent public health and personal health care workforce Evaluate effectiveness, accessibility, and quality of personal and population-based health services Conduct research to attain new insights and innovative solutions to health problems

Adapted from Essential Public Health Services Work Group, Centers for Disease Control and Prevention. (1995). *The essential services of public health.* Washington, DC: The Association.

The Institute of Medicine study identified three **core functions of public health**. Subsequently, the Essential Public Health Services Work Group (1995) identified 10 **essential public health services** necessary to meet these 3 core functions (Table 29-1). Both the core functions and 10 essential services focused on population-based care as opposed to direct health care to individuals—for example, communicable disease surveillance as opposed to home health care to an ill individual. The following are identified as critical public health responsibilities:

- Preventing epidemics and the spread of disease
- Protecting against environmental hazards
- Preventing injuries
- Promoting and encouraging healthy behaviors and mental health
- Responding to disasters and assisting communities in recovery
- Ensuring the quality and accessibility of health services (Essential Public Health Services Work Group, 1995)

Since 1988, and in response to the Institute of Medicine report, public health practice has made substantial change. There is an emphasis on population-based care and the development of coalitions and partnerships to provide health care to populations. *Healthy People 2010* added additional public health objectives, and made improvement of the public health infrastructure a key objective.

Funding for public health functions remains a problem. All governmental agencies combined spent $56.6 billion to provide essential public health services in 2005 (Catlin et al., 2007). Today, public health funding remains low, between 1% and 4% of the total health care budget (Hunt & Knickman, 2008; Levit et al., 2003; Turnock, 2004). Most funding (52%) is provided by state and local governments, and the remainder by the federal government, fees, and other sources (National Association of County and City Health Officials [NACCHO], 2006). Despite a renewed emphasis on population-focused care, only 24% of public health funds is used for population-based public health services. The remaining 76% is spent on providing direct individual care or linking people to direct care. Turnock (2004) estimates the amount of all government funds spent on population-based care at $62.06 per person per year, a very minimal amount.

Despite sporadic funding and changes in the focus of care, public health efforts have produced significant success in the 20th century. The Centers for Disease Control and Prevention (CDC) (1999) has identified the following 10 great public health achievements:

- Vaccinations
- Motor vehicle safety
- Safer workplaces
- Control of infectious diseases
- Decline in deaths from coronary artery disease and stroke
- Safer and healthier foods
- Healthier mothers and babies
- Family planning
- Fluoridation of drinking water
- Recognition of tobacco as a health hazard

Much of the improvements in these 10 health areas are the result of state and local health departments.

IMPACT OF TERRORISM ON PUBLIC HEALTH RESPONSIBILITIES

September 11, 2001, brought renewed resolve to the effort to improve public health surveillance and infrastructure. The anthrax attack that same year solidified interest in improving public health population-based functions. Federal funding past 9/11 increased in the area of disease surveillance and emergency preparedness. However, in subsequent years federal monies were reduced from $918 million in 2002 to $711 million in 2006 (Landers, 2007). Federal monies have improved since 2006. For example, in 2007 state health departments received approximately $896.7 million in federal funds to prepare for and respond to terrorism, infectious disease outbreaks, and other public health threats and emergencies (U.S. Department of Health and Human Services [USDHHS], 2007). For 2008 the funding proposals would increase to $919 million, the same level of funding as in 2002 (NACCHO, 2007).

All 50 SHAs indicate persistent problems with resource allocation, staffing, and surveillance (National Governors Association, 2003). The federal government has added responsibilities for emergency preparedness to SHAs without consistently funding these responsibilities. As a result, SHAs have had to reassign resources and personnel from other program areas, thus reducing services in those areas

(Bashir et al., 2007; Morbidity and Mortality Weekly Reports [MMWR], 2005). This has exacerbated problems inherent in pubic health services and programs. The Institute of Medicine (IOM, 2003a) issued a second study titled *The Future of the Public's Health in the 21st Century,* which provides additional recommendations for strengthening the public health system in the United States. The CDC (2000) status report to the U.S. Senate indicated the following three critical areas for improvement necessary to strengthen the public health infrastructure:

- Skilled public health workforce
- Robust information and data systems
- Effective health departments and laboratories

It is important to review the present state of public health in the United States in the wake of current events and in light of the concerns and recommendations from the public health community. State and local health departments are the essential units of public health service delivery and the subject of this chapter.

STRUCTURE AND RESPONSIBILITIES OF THE STATE HEALTH AGENCY

Each of the 50 states has a SHA, usually called the state health department. The structures of these agencies vary dramatically (IOM, 1988). Half of the states have freestanding, independent health agencies. There is a movement toward integration into a larger **"superagency"** such as a health and human services department (Beitsch et al., 2006). Between 1990 and 2000, six additional freestanding state health departments were merged into superagencies (Figure 29-1). Chapter 3 has an organizational chart for a state superagency with health responsibilities. Figure 29-2 is an example of the organizational structure and functions of a state health department.

The chief executive of an SHA is the state health officer/director. Most are political appointees, serving at the discretion of the state's governor. Many are physicians. In some states, the health code requires a physician to serve as the health officer; in most it has been a matter of tradition. Beitsch and colleagues (2006) found that fewer states are requiring a medical degree for the state health officer/director and more than one third of states do not have any specific degree requirement.

A state health agency either provides or funds direct client services for select populations, usually the economically disadvantaged (for example, low-income pregnant females or young children). They may also administer care for institutional populations, such as the elderly (nursing homes) or mentally ill (state mental hospitals). The IOM (1988) has made it clear that the states are the central force in maintaining public health. Most states meet these requirements and their

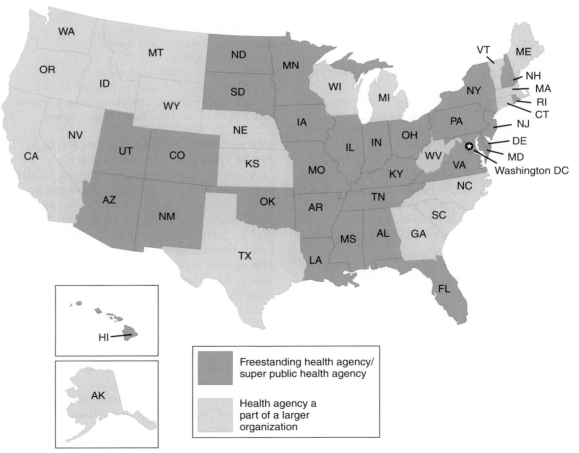

FIGURE 29-1 State public health agencies by type. (Data from Association of State and Territorial Health Officials. Retrieved December 24, 2003, from http://www. statepublichealth.org/?template5query-new.php; and National Governors Association. [2003]. *Reorganizing state health agencies to meet changing needs: State restructuring efforts in 2003.* Washington, DC: Author.)

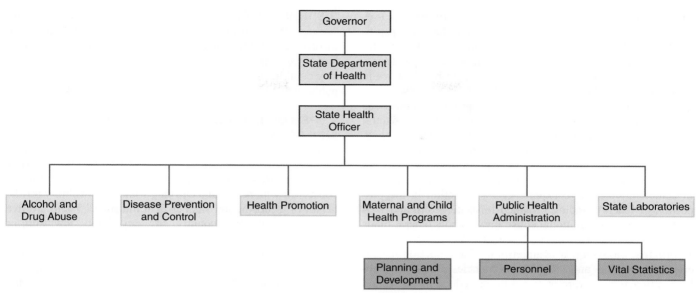

FIGURE 29-2 An example of a state health department organizational chart.

other assigned obligations through the combined efforts of the SHA and local health departments. In most instances, the SHA assists, delegates, and/or oversees local health departments. The services provided by state and local health departments are a mix of direct health care to select populations and core public health functions to communities (Box 29-1). Other state and local agencies may assume primary responsibility for some portion of these services, such as mental health, professional and institutional licensure, and environmental health. Beitsch et al. (2006) report that more states have increased emphasis on health planning and development, quality improvement and performance management, bioterrorism preparedness, and emergency medical services' oversight.

FUNDING OF STATE HEALTH AGENCIES

Most funding for SHAs comes from public tax dollars provided by the state and federal government. States vary in the degree to which they fund public health and population-focused activities. The National Association of State Budget Officers (NASBO) and Reforming State Groups (NASBO and

---

Box 29-1 | **Public Health Programs Funded by State and Local Health Departments**

Direct Public Health Services
Pharmaceutical assistance for the elderly
Chronic disease hospitals and programs
Hearing aid assistance
Adult daycare for persons with Alzheimer's disease
Health grants
Maternal and child health
Medically handicapped children
Women, Infants, and Children (WIC) programs
Pregnancy outreach and counseling
Chronic renal disease treatment programs
STD screening and/or treatment
AIDS treatment
Blood pressure screening
Breast and cervical cancer treatment
Tuberculosis (TB) programs
Emergency health services
Adult genetics programs
Phenylketonuria (PKU) testing

State Facility-Based Services
Schools for the blind
Schools for the deaf

Mental health hospitals
Facilities for the developmentally disabled
Substance abuse facilities
Veterans' homes
Rehabilitation facilities

Community-Based Services
Food service inspection and licenses
Rehabilitation services
Alcohol and drug abuse treatment
Mental health community services
Developmental disabilities community services

Population Health Expenditures
Prevention of epidemics and the spread of disease, including adult and child immunization programs and communicable disease surveillance
Environmental health surveillance
Injury prevention/control
Promotion of chronic disease control and encouragement of healthy behaviors including tobacco use prevention
Disaster preparation
Disaster response
Health infrastructure

Data from National Association of State Budget Officers. (2003). *2000-2001 State health care expenditure report.* Washington, DC: NASBO, Reforming States Group, and Milbank Memorial Fund; and National Association of County and City Health Officials (2006). *2005 National profile of local health departments.* Washington, DC: Author.

Reforming State Groups, 2003) report public health expenses varied from 0.8% to 33.2% of a state's total health expenditures. In 2004 public health expenditures for all activities including SHAs were $47 billion. Public health expenditures represented only 4% of the $1.2 trillion spent by all states in 2004 (NASBO, 2005; U.S. Bureau of the Census, 2004).

State budgets for health and welfare programs have been squeezed by several factors. In the past 3 decades, federal funding to SHAs has been reduced and concentrated in block grants. This action by the federal government was intended to give states more control over their programs as well as put limits on federal spending for health and welfare programs. In actuality, states have experienced a reduction in the proportion of federal funding provided for state health and welfare programs and additional constraints on how federal funds are spent (Fee & Brown, 2002; Chapter 4). Turnock (2004) reports that block grants resulted in a 25% reduction in federal funds to state and local health agencies. Funds for public health activities were included in the reductions in federal support. At the same time, state sources of money (the state tax base) were strained. State income sources have not kept up with state responsibilities, initially because of a downturn in the economy and more recently a result of tax reform efforts and pressures to improve disaster preparedness and response (NACCHO, 2007). Consequently, SHAs have experienced budget cuts and staffing reductions, and have had to reduce services to individuals and communities.

LIAISON OF STATE AND LOCAL PUBLIC HEALTH AGENCIES

Each state specifies its relationship with **local health departments (LHDs),** with some states being more centralized than others. The SHA coordinates efforts of all the local departments (for example, oversight of communicable disease reporting and control) and provides some of the funding for the LHDs. In some states, the LHD is an agency within the SHA; however, most LHDs are more autonomous, either consulting with the state or directly planning programs and setting health policy for the communities they serve. In most states with LHDs, **direct health care services** are primarily provided at the local level.

SHAs may provide some direct care, but they are more involved in the development and oversight of health-related regulations, coordination of statewide health assessments, and monitoring the health of special-risk populations. Although both state and local health departments provide vital services to guard the public's health, the more visible services are provided at the local level. LHDs provide most of the direct care to clients and communities.

STRUCTURE AND RESPONSIBILITIES OF LOCAL PUBLIC HEALTH AGENCIES

Local health departments obtain their authority through state law and additional local ordinances. Whatever the organizational structure, it is LHDs that directly provide public health services to community residents.

Each LHD carries out the three core functions of public health (see Table 29-1). *Healthy People 2010* specifically listed these core functions as objectives for local health departments. *Healthy People 2010* (U.S. Department of Health and Human Services

[USDHHS], 2000) increases the emphasis on public health, stressing the need for both state and local health department involvement in improving public health infrastructure, data collection, and service to the population and risk groups. The three core public health functions serve as the foundation for these new public health objectives (see the *Healthy People 2010* box).

TYPES OF LOCAL PUBLIC HEALTH DEPARTMENTS

A LHD has been defined by the National Association of County and City Health Officials (NACCHO, 1995, p. 13) as "an administrative or service unit of local or state government concerned with health and carrying some responsibility for the health of a jurisdiction smaller than the state." There are five major types of LHD: country, city, city-county, township, or multi-county/region. County LHDs are the most common type. Multi-county health departments are the least common. Multi-county health departments span large geographic areas and are more common in the western United States. For example, the Northeast Colorado Health Department serves six counties in Colorado. **Website Resource 29A** provides several examples of the organizational charts for different types of local public health agencies (LPHAs).

NACCHO reports the following information concerning LHDs:

* There are 2864 LHDs in 49 states and the District of Columbia. Rhode Island does not have a LHD.
* Two thirds of the LHDs serve jurisdictions of less than 50,000 people, and 6% serve populations of 500,000 or more (Figure 29-3).
* Fifty-nine percent of LHDs are county based.
* Sixty percent of LHDs have 25 or fewer full-time employees. Metropolitan LHDs have more employees than nonmetropolitan LHDs.
* Ninety-five percent of LHDs report employing full- or part-time registered nurses either directly or through contracted services (NACCHO, 2006).

FUNDING SOURCES

The funding source for LHDs is a combination of local, state, and federal funds (Figure 29-4). In addition, LHDs may collect fees from clients who receive direct personal health care services and from regulatory or licensing fees. For example, a health department responsible for inspecting restaurants to ensure food safety may collect fees as part of the food permit process.

Budgets for LHDs range from $10,000 to $1 billion (NACCHO, 2006). LHD budgets represent less than 1% of the total national health care budget (see Chapter 3). Local public health costs are estimated at approximately $23 to $32 per community resident (NACCHO, 2006). For the most part, LHDs that serve larger populations have bigger budgets and are more reliant on state and local funding and less on Medicare and Medicaid (Figure 29-5). Half of all LHDs have budgets of $1 million or less per year (NACCHO, 2006).

Local Funds

Revenue coming from local sources is primarily from taxes or a levy. A levy is a mechanism for raising money through the ballot box. It is similar to a bond issue in that it is a determined percentage of the local property tax or a local income tax approved by voters. Because general tax money fluctuates with

■ HEALTHY PEOPLE 2010 ■
Objectives for Public Health Infrastructure: State and Local Health Departments

1. Increase the proportion of federal, tribal, state, and local health agencies that have made information available for internal or external public use in the past year based on health indicators related to *Healthy People 2010* objectives. (Developmental; no current baseline.)

2. Increase to 100% the proportion of major national data systems that use geocoding to promote nationwide use of geographic information systems (GIS). (Baseline: 50% of major national health data systems are geocoded in 2000.)

3. Increase to 100% the proportion of population-based *Healthy People 2010* objectives for which national data are available for all population groups identified for the objective. (Baseline: 13% of the objectives have national data for select populations in 2004.)

4. Increase the proportion of tribal and local agencies that incorporate core competencies in the essential public health services into job descriptions and performance evaluations. (Developmental; no current baseline.)

5. Increase by 10% the proportion of tribal, state, and local public health personnel who receive continuing education consistent with the core competencies in essential public health services. (Tribal, developmental with no current baseline; state public health personnel, 13%; local public health personnel, 15% in 2000.)

6. Increase to 50% the proportion of state and local public health systems that meet national performance standards for essential public health services. (Baseline: 9% of state systems and 12% of local public health systems in 2004.)

7. Increase the proportion of tribal, states (100%), and local health agencies (80%) that have implemented a health improvement plan and increase the proportion of local jurisdictions that have a health improvement plan linked with their state plan. (Tribal, developmental with no current baseline; states and District of Columbia, 78% in 1997; local jurisdictions, 32% in 1993; local plans linked to state plans, developmental with no current baseline.)

8. Increase the proportion of tribal, state, and local public health agencies that provide or ensure comprehensive laboratory services to support essential health services. (Baseline: 90% disease control, 31% environmental protection, 29% emergency response, 2% food safety in 2004. 2010 goals: 98% disease control, 70% environmental protection, 65% emergency response, 50% food safety.)

9. Increase the proportion of tribal, state, and local public health agencies that provide or ensure comprehensive epidemiology services to support essential public health services. (Developmental; no current baseline.)

10. Increase the proportion of federal, tribal, state, and local public health agencies that conduct or collaborate on population-based prevention research. (Developmental; no current baseline.)

From U.S. Department of Health and Human Services. (2000). *Healthy People 2010: Understanding and improving health* (2nd ed.). Washington, DC: U.S. Government Printing Office; and U.S. Department of Health and Human Services. (2006). *Healthy People 2010: Midcourse review.* Washington, DC: U.S. Government Printing Office.

the strength of business and industry in the community, a levy must be placed on the ballot periodically for voter approval.

Many states have a legislatively allocated LHD subsidy of a few cents to a few dollars per capita. This subsidy is derived from a state's general fund, which comprises taxes, fees collected, and grant monies that do not have a specified

expenditure. This is not sufficient to support LHD programs but is important in the total financial scheme.

Although most LHDs collect fees, these fees account for a small portion (6%) of the total budget (NACCHO, 2006). The larger the LHD, the more likely it is to collect fees for services. Fees are collected for most health, environmental,

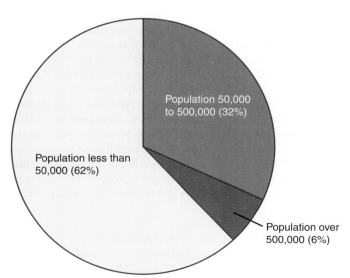

FIGURE 29-3 Distribution of the local health departments by the reported population of their jurisdiction. (Data from National Association of County and City Health Officials. [2006]. *2005 National profile of local health departments.* Washington, DC: NACCHO.)

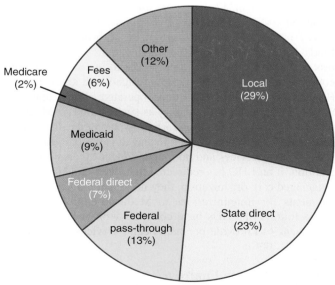

FIGURE 29-4 U.S. local health department funds by source: 2005. (Data from National Association of County and City Health Officials. [2006]. *2005 National profile of local health departments.* Washington, DC: NACCHO.)

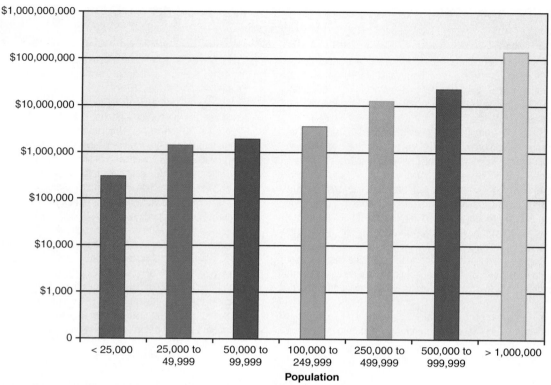

FIGURE 29-5 U.S. local health department average annual expenditures by size of population served. (Data from National Association of County and City Health Officials. [2006]. *2005 National profile of local health departments.* Washington, DC: NACCHO.)

counseling, and birth and death registration services. Many nursing services also have a service fee. A sliding fee scale is used to determine what percentage of the fee the client will pay based on the client's financial assets. Generally, service fees are not sufficient to fully cover the cost, but if a client cannot pay, service is not denied. If a client has a third-party payer (e.g., Medicaid or private health insurance), some departments will bill that source or provide the client with a receipt to file for reimbursement. Fees may be used within the department to partially support health and environmental services. Such money might also become part of the jurisdiction's general funds. Medicare and Medicaid funding sources are becoming less available as direct health services to at-risk populations continue to be contracted out to managed care organizations. For example, many LHDs once operated clinics that provided care to sick children, and, as such, collected Medicaid fees for treating those children who were Medicaid eligible. Most LHDs now contract with managed care organizations to provide such services and no longer collect Medicaid fees. In addition, if an LHD has redirected their well-child services to a managed care organization, they no longer collect Medicaid payments for immunizations to Medicaid-eligible children. Three fourths of LHDs have contracts with at least one private agency to provide personal health services (Gollust and Jacobson, 2006).

Federal and State Funds

State and federal monies account for almost 36% of LHD funds (NACCHO, 2006). Some of the state money is passed from the federal government. These federal funds are intended to finance certain programs or services, and the states act as the oversight authority for the federally supported services.

Impact of Federal and State Budgets on LHDs. The federal and state portion of the LHD budget has increased approximately 3% since 2001 (NACCHO, 2001, 2006). Since inflation has averaged 2.6% per year each year during that time frame (Bureau of Labor Statistics, 2007), the actual impact has been a reduction in funding from those sources. Funding allocations are the result of changing government policies and shrinking tax revenues. The federal block grant process has limited funding to programs administered by both state and local health departments (Chapter 4). Federal block grants and cutbacks in other federal health-related funding have stressed state government budgets. States have been forced to assume more responsibility for health and welfare programs. These changes have a domino effect as federal reductions in contributions to state budgets force states to provide fewer dollars to local departments for which most of the public health care services are provided. Finally, the economic recession of the late 1990s and early 2000s and the shrinking value of property have reduced tax revenues, impacting both budget and service at all three levels of government.

IMPACT OF FUNDING VARIATION

Most LHDs rely on several funding sources; some may attach specific conditions to the use of funds. The cost to the department of the restrictions and accountability imposed by the grantor may exceed the benefits obtained with the money. Staff hired with grant money must work on that program only, or the work time of the numbers of people providing part-time services must equal the full-time equivalent. When money is no longer available or is cut, jobs paid by those funds may be lost. Some funds cannot be used for rental space, building, or equipment purchases. If equipment can be purchased, those items may be claimed by the funding sources when money allocation is terminated. Reports and data for federal or state money, which must be collected and reported in a set format, frequently duplicate data collected at the local level—all in a different format. Nursing and other personnel may spend time in producing redundant paperwork rather than providing services to clients and communities.

Local health department costs—salaries, supplies, equipment, and benefits—increase annually. However, the amount of appropriations often remains the same over time or is reduced. Thus, the degree to which this money actually supports local services is decreased. In the difficult economy of the late 1990s through the mid 2000s, the demand for public health nursing services has increased. Local health departments are continually challenged to be innovative, creative, flexible, and available.

At one time, LHDs tried to avoid having nursing and/or other staff on time-limited, or "soft," money, but currently, staff may be paid by two or three funding sources. This is where the full-time-equivalent factor enters the equation. Community health nursing administrators address difficult questions as they modify budgets. What components of a perinatal or child health program can be financed by other money when a funding source ends or decreases? When child health funds do not keep pace with costs, how can sufficient child health services be incorporated into the Women, Infants, and Children (WIC) program? Similar questions arise for all public health nursing services. With flexible hours and flexible staffing, two part-time employees can fill a full-time position. If possible, other types of employees, such as nursing assistants, may be hired to perform nonnursing tasks and allow more efficient use of nursing time.

IMPACT OF LEGISLATION

The funding sources discussed previously are considered legislative, except for foundations. State and federal agencies and programs have evolved through legislation. The appropriations are made or withheld based on state and federal budget emphases, the interests and power of legislators, and the demands of lobbying groups and constituents.

Both federal and state legislatures and agencies are skilled at passing health-related bills or issuing health-related directives without appropriate funds to implement the program. One example involves the use of the WIC program to monitor childhood immunizations. Studies indicate that linking WIC and children's immunization services is an effective strategy (Briss et al., 2000; Hutchins et al., 1999). Children seen for WIC services were reviewed to determine immunization status. Those found deficient were either immunized at the WIC center or referred to other sources for immunization. The costs of providing these services at each WIC site ranged from $19,500 to $60,300, depending on staff requirements. The preliminary studies were done with grant money. In 2000 a Presidential directive required the WIC program to implement immunization screening and referral at all WIC sites (Shefer et al., 2002). No additional money was allocated for the additional staffing and administrative requirements.

Public health employees are becoming more effective working with legislators. Public health nurses, environmentalists, administrators, and other staff working with programs such as substance and alcohol abuse, human immunodeficiency virus (HIV) testing, and acquired immunodeficiency syndrome (AIDS) case coordination organize networks to initiate, support, or oppose legislation that will adversely affect LHDs and communities. For example, in a number of states, public health professionals have been highly effective in guiding and supporting specific HIV testing and AIDS legislation. The bills afford protection for health care workers by the availability of HIV tests and employment security if that test is positive. Public health advocates have been equally effective in opposing broad AIDS legislation that would compromise an individual's privacy, employment, and/or health insurance coverage (Roseau & Reomer, 2002).

GEOGRAPHIC VARIATIONS IN SERVICES AND FUNDING

As noted earlier, most local public health programs serve populations of 50,000 or less. All the factors noted within this chapter heavily influence the needs of and services for rural areas and small towns in the United States.

Medical personnel and health services are often concentrated in urban areas and in group medical practices in the United States. Group practices afford individuals access to the care they may need, be it family medicine, internal medicine, or other specialty represented in a group practice. This sounds beneficial to the client. This geographic maldistribution of physicians has led to inner-city and rural areas being medically underserved, although there has been a slight improvement in physician supply in rural areas (Smart, 2006). These areas may attract only the single-specialty physician, who may practice alone in communities with great needs. Some communities with populations of 15,000 to 30,000 have only one physician. Even the state health department may not have clinics in inner-city areas or some rural communities. Transportation problems and appointment times that conflict with employment can be added barriers (see Chapter 32).

Public health nurses in rural communities and city health departments provide wide-ranging wellness care and health screening to detect potential problems. Education regarding health-promotion and lifestyle adaptations that reduce risks to good health is an important component. Nurse practitioners monitor and/or treat illnesses and chronic diseases depending on the support of the department's medical director and on community needs. Because most public health nurses are long-term residents of their community, they know their community.

Some state health departments, through maternal and child health programs, may provide itinerant multidisciplinary teams of specialists for diagnosis and treatment of infants and children with disabilities. The local public health nursing staff provides follow-up, case management, and continuing family and client support and guidance.

STAFFING OF LOCAL PUBLIC HEALTH AGENCIES

The LHDs may have a staff as small as one public health nurse, one environmentalist (sanitarian), and one part-time health director, or it may employ hundreds of employees to meet major city and jurisdiction health and environmental needs. The staff may comprise public health nurses, nurses in expanded roles (e.g., nurse practitioners), nutritionists, environmentalists, health educators, a biostatistician, clerical and laboratory staff, nursing or home health aides, counselors for alcohol and substance abuse, the health director, physicians, and various administrative staff. States also vary regarding whether the chief administrative officer is required to be a physician. The duties of public health personnel are both direct individual and population-focused care.

A health department may be a combined agency, having both wellness services and home health services for the ill and disabled. Combined agencies may employ or contract for physiotherapists, home care aides or nursing assistants, nutritionists, social workers, speech or occupational therapists, and others.

Public Health Nurses

Previous chapters have dealt with the definition and scope of community/public health nursing and its many facets for nursing practice (see Chapters 1 and 2). Aside from administrative staff, community/public health nurses are the single largest professional staff in LHDs (Kennedy et al., 2000; NACCHO, 2006). This has been true since the 1920s, when many local governments (counties, cities, or multi-county regions) developed health departments to promote the health of the people residing in their jurisdictions. Although the terms community health nurse and public health nurse are used interchangeably, nurses working for government-sponsored (public) entities often prefer the original name, public health nurse (see Chapter 2).

Public health nurses were and are professionals who attempt to develop healthful communities through population-based practice. An ecologic approach toward public health nursing recognizes the influence of determinants of health on multiple layers including individuals, families, communities, organizations, and social systems (ANA, 2007). Public health nurses may simultaneously target individuals, families, communities, or systems with their interventions, as the focus of their work is the population as a whole. Public health nurses emphasize primary prevention of "illness, injury or disability, the promotion of health, and maintenance of the health of populations" (American Public Health Association [APHA], 2007). The area of public health nursing will be addressed in greater detail later in this chapter.

Environmental Sanitarians

Environmental sanitarians are concerned with safe air, water, food, and housing. They conduct routine sampling of air and private water sources and inspect restaurants, dairies, and food processing sites. Sanitarians provide environmental education, enforce environmental laws, and respond to complaints. They may collect residential paint samples for lead analysis and address noise, unsafe dwellings, rodent control, and hazardous wastes.

Biostatisticians and Epidemiologists

Biostatisticians and epidemiologists apply their knowledge of statistics and the natural history of diseases to describe the health of communities, explore the causes of specific disease outbreaks, predict health hazards, and evaluate interventions. These health specialists are employed primarily at the state level or by larger LHDs. In response to terrorism and emergency preparedness, federal funding rapidly increased the number of epidemiologists at the state level between 2001

and 2004. However, state public health officials estimate that 45.3% more epidemiologists are needed nationwide to fully staff terrorism preparedness programs (MMWR, 2005).

Environmental issues and communicable disease control remain LHD mandates and priorities. Food and water sanitation and vector control exist alongside such modern concerns as hazardous waste management and swimming pool inspections. When a food-borne or water-borne disease is reported, the public health nurse and environmentalist work together to discover the source, follow-up with people reporting illness or symptoms, refer them for medical treatment, and get the problem under control.

SERVICES PROVIDED BY THE STATE HEALTH AGENCY AND THE LOCAL HEALTH DEPARTMENT

As previously stated, SHAs and LHDs are partners in ensuring the public health of their citizens. According to the Association of State and Territorial Health Officials (ASTHO) (2007), the main services provided to meet that goal are as follows:

- Collect vital statistics and analyze statistics.
- Control infectious disease.
- Ensure environmental health and safety.
- Provide health education.
- Provide laboratory facilities.
- Ensure occupational health.
- Provide health care delivery.
- Ensure emergency and disaster preparedness.
- Provide maternal and child health care.
- Prevent chronic diseases.
- Control injuries.
- Provide mental health and substance abuse services.

Most of the services are coordinated. The collection of *vital statistics,* for example, begins at the local level. The state collects individual local reports and coalesces this information into a report of the statewide status of births, deaths, marriages, and so on. Many of the other services provided by state and local health agencies are discussed later.

PERSONAL HEALTH CARE

In addition to population-based health care such as control of communicable diseases and injuries, promotion of wellness and reduction of risks to health, and provision of home health care, community data may also dictate the need for primary care. *Primary care* is the provision of personal health services to individuals and family members, including screening and referral, health maintenance, long-term management of chronic disease, and care for acute illnesses.

In the early 1980s, as a response to increases in the number of medically uninsured and underinsured people, more health departments became directly involved in providing primary care services. Starting in the early 1990s, LHDs began to reassess and redefine their role in health care delivery in line with the IOM recommendations. A renewed focus on **population-based health services** has resulted in a reduction in direct personal health care by LHDs. Today, LHDs still provide direct care, although many are attempting to redirect these types of services to other organizations such as managed care (Gollust & Jacobson, 2006). For example, the state of Maryland redirected its well-child and sick-child care to specially contracted managed care organizations. The managed care organizations are paid to provide specific screening and immunization services for well-children. They also provide specific illness and rehabilitative services up to a certain dollar amount for children with health problems. Some of the state and local public health nurses act as case managers to oversee and coordinate additional services for children with special needs.

Redirecting or eliminating direct personal health care services is influenced by the geographic area and availability of other health care resources. Nonmetropolitan areas are more likely to have problems finding alternative sources for direct care. In 2005, 28% of LHDs provided home health care services to community members, a 26% decline since 1993 (NACCHO, 2001, 2006). However, twice as many nonmetropolitan LHDs still provide home health care as do metropolitan LHDs.

Figure 29-6 illustrates the types of direct care provided by various LHDs. Aside from screening services, the bar graph shows that personal services are provided by fewer LHDs today than in 1993 (NACCHO, 1995, 2001). For example, HIV/AIDS treatment was provided by 32% of LHDs in 1993, and only 26% still provide direct care in 2005. Family planning services were provided by 68% of LHDs in 1993 and 58% in 2005 (NACCHO, 1995, 2006).

Clients are being redirected to other health care providers for services discontinued by LHDs. Some important areas of investigation related to these changes in service focus include the following questions:

- Are alternative health care providers available for services dropped from LHDs?
- If clients are redirected to other providers, are they receiving similar, better, or worse services than those previously provided by the LHD?
- What is the financial consequence of redirected services? In other words, are clients now required to pay for services previously provided by LHDs on a sliding scale or at no cost? If so, are clients using services or do they discontinue care?

Many of the personal services by LHDs are supported, in part, by federal and state funds. State and federal requirements often demand a combination of several types of services within the programs they help fund. In the co-funded programs, you see elements of personal health care, communicable disease control, and health-education types of services provided by public health agencies.

PROGRAMS SUPPORTED BY FEDERAL AND STATE FUNDS

It must be remembered that types of appropriations and funds change over time. Federal and state governments may appropriate money differently during each legislative session. As health care reform evolves, some or all of the following programs will be discontinued, change by title or how appropriated, and/or incorporated into new plans.

Women, Infants, and Children Supplemental Food Program

In this program, money supplied by the U.S. Department of Agriculture is funneled through state departments of health to LHDs or other community agencies that administer the program and provide the services. This program provides direct services in the form of supplemental foods and infant formula, as well as nutrition education. The WIC program has resulted in healthier mothers, infants, and children. WIC is still administered directly by 67% of LHDs (NACCHO, 2006).

Centers for Disease Control and Prevention Funds

Federal and state funds are allocated for biologicals for childhood immunization programs and for influenza vaccines for elderly persons. Health departments may pay a nominal cost for the influenza vaccine; immunization is generally limited to medically indigent elderly individuals and those with chronic lung and heart diseases. Since 1993, Medicare has expanded payments for vaccines for all individuals with Medicare Part B coverage. Currently, Medicare will pay for influenza, pneumonia, and hepatitis B vaccinations, but not the vaccine for shingles (Centers for Medicare and Medicaid Services [CMS], 2007). These immunization services are directly billed to Medicare. The state usually does not charge for biologicals used to immunize children.

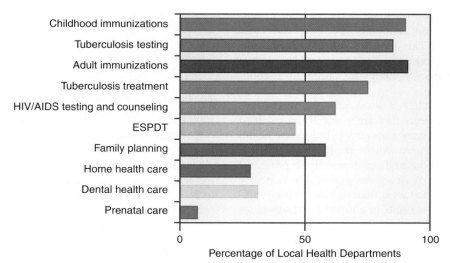

FIGURE 29-6 Most common personal health care services, provided by percentage of providing local health departments (LHDs) in 2005. *EPSDT*, Early and periodic screening, diagnosis, and treatment. (Data from National Association of County and City Health Officials. [2006]. *2005 National profile of local health departments*. Washington, DC: NACCHO.)

AIDS and HIV education and screening programs receive funding through state or federal competitive grants or direct appropriation. Interested community groups or agencies are encouraged to form cooperative agreements or consortia to avoid duplication of services. Much of this money funds HIV laboratory costs and the test materials necessary to obtain blood specimens and transport them to the laboratory. The money also supports AIDS/HIV counselors who assist HIV-positive clients with support and access to additional evaluation.

One example of a CDC-funded program is "Advancing HIV Prevention: New Strategies for a Changing Epidemic" (MMWR, 2003a). It is an effort to reduce barriers to early diagnosis of HIV and to increase access to quality medical care, treatment, and ongoing prevention services. CDC helps fund comprehensive local and state programs, which include the partner counseling and referral services as a means of identifying undiagnosed HIV.

In some states and health departments, CDC money funds disease investigation staff who track contacts of persons infected with specific sexually transmitted diseases (STDs), including syphilis, gonorrhea, and HIV. Contact follow-up is important epidemiologically for STD treatment, but reductions in federal and state funds and investigator staff have altered this component. State laws and health department regulations may also preclude investigations. Treatment medications for gonorrhea or other STDs may be provided free, at reduced cost, or at full cost. Some LHDs will provide prescriptions, but clients are expected to fill the prescription at their own expense.

Tuberculosis (TB) money increased in the 1980s and 1990s with the increased incidence and prevalence of tuberculosis and the advent of multi–drug-resistant strains and special risk populations. In the 2000s, tuberculosis funding has been strained by the new burdens on public health, and many LHDs report funding reductions (Tougher times strike more TB programs as budget axes fall: Immigrants, indigent, recession contributing causes, 2002). Increases in multi–drug-resistant TB and the introduction of extensively multi–drug-resistant TB have further strained the budgets for TB control programs.

Health and Human Services Funds

Health-promotion and risk reduction money has generally been competitive funds used for high blood pressure screening, referral, and follow-up; smoking cessation; and other risk-assessment activities. This money is targeted for health-education initiatives and frequently is used to provide financial support to targeted community groups for professional counseling services.

Federal substance and alcohol abuse program funds have been available for some years and are generally augmented by state money. The funds may come through the state health department or the state department of mental health. Some states have combined alcohol and substance abuse programs into a separate department of alcohol/mental health. Certainly both mental and physical factors influence how well an individual and his/her family succeeds in efforts to end substance abuse. Extensive community education is an important component of these programs, both to prevent the development of abusive behaviors and to assist the client, family, and community in dealing with substance abuse. Public health nurses, psychologists, counselors, and health educators form the nucleus for intervention (see Chapter 25).

Maternal/Child Health Block Grant

Federal Child and Family Health Services money is funneled through state health departments and may be augmented by state maternal/child health funds. The goal is to support comprehensive health assessment services, appropriate education and counseling, referrals, and follow-up for pregnant women and their infants and children. The money may go to the health department, to other agencies, or to consortia and cooperatives formed between local agencies and the health department. Money is limited; the more agencies involved, the more limited the support is for any one component or agency. Comprehensive services are defined by the grantor and vary from state to state. Grants must be renewed annually, and the grant award usually does not keep pace with inflation.

Health care reform and the greater use of managed care continue to change the way funds for maternal and child health services are used. In 1994 federal money was added for childhood immunizations. Mandatory and/or voluntary enrollment in managed care for pregnant women and children in the Medicaid program continues on a state-by-state basis.

Special initiative maternal/child health funds also require competitive grant proposals, which allow any interested state or local health department or appropriate agency to apply for this money. Each year, a focus is selected, such as adolescent pregnancy or early childhood intervention. The emphasis of the intervention is based on community and/or agency perceptions of local health problems and innovative ideas to address them. The federal or state agency administering the money reviews the submitted proposals and selects those to be funded. This is time- and amount-limited money. It is not intended to subsidize established services but may be used to add a new service to a population that is being served or to begin a completely new program targeted to a special population.

Concerned with the use of tobacco during pregnancy, one funding effort aimed at reducing or eliminating smoking behavior in pregnant women during pregnancy. One county developed and submitted for funding a protocol for health education on tobacco risk and smoking cessation support for their prenatal clients. Community health nurses involved in the maternal/child program developed the teaching model, identified support personnel to help with the smoking cessation program, and enrolled approximately 150 pregnant women in the program. During participation in the program, 50% were able to stop smoking and another 25% reported cutting consumption by about 50%. The county health department is considering methods to continue the program once grant funding ends.

Crippled/handicapped children's program money became available in the mid-1930s to support detection, medical treatment, and ongoing follow-up of a broad range of physically and medically handicapping conditions in newborns and children up to 21 years of age. Orthopedic appliances, orthodontic devices (after cleft palate repair), hearing aids, and any therapist consultations necessary for appropriate treatment are some of the services available with this program. The program, originally the Crippled Children's Program, has been renamed Services for Children with Special Health Care Needs. There are financial and other eligibility criteria, which are generally determined by the state health department. Public health nurses often provide case management for these children and their families. Some states have expanded funding to pay for all services that public health nurses provide to eligible families. Public health nursing visits to homes, schools, or other places are currently being reimbursed at rates commensurate with the degree of comprehensiveness, assistance, and advocacy necessary for the family and/or child with a disability. Some states have redirected these personal health care services to managed care organizations with case management by public health personnel.

Lead poisoning program funds come from the federal government through the state for education (of family, community, and LHD personnel), detection, and limited emergency housing abatement for childhood lead poisoning. For example, Claudia Smith, a member of the Community Health Nursing Department, University of Maryland, developed a proposal for lead abatement in high-risk homes in one metropolitan area. She was awarded a 1-year grant from the U.S. Department of Housing and Urban Development, and was able to provide lead abatement services to low-income city residents. The CDC also funds state and local programs to develop childhood lead poison prevention programs and surveillance programs (MMWR, 2003b). Many child health programs include blood lead screening for children ages 9 months to 6 years and parent education. Some local health departments are designated teaching centers. A public health nurse and an environmentalist work with LHD personnel in designated counties to help establish blood lead screening and education programs.

Other Funds

There has been federal and state money for other health department programs, such as air quality control and care at corrections' facilities. Public health nursing may be involved, depending on the services to be provided. Medicaid and Medicare reimburse for specific services to individuals. Federal programs, including Medicaid and Medicare Part B, reimburse for nursing services provided by nurse practitioners and certified nurse-midwives, especially in rural areas.

Medicaid

Title XIX money consists of both federal and state funds reimbursed to LHDs. The client must meet Medicaid financial and other eligibility criteria. Medicaid reimbursement to service providers for medical or wellness-centered care may vary by state (see Chapter 4). The priority populations are pregnant women, infants, and children (2 through 18 years of age) and some older adults who need chronic disease treatment or nursing home care. These priority populations were selected because they are unable to afford health care and are vulnerable to conditions that are expensive to treat if not prevented. For example, provision of prenatal care and nutrition increases the likelihood of a healthy infant and reduces the need for expensive neonatal intensive care services. Medicaid funds are frequently administered through state departments of human services with health maintenance services monitored by state health departments. Many states and LHDs have contracted with managed care organizations to provide services, although 36% of LHDs still directly provide prenatal care to clients (NACCHO, 2006).

The Early Periodic Screening, Diagnosis, and Treatment (EPSDT) program is an example of Medicaid-funded health-promotion services for children. Infants and children are entitled to physical examinations, immunizations, screening tests, health histories, nutrition assessment (referral to WIC and/or interim WIC visits as appropriate), and anticipatory guidance at specified age levels from birth to 18 years. Although EPSDT services have been redirected away from LHDs, 46% of LHDs still provide direct EPSDT care (NACCHO, 2006).

Medicare

Medicare money is a reimbursement source for combined agencies providing home health care. Physician-ordered services provided by public health nurses; physical, occupational, and speech therapists; and home health aides are reimbursable for specified time periods at specified payment levels. Medicare funds reimburse physician-provided primary care, specified diagnostic tests, and hospitalization for elderly persons. In 1992 Congress broadened Medicare coverage to pay for mammograms at specified intervals for women ages 65 years and older. Some LHDs (28%) provide home health care services and many others offer screening services for mammograms, which are reimbursed by Medicare.

Foundations

Foundations are philanthropic groups (formed by businesses, individuals, or industries) that support research and service proposals reflecting the emphases of the foundation. They may be national in focus, such as the Kellogg and Robert Woods Johnson trusts, or local. Foundations encourage competitive proposals that must meet certain guidelines. They can be excellent sources of funds for research or small local efforts.

ENVIRONMENTAL HEALTH SERVICES

An important area of public health is control of environmental hazards. In most locales, the LHD is the agency that oversees environmental conditions such as sewage disposal, air and water quality, and vector control (Figure 29-7). In some instances, another agency may be responsible for local oversight. Depending on organization and funding, the SHA may or may not be the agency to which the LHD reports on environmental issues. Sometimes the environmental functions may be part of another state agency or a stand-alone agency responsible only for environmental concerns. In addition to the services listed in Figure 29-7, LHDs may be the primary agency for other types of monitoring and inspections, including the following:
- Food restaurants
- Processing and milk suppliers
- Swimming pool inspections
- Nursing home inspections
- Schools/daycare centers
- Campgrounds/RVs/mobile homes
- Smoke-free ordinances
- Solid waste disposal sites
- Cosmetology businesses (tanning salons, tattoo parlors, barber and beauty shops)

Even if not the responsibility of LHDs, these types of facilities are usually monitored by some local authority.

LABORATORY SERVICES

Laboratory services include monitoring samples taken by environmental health personnel, as well as specimens from those receiving direct health care services or involved in communicable disease surveillance. Water samples are tested for parasites

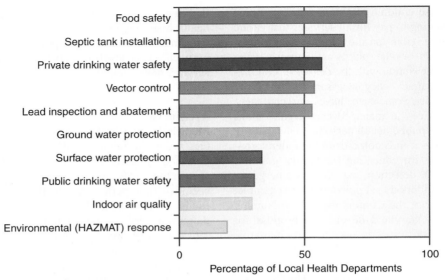

FIGURE 29-7 U.S. local health department (LHD) selected environmental services: 2005. (Data from National Association of County and City Health Officials. [2006]. *2005 National profile of local health departments.* Washington, DC: NACCHO.)

and other contaminants. Blood and other human samples are tested for communicable diseases. Radiographic testing is employed to monitor tuberculosis clients. The laboratories also provide genetic screening tests. In some jurisdictions, SHAs rather than LHDs operate the laboratory. In either case, the services provided protect the public's health. Laboratories may also offer testing services to other groups and organizations in the community on a fee-for-service basis. Laboratory services is one of the areas identified by *Healthy People 2010* as needing improvement.

OCCUPATIONAL HEALTH

The Occupational Safety and Health Act of 1970 allowed states oversight responsibilities; however, state standards must meet or exceed federal standards for occupational safety and health. Unless it is a superagency, the SHA is not the primary agency monitoring occupational health issues. When the SHA is not the primary agency, they are usually involved in a consultative fashion to help with issues such as identifying the health effects of exposure, conducting epidemiologic studies to identify causes of health problems, and monitoring health status in exposure situations.

LHDs have even less oversight responsibility than SHAs, although they are frequently the initial contact point for complaints. Approximately 12% of LHDs provide occupational safety and health services (NACCHO, 2006). More frequently, state and local agencies receive complaints and refer them to the appropriate oversight agency. Sometimes on-site investigations are warranted because they involve environmental issues, such as food storage or water safety, that are more frequently the purview of the LHD.

EVOLUTION OF PUBLIC HEALTH NURSING IN OFFICIAL AGENCIES

Public health nursing preceded the widespread development of LHDs. In the late 1800s, Lillian Wald coined the term *public health nurse*. This term was appropriate not only because the nurse worked on behalf of the public, but also because

"she was to create a public sphere that drew upon the diversity of cultural beliefs and societal demands of the populace" (Reverby, 1993, p. 1662). Local health departments expanded in part because of the successes of both public health nurses working in voluntary agencies and sanitary reformers. Local governments desired to provide such services for their communities to protect the health of the public.

Public health nursing, at its inception, focused on sick people and those who were living in poverty and on indigent pregnant and postpartum women and their newborns. These nurses worked primarily in visiting nurse associations and were not affiliated with those first health departments (see Chapter 2). Los Angeles (in 1898) and New York City (in 1908) began to employ nurses who would formally carry out public health nursing responsibilities (Pickett & Hanlon, 1990). This work continued to center on the poor and on control of communicable diseases, such as tuberculosis. Public health nurses performed nursing assessments, health and social histories, and health and risk reduction education, and they also provided home health care.

With the passage of the Shepard-Towner Act in 1921, providing for complete birth registration (Last & Wallace, 1992), maternal and child health services became a mainstay of public health nursing in SHAs and LHDs. In the intervening years, numerous programs and services have been added.

EXTERNAL INFLUENCES ON PUBLIC HEALTH NURSING

Historically, public health nursing has responded to changing social, cultural, political, and economic influences. The landmark IOM (1988) study provided a catalyst for change in the role of public health nurses. Change has also been influenced by an increasing emphasis on performance outcomes, the threat of bioterrorism, and the emergence of new communicable diseases. In response to these issues, public health nursing practice is changing to an increased emphasis on population-focused care.

Public health nursing positions are financed through a variety of sources: local taxes; state and federal appropriations, grants, and contracts; fees and reimbursements for services; and private grants and donations. Some funding received by local agencies is designated for specific programs or projects and often cannot be used to support specific positions. Because most nursing functions do not generate funds, nursing positions are sometimes in jeopardy when budgets are low (Gebbie et al., 2002).

PUBLIC HEALTH NURSING PRACTICE

Public health nursing is defined as the practice of promoting and protecting the health of populations using the knowledge from nursing, social, and public health sciences (APHA, Public Health Nursing Section, 1996). Public health nursing is clarified and differentiated from other types of nursing by adherence to all eight of the Tenets of Public Health Nursing (Quad Council of Public Health Nursing Organizations, 1999). Public health nursing expands basic nursing theory and practice, which focuses on an individual or family, to a focus on *populations*. Population focus distinguishes public health nursing from other specialty areas. The public health nurse may provide care to an individual or family, but the ultimate beneficiary of the care is the population. For example, the public health nurse may teach a client with tuberculosis about the disease and observe the client taking medication. However, the ultimate intent and beneficiary of care are the people of the community who are protected from contracting the disease. Box 29-2 lists the basic tenets of public health nursing.

The Association of State and Territorial Directors of Nursing (ASTDN) has developed a Public Health Nursing Practice Model (Figure 29-8) to illustrate how public health nurses take the concepts of basic nursing and link them with the public

| Box 29-2 | **Tenets of Public Health Nursing** |

- The client or unit of care is the population.
- The primary obligation is to achieve the greatest good for the greatest number of people or the population as a whole.
- The processes used by public health nurses include working with the client as an equal partner.
- Primary prevention is the priority in selecting appropriate activities.
- Public health nursing focuses on strategies that create healthy environmental, social, and economic conditions in which populations may thrive.
- A public health nurse is obligated to actively identify and reach out to all who might benefit from a specific activity or service.
- Optimal use of available resources to assure the best overall improvement in the health of the population is a key element of the practice.
- Collaboration with a variety of other professions, populations, organizations, and other stake holders is the most effective way to promote and protect the health of the people.

Reprinted with permission from American Nurses Association. *Public health nursing: Scope and standards of practice.* Copyright 2007, Nursebooks.org, Silver Spring, MD.

health and population concepts to practice the specialty of public health nursing (ASTDN, 2000). The core of the model is the art and science of nursing practice and includes the nursing process components of assessment, diagnosis, planning, intervention, and evaluation. The middle ring of the model represents the core public health functions—assessment, policy development, and assurance. These core functions are defined

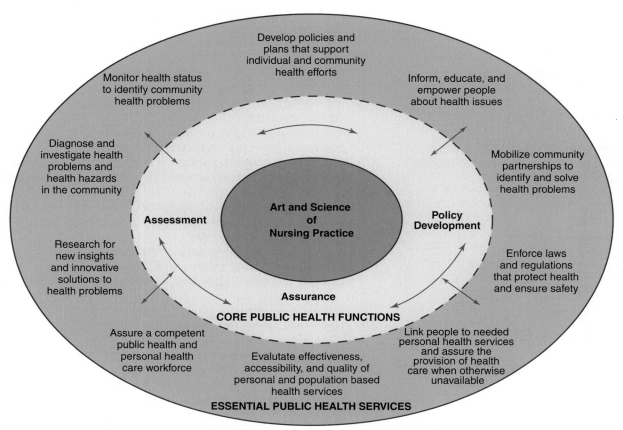

FIGURE 29-8 Public Health Nursing Practice Model. (Reprinted with permission from American Nurses Association. *Public health nursing: A partner for healthy populations.* Copyright 2000, Nursebooks.org, Silver Spring, MD.)

as the governmental role in protecting and promoting the health of the public. The outer ring represents the essential public health services. These essential services clarify and describe how the core functions are accomplished. Essential public health services are provided by multidisciplinary public health professionals, including public health nurses. Table 29-2 provides examples of public health nursing activities performed to accomplish the essential services.

Several other public health nursing practice models have been developed to describe the work of public health nurses. One model is the Minnesota Interventions Wheel, more commonly referred to as "The Wheel." The model is grounded in community assessment, considers determinants of health, and emphasizes prevention (Keller et al., 2004). The Wheel consists of 3 levels of practice (individual, community, and systems) and 17 nursing interventions that target change in "attitudes, knowledge, beliefs, practices and behaviors" (ANA, 2007) at the different practice levels to contribute to the improvement of a population's health. The Intervention Wheel has been a major influence on public health nursing practice across the country and is being used to assess and document public health nursing work with communities, systems, and individuals (Keller et al., 2004).

TABLE 29-2   Examples of Public Health Nursing Activities for the Ten Essential Services

Essential Public Health Service	Public Health Nursing Activities
Monitor health status to identify community health problems	Participate in community assessment* Review birth records to identify individuals or groups that may be at high risk Identify potential environmental hazards*
Diagnose and investigate health problems and health hazards in the community	Understand and identify determinants of health and disease* Review and monitor communicable disease reports Participate in case identification and treatment of communicable diseases* Use knowledge of environmental health hazards when observing the community
Inform, educate, and empower	Develop and implement educational plans for individuals and families* Provide information to policy makers about needs of special populations Advocate for and with under-served and disadvantaged populations* Provide education about health and public health issues to the community
Mobilize partnerships to identify and solve health problems	Form relationships and interact with providers in the community Convene and participate in community groups to address needs of special populations Teach community members about health issues
Develop policies and plans that support individual and community health efforts	Participate in community and family decision making* Provide information and advocate for the interests of special populations when developing policies.* Develop programs and services to meet needs of high-risk populations* Participate in emergency response planning and training
Enforce laws and regulations	Implement ordinances that protect the environment* Work with public health team to enforce food safety regulations Regulate and support care and treatment of dependent populations such as children and elderly* Provide education to regulated facilities and providers such as child care facilities
Link people to needed personal health services and ensure the provision of health care when otherwise unavailable	Provide clinical preventive services to high-risk populations Link clients and families to clinical care and other services in the community Establish programs and services to meet special needs not available elsewhere in the community Provide clinical surveillance and identification of communicable disease* Participate in provider coalitions and meetings to educate about community needs*
Assure a competent workforce	Participate in continuing education* Maintain client record systems and community documents* Establish and maintain procedures and protocols for care* Develop or participate in quality assurance activities, such as record audits and clinical guidelines*
Evaluate health services	Collect data and information on community interventions* Identify unserved and under-served populations in the community* Review and analyze data on the health status of the community* Conduct surveys or observe high-risk populations to evaluate needs
Research for new insights and innovative solutions to health problems	Implement nontraditional interventions and programs* Participate in collection of information and research activities Develop relationships with academic institutions and faculty* Use evidence-based information to make decisions

*Activities from Association of State and Territorial Directors of Nursing (ASTDN). (2000). *Public health nursing: A partner for healthy populations.* Washington, DC: American Nurses Publishing.

EDUCATIONAL PREPARATION

The baccalaureate degree in nursing is the educational standard for entry-level public health nursing. Master's level education is assumed for the nurse specialist level with specific expertise in population-focused care (ANA, 2007). A baccalaureate degree in nursing is considered to be preferred by most LHDs. However, the realities of the nursing shortage and the intense competition for baccalaureate-prepared nurses force many agencies to fill positions with nurses with different educational backgrounds (Quad Council, 2006). Recent data indicate that half of all practicing public health nurses are educated at the associate or diploma level (IOM, 2003b).

A graduate education in public health or nursing is considered the standard for supervisory or leadership positions (IOM, 2003b). Some management and business courses are useful. The National League for Nursing and the American Nurses Association encourage advanced practice and advanced degrees.

Nurses working in public health must actively participate in ongoing continuing education in order to function effectively and ensure quality practice in the context of rapid social and practice changes. All public health nurses are expected to be lifelong learners. Some of the most important areas of continuing education are identified in Box 29-3. In addition to specific knowledge areas, it is essential that public health nurses have the ability to work independently as well as with colleagues and the public to provide effective population-based community care.

Baccalaureate and higher nursing education remains economically and geographically inaccessible for many nursing candidates, but opportunities for such education are growing for diploma or associate degree nurses who desire baccalaureate or master's level education. Equally important have been continuing education opportunities that include subjects pertinent to community health, such as environmental assessment, community assessment, community health planning and development, coalition building and leadership, communication, cultural

---

Box 29-3 Suggested Course Content for Public Health Nursing Continuing Education

Nursing process, public health process, systems thinking
Core functions of public health, essential services
Public health in America, history, legal basis, ethics, values
Community health assessment
Program planning and evaluation
Community mobilization, systems thinking
Communication skills
Partnership development
Leadership skills
Environmental health, risk assessment, and communications
Applied epidemiology
Data analysis for public health
Quality and outcomes evaluation
Informatics/communication technology
Politics of health policy
Health economics
Conflict resolution, negotiation, change theory

From Gebbie, K., & Hwang, I. (2000). Preparing currently employed public health nurses for changes in the health system. *American Journal of Public Health, 90*(5), 719.

---

competency, evaluation, and health-education strategies. These programs may be sponsored by collegiate nursing continuing education departments. Community health nursing faculty and LHD staff are often the speakers or leaders for programs that address public health nursing issues. Specialty certification in public health nursing is available from the American Nurses Association Credentialing Center (ANA Credentialing Center, 2007) for the public health/community health clinical nurse specialist.

STANDARDS OF PRACTICE

The 2007 American Nurses Association (ANA) publication *Public Health Nursing: Scope and Standards of Practice* outlines the public health registered nurse's professional role through 16 standards of practice and professional performance (see Chapter 1). This ANA work incorporates the 1986 *Standards of Community Health Nursing* as well as the Quad Council's *Scope and Standards of Public Health Nursing Practice* published in 1999. The Quad Council is comprised of representatives from the American Nurses Association; the American Public Health Association, Public Health Nursing Section; the Association of Community Health Nursing Educators; and the Association of State and Territorial Directors of Nursing. The scope and standards provide guidance and define and direct public health professional nursing practice in all settings, including the role of the advanced practice public health nurse. Additionally, consistent application of the scope and standards sets a framework for future public health nursing practice, education, and research (ANA, 2007).

POPULATION-BASED PLANNING

Efficient and effective care to populations requires strategic planning. With the advent of the *Healthy People 2000* objectives (USDHHS, 1990), national objectives covering all areas of health and the environment challenged public health personnel to involve their state and local communities in exploring what good health and wellness mean. The objectives encompassed traditional facets of public health as well as the concerns of AIDS and HIV infection, violence in the community, and dental care. *Healthy People 2010* continues the focus on population-based health planning and stresses the importance of improving the public health infrastructure.

The SHAs and LHDs choose objectives pertinent to their communities and develop action plans and methods to accomplish the objectives. These plans contribute to development and maintenance by communities, families, and individuals of behaviors and lifestyles to achieve and maintain healthy lives. Two thirds of all LHDs have established long-term plans using a planning model. Two of the most common models are Mobilizing Action through Partnerships and Planning (MAPP) and the Assessment Protocol for Excellence in Public Health (APEX-PH).

Mobilizing Action through Partnerships and Planning (MAPP)

The **MAPP Model** is a strategic approach to community health improvement to help communities improve health and quality of life through community-wide strategic planning (Figure 29-9). Using MAPP, communities

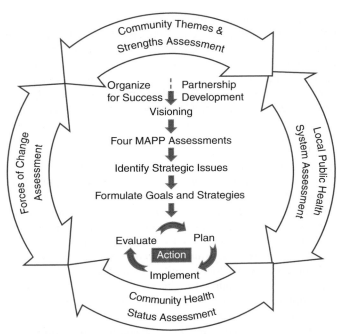

FIGURE 29-9 MAPP Model. (Redrawn from National Association of County and City Health Officials. [2004]. *Mobilizing Action through Partnership and Planning.* Washington, DC: Author.)

seek to achieve optimal health by identifying and using their resources wisely, taking into account their unique circumstances and needs, and forming effective partnerships for strategic action. The MAPP tool was developed by the National Association of County and City Health Officials (NACCHO) in cooperation with the Public Health Practice Program Office, Centers for Disease Control and Prevention (NACCHO, 2004).

MAPP places emphasis on an assessment process that is community driven and owned. MAPP also assesses the capacity of the entire public health system and infrastructure to deliver health services. MAPP uses the following seven principles: systems thinking, dialogue with diverse perspectives, shared vision for a healthy future, quantitative and qualitative data, partnership and collaboration, strategic thinking and celebration of successes.

Assessment Protocol for Excellence in Public Health (APEX-PH)

APEX-PH is another tool for community and organizational assessment that allows for identification of local needs and development of practical objectives (NACCHO, 1995, 2001). APEX-PH has two components: internal assessment of the agency and community assessment of health needs.

The APEX-PH community assessment of health needs program involves the health agency, community leaders, and consumers in priority setting, policy development, and assurance that identified needs are met. The second component of APEX-PH, internal assessment, helps local agencies review organizational structure and its effectiveness in meeting health objectives. For the most part MAPP has replaced the APEX-PH tool, components of which are present in the MAPP Model.

Management by Objectives

Many health departments take components of the *Healthy People* objectives and translate them into manageable action plans for their own locale by establishing management objectives and results.

Heart disease and cerebral vascular accidents were the leading causes of adult deaths in Akron, Ohio. As good public health practice, nurses performed blood pressure checks for most adult clients along with the services requested by the clients. Over the years, the health department has also made blood pressure screening available at the Bureau for Employment Services, the county department of human services, barber shops in black neighborhoods, health fairs, and other sites where high-risk populations can be screened. Those with hypertension are referred to the health department for additional blood pressure monitoring and referral, diagnostic work-up, treatment, and follow-up as appropriate. The objectives and methods for this hypertension program have developed as the program evolved over 7 to 8 years. The program is ongoing. Objectives and methods are reviewed quarterly and revised annually by the nursing management staff and the director of health. **Website Resource 29B** provides a step-by-step implementation program and objectives for a hypertension program.

ORGANIZATION OF SERVICES AND STAFF

Nursing assignments in LHDs are determined by the agency and community needs, complexity of services, number of nursing programs, number of staff, and availability of grant funds. Public health nurses may be assigned as generalists across several health department programs or as specialists in one specific program, such as child health or adult health.

Generalized Practice

Traditionally, nurses in local health have been generalists. All nurses were oriented in and responsible for all services. This remains true in small departments with limited staffs. Public health nurses provide clinic, home visit, community education, school, and civic activities within their jurisdiction. They participate in community needs' assessments and in quality assurance activities, and they serve as case managers with families and the varied resources involved in client care. Assignments may be geographically determined according to the available public health nurses among the population served. Each public health nurse has greater expertise and interest in some programs than in others; colleagues collaborate with each other for consultation and assistance.

Alice Archer is a generalized public health nurse working with the York County Department of Health. She is assigned to clinics 2 days a week. One clinic is a sexual disease clinic and the other is an HIV/AIDS screening clinic. One day a week she reviews charts and communicable disease surveillance reports to assist in collecting communicable disease tallies sent to the state health agency and reported to the Centers for Disease Control and Prevention. The other 2 days are spent in home visits as part of the prenatal services provided in her county. She home visits pregnant women and new mothers, who are seen for prenatal and postnatal care by the health department. Her agency continues to provide this direct care to clients who have no other means of receiving prenatal care.

Program-Specific Practice

As public health nursing practice becomes more comprehensive and specialized, generalization in work assignments is less feasible. Nurses may elect assignments or be assigned by specific population group; by geographic area; by programs such as adult, maternal, or child health services or home health care; or by combinations of these. Expanded practice nurses in pediatrics, geriatrics, and family health have also found a niche in many public health agencies, particularly large ones. The variety of public health nursing activities and settings is discussed later. The wisdom of using nurses' special interests and skills has led some agencies to pay part or all of the costs of nurse practitioner education or to develop job classifications for the expanded roles of the nurse.

> Jane Elders is a nurse practitioner working with the Los Palso Health Department. The health department services a geographic area with few health care providers. The health department had used contracted physicians to staff their STD clinic. During the past few years, the health department has had difficulty arranging for physician coverage in the clinic. Jane has worked for the health department for 10 years, primarily in communicable disease control. The health department approached Jane and asked her if she would be interested in becoming a nurse practitioner if the health department would fund her education. The health department would expect Jane to work as a nurse practitioner in the STD clinic for at least 4 years, to pay back her educational expenses. Jane completed her nurse practitioner program in 2 years and now staffs the STD clinic and also teaches health and sexual education courses in the local secondary school.

ACTIVITIES AND RESPONSIBILITIES

Public health nurses in LHDs are responsible for working with other professionals and community residents to assess the health needs of the population within their jurisdiction. They describe the population's health status and identify the degree to which there are resources available to address the health problems and issues. Public health nurses are experts in identifying health needs that can be addressed through nursing care. They develop, implement, and evaluate nursing services for primary, secondary, and tertiary levels of prevention (Box 29-4).

All of the responsibilities discussed in Chapter 1 are carried out in some measure by public health nurses. Education, screening and case finding, advocacy, and the development of new services all occur in partnership with the community. In addition, nurses actively work with members of the community to develop and maintain coalitions to address health issues.

Nurses in LHDs have traditionally focused on health promotion; health protection; lifestyle adaptation to maintain health; and detection, referral, and treatment for health problems. Specific interventions may be focused on an individual, on the community as a whole, or on vulnerable populations, such as elderly persons, pregnant adolescents, or males susceptible to hypertension. In larger health departments, education efforts are frequently multidisciplinary, with staff from nursing, health education, and nutrition and/or other health department staff providing expertise. In many LHDs, nurses work with communicable disease prevention, including surveillance, contact tracing, and treatment. Nurses may also be responsible for planning and evaluating programs, writing grant applications, and performing quality improvement activities.

BOX 29-4 Public Health Nursing Services by Levels of Prevention

Primary Prevention

Coalition-building to conduct a community assessment

Partnering with community agencies to plan courses of action for needs identified in the assessment

Prenatal care clinics

Family planning clinics

Health education for health promotion and risk reduction

Identification of those at risk for communicable diseases

Identification of those at risk for alcohol and drug abuse and other mental health problems

Immunizations (education campaigns and clinics)

Anticipatory guidance for parents regarding childcare and parenting

Safety and environmental education

Home visits for health promotion for pregnant women, new parents, and frail, elderly individuals

School health promotion, especially regarding substance abuse, pregnancy, and violence prevention

Worker health-promotion programs

Inspection and licensing (nursing homes and daycare centers)

Secondary Prevention

Health screening, case finding, and referral (e.g., hypertension and communicable diseases)

Health screening, case finding, and referral for alcohol and drug abuse and other mental health problems

Health screening, case finding, and referral for children with developmental delays and disabilities

Outreach during home visits and at work sites and schools to identify targeted populations, such as pregnant women, adolescents, and chronically ill and disabled persons

Contact investigation for communicable diseases

Clinics for sexually transmitted diseases

Clinics for tuberculosis

Treatment for specific illnesses (e.g., medications for sexually transmitted diseases based on medical orders and treatment protocols)

Primary care clinics

Clinics for the homeless

Environmental surveillance

Tertiary Prevention

Case management for disabled children

Case management for disabled adults

Case management for frail, elderly individuals

Home health care

Geriatric evaluations before institutional placement

Adult medical daycare

Compiled by C. M. Smith, University of Maryland.

Local agencies are increasingly involved in preparing for emergencies and disasters, both natural and man-made. The nurses working in LHDs have important roles in planning and responding to emergencies. The specific role of the nurse will vary depending on the type of emergency and the agency where the nurse is employed, and in many cases the nurse may assume a leadership position. As such, public health nurses should be familiar with the core competencies for public health workers, leaders/administrators, and technical and support staff related to emergency readiness (Columbia University School of Nursing, Center for Health Policy, 2002) (Box 29-5).

SETTINGS AND POPULATIONS

Public health nurses have always worked in homes, occupational settings, schools, and clinics. Currently, public health nurses in some locales have expanded practice into other sites, such as recreation centers, prisons, medical daycare centers, and wellness centers. Public health nursing services also may be provided in group or transitional housing for people with physical disabilities or developmental delays or those returning to the community after hospitalization for mental illness, imprisonment, or other social and health problems.

Clinics

Traditionally, public health nurses have targeted populations that are underserved or that have higher than average morbidity and mortality. Health department clinics usually target specific populations, such as women of childbearing years (maternity and family planning clinics), children and adolescents (well-child clinics and clinics for children with disabilities), and adults

(primary care and wellness centers). Such clinics may complement private-sector personal health services or be the only health services in medically underserved communities.

Public health nurses often manage these clinics as well as provide population-based and, often, direct client services. Public health nurses collaborate and partner with other community agencies to gather assessment information, and organize appropriate population-based interventions to address community health concerns. They also organize and evaluate nursing services, supervise nursing assistants and volunteers, document client records, and collect information about the numbers of persons served at the site. Box 29-6 lists some direct care activities performed by public health nurses in primary care clinics. As noted earlier in this chapter, direct client services are being redirected to other health care providers as LHDs increase their population-focused practice.

Prison Facilities

Health services for prisoners may be provided by the health department. Services may be provided at the prison facility as part of broad community services or through a contract for public health nursing, physician, or other practitioner time. The nurse performs appropriate screening tests, which may include a tuberculin test, HIV screening, blood and other body

---

Box 29-5 Emergency Preparedness: Core Competencies for All Public Health Workers

Describe the public health role in emergency response in a range of emergencies that might arise.

Describe the chain of command in emergency response.

Identify and locate the agency emergency response plan (or pertinent portion of plan).

Describe his/her functional roles in emergency response and demonstrate his/her roles in regular drills.

Demonstrate correct use of all communication equipment used for emergency communication.

Describe communication roles in emergency response:
- Within the agency using established communication systems
- With the media
- With the general public
- Personal (with family, neighbors)

Identify limits to own knowledge/skill/authority and identify key system resources for referring matters that exceed these limits.

Recognize unusual events that might indicate an emergency and describe appropriate action (e.g., communicate within the chain of command).

Apply creative problem solving and flexible thinking to unusual challenges within his/her functional responsibilities and evaluate effectiveness of all actions taken.

From Columbia University School of Nursing, Center for Health Policy. (2002). *Bioterrorism and emergency readiness: Competencies for all public health workers.* Atlanta: Centers for Disease Control and Prevention.

Box 29-6 Public Health Nursing in a Primary Care Clinic

Interview to learn the reason for the visit and determine the severity of the problem.

Obtain a health history, including sexual activity and birth history as appropriate.

Review affected body systems.

Obtain appropriate blood and body fluid specimens for laboratory analysis.

Conduct a risk assessment (see Chapter 19).

Discuss screening tests that are relevant based on risk assessment and standard recommendations, such as the following:
- Pelvic examination and Pap smear for women, as indicated
- Breast examination and breast self-examination teaching as necessary with mammogram education and/or referral
- Testicular examination education
- Discussion of HIV/AIDS risks and anonymous or confidential blood test
- Tuberculin skin testing as appropriate
- Blood pressure screening and history of hypertension, medication, and/or care source

Administer immunizations, medication, or other treatments as medically ordered.

Discuss contraindications, possible reactions, and any accompanying food or lifestyle adaptations while taking medications or participating in other treatment.

Obtain feedback from the client to determine what she or he has understood about the diagnosis, treatment, education, and planned follow-up.

If this is a clinic visit for a communicable disease, especially a sexually transmitted disease, provide a time for a test of cure and the clinic telephone number so the client may call and, with a coded request, receive culture test results. For specific illnesses, home visits may be conducted to trace contacts.

fluid specimens for tests and cultures, and vision and hearing tests. Immunizations, minor illness treatment, and medications for control of health problems (e.g., hypertension, epilepsy) are provided as ordered by the physician or nurse practitioner. Chapter 21 provides additional information on health issues of the prison population.

Work Sites

Some local health agencies are involved with industries and businesses (see Chapter 9). Nursing and health-education staffs provide education, risk assessment, and screening programs to promote healthier employee lifestyles and reduce employees' health risks. Employees benefit personally, and sometimes benefit by a reduction in their co-payment for health insurance. Employers benefit through better health insurance coverage, perhaps at a reduced cost, and less employee time away from work resulting from illness or injury. The types of service provided depend on employer/employee decisions and on the content of the contract or letter of agreement with the local health department.

Other Service Sites

Shelters for the homeless, nutrition sites for elderly persons, and daycare or Head Start centers are also places where public health nursing may take place. This may involve obtaining health and risk assessment histories or providing group teaching or one-on-one counseling. Specific screening and immunization services may be provided, such as tuberculin tests and blood pressure screening for staff and clients in a homeless shelter or blood pressure screening at a senior citizen meal center. Immunizations may include hepatitis B, influenza, pneumococcal, or tetanus-diphtheria vaccines. With expanded role nursing, primary care in shelters, apartments for elderly persons, or group homes for developmentally delayed clients has become possible through agency contracts or volunteer programs.

One area not often a part of general public health nursing involves mental health counseling and care. Nurses recognize persons with mental disorders and use the resources of their community for education, referral, and/or networking (see Chapters 25 and 33). If the health department has an alcohol and/or substance abuse program, one or some of the counselors may be licensed psychologists, psychiatric social workers, or psychiatric mental health nurse specialists. Public health nurses find these colleagues to be good consultants for assistance in developing alternatives for and with their clients. With the number of people needing mental health services steadily growing and local agencies stretched to their maximum, alternative service avenues must be explored. Additional preventive mental health programs are needed to address public health concerns such as substance abuse, teenage pregnancy, violence, mental illness, and the stresses of homelessness.

The clinical psychiatric/mental health nurse specialist is an asset to community public and mental health agencies, as she or he can guide the nurses or other staff in ways to detect, approach, and assist those with mental illnesses to seek and use counseling and treatment programs. The nurse specialist has skills for individual and group counseling and for working with the staff of group homes or homeless shelters in concert with other professionals. These programs focus on ways to help individual clients achieve socially appropriate behavior, a feeling of self-worth, and greater independence.

FUTURE TRENDS AND ISSUES IN PUBLIC HEALTH AND PUBLIC HEALTH NURSING

Public health made remarkable improvement in the lives of Americans in the 20th century including an increase in life expectancy of 30 years, in part due to a dramatic drop in infant mortality (USDHHS, 2000). Much of this progress was due to improved sanitation, communicable disease control, vital statistics, and services for infants and children. Some of the new challenges in public health closely resemble the enemies of the previous century, including reemergence of infectious diseases, tobacco-related diseases, maternal and infant morbidity and mortality, unintentional injuries, cardiovascular diseases, and food safety (Turnock, 2004). Additionally, health disparities across gender, race or ethnicity, education or income, disability, geographic location, or sexual orientation present challenges to advances in the public's health in the 21st century (USDHHS, 2000).

The IOM report *The Future of the Public's Health in the 21st Century* (IOM, 2003a) examined the current status of public health and concurs with many of the previous recommendations. The study recommends changes in the following areas:

- Adopting a focus on population health that involves multiple determinants of health
- Strengthening the public health infrastructure
- Building partnerships
- Developing a system of accountability
- Emphasizing evidence-based practice
- Improving communication between government agencies responsible for public health

This IOM report emphasizes that governmental public health agencies must build and maintain partnerships with other organizations and sectors of society to achieve the *Healthy People 2010* goal of *healthy people in healthy communities* (USDHHS, 2000). The participation of the entire public health system is necessary to ensure the health of the population. The IOM report describes the public health system as: the governmental public health infrastructure, communities and community based organizations, the health care delivery system, academia, employers and business, and the media (Figure 29-10).

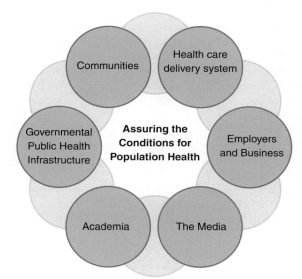

FIGURE 29-10 The Intersectoral Model of a public health system. (From the Institute of Medicine. [2003a]. *The future of the public's health in the 21st century.* Washington, DC: The National Academy Press.)

Tilson and Berkowitz (2006) outlined six major policy challenges for public health in the 21st century: public health infrastructure, agreement on the essential services, a heightened level of preparedness, the public health workforce, accountability and measurement, and the public health research agenda. State and LHDs are addressing accountability and performance measurement in a variety of ways including evaluation of programmatic and agency-wide impacts (ASTHO, 2007). Emerging public health standards, workforce competencies, and accreditation models strive to provide a link toward improved population health through standardization, effectiveness, and efficiency (Ogalla & Cioffi, 2007). While more research is needed to link accreditation and performance assessment to community health improvement outcomes, several projects and processes (such as the Turning Point Performance Management Collaborative) have demonstrated success in improving structures and processes resulting in positive health outcomes (Joly et al., 2007).

The social justice foundation of the nursing profession (Bekemeier & Butterfield, 2005) and the ecologic methodologies advocated by public health nursing leaders (ANA, 2007) place public health nurses at the local level in key positions to make substantial contributions to the health of the population. Successful collaboration and communication between public health nurses and community partners in the public and private sectors will continue to be vital to achieving sustainable community and system changes. As such, state and LHDs will continue to seek partnerships with the private sector (IOM, 2003a; Turnock, 2004). Such partnerships often decrease the role of public nurses in direct care, whenever possible, and place efforts on improving the health status of whole communities (Avila & Smith, 2003).

Public health nursing will adapt to the trends in public health by changing roles and functions and learning new skills. As public health agencies shift from a focus on providing clinical care to ensuring population health, public health nurses will become more involved in advocacy, social marketing, community assessment, collaboration, and coalition building to ensure local public health nurses are visible and active in the community.

The prevention of chronic diseases and disability will become a bigger priority and place an increased emphasis on primary prevention. Prevention requires new interventions that address the multiple determinants of disease, including the political, environmental, and societal impacts on the health status of populations (Bekemeier & Butterfield, 2005). To promote prevention, public health nurses will be at the forefront in developing health-education programs, educating policy makers, and collaborating with other public health professionals, to advocate for systems' changes that are congruent with the social justice values of the nursing profession.

CASE STUDY Investigation and Follow-up for Communicable Disease Exposure

Tuberculosis can be a very frightening diagnosis, particularly among Alaska Native communities in rural Alaska. In generations past, people who were infected with TB had been taken from their villages and placed in TB sanatoriums miles away from their families, often in other states. Frequently, individuals died of the disease away from their community. The fear of TB and the fear of the consequences of both the disease and the treatment are profound in many of these communities.

A public health nurse working with a small, Alaska Native community received a report of two active pulmonary tuberculosis (TB) cases. The public health nurse serving the area travels to multiple villages in the region, and does not live in the village. Therefore the nurse began to work on developing a process through the village Community Health Aide and Indian Health Services in the region to complete directly observed therapy (DOT) of the clients taking their medication.

The nurse then travelled to the village and made home visits to begin contact investigation through priority ranking according to risk. High-priority contacts between both families included two spouses and a total of five children, ages 1, 3, 4, 7, and 10 years. The nurse coordinated TB skin testing and chest x-rays, and worked with the community health aide (who communicates daily with a physician) to begin the contacts on preventive medication.

A high number of moderate-priority individuals were also contacted, but would not come in for screening. The nurse realized that in order to assess the extent of both latent and newly exposed individuals in the community, a partnership with the village elders was essential to assist the community to grieve for those who were lost to TB in the past, and to address the fear about TB coursing through the community. The elders called a village meeting and the nurse was able to assist the community in acknowledging the struggles they had in the past with TB. The nurse was simultaneously able to raise awareness of the continued threat of TB and encourage people to attend screening the following day to quickly address the threat of TB reemerging in the community. As a result of this culturally sensitive intervention, the following day approximately 95% of the village residents attended screening for TB.

Several people in the village had positive skin tests and received x-rays and preventive therapy. The achievement demonstrated in the community for screening, raising awareness, and educating the residents about TB was so successful that the recommendation was made by both the tribal health providers and epidemiologists to integrate this culturally sensitive approach to other instances of TB outbreaks in Alaska Native villages.

WEB See **Critical Thinking Questions** for this Case Study on the book's website.

KEY IDEAS

1. There are 3 core functions of public health and 10 essential services that public health agencies must perform to meet the core functions.

2. The states have the primary responsibility for ensuring the health of citizens; the lead agency for health concerns is the state health agency or department.

3. State and local health departments are engaged in a partnership to provide health care services to citizens and communities. Population focus rather than individual care is the concern of public health agencies.

4. Funds for state health departments come predominantly from state and federal tax money. Funds for local health agency programs come from local tax money, but varied federal, state, and private funds might also be used.

5. Legislation and funding influence the ability of public health agencies to provide essential services.

6. Public health nursing is multifaceted, providing assessments, service, advocacy, counseling, and caring for individuals, families, and the community.

7. The emphases for nurses in local public health agencies vary according to community needs; what is already available for specific populations; federal, state, and local mandates; and funds for service provision.

8. Communicable disease control was a major emphasis in the formative days of public health nursing. Some diseases are no longer a threat, whereas others remain so. New diseases, such as HIV and severe acute respiratory syndrome (SARS), have evolved. Control, education, investigation, and prevention will remain key emphases.

9. The standards of public health nursing and the components/concepts of this nursing specialty will continue to evolve to remain relevant to the changing responsibilities of the public health nurse. A baccalaureate education, because it includes elements of family- and community-focused care, is the standard for community health practice.

10. Public health nursing is becoming more comprehensive and the sites for services more varied than the traditional homes, schools, and clinics of the past.

LEARNING BY EXPERIENCE AND REFLECTION

1. Contact your state or local health department and ask what programs exist, what services are offered, how the department reaches out to the community, how its work is funded, and what fees are charged for services.

2. Talk with your legislators and determine what they know about pending health legislation and about state and local health department mandates, funding, and personal health services. Become a resource for the legislators.

3. Select an objective from *Healthy People 2010* (U.S. Department of Health and Human Services, 2000) and develop an intervention plan.

4. Obtain an entry-level public health nurse job description from a local public health agency.

5. Consider the qualifications for question 4; if you have questions about them, ask for clarification.

6. Explore your own previous feelings and knowledge about local public health agencies. Did you know there was a health department? Did you know the populations it serves? What can be done to increase the visibility of public health nurses to the public?

COMMUNITY RESOURCES FOR PRACTICE   *WEB*

American Nurses Association (ANA)
American Public Health Association (APHA)
Association of State and Territorial Directors of Nursing (ASTDN)
Association of State and Territorial Health Officers (ASTHO)
PublicHealth.Medscape.com (a joint venture between APHA and Medscape)
Centers for Disease Control and Prevention (CDC)
National Association of County and City Health Officials (NACCHO)
National League for Nursing

STUDY AIDS   http://evolve.elsevier.com/Maurer/community/

Visit the Evolve website for this book to find the following study and assessment materials:

- Quiz
- Web Scenario
- Critical Thinking Questions and Answers for Case Studies

- Care Plans
- *Healthy People* Updates
- Glossary

WEBSITE RESOURCES

WEB

These items supplement the chapter's topics and are also found on the Evolve site:

29A: Examples of Health Department Organizational Charts

29B: Management by Objectives: A Nursing Plan to Detect and Control Hypertension

REFERENCES

American Nurses Association. (1986). *Standards of community health nursing practice.* Washington, DC: Author.

American Nurses Association. (2007). *Public health nursing: Scope and standards of practice.* Silver Spring, MD: Author. Available at *http://nursesbooks.org.*

American Nurses Association Credentialing Center. (2007). *Certification and renewals.* Retrieved September 22, 2007, from *http://www.nursecredentialing.org/.*

American Public Health Association, Public Health Nursing. (2007). *Public health nursing section: Overview.* Retrieved September 10, 2007, from *http://www.apha.org/membergroups/sections/aphasections/phn/.*

American Public Health Association, Public Health Nursing Section. (1996). *The definition and role of public health nursing.* Washington, DC: Author.

Association of State and Territorial Directors of Nursing. (2000). *Public health nursing: A partner for healthy populations.* Washington, DC: American Nurses Publishing.

Association of State and Territorial Health Officials. (2007). *Innovations in public health: Understanding state public health.* Washington, DC: Author.

Avila, M., & Smith, K. (2003). The reinvigoration of public health nursing: Methods and innovations. *Journal of Public Health Management Practice, 9*(1), 16-24.

Bashir, Z., Johnson, V., & Leep, C. J. (2007). *Local impact of changes to federal funding for public health emergency preparedness activities (abstr no. 153134).* Washington, DC: American Public Health Association.

Beitsch, L., Brooks, R. G., Grigg, M., et al. (2006). Structure and functions of state public health agencies. *American Journal of Public Health, 96*(1), 167-172.

Bekemeier, B., & Butterfield, P. (2005). Unreconciled inconsistencies: A critical review of the concept of social justice in 3 national nursing documents. *Advances in Nursing Science, 2*(28), 152-162.

Briss, P. A., Rodewald, L. E., Hinman, A. R., et al. (2000). Review of evidence: Intervention to improve vaccination coverage in children, adolescents, and adults. *American Journal of Preventive Medicine, 18*(15), 97-140.

Bureau of Labor Statistics. (2007). *Consumer price index for all urban consumers (CPI-U): U.S. city average by expenditure category and service group (Table 1-A).* Retrieved October 8, 2007, from *http://www.bls.gov/cpi/cpid01av.pdf* (note each year is a different URL, e.g., cpid02, 03, 04, 05, 06).

Catlin, A., Cowan, C., Heffler, S., Washington, B., National Health Expenditure Accounts Team. (2007). National health spending in 2005: The slowdown continues. *Health Affairs, 36*(1), 142-153.

Centers for Disease Control and Prevention. (1999). Achievements in public health, 1900-1999: Changes in the public health system. *Morbidity and Mortality Weekly Report, 48*(50), 1141-1147.

Centers for Disease Control and Prevention. (2000). *Preparedness of the public health infrastructure: A status report. Prepared for the Appropriations Committee of the U.S. Senate.* Washington, DC: Author.

Centers for Medicare and Medicaid Services. (2007). *Medicare and you 2007.* Baltimore, MD: Author.

Columbia University School of Nursing, Center for Health Policy. (2002). *Bioterrorism and emergency readiness: Competencies for all public health workers.* Atlanta: Centers for Disease Control and Prevention.

Essential Public Health Services Work Group. (1995). *The essential services of public health.* Washington, DC: Centers for Disease Control and Prevention.

Fee, E., & Brown, T. M. (2002). The unfulfilled promise of public health: Déjà vu all over again. *Health Affairs, 21*(6), 31-43.

Gebbie, K., & Hwang, I. (2000). Preparing currently employed public health nurses for changes in the health system. *American Journal of Public Health, 90*(5), 719.

Gebbie, K., Medrrill, J., & Tilson, H. H. (2002). The public health workforce: Without a competent workforce, a public health agency is as useless as a new hospital with no health care workers. *Health Affairs, 21*(6), 57-67.

Gollust, S., & Jacobson, P. (2006). Privatization of public services: Organizational reform efforts in public education and public health. *American Journal of Public Health, 96*(10), 1733-1739.

Hunt, K. A., & Knickman, J. R. (2008). Financing for health care. In S. Jonas & A. R. Kovner (Eds.), *Health care delivery in the United States* (8th ed., pp. 46-72). New York: Springer.

Hutchins, S. S., Rosenthal, J., Eason, P., et al. (1999). Effectiveness and cost effectiveness of linking the special supplemental program for Women, Infants, and Children (WIC) and immunization activities. *Journal of Public Health Policy, 20*(4), 408-423.

Institute of Medicine. (2003a). *The future of the public's health in the 21ˢᵗ century.* Washington, DC: The National Academy Press.

Institute of Medicine. (2003b). *Who will keep the public healthy? Educating public health professionals for the 21ˢᵗ century.* Washington, DC: The National Academy Press.

Institute of Medicine, Committee for the Study of the Future of Public Health. (1988). *The future of public health.* Washington, DC: National Academy Press.

Joly, B. M., Polyak, G., Davis, M. V., et al. (2007). Linking accreditation and public health outcomes: A logic model approach. *Journal of Public Health Management Practice, 13*(4), 349-356.

Keller, L. O., Strohschein, S., Schaffer, M. A., et al. (2004). Population-based public health interventions: Innovations in practice, teaching, and management, Part II. *Public Health Nursing, 21*(5), 469-487.

Kennedy, V. C., Quill, B. C., & Wiltshire, A. D. (2000). *Final report: NACCHO public health workforce development project.* Washington, DC: National Association of County and City Health Officials.

Landers, S. J. (2007). *Federal funding cuts could threaten public health progress. AMNews, October 1, 2007.* Retrieved October 8, 2007, from *http://www.ama-assn.org/amednews/2007/10/01/hlsb1001htm.*

Last, J. M., & Wallace, R. B. (1992). *Public health and preventive medicine* (13th ed.). Norwalk, CT: Appleton & Lange.

Levit, K., Smith, C., Cowan, C., et al. (2003). Trends in U. S. health care spending, 2001. *Health Affairs, 22*(1), 154-172.

Morbidity and Mortality Weekly Reports. (2003a). Partner counseling and referral services to identify persons with undiagnosed HIV—North Carolina 2001. *Morbidity and Mortality Weekly Reports, 52*(48), 1181-1183.

Morbidity and Mortality Weekly Reports. (2003b). Surveillance for elevated blood lead levels among children—United States 1997-2001. *Morbidity and Mortality Weekly Reports, 52*(SS-10).

Morbidity and Mortality Weekly Reports. (2005). Brief report: Terrorism and emergency preparedness in state and territorial public health departments—United States, 2004. *Morbidity and Mortality Weekly Report, 54*(18), 459-460.

National Association of County and City Health Officials. (1995). *1992-1993 National profile of local health departments.* Washington, DC: Author.

National Association of County and City Health Officials. (2001). *Local public health agencies infrastructure: A chartbook.* Washington, DC: Author.

National Association of County and City Health Officials. (2004). *Mobilizing Action through Partnerships and Planning.* Washington, DC: Author. Available at *http://mapp.naccho.org/mapp_introduction.asp.*

National Association of County and City Health Officials. (2006). *2005 National profile of local health departments.* Washington, DC: Author.

National Association of County and City Health Officials. (2007). *Public health preparedness: State and local capacity-building.* Washington, DC: Author. Available at *htttp://www.NACCHO.org.*

National Association of State Budget Officers. (2005). *2003-2004 State expenditure report.* Washington, DC: Author.

National Association of State Budget Officers and Reforming State Groups. (2003). *2000-2001 State health care expenditure report.* Washington,

DC: NASBO, Reforming States Group, and Milbank Memorial Fund.

National Governors Association. (2003). *Reorganizing state health agencies to meet changing needs: State restructuring efforts in 2003*. Washington, DC: Author, Center for Best Practices.

Ogalla, C., & Cioffi, J. P. (2007). Concerns in workforce development: Linking certification and credentialing to outcomes. *Public Health Nursing, 24*(5), 429-438.

Pickett, G., & Hanlon, J. (1990). *Public health administration and practice* (9th ed.). St. Louis: Mosby.

Quad Council of Public Health Nursing Organizations. (1999). *Scope and standards of public health nursing practice*. Washington, DC: American Nurses Publishing.

Quad Council of Public Health Nursing Organizations. (2006). *The public health nursing shortage: A threat to the public's health*. Washington, DC: American Nurses Association.

Reverby, S. (1993). From Lillian Wald to Hillary Rodham Clinton: What will happen to public health nursing? *American Journal of Public Health, 83*(12), 1662-1663.

Roseau, P. V., & Reomer, R. (2002). *Ethical issues in public health and health services*. In S. J. Williams & P. R. Torrens (Eds.), *Introduction to health services* (6th ed.; pp. 392-413). Boston: Delmar.

Shefer, A. M., Fritchley, J., Stevenson, J., et al. (2002). Linking WIC and immunization services to improve preventive health care among low-income children in WIC. *Journal of Public Health Management, 8*(2), 56-65.

Smart, D. R. (2006). *Physician characteristics and distribution in the US; 2006 edition*. Chicago: The American Medical Association.

Tilson, H., & Berkowitz, B. (2006). The public health enterprise: Examining our twenty-first century policy challenges. *Health Affairs, 25*(4), 900-910.

Tougher times strike more TB programs as budget axes fall: Immigrants, indigent, recession contributing causes. (2002). *TB Monitor, 9*(10), 109-112.

Turnock, B. J. (2004). *Public health: What it is and how it works* (3rd ed.). Sudbury, MA: Jones & Bartlett.

U.S. Bureau of the Census. (2004). *Government expenditures for health services and supplies 1991-2004* (Table 124). Retrieved October 23, 2007, from *http://www.census.gov/compendia/statab/tables/0705124.xls*.

U.S. Department of Health and Human Services. (1990). *Promoting health preventing disease: Year 2000 objectives for the nation. Summary report*. Washington, DC: U.S. Government Printing Office.

U.S. Department of Health and Human Services. (2000). *Healthy People 2010 objectives: Understanding and improving health* (2nd ed.). Washington, DC: U.S. Government Printing Office.

U.S. Department of Health and Human Services. (July 17, 2007). *HHS announces $896.7 million in funding to states for public health preparedness and emergency response*. Retrieved October 8, 2007, from *http://www.hhs.gov/news/press/2007pres/07/pr20070717c.html*.

SUGGESTED READINGS

American Nurses Association. (2007). *Public health nursing: Scope and standards of practice*. Silver Spring, MD: Author. Available at *http://nurses-books.org*.

Avila, M., & Smith, K. (2003). The reinvigoration of public health nursing: Methods and innovations. *Journal of Public Health Management Practice, 9*(1), 16-24.

Baker, E. L., & Koplan, J. P. (2002). Strengthening the nation's public health infrastructure: Historic challenge, unprecedented opportunity: It takes a system that is competent to handle routine public health situations to handle the emergencies. *Health Affairs, 21*(6), 15-27.

Beitsch, L., Brooks, R. G., Grigg, M., et al. (2006). Structure and functions of state public health agencies. *American Journal of Public Health, 96*(1), 167-172.

Berkowitz, B., Dahl, J., Guirl, K., et al. (2001). *Public health nursing leadership*. Washington, DC: American Nurses Publishing.

Canter, J. C., Schoen, C., Belloff, D., (2007). *Aiming higher: Results from a state scorecard Commonwealth Fund Commission on a high performance health system*. New York: The Fund.

Freeman, R. (1957). *History of public health nursing*. Philadelphia: W.B. Saunders.

Gardner, M. S. (1936). *Public health nursing* (3rd ed.). New York: Macmillan

Gollust, S., & Jacobson, P. (2006). Privatization of public services: Organizational reform efforts in public education and public health. *American Journal of Public Health, 96*(10), 1733-1739.

Institute of Medicine. (2003). *The future of the public's health in the 21st century*. Washington, DC: The National Academy Press.

Kuss, T., Proulx-Girouard, L., Lovitt, S., et al. (1997). A public health nursing model. *Public Health Nursing, 14*(2), 81-91.

Lipson, D. J. (1997). *State roles in health care policy: Past as prologue?* In T. J. Litman & L. S. Robins (Eds.), *Health politics and policy* (3rd ed.). Boston: Delmar.

Millio, N. (2000). *Public health in the market: Facing managed care, lean government, and health disparities*. Ann Arbor: University of Michigan Press.

Rawding, N., & Wasserman, M. (1997). *The local health department*. In F. D. Scutchfield & C. W. Keck (Eds.), *Principles of public health practice* (pp. 87-100). Boston: Delmar.

Turnock, B. J. (2004). *Public health: What it is and how it works* (3rd ed.). Sudbury, MA: Jones & Bartlett.

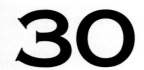

School Health

Sara Groves and Joan E. Kub

FOCUS QUESTIONS

What is the history of school health nursing? What can we learn from the past in defining the future of school nursing?

What are the eight components of a coordinated school health model?

How are school health programs organized and regulated?

What are the roles of the school nurse in the various components of school health?

What professional standards guide the practice of school nurses?

What are the common health concerns of school-aged children, and what interventions are provided within school settings?

What are the future trends in school health?

How can schools contribute to the accomplishment of the objectives set forth in *Healthy People 2010?*

CHAPTER OUTLINE

KEY TERMS

Comprehensive health education advisory committee

Comprehensive school health education

Coordinated school health program

Federal Educational Rights and Privacy Act (FERPA)

Handicapped Infant and Toddler Program

Health services

Healthy school environment

Individualized education program (IEP)

Individualized family service plan

Individuals with Disabilities Education Act

No Child Left Behind Act

Public Law 94-142

School-based health centers (SBHCs)

School nursing

Health problems facing American children and adolescents have changed dramatically since World War II from those that involve contagious diseases to problems that are primarily related to health behavior. Although mortality rates among adolescents and young adults have fallen dramatically during the past two decades, health risk behaviors contributing to mortality and morbidity continue to be worrisome (Brener et al., 2007). In the United States, approximately three fourths of all deaths among adolescents aged 15 to 19 are related to injuries, including homicide, suicide, and unintentional injuries (Childstats.gov, 2007). High-risk behaviors that contribute to the leading causes of mortality include driving a car after drinking alcohol, carrying weapons, and using alcohol or marijuana (Centers for Disease Control and Prevention [CDC], 2006a). With regard to morbidity, the proportion of children who suffer from a chronic health condition is estimated to be between 22% and 44%, depending on how chronic illness is defined (Van der Lee et al., 2007). For example, there is an expanding population of schoolchildren, between 12 and 18 million, with chronic health conditions such as asthma, diabetes, cancer, and cystic fibrosis (Trossman, 2007). In addition, one of the greatest public health challenges is the increasing percentage of overweight children (Childstats.gov, 2007). Behaviors that contribute to morbidity in children include tobacco use; use of alcohol and other drugs; sexual activities that lead to unintended pregnancy and sexually transmitted diseases (STDs), including human immunodeficiency virus (HIV) infection; unhealthy dietary choices; and physical inactivity.

School nurses have played a significant role in school health for over a century. In 1999, the National Association of School Nurses (NASN) defined **school nursing** as "a specialized practice of professional nursing that advances the well-being, academic success, and lifelong achievement of students. To this end, school nurses facilitate positive student responses to normal development; promote health and safety; intervene with actual and potential problems; provide case management services; and actively collaborate with others to build student and family capacity for adaptation, self-management, self-advocacy, and learning" (NASN, 2002, p. 1).

HISTORICAL PERSPECTIVES OF SCHOOL NURSING

The NASN celebrated the 100th anniversary of school nursing in October 2002. The beginnings of school health services can actually be traced back to the nineteenth century when nurses provided their services in schools in Europe. The attention of these nurses was focused on both nutritional problems and improvement of sanitary conditions (Wold & Dagg, 1981).

In the United States, communicable diseases were influential in the development of school nursing. In 1894, Boston established school health services to identify and exclude students with communicable diseases (Wold & Dagg, 1981). A demonstration project, initiated by Lillian Wald in New York City in 1902, shifted the focus of school nursing. In an effort to reduce school absences, Lina Rogers Struthers, the first school nurse, was placed in a school, where she drafted protocols for specific illnesses (Hawkins et al., 1994; Schumacher, 2002; Vessey & McGowan, 2006). Struthers investigated children's absences from school, and within 1 year, school absences dropped by 90% (Kennedy, 2003). As a result, more school nurses were placed in the schools of New York, and the practice soon spread coast to coast, from Boston to Los Angeles (Vessey & McGowan, 2006).

Throughout the succeeding decades, school health programs expanded (Veselak, 2001). During the 1920s and 1930s, the focus of school health programs was threefold: (1) medical inspections to prevent the spread of contagious diseases, (2) medical examinations for all children to ensure child health, and (3) incorporation of health education into the curriculum to teach students responsible health behaviors (Wold & Dagg, 1981). Concerns of the school nurses at that time also included providing a hygienic school, promoting fresh air, addressing child labor, and improving diets ("Changing times, changing needs, changing programs," 1952).

School nursing became more public health oriented during the 1940s and 1950s. Approximately half of all community/public health nurses were employed in school health at that time (Wold & Dagg, 1981). This public health orientation provided a more family-centered approach to care. Nurses provided health guidance and consultation with an emphasis on health promotion. The health team, a collaboration between nurses and teachers, evolved during this period.

The years since 1970 have been both innovative and precarious (Wold & Dagg, 1981). The concept of the school nurse practitioner, developed in 1970, allowed for an expansion of the nurse's skills in the areas of history taking, physical appraisal, and developmental assessment (Igoe, 1975). An increasing emphasis was placed on primary care in the school setting and community involvement in program development (Hawkins et al., 1994). School-based health centers grew rapidly from their initial introduction in the late 1960s and expanded in the 1990s (Gustafson, 2005). Today, school nurses are being challenged to expand their scope of practice, to manage the more complex health problems of some students, and to be instrumental in integrating new health care delivery models into the school setting (Lear, 2002; Trossman, 2007).

Since the early 1900s, the development of school health has been influenced by multiple external forces. These forces have included developments within public health, nursing, pediatrics, education, and the political arena. Social and legislative initiatives have also shaped the development of this specialty. All of these factors continue to influence the scope of school nursing practice. The future of school nursing will depend on the ability of nurses to respond to new opportunities and changing political and funding environments. One of those challenges is to determine the role for school nursing in the health-promoting school (Whitehead, 2006).

COORDINATED SCHOOL HEALTH AND ITS COMPONENTS

During the twentieth century, the roles of the school nurse and the school health team evolved based on the needs of school-aged children. The traditional school health approach in the 1980s encompassed three domains: health services, health education, and the environment. In the twenty-first century, an even broader, more comprehensive coordinated school program is being advocated (Figure 30-1). The objectives of

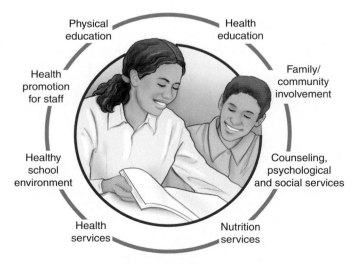

FIGURE 30-1 A coordinated school health model and its components. Redrawn from Centers for Disease Control and Prevention. [2003]. *About the program: School health defined.* Retrieved September 6, 2007 from *http://www.cdc.gov/HealthyYouth/CSHP.*

Healthy People 2010 (U.S. Department of Health and Human Services [USDHHS], 2000a) support school-based education, health promotion, physical activity, and care services (see the *Healthy People 2010* box on this page).

The **coordinated school health program** consists of a broad spectrum of school-related activities and services. It includes the three traditional areas of health services, health education, and the school environment, and five other components, including physical education and other physical activity programs; nutrition services; school counseling, psychologic, and social services; family/community involvement; and faculty and staff health promotion (Allensworth & Kolbe, 1987; Brener et al., 2006; CDC, 2007a; Kann et al., 1995). The definitions of these components are presented in Table 30-1 and are described in the following sections.

HEALTH EDUCATION

The focus in the twenty-first century is on health promotion and the effects of individual behavior on health status, including poor eating habits; physical inactivity; substance use; behaviors that result in unintentional and intentional injuries; and sexual behaviors that result in HIV infection, other sexually transmitted diseases, or unintentional pregnancy. Key elements of **comprehensive school health education** include (1) a documented, planned, and sequential program of health instruction for students in grades kindergarten through 12; (2) a curriculum that addresses and integrates education about a range of categorical health problems; (3) activities that help young people develop skills to avoid health problems; (4) instruction for a prescribed amount of time at each grade level; (5) management and coordination by an education

---

■ HEALTHY PEOPLE 2010 ■
Sample Objectives for Improving Health Related to School Nursing

1. Increase the proportion of middle, junior high, and senior high schools that provide school health education to prevent health problems in the following areas: unintentional injury; violence; suicide; tobacco use and addiction; alcohol and other drug use; unintended pregnancy, HIV/AIDS, and STDs; unhealthy dietary patterns; inadequate physical activity; and environmental health.

Education Area	Target 2010	Baseline in 1994
All components listed above	70% of schools	28% of schools
Unintentional injury	90%	66%
Violence	80%	58%
Suicide	80%	58%
Tobacco use and addiction	95%	86%
Alcohol and other drugs	95%	90%
Unintended pregnancy, HIV/AIDS, and STDs	90%	65%
Unhealthy dietary patterns	95%	84%
Inadequate physical activity	90%	78%
Environmental health	80%	60%

2. Increase the proportion of the nation's elementary, middle, junior high, and senior high schools that have a nurse-to-student ratio of at least 1:750

Type of School	Target 2010	Baseline in 1994
Senior high schools	50% of schools	26% of schools
Middle and junior high schools	50%	32%
Elementary schools	60%	53% (in 2000)

3. Increase to 100% the proportion of the nation's elementary, middle, junior high, and high schools that have official school policies ensuring the safety of students and staff from environmental hazards, such as chemicals in special classrooms, poor indoor air quality, asbestos, and exposure to pesticides (baseline: 94% of schools in 2000).

4. Reduce to 32% physical fighting among adolescents in schools (baseline: 36% of students in grades 9 to 12 fought in 1999).

5. Increase the proportion of school-based health centers with an oral health component to 15% applying dental sealants and 11% providing dental care (baseline: 12% provided sealants and 9% provided dental care in 2001-2002).

6. Increase the proportion of the nation's public and private schools that require daily physical education for all students.

Type of School	Target 2010	Baseline in 1994
Middle and junior high schools	9.4% of schools	6.4% of schools
Senior high schools	14.5%	5.8%

7. Increase to 50% the proportion of adolescents who participate in daily school physical education (baseline: 29% of students in grades 9 to 12 in 1999).

8. Increase to 50% the proportion of adolescents who spend at least 50% of school physical education class time being physically active (baseline: 38% of students in grades 9 to 12 in 1999).

9. Increase to 50% the proportion of the nation's public and private schools that provide access to their physical activity spaces and facilities for all persons outside of normal school hours (that is, before and after the school day, on weekends, and during summer and other vacations) (baseline: 35% of schools in 2000).

10. Reduce to 2 days the number of school or work days missed by persons with asthma due to asthma (baseline: 6.1 days missed in 2002 for persons aged 5 to 64 years).

11. Increase to 100% the proportion of smoke-free and tobacco-free environments in schools, including all school facilities, property, vehicles, and school events (baseline: 37% of middle, junior high, and high schools were smoke free and tobacco free in 1994).

12. Increase adolescents' disapproval of smoking.

Grade Level	Target 2010	Baseline in 1998
Eighth grade	95% of students	80% of students
Tenth grade	95%	75%
Twelfth grade	95%	69%

From U.S. Department of Health and Human Services. (2000). *Healthy people 2010: Understanding and improving health* (2nd ed.). Washington, DC: U.S. Government Printing Office.

| TABLE 30-1 | Definitions of the Components of a Coordinated School Health Program |

Component	Definition
Health education	A planned, sequential, K-12 curriculum that addresses physical, social, mental, and emotional dimensions of health.
Physical education	A planned, sequential K-12 curriculum to address physical fitness, movement, rhythms, dance, sports (individual, dual, and team), tumbling, and gymnastics, and aquatics.
Health services	Services to students to appraise, protect, and promote health. These are designed to ensure access or referral to primary care, prevent and control disease and health problems, provide emergency care, provide a safe environment, and provide educational and counseling opportunities for promoting health.
Nutrition services	Access to a variety of nutritious appealing meals that meet the health and nutrition needs of students.
Health promotion for staff	Activities focused on improving the health of faculty/staff through assessments, health education, and health-related physical activities.
Counseling and psychological services	Services to improve students' mental, emotional, and social health.
Health school environment	Physical and aesthetic surroundings and the psychosocial climate and culture of the school.
Parent/community involvement	An integrated approach that would include school health advisory councils, coalitions, and constituencies to build the program.

Adapted from Centers for Disease Control and Prevention (CDC). (2007). *About the program: School health defined.* Available online at www.edc.gov/HealthyYouth/CSHP/.

professional; (6) instruction from teachers who are trained to teach the subject; (7) involvement of parents, health professionals, and community members; and (8) periodic evaluation (CDC, 2005a).

Progress toward comprehensive school health education was monitored in the School Health Policies and Programs Study 2000 (SHPPS) (Kann et al., 2001). SHPPS is the largest and most comprehensive study of school health policies and programs at the state, district, school, and classroom levels nationwide. Data were collected in 1994, 2000, and again in 2006. As of the publication of this book, results are not yet available for 2006. In 2000, the study found that although most states and districts require health education, the percentage of schools requiring health education at the given grade level decreased from grades 6 through 12. Classroom instruction on specific health topics did not consistently reflect school-level goals, objectives, and expected outcomes for health education. SHPPS researchers concluded that health education teachers need more effective health education curricula, effective teaching materials, and appropriate staff development to provide instruction that more closely reflects the National Health Education Standards (CDC, 2005b; Kann et al., 2001).

Health Curricula

Health curricula traditionally have been organized around broad content areas. An additional focus is on teaching critical health skills with the aim of improving healthy behaviors and reducing unhealthy ones. Strategies need to be geared toward negating harmful media messages and emphasizing skills that promote adoption of health-enhancing behaviors (refusal skills, problem solving, decision making, media analysis, assertiveness skills, communication, coping strategies for stress, and behavioral contracting).

State education agencies and local school districts can use the national standards to make decisions about which lessons, strategies, and activities to include in health curricula. The majority of states and districts require certain topics to be taught. These topics include accident or injury prevention,

prevention of alcohol and other drug use, HIV infection prevention, healthy nutritional and dietary behavior, physical activity and fitness, pregnancy prevention, STI prevention, suicide prevention, tobacco use prevention, and violence prevention (CDC, 2005a). In addition, over 80% of states and districts require schools to teach health education at all three levels—elementary, middle/junior high, and senior high. A comprehensive school health program using these standards will most likely show evidence of the following:

- Health content that is introduced in the early grades and reinforced in later grades
- Student assessments that measure skill acquisition as well as knowledge
- Use of performance indicators that define what a student is able to do at different grade levels
- Provision of a minimum of 50 hours of health education at every grade level

Curriculum planning and development should accommodate to the unique local needs and preferences of each community. This is a critical step in increasing support from and awareness of the community. Lohrmann and Wooley (1998) have suggested that several steps can be implemented to achieve this support: (1) creation of a **comprehensive health education advisory committee** that includes parent representation; (2) holding of awareness sessions for the school board, school staff, and community members; and (3) development of a plan for funding that involves school personnel, families, students, related community agencies, and businesses.

Curriculum Implementation

Implementing a curriculum for health education requires teaching strategies that are effective in increasing knowledge, changing attitudes, and influencing health-related behavior. Suggested strategies include the following (Nastasi & Clements, 1991; Seffrin, 1990):

- The use of discovery approaches, with opportunities for hands-on experiences

- The use of student learning stations, small work groups, and cooperative learning techniques
- Cross-age and peer teaching, especially regarding drug use
- The use of positive approaches that emphasize the value of good health and normal growth and development
- An emphasis on the affective domain (e.g., self-esteem and self-efficacy)

The use of information technologies as a teaching tool, team building and collaborative planning between elementary teachers and colleagues, and strategies that foster family involvement in students' health education help improve the effectiveness of health education (Lohrmann & Wooley, 1998).

PHYSICAL EDUCATION

Physical activity promotes positive health behaviors and psychologic well-being. Regular physical activity decreases premature mortality and risk of chronic disease. The benefits of regular physical activity include building and maintaining healthy bones, reducing the risk of developing obesity and chronic illnesses, and reducing feelings of depression and anxiety (CDC, 2006b). Several *Healthy People 2010* objectives emphasize the importance of physical education in schools to promote and sustain physical activity. The SHPPS study in 2000 identified a decrease in physical activity in schools and recommended an increase in the quantity and quality of activities to meet the objectives for 2010 (Burgeson et al., 2001; Lowry et al., 2001). Using the School Health Index (a self-assessment and planning tool developed by the Centers for Disease Control and Prevention [CDC] in 2000) and SHPPS data, Brener and colleagues (2006) found that only 8% of the elementary schools had the recommended minimum of 150 minutes of physical education per week and only 6.2% of the middle schools had the recommended minimum of 225 minutes per week.

According to guidelines developed by the CDC (1997), physical education should be taught by state-certified teachers and provided daily for all students in sequential courses. Students should spend 50% of class time in moderate to vigorous activity, and physical activity outside of formal physical education classes and interscholastic sports is encouraged. The goal of physical education is to improve knowledge, positively change behavior and attitudes, and promote lifelong physical activity. Schools can use the *Physical Education Curriculum Analysis Tool* recently developed tool by the CDC to help assess the extent to which their curricula reflect the national physical education standards of the National Association for Sport and Physical Education and other characteristics of effective physical education programs (Brener et al., 2006; CDC, 2007b).

HEALTH SERVICES

Health services are critically important to the welfare of students and very important to the educational mission of schools (Brener et al., 2001). Three core functions of school health services are the following (Duncan & Igoe, 1998):

- Direct client care, such as screening, diagnosis, and treatment, including the administration of medications, provision for emergency care, and counseling
- Referrals and linkages with other health providers
- Health promotion and disease-prevention education

Models for health services vary depending on the needs of the students and the resources available in the school and community. Three models of care are traditional basic care, expanded school health services, and comprehensive primary care services (Allensworth, 1994). The first two models vary in the degree to which mental health, counseling, and social services are included (Brener et al., 2001). Nurses are critical to these functions. There are currently an estimated 45,000 school nurses employed in the United States, which results in a ratio of one school nurse to 1155 students (American Federation of Teachers [AFT], nd). The recommended ratio is one nurse for every 750 students with an ultimate goal of at least one nurse in every school (Trossman, 2007). A lower ratio is needed for student populations that confront greater physical and mental health challenges in learning: 1:225 for mainstreamed students and 1:125 for the severely and profoundly handicapped (NASN, 2006a).

Comprehensive primary care services are provided in **school-based health centers (SBHCs)** or in other locations, such as school-linked or community health centers (Brindis et al., 2003; Fothergill & Ballard, 1998). The number of SBHCs has increased from 200 in 1990 to 1500 in 2004 (Chmelynski, 2004). The comprehensive SBHC, which provides primary preventive health care, acute care, reproductive health services, mental health services, and health education, is one approach to address the lack of health insurance that exists among 22% of adolescents 12 to 21 years of age (Fox et al., 2007). A survey of 806 SBHCs found that clinics now operate in diverse areas and serve students in grades K through 12, and close to 73% of the clinics bill Medicaid and other third-party insurers for student-provider encounters (Brindis et al., 2003).

NUTRITION SERVICES

Healthy eating in children and adolescents is essential for positive growth and development, intellectual development, and prevention of nutrition-related health problems, such as obesity, iron deficiency anemia, dental caries, and eating disorders. The essential functions of school nutrition services are to provide adequate access to a variety of culturally and nutritionally appropriate foods, to provide nutrition education to empower students as consumers, and to assess and intervene when nutritional problems are identified. Nutrition services must be integrated in the school, encouraging communication among the cafeteria, health services, and the classroom with input also from the physical education staff, families, and community organizations (Caldwell et al., 1998; CDC, 2007a).

In 2004, nationwide 17.4% of adolescents 12 to 19 years of age were overweight, a percentage that has tripled since 1980 (Ogden et al., 2006). Data from the 2003-2004 National Health and Nutrition Examination Survey (NHANES) indicated that the prevalence of overweight children (aged 6 to 11 years) increased from 4.2% in 1963 to 1965 to 18.8% in 2003 to 2004 (CDC, 2007a). Trends in children's eating patterns show especially low intake of fruits and dairy products, excessive intake of total and saturated fats, and diets very high in added sugar (Mathematica Policy Research, 2001). Based on the Youth Risk Behavior Survey (YRBS) in 2005, only 20.1% of all students ate five or more servings per day of fruits and vegetables. When this percentage is broken down by race, 18.6% of white students, 22.1% of black students, and 23.2% of Hispanic students ate five or more servings (CDC, 2006a). During the 1990s, schools began to offer competitive food products in addition to the school meal program. Schools provide competitive foods to meet student preferences, to gain added revenue when school food services must be self-supporting, to get additional discretionary income from exclusive contracts with soft-drink companies, and to meet student needs when food preparation and serving space is limited with inadequate meal periods. Today, professional nutrition, health, and education organizations are concerned with the increasing prevalence of these competitive foods, and the impact of their consumption on children's health (Jones et al., 2003; Watkins, 2001). Food delivery options include vending machines, school stores, snack bars, and à la carte foods in the cafeteria. Competitive foods have been found to be low in nutritional density and high in fat, sugar, and calories; the availability of competitive foods tends to stigmatize participation in the school meal program and can affect the viability of these programs; and the availability of competitive foods conveys a mixed nutritional message when children are taught the value of healthy food choices. The NASN encourages school nurses to provide nutrition education and role modeling and to work with schools, parents, and the community to send a consistent message by providing healthy foods and beverages in all school vending machines, school stores, and snack bars (NASN, 2007).

> Jim Powell is a school nurse assigned to Adamsville High School. Two years ago, the school board opted to allow the use of vending machines for soda and snacks outside the cafeteria. Since that time, the school meal program has served fewer meals to students. Several parents complained to Jim. Jim also observed students using the vending machines as their sole source of nutrition. Jim brought this issue to the attention of the School Health Services Committee of which he is a member. Other members were also concerned. A poll of parents revealed support for changes to the vending machines. The committee investigated and found a company willing to provide vending machines with healthy snack choices, such as fruit and juices. The machines were changed during the summer months. Students still have food choices, but the options are more nutritious.

COUNSELING, PSYCHOLOGIC, AND SOCIAL SERVICES

Historically, school-based mental health services focused on students with special educational needs; more recently, there is a recognition of the need to be concerned with the overall mental health and social needs of all children. In the population of children aged 9 to 17 years, 21% have signs and symptoms of a psychiatric disorder defined by the *Diagnostic and Statistical Manual of Mental Disorders (DSM-IV)* (American Psychiatric Association, 2000) during the course of 1 year (Adelman, 1998; USDHHS, 2001). Mental health services may be fully integrated into the school or may be offered in the context of primary health care in SBHCs. An expanded school mental health framework includes prevention, assessment, treatment, and case management of students in special and general education (Weist & Christodulu, 2000). Services can be focused on individuals, groups, or institutions (school environment). Nurses, certified school counselors, psychologists, and social workers provide these services in schools.

HEALTHY SCHOOL ENVIRONMENT

The **healthy school environment** has both physical and psychosocial aspects. The school environment includes the 120,000 public and private school buildings, school grounds, and all the events related to school activities, including getting to and from school. This environment involves physical conditions such as noise, sanitation, temperature, heating, and lighting. It includes safety for sports, activities in the building, extracurricular activities, and transportation. It also incorporates safety in the immediate areas surrounding the school (Geller et al., 2007). Several excellent tools are available on the Internet to assist schools in maximizing their environment. The *Healthy School Environments Assessment Tool* (HealthySEAT) from the Environmental Protection Agency (EPA) contains a fully integrated environmental health and safety checklist and can be adapted to reflect state and local requirements and policies (U.S. EPA, 2007). Healthy Schools Network is a national organization that works to ensure a healthy school environment for every child and has suggestions for assessments and interventions (Healthy Schools Network, 2007).

A recent study of 60 elementary schools found several factors to be important in the exacerbation of asthma in the classroom (Tortolero et al., 2002). These included less than optimal fresh air exchange, poor air quality, and high levels of dust mites and mold spores in dust samples taken in the classrooms. Detectable levels of cockroach allergen were also found in all of the schools studied. Box 30-1 lists common sources of allergens in classrooms. The Community Resources for Practice section at the end of the chapter provides resources for nurses and school personnel interested in learning more about healthy school environments, including resources on drinking water, pest management, air quality, and environmental education.

A healthy psychosocial school environment encompasses both physical and psychologic safety. It includes a tobacco- and substance-free environment. Effective policies can help to

---

BOX 30-1   Common Classroom Sources of Allergens

- Pets
- Chalk dust and erasers
- Food odors
- Particle-board furniture
- Fragrance emitters
- Cosmetics, hair spray, nail polish, and perfume
- Fabric softeners
- Magic Markers
- Paints, glues, solvents, and science chemicals
- Insecticides
- Floor wax
- Ammonia-, phenol-, and chlorine-containing cleaning products
- Carpeting
- Gas heat
- Ozone emitters
- Outdoor contaminants: pollens, motor vehicle exhaust, sewage, and bus stop odors
- Ceiling tiles
- Tobacco smoke
- Mold growth and dust on books
- Flowering plants

From Robbins, A. (1995). Creating an allergy free classroom. In N. L. Miller (Ed.), *The healthy school handbook: Conquering the sick building syndrome and other environmental hazards in and around your school* (p. 329). Washington, DC: National Education Association.

create a safe environment. The CDC's Guidelines for School Health Programs to Prevent Tobacco Use and Addiction, for example, prohibit tobacco use by students, all school staff, and visitors on school property, in school vehicles, and at school-sponsored functions away from school (CDC, 2002a). Student and staff exposure to violence in the schools is an increasing problem. Prevention of injuries and assurance of a violence-free environment inside and outside school buildings are important. In 2001, the CDC issued guidelines to prevent unintentional injuries and violence (CDC, 2001). Box 30-2 lists the CDC recommendations.

HEALTH PROMOTION FOR STAFF

Some 6 million adults are employed by public school systems in the United States; half are teachers (U.S. Department of Education, 2005). Working with staff members to protect their health and to develop healthy behaviors is an important contribution of the school nurse. Health promotion activities improve productivity, increase staff morale, decrease absenteeism, and reduce health insurance costs (School Employee Wellness, 2006). Healthy staff members are excellent role models for students. Some examples of staff health promotion activities include maintaining a health promotion library stocked with books on stress, conducting on-site smoking cessation classes with a quitters' support group, and holding classes on defensive driving, first aid, and cardiopulmonary resuscitation (CPR). The Directors of Health Promotion and Education, in cooperation with several other agencies, has developed the manual *School Employee Wellness: A Guide for Protecting the Assets of Our Nation's Schools,* which includes tools and resources to help schools develop their own staff wellness programs. The manual and other information sheets can be downloaded free from *http://www.schoolempwell.org.*

FAMILY/COMMUNITY INVOLVEMENT

Schools are not isolated entities. Enhancing the health of students requires an integrated approach in working with families and communities. Support for a school program can be achieved through the efforts of school health advisory councils, coalitions, and broadly based constituencies for school health (CDC, 2007a). SHPPS found that 45.1% of districts and 65.5% of schools have school health councils. SHPPS also identified many barriers to family and community involvement. These included a lack of time, language difficulties, and a lack of knowledge and awareness of the different cultures served by the school and community (Brener et al., 2001). Joyce Epstein and colleagues (2002) have created a useful research-based handbook to guide schools, parents, and community partners in determining best how to plan, implement, evaluate, and improve family and community interactions with schools.

ORGANIZATION AND ADMINISTRATION OF SCHOOL HEALTH

Most nations have centralized school systems in which a national ministry prescribes curricula. That is not the case in the United States, where public education is decentralized.

PATTERNS OF ORGANIZATION AND MANAGEMENT OF SCHOOL HEALTH PROGRAMS

Education is primarily the responsibility of local and state governments. The federal government enacts laws that impact education, but provides little of the funding for educational programs. School health is also, for the most part, a local and state responsibility. There is some concern that the new federal law, the **No Child Left Behind Act,** discussed later in this chapter, will divert funding from health services and physical education.

At the local level, each school adopts, implements, and organizes the components of a coordinated school health program. This involves a multidisciplinary team, including the school nurse, health educator, physical educator, school counselors, physical therapist, speech therapist, school social workers, school psychologists, food service staff, parents, police liaisons, clerical staff, bus drivers, custodial staff, and older students. Teachers, support staff, and representatives of community organizations are equally important as partners in the development and implementation of a coordinated school health program.

The school health program needs the support of the local community and school district. To guarantee long-term sustainability, support from the leadership in the district and the school board is key. Programs will differ from school to school and district to district. Each district will have certain mandated elements (e.g., vision and hearing screening, physical education), and other components dictated by the child's age, the environment, and geographic location. Other elements will be identified, modified, or emphasized based on the individual school's health team assessment (Fetro, 1998).

> **Box 30-2** **School Health Recommendations to Prevent Unintentional Injuries, Violence, and Suicide**
>
> 1. Establish a social environment that promotes safety and prevents unintentional injuries, violence, and suicide.
> 2. Provide a physical environment, inside and outside school buildings that promotes safety and prevents unintentional injuries, violence, and suicide.
> 3. Implement health and safety education curricula and instruction that help students develop the knowledge, attitudes, behavioral skills, and confidence needed to adopt and maintain safe lifestyles and to advocate for health and safety.
> 4. Provide safe physical education and extracurricular physical activity programs.
> 5. Provide health, counseling, psychologic, and social services to meet the physical, mental, emotional, and social health needs of students.
> 6. Establish mechanisms for short- and long-term responses to crises, disasters, and injuries that affect the school community.
> 7. Integrate school, family, and community efforts to prevent unintentional injuries, violence, and suicide.
> 8. For all school personnel, provide regular staff development opportunities that impact the knowledge, skills, and confidence to effectively promote safety and prevent unintentional injury, violence, and suicide, and support students in the efforts to do the same.
>
> From Centers for Disease Control and Prevention. (2001). School health guidelines to prevent unintentional injuries and violence. *Morbidity and Mortality Weekly Report, Recommendations and Reports, 50* (RR-22), 1-46.

The organizational component of nursing services varies among schools and districts. Community/public health nurses in school health settings are most often employed by a board of education or board of health. In addition, nurses hired through a board of health may be assigned to specialized services in schools or to generalized nursing services with occasional assignments in the school setting. Some innovative approaches to hiring include the use of agency nurses to fill school nurse positions, the hiring of school nurses by parent/teacher/student associations, contracting with local hospitals and health maintenance organizations, and the assignment of special project nurses funded by private or government grants. All school nurses have some accountability to school administrations as well as to the organization responsible for their hiring.

LEGISLATIVE AND ADMINISTRATIVE REGULATIONS

School health programs vary markedly across the United States. Local schools primarily define their programs, but are influenced by federal, state, and local regulations. Federal requirements focus on protecting children, families, and employees and providing services to children with disabilities (Lear, 2002; Thackaberry, 2003). The federal laws governing school health programs include the following:

- Occupational Safety and Health Act (OSHA) of 1970
- Rehabilitation Act of 1973, Section 504
- Family Educational Rights and Privacy Act (FERPA) of 1974
- Education for All Handicapped Children Act (EHA) of 1975
- Americans with Disabilities Act (ADA) of 1990
- Individuals with Disabilities Education Act (IDEA) of 1990 (a revision and renaming of the EHA); amended in 1997 and amended again in 2004 to the Individuals with Disabilities Education Improvement Act (IDEIA)
- Health Insurance Portability and Accountability Act (HIPAA) of 1996
- No Child Left Behind Act of 2001

The Occupational Safety and Health Administration (OSHA) imposes requirements on the workplace to promote safety for employees, including school employees. In the schools, requirements include implementation of the following (U.S. Department of Labor, 2007):

- Universal precautions and compliance to prevent contact with blood or potentially infectious materials
- Engineering controls and work practice controls to eliminate or minimize harmful exposure to employees
- Hepatitis B vaccination for all employees who may have exposure to blood or potentially infectious materials and postexposure evaluation and follow-up

Section 504 of the Rehabilitation Act of 1973 (Public Law 93-112) protects the rights of individuals with disabilities to participate in programs that receive federal money. The Office of Civil Rights is responsible for overseeing compliance with Section 504. The law ensures that federally assisted programs and activities are operated without discrimination on the basis of disabilities and that reasonable accommodation to the disability of students and employees are made (see Chapters 26 and 27). A free and appropriate education must meet the individual needs of students who qualify as handicapped and can consist of special or regular education. A handicap covered by Section 504 must be severe enough to result in the student's having a substantial limitation in carrying out one or more major life activities (e.g., breathing, walking, talking, seeing, and hearing), having a record of having such an impairment, or being regarded as having such an impairment (Lear, 2002; Moses et al., 2005; Thackaberry, 2003).

In 1975 the Education for All Handicapped Children Act (EHA), known as **Public Law 94-142,** was enacted. This law gives all students between 6 and 18 years of age the right to a "free and appropriate public education" in the least restrictive environment possible, regardless of their physical or mental disabilities. The 1986 amendments to the EHA contained in Public Law 99-457 expanded the eligible population to include preschool students from birth to 5 years of age. This law created two new federal programs: the **Handicapped Infant and Toddler Program** and the Preschool Grants Program. The Handicapped Infant and Toddler Program, for children from birth to 3 years of age, was established to reduce the potential for developmental delays, minimize institutionalization of children with disabilities, help families meet the special needs of their children, and reduce the cost to society. Under the Preschool Grants Program, state educational agencies must provide free and appropriate education for all children with disabilities beginning at age 3 years (Zantal-Wiener, 1998).

In 1990, the **Individuals with Disabilities Education Act** (IDEA; Public Law 105-17) succeeded the EHA. In 1997 Congress passed amendments to the IDEA further defining the responsibility of school districts to provide students aged 3 to 21 years with disability participation in the general curriculum. These called for the development of an **individualized education program (IEP)** for each student with a disability that identifies the special education and related services the student needed. The law's definition of the IEP team did not specify the inclusion of a nurse. In 2004 the IDEA was reformed to the Individuals with Disabilities Education Improvement Act (IDEIA). School districts must continue to educate disabled children in the least restrictive environment possible, keeping them in the regular classrooms if it does not interfere with their educational performance. When special education services are needed, a multidisciplinary team including the school nurse meets to determine eligibility and necessary services. The health services necessary for a child to participate safely and fully in the school are determined and are reflected in an IEP for children aged 5 to 21 years and in an **individualized family service plan** for children aged 3 to 5 years (NASN, 2006b). Many school districts face seemingly insurmountable tasks in meeting their responsibilities for providing related services to the 6.8 million U.S. school-aged children with disabilities (U.S. Department of Education, 2006). Districts are deterred by a lack of adequate funds and a shortage of trained personnel. Clear documentation of the specific needs of the student in the IEP is imperative, and parents and schools must become partners in developing strategies for increased funding to provide services for students. Interdisciplinary and interagency collaboration must be achieved, and new, creative planning must be accomplished to use all school and community resources to help students with disabilities feel valued as members of the community. The Americans with Disabilities Act of 1990 extends the Public Accommodation Act to include individuals with disabilities. This allows people with disabilities to have equal access to and opportunity to use and enjoy facilities and programs. This act extends the requirements to even some private school health programs and provides coverage to children who were not included in Section 504 of the Rehabilitation Act (Lear, 2002).

Confidentiality of school records is ensured under the **Federal Educational Rights and Privacy Act (FERPA).** FERPA protects the privacy of student records by limiting access to parents, students over age 18 or emancipated minors, and educators who have a legitimate educational interest. FERPA privacy provisions also address the need to keep records in locked cabinets, to protect computer records with passwords, and to be vigilant about the illegal use of health sign-in logs (Thackaberry, 2003). School nurses must be aware of the laws and use judgment in recording information obtained from the student. It should be noted that school-based health clinic and health center records, records connected with treatment of a student in a federally assisted program for drug or alcohol abuse, and records connected with child abuse or neglect are not considered part of the education records.

The Health Insurance Portability and Accountability Act (HIPAA) protects the privacy of an individual's health information, including name, medical diagnoses, and treatment. All records from SBHCs fall directly under HIPAA regulation. There continues to be concern and clarification about the interaction between HIPAA and FERPA, which regulates information such as immunization records and records of mandated physical examinations (Bergren, 2004; Cohn, 2007; U.S. Department of Education, 2007). All schools do exchange information with multiple health care providers who must meet HIPAA requirements. Therefore, the *release of information* forms should meet the HIPAA criteria, including closely defined use of the permission form, ability to revoke the permission form, and limitation on who can receive the information. The nurse must protect information that allows the client to be identified in written, verbal, and electronic transfer of information (Schwah, 2005).

The new federal law the *No Child Left Behind Act* of 2001 has several major provisions that focus on increasing accountability for student progress and achievement. This act ensures that parents, citizens, educators, administrators, and policy makers have information about the local schools and their ability to meet the academic needs of their students. The information is to be used at the state and local levels to improve elementary and secondary school performance and to guarantee that no child is trapped in a failing school. Many of the components of this law support the role functions of the school nurse: promoting school attendance and high school graduation through health education and health services, keeping the environment safe, providing counseling, guaranteeing a coordinated school health program, engaging in advocacy, and working with a multidisciplinary team (Constante, 2006). It is unclear at this time what effects the new increased emphasis on academic performance and measurement of performance will have on school health. There is concern that these new requirements will drain funds and time from health education programs, perhaps eliminating or reducing the time spent in physical education. A benefit is that these changes support efforts to keep the schools safe and drug free. Schools must report school safety statistics, and funding under the Federal Safe and Drug-Free Schools and Communities program must be used to implement effective drug and violence prevention programs (U.S. Department of Education, 2003).

State laws vary from state to state. Some mandated responsibilities of health service programs include overseeing school entrance requirements (immunizations and physical examinations), performing health screenings, developing nursing care plans for children with disabilities, and providing emergency care. The state statutes frequently are recommended by the health department and enforced by the local school administration and the health department. Other examples of state requirements include Board of Nursing registered nurse (RN) licensure and, when relevant, school nurse and health education certification. Each state requires the reporting of suspected child abuse (Thackaberry, 2003). Most states identify health services that can be delegated to nonnursing staff members. School personnel, by and large, have no training in health-related fields and never anticipate having to perform health care procedures when they prepare to become teachers or school employees. School staff are with the students for most of the day and are the primary caretakers. It is imperative that all members of the team—teachers, paraprofessionals, other classified personnel, and related service providers—be trained to participate in appropriate procedures and activities and know when to call or contact the school nurse or secure emergency assistance.

RESPONSIBILITIES OF THE SCHOOL NURSE

The scope of practice of school nursing has been significantly influenced by the evolution of specialty practices within the broad field of nursing. Nurses within a specialty acquire the philosophy, goals, and qualifications and specific education needed by its practitioners.

Traditionally, the school nurse has been viewed from a limited perspective as a case finder and provider of basic health services to the student population. Economic changes, legislation, and the growing costs of health care have led a large segment of our population to rethink the role of the school nurse. Children from low-income families frequently have unmet health care requirements. The school nurse may be pressed into service as the primary health care provider. Changes in public law have mainstreamed students with disabilities into the general school population. In the past, these disabled students were educated in special environments. Now, school nurses find themselves tasked with ensuring optimum health awareness and wellness of a very diverse student population, the school staff, and the community.

A new paradigm for school nursing is emerging, one that incorporates a new value structure of prevention and enhances the enormous diversity in the role and function of the practicing school nurse. This expanded role includes program management, interdisciplinary collaboration, health education, health counseling, school-community coordination, and research.

EDUCATIONAL PREPARATION AND CERTIFICATION

School nurses should have academic credentials comparable to those of other faculty members in the school. The NASN has determined that the minimum qualification for the professional school nurse at the entry level of school nursing is a baccalaureate degree and licensure as an RN. Nurses in certain states also need to meet state certification requirements. The National Board of Certification of School Nurses (NBCSN) offers a voluntary national certification examination for school nurses that confirms that the nurse meets a national standard of preparation, knowledge, and practice in the field of school nursing. Eligibility to take the examination requires a current RN license, a bachelor's degree, current employment in school health services or school-related services, and a recommended 3 years of experience as a school nurse (NBCSN, nd).

Advanced practice RNs provide valuable services to students through expanded school health services. Clinical nurse specialists in community health with organizational and policy skills have the ability to assess, implement, and evaluate school health programs. School nurse practitioners and pediatric nurse practitioners have the ability to diagnose and manage most common illnesses, providing primary health care on site at the school. The NASN supports these advanced practice roles to broaden the health service so that more health needs are met and the education of the students is thereby improved (NASN, 2003a).

STANDARDS OF PRACTICE

School nurses are professionals who are accountable for practicing in accordance with the Standards of Professional School Nursing Practice. The purpose of the standards of school nursing practice is to fulfill the profession's obligation to provide a means of improving the quality of care. The current school nursing standards have evolved over a 20-year period from numerous documents published by the American Nurses Association (ANA), the NASN, and the Western Interstate Commission on Higher Education and are available *WEB* on this book's website as **Website Resource 30A.**

ROLES OF THE SCHOOL NURSE

The NASN recently outlined and defined roles of the school nurse (NASN, 2005a). These roles include the following:

- Provider of direct health care to students and staff
- Leader for the provision of health services
- Health screener and source of referrals for health conditions
- Promoter of a healthy school environment
- Promoter of health
- Leader for health policies and programs
- Liaison between school personnel, family, community, and health care providers

School nurses provide interventions directed toward all levels of prevention, and positive health outcomes are expected among students, teachers, other school personnel, and the families of students.

Provider of Direct Health Care to Students and Staff

The school nurse provides direct care to students and staff who have been injured or are suffering from acute illness (NASN, 2002). This requires knowledge of first aid, management of emergencies, community resources, and referral and follow-up procedures. The school nurse also deals with chronic health problems. The prevalence of chronic illness varies widely depending on definition. The National Survey of Children with Special Health Care Needs found that 12.8% of children (9.4 million) have chronic conditions with special health care needs (USDHHS, 2004). Nurses can help children with chronic health problems succeed by providing emotional support and direct care, including performing technical procedures and administering prescription medications. Erickson and colleagues (2006) note that chronic conditions are complex and require an integrated system, and have developed a comprehensive community-based model to help students remain healthy, stay in school, and be able to learn.

The administration of prescription medications is one of the most common health activities performed in schools and is critical to keeping children in school. It is estimated that 5.6% to 5.8% of U.S. schoolchildren receive medication every day (McCarthy et al., 2000). The number of children requiring medication has grown, and school nurses are often required to delegate medication administration to unlicensed assistive personnel (Johnson & Hayes, 2006). School districts must develop policies and procedures to address medication administration in accordance with federal and state laws and guidelines that are outlined by the NASN position statement (2003b). The ANA recently published a position statement concerning school health. In this statement, the ANA "supports the development and dissemination of instructional curricula to assist school nurses in educating non–health care providers to competently perform delegated tasks in an educational setting" (ANA, 2007, p. 9). It also supports the dissemination of consistent information on delegation to school nurses that reflects the legal requirements of their states as well as the professional standards required of professional RNs.

Leader for the Provision of Health Services

The school nurse is the health care expert in the school environment. He or she is responsible for assessing the health care services program and developing a plan to meet all health needs. This leadership role includes developing a plan for responding to emergencies and disasters, including natural disasters, school-related violence, and bioterrorism. The NASN has issued several position statements that address emergency preparedness and bioterrorism emergency preparedness (NASN, 2005a). School nurses should be trained in triage and prepare staff to administer first aid and nursing care in a disaster (Doyle, 2003; NASN, 2004a). A comprehensive school crisis plan includes (1) prevention activities, (2) intervention if a crisis occurs, and (3) follow-up of all persons affected (Poland, 2003). In a national random survey 86.3% of the schools had a response plan, but only a little over half had a prevention plan, a little over a fifth had a plan for children with special needs, and a quarter had plans for postdisaster counseling (Graham et al., 2006). The school nurse is well placed for surveillance and assessment of chemical and radiologic exposure, can provide education about these threats, is positioned on the front line when an emergency does occur, and can participate in short- and long-term recovery phases (NASN, 2005a).

In some school districts, school nurses have responsibility for many different schools and might not be available when an emergency arises, such as the need for first aid, medication administration, or even CPR. The nurse is responsible for ensuring that designated school personnel are capable of providing such services. It is critical that the delegation of care to an unlicensed person be appropriate within the requirements of both the state nurse practice act and the administrative policy of the district. In delegating, the nurse must train and supervise the delegatee and monitor the health outcome of the student. The training must be documented, and ongoing evaluation by the RN is required (NASN, 2006c).

Promoter of a Healthy School Environment

The nurse is concerned with both the physical and emotional safety of the school community. Activities to ensure physical safety include monitoring immunizations, reporting communicable diseases, providing the leadership for conducting blood-borne pathogen in-service training, implementing measures to control infectious diseases, and ensuring good indoor air quality. In examining hazards in the school building there is a fine balance between maximizing educational learning experiences in the classroom and minimizing the potential dangers, especially in the science laboratory and in physical education (Geller et al., 2007). Issues related to the emotional environment include the extent of violence or bullying, crowding, and overstimulation in the school (Geller et al., 2007; NASN, 2005b).

Injuries on playgrounds are a particular problem for children, especially those younger than 5 years. It is again important for the nurse to encourage creativity and exercise while keeping the environment safe. Falls account for more than three quarters of playground injuries, with 3% requiring hospitalization (Safe Kids USA, 2006). School nurses can play a significant role in addressing this issue through several interventions, including the development of a safety assessment guide, in-service training for teachers and playground monitors, and a student-oriented program to improve safe behavior.

Promoter of Health

The school nurse provides health education by directly teaching students or by assisting in the development of the health education curriculum (NASN, 2005b). The school nurse has a unique opportunity in the educational setting to facilitate maintenance of or change in health attitudes, values, beliefs, and behavior in a captive audience. The nurse may provide the following (NASN, 2005b):

- Informal health teaching for students, staff, and parents
- Formal health teaching in a classroom setting
- Health teaching support for the classroom teacher, such as providing materials, resources, and expertise
- Formal in-service health education
- Curriculum planning and development
- Health promotion programs, such as health fairs, staff wellness programs, and consultation

School nurses engage in health education on many levels. Informal activities capitalize on the teachable moment when a student expresses a desire or need to learn about wellness, whereas the formal approach to health education is a systematic process of assessment of learner needs, exploration of learner readiness, development of planned outcomes, development and implementation of a teaching plan, and evaluation of learner outcomes and teacher effectiveness.

The 1991 federal standard issued by OSHA of the U.S. Department of Labor mandates that all staff members who might be at risk for occupational exposure to blood-borne pathogens be instructed annually on universal precautions. The nurse is the ideal person to plan and implement the in-service program. Accurate health education material helps allay staff concerns and fears about dealing with body fluid spills.

Leader for Health Policies and Programs

The school nurse uses biostatistical data to determine the extent and distribution of specific health problems and to set priorities for program planning. The school nurse also participates in and provides leadership to coordinated school programs, crisis and disaster management teams, and school health advisory councils (NASN, 2002).

For students with special needs, the school nurse is knowledgeable about the federal laws that afford these students a free and appropriate education in the least restrictive environment. The nurse functions as an advocate for students and families while facilitating normalization of the students' educational experience.

School nursing research is necessary to justify practice and develop new knowledge. Outcome research is important. Currently, the results, costs, and benefits of school nursing services are not well understood, and there is a need to document the type, extent, and effectiveness of nursing interventions (Brener et al., 2001; Stock et al., 2002). School nurses need to initiate research studies and test new approaches and concepts that will clarify and strengthen their contributions in the area of school health.

Liaison between School Personnel, Family, Community, and Health Care Providers

The mores, belief systems, values, and resources of the community in which students and families live are a primary concern of the school nurse. A successful school nurse seeks community input at each level of health services program planning, because community groups are more interested in supporting initiatives if they have participated in the planning of the program. To facilitate community-school interactions, the nurse should be involved in community groups, agencies, and coalitions (NASN, 2002).

The school nurse is also a case manager. An identifiable population for case management is "included" students with IEPs. These students are developmentally disabled but attend regular classrooms. Other students who benefit from case management are those with HIV infection or acquired immunodeficiency syndrome (AIDS), previous closed-head injuries, or transplants; students who are technologically dependent; and students who are severely compromised by an acute illness or an acute exacerbation of a chronic illness (see Chapter 27). Other groups that are candidates for case management are obese children and pregnant adolescents.

Screener and Source of Referrals for Health Conditions

Routine health screenings are performed in schools. Assessments include measurement of weight for height, vision, hearing, and blood pressure, and scoliosis screening. When planning a state-mandated program, the school nurse should be familiar with the state laws governing screenings and the specific disease conditions included. Screening requires follow-up to confirm diagnosis and appropriate treatment. The school nurse can develop strategies to assist families overcome barriers to increase follow-up on positive screening findings (Kimel, 2006). Schools are ideal places to conduct health screenings because of their captive audience and the opportunity for easy detection, diagnosis, and treatment of health conditions (see Chapter 19). It is important to be aware that children who are at risk may be omitted from screening because they are absent from school or their parents refuse to allow screening.

COMMON HEALTH CONCERNS OF SCHOOL-AGED CHILDREN

School nurses are in a unique position to help children achieve and maintain a high level of wellness. This section discusses some of the most common health problems of school-aged children and adolescents encountered by school nurses and other school personnel.

DRUG AND ALCOHOL USE

In 2005, data from the YRBS indicated that 43.3% of the surveyed students had imbibed alcohol, 20.2% had used marijuana, and 2.1% had injected an illegal drug during their lifetime (CDC, 2006a). Nationwide, 7.6% had used a form of cocaine, and 12.4% had sniffed glue, breathed the contents of aerosol cans, or inhaled paints or sprays to get high during their lifetime (CDC, 2006a).

School nurses can be instrumental in implementing comprehensive programs to address these problems. Nurses can survey the extent of the problem in the school and community, identify those children at risk, and develop appropriate interventions. Some common risk factors for adolescent drug use include academic failure, a low degree of commitment to education, and a low level of attachment to teachers and schools. From a primary prevention perspective, nurses can also be effective in identifying those children exposed to substance abuse in their families.

Drug abuse prevention programs are critical for grades K through 12, with a particular focus on middle school. Programs can be categorized as one of the following (Walsh, 1997):

- Universal programs that are focused on everyone in a given population
- Selective interventions that are recommended for adolescents who are members of high-risk groups (i.e., youth whose parents use drugs)
- Indicated interventions designed for youth who are displaying characteristics of having a problem (e.g., drug use, drop out of school)

Effective prevention curricula components include social resistance skills training and training in broader personal and social skills within the context of comprehensive health education (Dusenbury & Falco, 1995).

Achieving reductions in tobacco, alcohol, and illicit drug use will take a comprehensive approach to substance abuse prevention (see Chapter 25). The National Institute on Drug Abuse (NIDA) has published the document *Preventing Drug Use among Children and Adolescents: A Research-Based Guide for Parents, Educators, and Community Leaders* (2003). It lists universal, selective, and indicated programs that have proven to be effective with different groups of children. The Task Force on Community Preventive Services conducted a systematic review of published scientific data concerning the effectiveness of these programs and found strong evidence that universal school-based programs decrease rates of problem behavior, violence, and aggressive behavior among school-aged children (Hahn et al., 2007). The CDC has also issued guidelines for tobacco use prevention that have been recently modified to address all addictions (Wenter et al., 2002) (Box 30-3).

BOX 30-3 Recommendations for School Substance Use Prevention Programs

1. Develop and enforce a school policy on substance use.
2. Provide education on short- and long-term negative physiologic and social consequences of substance use, social influences on substance use, peer norms regarding substance use, and refusal skills.
3. Provide substance use prevention education in grades K through 12; this instruction should be especially intensive in junior high or middle school and should be reinforced in high school.
4. Provide program-specific training for teachers.
5. Involve parents or families in support of school-based programs to prevent substance use.
6. Support cessation efforts among students and school staff who use substances.
7. Assess the substance use prevention program at regular intervals.

From Wenter, D. L., Ennett, S. T., Ribisl, K. M., et al. (2002). Comprehensiveness of substance use prevention programs in U.S. middle schools. *Journal of Adolescent Health, 30,* 456.

CIGARETTE USE

The 2005 YRBS found that, nationwide, 23.0% of students had smoked cigarettes at least once in the previous month, and 9.4% of the students had smoked cigarettes on 20 of the 30 preceding days (CDC, 2006c). The CDC recently analyzed cigarette use trends among high school students as evidenced in the YRBS data for 1991 to 2005. The analysis found that cigarette smoking increased during most of the 1990s and then decreased significantly from the late 1990s to 2003, but the prevalence was unchanged from 2003 to 2005 (CDC, 2006c). To achieve the *Healthy People 2010* objectives, the downward trend will have to resume.

School nurses are in a position to address both tobacco use cessation and the prevention of tobacco use. Successful components of smoking prevention programs include a focus on skills training, involvement of the community in creating the program and disseminating the messages, and development of long-term programming to ensure adequate delivery of prevention measures (Wiehe et al., 2005). This includes interventions designed to help students develop refusal skills, cope with peer pressure, and avoid or cope with cues for smoking behavior (Nabors et al., 2007; Wiehe et al., 2005).

In 2002, the CDC identified two programs that show evidence of reducing tobacco use (Collins et al., 2002). They are Life Skills Training (Botvin & Eng, 1982; Hahn et al., 2002) and Project Toward No Tobacco Use (Dent et al., 1995). A recent study found that school nurses and school nurse practitioners were able to effectively address prevention among youth using the life skills curriculum (Tingen et al., 2006). In another study, school nurses delivered a four-session cessation intervention and reported an increased short-term abstinence rate among the students (Pbert et al., 2006).

SEXUALLY TRANSMITTED DISEASES

The 2005 national school-based YRBS revealed that 46.8% of all high school students had had sexual intercourse during their lifetime, a decrease from 53.1% in 1995 (see Chapter 24). Among currently sexually active students (33.9%) nationwide, 62.8% reported that they or their partner used a condom during the last sexual intercourse, and 17.6% reported that either they or their partner had used birth control pills before their last sexual intercourse (CDC, 2006a). Among teens who reported on their most recent sexual encounter, 83% of teen females and 91% of teen males used contraceptives. The female teen pregnancy rate has decreased 36% since its high in 1990 (Alan Guttmacher Institute, 2006a). Of the currently sexually active students, 23.3% had used drugs or alcohol at last sexual intercourse. Of sexually active students, 14.3% had had sex with four or more sex partners. Nationally, 87.9% of students reported being taught in school about HIV/AIDS, and 11.9% had been tested for HIV (CDC, 2006d).

These behaviors place adolescents at risk for STDs. Each year there are approximately 19 million cases of STDs, with half occurring among young people aged 15 to 24 years (CDC, 2007c). Infection with *Chlamydia trachomatis* and human papillomavirus (HPV) are more common in adolescents. The majority of HPV infections are self-limiting and without clinical symptoms, but persistent infection with oncogenic types can cause cervical cancer in women. In March 2007, the CDC's Advisory Committee on Immunization Practices recommended routine vaccination of girls aged 11 to 12 years with three doses of quadrivalent HPV vaccine. The vaccination series can be started as young as age 9 years (Advisory Committee on Immunization Practices, 2007). Half of all new HIV infections in the United States are among people younger than age 25, and most are infected sexually. Although AIDS incidence is declining, there has not been a comparable decline in the number of newly diagnosed cases of HIV infection in adolescents. Adolescent females are at greater risk than adolescent males (CDC, 2007c).

According to the CDC's School Health Policies and Program Study in 2000, 73% of schools have adopted policies on students with HIV/AIDS, and 64% of schools have adopted policies on faculty and staff with HIV/AIDS (National Association of State Boards of Education, 2001). Brown and Simpson (2000) argue that to cause no harm and promote good, school nurses have an ethical responsibility to educate adolescents about STDs and HIV infection and about strategies to prevent the spread of these diseases. School nurses can play an important role in meeting the challenges of the AIDS epidemic. Nurses can be instrumental in the implementation of broad-based prevention programs that incorporate theory and research. The CDC has identified effective and efficient school-based programs that work to reduce health risk (CDC, 2007a; Collins et al., 2002). Several programs focus on reducing initiation of intercourse, understanding AIDS, and making safer choices. National, state, and local decision makers are encouraged to implement HIV prevention programs that include policy, staff development, curriculum, and measurement of student outcomes (Lohrmann et al., 2001). Several studies have shown that peer education programs have changed teen sexual behavior, and school nurses can play a role in planning, implementing, and evaluating such programs (Mahat et al., 2006; Mason, 2003).

TEENAGE PREGNANCY

Childbearing during adolescence is another potential consequence of high-risk sexual behavior (see Chapter 24). Between 1991 and 2005, the teen birth rate declined significantly. The rate has fallen more than 40% since 1991 in teens 15 to 17 years

of age and to a lesser extent in teens 18 to 19 years. The birth rate continues to decline in teens (15 to 17 years). In 2005 the birth rate was 21 births per 1000 in 15- to 17-year-old females and 40.4 per 1000 in all teens aged 15 to 19 years (Hamilton et al., 2006). The birth rate for black, non-Hispanic adolescents has dropped 60% (Childstats.gov, 2007). However, birth rates among U.S. teenagers remain more than twice the rate in Canada and more than seven times the rate in the Netherlands (Planned Parenthood, 2006).

Teen pregnancy is a complex problem impacted by multiple factors that include the influence of individuals, family, school, faith community, and numerous other institutions. Introducing programs into the schools, although helpful, may yield only modest results. In selecting a program, it is important to review any documentation of program effectiveness so that time and funds may be used wisely. Currently, the federal government has placed an emphasis on abstinence-only education programs (see Chapter 24). To date there is little evidence that abstinence-only programs have been more effective than other programs at reducing sexual activity, STDs, or pregnancy among teens (Bleakley et al., 2006, USDHHS, 2007). Comprehensive sex education programs that include information about contraceptives and their correct use as well as STDs and the risk of multiple sex partners appear to be a more effective strategy. Comprehensive sex education programs have been found to delay the onset and reduce the frequency of sexual activity as well as increase the use of contraceptives and decrease the rate of pregnancy among sexually active teens (Alan Guttmacher Institute, 2006b; Bleakley et al., 2006).

School-based clinics are another approach for working with adolescents in middle and high schools. School-based clinics that specifically target sexually active teens have been shown to decrease the teen pregnancy rate (Ricketts, 2006). Currently, however, increased condom use is not consistently seen even when condoms are available in the school or in school-based clinics (Kings County Health Department, 2003; Kirby, 2001).

VIOLENCE

Violence is a significant public health issue. In 2003, 5570 young people aged 10 to 24 years were murdered—an average of 15 each day. Of these victims, 82% were killed with firearms. In 2004, more than 750,000 young people aged 10 to 24 years were treated in emergency departments for injuries due to violence (CDC, 2006e). School-related violence and safety concerns have also taken on more meaning since the occurrence of several high-profile school shootings. In the 2005 YRBS, 6.0% of the students stated that they had missed 1 day in the preceding 30 days because they felt unsafe at school, 6.5% of the students nationwide admitted carrying a weapon on school property, 13.6% of the students had been in a physical fight on school property, and 7.9% of the students had been threatened or injured with a weapon (CDC, 2006a).

The prevalence of lifetime, past-year, and current physical violence in dating relationships among middle and high school students varies in different studies, but ranges from 9% to 46% (Glass et al., 2003). Clinical implications for school nurses include the need for routine screening, lethality assessments, and interventions that assist in ensuring safety and access to resources.

Child maltreatment is another form of violence that has also reached epidemic proportions. Such maltreatment can consist of physical and psychologic abuse and neglect and sexual abuse. The school nurse plays a very important role in the early identification of abuse, reporting of actual or suspected cases, and early intervention (see Chapter 23).

There has been an increased awareness of the impact of bullying on students since the occurrence of several high-profile shootings in schools (see Chapter 23). An estimated 30% of sixth- to tenth graders in the United States were found to be involved in bullying other children (Bauer et al., 2007). Bullying creates a multitude of problems for children. Both bullied and bullying young people are more likely to be involved in fights and carry weapons in school (Fox et al., 2003; Nansel et al., 2003). Other studies have identified other health issues associated with those who are the target of bullying, including somatic pains, loneliness, depression, and increased drug and alcohol use (Fekkes et al., 2004; Kim et al., 2005; Sullivan et al., 2006).

Violence prevention programs are established in many schools. The Olweus Bullying Prevention Program, for example, is a widely disseminated program. Recent findings of an evaluation of this program found mixed positive effects varying by gender (Hickman et al., 2004). In 1996, the Center for the Study and Prevention of Violence at the University of Colorado launched an initiative to identify programs that are effective. Eleven model programs, called *Blueprints,* were identified as being effective, and 21 other programs were identified as promising programs (Center for the Study and Prevention of Violence, 2004). Information about these programs can be found on the center's website (see Community Resources for Practice at the end of the chapter).

The CDC published strategies to address unintentional injuries, violence, and suicides in 2001 in *Morbidity and Mortality Weekly Report (MMWR), Recommendations and Reports.* One of the most important strategies outlined by the CDC is that of establishing a social environment that promotes safety and prevents unintentional injuries, violence, and suicide (CDC, 2001).

MENTAL HEALTH

Mental health programs in schools include a range of programs focused on adolescent development, self-esteem, depression, suicide, and coping. It is generally recognized that the school is a primary site for the prevention and treatment of child and adolescent psychologic problems (Bruns et al., 2004; Weist, 1999). With the multiple pressures and stresses affecting children, many potential needs can be identified by teachers and staff. Teachers may observe decreased attendance, poor performance, or attitude problems that may signify underlying mental health issues. Teenagers may display behavior problems, withdrawal, or somatic complaints. The 2005 YRBS found that during the 12 months before they were surveyed, 28.5% of the students felt so sad or hopeless for 2 weeks or more in a row that they stopped usual activities (CDC, 2006a). Although sadness is only one symptom of depression, it is important to recognize that at least 10% of teens experience an episode of major depression (National Mental Health Information Center, 2003). School nurses have opportunities to assess children's emotional health when children come with somatic complaints, which in many cases are the presenting symptoms of mental health problems. It is the responsibility of the nurse to be aware of signs of depression and to know the resources in the community (Davis, 2005).

Other mental health problems that are frequently seen are attention-deficit/hyperactivity disorder (ADHD), anxiety disorders, eating disorders, substance abuse, physical and sexual abuse, aggressive or violent tendencies, suicide attempts, and conflicts regarding sexual behavior. It is estimated that 5% to 10% of children worldwide suffer from ADHD, which often results in academic and social dysfunction (Biederman, 2005; Faraone et al., 2003). Overall, it is estimated that of the population of 9- to 17-year-olds, 21% experience signs and symptoms meeting the *DSM-IV* criteria for a mental disorder (USDHHS, 1999).

Schools seem to function as a significant source of mental health care for children. Although only 16% of all children receive any mental health services overall, 70% to 80% of these receive that care in a school setting (Burns et al., 1995; Rones & Hoagwood, 2000). In fact, 83% of schools report providing case management for students with behavioral or social problems (Brener et al., 2000). This has many implications for school nurses, putting them in the position to identify problems early on, to promote mental health, and to make referrals for mental health services (DeSocio & Hootman, 2004).

Suicide Attempts

Suicide is the third leading cause of death among young people 15 to 24 years of age. The suicide rate among adolescents aged 15 to 19 years is 8.2 per 100,000 and among children aged 10 to 14 years it is 1.5 per 100,000 (National Institute of Mental Health, 2006). In 2005, 8.4% of high school students reported making at least one suicide attempt (10.8% of females and 6.0% of males), 13% made a suicide plan, and 16.9% seriously considered attempting suicide (CDC, 2006a). Risk factors for suicide include mental disorders such as depressive disorders and substance abuse, family discord, arguments with a boyfriend or girlfriend, school-related problems, hopelessness, and contact with the juvenile justice system.

The Best Practices Registry for suicide prevention, a collaboration between the Suicide Prevention Resource Center and the American Foundation for Suicide Prevention, has been developed. The registry is funded by the Substance Abuse and Mental Health Services Administration. There are six school-based suicide prevention programs that have been identified as either effective or promising. These include C-Care Cast, Columbia University Teen Screen, Lifelines, Reconnecting Youth, SOS Signs of Suicide, and Zuni Life Skill Interventions (Suicide Prevention Resource Center & American Foundation for Suicide Prevention, nd).

DERMATOLOGIC DISORDERS

Skin conditions remain a significant focus of school nursing practice. Nurses must allay fears among school personnel, students, and parents concerning the communicability and transmission of these conditions while providing emotional support. Assisting the student and the family to comply with medical treatment may reduce the severity of the condition. It is important for school nurses and other staff members to recognize the sensitivity of students concerning any skin disorder that may affect their physical appearance or cause their exclusion from school.

Public health laws in most states require exclusion of students who may have conditions or symptoms that are suspected of being communicable. However, school health professionals recognize that there are degrees of contagiousness, and discretion is used in complying with these laws or regulations. For conditions such as tinea capitis, impetigo, and infection with herpesvirus types 1 and 2, it is not usually necessary to immediately exclude the student from school. The school nurse should communicate with parents through notes or telephone calls at the end of the school day, requesting that the student be seen by his or her usual provider of medical care before returning to school. Scabies and pediculosis present no emergency to the child or the school population, and pediculosis should not interrupt a child's education through school exclusion (NASN, 2004b; Sciscione & Krause-Parello, 2007).

Alberta Wilson, the school nurse, discovers that a student, Robert, has pediculosis (head lice). She advises Robert not to share combs and hats, because they are prime means of spreading the infestation. Ms. Wilson calls Robert's parent to advise on treatment, including the use of pediculicidal shampoo and the removal of nits (lice eggs). Ms. Wilson advises school staff to watch for other students who scratch their heads more than usual. The school received numerous telephone calls from concerned parents. With the consent of the school district, Ms. Wilson develops an informational letter on head lice to be sent to all concerned parents. Ms. Wilson assures all persons involved (staff, parents, Robert) that lice infestation is a nuisance condition, not a major health threat.

Fungal Infections

Pathogenic fungi can invade the skin superficially or deeply. Superficial skin invasions are most commonly seen in the school-aged child and may be due to the sharing of objects such as caps, combs, socks, and shoes. Shallow fungal infections affect the skin, hair, and nails.

Tinea corporis begins as small red, colorless, or depigmented circles that get progressively larger. The center of the circle heals as the area grows larger. The borders of the circle are frequently elevated and either scaly and dry or moist and crusty. There may be mild pruritus and pain. *Tinea capitis* (ringworm of the scalp) is the most common cutaneous mycosis in children between the ages of 3 and 7 years and is twice as common in males. *Trichophyton tonsurans* is the major etiologic agent, and the lesions are characterized by the presence of broken hairs at the follicular line; inflamed, circumscribed, pustular or scaly dry patches; and possibly even bald areas. *Microsporum canis* is a less common agent and produces inflammatory papules and pustules. A Wood lamp is effective for screening for *M. canis*, but *T. tonsurans* does not fluoresce (Brodell & Vescera, 2002). *Tinea capitis* is transmitted from person to person and through spores on fomites. Sharing of sports equipment, such as helmets and exercise mats, and personal items, such as combs and barrettes, should be avoided. When incidence is 15% or higher, routine screening may be appropriate. *Tinea capitis* is treated with oral griseofulvin. Treatment for *tinea corporis* includes systemic and topical antifungal agents (Lewis & Bear, 2002; MedlinePlus, 2007).

Bacterial Infections

The skin normally harbors a variety of bacteria. The degree of their pathogenicity depends on variables such as the integrity of the skin, the immune and cellular defenses of the host, and the toxigenicity and invasiveness of the organism. Impetigo is an example of a bacterial infection caused by *Staphylococcus aureus* or *group A beta-hemolytic streptococci,* which can appear after minor trauma or another skin lesion. The resulting highly contagious infection is characterized by pruritus with honey-colored, crusted lesions. The lesions tend to spread peripherally. Treatment includes careful removal of the crusts with soap and water and topical application of an antibiotic ointment. Systemic administration of antibiotics may be used when lesions are extensive (Mayo Clinic Staff, 2007).

Viral Infections

Some viral infections common to school-aged children include verruca (warts), herpes simplex due to herpesvirus type 1 (cold sores) and type 2 (sexually transmitted lesions), herpes zoster (shingles), rubeola (10-day measles), rubella (3-day measles), and varicella zoster (chickenpox). Most of the communicable diseases of childhood and adolescence are associated with rashes, and each rash is characteristic. Treatment is usually symptomatic for pain and discomfort. The goal of therapy in viral illnesses is to prevent secondary infection. Various topical applications are used as palliative therapy. Steroid ointments should not be used, but antibiotic ointment may be used if secondary infection occurs. Antiviral drugs, such as acyclovir (Zovirax), have been used in the treatment of infections caused by herpesvirus types 1 and 2. Sun protection, including sunscreen, is important to prevent recurring herpes simplex due to type 1 herpesvirus. Aspirin should not be given for viral infections because of the potential for the development of Reye's syndrome. Verruca tends to disappear spontaneously, but the growth may be surgically removed or treated with caustic solutions.

Allergic Conditions

Atopic dermatitis (eczema) is a chronic inflammation of the skin that usually begins in infancy. The term refers to a descriptive category of noncontagious dermatologic diseases and not to a specific etiology. The primary symptoms are pruritus and acute epidermal and dermal edema, with vesicles on the face, scalp, trunk, and limbs. Chronic changes characterized by dry flaky skin, secondary fissures, or lichenification are found. Atopic dermatitis has a prevalence rate of 15% in the United States. The three goals of treatment are to heal the skin, treat the symptoms, and prevent flares. New medications known as immune modulators can be used in children older than 2 years of age. Contact dermatitis is an inflammatory reaction of the skin to direct contact with a chemical substance that evokes an allergic hypersensitivity. In both types of dermatitis, reducing exposure to suspected allergens may improve the dermatitis. Treatment of the lesions may also consist of topical corticosteroids for prevention or relief of inflammation and antihistamines to reduce pruritus. Systemic corticosteroids and oral antibiotics may be needed for extensive dermatitis (National Institutes of Health, 2003).

Skin Cancer

Schools can be instrumental in reducing children's exposure to ultraviolet radiation. Skin cancer is now the most common cancer in the United States, and *80% of lifetime sun exposure occurs in childhood and adolescence* (Task Force on Community Preventive Services, 2004; Tillotson, 2006). The CDC has identified guidelines for schools to implement to reduce skin cancer risks through education and appropriate school policies, changes in attitudes, and alteration of environments to reduce exposure to ultraviolet rays. To be successful, such a program needs to include family members and the school staff (CDC, 2002b; NASN, 2005c).

RESPIRATORY CONDITIONS

Acute conditions of the respiratory tract are a common cause of illness in school-aged children. Most upper respiratory infections are caused by viruses and may be self-limiting. However, secondary infections, such as otitis media, acute bronchitis, influenza, and pneumonia, can cause serious complications.

Asthma

Asthma is a major public health problem, and its incidence continues to increase in the United States. More than 6.5 million children currently suffer from asthma (National Center for Health Statistics, 2007). Among students who participated in the YRBS, 17.1% reported having been told that they had asthma sometime in their lives, whereas 14.5% reported it in the 12 months preceding the survey (CDC, 2006f). Asthma accounts for the most absences from school (average of 7.6 days per year), hospital admissions, and emergency department visits for school-aged children. The environment (crowding, poverty, residence in inner cities, and air pollution), environmental tobacco smoke, birth history (prematurity and bronchopulmonary dysplasia), and family history of asthma are all associated with the disease.

Asthma accounts for 14 million lost school days and an estimated $14.7 billion dollars in treatment costs per year for children under 18 years of age (American Lung Association, 2006; 2007). Absence because of asthma is not related exclusively to the severity of the health problems; psychosocial difficulties, frequent physician visits, and activity limitations may also contribute. The reason for the alarming increase in asthma rates is unclear, but increased exposure to environmental irritants and pollutants may be the major culprit. Secondhand smoke may worsen the condition of an estimated 200,000 to 1 million asthmatic children (American Lung Association, 2006). Environmental factors that frequently trigger asthmatic episodes can be addressed in the home, but addressing such factors in the school setting may present difficulties, because air temperature, humidity, and odors from hair sprays, perfumes, and chemicals are not as easily controlled in the school.

Peak flow monitoring of air expelled from the lungs can predict when an asthma episode is likely to occur. The peak flow meter is an invaluable tool in the school setting. It provides information to the school nurse and the student about lung function. It also allows an objective assessment of whether the asthma is under control, whether medication is needed to prevent an attack, and whether the medication is effective. Peak flow monitoring allows the student to alter exercise levels in physical education classes to prevent attacks. Periodic monitoring of the peak flow helps the nurse assess trends in the school-aged child and recognize when the risk of an asthma attack is present. Ideally, each child should have his or her own peak flow meter. One meter may be sufficient for all students, however, as long as individual disposable mouthpieces are used. The instrument and nondisposable mouthpieces should be washed and air-dried between uses.

The school nurse should become involved in the management of asthma in the school-aged child. The nurse can promote a close, cooperative relationship with the student, the family, and the usual source of medical care, which will enhance the student's ability to benefit from his or her educational experience. Currently, there are programs in the schools to reduce asthma exacerbations (Lwebuga-Mukasa & Dunn-Georgiou, 2002), identify environmental allergens and irritants (Cicutto et al., 2006; Tortolero et al., 2002), provide computer-based student education about asthma (Yawn et al., 2000), and reduce asthma absences and hospitalizations (Levy et al., 2006; Splett et al., 2006). The CDC (2006f) has proposed strategies for addressing asthma in a coordinated school health program (Box 30-4). Not all strategies are appropriate for every school. The school and the district should determine what are the highest priorities. The CDC has expertly outlined how each of these strategies can be implemented (CDC, 2006f). In addition, a school toolkit that provides guidance to the school nurse can be found at the American Lung Association website (see Community Resources for Practice at the end of the chapter).

COMMUNICABLE DISEASE AND INFECTION CONTROL

Since the advent of immunization, the incidence of common childhood communicable diseases has declined. Complications from these infections have been reduced through the use of antibiotics and antitoxins. Nevertheless, communicable diseases are a leading cause of childhood morbidity and school absences. Students with signs and symptoms of these diseases are usually excluded from the school setting for the period of communicability and readmitted in accordance with the recommendations of their usual source of medical care, the state epidemiologic and disease control program, and the local school district policy. Children with mild illnesses can still attend school. Excluding children when it is unnecessary may result in work loss by parents, unnecessary visits to the pediatrician, and unneeded treatment with antibiotics. For additional information, refer to Chapter 8.

NUTRITIONAL CONSIDERATIONS

Dietary factors are associated with 4 of the 10 leading causes of death: coronary heart disease, some types of cancer, stroke,

---

BOX 30-4 CDC Strategies for Addressing Asthma

1. Establish management and support systems for asthma-friendly schools.
2. Provide appropriate school health and mental health services for students with asthma.
3. Provide asthma education and awareness programs for students and school staff.
4. Provide a safe and healthy school environment to reduce asthma triggers.
5. Provide safe, enjoyable physical education and activity opportunities for students with asthma.
6. Coordinate school, family, and community efforts to better manage asthma symptoms and reduce school absences among students with asthma.

From Centers for Disease Control and Prevention. (2006). *Healthy youth! Asthma: Strategies for addressing asthma within a coordinated school health program.* Atlanta: Centers for Disease Control and Prevention, National Center for Chronic Disease Prevention and Health Promotion. Retrieved August 8, 2007 from *http://www.cdc.gov/HealthyYouth/asthma/strategies.htm.*
CDC, Centers for Disease Control and Prevention.

and type 2 diabetes (USDHHS, 2000a). Therefore, preventive efforts to change behaviors to protect from future illnesses should begin at school age. Children who learn good nutritional practices can be proactive and take responsibility for developing healthy bodies. Proper nutrition is also important for the mental development of individuals (see Chapter 21).

Children receive mixed messages about diet and nutrition. Families and some school systems encourage children to "stay healthy and eat right" but provide meals that are high in fat and cholesterol and low in needed complex carbohydrates and dietary fiber. Vending machines in schools often provide nutritional choices that are high in fat and carbohydrates. Television networks advertise foods that contain empty calories during programming for children.

Healthy People 2010 stresses nutritional education targeted at school-aged children. Essential topics should increase student knowledge about nutrition, shape attitudes, and develop skills to plan, prepare, and select healthy meals. The program content should include such things as reading food labels, increasing fruit and vegetable consumption, eating foods low in saturated and total fat, and eating foods high in calcium. Physical activity, started at an early age, should be emphasized (USDHHS, 2000a). Schools can provide healthful foods in the school breakfast and lunch programs; physical education can teach fitness activities that can be maintained for life; and classroom instruction can address knowledge, attitudes, and beliefs. However, parents appear to have the greatest influence in changing poor eating behaviors, because they have control over food purchasing, food preparation, peer support among family members, and modeling of positive eating behaviors. If parents are to assist in changing behavior in children, accurate knowledge about food consumption and the health consequences of certain eating patterns is needed. School nurses can provide information to parents about healthy nutrition.

Obesity

Obesity, now defined as an epidemic, is the fastest growing public health problem in the United States. Once a person is overweight, it is difficult both to lose weight and to maintain the weight loss (Wechsler et al., 2004). Primary prevention through integrated nutrition education and physical education should be a focused school health intervention in a coordinated school health program (see the *Healthy People 2010* box on page 762). Appropriate nutritional intake, decreased sedentary behavior, and increased physical activity need to be lifelong family goals encouraged by school intervention programs.

The nurse should be involved in developing school policies that promote lifelong physical activities and healthy eating patterns. Daily physical education and a high-quality comprehensive health education program are important components. The nurse should encourage faculty and staff also to be physically active. Extracurricular activities at school or in the community with the support of staff, families, and the community should to be encouraged (American Obesity Association, 2007; Austin et al., 2006; Cole et al., 2006; Mauriello et al., 2006). Robinson and colleagues (2003) found that providing dance classes as an after-school activity, as well as family intervention, reduced television viewing and weight gain in African American girls. The Child and Adolescent Trial for Cardiovascular Health (CATCH) is an evidenced-based program targeting many aspects of a coordinated school health program, including physical education, food service, and a home component. The program lends itself to adaptation for minority and low-income schools (Coleman et al., 2005).

Type 2 diabetes in school-aged children is also identified as an epidemic. Inactivity and overeating are causes. Children spend many hours in front of computers and television sets and eat supersized portions of high-calorie food. Complications of diabetes (kidney failure, blindness, cardiovascular disease, and amputation) will occur at younger ages and become a serious public health threat. School nurses can be instrumental in promoting healthy changes, such as increased physical activity and consumption of properly proportioned nutritious food. Diabetes is a complex problem that needs major, sustained societal efforts to solve (DiabetoValens.com, 2003; Shaw-Perry et al., 2007).

Eating Disorders

Both anorexia nervosa and bulimia nervosa are characterized by disturbed eating patterns, a preoccupation with weight, and excessive self-evaluation of weight and shape. The overall lifetime prevalence of anorexia nervosa is 0.5% to 1% of adolescents (Eating Disorders Coalition, 2007). Although it is commonly associated with girls and women, males also suffer from anorexia nervosa, especially males involved in sports that focus on leanness (Hatmaker, 2005). Anorexia nervosa has the highest mortality rate of any psychiatric disorder. In the school setting, the anorectic student may be identified as one who has a marked disturbance in body image but regards his or her appearance as normal. These students attempt to hide their appearance by wearing bulky clothing. They may be preoccupied with food (e.g., hoarding snacks, preparing food for others, and obsessively conversing about food). They tend to increase their physical activity, and females may have primary or secondary amenorrhea.

In a recent study of 18- to 25-year-old females, lifetime bulimia nervosa was diagnosed in 4.6% of the subjects (Favaro et al., 2003). Bulimia can be one of two types: purging or nonpurging. Nonpurging bulimia is characterized by alternating periods of binge eating and weight-loss behaviors such as fasting or excessive exercise, but without purging (Striegel-Moore & Franko, 2003; Striegel-Moore et al., 2003). Purging bulimia is characterized by self-induced vomiting or the misuse of laxatives, diuretics, or enemas. There may be wide fluctuations in weight accompanied by depression and overconcern about body weight and shape. A recent review found high rates of comorbid psychopathology among women with eating disorders (O'Brien & Vincent, 2003). Major depression is common in individuals with both anorexia and bulimia, and obsessive-compulsive disorder is common with those with anorexia.

Eating disorders are some of the most difficult of all adolescent disorders to treat. The approach must be multidisciplinary, with input from the primary physician, psychiatrist, school nurse, nutritionist, family members, and peers. The focus must include reinstitution of normal nutrition, resolution of disturbed patterns of family interactions, and individual psychotherapy to correct deficits and distortions in psychologic functions. School health personnel must be patient and understanding and provide opportunities for acceptance and the development of a positive self-image. Physical manifestations should be monitored in students, because serious illness or death can occur. School nurses are a link joining the student, parent, treatment team, and teachers.

The role of school-based programs in the prevention of eating disorders has become the focus of several authors worldwide. Strategies have included methods to build self-esteem, peer involvement, parental involvement, identification of high-risk girls, and teaching of students to deconstruct body image ideals. It is critical to choose school-based programs that will do no harm by introducing students to beliefs, attitudes, and behaviors known to precede eating problems (O'Dea & Maloney, 2000).

DENTAL HEALTH

Dental caries is the single most common chronic childhood disease in the country, five times more common than asthma. Of children in preschool (2 to 3 years old) almost one fifth have at least one tooth with untreated caries. Of younger school-aged children (5 to 7 years old) more than half either have caries or a filling in a primary tooth. Of all children 5 to 17 years of age almost 60% have caries (American Academy of Pediatrics, 2007). There is also disparity in dental health, with 25% of school-aged children experiencing 75% of all dental decay. The two groups most likely to have decay are children living below the poverty level and children with disabilities and special needs. *Healthy People 2010* noted that 6- to 8-year-olds had the same amount of tooth decay in 2000 as in 1986. Childhood decay may be the result of dental infection transmitted from the mother to the child, frequent and consistent exposure to carbohydrates (snacks, soft drinks, hard candies, foods that adhere to the teeth), and omission of or delay in brushing and flossing. Oral disease and the consequences lead to the loss of 51 million school hours each year (Simoyan & Badner, 2002).

There is great need for dental health education. Many physicians do not conduct basic examinations of the mouths of children or provide parents with counseling and referral to a dentist for care. Children entering school programs for the first time should undergo oral health screening, referral, and follow-up for the necessary diagnostic, preventive, and treatment services. The prevention of dental disorders is largely dependent on family commitment. School health personnel can address and improve dental health education and services in the schools and encourage good oral hygiene practices. The school nurse can help increase parental attention to dental issues through the dissemination of information to parents at workshops or in one-to-one parent conferences (USDHHS, 2000b).

The school nurse can develop and deliver health education in dental health, including education on such topics as the need for regular dental checkups, good oral hygiene (proper brushing and the use of dental floss), and sound nutrition practices (restricting cariogenic foods). Early and lifelong commitment to dental health behaviors (e.g., keeping dental appointments and following through on recommended treatments and practices) should be encouraged.

FUTURE TRENDS AND ISSUES IN SCHOOL HEALTH PROGRAMS

There is a consensus that health promotion and education efforts should be centered in and around schools. The schools are the "workplace" for nearly one fifth of the U.S. population. It is clear that the school environment affects the lives of students' families as well as the entire community. Therefore, it is imperative that a school health program provide health promotion activities to address health and social problems that adversely affect learning and productivity. To accomplish this end, there is a need to address the educational, psychosocial, and health needs of students by developing effective health promotion programs that take into consideration the leading causes of morbidity and mortality related to behavior. It is believed that schools could be one of the most efficient means of addressing four main risk factors for chronic disease: tobacco use, unhealthy eating patterns, inadequate physical activity, and obesity (Kolbe et al., 2004). There is evidence that the School Health Index can be used to guide self-assessments, planning of programs, and actual implementation of health promotion programs (Austin et al., 2006; CDC, 2002c).

To accomplish these goals, schools can be expected to collaborate with many components of the community. There will be an increased emphasis on building coalitions with the community (businesses and churches) to address the health needs of students. The concept of the health-promoting school worldwide adheres to similar principles that, in turn, were shaped by the 1986 Ottawa Charter for Health Promotion of the World Health Organization (World Health Organization, 1986). These principles include building healthy public policy, creating supportive environments, strengthening community action, developing personal skills, and reorienting health services (St. Leger, 1999). There is also a need to collaborate with youth to help identify unrecognized needs and to then shape programs to meet those needs (Mandel & Qazilbash, 2005).

There is an increased interest is assuring that these health promotion efforts are evidenced based, and this will undoubtedly continue into the future. Evidenced-based nursing care is the standard of health care practice that is being recommended by nursing overall. There is a need now to develop evidenced-based practice guidelines specific to school nursing. The first step is to identify existing guidelines that are appropriate for school nurses. In addition, there is a need to develop new evidenced-based practice guidelines specific to school nurses and educators addressing health issues in schools. The University of Iowa has established a center to develop these guidelines (Adams & McCarthy, 2007). Other resources that may be helpful are listed in Community Resource for Practice at the end of the chapter.

School nurses are going to be increasingly challenged not only to use evidenced-based protocols but also to show evidence that their efforts have had an impact on the overall health status of children, thereby optimizing the opportunity to learn. There is a continued need to support practice roles for school nurses based on the Standards of Professional School Nursing Practice (Rice et al., 2005). Some other mechanisms to assure the level of competency needed in school nursing include a requirement for continuing education and the establishment of a differentiated practice model that includes three levels of practitioner: generalist, master's prepared, and school nurse policy analyst. Each level is characterized by an increased degree of responsibility (Keller & Ryberg, 2004; Vought-O'Sullivan et al., 2006). There is also a move to convert to electronic records, sometimes using the diagnoses, interventions, and outcomes of the North American Nursing Diagnosis Association, Nursing Interventions Classification, and Nursing Outcomes Classification (Lunney, 2006). These approaches have the potential to increase the links with other systems of care as well as to provide data to support evidenced-based school nursing practice, policy development, and communication of the value of school nursing practice to stake holders.

We are living in a time of great change, marked by a need for a global perspective in school nursing (Denehy, 2006). This demands a knowledge of the health concerns around the world and a sharing of school perspectives with other nurses around the globe. The population of students in the United States, for example, is becoming more diverse, and immigration results in the need for school nurses to increase their knowledge of the cultural heritage of many groups. This knowledge will have to encompass the political or economic events in these families' lives as well as their religious beliefs, health beliefs, practices, and cultural traditions (Denehy, 2006).

There continues to be a need to address the reality of a decrease in fiscal resources at the federal, state, and local levels for these stake holders. Since the 1970s, school nurses have been faced with budgetary cuts that have resulted in a loss of job security. This trend became especially strong in the early 1990s with budgetary deficits at all levels of the government and in the private sector. Efforts continue to reduce the increasing costs of health care, and in a cost-containment environment, school nurses are not exempt from further cutbacks. School health services, including SBHCs, are no exception either. It will be critical to bridge with potential community partners to guarantee the viability of health centers (Geierstanger et al., 2004; Gustafson, 2005).

If school nursing is to survive and continue to grow, efforts must be made to secure funding and to justify the existence of school health programs. One important means of justifying the existence of school health programs is to determine how activities contribute to improving student academic performance (Geierstanger et al., 2004; O'Rourke, 2005). In addition, funding will have to be sought in the public sector through lobbying efforts at the federal, state, and local levels. In the public and private sectors, efforts must also be made to creatively seek funding to address the special needs of children. Managed care organizations might provide a mechanism for increasing resources, and work can continue on developing reasonable and cost-effective models for reimbursement to schools. In addition, it is critical to remember that school nurses are beneficial not only for the students but staff and faculty as well. Creative approaches to reimbursing nurses will require thinking "outside the box" (Perrin et al., 2002).

Innovative programs and responses to opportunities can help not only to secure funds but also to provide the means to evaluate creative approaches to meeting the needs of children. Answers to the following questions are crucial to that effort and to the survival of school nursing:

- Is nursing care making a difference?
- How are the children and adolescents most in need being served?
- What are the health and education benefits that result from school health nursing services?
- How can school nurses most effectively address the complex behavioral and psychosocial risk factors associated with morbidity and mortality in today's adolescents?
- What are the complex legal and moral liabilities surrounding the provision of care by nonmedical personnel?

The future of school nurses depends on innovation, research, and the ability of school nurses to convince communities of the value of their interventions to children and adolescents who are often forgotten and underserved.

KEY IDEAS

1. Comprehensive school health programs must play an important role in promoting the health of children and adolescents. This comprehensive approach will have to include factual knowledge, attitudes, and skill development with respect to health. Additional components of a comprehensive approach for the twenty-first century will include school and community linkages and employee wellness programs.

2. There are eight components of a coordinated school health program. These are health services; health education; provision of a safe and healthy environment; nutrition services; physical education; counseling, psychologic, and social services; health promotion for staff; and parent and community involvement.

3. School health programs are largely under the jurisdiction of state mandates and laws, which results in variation among school health programs across the United States.

4. The responsibilities of the school nurse have evolved from serving a limited function to fulfilling expanded roles that include school nurse practitioner, manager of a school-based clinic, provider in a comprehensive wellness center, and case manager.

5. School nurses function according to standards that can be found in *School Nursing: Scope and Standards of Practice* (American Nurses Association & National Association of School Nurses, 2005). These standards provide direction and a framework for professional school nursing practice.

6. Common functions of the school nurse include providing direct care to students and staff; promoting a healthy environment; promoting health through health education; serving as a liaison between school personnel, family, community, and health care providers; and providing screening and referral for health conditions.

7. It is imperative that school health programs provide health promotion activities for children and families. Many of the objectives of *Healthy People 2010* can be directly attained or advanced by schools.

8. The activities of school nurses influence the mortality and morbidity of children. Problems that must be effectively addressed by school nurses include violence, mental health, substance abuse, accidents, sexually transmitted diseases, pregnancy prevention, and chronic and other physical health problems. Interventions must focus on reduction of high-risk behavior and promotion of healthy lifestyles.

9. There is increasing optimism about the role of schools in promoting the health of children. In the twenty-first century, an opportunity exists for change and innovation in establishing partnerships among schools, families, and communities. This will result in an increased emphasis on policy planning and the need to creatively approach the financing of school health programs.

CASE STUDY Experiences as a School Nurse

Mr. W., a social studies teacher, has just finished going over a classroom drill when he notices that Susan is not looking well. As he moves toward her desk, her arms and legs begin to jerk. He quickens his pace to keep her from falling out of her chair. As he reaches her desk and provides support, he calls to John to press the intercom button at the front of the room. The office asks what is wrong. Mr. W. says that the school nurse is needed immediately. In a calm voice, he reassures the class that Susan will be fine.

In the back of his mind, he is thinking how fortunate he is to have heard a lecture on seizures at the faculty meeting 3 months earlier. "Don't try to stop the movements; protect the student from injury; remain calm," he recalls the school nurse saying. The policy handout *Care of a Student Having a Seizure* was just redistributed at midyear. He remembers thinking that he would never use it, but he is glad he read it.

The school nurse arrives at the classroom door, assesses the situation, and instructs Mr. W. to help place Susan on her side on the floor. Mr. W. then instructs the class to move to an adjacent vacant classroom. Susan's color is poor, but her respirations are within the normal rate.

Fortunately, the last student leaves the room before Susan loses bladder control. After 2 minutes, Susan's seizure stops, and she is moved to the health suite. Although the nurse is aware of Susan's diagnosis of epilepsy, this is Susan's first seizure during school.

Susan is assessed at regular intervals during her recovery period. Susan's mother is notified and assured that her daughter is in no danger. Arrangements are made for a change of clothing to be brought to the school. After about an hour, Susan is alert; her main concern is what her classmates are going to think about her. Arrangements are made to provide information about epilepsy to her classmates during the next period, and the school nurse and Susan will allow her classmates an opportunity to talk. Susan is glad that her classmates did not witness her loss of bladder control and asks how

Mr. W. knows so much about epilepsy. The school nurse uses material from the Epilepsy Foundation to educate Susan's peers. About a week later, the school nurse sees Susan in the lunchroom, and with a subtle wave, Susan indicates she is doing well.

Mrs. H., an English teacher, is waiting to have her blood pressure checked. During the faculty wellness blood pressure screening program, Mrs. H. was referred to her physician. Since that time, she has been taking antihypertension medication. Routine blood pressure checks by the school nurse assist Mrs. H. in maintaining her level of wellness. The faculty wellness program is a natural adjunct to the health services program, because a healthy faculty provides students with a better educational program.

As the nurse finishes recording Mrs. H.'s blood pressure, in walks Thomas, a student with asthma. Thomas is acutely short of breath, diaphoretic, pale, and anxious. The school nurse takes a reading with the peak flow meter and administers the prescribed medication via an inhaler. As for all children with a chronic health condition, the nurse, in collaboration with the primary health care provider and the parents, has developed a plan of care. After the medication begins to take effect, an additional peak flow reading is obtained. Thomas's condition improves, and he becomes less anxious and returns to class within 30 minutes.

The preceding examples illustrate the role of the school nurse in meeting the health needs of a varied school population. It is important to visualize school nurses in the roles of caregiver, health counselor, advocate, consultant, collaborator, educator, and researcher to realize their value to the school community. Because new models for school health are evolving, school nurses must document and promote their services to students, parents, school staff members, and local and state legislators who may control funding sources. The school nurse remains the most cost-effective community resource for maintaining a high level of wellness in school-aged children.

Courtesy Robert Mehl, BSN, RN, school nurse, Baltimore County Public Schools, Towson, Maryland.

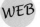

See **Critical Thinking Questions** for this Case Study on the book's website.

LEARNING BY EXPERIENCE AND REFLECTION

1. Spend a day with a school nurse or school nurse practitioner. Observe the nurse interacting with children of various ages. Note the health problems of the students identified by the nurse. What interventions did the nurse provide?
2. Interview a school nurse regarding her or his perception of the role of the nurse in the school. What frustrations and rewards does the nurse experience?
3. Interview school-aged children to determine their perception of health and wellness and of health promotion in their schools. What services are provided? How satisfied are these children with their school health programs? How do their perceptions of health and wellness vary with age?
4. Write an essay on your perception of the concept of comprehensive school health. What should be the components

of a comprehensive school health program? Share your reflections with a school health team member to compare your ideas with an existing program.
5. Interview a school nurse to discuss ethical problems that arise in the school setting. How are ethical issues resolved?
6. Interview a school nurse regarding the care of high-risk children in the school setting (e.g., children with AIDS or disabilities). What barriers exist in caring for these children? How is the nurse involved in educating the school and the community about the needs of these children?
7. Review the health curriculum for a local school system. How does the curriculum address the indicators of child well-being and the *Healthy People 2010* objectives?
8. Review current federal, state, or local legislation related to school health services, education, or the environment.

COMMUNITY RESOURCES FOR PRACTICE

Information about each of the following organizations can be found on its website, which can be accessed through this book's website at *http://evolve.elsevier.com/Maurer/community/*.

Healthy School Environments

American Lung Association
Beyond Pesticides
Children's Environmental Health Network
Environmental Protection Agency
National Clearinghouse for Education Facilities

Alcohol, Tobacco, and Drug Use

American Legacy Foundation
Children of Alcoholics Foundation
Substance Abuse and Mental Health Services Administration

Chronic Diseases

Children's Health Fund—Healthy K.I.D.S.
Internet Resources for Special Children (IRSC)
National Education Association Health Information Network (HEA/HIN)
National Institute of Diabetes and Digestive and Kidney Diseases (NIDDK)
School Nurses Allergy and Asthma Tool Kit

Teen Sexuality

National Campaign to Prevent Teen Pregnancy

Children's Mental Health

Center for the Study and Prevention of Violence, Blueprints for Violence Prevention program
National Institute of Mental Health
National Youth Violence Prevention Resources Center
National Mental Health Association (NMHA)

Health Education—Prevention and Promotion of Health

Children's Health Fund—Healthy B.A.S.I.C.S.

School Health

Division of Adolescent and School Health, Centers for Disease Control and Prevention
Guidelines for Emergency Medical Care in School (publication of the American Academy of Pediatrics)
National Association of School Nurses
National Assembly on School-Based Health Centers
School Health Resource Services (SHRS)

Evidenced-Based Guidelines

Evidence-based guidelines provide summaries of evidence and recommendations for practice from government agencies, professional organizations, and convened expert panels.
Guide to Clinical Preventive Services (U.S. Preventive Services Task Force)—Collection of summaries with associated supporting documentation evaluating preventive measures for a variety of clinical services, including health screenings, immunizations, and counseling.
Guide to Community Preventive Services (Task Force on Community Preventive Services)—Collection of summaries and recommendations detailing the effectiveness, economic efficiency, and feasibility of interventions on a number of health topics.
Morbidity and Mortality Weekly Report, Recommendations and Reports (CDC)—Published reports outlining policy statements for prevention and treatment in all areas within the CDC's scope of responsibility.
National Guideline Clearinghouse (Agency for Healthcare Research and Quality)—Comprehensive, searchable collection of evidence-based clinical practice guidelines.
National Registry of Evidence-Based Programs and Practices (Substance Abuse and Mental Health Services Administration)—Searchable database of interventions for the prevention and treatment of mental and substance use disorders

STUDY AIDS   http://evolve.elsevier.com/Maurer/community/

Visit the Evolve website for this book to find the following study and assessment materials:

- Quiz
- Web Scenario
- Critical Thinking Questions and Answers for Case Studies

- Care Plans
- *Healthy People* Updates
- Glossary

WEBSITE RESOURCES

These items supplement the chapter's topics and are also found on the Evolve site:

30A: Standards of School Nursing Practice

REFERENCES

Adams, S., & McCarthy, A. (2007). Evidence-based practice guidelines and school nursing. *Journal of School Nursing, 23*(3), 128-136.

Adelman, H. (1998). School counseling, psychological, and social services. In E. Marx, S. Wooley, & D. Northrop (Eds.), *Health is academic: A guide to coordinated school health programs* (pp. 42-168). New York: Teachers College Press.

Advisory Committee on Immunization Practice. (2007). Quadrivalent human papillomavirus vaccine. *Morbidity and Mortality Weekly Report, Recommendations and Reports, 56*(RR-2), 1-24.

Alan Guttmacher Institute. (2006a). *In brief: Facts on American teens' sexual and reproductive health.* Retrieved August 3, 2007 from *http://www.guttmacher.org/pubs/fb_ATSRH.html.*

Alan Guttmacher Institute. (2006b). *Sex education: Needs, programs, and politics.* Retrieved February 2, 2007 from *http://www.guttmacher.org/presentations/ed_slides.html.*

Allensworth, D. D. (1994). School health services: Issues and challenges. In P. Cortese & K. Middleton (Eds.), *The comprehensive school health challenge: Promoting health through education* (Vol. 1, pp. 179-212). Santa Cruz, CA: ETR Associates.

Allensworth, D., & Kolbe, L. (1987). The comprehensive school health program: Exploring an expanded concept. *Journal of School Health, 57*(10), 409-412.

American Academy of Pediatrics. (2007). *Children's health topics: Oral health.* Retrieved August 5, 2007 from *http://www.aap.org/healthtopics/oralhealth.cfm.*

American Federation of Teachers (AFT). (nd). Every child needs a school nurse. Retrieved May 16, 2008 from *http://www.aft.org/topics/school-nurses.*

American Lung Association. (2006). *Asthma and children fact sheet.* Retrieved August 8, 2007 from *http://www.lungusa.org/site/apps/nl/content3.asp?c=dvLUK9OOE&b=2058817&content_id={05C5FA0A-A953-4BB6-BB74-F07C2ECCABA9}&notoc=1.*

American Lung Association. (2007). *Asthma in children fact sheet.* Retrieved May 5, 2008 from http://www.lungusa.org/site/apps/n1/content3.asp?c=duLUK90OE&b=205

American Nurses Association. (2007). *Position statement: Assuring safe, high quality health care in pre-K through 12 educational settings.* Retrieved August 1, 2007 from *http://www.nursingworld.org/readroom/position/practice/AssuringSafeHealthCarePreK.pdf.*

American Nurses Association & National Association of School Nurses. (2005). *School nursing: Scope and standards of practice.* Silver Spring, MD: Author.

American Obesity Association. (2007). *Childhood overweight.* Retrieved August 8, 2007 from *http://www.obesity.org/.*

American Psychiatric Association. (2000). *Diagnostic and statistical manual of mental disorders, text revision* (4th ed.). Washington, DC: Author.

Austin, S., Bauer, K., Patel, A., et al. (2006). Swimming upstream: Faculty and staff members from urban schools in low-income communities describe their experience implementing nutrition and physical activity initiatives. *Preventing Chronic Disease, 3*(2), A37.

Austin, S. B., Fung, T., Cohen-Bearak, A., et al. (2006). Facilitating change in school health: A qualitative study of experiences using the School Health Index. *Preventing Chronic Disease, 3*(2), A35.

Bauer, N. S., Lozano, P., & Rivara, F. P. (2007). The effectiveness of the Olweus Bullying Prevention Program in public middle schools: A controlled trial. *Journal of Adolescent Health, 40*(3), 266-274.

Bergren, M. (2004). HIPAA-FERPA revisited. *Journal of School Nursing, 20*(2), 107-112.

Biederman, J. (2005). Attention-deficit/hyperactivity disorder: A selective overview. *Biological Psychiatry, 57*, 1215-1220.

Bleakley, A., Hennessy, M., & Fishbein, A. (2006). Public opinion on sex education in U.S. schools. *Archives of Pediatrics and Adolescent Medicine, 160*(11), 1151-1156.

Botvin, G., & Eng, A. (1982). The efficacy of a multicomponent approach to the prevention of cigarette smoking. *Preventive Medicine, 11*(2), 199-211.

Brener, N. D., Burstein, G. R., DuShaw, M. L., et al. (2001). Health services: Results from the School Health Policies and Programs Study 2000. *Journal of School Health, 71*(7), 294-305.

Brener, N. D., Kann, L., Garcia, D., et al. (2007). Youth risk behavior surveillance—Selected steps communities, 2005. *Morbidity and Mortality Weekly Report, Surveillance Summaries, 56*(2), 1-16.

Brener, N.D., Martindale, J., & Weist, M. D. (2000). Mental health and social services: Results from the School Health Policies and Programs Study 2000. *Journal of School Health, 7*(7), 305-312.

Brener, N. D., Pejavara, A., Barrios, L. C., et al. (2006). Applying the School Health Index to a nationally representative sample of schools. *Journal of School Health, 76*(2), 57-66.

Brindis, C. D., Klein, J., Schlitt, J., et al. (2003). School-based health centers: Accessibility and accountability. *Journal of Adolescent Health, 32S*, 98-107.

Brodell, R. T., & Vescera, G. (2002). Black-dot tinea capitis. *Postgraduate Medicine Online, 114*(4). Retrieved from *http://www.postgradmed.com/issues/2002/04_02/pd_brodell.htm.*

Brown, E., & Simpson, E. (2000). Comprehensive STD/HIV prevention education targeting US adolescents: Review of ethical dilemma and proposed ethical framework. *Nursing Ethics, 7*(4), 339-349.

Bruns, E. J., Walrath, C., Glass-Siegel, M., et al. (2004). School-based mental health services in Baltimore: Association with school climate and special education referrals. *Behavior Modification, 28*(4), 491-512.

Burgeson, C., Wechsler, H., Brener, N., et al. (2001). Physical education and activity: Results from the School Health Policies and Programs Study 2000. *Journal of School Health, 71*(7), 279-293.

Burns, B. J., Costello, E. J., Angold, A., et al. (1995). *Health Affairs, 14*(3), 149-159.

Caldwell, D., Nestle, M., & Rogers, W. (1998). School nutrition services. In E. Marx, S. Wooley, & D. Northrop (Eds.), *Health is academic: A guide to coordinated school health programs* (pp. 195-223). New York: Teachers College Press.

Center for the Study and Prevention of Violence, Institute of Behavioral Science. (2004). *Blueprints for violence prevention overview.* Retrieved August 9, 2007 from *http://www.colorado.edu/cspv/blueprints.*

Centers for Disease Control and Prevention. (1997). Guidelines for school and community programs to promote lifelong physical activity among young people. *Morbidity and Mortality Weekly Report, Recommendations and Reports, 46*(RR-6), 1-36.

Centers for Disease Control and Prevention. (2001). School health guidelines to prevent unintentional injuries and violence. *Morbidity and Mortality Weekly Report, Recommendations and Reports, 50*(RR-22), 1-46.

Centers for Disease Control and Prevention. (2002a). Trends in cigarette smoking among high school students—United States, 1991-2001. *Morbidity and Mortality Weekly Report, 51*(19), 409-412.

Centers for Disease Control and Prevention. (2002b). Guidelines for school programs to prevent skin cancer. *Morbidity and Mortality Weekly Report, Recommendations and Reports, 51*(RR-4), 1-16.

Centers for Disease Control and Prevention. (2002c). *School health index: A self assessment and planning guide.* Atlanta: Department of Health and Human Services.

Centers for Disease Control and Prevention. (2003). *About the program. School health defined.* Retrieved September 5, 2007 from *http://www.cdc.gov/HealthyYouth/CSHP.*

Centers for Disease Control and Prevention. (2005a). *Healthy youth! Coordinated School Health Programs: Comprehensive health education.* Retrieved July 7, 2007 from *http://www.cdc.gov/HealthyYouth/CSHP/comprehensive_ed.htm.*

Centers for Disease Control and Prevention. (2005b). *SHPPS 2000.* Retrieved June 25, 2007 from *http://www.cdc.gov/HealthyYouth/shpps/overview/index.htm.*

Centers for Disease Control and Prevention. (2006a, June 9). Youth risk behavior surveillance. United States: 2005. *Morbidity and Mortality Weekly Report, Surveillance Summaries*, 55(SS-5), 1-108.

Centers for Disease Control and Prevention. (2006b). *Healthy youth! Health topics: Physical activity*. Retrieved July 28, 2007 from *http://www.cdc.gov/HealthyYouth/physicalactivity/facts.htm.*

Centers for Disease Control and Prevention. (2006c). Cigarette use among high school students—U.S., 1991-2005. *Morbidity and Mortality Weekly Report*, 55(26), 724-726.

Centers for Disease Control and Prevention. (2006d). *CDC HIV/AIDS fact sheet: HIV/AIDS among youth*. Retrieved August 3, 2007 from *http://www.cdc.gov/hiv/resources/factsheets/youth.htm.*

Centers for Disease Control and Prevention, National Center for Injury Prevention and Control. (2006e). *Web-based Injury Statistics Query and Reporting System (WISQARS)* (interactive online database) (cited 2006 Feb 8). Retrieved May 12, 2008 from *http://www.cdc.gov/ncipc/wisqars.*

Centers for Disease Control and Prevention. (2006f). *Healthy youth! Asthma: Strategies for addressing asthma within a coordinated school health program*. Atlanta: Centers for Disease Control and Prevention, National Center for Chronic Disease Prevention and Health Promotion. Retrieved August 8, 2007 from *http://www.cdc.gov/HealthyYouth/asthma/strategies.htm.*

Centers for Disease Control and Prevention. (2007a). *Healthy youth! Coordinated school health programs*. Retrieved June 20, 2007 from *http://www.cdc.gov/healthyyouth/CSHP/.*

Centers for Disease Control and Prevention. (2007b). *Healthy youth! Physical Education Curriculum Analysis Tool (PECAT)*. Retrieved July 28, 2007 from *http://www.cdc.gov/HealthyYouth/PECAT/index.htm.*

Centers for Disease Control and Prevention. (2007c). *Healthy youth! Health topics: Sexual risk behaviors*. Retrieved July 31, 2007 from *http://www.cdc.gov/healthyyouth/sexualbehaviors/index.htm.*

Changing times, changing needs, changing programs (Editorial). (1952) *Public Health Nursing*, 44(4), 171-172. Reprinted in *Public Health Nursing*, 2005, 22(3), 267-268.

Childstats.gov. (2007). *America's children: Key national indicators of well-being, 2007*. Retrieved August 3, 2007 from *http://www.childstats.gov/americaschildren/highlights.asp.*

Chmelynski, C. (2004). *More districts see benefits of school-based health clinics*. Retrieved July 28, 2007 from *http://www.nsba.org/site/doc_sbn.asp?TRACKID=&VID=58&CID=1140&DID=34823.*

Cicutto, L., Conti, E., Evans, H., et al. (2006). Creating asthma-friendly schools: A public health approach. *Journal of School Health*, 76(6), 255-258.

Cohn, S. (2007). *Re: Improving the interaction of FERPA and the HIPAA Privacy Rule with regard to school health records* [Letter]. Retrieved July 14, 2007 from *http://www.ncvhs.hhs.gov/070621lt1.pdf.*

Cole, K., Waldrop, J., D'Auria, J., et al. (2006). An integrative research review: Effective school-based childhood overweight interventions. *Journal of the Society of Pediatric Nurses*, 11(3), 166-177.

Coleman, K., Tiller, C., Sanchez, J., et al. (2005). Prevention of the epidemic increase in child risk of overweight in low-income schools. *Archives of Pediatrics and Adolescent Medicine*, 159(3), 217-224.

Collins, J., Robin, L., Wooley, S., et al. (2002). Programs-that-work: CDC's guide to effective programs that reduce health-risk behavior of youth. *Journal of School Health*, 72(3), 93-100.

Constante, C. (2006). School health nursing services role in education: The No Child Left Behind Act of 2001. *Journal of School Nursing*, 22(3), 142-147.

Davis, N. M. (2005). Depression in children and adolescents. *Journal of School Nursing*, 21(6), 311-317.

Denehy, J. (2006). Moving toward a global perspective of school nursing. *Journal of School Nursing*, 22(5), 247-249.

Dent, C., Sussman, S., Stacy, A., et al. (1995). Two-year behavior outcomes of project Towards No Tobacco Use. *Journal of Consulting and Clinical Psychology*, 63(4), 676-677.

DeSocio, J., & Hootman, J. (2004). Children's mental health and school success. *Journal of School Nursing*, 20(4), 189-196.

DiabetoValens.com. (2003). *Type II diabetes—Kid's epidemic*. Retrieved September 24, 2003 from *http://my.diabetovalens.com/diab_kids/epidemic.asp.*

Doyle, J. (2003). Disaster preparedness: Are you ready? *NASN Newsletter*, 18(3), 11-14.

Duncan, P., & Igoe, J. B. (1998). School health services: Issues and challenges. In E. Marx, S. Wooley, & D. Northrup (Eds.), *Health is academic: A guide to coordinated school health programs* (pp. 169-194). New York: Teachers College Press.

Dusenbury, L., & Falco, M. (1995). Eleven components of effective drug abuse prevention curricula. *Journal of School Health*, 65(10), 420-425.

Eating Disorders Coalition. (2007). *Eating disorder statistics*. Retrieved August 9, 2007 from *http://www.eatingdisorderscoalition.org/reports/FactSheet9Million.pdf.*

Epstein, J., Sanders, M., Simon, B., et al. (2002). *School, family and community partnership: Your handbook for action* (2nd ed.). Thousand Oaks, CA: Corwin Press.

Erickson, C. D., Splett, P. L., Mullett, S. S., et al. (2006). The health learner model for student chronic condition management—Part 1. *Journal of School Nursing*, 22(6), 310-318.

Faraone, S. V., Sergeant, J., Gillberg, C., et al. (2003). The worldwide prevalence of ADHD: Is it an American condition? *World Psychiatry*, 2, 104-113.

Favaro, A., Ferrara, S., & Santonastaso, P. (2003). The spectrum of eating disorders in young women: A prevalence study in a general population sample. *Psychosomatic Medicine*, 65(4), 701-708.

Fekkes, M., Pijpers, F. I. M., & Verloove-Vanhorick, S. P. (2004). Bullying behaviour and associations with psychosomatic complaints and depression in victims. *Journal of Pediatrics*, 144, 17-22.

Fetro, J. (1998). Implementing coordinated school health program in local schools. In E. Marx, S. Wooley, & D. Northrop. *Health is academic: A guide to coordinated school health programs* (pp. 15-42). New York: Teachers College Press.

Fothergill, K., & Ballard, E. (1998). The school-linked health center: A promising model of community-based care for adolescents. *Journal of Adolescent Health*, 23, 29-38.

Fox, J., Elliot, D., Kerlikowske, R., et al. (2003). Bully prevention is crime prevention. *Public Health Reports*, 121(4), 419-427.

Fox, H., Limb, S., & McManus, M. (2007). *The public health insurance cliff for older adolescents*. Retrieved August 7, 2007 from *http://www.incenterstrategies.org/jan07/factsheet4.pdf.*

Geierstanger, S. P., Amaral, G., Mansour, M., et al. (2004). School-based health centers and academic performance: Research, challenges, and recommendations. *Journal of School Health*, 74(9), 347-352.

Geller, R., Rubin, I., Nodvin, J., et al. (2007). Safe and healthy school environments. *Pediatric Clinics of North America*, 54, 351-373.

Glass, N., Fredland, N., Campbell, J., et al. (2003). Adolescent dating violence: Prevalence, risk factors, health outcomes, and implications for clinical practice. *Journal of Obstetric, Gynecologic, and Neonatal Nursing*, 32, 1-12.

Graham, J., Shirm, S., Liggin, R., et al. (2006). Mass-casualty events at schools: A national preparedness survey. *Pediatrics*, 117(1), e8-e15.

Gustafson, E. M. (2005). History and overview of school-based health centers in the US. *Nursing Clinics of North America*, 40, 595-606.

Hahn, R., Fuqua-Whitley, D., Wethington, H., et al. (2007). The effectiveness of universal school-based programs for the prevention of violent and aggressive behaviour. *Morbidity and Mortality Weekly Report, Recommendations and Reports*, 56(RR-7).

Hahn, E. J., Noland, M. P., Rayens, M. K., et al. (2002). Efficacy of training and fidelity of implementation of the life skills training program. *Journal of School Health*, 72(7), 282-288.

Hamilton, B. E., Martin, J. A., & Ventura, S. J. (2006). *Births: Preliminary data for 2005*. Hyattsville, MD: National Center for Health Statistics.

Hatmaker, G. (2005). Boys with eating disorders. *Journal of School Nursing, 21*(6), 329-332.

Hawkins, J. W., Hayes, E. R., & Corliss, C. (1994). School nursing in America 1902-1904: A return to public health nursing. *Public Health Nursing, 11*(6), 416-425.

Healthy Schools Network. (2007). *Home page.* Retrieved July 5, 2007 from *http://www. healthyschools.org.*

Hickman, L. J., Jaycox, L. H., & Aronoff, J. (2004). Dating violence among adolescents: Prevalence, gender distribution, and prevention program effectiveness. *Trauma, Violence, and Abuse, 5*(2), 123-142.

Igoe, J. (1975). The school nurse practitioner. *Nursing Outlook, 23*, 381.

Johnson, P. E., Hayes, J. M. (2006). Medication use in schools. *American Journal of Health-System Pharmacy, 63*, 1277-1285.

Jones, S. E., Brener, N., & McManus, T. (2003). Prevalence of school policies, programs, and facilities that promote a healthy physical school environment. *American Journal of Public Health, 93*(9), 1570-1575.

Kann, L., Brener, N. D., & Allensworth, D. D. (2001). Health education: Results from School Health Policies and Programs Study 2000. *Journal of School Health, 71*(7), 266-278.

Kann, L., Collins, J., Pateman, B., et al. (1995). The School Health Policies and Programs Study (SHPPS): Rationale for a nationwide status report on school health programs. *Journal of School Health, 65*(8), 291-294.

Keller, T., & Ryberg, J. (2004). A differentiated practice model for school nursing. *Journal of School Nursing, 20*(5), 249-256.

Kennedy, M. S. (2003). School nursing: A successful experiment: Celebrating 100 years of service. *American Journal of Nursing, 103*(2), 102-103.

Kim, Y. S., Koh, Y., & Leventhal, B. (2005). School bullying and suicide risk in Korean middle school students. *Pediatrics, 115*(2), 357-363.

Kimel, L. (2006). Lack of follow up exams after failed school vision screenings: An investigation of contributing factors. *Journal of School Nursing, 22*(3), 156-162.

Kings County Health Department. (2003). *Public health announces dramatic decline in teen pregnancies, births, and abortions in Seattle and Kings County.* Retrieved September 20, 2003 from *http://www.mereokc.gov/health/yhs.*

Kirby, D. (2001). *Emerging answers: Research findings on programs to reduce teen pregnancy (summary).* Washington, DC: National Campaign to Prevent Teen Pregnancy.

Kolbe, L., Kann, L., Patterson, B., et al. (2004). Enabling the nation's schools to help prevent heart disease, stroke, cancer, COPD, diabetes, and other serious health problems. *Public Health Reports, 119*, 286-302.

Lear, J. G. (2002). Schools and adolescent health: Strengthening services and improving outcomes. *Journal of Adolescent Health, 31*, 310-320.

Levy, M., Heffner, B., Stewart, T., et al. (2006). The efficacy of asthma case management in an urban school district in reducing school absences and hospitalizations for asthma. *Journal of School Health, 76*(6), 320-324.

Lewis, K., & Bear, B. (2002). *Manual of school health* (2nd ed.). St. Louis: Saunders.

Lohrmann, D., Blake, S., Collins, T., et al. (2001). Evaluation of school-based HIV prevention education programs in New Jersey. *Journal of School Health, 7*(6), 207-212.

Lohrmann, D. K., & Wooley, S. F. (1998). Comprehensive school health education. In E. Marx, S. Wooley, & D. Northrop (Eds.), *Health is academic: A guide to coordinated school health programs* (pp. 43-66). New York: Teachers College Press.

Lowry, R., Wechsler, H., Kann, L., et al. (2001). Recent trends in participation in physical education among US high school students. *Journal of School Health, 71*(4), 145-152.

Lunney, M. (2006). NANDA diagnoses, NIC interventions, and NOC outcomes used in an electronic health record with elementary school children. *Journal of School Nursing, 22*(2), 94-101.

Lwebuga-Mukasa, J., & Dunn-Georgiou, E. (2002). A school based asthma intervention program in the Buffalo, New York, schools. *Journal of School Health, 72*(1), 27-33.

Mahat, G., Scoloveno, M., Ruales, N., et al. (2006). Preparing peer educators for teen HIV/AIDS prevention. *Journal of Pediatric Nursing, 21*(5), 378-384.

Mandel, L. A., & Qazilbash, J. (2005). Youth voices as change agents: Moving beyond the medical model in school-based health center practice. *Journal of School Health, 75*(7), 239-242.

Mason, H. (2003). *Peer education: Promoting healthy behaviors.* Washington, DC: Advocates for Youth.

Mathematica Policy Research. (2001). *Changes in children's diets: 1989-91 to 1994-96. Final report submitted to the U.S. Department of Agriculture.* Princeton, NJ: Mathematica Policy Research Inc.

Mauriello, L., Driskell, M., Sherman, K., et al. (2006). Acceptability of a school-based intervention for the prevention of adolescent obesity. *Journal of School Nursing, 22*(5), 269-272.

Mayo Clinic Staff. (2007). *Skin: Impetigo. Mayo Clinic.com.* Retrieved August 3, 2007 from *http://www.mayoclinic. com/health/impetigo/DS00464.*

McCarthy, A. M., Kelly, M. W., & Reed, D. (2000). Medication administration practices of school nurses. *Journal of School Health, 70*(9), 371-376.

MedlinePlus. (2007). *Medical encyclopedia: Tinea corporis.* Retrieved August 3, 2007 from *http:// www.nlm.nih.gov/medlineplus/ency/ article/000877.htm.*

Miller, N. (Ed.). (1995). *The healthy school handbook.* Washington, DC: National Education Association.

Moses, M., Gilchrest, C., Schwab, N. (2005). Section 504 of the Rehabilitation Act: Determining eligibility and implications for school districts. *Journal of School Nursing, 21*(1), 48-58.

Nabors, L., Iobast, E. A., & McGrady, M. E. (2007). Evaluation of school-based smoking prevention programs. *Journal of School Health, 77*(6), 331-333.

Nansel, T. R., Overpeck, M. D., Haynie, D. L., et al. (2003). Relationships between bullying and violence among U.S. youth. *Archives of Pediatrics and Adolescent Medicine, 157*, 348-353.

Nastasi, B., & Clements, D. (1991). Research on cooperative learning: Implications for practice. *School Psychology Review, 20*(1), 110-131.

National Association of School Nurses. (2002). *Issue brief: School health nursing services, role in health care.* Retrieved August 7, 2007 from *http://www.nasn.org/Default.aspx?tabid=279.*

National Association of School Nurses. (2003a). *Position statement: The role of the advanced practice registered nurse.* Retrieved August 7, 2007 from *http://www.nasn.org/Default. aspx?tabid=197.*

National Association of School Nurses. (2003b). *Position statement: Medication administration in the school setting.* Retrieved August 7, 2007 from *http://www.nasn.org/Default.aspx?tabid=230.*

National Association of School Nurses. (2004a). *AHA scientific statement: Response to cardiac arrest and selected life-threatening medical emergencies: The medical emergency response plan for schools.* Retrieved July 14, 2007 from *http://www.nasn.org/Portals/0/statements/ jointstatementcardiac.pdf.*

National Association of School Nurses. (2004b). *Position statement: Pediculosis in the school community.* Retrieved August 2, 2007 from *http://www.nasn.org/Default.aspx?tabid=237.*

National Association of School Nurses. (2005a). *School nurse role in bioterrorism emergency preparedness and response.* Retrieved July 14, 2007 from *http://www.nasn.org/Default. aspx?tabid=205.*

National Association of School Nurses. (2005b). *Position statement: Environment impact concerns in the school setting.* Retrieved July 29, 2007 from *http://www.nasn.org/Default. aspx?tabid=293.*

National Association of School Nurses. (2005c). *Position statement: The school nurse and sun protection.* Retrieved August 5, 2007 from *http://www.nasn.org/Default.aspx?tabid=251.*

National Association of School Nurses. (2006a). *Position statement: Caseload assignments.* Retrieved August 20, 2007 from *http://www. nasn.org/Default.aspx?tabid=209.*

National Association of School Nurses. (2006b). *Issue brief: Individuals with Disabilities Education Act (IDEA): Management of children in the least restrictive environment.* Retrieved July 14, 2007 from *http://www.nasn.org/Default. aspx?tabid=274.*

National Association of School Nurses. (2006c). *Position statement: Delegation.* Retrieved August 7, 2007 from *http://www.nasn.org/Default.aspx?tabid=349.*

National Association of School Nurses. (2007). *Resolution: Vending machines and healthy food choices in school.* Retrieved July 2, 2007 from *http://www.nasn.org/Portals/0/statements/resolutionvending.pdf.*

National Association of State Boards of Education. (2001). Results from CDC's School Health Policies and Programs Study 2000. *Policy Update, 9*(11), 1-2. Retrieved May 12, 2008 from *http://www.nasbc.org/nw_resources_section/policy_yslater/PU_CDC_School_Health_2000_Results_12.01.pdf.*

National Board of Certification of School Nurses. (nd). *Examination: Eligibility.* Retrieved July 29, 2007 from *http://www.nbcsn.com/examdefault.htm#eligibility.*

National Institute on Drug Abuse. (2003). *Preventing drug abuse among children and adolescents: A research-based guide for parents, educators, and community leaders.* Washington, DC: NIH Publications.

National Center for Health Statistics. (2007). *Asthma prevalence, health care use, and mortality: United States 2003-05.* Retrieved August 20, 2007 from *http://www.cdc.gov/nchs/products/pubs/pubd/hestats/ashtma03-05/asthma03-05.htm.*

National Institute of Mental Health. (2006). *Suicide in the U.S.: Statistics and prevention.* Retrieved August 8, 2007 from *http://www.nimh.nih.gov/publicat/harmsway.cfm#children.*

National Institutes of Health, National Institute of Arthritis and Musculoskeletal and Skin Disease. (2003). *Atopic dermatitis.* Retrieved August 9, 2007 from *http://www.niams.nih.gov/hi/topics/dermatitis/index.html.*

National Mental Health Information Center. (2003). *Major depression in children and adolescents.* Substance Abuse and Mental Health Services Administration. Retrieved September 22, 2007 from *http://mental-health.samhsa.gov/publications/allpubs/CA-0011/default.asp.*

O'Brien, K. M., & Vincent, N. K. (2003). Psychiatric co-morbidity in anorexia and bulimia nervosa: Nature, prevalence, and causal relationships. *Child Psychology Review, 23,* 57-74.

O'Dea, J., & Maloney, D. (2000). Preventing eating and body image problems in children and adolescents using the health promoting schools framework. *Journal of School Health, 70*(1), 18-21.

Ogden, C., Carroll, M., Curtin, L., et al. (2006). Prevalence of overweight and obesity in the United States, 1999-2004. *Journal of the American Medical Association, 25,* 1549-1555.

O'Rourke, T. W. (2005). Promoting school health—an expanded paradigm. *Journal of School Health, 75*(3), 112-114.

Pbert, L., Osganian, S. K., Gorak, D., et al. (2006). A school nurse-delivered adolescent smoking cessation intervention: A randomized controlled trial. *Preventive Medicine, 43,* 312-320.

Perrin, K. M., Goad, S. L., & Williams, C. (2002). Can school nurses save money by treating school employees as well as students? *Journal of School Health, 72*(7), 305-306.

Planned Parenthood. (2006). *Pregnancy and child-bearing among U.S. teens.* Retrieved August 2, 2007 from *http://www.plannedparenthood.org/news-articles-press/politics-policy-issues/teen-pregnancy-sex-education/teen-pregnancy-6239.htm.*

Poland, S. (2003). Key players in crisis planning, response, and prevention. *NASN Newsletter, 18*(1), 25-26.

Rice, S. K., Biordi, D. L., & Zeller, R. A. (2005). The relevance of standards of professional school nursing practice. *Journal of School Nursing, 21*(5), 293-298.

Ricketts, S. (2006). School-based health centers and the decline in black teen fertility during the 1990's in Denver, Colorado. *American Journal of Public Health, 96*(9), 1588-1592.

Robbins, A. (1995). Creating an allergy free classroom. In N. L. Miller (Ed.), *The healthy school handbook: Conquering the sick building syndrome and other environmental hazards in and around your school* (p. 329). Washington, DC: National Education Association.

Robinson, T., Killen, J., Kraemer, H., et al. (2003). Dance and reducing television viewing to prevent weight gain in African American girls: The Stanford GEM pilot study. *Ethnicity and Disease, 13*(1, suppl 1), 565-577.

Rones, M., & Hoagwood, K. (2000). School-based mental health services: A research review. *Clinical Child and Family Psychology Review, 3*(4), 223-241.

Safe Kids USA. (2006). *Seasonal safety: No. 1 cause of injury in elementary school: Playground accidents.* Retrieved July 29, 2007 from *http://www.usa.safekids.org/tier3_cd.cfm?content_item_id=23310&folder_id=301.*

School Employee Wellness. (2006). *A guide for protecting the assets of our nation's schools.* Retrieved July 6, 2007 from *http://www.schoolempwell.org.*

Schumacher, C. (2002). Lina Rogers: A pioneer in school nursing. *Journal of School Nursing, 185,* 247-249.

Schwah, N. (2005). HIPAA and schools: Fact sheet. *NASN Newsletter, 20*(1), 6-7.

Sciscione, P., & Krause-Parello, C. (2007). No-nit policies in schools: Time for change. *Journal of School Nursing, 23*(1), 13-20.

Seffrin, J. (1990). The comprehensive school health curriculum: Closing the gap between state-of-the-art and state-of-the-practice. *Journal of School Health, 60*(4), 151-156.

Shaw-Perry, M., Horner, C., Trevino, R., et al. (2007). NEEMA: A school-based diabetes risk prevention program designed for African-American children. *Journal National Medical Association, 99*(4), 368-375.

Simoyan, O., & Badner, V. (2002). Implementing a school-based dental health program: The Montefiore Model. *Journal of School Health, 72*(6), 262-264.

Splett, P. L., Erickson, C. D., Belseth, S. B., et al. (2006). Evaluation and sustainability of the healthy learners asthma initiative. *Journal of School Health, 176*(6), 276-282.

St. Leger, L. H. (1999). The opportunities and effectiveness of the health promoting primary school in improving child health—A review of the claims and evidence. *Health Education Research, 14*(1), 51-69.

Stock, J., Larter, N., Kieckehefer, G. M., et al. (2002). Measuring outcomes of school nursing services. *Journal of School Nursing, 18*(6), 353-359.

Striegel-Moore, R. H., Dohm, F.A., Kraemer, H. C., et al. (2003). Eating disorders in white and black women. *American Journal of Psychiatry, 160*(7), 1326-1331.

Striegel-Moore, R. H., & Franko, D. L. (2003). Epidemiology of binge eating disorder. *International Journal of Eating Disorders, 34*(S), 19-29.

Suicide Prevention Resource Center & American Foundation for Suicide Prevention. (nd). *Section 1b: SPRC/AFSP evidenced-based practices project.* Retrieved August 8, 2007 from *http://www.sprc.org/featured_resources/bpr/ebpp.asp.*

Sullivan, T. N., Farrell, A. D., & Kliewer, W. (2006). Peer victimization in early adolescence: Association between physical and relational victimization and drug use, aggression, and delinquent behaviors among urban middle school students. *Development and Psychopathology, 18,* 119-137.

Task Force on Community Preventive Services. (2004). Recommendation to prevent skin cancer by reducing exposure to ultraviolet radiation. *American Journal of Preventive Medicine, 27*(5), 467-470.

Thackaberry, J. (2003). School health law: What private school nurses need to know. *NASN Newsletter, 18*(3), 21-22.

Tillotson, B. (2006). Encouraging sun safety for children and adolescents. *Journal of School Nursing, 22*(3), 136-141.

Tingen, M. S., Waller, J. L., Smith, T. M., et al. (2006). Tobacco prevention in children and cessation in family members. *Journal of the American Academy of Nurse Practitioners, 18,* 169-179.

Tortolero, S. R., Bartholomew, L. K., Tyrrell, S., et al. (2002). Environmental allergens and irritants in schools: A focus on asthma. *Journal of School Health, 72*(1), 33-39.

Trossman, S. (2007). Issues up close: Is the school nurse in? ANA promotes strategies to help meet students' health and safety needs. *American Nurse Today, 2*(8), 38-40.

U.S. Department of Education. (2003). *Overview: Fact sheet on the major provisions of the conference report to H.R.1, the No Child Left Behind Act.* Retrieved August 7, 2007 from *http://www.ed.gov/nclb/overview/intro/factsheet.html.*

U.S. Department of Education. (2006). *Overview: OSER: Office of Special Education and Rehabilitative Services*. Retrieved July 14, 2007 from *http://www.ed.gov/about/offices/list/osers/osep/index.html*.

U.S. Department of Education. (2007). *Family educational rights and privacy (FERPA)*. Retrieved July 14, 2007 from *http://www.ed.gov/policy/gen/guide/fpco/ferpa/index.html*.

U.S. Department of Education, National Center for Education Statistics. (2005). *Overview of public elementary and secondary students, staff, schools, school districts, revenues, and expenditures: School year 2004-05 and fiscal year 2004*. Retrieved July 7, 2007 from *http://nces.ed.gov/pubs2007/overview04/tables/table_4.asp?referer=list*.

U.S. Department of Health and Human Services. (1999). *Mental health: A report of the Surgeon General, executive summary*. Rockville, MD: U.S. Department of Health and Human Services, Substance Abuse and Mental Health Services Administration, Center for Mental Health Services, National Institutes of Health, National Institute of Mental Health.

U.S. Department of Health and Human Services. (2000a). *Healthy people 2010: Understanding and improving health* (2nd ed.). Washington, DC: U.S. Government Printing Office.

U.S. Department of Health and Human Services. (2000b). *Oral health in America: A report of the Surgeon General—Executive summary*. Rockville, MD: National Institutes of Health, National Institute of Dental and Craniofacial Research.

U.S. Department of Health and Human Services. (2007). *Impact of four Title V, Section 510 abstinence education programs: Final report*. Washington, DC: U.S. Government Printing Office.

U.S. Department of Health and Human Services, Federal Interagency Forum on Child and Family Statistics. (2001). *America's children: Key national indicators of well-being, 2001*. Washington, DC: U.S. Government Printing Office.

U.S. Department of Health and Human Services, Health Resources and Services Administration, Maternal and Child Health Bureau. (2004). *The National Survey of Children with Special Health Care Needs chartbook 2001*. Rockville, MD: U.S. Department of Health and Human Services.

U.S. Department of Labor. (2007). *OSHA facts— August 2007*. Retrieved August 7, 2007 from *http://www.osha.gov/as/opa/oshafacts.html*.

U.S. Environmental Protection Agency, Office of Children's Health. (2007). *HealthySEAT: Healthy school environments assessment tool*. Retrieved July 4, 2007 from *http://epa.gov/schools/healthyseat/*.

Van der Lee, J., Mokkink, L. B., Grootenhuis, M. A., et al. (2007). Definitions and measurement of chronic health conditions in childhood. *Journal of the American Medical Association, 297*(24), 2741-2751.

Veselak, K. E. (2001). Historical steps in the development of the modern school program. *Journal of School Health, 71*(8), 369-372.

Vessey, J. A., & McGowan, K. A. (2006). A successful public health experiment: School nursing. *Pediatrics, 32*(3), 255-256.

Vought-O'Sullivan, V., Meehan, N. K., Havice, P. A., et al. (2006). Continuing education: A national imperative for school nursing practice. *Journal of School Nursing, 22*(1), 2-8.

Walsh, E. (1997). Prevention of adolescent substance abuse: Choosing and implementing a program. *Journal of Addiction Nursing, 9*(4), 173-181.

Watkins, S. (2001). *Foods sold in competition with USDA school meal programs*. Report to Congress on January 12, 2001. Alexandria, VA: U.S. Department of Agriculture, Food and Nutrition Service.

Wechsler, H., McKenna, M., Lee, S., et al. (2004, December). The role of schools in preventing childhood obesity. *The State Education Standard, 15*(2), 4-12.

Weist, M. D. (1999). Challenges and opportunities in expanded school mental health. *Clinical Psychology Review, 19*, 239-253.

Weist, M. D., & Christodulu, K. V. (2000). Expanded school mental health programs: Advancing reform and closing the gap between research and practice. *Journal of School Health, 70*(5), 201-205.

Wenter, D. L., Ennett, S. T., Ribisl, K. M., et al. (2002). Comprehensiveness of substance use prevention programs in U.S. middle schools. *Journal of Adolescent Health, 30*, 455-462.

Whitehead, D. (2006). The health-promoting school: What role for nursing? *Journal of Clinical Nursing, 15*, 264-271.

Wiehe, S. E., Garrison, N. M., Christakis, D. A., et al. (2005). A systematic review of school-based smoking prevention trials with long term follow-up. *Journal of Adolescent Health, 36*, 162-169.

Wold, S., & Dagg, N. (1981). School nursing: A passing experiment? In S. Wold (Ed.), *School nursing* (pp. 3-19). North Branch, MN: Sunrise River Press.

World Health Organization. (1986). *Ottawa Charter for Health Promotion*. Geneva: Author.

Yawn, B., Algatt-Bergstrom, P., Yawn, R., et al. (2000). An in-school CD-ROM asthma education program. *Journal of School Health, 70*(4), 153-159.

Zantal-Wiener, K. (1998). Preschool services for children with handicaps. *ERIC Digest 450*. Retrieved October 10, 2003 from *http://www.ericdigests.org/pre-928/preschool.htm* .

SUGGESTED READINGS

American Nurses Association & National Association of School Nurses. (2005). *School nursing: Scope and standards of practice*. Silver Spring, MD: Author.

Barnes, S. P., Torrens, A., George, V., et al. (2007). The use of portfolios in coordinated school health programs: Benefits and challenges to implementation. *Journal of School Health, 77*(4), 171-179.

Birnbaum, A. S., Lytle, L. A., Perry, C. L., et al. (2003). Developing a school functioning index for middle schools. *Journal of School Health, 73*(6), 232-238.

Centers for Disease Control and Prevention. (2001). *State-level school health policies and practices: A state-by-state summary from the School Health Policies and Programs Study 2000*. Atlanta: U.S. Department of Health and Human Services.

Hallfors, D., Cho, H., Sanchez, V., et al. (2006). Efficacy vs effectiveness trial results of an indicated "model" substance abuse program: Implications for public health. *American Journal of Public Health, 96*(12), 2254-2259.

Igoe, J. (1995). School health: Designing the policy environment through understanding. *Nursing Policy Forum, 1*(3), 12-36.

Igoe, J. (1994). School nursing. *Nursing Clinics of North America, 29*(3), 443-458.

Institute of Medicine. (1997). *Schools and health: Our nation's investment*. Washington, DC: National Academy Press.

Schainker, E., O'Brien, M. J., Fox, D., et al. (2005). School nursing services. *Archives of Pediatrics and Adolescent Medicine, 159*, 83-87.

Silkworth, C., Arnold, M., Harrigan, J., et al. (Eds.). (2005). *Individualized healthcare plans for the school nurse*. North Branch, MN: Sunrise River Press.

Taras, H., & Potts-Datema, W. (2005). Chronic health conditions and student performance at school. *Journal of School Health, 75*(7), 255-266.

Home Health Care

*Robyn Rice**

FOCUS QUESTIONS

What is the relationship between community/public health nursing and home health care nursing?

What are the responsibilities of the home health care nurse relative to other members of the home health care team?

What are the major sources of reimbursement for home health care, and how are agencies paid for service (prospectively or retrospectively)?

In what ways do third-party payers influence care that is provided in the home?

How does the application of universal precautions in the home differ from their application in the hospital?

What is the impact of managed care on home health care?

What are the rights and responsibilities of individuals who receive home health care and their families?

What is the philosophy of hospice?

CHAPTER OUTLINE

Definitions
Standards and Credentialing
Current Status of Home Health Care
 Types of Agencies
 Types of Services
 Reimbursement Mechanisms
 Types of Home Care Providers
Responsibilities of the Home Health Care Nurse
 Direct Care

Documentation
Coordination of Services and Case
 Management
Determination of Financial Coverage
Determination of Frequency and Duration
 of Care
Client Advocacy
Issues in Home Care
 Infection Control
 Management of Care

Quality of Care
Home Health Care and *Healthy People 2010*
Advance Medical Directives
Patient Rights and Responsibilities
Hospice Home Care
 Medicare Hospice Benefit

KEY TERMS

Deemed status
Home health care nursing
Home health care
Homebound status

Hospice
Medicare certification
Outcome Assessment and Information Set (OASIS)

Skilled service
Visiting nurse associations (VNAs)

Home health nurses make up the largest number of nurses in community health work settings (U.S. Department of Health and Human Services [USDHHS], 2006b). Care of the ill in their homes was an integral part of public health nursing at its inception in the United States (see Chapter 2) and there are numerous reasons that home health care will continue to grow. Advances in technology allow equipment to move from hospitals to homes, which allows more complex home health care. Health care policies aimed at cost containment in health services encourage care in less expensive settings, including homes. Public demand for quality health care continues.

This chapter describes ways in which home health care nursing incorporates principles of nursing practice that are both old and new. Home health care is intricately bound to government and health care provider policy regulating reimbursement of services; yet, home health care nursing blends concepts of community/public health nursing with diseased-focused care that is holistic.

---

* This chapter incorporates material written for previous editions by Paula Milone-Nuzzo.

Trends and statistics reveal the nature and future of home health care. For example, the National Association for Home Care (NAHC) reports that approximately 7.6 million people in the United States require some form of home health care (NAHC, 2007). More than two thirds (68.6%) of home health care recipients are over age 65. Almost two thirds (64%) of home health care recipients are women. Conditions most frequently requiring home health care are diabetes, heart failure, chronic ulcer of the skin, osteoarthritis, and hypertension. Medicare remains the largest single payer of home health care services. The USDHHS reports that we can expect to see a very dramatic increase both in the absolute number of elderly persons and in the proportion of elderly persons in the population. The most rapid increases in the number and share of persons 85 years and older will occur between 2030 and 2050, when the baby boom cohort reaches these ages (USDHHS, 2007). The cumulative growth of the population 85 years and older from 1995 to 2050 is expected to be over 400%, and this group will make up nearly 5% of the population in 2050 compared with 1.4% today. In addition, data indicate that as more patients and families are educated about the many benefits of hospice care, its use will grow as an attractive alternative to facing death in a clinical setting (Hospice Association of America, 2007). Hence, home care in all its forms will likely play a significant role in future U.S. health care.

Home care is not a new concept in health care. Community/public health nursing began with the offering of services to sick poor persons in their homes. As early as 1859, William Rathbone of Liverpool, England, set up a system of visiting nurses after a nurse cared for his wife at home before her death. With the help of Florence Nightingale, Rathbone started a school to train visiting nurses at the Liverpool Infirmary. The graduates were prepared to help the sick poor in their homes.

In the late 1800s, the United States experienced rapid urban growth fueled by large waves of immigration to America. Poor living and working conditions gave rise to problems of hygiene and communicable diseases. **Visiting nurse associations (VNAs)** were developed in the United States by philanthropists, usually wealthy women who wanted to assist the poor in improving their health. Like their counterparts in England, VNAs focused their services almost exclusively on ill people who were poor.

The first VNA in the United States was established in 1885 in Buffalo, New York, and was followed closely by VNAs in Boston and Philadelphia. At this time, agencies operated on private contributions. By the early 1900s, care of the ill and the disabled in their homes was the traditional form of health care for most people.

From the late 1800s to the mid-1960s, VNAs were established across the country in major cities and small towns (see Chapter 2). In 1965, home health care changed dramatically with the passage of Medicare legislation through the Social Security Act. VNAs that had previously served the health needs of the poor were used more frequently, because home health care was a benefit provided to all elderly patients who participated in Medicare. The passage of the Medicare legislation thus forced home health care to change from a "mom-and-pop" industry to a business. No longer did agencies rely on the charitable giving of wealthy men and women for the money needed to provide care. Care also was no longer provided primarily to the sick poor. Medicare legislation changed the populations that received home health care as well as the system of paying for that care. In 2000, there was another significant change in the reimbursement system for home health care that dramatically altered the way home health care services are delivered. This change is discussed in the section on reimbursement for home health care services.

In 1967, there were about 1750 Medicare-participating home health care agencies in the United States; most of these were VNAs and public agencies. In 1995, there were more than 9100 Medicare-certified home health care agencies, the largest percentage of which were proprietary agencies (freestanding, for-profit home health care agencies), followed by hospital-based agencies. The VNAs that provided many free visits continued to inherit the indigent patient population, while experiencing a loss of paying patients to these proprietary and hospital-based agencies. It is believed that the decline in voluntary or nonprofit agencies was related to an inability to compete with the tremendous resources of hospital-based agencies as well as the difficulties in adhering to the numerous federal and state regulations. However, the quality of VNA services and the dedication of VNAs to their communities continue to be well respected and much emulated.

In the early 1980s, in an attempt to curb the increasing costs of hospitalization, a nationwide system of reimbursement of hospitals according to diagnosis-related groups (DRGs) was phased in over a 4-year period. A significant result of the DRG system was a decrease in the length of clients' hospital stays and an increased demand for home health care to provide care to clients while they were still recovering from surgery or an illness.

Changes in the current health care market toward managed care parallel in magnitude and scope the changes that took place when the Medicare legislation was passed. These changes in health care have had a significant impact on the way the home care system has developed and the way in which home care nurses provide care. The impact of managed care on home care is discussed later in this chapter.

Home health care continues to be viewed as not only the most preferred way to provide care to clients but also the most cost effective. The *Nursing Home without Walls (NHWW)* program in New York state was designed to provide home health care services to eligible clients to prevent institutionalization in nursing homes. The cost of services for clients in the NHWW program has consistently been half of the cost of corresponding institutional care (NAHC, 2003).

Medical technology has been developed so that clients can receive more complex, highly technologic care at home. Bulky equipment that was difficult and impractical for use in the home has been modified so that it is smaller, portable, and user friendly. For example, clients can receive continuous parenteral nutrition using a feeding system that is stored in a pouch resembling a fanny pack. Patient-controlled analgesia pumps that resemble a beeper can be worn by clients on their belt straps. This new technology has enabled some clients to maintain daily activities, including work and school.

Advances in telehealth have also moved forward the delivery of home health care nursing to clients (Arnaert & Delesie, 2007). Telehealth is the use of remote computer equipment to monitor the condition of a client and relay information over a telephone line or wireless connection back to a central nursing station. Clients can use sensing devices to monitor blood pressure, respirations, pulse, arterial oxygen saturation, weight, and such and have that data transmitted to the home care nurse regularly and as needed, based on the client's condition. Telehealth has had an impact on client hospitalization and emergency department visits as well as nurse performance, satisfaction, and retention (Tweed, 2003). Most importantly, telehealth and its ultimate expression, telecare, places the home health nurse and patient/family in a virtual environment of care that we are just beginning to understand (Rice, 2003).

In addition, clients and caregivers have recognized the positive therapeutic effect that home care can have on the client. No matter how receptive hospital staff may be, the hospital environment is foreign and antiseptic. Adults who are ill may be comforted by the familiarity of their homes and their control over the environment. For children, the ability to remain an integral part of the family in the presence of severe illness is critical to their development.

For some clients, home care prevents the need for admission to a hospital or nursing home. Other clients enter an inpatient setting and return to their homes to receive home care after hospitalization. An understanding of the home health care system is essential to effectively and economically assist clients through the continuum of care from home to hospital and back to home again.

DEFINITIONS

The term *home health care* conjures up a variety of images. Many professional organizations involved in home health care, such as the NAHC, have developed their own definitions of home health care. Traditionally, **home health care** includes an arrangement of services provided to people in their places of residence. The following comprehensive definition has been offered by Warhola (1980):

> Home health care is that component of a continuum of comprehensive health care whereby health services are provided to individuals and families in their places of residence for the purpose of promoting, maintaining, or restoring health, or of maximizing the level of independence, while minimizing illness. Services appropriate to the needs of the individual patient and family are planned, coordinated, and made available by providers organized for the delivery of home care through the use of employed staff, contractual arrangements, or a combination of the two patterns.

Home health care services can be classified into two broad categories: professional and technical. *Professional home health care* is practice driven—that is, the boundaries of practice are determined by legal and professional standards with a basis in scientific theory and research. This type of home care is provided by professionals with licenses, certifications, or special qualifications. Home health care nursing is an example of professional home health care (Humphrey & Milone-Nuzzo, 2000).

Technical home health care is product driven, sometimes with a zeal for bottom-line profits. These providers do not always have standards or regulations that guide their practice. Instead, they follow reimbursement guidelines outlining their payments. Technical home health care providers include durable medical equipment suppliers.

Both types of home health care providers are necessary to ensure comprehensive care to clients. If a client needs oxygen therapy in the home, a supplier is needed to provide equipment such as the oxygen tank and nasal cannula and to service the equipment on a regular basis. The home health care nurse makes home visits to assess the client's respiratory status and observe for any side effects of the therapy. The home health care nurse is also involved in instructing the client and family about the special precautions that must be taken when a client is receiving oxygen in the home. Either provider alone could not meet the client's total health care needs. Through their collaboration, however, the client can be maintained safely and effectively in his or her own home.

The roots of home health care nursing can be found in the proud heritage of public health nursing. The initial focus of the American public health nurse was on caring for the sick in the home and preventing disease. An emphasis on health promotion and disease prevention with groups rather than individuals began to emerge in the 1930s. Grounded in the concepts and theory of public health, a specialty called *community/public health nursing* developed. The Quad Council of Public Health Nursing Organizations has defined public health nursing as more than generic nursing carried out in a nonhospital setting. It is a "synthesis of nursing practice and public health practice applied to promoting and preserving the health of populations" (American Nurses Association [ANA], 2007, p. 72). Inherent in the practice of community/public health nursing is health promotion and disease prevention for population groups, with a family-centered focus. Consideration is given to the environmental, social, and personal factors that affect the client's health.

The theory and principles that form the foundation for the practice of community/public health nursing are also the foundation for home health care nursing. The client's family, which can be defined as any significant other of the client, is an integral part of home health care. Family-centered care is critical as the home care provider shifts the responsibility for care from the professional to the patient or the significant other. The individual client as part of the family is influenced by the activities of the family. In addition, the client's illness in some way affects the other members of the family. **Home health care nursing,** as a subspecialty of community health nursing, is defined as the provision of nursing care to acute and chronically ill and well clients of all ages in their homes while integrating public health nursing principles that focus on health promotion and on environmental, psychosocial, economic, cultural, and personal health factors that affect an individual's and family's health status (Humphrey & Milone-Nuzzo, 2000).

STANDARDS AND CREDENTIALING

The American Nurses Association (ANA, 2008) has developed standards of practice for home health care to fulfill the profession's obligation to provide a means for assessing quality of care and to develop measures for improvement of care. Standards reflect the current state of knowledge in the field and are the basis for characterizing, measuring, and providing guidance in achieving quality care. The home health care standards are grounded in the nursing process and are based on the ANA standards for community health nursing. The standards for care, without their interpretive statements, are presented in Box 31-1.

BOX 31-1   **American Nurses Association Home Care Nursing Standards**

Standards of Care

Standard 1: Assessment
The home health nurse collects comprehensive data pertinent to the patient's health or situation.

Standard 2: Diagnosis
The home health nurse analyzes the assessment data to determine the diagnoses or issues.

Standard 3: Outcomes Identification
The home health nurse identifies expected outcomes in a plan individualized to the patient and the situation.

Standard 4: Planning
The home health nurse develops a plan that prescribes strategies and alternatives to attain expected outcomes.

Standard 5: Implementation
The home health nurse implements the individualized patient plan.

Standard 6: Evaluation
The home health nurse evaluates progress toward attainment of outcomes.

Standards of Professional Performance

Standard 7: Quality of Care
The home health nurse systematically evaluates the quality and effectiveness of nursing practice.

Standard 8: Education
The home health nurse attains knowledge and competency that reflects current nursing practice.

Standard 9: Performance Appraisal
The home health nurse evaluates one's own nursing practice in relation to professional practice standards and guidelines, relevant statutes, rules, and regulations.

Standard 10: Collegiality
The home health nurse interacts with peers and colleagues and contributes to their professional development.

Standard 11: Collaboration
The home health nurse collaborates with the patient, family, and others in the conduct of nursing practice.

Standard 12: Ethics
The home health nurse integrates ethical principles into all areas of practice.

Standard 13: Research
The home health nurse integrates research findings into practice.

Standard 14: Resource Utilization
The home health nurse considers factors related to safety, cost, and impact on practice in the planning and delivery of nursing services.

From American Nurses Association. (2008). *Home health nursing: Scope and standards of practice.* Silver Spring, MD: Nursebooks.org. Reprinted with permission.

The role of the generalist includes teaching, providing direct care to clients, managing resources needed to provide care, collaborating with other disciplines in the provision of that care, and supervising ancillary personnel. The role of the advanced practice nurse in home care includes such activities as provision of direct care to clients with complex conditions, consultation with other providers, development and evaluation of agency policy, and staff development. The advanced practice role also focuses on supporting and developing the system within which home care services are delivered (ANA, 2008).

Certification is a means to recognize professional nurses' accomplishments in well-defined clinical or functional areas of nursing. The ANA offers certification in three areas: generalist, clinical specialist, and nursing administrator. Each area has a specific focus, and the examinations are based on content from that area of specialization.

In 1992, the American Nurses Credentialing Center (ANCC) approved a certification in home health care at the generalist level of practice (Home Health Nurse). The first certification examination was offered in 1993. In October 1996, the ANCC offered an advanced practice certification examination for the home care clinical specialist (Home Health Nursing CNS). This certification recognizes the need for a home care clinical specialist to engage in research, management, education, and consultation as well as to provide direct care in the home. Examinations for both Home Health Nurse and Home Health Nursing CNS were retired in 2005 (ANCC, 2007). Currently, those already certified

can renew their certification through professional development and practice hours. Certification as a Home Health Nurse is not available for new applicants (ANA, 2008).

CURRENT STATUS OF HOME HEALTH CARE

Although home health care providers have been delivering high-quality health care to clients in their homes since the late 1800s, most growth in home health care nursing has taken place since 1970. As described earlier, this growth is due in part to the enactment of Medicare legislation in 1965, and current growth is largely due to the influence of managed care and technology. There are many different types of home care agencies that provide various services to clients in their homes. The regulations for operation of such an agency differ from state to state and depend on the type of services provided by the agency. Through licensure law, the states set specific rules and requirements for staffing, policies, and practices and establish minimal operating standards for various programs and services. If the home health agency meets the legal conditions set out in the licensure law, it is granted a license; if not, it cannot operate in that state.

In some states, only those agencies that provide professional services are required to have a license. For example, agencies that provide skilled nursing or physical therapy services need a license, whereas agencies that provide unskilled service or custodial care (e.g., companion services) do not need a license for operation.

For an agency to be reimbursed by Medicare for services provided to clients, it must be Medicare certified. In 2006, there were more than 8800 Medicare-certified home health care agencies (NAHC, 2007). **Medicare certification** means that the agency meets the *conditions of participation (COPs)*, which are outlined in rules, standards, and criteria established by the federal government. These regulations dictate things such as the type and number of personnel, agency structure, and billing methods. For example, the administrator of a home health agency must be a licensed physician or a registered nurse with at least 1 year of supervisory experience in a home health agency. Because it is a federal program, the requirements for Medicare certification are consistent across the country. Medicare certification is required even in those states that require licensure for home care agencies. To maintain Medicare certification, an agency is required to periodically undergo an unannounced site visit by an external evaluator who reviews the agency's records and makes home visits to determine that the conditions of participation are being maintained.

State licensure laws are usually written to identify the minimum standard for patient safety and quality of care that an agency must achieve. Medicare certification standards are slightly more rigorous than licensure standards and regulations. Agencies that want to further define the quality of their services to their clients and the community may also seek voluntary *accreditation,* which is a rigorous process in which an agency seeks to be evaluated on the basis of comprehensive criteria that influence the quality of care. The cost of this process is assumed by the home health care agency. An agency that is accredited seeks to demonstrate to consumers that it far exceeds the minimum standards for operation and has achieved a standard of excellence that is superior to that of its nonaccredited competitors.

There are two accreditation programs for home health care agencies in the United States: the Community Health Accreditation Program (CHAP), administered through the National League for Nursing, and the Home Care Accreditation Program of the Joint Commission (formerly the Joint Commission on Accreditation of Healthcare Organizations, or JCAHO). Both programs require the agency to conduct a thorough self-evaluation based on identified objectives and to compile a self-evaluation report that is reviewed by a group of professionals. An unannounced, on-site survey is also conducted by peer reviewers as part of the review process. Based on review of the self-evaluation report and the site visit, which includes home visits to clients, the accrediting agency (either CHAP or the Joint Commission) determines whether the agency will be accredited.

A home health care agency accredited by CHAP or the Joint Commission is considered to have **deemed status,** which refers to the Medicare conditions of participation. Because accreditation standards are more rigorous than the Medicare conditions of participation, an agency that meets accreditation standards is deemed to have met the Medicare standard as well. Therefore, an accredited agency would have to undergo only the accreditation site visit, which includes the assessment for continued Medicare certification.

TYPES OF AGENCIES

Currently, there are many different types of home health care agencies. In the early days of home health care, services were

likely to be delivered by a nurse from a VNA. In some parts of the country, this continues to be true. In most of the country, however, the mix of home health care agencies more commonly includes other types of agencies, such as official, proprietary, and hospital-based agencies.

Official Agencies

Official or *public agencies* are supported by tax dollars and are given power through statutes enacted by legislation. An example of an official agency involved in home health care is a state or local health department with a nursing division. Home health care services (care of the sick) and traditional public health nursing services (preventive care) may be combined in the same nursing division of the health department.

There has been a gradual decline in the number of local health departments with certified home health care agencies. Increased competition from other agencies left health departments with the task of caring only for those people unable to pay for services. More importantly, the growth of public health problems, such as bioterrorism and maternal and child health needs in high-risk populations, has necessitated that official agencies focus their energy and resources on the public health needs of the community.

Voluntary Agencies

Voluntary home health care agencies are governed by a volunteer board of directors and are supported primarily by nontax funds such as donations, endowments, United Way contributions, and reimbursements from third-party payers (e.g., Medicare, Medicaid, and private insurance). They are considered to be community based because they provide services within a well-defined community or geographic location.

Because voluntary agencies have a charitable mission and are nonprofit, they are tax exempt. Nonprofit status is not exactly what the name implies. An agency that is nonprofit must operate in a fiscally responsible manner designed to either break even or end the year with a surplus. Nonprofit status means that the accrued profit goes back into the functioning of the agency to support its mission in the form of free client care, staff development, or capital expenditures. A nonprofit agency that continually runs a fiscal deficit will soon be out of business. An example of a voluntary agency is a VNA.

Private Agencies

Private home health care agencies can be either for profit or not for profit. Private not-for-profit home health care agencies are governed by either a board of directors or the agency's owner.

Most private agencies are proprietary, which means they plan to make a profit on the home care they provide. Proprietary agencies make up the largest percentage of home health care agencies in the country. These agencies can be locally owned or part of a national or international chain. Unlike in voluntary agencies, the profit made on home care goes to either the stockholders of the corporation or the owners of the company and therefore is not tax exempt. There is no requirement that the profits be returned to the agency. The stockholders or the owners determine how these profits are allocated.

Hospital-Based Agencies

Hospitals began entering the home health care industry in large numbers in the 1980s to maintain clients within their health care systems, provide a more comprehensive program of health services, and increase revenue. In a managed care framework, hospital-based home care agencies allow close collaboration to facilitate the movement of the client across the health care continuum. A hospital-based home health care agency is governed by the sponsoring hospital's board of directors and receives most of its referrals from the sponsoring hospital.

Home Care Aide Agencies

A home care aide agency provides paraprofessional services such as homemaking, companionship, or custodial care to clients. These agencies are usually privately owned and receive direct payment from a client or a private insurance company.

Certified Hospice Agencies

Many communities have home health care agencies that provide hospice care to the terminally ill in the community. These agencies have received certification from the federal government as a Medicare hospice provider. Hospice home care has grown as a result of a trend toward providing terminal care in the home. In 2006, there were over 3000 Medicare-certified hospices (NAHC, 2007). Some hospice agencies are freestanding and serve only hospice clients, whereas others are part of a larger organization such as a VNA. Reimbursement for hospice care is provided by Medicare, Medicaid in most states, and private insurance companies.

TYPES OF SERVICES

Home care services are traditionally divided into three categories of service: care of the ill, public health (also known as preventive care), and specialized home care services (e.g., high-technology care). Although each category is unique, the categories are not mutually exclusive either in theory or in practice. In theory, they are not mutually exclusive because high-technology care, such as care for a ventilator-dependent client, may also be part of the program for care of the ill. In practice, when a home care nurse visits a 50-year-old woman who needs wound care, the nurse provides instruction about the need for routine preventive health care measures (e.g., mammogram and Pap smear test) in addition to performing the wound care.

Care of Ill Persons

The care of ill persons is the largest program in home health care. As the term implies, these care recipients are ill and require services to improve their health outcome or prevent hospitalization. Most of the care for qualified clients is covered by a third-party payer, such as Medicare, Medicaid, or a private insurance company.

Public Health Services

Public health services focus on the promotion of health and the prevention of disease. They include such services as instruction for a new mother in how to care for an infant, physical examinations for children, and diet teaching for the elderly. Although VNAs were founded on the principles of public health services, most home health care agencies *do not* provide traditional public health services. Traditional third-party payers do not reimburse home health care agencies for care that is exclusively preventive. The home care agencies that do provide public health services usually fund these programs through money donated to them from the jurisdiction in which the services are provided or through private donations or grants.

Specialized Home Care Services

Specialized home care practice includes such programs as high-technology home care, pediatric care, psychiatric mental health care, cardiac care, pediatric high-technology care, and hospice care. High-technology home care has grown in direct response to shortened hospital stays of clients and the need to reduce health care costs related to treatment in the hospital. Technology that was previously available only in the hospital has been adapted for use in the home. For example, clients who would previously have had to remain hospitalized to receive long-term antibiotic therapy can now receive it at home as a result of changes in infusion technology.

However, not all clients or situations are suited for high-technology home health care. Discharging a client who requires high-technology care to the home requires thorough assessment of the client, the caregiver, and the home environment. This can be accomplished through the collaborative efforts of the discharge planner in the hospital and the home care nurse who will be involved after discharge. Before the client is discharged, decisions must be made and plans developed. To evaluate the client's suitability for discharge home, the home health care nurse and the discharge planner in the hospital should discuss the following questions before the client is discharged (Humphrey & Milone-Nuzzo, 2000):

- What kinds of services or care does the individual client/family need or want?
- What is the client's and caregiver's understanding of the specified therapy, and what are their roles in performing the therapy?
- Is it safe to perform the therapy in the home, and does the client have the means to perform the therapy safely?
- Do the client and caregiver have the willingness and commitment to become involved in the client's therapy?
- What is the availability of equipment, supplies, and expertise?
- What is the availability of financial resources to pay for the proposed services?

Pediatric programs can focus on providing short-term care to the acutely ill child (e.g., total parenteral nutrition for a child after bowel surgery) or providing long-term care to the chronically ill child (e.g., home ventilator care for a child with a respiratory condition). Whatever the need, there is significant benefit to providing care to children in the home rather than in an institution. Unlike in the hospital setting, at home a child's development tends to advance, even in the presence of a debilitating or chronic illness. In addition, children at home have fewer infections, and socialization occurs more rapidly (McEvoy, 2003). The appearance of normalcy has a positive impact on the ill child as well as on other family members. Funds for pediatric home care come from Medicaid, private insurance carriers, local community organizations, and private foundations or state entitlement programs (see Chapter 27).

Some home health care agencies deliver psychiatric and mental health services to clients in their homes. Medicare guidelines for the reimbursement of care for psychiatric clients require that the client be under the care of a physician (not necessarily a psychiatrist), that the evaluation and psychotherapy needed by the client require the care of a nurse with psychiatric training, and that the client meet all the requirements for Medicare home care services, which include being home-bound and needing intermittent, part-time care that is reasonable and necessary (Freed, 2006). Many home care agencies have developed psychiatric home care programs for both children and adults to meet the increasing demand for psychiatric care in the home.

> Mrs. Jones is an 86-year-old client with increasing dementia. She is alert and oriented enough to be able to voice her strong desire to stay in her home. She is homebound and is able to perform her activities of daily living. Yet she is unsure about how and when to take her medications. She also has unstable hypertension that needs to be assessed and managed by a skilled nurse. Mrs. Jones is seen by the psychiatric nurse daily as part of the psychiatric care program. In addition to providing a psychiatric evaluation, the nurse helps Mrs. Jones with her medications and assesses and manages her hypertension. These services allow Mrs. Jones to remain in her home for as long as she is safe there.

Other specialty programs such as cardiac or oncology programs are often developed in response to identification of a large number of clients (population) with a particular problem or need by the referral source or the managed care company with which the agency contracts. These specialty programs generally consist of a defined set of services and identified client outcomes, with a price designated for the package of services. Often, the package involves some level of specialty nursing practice for the design of the plan of care. Hospice home care as a specialty service is described in detail later in this chapter.

REIMBURSEMENT MECHANISMS

Home health services are reimbursed by both commercial and government third-party payers as well as by individuals. Government third-party payers include Medicare, Medicaid, the Civilian Health and Medical Program of the Uniformed Services (now TRICARE), and the Veterans Administration system. These government programs have specific conditions that must be met for services to be covered. Commercial third-party payers include insurance companies, health maintenance organizations (HMOs), preferred provider organizations, and case management programs. Commercial insurers often allow for more flexibility in their requirements than does Medicare. For example, the home care nurse may negotiate with an insurance company to obtain needed services for the client in the home, based on the cost effectiveness of the home care plan.

Home care costs may be reimbursed either after the services are provided (i.e., retrospective reimbursement) or before the services are delivered based on the anticipated cost of providing care (prospective payment) (see Chapter 4). In the retrospective payment method, an agency makes a determination about the client's care needs, provides the needed care within the agency's interpretation of the guidelines of the third-party payer, and then bills the payer for the services delivered. At times, third-party payers will question or deny payment for the care provided. If it is determined that the provided care is not reimbursable, the agency must assume financial responsibility for that care.

In a prospective payment model, the agency is reimbursed based on the anticipated cost of providing care. Using a variety of factors, the average or usual cost of the care for a client is calculated. The agency is paid a set amount following the admission of that client to service. The agency that provides care efficiently and discharges the client to self-care in a shorter number of visits than expected reaps the financial rewards. If it takes more visits than anticipated, the agency has to provide the care and assume the financial costs.

Medicare

Medicare is a federal insurance program for the elderly (older than 65 years), persons with end-stage renal disease, and persons disabled for more than 24 months in the United States. Because it is a federal program, procedures and qualifying criteria should not vary significantly from state to state. To be eligible for this program, a person or his or her spouse must have contributed to Social Security through payroll deductions. The Centers for Medicare and Medicaid Services (CMS), formerly called the Health Care Financing Administration (HCFA), a department of the federal government, regulates payments for services under Medicare (see Chapters 3 and 4). The rules developed by CMS that guide the Medicare program are detailed in the *The Home Health Agency Manual (Publication 11) (1978; revised 1997)*. CMS contracts with insurance companies to process the Medicare claims submitted by home care agencies; these insurance companies are called *fiscal intermediaries (FIs)*. The United States is broken into 10 geographic regions, each with its own fiscal intermediary.

In 1997, the Balanced Budget Act (Public Law 105-33) (U.S. Congress, 1998) mandated a prospective payment system for home health agencies beginning in October 2000. In the prospective payment model of home care, each client is assessed on admission by the home care nurse or physical therapist using a set of standardized criteria called the **Outcome Assessment and Information Set (OASIS)** (HCFA, 1999) (Box 31-2). This instrument consists of many questions, of which 19 are used to determine the home health resource group

---

Box 31-2   Outcome and Assessment Information Set (OASIS)

The OASIS data set is a home health assessment tool required by Medicare. It has been developed as a tool for outcome assessment, and OASIS data are required for all Medicare and Medicaid patients (except hospice patients, obstetric patients, and patients under age 18). OASIS questions have the notation M0 or M00 before or after the question. If the notation appears before the question, the information is required; if after, it is optional. OASIS data cannot be submitted electronically, as required, unless they are "locked." The assessment data will not lock if these required questions are not answered. The assessment must be completed by a registered nurse, physical therapist, occupational therapist, or speech therapist.

OASIS data are required at the following times:
- Start of care
- Recertification
- Discharge
- Transfer (to hospital or skilled nursing facility)
- Resumption of care
- Any time there is a significant change in the patient's condition

OASIS is a dynamic instrument, and home health care agencies should use the most recent version, which may be obtained from the OASIS website at *http://www.cms.hhs.gov/oasis*.

(HHRG) in which the client will be placed. These OASIS items are based on the clinical, functional, and service needs of the client. A specified dollar amount is attached to each of the 80 possible HHRGs based on the anticipated complexity of the clinical situation. For example, for care of clients in one HHRG, the reimbursement to the home care agency may be $2100, but for those in a different HHRG, which represents a more complex clinical situation, the reimbursement to the clinical agency may be as high as $5000.

Agencies are reimbursed for admitted clients based on the HHRG to which the clients are assigned on admission. There are some intricacies to the system that are beyond the scope of this chapter that have to do with adjustments to reimbursement if the client goes into the hospital soon after being admitted to home care or if the client's condition substantially changes over the course of the home care episode. It is critically important that the home care nurse know how to assess a client's clinical, functional, and social dimensions of care using the OASIS instrument, because these assessments determine the revenues generated by the agency (Fazzi, 2006).

In a Medicare managed care model, the Medicare client enrolls with an HMO provider to receive care. The HMO makes specific arrangements with one home care agency or a group of agencies to provide care when needed. The home care agency may be paid a capitated rate; that is, a set amount based on the number of people enrolled in the managed care program. For example, if the home care agency is responsible for 100 clients and is paid $10 per client per month, the income to the home care agency will be $1000 per month. If 1000 people enroll in the HMO, then the home care agency will be paid $10,000 per month. The home care agency is responsible for providing care to the enrollees who need home care services. It is anticipated that many of those enrollees will remain healthy and will not require home care services. Home care nurses are responsible not only for treating those people who are sick but also for making sure the healthy enrollees stay well.

Criteria for Reimbursement under Medicare. There are five criteria a client must meet to be eligible for Medicare home care services:

1. **Homebound.** A client must be considered essentially homebound to be eligible for home care benefits under Medicare. **Homebound status** means that the client has difficulty with mobility and can leave the home only with considerable and taxing effort. The client is considered homebound if home absences are rare and of short duration and largely for the purpose of receiving medical care (Zuber, 2002). The criteria for homebound status may also be considered met if the client attends adult daycare and the purpose of attending is related to the client's receipt of medical care.

2. **Completed plan of care.** The plan of care for Medicare clients must be completed on CMS (formerly HCFA) forms 485, 486, and 487. These federal government forms require very specific information regarding the client's diagnosis, prognosis, functional limitations, medications, and types of services needed. The home health care nurse often has the primary responsibility for ensuring that these forms are completed appropriately.

3. **Skilled services.** To qualify for home care services under Medicare, the client must be in need of a **skilled service.** In the home, skilled services are provided by a nurse, a physical therapist, or a speech therapist. Medical social work

and home care aide services are considered to be dependent services and therefore are reimbursed under Medicare only if they are combined with one of the skilled services. Occupational therapy is not considered a skilled service for initiating care. After the skilled service has discharged the client, however, occupational therapy can serve as the qualifying service for other dependent services in the home. Reimbursement for occupational therapy in the home depends on the inherent complexity of the service and the condition of the client.

Skilled nursing service encompasses four major areas: skilled observation and assessment, teaching, management and evaluation of the plan of care, and skilled procedures. Skilled observation and assessment may include assessment of a congestive heart failure patient for the early signs of pulmonary edema. Teaching, one of the most common interventions performed by the home care nurse, may include instructing a patient with newly diagnosed diabetes about his or her diet. The teaching plan must include new information, not just a reinforcement of material about which the client has already been instructed. Management and evaluation of the plan of care involve the professional nurse's supervision of the delivery of care by multiple caregivers, both professional and nonprofessional. Skilled procedures include interventions such as wound care or dressing changes.

4. **Intermittent and part-time service.** Medicare specifies that home care services be provided on an intermittent basis, usually a few hours per day for several days per week for a specified length of time. It is anticipated that clients requiring more than intermittent and part-time care could be cared for more cost effectively in a setting other than the home (e.g., a nursing home).

5. **Reasonable and necessary.** Under Medicare, services provided to a client must be considered "reasonable and necessary." This term refers both to the nursing care clients receive to effect a positive health outcome and the frequency with which that care is provided. Medicare regulations, as they appear in *The Home Health Agency Manual* (Section 705) state that a service is considered reasonable and necessary if the following criteria are met (Zuber, 2002):
   - It is appropriate to the client's diagnosis.
   - It meets generally accepted professional standards.
   - It requires the skills of a professional to perform to ensure safety and meet legal requirements.

The decision about whether these criteria are met is based on the client's health status and medical needs as reflected in the plan of care and the medical record. For example, daily visits may not be deemed reasonable for a client who requires twice-weekly blood glucose level determinations. Similarly, if a care plan has been ineffective over a long period of time, continuation of that care plan would not be considered reasonable. Therefore, comprehensive documentation by the home health care nurse is essential to validate that the care provided is both reasonable and necessary.

Medicaid

Medicaid is an assistance program for the poor and some disabled. Unlike Medicare, Medicaid is jointly sponsored by the federal government and the states; therefore Medicaid coverage differs from state to state (see Chapters 3 and 4).

These differences can often be dramatic and in some cases are dependent on the state's financial health. Eligibility for Medicaid is based on income and assets and is not contingent on any previous payments to the federal or state government.

Unlike Medicare, Medicaid covers both skilled and unskilled care in the home and does not require that the client be homebound. To qualify for home care benefits under Medicaid, the client must meet income eligibility requirements, the client must have a plan of care signed by a physician, and the plan of care must be reviewed by a physician every 60 days.

Many states are also changing the way care is reimbursed for the Medicaid population. For example, in Connecticut, the care of women and children receiving Medicaid benefits has been converted to a managed care model of reimbursement. Other populations of Medicaid clients will be transitioned into managed care in an effort to control costs and ensure high-quality care for clients in all phases of health care delivery, including home care.

Commercial Private Payers

Many commercial insurance companies are involved in health insurance for individuals or groups. These local or national companies often write policies that include a home care benefit. Commercial insurers often cover the same services covered by Medicare in addition to covering preventive, private duty, and supportive services such as those provided by a home health aide or homemaker (discussed later).

Commercial insurance often has a maximum lifetime benefit specified as part of the policy. Because of the high cost of high-technology care, more patients reach this maximum and face the loss of coverage. This has resulted in the development of case management programs administered by insurance companies. The case manager projects the client's long-term needs and costs of care and develops a plan with the client to meet those needs in a cost-efficient manner. Consideration is given to the life expectancy of the client in relation to the maximum lifetime benefit.

TYPES OF HOME CARE PROVIDERS

Interdisciplinary collaboration is a hallmark of home health care practice. The home health care team is made up of several, if not all, of the home health care providers discussed in this section. The client's needs mandate the home care providers who will be part of the home health care team. The standards of home health nursing practice specify that the home health care nurse is responsible for initiating collaboration with other providers (ANA, 2008). In addition, collaboration is mandated as part of the conditions of participation for those agencies that are Medicare certified (Medicare Conditions of Participation, 1996).

The role of the professional in home health care involves both the provision of direct care to clients and consultation with other professionals and paraprofessionals involved in care. For example, a client needing skilled nursing service for a dressing change and assessment of a leg wound may also need some range-of-motion exercises for the affected extremity. If this is an uncomplicated clinical situation, the home care nurse may ask the physical therapist to suggest some exercises that can be done by the client instead of having the physical therapist make a home visit.

Home Health Care Nurse

Nursing services are the most frequently provided skilled service in the home. Nursing care in the home is provided by a registered nurse or a licensed practical nurse, is authorized by a physician, and is based on the client's needs. A registered nurse may make an initial visit to a client to obtain an assessment without a physician's order but must receive physician approval and direction for follow-up care to be delivered.

Advanced practice nurses (nurse practitioners, clinical nurse specialists, and nurse-midwives) are being integrated into home care practice because of the complexity of the health care being delivered in the home. Advanced practice nurses can provide direct care to patients with complex conditions or serve as an expert consultant to the home care nurse. In addition, they can provide for staff development through education and case analysis. By integrating advanced practice nurses into home care, agencies are hoping to raise the quality of clinical practice and improve patient outcomes (Milone-Nuzzo, 2003).

Primary Physician

Clients receiving care in the home must be under the current care of a physician or an osteopath. Although physician home visits were once a widespread practice, physicians in the United States rarely make them anymore. The current role of the physician in home care is to provide information to the home care provider regarding the medical condition of the client, to serve as a resource to other home care providers, and to certify a plan of treatment. The plan of treatment must be reviewed by the physician at least every 60 days, with more frequent review if a change in the client's situation warrants it.

Physical Therapist

The focus of the physical therapist in home care is on improving the client's ability to use his or her large muscle groups. Physical therapists provide maintenance, preventive, and restorative treatment in the home for clients of all ages with varying diagnoses. The body systems most likely to be associated with the need for home physical therapy are the musculoskeletal, neurologic, and cardiopulmonary systems. Physical therapists focus on gross motor skills, the lower extremities, and the respiratory system. For example, a client with chronic obstructive pulmonary disease may have home visits by the physical therapist for postural drainage.

Occupational Therapist

The occupational therapist helps the client acquire the skills necessary to perform the activities of daily living. Occupational therapists focus most of their interventions on the upper extremities and on the fine muscle skills needed to perform functional activities, such as eating and dressing. In addition to teaching self-care activities, the occupational therapist is involved in assessing the home for safety and suggesting modifications for improving the client's ability to function independently. These modifications may include installation of adaptive equipment, such as a grab bar in the bathtub, or modification of existing structures in the home to make self-care possible. For example, the occupational therapist may suggest modifications to a kitchen to allow the client to prepare his or her own meals; these might include installation of a sink that allows a wheelchair to fit under it or cabinets that have easily accessed pulls.

Speech Therapist

The speech therapist (speech-language pathologist) works with clients who have difficulty with communication, both expressive and receptive. The speech therapist's goal is to help the client develop optimal communication skills. Speech therapists may also work with clients who are experiencing difficulty in swallowing.

Medical Social Worker

The medical social worker helps clients and families deal with the social and emotional issues associated with illness and long-term care. Often families are unprepared for the adjustments required to care for an ill member. The social worker can be helpful in easing this transition to the caregiver role. Traditionally, social workers have helped clients identify health and social service needs and have made referrals to community agencies that address those needs. In home care, the social worker also assists clients with applications for services and provides financial assistance information.

Home Care Aide

The home care aide is a paraprofessional providing services ranging from basic housekeeping to complex personal care. Services performed by the home care aide typically include ensuring a clean, healthy home environment; shopping and preparing meals; and grooming, bathing, and performing other personal care services.

Supervision of paraprofessionals, such as home care aides, is primarily the responsibility of the home health care nurse. If the home health care nurse is not directly involved in the client's care, the nurse can delegate this supervisory responsibility to a professional such as the physical therapist or speech therapist. Medicare mandates that the home care aide be supervised every 2 weeks, which means that the home care nurse visits the client's home either when the home care aide is present to observe the aide providing care or when the aide is absent to assess the relationship between the aide and the client (HCFA, 1989). Licensure requirements vary from state to state regarding the frequency of supervision for clients not covered by Medicare.

Business Office Staff

Business office staff include the bookkeepers, clerks, and computer operators who prepare bills, track reimbursements, and maintain the agency's database. The business office is integral to an agency's ability to deliver home care services to clients. A home health agency cannot function without an efficient business office staff that works effectively with the clinical staff. The relationship between the business office staff and the clinical staff is unique in home care. Professional staff must have an understanding of the financial aspects of the client's care and provide information to the business staff so that reimbursement can be obtained for the services provided.

RESPONSIBILITIES OF THE HOME HEALTH CARE NURSE

Although there is a great deal of similarity between the roles and functions of inpatient care nurses and those of home care nurses, there are some unique aspects of practice in the home. This section focuses on the differences in nursing practice between home care and inpatient care.

DIRECT CARE

Direct care is defined as the actual nursing care that is provided to clients in their homes (Humphrey & Milone-Nuzzo, 2000). Nursing care may involve assessment of physical or psychosocial status, performance of a skilled intervention, or teaching. In performing assessments and skilled interventions, the home health care nurse must give consideration to the 24-hour needs of clients. Integration of the client, family, and caregiver into the care plan is essential to ensure continuity of care during the time the nurse is not in the home. Home health care nurses provide care on a short-term, intermittent basis. Most care provided in the home is the responsibility of someone other than the nurse. Therefore, teaching becomes the most common intervention performed by home health care nurses. Nurses are responsible for providing the client and family with the necessary knowledge and skills to provide safe care between home visits by nurses and after discharge from the home care agency.

The home health care nurse is not routinely involved in the client's personal care (e.g., bathing, hair washing, or linen changing). Although these activities are considered essential to the client's recovery, the responsibility for performing these tasks on a routine basis is assigned to the home care aide or the client's family member. However, this does not mean that the home health care nurse never provides personal care to the client. For example, the home health care nurse may make a home visit to a client who is in need of help with his or her personal hygiene. The nurse performs these tasks in addition to performing the skilled care that was the purpose of the visit. The home health care nurse, together with the client,

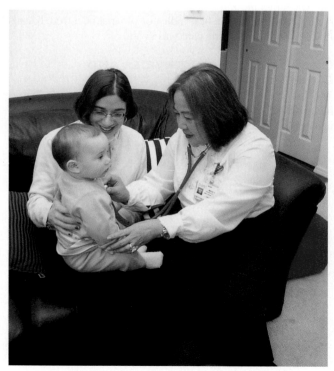

Home health nurse visiting a mother and infant checks the baby's heart rate.

then determines whether continued personal care assistance is needed. If so, the nurse makes arrangements for those needs to be met.

DOCUMENTATION

Documentation of care is just as important a responsibility of the home care nurse as is provision of direct care. The time and effort a home health care nurse must spend on documentation to meet reimbursement and regulatory requirements are difficult to comprehend. In addition to addressing regulatory and reimbursement requirements, the purpose of documentation is to convey the clinical course of care for the client. Many agencies already have developed strategies to reduce the amount of time a home care provider must spend on documentation. These include the use of voice-processing systems for charting home visits, the implementation of computerized care plans and documentation systems using point-of-service technology, and the use of flow sheets, critical paths, or standardized care plans.

Documentation in home health care serves several purposes. As in the inpatient setting, the documentation in the record is a written account of the client's history, status, and progress. The written record is the basis for planning individualized care and serves to communicate information to all health professionals involved in the client's care. Specifically in home care, third-party payers use the client record as a tool to justify payments (Turnbough-Hill & Rice, 2006). The payer not only inspects the record for the number of home visits made but also may examine the services provided to determine whether they are appropriate to meet the determined goal. The home care record also is one of the many documents examined in the total quality improvement program of an agency. Record reviews are an important tool for assessing the quality of care provided by the home health care team. In addition, accurate documentation is the key to the nurse's and agency's protection from liability. If there is a question about the type, amount, or quality of care a client received, the written record is viewed as the best indicator of what occurred, because it was written at the time care was given.

COORDINATION OF SERVICES AND CASE MANAGEMENT

The home health care nurse is responsible for coordinating the services of the other professionals and paraprofessionals involved in the client's care. Central to the role of case manager

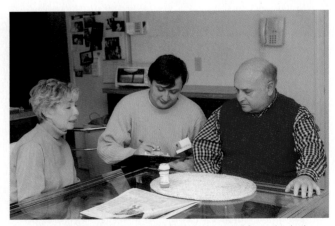

Nurse visiting an older couple in their home documents information in the man's medication chart.

is the ability to assess the client's needs, determine priority of needs, identify how those needs can be met, and implement a plan for meeting the identified needs. In addition, the home care nurse is the primary contact with the client's physician, reporting changes in the client's condition and securing changes in the plan of care.

As the care coordinator, the home health care nurse must have current information about the services provided by all caregivers in the home and the response to those services. Case conferences are conducted regularly among professionals and paraprofessionals to share information, discuss problems, and plan a course of action to achieve the best possible outcome for the client. Medicare mandates that case conferences occur every 60 days when care providers from more than one discipline are involved in the client's care. A written summary of each client's case conference must be sent to the primary physician for review. At times, the client or caregivers are included in the case conference. Case conferences can occur over the telephone with professional care providers who are not affiliated with the home care agency from which the client is receiving most of his or her care (known as the primary home care agency).

Many times clients need services not provided by the primary home care agency. As coordinator of care, the home care nurse must be knowledgeable about the many community resources existing to meet the needs of clients in their homes. A *community resource* is any agency, organization, program, or individual that delivers a service to residents in the community. To keep a record of the many resources in a community, a home health care nurse may begin a community resource file. This file consists of a small box of index cards, notebook, or personal electronic device (personal digital assistant, or PDA) in which the home health care nurse collects information about community resources. When a resource is identified, the home health care nurse records the name of the agency, contact person, hours of operation, telephone number, eligibility requirements, and cost of services. This information can be filed according to the service provided for future reference in working with clients. Information about community resources can be found in the yellow pages of the local telephone directory or the directory of organizations and services for the community. National resources also provide useful information about home health nursing practice and client care (see Community Resources for Practice at the end of the chapter).

DETERMINATION OF FINANCIAL COVERAGE

A unique aspect of the role of the home health care nurse is involvement in the financial aspects of delivering care to the client. The home health care nurse must know who is going to pay for services from the first visit to the time of discharge. At the time of admission, the home health care nurse determines the type of services needed based on the assessment and the physician's orders. The home health care nurse must also determine the source of payment (Medicare, Medicaid, private insurance, or client) for the necessary care. If the client does not have a fee source for the care needed, it becomes the responsibility of the agency to determine whether the client will receive the care free of charge or at a reduced cost. Many agencies have a sliding fee scale, which means that the charge for the services is based on the client's ability to pay. Determining the ability to pay includes reviewing the client's income and assets.

DETERMINATION OF FREQUENCY AND DURATION OF CARE

The home health care nurse is responsible for determining both the frequency and the duration of client care. *Frequency of care* is defined as how often home visits are made to the client in a specified period of time. *Duration of care* is defined as the length of time the client receives home care services. In collaboration with the physician, the home care nurse must determine whether the client needs daily, biweekly, weekly, or monthly home visits. As the care is provided and the client's clinical status improves, the home health care nurse, in collaboration with the physician, must determine whether the frequency of visits should be reduced and when to discharge the client from the care of the agency. Many organizations have standardized care plans for certain diagnoses that outline the expected frequency and duration of care. The prescribed number and length of home visits will not be appropriate for all clients, however. The condition of the client, the needs of the client and the family, and any reimbursement regulations are significant variables in determining the frequency and duration of care.

CLIENT ADVOCACY

Although the role of advocate is not unique to home health care nursing, the context in which the home health care nurse carries out this role requires additional knowledge about health care finance. Many client advocacy responsibilities center around helping clients to negotiate the complex medical care system. This may involve assisting the client in interpreting hospital bills or organizing receipts for submission to the insurance company. Although this may not seem significant, the stress caused by these financial matters may prohibit the client from learning the information necessary for successful recovery from his or her illness.

ISSUES IN HOME CARE

INFECTION CONTROL

Universal precautions are as important in the provision of care to clients in the home as they are in the provision of care in the intensive care unit of the hospital. Because of shortened hospital stays, many clients with communicable diseases and multiple invasive devices are being cared for in the home by home care nurses. Two major concerns for the home care nurse in caring for any client in the home are the following:

1. How can infection be prevented in a client who is debilitated and may be immunocompromised?
2. How can the nurse, family, and community be protected from a client who has a communicable disease?

   The home setting provides some unique challenges for the control of communicable disease and the prevention of infection. In some cases, the home may lack the facilities to implement optimal infection control measures; for example, a client with hepatitis A may live in a rooming house with shared bathroom facilities. In other cases, family members may be unwilling or unable to implement the necessary precautions to protect themselves from a communicable disease. The unique nature of the home as the setting of care necessitates the development of unique solutions to the problems faced by the home health care nurse.

Universal Precautions

In 1996, the Hospital Infection Control Practices Advisory Committee of the Centers for Disease Control and Prevention issued recommendations for isolation precautions in hospitals. These principles can also be used in home care. The term *standard precautions* is used to indicate the combined principles of universal precautions and body substance isolation. Standard precautions describe the basic protective measures to be used with all patients and incorporate the basic principles of infection control to minimize the risk of transmission of potentially infectious pathogens from both recognized and unrecognized sources (Rice, 2006). Strategies to reduce the transmission of infectious diseases are outlined in Box 31-3. Because the medical history or physical examination is unreliable in identifying those clients with a bloodborne pathogen, standard precautions should be used consistently with all clients, regardless of diagnosis.

Measures to Control the Spread of Communicable Disease

The presence of a family member with a communicable disease need not be a hazard for the other members of the household or the community. The role of the home health care nurse is to instruct the client and family regarding measures to control the spread of the communicable disease and to provide information to allay the fears of the family in the caregiving process. Isolation precautions in the home should be based on common sense and an understanding of the method of transmission of the communicable disease. The guidelines in Box 31-4 can be followed in the home to control the spread of communicable disease (also see Chapter 8).

Measures for the Immunocompromised

To reduce the possibility of a nosocomial infection, the immunocompromised client is often cared for in the home setting. The inability of the client to fight off infection may be caused by many conditions, including acquired immunodeficiency syndrome (AIDS), chemotherapy, or genetic absence of an antibody. Clients can take the following special precautions in the home to prevent the development of infectious diseases (Rice, 2006):

- Keep a clean kitchen and bathroom.
- Maintain an optimal nutritional status.

BOX 31-3   Principles of Standard Precautions to Prevent Transmission of Infectious Disease

1. Assume that all patients are infectious for HIV and other bloodborne pathogens.
2. Be immunized for hepatitis B virus.
3. Wash hands frequently. Wearing gloves does not negate the necessity of handwashing.
4. Use protective barriers to prevent percutaneous exposure to blood and other potentially hazardous body fluids.
5. Properly disinfect work areas, equipment, and clothing.
6. Properly dispose of contaminated waste and sharp objects.
7. Properly secure and transport blood and other laboratory specimens.
8. Document exposure and report to employer, who is required to report occupational injuries to the federal government.

Box 31-4 **Guidelines to Control the Spread of Communicable Disease in Homes (Includes Persons with HIV/AIDS)**

1. Everyone should wash hands with soap and water before and after using the bathroom, before handling food, and before and after giving patient care.
2. Everyone should cover their mouth and nose when coughing or sneezing to prevent the spread of germs. Turn your head to avoid droplets from coughs or sneezes.
3. Everyone should avoid sharing articles such as combs, razors, towels, and toothbrushes.
4. Everyone should refrigerate milk and other perishable foods. Cook food thoroughly. Do not share food from the same plate. Wash the patient's dishes in a dishwasher or wash them last by hand with hot water and soap.
5. If the illness is transmitted by the gastrointestinal route, the patient should not prepare food until he or she has had at least two negative stool cultures 24 hours apart and completed antibiotics at least 24 hours ago (Chin, 2000).
6. If the illness is transmitted by the respiratory route, provide a separate room for the patient if possible. Air out the room if possible.
7. Bathrooms may be shared if good hygiene is practiced. Use liquid soap in the bathroom. Wash and disinfect bathroom surfaces at least once a day. Flush wastes down the toilet, and clean any fecal contamination and commodes with a household disinfectant. "If you have an outdoor toilet, place 3 to 4 cups of lime in the toilet weekly" (Rice, 2000, p. 95).
8. Launder soiled linens and clothing separately "in the family washer using the hot cycle, detergent, and 1 cup of bleach, then dry in the family dryer on the hot cycle" (Humphrey & Milone-Nuzzo, 2000, pp. 3:8-3:9).
9. The family should wear clean, disposable gloves (a) when changing dressings of an infected or draining would or (b) if in contact with the patient's blood, wound drainage, open areas of the skin, feces, urine, or other bodily fluids.
10. Wear utility gloves to clean up spills of patient blood or urine with 10% bleach solution. Mix 1 part bleach and 9 parts water daily. Throw away unused bleach solution at the end of the day.
11. Bag patient trash separately in a leak-proof bag.

Data adapted from Chin, J. (2000). *Control of communicable diseases manual* (17th ed.). Washington, DC: The American Public Health Association; Humphrey, C. J., & Milone-Nuzzo, P. (2000). *Manual of home care nursing orientation* (pp. 3:8-3:9). Gaithersburg, MD: Aspen; and Rice, R. (2000). *Manual of home health nursing procedures* (2nd ed.; pp. 95-96). St. Louis: Elsevier.

- Avoid cleaning birdcages and cat litter boxes and avoid areas containing dog excreta, because excreta contain a high level of fungi and bacteria.
- Maintain personal hygiene and cleanliness by showering or bathing daily or, for the elderly, on an appropriate schedule.
- Prevent injury to the rectal mucosa by avoiding the use of rectal thermometers, rectal suppositories, and enemas, and straining at stool.
- Assess for signs of infection frequently by taking the temperature at the same time of the day every day. Report a temperature higher than 100° F and report any signs or symptoms of infection (e.g., cough with or without sputum, fever, burning on urination, urgency or frequency of urination, or cloudy urine).
- Use a soft toothbrush and clean the mouth and teeth after every meal.
- Conserve energy and maintain adequate periods of sleep and rest.
- Limit visitors, check visitors for communicable diseases, and avoid crowded places.
- Avoid cut flowers and house plants. Water standing for long periods of time can be a medium for the growth of bacteria. If cut flowers are in the home, changing the water and cleaning the vase frequently will reduce the chance of infection.

MANAGEMENT OF CARE
Integration of Providers

In a managed care framework, insurance companies are seeking ways to streamline their overhead costs and improve the efficiency of operations. One way in which managed care organizations (MCOs) have sought to meet that objective is through vertical and horizontal integration. Vertical integration allows MCOs to contract with a health care delivery system for all the services needed for a client across the continuum of care. For example, a vertically integrated network might include an

acute care hospital, a subacute care facility, physician practices, a nursing home, and a home care agency. The vertically integrated health system contracts with an MCO to provide the full spectrum of care to people in the plan. A client is seen in the most appropriate setting because the incentive is to provide the needed care in the most cost-effective setting possible.

Horizontal integration allows home care providers to form formal or informal coalitions to expand their geographic coverage area or the types of services provided. The integration is between providers of similar services rather than providers of different health care services, as is characteristic of vertical integration models. Expanded geographic coverage provides the benefit of efficiency in contracting for services for enrollees. A horizontally integrated network that provides statewide coverage can provide for all the home care needs for the people enrolled in a managed care plan.

Home health care practice has long been based on a close relationship between the home care provider and the physician responsible for approving the plan of care for the client. This relationship will need to be nurtured and strengthened in a managed care environment.

Management of Care and Cost

Home health care nurses have a long history of managing the care they provide to clients. In the traditional Medicare model, the home care nurse develops the plan of care (CMS Form 485) and sends it to the physician for approval. The home health care nurse determines the number of visits needed by the client, restricted only by the Medicare reimbursement criteria that relate to the reasonableness and necessity of care.

The management of care under a prospective payment system requires that the home care nurse manage the care by balancing both clinical and economic demands (Crossen-Sills et al., 2007). For example, a home health care nurse may be accustomed to providing approximately eight visits to a client newly diagnosed with diabetes to accomplish the teaching needed for self-management. In a prospective payment framework, one might be encouraged to accomplish in three visits what previously took eight. New strategies are needed to provide the necessary care in a reduced number of visits. The home health care nurse may be creative in using videos as a teaching and reinforcement tool. Printed material with pictures may substitute for comprehensive verbal instructions. There may be opportunities for group teaching that not only provides peer support for learning but also is an economical way to teach numbers of clients.

Need for Data

The need for reliable and consistent data related to home care practice has never been greater than it is today. Agencies that are unable to determine the costs for the services provided or for an episode of care will be unable to be efficient under the Medicare prospective payment system or effectively negotiate managed care contracts. Inability to accurately portray the unique characteristics of the home care population served puts the agency at risk of overlooking the need for additional home visits. For example, recognizing that the population the agency serves includes a significant number of elderly people (over age 85) is only half the picture. What are the utilization patterns of this population? What are the common diagnoses and comorbidities that influence return to self-management? How has care been provided to these clients in the past? The answers to these questions factor into the planning of care for this population. Many home health care agencies, however, still do not have the data collection capabilities necessary to answer these questions.

Although the need for data for individual agency decision making is paramount, the need to compare or benchmark one agency with another is also important. The comparison of agencies in a particular region requires that agencies collect data that are comparable across settings. This means that the definition of data elements must be similar from one agency to the next. This is accomplished in home care through the collection and reporting of OASIS data.

In the fall of 2003, the home care industry was the subject of a new program initiated by the Centers for Medicare and Medicaid Services (CMS) called *Home Care Compare*. In this program, several key variables indicative of the quality of home care are used to measure agency outcomes against each other. As with nursing homes, the CMS takes out full-page ads in the newspapers of the region telling consumers how home care agencies fared with regard to patient outcomes related to these variables. For example, one of the variables CMS might choose to report on is "ability to ambulate independently." All home care agencies in a region are compared on patient outcomes related to this variable. Agency A might achieve a 65% success rate on this variable, whereas Agency B might achieve only a 20% rate. The hope is that patients and families will be better decision makers in choosing their home care providers when armed with this information. Agencies with the most positive patient outcomes will be portrayed to the public in a more positive light and therefore will be, in theory, the more requested home care agency. For all these reasons, agencies have invested heavily in assessing and improving the quality of care received by a patient or groups of patients.

Measurement of client satisfaction is another essential dimension in demonstrating the strength of an agency. Several standardized client satisfaction instruments exist to allow comparison along this dimension. In addition to measuring the satisfaction of the consumers of the care that is provided, it is essential to examine the satisfaction of the customers who provide the agency with referrals. In home care, customers include MCOs, physicians, hospitals, subacute facilities, and patients and families who self-refer for services. Do these customers know about the home care agency? Do they know the special services it provides? Is it easy to refer to this agency? What agency do they think of when home care is needed and why? All this information factors into administrative decision making about where to put agency resources for improvement.

Integration of Prevention

With all its perceived problems, one characteristic of a managed care system is the incentive to keep people healthy; the system does not benefit when people get ill. Therefore, a true managed care plan emphasizes prevention of problems. In the fee-for-service world, providers wait until a person presents with a problem and then make a profit from treating the person.

Including health promotion in the home health care practice is essential for home health care nurses working in a prospective payment environment. When agencies get reimbursed for the acute care of clients, we begin to think of the client as the "wound" or the "congestive heart failure," ignoring the other dimensions of the client where acute problems may not exist. The home health care plan focuses on interventions directed toward the patient's medical problems, with little attention to the whole individual. We are taught to provide holistic care to clients, yet health promotion is rarely included in the home care plan.

One way to keep people healthy is to prevent the onset of a disease through positive changes in health habits, immunizations, and injury prevention. For home health care nurses, this means treating the problem for which the patient is referred and also looking for ways to help the patient develop positive health habits. Integrating health promotion interventions may seem difficult at first. The biggest obstacle perceived by home health care nurses is the time it takes to include appropriate instruction in the home visit. Time does not have to be the factor that prohibits home care nurses from addressing health promotion with their patients. A visit implementing a plan of care that integrates prevention of problems may take only a few more minutes than a traditional home visit. By integrating health promotion into the home care practice, nurses are better able to meet the needs of clients and improve the quality of home care delivery.

Technology

Technology has changed the way home care is provided and will continue to affect the delivery of services in a managed care system (Rice, 2003). Because the documentation of care is essential to verify that care was provided and to describe the outcome of that care, point-of-care hand-held computer devices are being used to reduce the burden and associated time for documentation. New approaches called *telehealth* have made their way into the home health care market. For example, computers with two-way viewing placed in a client's home allow the home health care nurse to make a "home visit" without leaving the office. The nurse calls the client on the telephone and asks him or her to perform certain functions. The data are immediately transmitted to the nurse in the office via telephone lines. The nurse might instruct the client to insert his or her arm in the sleeve attached to the home monitoring device. This sleeve takes the blood pressure and transmits the data to the nurse. The nurse might also ask the client to place the stethoscope on the chest so an apical pulse can be heard. The nurse can view placement of the stethoscope and instruct the client if it is incorrectly placed.

QUALITY OF CARE

Although the home health care industry has become more business-like, creating new financial arrangements that maximize income-generating potential, interest in the quality of care has remained paramount. As the number of home care agencies has increased, competition has become intense, particularly in urban areas. Home health care agencies are seeking to excel in this competitive market through accreditation or other visible means of ensuring excellence in the care they provide. This competitive climate has had a direct impact on the examination of quality care in the home care arena.

In the assessment of the quality of care, home health care agencies must first identify who is the customer and who is the consumer of care. In home care, these are often different people. The *customer* is the person who refers the client to the home health care agency. This may be the client's physician, the family of the client, or the discharge planner in the hospital that discharged the client. In some cases, the customer may be the individual client. The *consumer* is the recipient of the home care. This is the individual client, family, or significant other who receives the care provided by the home care agency. Recognizing that the consumer and the customer are often different, the home care agency must demonstrate quality care to both. Perceptions of quality of care may differ between the consumer and the customer. For example, the physician (customer) may be mainly interested in avoiding rehospitalization or infection, whereas the client (consumer) may define quality in terms of the promptness of the home care aide in arriving for the scheduled visit. Customer and consumer satisfaction is essential to a home health care agency's survival. Providing quality care means meeting or exceeding the customer's and consumer's expectations in every encounter.

Development of the mechanisms to assess quality of care in the home care setting has been slow compared with development of such mechanisms in the institutional setting. The following issues affect the ability to assess home health care quality:

- Home health care providers are limited in their ability to influence the patient care environment.
- Home health care patients typically receive other types of care in the community in addition to formal home health care.
- Clients' goals vary considerably, even among those with like conditions or illnesses.
- Data for quality measurement in home health care are difficult to acquire, because large-scale studies are difficult to do in the home.

The new focus on quality represents a shift in focus from assessment and monitoring to customer and consumer satisfaction and outcomes of care. The standardized OASIS data, discussed previously in this chapter, provide a basis for outcome-based quality improvement.

HOME HEALTH CARE AND *HEALTHY PEOPLE 2010*

Home health care is traditionally thought of as illness care in the home. Most care given to clients is precipitated by an acute illness, but treatment of the presenting problem is only part of the responsibilities of the home care nurse. Although home health care is provided primarily for care of ill people, health promotion, disease prevention, and early diagnosis should be part of each contact with a client or family.

In the early 1990s, the USDHHS developed *Healthy People 2000,* a statement of the nation's health objectives for the year 2000. Accompanying that document was *Healthy Communities 2000*, which provided comprehensive goals and objectives to encourage community leaders to work together to improve the health, environment, and quality of life of communities (American Public Health Association [APHA], 1991).

Objective 21 of *Healthy Communities 2000* relates to clinical preventive services in the community. The model goal for this objective states,

> *The community will promote, achieve, and maintain optimum health for all residents through the provision of primary health care services, including clinical preventive primary health care services and home health care. (APHA, 1991)*

This objective deals specifically with many aspects of home health care, including the availability and accessibility of all types of high-quality home care services for all members of the community. Community awareness of the multidisciplinary home health care services that are available is also included in this objective. The importance of providing home health care that is responsive to the many different populations in the community (e.g., hospice clients, chronically ill persons, and the elderly) is defined by this objective.

Home health care nurses are in the position to implement this objective and the objectives of *Healthy People 2010* (USDHHS, 2000, 2006a) in their clinical practice with clients and families in the community (see the *Healthy People 2010* box). Based on the developmental needs or situational issues the client is confronting, the home health care nurse can include relevant health promotion teaching or guidance in the care plan.

Although clients receiving home care are required to have a medical provider, not all physicians routinely assess for risky health behaviors and provide appropriate counseling and referral. Professional home health nurses can routinely include these assessments in the client histories taken on admission to home health services. For example, the home health care nurse may include teaching about the need for mammography for all female clients and their female caregivers aged 40 years and older. The nurse may include in the teaching a brochure listing all the community agencies that provide this service and the related cost. Another example of health promotion is to include dietary teaching about fat reduction for all clients and their caregivers.

The concept of family-focused care goes beyond integrating the family into the established care plan of the individual client. To integrate the *Healthy People 2010* objectives into the community, the home health care nurse may identify specific needs of family members and address those needs during a home health visit to the client. For example, while making home health visits to a woman for wound care, the home health

■ HEALTHY PEOPLE 2010 ■
Selected Objectives for Assessment, Counseling, and Referrals by Home Care Providers

1. Increase the proportion of persons appropriately counseled about health behaviors during a physician visit in the past year.

Health Behavior	2010 Objective	2002 Baseline
Diet and nutrition	56%	43%
Smoking cessation	72%	66%
Reduced alcohol consumption	17%	11%
Physical activity/exercise	54%	45%

2. Increase to 85% the proportion of physicians and dentists who counsel their at-risk patients about tobacco use cessation, physical activity, and cancer screening (current baseline: 22% to 59% of providers in 1996).
3. Increase to 60% the proportion of persons with diabetes who receive formal diabetes education (baseline: 45% in 1998).
4. Increase to 91% the proportion of persons with diabetes who have at least an annual foot examination (baseline: 68% in 1998).
5. Reduce the hospitalization of older adults with congestive heart failure as the principal diagnosis.

Age	2010 Objective/1000 Population	1997 Baseline/1000 Population
65-74 years	6.5	13.2
75-84 years	13.5	26.7
85+ years	26.5	52.7

6. Increase to 95% the proportion of patients who receive verbal counseling from prescribers and pharmacists on the appropriate use and potential risks of medications (baseline: 24% of prescribers and 14% of pharmacists in 1998).
7. Increase to 13% the proportion of adults with doctor-diagnosed arthritis who have had effective evidence-based arthritis education as an integral part of management of their conditions (baseline: 11% in 2002).
8. Increase the number of primary care facilities that provide mental health treatment on site or paid by referral to 68% of primary care facilities funded by the Health Resources and Services Administration (HRSA) (baseline: 62% of HRSA facilities in 2000).
9. Increase to 56% the proportion of children and adults who use the oral health care system each year (baseline: 44% of persons aged 2 years and older in 1996).
10. Increase vision rehabilitation to 15.5% and the use of visual and adaptive devices in persons with visual impairments to 26% (baseline: 14% use rehabilitative services and 22% use visual and adaptive devices in 2002).
11. Increase the proportion of adults aged 20 to 69 years with hearing loss who have ever used a hearing aid to 155 per 1000 of population (baseline: 149.6 per 1000 in 2001).
12. Reduce the proportion of persons with long-term care needs who do *not* have access to the continuum of long-term care services.

Health Need	2010 Target	2001 Baseline
Home health care	7.7%	9.6%
Adult daycare	2.3%	2.9%
Assisted living	1.8%	3.3%
Nursing home care	0.8%	1.1%

From U.S. Department of Health and Human Services. (2000). *Healthy people 2010: Understanding and improving health* (2nd ed.). Washington, DC: U.S. Government Printing Office; and U.S. Department of Health and Human Services. (2006). *Healthy people 2010: Midcourse review.* Washington, DC: U.S. Government Printing Office.

care nurse may observe that the spouse is a heavy smoker. Discussion of smoking cessation may reveal that the spouse desires to stop but feels he needs assistance. The home health care nurse may provide the necessary information and external motivation for seeking help with smoking cessation.

The use of the *Healthy People 2010* objectives is consistent with professional home health care. Ethically, there may be a conflict between the professional care needed by the client and the efficient, reimbursable care demanded by the home care agency. The professional nurse can use the standards of home health care practice (ANA, 2007a) as a guide for assessing the types of interventions that are appropriate in the home health care setting. Nurses must remain committed to prevention as an integral part of their nursing care of ill clients at home (Bohny, 1997).

ADVANCE MEDICAL DIRECTIVES

There is growing evidence that clients should have a voice in decision making regarding treatment options and the refusal of medical care. This is uncomplicated when people are alert and can make their wishes known to their primary care providers. In January 1993, the advance medical directive was initiated to clearly identify a course of medical action in a situation in which the client is unable to make decisions and communicate those decisions to the primary care provider.

The *advance medical directive* is a document that indicates the wishes of the client regarding various types of medical treatment in representative situations. There are two types of advance medical directive: a living will and a health care proxy, also called a durable power of attorney for health care. Either type of directive would come into effect only if the client becomes incapacitated and unable to make decisions; both are subject to change at any time.

Living wills are used by people to record their decisions to decline life-prolonging treatment if they become hopelessly ill. The living will indicates the circumstances under which it should be implemented and the care that should be provided if these circumstances arise. A *health care proxy (durable medical power of attorney),* on the other hand, focuses on naming someone who will make health care decisions if the client becomes unable to make them. The proxy also incorporates knowledge of the client's wishes regarding care.

Each state has its own laws governing the circumstances under which advance directives are invoked, their content, and the procedures for executing them. **Website Resource 31A** presents an example of forms legal in one state. Home health care nurses should become aware of the law governing advance directives in the state in which they practice.

In 1990, the federal government passed the Patient Self-Determination Act (U.S. Congress, 1990). This act, which was part of the Omnibus Reconciliation Act of 1990, required that hospitals, skilled nursing facilities, home health agencies, health maintenance organizations, and hospices provide written information to patients about their option to accept or refuse medical or surgical treatment and to formulate advance directives in compliance with state law. This act also mandates that the health care provider document in the medical record whether clients have executed advance directives. A copy of the advance medical directive must be maintained in the client's record.

In response to this legislation, home health care agencies have provided education regarding advance directives to their direct care staff. As part of the process of admission to home health care, the home health care nurse must discuss advance directives with the client, including their meaning and use. The nurse must be careful not to influence the client concerning his or her choices and decisions. Each time a client enters a health care organization (hospital, nursing home, home care health agency), he or she is asked whether advance medical directives exist. Collaboration between providers will reduce the frequency with which a client will have to communicate his or her wishes about care.

PATIENT RIGHTS AND RESPONSIBILITIES

The Medicare conditions of participation require the home health agency to provide clients with written notification of their rights, either before they receive care or during the initial evaluation visit. In addition, the home health agency must keep written documentation showing that the agency has complied with this requirement (Medicare Conditions of Participation, 1996). The NAHC (1995) established a listing of patient rights for clients and families to inform them of the ethical conduct they can expect from home health care agencies. This document is widely used by such agencies (Box 31-5).

Some home health care agencies have adapted this bill of rights to include other rights specifically applicable to their clients. Others have added a list of responsibilities the patient and family must assume to receive home health care, such as notifying agency personnel of changes in health status or providing care in the absence of the home health care nurse.

Box 31-5   Home Care Bill of Rights

Home care clients have a right to be notified in writing of their rights and obligations before treatment begins and to exercise those rights. The client's family or guardian may exercise the client's rights when the client has been judged incompetent. Home care providers have an obligation to protect and promote the rights of their clients, including the following rights.

Clients and Providers Have a Right to Dignity and Respect
Home care clients and their formal caregivers have a right not to be discriminated against based on race, color, religion, national origin, age, sex, or handicap. Furthermore, clients and caregivers have a right to mutual respect and dignity, including respect for property. Caregivers are prohibited from accepting personal gifts and borrowing from clients.

Clients Have the Right:
- To have relationships with home care providers that are based on honesty and ethical standards of conduct
- To be informed of the procedure they can follow to lodge complaints with the home care provider about the care that is, or fails to be, furnished and about a lack of respect for property. (To lodge complaints with us, call _____.)
- To know about the disposition of such complaints
- To voice their grievances without fear of discrimination or reprisal for having done so
- To be advised of the telephone number and hours of operation of the state's home care hot line that receives questions and complaints about local home care agencies, including complaints about implementation of advance directive requirements. The hours are _____ _____ and the number is _____.

Decision Making
Clients Have the Right:
- To be notified in advance about the care that is to be furnished, the types (disciplines) of the caregivers who will furnish the care, and the frequency of the visits that are proposed to be furnished
- To be advised of any change in the plan of care before the change is made
- To participate in the planning of the care and in the planning of changes in the care, and to be advised that they have the right to do so

- To be informed in writing of rights under state law to make decisions concerning medical care, including the right to accept or refuse treatment and the right to formulate advance directives
- To be informed in writing of policies and procedures for implementing advance directives, including any limitations if the provider cannot implement an advance directive on the basis of conscience
- To have health care providers comply with advance directives in accordance with state law requirements to receive care without condition on, or discrimination based on, the execution of advance directives
- To refuse services without fear of reprisal or discrimination; the home care provider or the client's physician may be forced to refer the client to another source of care if the client's refusal to comply with the plan of care threatens to compromise the provider's commitment to quality care

Privacy
Clients Have the Right:
- To confidentiality of the medical records of information about their health, social, and financial circumstances and about what takes place in the home
- To expect the home care provider to release information only as required by law or authorized by the client and to be informed of procedures for disclosure

Financial Information
Clients Have the Right:
- To be informed of the extent to which payment may be expected from Medicare, Medicaid, or any other payer known to the home care provider
- To be informed of the charges that will not be covered by Medicare
- To be informed of the charges for which the client may be liable
- To receive this information, orally and in writing, before care is initiated and within 30 calendar days of the date the home care provider becomes aware of any changes in charges
- To have access, upon request, to all bills for service the client has received, regardless of whether the bills are paid out of pocket or by another party

Box 31-5	Home Care Bill of Rights—cont'd

Quality of Care

Clients Have the Right:

- To receive care of the highest quality
- In general, to be admitted by a home care provider only if it has the resources needed to provide the care safely and at the required level of intensity, as determined by a professional assessment; a provider with less than optimal resources may nevertheless admit the client if a more appropriate provider is not available, but only after fully informing the client of the provider's limitations and the lack of suitable alternative arrangements
- To be told what to do in the case of an emergency

The Home Care Provider Shall Ensure That:

- All medically related home care is provided in accordance with physicians' orders and that a plan of care specifies the services and their frequency and duration
- All medically related personal care is provided by an appropriately trained home care aide who is supervised by a nurse or other qualified home care professional

Client Responsibility

Clients Have the Responsibility:

- To notify the provider of changes in the condition (e.g., hospitalization, changes in the plan of care, symptoms to be reported)
- To follow the plan of care
- To notify the provider if the visit schedule needs to be changed
- To inform providers of the existence of, and any changes made to, advance directives
- To advise the provider of any problems or dissatisfaction with the services provided
- To provide a safe environment for care to be provided
- To carry out mutually agreed responsibilities

To satisfy the Medicare certification requirements, the Centers for Medicare and Medicaid Services requires that agencies:

1. Give a copy of the *Bill of Rights* to each patient in the course of the admission process
2. Explain the *Bill of Rights* to the patient and document that this has been done

To minimize confusion, the National Association for Home Care recommends that agencies have clients sign one form that shows that the client acknowledges all of the agency's policies and procedures (e.g., release of medical information, billing procedures).

From National Association for Home Care. (1995). *Home care bill of rights.* Washington, DC: Author.

Home health care agencies and home health care nurses often face difficult ethical dilemmas regarding the delivery of care to clients. At times, a client will require or desire care for which Medicare or private insurance will not pay. The home health care agency has to decide whether it will provide care to the client even if there is no reimbursement. Home health care agencies have written policies to guide the decision-making process. It may be the responsibility of the home health care nurse to find another community agency that can meet the client's needs at a cost the client can afford. Home health care agencies are prohibited from discharging clients from care because they are unable to pay for the services they need. If clients need services for which they are unable to pay, and there is no other agency willing to provide that care, the agency must continue to provide care until the clients no longer need care or referral can be made to another agency.

HOSPICE HOME CARE

Hospice is a philosophy of care rather than a place of care. Hospice programs are designed to provide palliative care to terminally ill clients in both the home and inpatient institutions. In 1983, legislation established a Medicare hospice benefit for terminally ill persons. Clients who meet specific admission criteria are allowed to waive their traditional Medicare benefit and receive the Medicare hospice benefit, which provides funding for services that more closely meet the needs of the terminally ill client.

In addition to teaching caregivers about physical care and providing such care, hospice nurses focus on the client's psychologic, social, and spiritual needs. Hospice services assist terminally ill persons, their caregivers, other family members, and friends to "accept the diagnosis, adjust to life with illness, and prepare for approaching death" (Humphrey & Milone-Nuzzo, 2000). Rather than cure, quality of life is emphasized. One of the primary outcomes of end-of-life care should be the experience of a good death on the part of the client and family (Kehl, 2006).

Hospice is a concept of care that is practiced anywhere and by anyone when support is offered to people who are dying. Hospice care unites the most up-to-date principles of pain control and symptom management with the centuries-old principles of compassionate, individualized care and concern for the dignity of the dying client. Specific, recognizable elements that are part of all hospice programs go beyond the basic medical care provided to the terminally ill client. The basic tenets of the hospice philosophy described by Sylvia Lack in 1978 continue to be the cornerstone of hospice care (Box 31-6).

MEDICARE HOSPICE BENEFIT

Like home health care agencies, hospice providers must bill for the services provided to their clients so they can remain fiscally solvent. The regulations and restrictions that are part of the traditional Medicare program are not well suited to the terminally ill client. The legislation of 1983 was passed to meet the needs of the terminally ill client more appropriately and economically.

For a client to be admitted to a hospice program, regardless of the payment source, certain admission criteria must be considered. For home care services, the usual admission criteria include the following:

- A diagnosis of a terminal illness. The client's terminal illness must be certified by the attending physician and the medical director of the hospice providing the care.

Box 31-6
Basic Tenets of the Hospice Philosophy

A comprehensive approach to care: Attention is given to the physiologic, psychosocial, sociologic, and spiritual needs of the client and the family, and continuity of care is maintained regardless of the setting.

Concentration on the family as the unit of service: Both the family and the client are the recipients of care.

An interdisciplinary team approach to care: The interdisciplinary team includes physicians, nurses, social workers, home health aides, specialized therapists, pastoral counselors, and clergy.

Utilization of direct service volunteers as part of the interdisciplinary team: Volunteers provide a variety of services, including respite care, meal preparation, and friendly visiting.

Concentration of care on the improvement of the quality of life, not the extension of life: Palliative care, care that is focused on the relief of symptoms, is the focus of hospice care.

Service availability 24 hours, 7 days a week: Round-the-clock availability of professional service is essential for both the client and the family.

Bereavement follow-up: Bereavement care is available to the family, usually for 1 year following the death of the client.

Data from Lack, S. (1978). *First American hospice.* New Haven, CT: Hospice.

- A prognosis of 6 months or less.
- Informed consent from the client to receive hospice services.
- A referral to the hospice by the client's attending physician.

When clients elect to use the Medicare hospice benefit (inpatient or home care), they must waive the traditional Medicare benefit. The hospice program is technically structured in periods. During their lifetimes, clients who are terminally ill may elect to receive hospice care for two 90-day periods with subsequent periods of 60-day recertification as needed.

The client elects to receive hospice care from a certified hospice provider for one of the periods defined by the hospice program. Clients may revoke their hospice election before the period has expired, thereby reinstating their eligibility for other Medicare benefits. For example, a client who is terminally ill may first decide that he or she only wants palliative care and elect the hospice Medicare benefit. Sixty days into the first 90-day period, the client may change his or her mind and decides to pursue aggressive curative therapy. The client can then transfer back to the traditional Medicare benefit and become eligible for all the traditional Medicare services.

By waiving the traditional Medicare benefit, the client becomes eligible to receive several services and resources that are unavailable through traditional Medicare. A client must meet all Medicare criteria for home care, except being homebound, to be eligible for the hospice Medicare benefit. The hospice Medicare benefit covers the following:

- Nursing, home health aide, and social work visits deemed necessary by the hospice care team
- Services, including pastoral care, dietary counseling, and other supportive programs
- Therapy services, such as physical therapy, deemed necessary by the hospice care team
- Prescription drugs related to the condition requiring hospice care covered at the rate of 95% of cost
- Durable medical equipment needed for hospice home care covered at 100% of cost

Unlike traditional home health care, which is reimbursed on a per-visit or prospective payment basis, hospice home care is reimbursed by Medicare on a per-day basis. Hospice home care agencies receive a per-diem payment regardless of the amount of care provided to the client. Clients in the early stages of the hospice experience may require few and infrequent services, whereas clients who are actively dying may use a multitude of services. In this way, hospices are able to balance the care demand of their clients in a financially responsible way. The federal government is now looking at ways to reimburse for hospice care under a prospective payment system (Hospice Association of America, 2007). How this plays out is yet to be determined.

KEY IDEAS

1. Home health care nursing practice has its foundation in the theory and concepts that guide community/public health nursing. Home health care nurses provide family-focused care to acutely and chronically ill clients of all ages.

2. Many types of agencies can provide home health care services to clients in the community. Some home health care agencies provide both professional and paraprofessional services, whereas others provide exclusively paraprofessional services.

3. Home health care services can include care of the ill client in the home, health promotion or disease prevention, and specialized home care services such as high-technology care, pediatric care, psychiatric care, or hospice care.

4. Home health care agencies are reimbursed for the services they provide by Medicare, Medicaid, other public funds, private insurance companies, client self-payment, and private donations. For a home care agency to receive reimbursement from Medicare, the client receiving care must meet certain eligibility requirements. Since October 2000, home health care provided under Medicare has been reimbursed primarily on a prospective, per-episode basis.

5. Although many professionals and paraprofessionals are members of the home health care team, the home health care nurse is primarily responsible for case management and coordination of the other professionals and paraprofessionals in the home to ensure that the client's health care needs are being met.

6. The ANA has developed standards of home health care practice that are designed to guide the delivery of home health care nursing service at both the generalist and specialist levels.

7. Infection control in home health care has two major components. Home health care providers must protect themselves from communicable diseases of clients and must protect the client, family, and community from the spread of communicable disease.

8. By focusing both on clinical and economic demands, managed care influences the relationships of home health care providers to physicians, insurers, and clients.

9. Total quality improvement involves the customers and consumers of home health care services and the outcomes of care provided in the home. OASIS data are used for outcome-based quality improvement.

10. Home health care nurses can operationalize the *Healthy People 2010* objectives in their clinical practice by including health promotion and disease prevention interventions in all care plans for acutely and chronically ill clients and their families.

11. Clients have both rights and responsibilities related to receiving home health care. The National Association for Home Care (NAHC) has published a list of client rights and responsibilities that is used by many home care agencies.

12. Hospice is a philosophy of care rather than a place of care. Medicare clients who elect to receive the hospice Medicare benefit can waive their traditional Medicare benefit to access services appropriate to the care of terminally ill clients.

CASE STUDY A Day in the Life of a Home Care Nurse

Jane Jones is a home health care nurse at the Hill Valley VNA, a nonprofit home health care agency serving a suburban population. She has worked in home care for 4 years. Before that, she was assistant head nurse on a cardiothoracic floor in the local community hospital. She left the hospital because she felt unable to practice nursing the way she believed it should be practiced. She found home health care to be an exciting alternative to the hectic pace of the acute care institution.

Jane arrives at the home health agency at 8:00 AM and reviews the cases she has scheduled. Her caseload for today includes five visits: two visits to perform daily dressing changes, one visit to perform a cardiac assessment for a client who is seen weekly, one visit to supervise a home care aide, and an admission visit to a client who is newly diagnosed with diabetes. Given that she has to do a new admission with all the accompanying paperwork, she considers five visits as her maximum for today. On days when she does not have a new admission or her scheduled visits are short, she will often make a sixth home visit, because the agency expects the nurses to make an average of 5.5 visits per day.

To plan her day, the first piece of information Jane needs is the time the home health care aide will be in the home. Her other visits must be scheduled around this time, because Jane must supervise the home health care aide at the client's home. Jane calls the home health care aide supervisor and learns that the aide is assigned to the client from 11 AM to 1 PM. Jane believes that she can make the two home health visits to do the dressing changes and then be at the client's home to supervise the home health care aide by 11:30 AM. Thus, the admission visit to the client with newly diagnosed diabetes and the home health visit to the client in need of a cardiac assessment are scheduled for the afternoon. If all goes as planned, Jane believes that she will be back in the office at 3 PM to complete documentation and make the necessary telephone calls.

Before she leaves, she calls all her clients and tells them the approximate time she will arrive at their homes. She also asks them if there have been any changes since her last home health visit. This helps her to determine whether she needs to plan anything different for today's home health visit. She assembles all the equipment she will need, because she will not return to the agency until the end of the day. Today she needs the agency's glucometer for the new diabetic client and the scale for the cardiac client. She stocks her bag with extra gloves, paper towels, and aprons. On her way out, she gives the receptionist a list of the clients she will see today, the approximate time of the home health visit, and the client's telephone number, so that anyone can contact her. At the home health care agency, she removes a pen and some change from her purse and

then locks it in the trunk, because she does not take her purse into the client's home or leave it visible in her car.

Her first two home health visits are relatively uneventful and are conducted as planned; the home health care aide supervision is scheduled for the third visit. However, when the home health care aide reached the client's home, the client was having difficulty breathing. The aide moved the client to a sitting position, which helped slightly. Jane arrives shortly after the home health care aide. Assessment of the client reveals severe dyspnea, elevated pulse, widening pulse pressure, and cyanosis around the mouth and in the nail beds. On auscultation, crackles are heard in all lung fields, and the client expectorates frothy sputum. The client has a history of congestive heart failure.

After reassuring the client and making her as comfortable as possible, Jane calls the primary physician. Jane relays the physical symptoms to the physician and asks if the client should be sent to the emergency department or the physician's office. Given the client's condition, the physician states that the emergency department is more appropriate. Because the client has no one to transport her, an ambulance is called. While waiting for the ambulance, Jane asks the home health care aide to pack some of the client's personal belongings in an overnight bag in case she is hospitalized. The home health care aide also makes sure the client has her Medicare card and the card from her supplemental insurance policy. Jane remains with the client, monitoring her physical status. The house is prepared for the client's absence by making sure all appliances are turned off and turning on some lights. Jane and the home health care aide stay with the client until the ambulance arrives. After the client leaves in the ambulance, Jane provides support to the home health care aide for her activities with this client.

After her lunch break, Jane proceeds with the two home health visits scheduled for the afternoon. Both visits proceed as planned, and Jane is ready to return to the home health care agency by 3 PM. After she returns to the agency, the major tasks of completing the documentation and case coordination begin. Her first task is to call the primary physician for the client she admitted to care by the home health care agency today. The client had been discharged from the hospital with orders for skilled care to teach him about his diabetic diet. During her visit with the client, Jane noted that he needs assistance with his personal care because of his weakness and instability. The physician is notified about this problem, and a home health care aide is requested for 2 hours per day, twice a week.

Jane also needs to call the state-subsidized pharmacy program on behalf of her cardiac client. During her home health visit today, the client informed Jane that she had received a letter stating that she would no longer be eligible for her medication subsidy. Without

Continued

CASE STUDY A Day in the Life of a Home Care Nurse—cont'd

the subsidy, the client will be unable to afford the expensive cardiac medications she is taking. The client tried several times to find out why her subsidy had been discontinued but did not understand the reason for this change. Jane said she would try to find out why the client's subsidy was changed. Jane also calls the hospital emergency department to see if her client was admitted to the inpatient facility.

Jane tries to reach the physical therapist involved with one of her clients. Jane changes the dressing for the large burn on the leg, and the therapist provides gait training and range of motion to the affected extremity. During her home visit today, Jane noted that the client was not using his crutches correctly. Because the physical therapist is at the agency, she and Jane have a case conference

regarding this and determine that the therapist will instruct the client again on the proper use of crutches.

After the telephone calls and the case conference with the physical therapist, Jane completes the documentation that is a large part of her job. An admission visit requires completion of the OASIS and other governmental forms, the social and physical databases, and many other forms that provide data for subsequent visits. Jane also must document the home visits, telephone calls, and case conference in her clients' service records. Finally, she completes her time sheet for the day and checks her calendar for tomorrow. Seven visits are scheduled. It looks like she will need some help tomorrow, so she informs her supervisor of this before she leaves.

 See **Critical Thinking Questions** for this Case Study on the book's website.

LEARNING BY EXPERIENCE AND REFLECTION

1. Arrange to spend a day with a home health care nurse. Notice the types of clients for whom care is provided, the family-centered approach to care, and the interventions used by the nurse. Identify the unique aspects of providing care to clients in their homes.

2. Interview an elderly client who has recently received home care to assess his or her perceptions of the experience. Try to determine what services were needed that were not covered by Medicare. Also, assess the client's perceptions of the benefits of home care.

3. Interview a family who has received hospice services. How was the care helpful?

4. Review the health care records used in a home health agency, including the standard Medicare CMS (formerly HCFA) forms 485, 486, and 487. Identify ways nurses in that agency have increased the efficiency of their recording. Explore how OASIS data are electronically reported.

5. Interview a legislator from your state who is interested in health care reform. Discuss the future role of home care in the proposals for reforming the American health care system. Discuss how these changes will affect the delivery of health care in general and home health care specifically.

6. Ask a home health care nurse to discuss a clinical situation in which she or he had to make a difficult ethical decision. This may include a decision to discharge a client who is unsafe in the home, to discharge a Medicare client who continues to need nursing care but is no longer homebound, or to terminate services because of inability to pay. Discuss the process the nurse went through to make the decision and its impact on her or his professional development.

7. Observe a home health care nurse making a home visit and a hospice nurse making a home visit. Compare and contrast the similarities and differences. Discuss the similarities and differences with the two nurses and ask for their impressions about your observations.

8. Explore your state's laws governing advance directives. Obtain or develop forms for a living will and a durable power of attorney for health care that are consistent with

the state law. Consider whether you wish to complete such forms for yourself. Do you need any additional information before completing the forms? If so, from whom?

COMMUNITY RESOURCES FOR PRACTICE

Information about each of the following organizations is found on its website, which can be accessed through this book's website at *http://evolve.elsevier.com/Maurer/community/*.

Alzheimer's Disease and Related Disorders Association
American Association of Retired Persons
American Cancer Society
American Diabetes Association
American Foundation for the Blind
American Heart Association
American Public Health Association
Independent Living for the Handicapped
Injury Control Center
International Hearing Society Hearing Aid Helpline: 800-521-5247
The Joint Commission (formerly Joint Commission on the Accreditation of Healthcare Organizations)
National Association for Home Care
National Center for Complementary and Alternative Medicine
National Center for Health Statistics, Clearinghouse on Health Indexes
National Clearinghouse for Alcohol and Drug Abuse Information
National Clearinghouse for Mental Health Information
National Clearinghouse on Child Abuse and Neglect Information
National Heart, Lung, and Blood Institute
National Hospice Organization
National Institute on Adult Day Care
National League for Nursing
National Multiple Sclerosis Society
National Rehabilitation Information Center (NARIC)
National Institute for Occupational Safety and Health
OASIS website
Public Health Service AIDS Information Hotline ([800] 342-AIDS)
Rehabilitation Services Administration
Sex Information and Education Council of the United States
Visiting Nurse Associations of America

STUDY AIDS　http://evolve.elsevier.com/maurer/community/

Visit the Evolve website for this book to find the following study and assessment materials:

- Quiz
- Web Scenario
- Critical Thinking Questions and Answers for Case Studies
- Care Plans
- *Healthy People* Updates
- Glossary

WEB

WEBSITE RESOURCES

These items supplement the chapter's topics and are also found on the Evolve site:

31A: Advance Medical Directive

REFERENCES

American Nurses Association. (2007). *Public health nursing: Scope and standards of practice*. Silver Spring, MD: Author.

American Nurses Association. (2008). *Home health nursing: Scope and standards of practice*. Silver Spring, MD: Nursebooks.org.

American Nurses Credentialing Center (ANCC). (2007). *Certification and certification renewal news and announcement archive*. Silver Spring, MD: Author. Retrieved May 9, 2008 from *http://www.nursecredentialing.org/cert/archives/index.htm*.

American Public Health Association. (1991). *Healthy communities 2000: Model standards* (3rd ed.). Washington, DC: Author.

Arnaert, A., & Delesie, L. (2007). Effectiveness of video-telephone nursing care for the homebound elderly. *Canadian Journal of Nursing Research, 39*(1), 20-36.

Bohny, B. J. (1997). A time for self-care: Role of the home healthcare nurse. *Home Healthcare Nurse, 15*(4), 281-286.

Centers for Medicare and Medicaid Services. (1978; revised 1997). *The home health agency manual (publication 11)*. Washington, DC: Author. Retrieved May 12, 2008 from *http://www.cms.hhs.gov/manuals/pbm/ItemDetail.asp?ItemID=CMS021914*.

Chin, J. (2000). *Control of communicable diseases manual* (17th ed.). Washington, DC: The American Public Health Association.

Crossen-Sills, J., Bilton, W., Bickford, M., et al. (2007). Home care today: Showcasing inter-disciplinary management in home care. *Home Healthcare Nurse, 25*(4), 245-252.

Fazzi, R. (2006). Best practice insights. Best practice ensuring OASIS accuracy. *Caring, 25*(5), 54-55.

Freed, P. (2006). The mental health patient. In R. Rice (Ed.), *Home care nursing practice: Concepts and applications* (4th ed.; pp. 425-442). St. Louis: Mosby.

Health Care Financing Administration. (1989, April). *Medicare home health agency manual* (Publication No. 11). Washington, DC: Author.

Health Care Financing Administration. (1999, January 25). Medicare and Medicaid programs:

Reporting Outcome and Assessment Information Set (OASIS) data as part of the conditions of participation for home health agencies. *Federal Register, 64*(15), 3747-3763.

Hospice Association of America. (2007). *Hospice facts and statistics*. Washington, DC: Author.

Humphrey, C. J., & Milone-Nuzzo, P. (2000). *Manual of home care nursing orientation*. Gaithersburg, MD: Aspen.

Kehl, K. (2006). Moving towards peace: An analysis of the concept of a good death. *American Journal of Hospice and Palliative Medicine, 23*(4), 277-286.

Lack, S. (1978). *First American hospice*. New Haven, CT: Hospice.

McEvoy, M. (2003). Culture and spirituality as an integrated concept in pediatric care. *MCN American Journal of Maternal and Child Nursing, 28*(1), 39-44.

Medicare Conditions of Participation: Home health agencies. (1996). *Federal Register, 54*(155).

Milone-Nuzzo, P. (2003). Clinical nurse specialists in home care. *Clinical Nurse Specialist, 17*(5), 234-235.

National Association for Home Care. (1995). *Home care bill of rights*. Washington, DC: Author.

National Association for Home Care. (2003). *State Licensure and Certificate of Need Survey*. Washington, DC: Author.

National Association for Home Care. (2007). *Basic statistics about home care*. Washington, DC: Author.

Rice, R. (2000). *Manual of home health nursing procedures* (2nd ed.). St. Louis: Elsevier.

Rice, R. (2003). *Telecaring: Home care nursing praxis and the discipline of nursing*. Unpublished doctoral dissertation, University of Colorado, Denver.

Rice, R. (2006). Infection control in the home. In R. Rice (Ed.), *Home care nursing practice: Concepts and applications* (4th ed.; pp 75-96). St. Louis: Mosby.

Turnbough-Hill, N., & Rice, R. (2006). Developing the plan of care and documentation. In R. Rice (Ed.), *Home care nursing practice: Concepts and applications* (4th ed.; pp 49-74). St. Louis: Mosby.

Tweed, S. (2003). Seven performance-accelerating technologies that will shape the future of home care. *Home Healthcare Nurse, 21*(10), 647-650.

U.S. Congress, Committee on Government Reform and Oversight. (1998). *Implementation of Public Law 105-33*. 105th Congress, Entry No. 98-18154. Washington, DC: U.S. Government Printing Office.

U.S. Congress, House. (1990). *Omnibus Budget Reconciliation Act of 1990: Patient Self-Determination Act*. House Resolution 5835, 101st Congress, Entry No. 95-09400. Washington, DC.

U.S. Department of Health and Human Services. (1990). *Healthy people 2000: National health promotion and disease prevention objectives*. Washington, DC: U.S. Government Printing Office.

U.S. Department of Health and Human Services. (2000). *Healthy people 2010: Understanding and improving health* (2nd ed.). Washington, DC: U.S. Government Printing Office.

U.S. Department of Health and Human Services. (2006a). *Healthy people 2010: Midcourse review*. Washington, DC: U.S. Government Printing Office.

U.S. Department of Health and Human Services. (2006b). *The registered nurse population: Findings from the March 2004 National Sample Survey of Registered Nurses*. Washington, DC: Division of Nursing, Bureau of Health Professions, Health Resources and Services Administration.

U.S. Department of Health and Human Services. (2007). *Statistics: Aging into the twenty-first century: Summary*. Retrieved May 9, 2008, from *http://www.aoa.gov/prof/statistics/future_growth/aging21/summary.asp*.

Warhola, C. (1980). *Planning for home health services: A resource handbook*. Washington, DC: U.S. Department of Health and Human Services.

Zuber, R. F. (2002). Assessing Medicare eligibility: Suggestions for improving processes. *Home Healthcare Nurse, 20*(7), 425-430.

SUGGESTED READINGS

Benefield, L. E. (2003). Implementing evidenced-based practice in home care. *Home Healthcare Nurse, 21*(12), 804-809.

Buhler-Wilkerson, K. (2002). No place like home: A history of nursing and home care in the U.S. *Home Healthcare Nurse, 20*(10), 641-647.

Carrico, R. M., & Niner, S. (2002). Multidrug resistant organisms—VRE and MRSA: Practical home care tips. *Home Healthcare Nurse, 20*(1), 23-29.

Crisler, K. S., Baillie, L. L., & Richard, A. A. (2000). Integrating OASIS data collection into a comprehensive assessment. *Home Healthcare Nurse, 18*(4), 249-254.

Evans, M. J., & Hallett, C. E. (2007). Living with dying: A hermeneutic phenomenological study of the work of hospice nurses. *Journal of Clinical Nursing, 16*(4), 742-751.

Fraiser, K. (2004). Decision-making and nursing case management. *ANS Advances in Nursing Science, 27*(3), 32-45.

Johnson, M. O. (2001). Meeting health care needs of a vulnerable population: Perceived barriers. *Journal of Community Health Nursing, 18*(1), 35-52.

Kouch, M. (2006). Managing symptoms for a good death. *Nursing, 36*(11), 58-64.

Krulish, L. H. (2000). When should I do an OASIS assessment? *Home Healthcare Nurse, 18*(4), 238-248.

Miller, K. E. (2002, December). Maintaining health in the elderly. *Home Health Care Consultant*, 18-23.

Mundinger, M. (1983). *Home care controversy: Too little, too late, too costly*. Rockville, MD: Aspen Systems Corporation.

Murashina, S., & Asahara, K. (2003). The effectiveness of the around-the-clock in-home care system: Did it prevent the institutionalization of frail elderly? *Public Health Nursing, 20*(1), 13-24.

Rice, R. (1999). Home health care. A little art in home care: Poetry and storytelling for the soul. *Geriatric Nursing, 20*(3), 165-166.

Ovington, L. G. (2001). Hanging wet-to-dry dressings out to dry. *Home Healthcare Nurse, 19*(8), 477-484.

Sandelowski, M. (2002). Visible humans, vanishing bodies, and virtual nursing: Complications of life, presence, place, and identity. *ANS Advances in Nursing Science, 24*(3), 58-67.

Sheeman, D. W. (2004). Palliative nursing: Nurse's stress and burnout: How to care for yourself when caring for patients and their families experiencing life-threatening illness. *American Journal of Nursing, 104*(5), 48-54.

Warrington, D. (2004). Effectiveness of a home-based cardiac rehabilitation for special needs patients. *Journal of Advanced Nursing, 41*(2), 121-126.

Wilson, J. S. (1996). National certification for home care nurses: Bird by bird. *Home Healthcare Nurse, 14*(10), 817-821.

Wooten, M. K., & Hawkins, D. (2001). Clean vs sterile: Management of chronic wounds. *Journal of Wound, Ostomy, and Continence Nursing, 28*(5), 24A.

Zander, K. (2002). Nursing case management in the twenty-first century: Intervening where margin meets mission. *Nursing Administration Quarterly, 26*(5), 58-67.

C
H
A
P
T
E
R

32 Rural Health

Angeline Bushy

FOCUS QUESTIONS

What do the terms *urban, rural, frontier, metropolitan, nonmetropolitan,* *and health professional shortage area* mean?

What at-risk populations live in rural areas? What are some of their special nursing care needs?

What factors affect accessibility, availability, and acceptability of health care services for rural residents?

What significant economic, social, and cultural factors affect rural community nursing?

How does rural community nursing differ from practice in more populated settings?

How does a community/public health nurse build a partnership with residents of a rural community?

CHAPTER OUTLINE

KEY TERMS

The U.S. Bureau of the Census estimates that there are 54 million people living in rural areas of the United States. They make up about one fifth (20%) of the total population but are spread out across four fifths (80%) of the land area. Although a few rural regions are experiencing a decline in population, since 1990 there has been a broad economic revival and population growth in many small towns across the 50 states (Office of Rural Health Policy [ORHP], 2002; U.S. Bureau of the Census, 2000; U.S. Department of Agriculture [USDA], 2006, 2007a, 2007b).

Concerns about rural health care services, especially in regions with insufficient numbers of all types of health care providers (designated as **health professional shortage areas [HPSAs]**), have become a national priority since the early 1990s. Those concerned with rural health delivery issues are

aware of the problems in recruiting and retaining qualified health professionals. Recently, more information has become available on the special challenges, problems, and opportunities of community health nursing in geographically large, sparsely populated areas (American Nurses Association, 1996; Burbank-Schmitt, 2006; Bureau of Health Professions, 2007; Gamm, 2007; National Rural Health Association [NRHA], 2004).

DEFINITIONS

The term *rural* is not easy to define because it means different things to different people. This diversity is a concern among policy makers, researchers, and health care providers alike, because it hampers a coordinated approach to understanding the demographics, epidemiology, and health-related problems of rural communities. A standardized definition of *rural* is needed for a more coordinated approach to describing clinical problems and addressing health care delivery issues in these settings. Most individuals include geographic and population factors as well as subjective perceptions in their idea of **rural** versus **urban** (Glasgow et al., 2004; Lee & Winters, 2006).

GEOGRAPHIC REMOTENESS AND SPARSE POPULATION

Several commonly used definitions for *rural* refer to the geographic size of an area in relation to its population density or the number of people per square mile. To establish some consensus of viewpoints, one pair of descriptors used by policy makers and program developers is **metropolitan** and **nonmetropolitan**. A *metropolitan* area is defined as a city or adjacent area having a total of 50,000 or more residents. Of the total U.S. population, 80.3% live in a metropolitan area, and 19.7% reside in rural areas (Coburn et al., 2007; ORPH, 2002; U.S. Bureau of the Census, 2000; USDA, 2006) (Figure 32-1).

Another set of definitions distinguishes among urban, suburban, rural, farm, and nonfarm residency. In these, *rural* refers to a community having fewer than 20,000 residents, and any community having a greater population is considered *urban*. Of the total U.S. population, approximately 20% live in rural areas, and approximately 5% live in towns of no more than 2500 residents. Fewer than 2% of the total U.S. population have a **farm residence;** that is, outside the city limits. Most farm residents are involved in agriculture. Another set of definitions classifies regions as urban, rural, and **frontier**. In some ways, these latter terms better illustrate the problems encountered by a few people living in a large geographic region.

A more specific definition of *rural* accounts for the distance and/or time to commute to an urban area to access health care services (e.g., more than 30 minutes or more than 20 miles). However, the factors of time and distance to access services also may be applicable to residents who live in inner cities or suburban areas. For research purposes, the rural-urban continuum offers a classification scheme that distinguishes metropolitan (metro) counties by the population size and nonmetropolitan (nonmetro) counties by the degree of urbanization associated

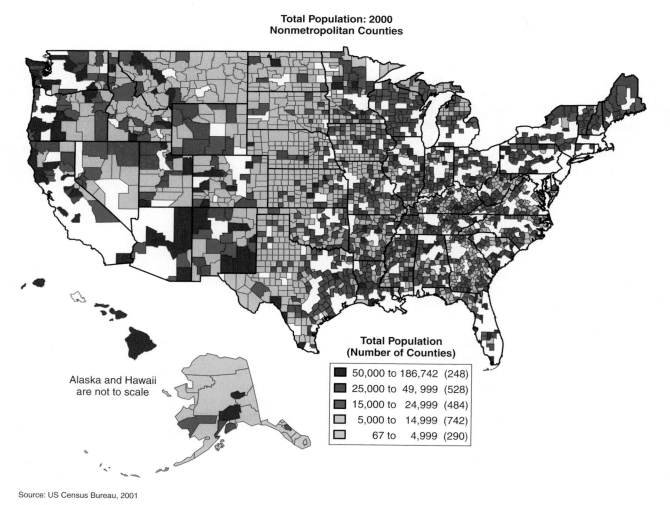

Total Population: 2000
Nonmetropolitan Counties

Total Population
(Number of Counties)

■	50,000 to 186,742 (248)
■	25,000 to 49,999 (528)
■	15,000 to 24,999 (484)
□	5,000 to 14,999 (742)
□	67 to 4,999 (290)

Alaska and Hawaii are not to scale

Source: US Census Bureau, 2001

Produced by North Carolina Rural Health Research and Policy Analysis Center, Cecil G. Sheps Center for Health Services Research, University of North Carolina at Chapel Hill.

Metropolitan areas are omitted. The New England County Metropolitan Area (NECMA) definition is used to classify nonmetropolitan counties in New England.

FIGURE 32-1 Total population: 2000 nonmetropolitan counties. (From U.S. Bureau of the Census & North Carolina Rural Health Research and Policy Analysis Center, Chapel Hill, NC. Retrieved May 28, 2007 from *http://www.shepscenter.unc.edu/research_programs/rural_program/mapbook2003/totalpopulation.pdf*.)

with adjacency to a metro area. This classification helps to address overlapping and inconsistent definitions of *rural* versus *urban* (Coburn et al., 2007; USDA, 2006; U.S. Department of Health and Human Services [USDHHS], 2007).

SUBJECTIVE PERCEPTIONS OF "RURAL"

Some Americans perceive rural areas as those not having access to cable television, whereas others think that any town with a major discount store is an urban center. However, there also are some rather grim rural scenes that are less obvious. For example, on American Indian reservations, most of which are located in rural areas, impoverishment is comparable with that in third world countries. In migrant labor camps, one-room shanties shelter two or more Mexican American families, toilet facilities are lacking, and workers suffer intense exposure to highly carcinogenic herbicides and pesticides. "Boom towns" that spring up overnight in energy-rich regions (i.e., areas with coal, oil, or precious metals) or in vacation-destination communities are not prepared to handle the social problems stemming from the massive influx of outsiders into long-established agricultural communities.

The "typical rural town" is hard to describe because of wide population and geographic diversity. A rural town in Utah is quite different from one in Alaska, Hawaii, or Tennessee. Likewise, there can be many differences among towns in the same state. Legislators' understanding of a rural area is usually based on the district they represent, and this often is reflected in their decisions.

Furthermore, the various terms used to describe and understand rural residency are relative. For instance, *small* communities with more than 25,000 population have some features that one expects to find in a large city, whereas residents in a community of fewer than 2000 perceive a town with 10,000 people as a city. Residents in geographically remote areas may not feel isolated because they perceive having urban services within easy reach, either through telecommunication or dependable transportation (Gamm, 2007; Gamm & Hutchison, 2004; Gamm et al., 2003a, 2003b; Monk, 2007).

RURAL ECONOMIC AND POPULATION PATTERNS

Another classification of rural areas created by the federal government provides greater specificity concerning a rural area's economic climate based on the principal industries in that area. The seven classes of nonmetropolitan counties, based on economic dependencies, are farming dependent, manufacturing dependent, mining dependent, specialized government, persistent poverty, federal lands, and recreational-retirement (USDA, 2006, 2007a, 2007b).

For example, manufacturing-dependent counties are characterized by a larger and more dense population, a higher proportion of households with a female head, and a greater proportion of African American residents. In contrast, farming-dependent counties are characterized by a smaller population, fewer persons per square mile, fewer households with female heads, and a higher proportion of elderly persons. This categorization, based on demographic characteristics, may also lend some insight into a particular community's health problems (e.g., elderly individuals with chronic illness, younger-than-average population with higher fertility rates, and specific types of occupational hazards and environmental risks, such

as farming and ranching with an increase in skin cancer). This approach, however, can falsely lead to a perceived homogeneity of the community, because little consideration is given to subpopulations (underrepresented groups) who also live there (Coburn et al., 2007; Gamm, 2007).

Recent demographic trends show that many nonmetropolitan areas experienced a substantial influx of new residents, especially in recreational and retirement counties. Counties experiencing the most rapid rural growth are found in states located in the intermountain west extending from Canada to Mexico, as well as in regions of the Ozarks, the lake country of the upper Midwest, Florida, the Blue Ridge Mountains, and along the outskirts of some thriving metropolitan suburbs. Population estimates reveal that some rural communities are expanding so rapidly with resettled urban residents that existing local infrastructures and public services are unable to keep pace with the growth. For instance, aging water, sewage, and communication systems; housing units; and schools are inadequate to handle the increased demands associated with the influx of local residents. However, approximately 25% of all nonmetropolitan counties continue to have a declining population. Disproportionately, communities with declining populations are located in the Great Plains, the Corn Belt, and the Mississippi delta and scattered among mining districts across the 50 states. Few data exist that describe either the short- or long-range impact on the health of rural communities caused by the rapid in-migration of formerly urban residents. A little more is known about the community impact of a declining population. Based on a review of the literature, one can project that traditional community dynamics will play a role in how long-time rural residents integrate new residents into their communities (ORHP, 2002; USDA, 2007b).

Consistent with national trends, there has been an increase in the proportion of racial minorities in rural areas, and they make up approximately 17% of the rural population (Bureau of Primary Health Care [BPHC], 2006; Gibbs, 2004; Kaiser Foundation, 2003; Probst et al., 2002). Although not much is known about residents of rural areas in general, even less is known about the subgroups and minorities who live there. Most health information about rural populations focuses on maternal, infant, and elderly populations; such information is easier to assess and monitor because of existing public services. However, there are regional differences as well as great variations in health status even within a given community. For example, some rural states in the upper Midwest and intermountain area report the best overall pregnancy outcomes. Within those same states, however, American Indians have the poorest outcomes, comparable with those of third world countries. Except for American Indians, many of whom receive care from the Indian Health Service (IHS, 2007a, 2007b, 2007c), we do not have adequate descriptions of the health status of rural minority populations. This is partially attributable to the very small numbers of rural minority group members, for whom data tend not to be broken out from large national data sets (ORHP, 2002).

Both out-migration and in-migration can create problems that, in many instances, a small town cannot solve because of the lack of resources. For example, population shifts disrupt long-established informal "helping networks," creating a need for unusual kinds of human services for localities, such as support services for abused women, parenting classes, and crisis intervention teams. Despite the need, public health programs, community nursing, and mental health services often are not available, accessible, or acceptable to target groups in rural areas.

STATUS OF HEALTH IN RURAL POPULATIONS

RURAL INITIATIVES: *HEALTHY PEOPLE 2010*

In general, rural areas can be described as "bipolar"—that is, most residents are either younger than 17 years or older than 65 years. In turn, the demographics are reflected in the health status and health care needs of residents in a particular community (see the *Healthy People 2010* box on this page). *Rural Healthy People 2010: A Companion Document to Healthy People 2010* (Gamm, 2007; Gamm & Hutchison, 2004; Gamm et al., 2003a, 2003b) has important implications for identifying and prioritizing the health care needs of rural residents. Consistent with *Healthy People 2010* (USDHHS, 2000), a number of at-risk populations are mentioned in this policy-guiding document, specifically migrant workers, blacks, American Indians and other American natives, Asians, and Pacific Islanders, as well as pregnant women, children, and the elderly. (Refer to Chapters 10 and 21 for additional information.) In spite of the contributions offered by this rurally focused initiative, there continues to be a serious gap in data on the health status of vulnerable and at-risk rural populations, particularly minorities (Gamm, 2007; ORHP, 2002; USDHHS, 2000, 2007).

In general, the literature indicates that, compared with urban Americans, rural people

- Have higher infant and maternal morbidity rates;
- Have higher rates of chronic illnesses, such as hypertension and cardiovascular disease;
- Experience problems associated with rural occupations, such as machinery accidents, skin cancer from sun exposure, and breathing problems from exposure to chemicals and pesticides;
- Have high rates of mental illness and stress-related diseases (especially among the rural poor);
- Are less likely to have health insurance with pharmacy coverage plans;
- Spend 25% more on prescription drugs than those in cities.

Rural Homelessness and Poverty

Homelessness is not unique to urban areas. People without homes are found in rural areas, too, and they face some rather unique health problems. For instance, rural homeless people often are families from the community who had their farms or businesses foreclosed. Sometimes they are able to continue living in their houses, depending on the law, but they no longer have a means of livelihood and therefore are without any income to purchase food or services. However, most are not able to remain in foreclosed properties and are truly homeless. Two major groups of rural homeless people are migrant workers and families who are poor (Brown & Swanson, 2003; Sawyer et al., 2006).

Migrant Workers. Migrant farmworkers travel from one work site to another in different states to seek employment in the agriculture industry. Many of them are documented immigrants, holding green cards that permit them to work in the United States. There are, however, a significant but imprecise number of migrant workers and seasonal workers (those who

■ HEALTHY PEOPLE 2010 ■
Rural Health Issues

1. Increase the proportion of persons who have access to rapidly responding prehospital emergency medical services (EMSs). Defined in rural areas as an interval of less than 10 minutes from the time an emergency call is placed to arrival on the scene for at least 80% of EMS responses (Baseline: populations covered by life support, 91%; by advanced life support, 77%; by helicopter transport services, 75%; by basic 911, 74%; living in areas with two-way communication between hospitals, 68% in 2002).

2. Reduce exposure to pesticides as measured by urine concentrations of metabolites used in agriculture.

| | 1988-1994 | |
Pesticide	Baseline	2010 Target
1-Naphthol (carbaryl)	36 mcg/g creatinine	25.2 mcg/g creatinine
Paranitrophenol (methyl parathion and parathions)	3.8 mcg/g	2.7 mcg/g
3,5,6-Trichloro-pyridinol (chlorpyrifos)	8.3 mcg/g	5.8 mcg/g
Isopropoxyphenol (propoxur)	1.6 mcg/g	1.1 mcg/g

3. Reduce deaths from agriculture work–related injuries to 16.3 per 100,000 workers (baseline: 23.2 per 100,000 workers in 1998).

4. Reduce work-related farm injuries resulting in medical treatment, lost time from work, or restricted work activity to 5.3 per 100 full-time workers (baseline: 7.6 per 100 workers in 1998).

5. Reduce occupational skin diseases or disorders among full-time workers to 47 new cases per 100,000 (baseline: 67 new cases per 100,000 full-time workers in 1997). *Note:* Agriculture, forestry, and fishing industries have the highest rate of diagnosed new cases; no data provided in *Healthy People 2010.*

6. Reduce new cases of work-related, noise-induced hearing loss (developmental; no baseline; agriculture workers have a high rate of hearing loss).

From U.S. Department of Health and Human Services. (2000). *Healthy people 2010: Understanding and improving health* (2nd ed.). Washington, DC: U.S. Government Printing Office; and U.S. Department of Health and Human Services. (2006). *Healthy people 2010: Midcourse review.* Washington, DC: U.S. Government Printing Office.

remain in one location throughout the year) who are undocumented aliens. As a group, generally they are Latinos who travel, work, live, and sleep together as they travel along one of several migrant streams starting and ending in Mexico and the Caribbean. The group often includes extended family members of several generations who live and travel in an older-model vehicle. They work for very low wages, and many send part of their salary to family members who remain in their country of origin. Migrant workers currently are receiving a great deal of national attention in discussions related to public assistance and health care. Policies regarding these federal initiatives have implications for public health. Additional information on migrant farmworkers can be found in the reference section and in Chapter 21 (BPHC, 2006; National Advisory Council on Migrant Health, 1993; USDA, 2007a).

The Poor. Poverty is on the rise in the United States, and racial and ethnic minorities have a higher prevalence of poverty and lower health status than whites (Gibbs, 2004). Economically depressed conditions in communities definitely affect the health status of the people who live there. For instance, unemployment and underemployment have left millions of Americans unable to afford medical insurance, which perpetuates the problem of lack of insurance or underinsurance among families (see Chapters 4 and 21). More than 50% of the medically underinsured live in nonurban areas. Forty percent of all rural families live below the poverty level. Although minority children represent only 20% of the rural population, they are more likely to live in poverty than their urban counterparts. These children experience substandard housing, poor sanitation, inadequate nutrition, contaminated water, and lack of public health services, particularly prenatal care, immunizations, health screening, and health education (Kaiser Foundation, 2003; NRHA, 2004; ORHP, 2002).

Prevention Behaviors

Overall, rural adults are less likely than urban adults to engage in preventive behaviors such as obtaining regular blood pressure checks, Pap smears, or breast examinations. Also, higher percentages of rural adults engage in risk behaviors such as smoking and not wearing seat belts, which have implications for their overall health status. Some experts speculate that these persistent lifestyle behaviors are associated with inadequate health promotion education by properly prepared health professionals, of which there are too few in rural areas. Still others speculate that the health-promoting information that is disseminated is not culturally appropriate for rural consumers. Consequently, the information that is distributed does not lead to behavior changes. More research is needed on the health beliefs and practices of rural communities to develop culturally and linguistically appropriate services for those communities (Gamm, 2007; Gamm & Hutchison, 2004; Gamm et al., 2003a, 2003b; USDHHS, 2007).

FAMILY SERVICES

Family planning and maternal, perinatal, and infant and child health care services are lacking in rural areas. As with the larger health system, maternal and infant health services in the United States are an ironic mixture of superb medical care for some segments and inadequate care for many minorities and economically deprived individuals. Like their metropolitan counterparts, poor rural families face significant barriers to adequate maternal and infant health care. However, rural families face additional problems, including greater travel distances and difficulty in maintaining comprehensive health services, especially for pregnant women, infants, and children.

Although many regional differences exist, generally there are higher rates of maternal and infant mortality and morbidity in rural areas than in urban areas, especially among racial minorities. This biostatistic reflects social, genetic, economic, and environmental factors that prevail in rural communities. For instance, social factors include a group's religious belief system regarding the appropriate time for a pregnant woman to seek professional prenatal services. A genetic factor is exemplified by the predisposition of African Americans to sickle cell anemia. Environmental factors include contaminated water, air pollution, or pesticide to which a migrant worker who is young and pregnant may be exposed. Less-than-optimal pregnancy outcomes, however, can also be attributed to impaired access to and availability of obstetric and pediatric providers and services (Gamm & Hutchison, 2004; Gamm et al., 2003a, 2003b; ORHP, 2002; Probst et al., 2002).

In recent years, there has been a marked reduction in the number of family planning, abortion, and maternal and child care providers and services in nonmetropolitan areas. Despite an overall increase in the number of obstetricians, pediatricians, and family/general practitioners in the United States, many children and pregnant women face a shortage of providers and services. This can be attributed partly to the high cost of malpractice insurance and partly to the fact that health care providers are not equitably distributed in rural geographic areas. This leaves some areas of the United States without any, or with an insufficient number of, health professionals (Bureau of Health Professions [BHPR], 2007; Burbank-Schmitt, 2006; Health Resources and Services Administration [HRSA], 2003; National Health Service Corps [NHSC], 2007; NRHA, 2004; Randolph et al., 2002).

In frontier regions of the United States, for example, some pregnant women must travel more than 150 miles one way to obtain care from an obstetrician. Traveling long distances for care also may be required for children with disabilities who live in rural environments, because specialists usually practice in urban areas. Consequently, pregnant women living in rural areas, especially minorities, are less likely to initiate care during the first trimester, and their children with special needs are less likely to receive rehabilitative and restorative care.

The closure of rural hospitals and their obstetric units has had an adverse effect not only on access to services but also on pregnancy outcomes. Hospital closures in rural areas often are associated with depressed local economies and inequitable prospective reimbursement policies. More recently, the development and expansion of large health care systems have also led to closures of small and rural hospitals.

For example, many large health care systems are buying out small hospitals and physician practices in rural communities. When these health care systems enter the community, local residents are told that outreach health care services will be provided to them. Because the numbers of rural residents are small and because the overall health of rural residents is poor, services to these communities are not as profitable as projected by the administrators of health care systems. Hence, to cut costs and improve profits, outreach services to rural communities in many cases are reduced or eliminated, which leaves already underserved communities with even fewer providers. The impact of health care systems on rural communities poses many unresolved and serious concerns. Data are currently being collected to assess the effects of this particular phenomenon on the health of rural communities (Centers for Medicare and Medicaid Services [CMS], 2007a, 2007b; Coburn et al., 2007; ORHP, 2002).

Women who live in communities with relatively few obstetric providers, for example, are less likely to deliver in their local community hospitals than are those who live in communities with a higher ratio of providers. Moreover, women who must leave "high-outflow" communities to deliver have been found to have a higher rate of complicated and premature births, which has been attributed to delays in seeking prenatal care early in pregnancy and inadequate health education (Coward et al., 2004).

Mothers and infants living in professionally underserved areas remain in the hospital longer after delivery than do those who have better access to obstetricians and pediatricians. Because of the distance of the hospital from their home and the potential need for emergency services, these women are not discharged as quickly as those who live closer. For example, a new mother who lives more than 100 miles from the hospital and must contend with ice and snow on a county road to reach her home is less likely to be discharged with her new infant after 24 hours than one who lives in the town in which the hospital is located.

Higher rates of maternal and perinatal mortality and morbidity among rural individuals cannot be attributed entirely to geographic distances and delays in securing health care, however. As mentioned earlier, rural areas suffer from higher rates of poverty and lower percentages of families with health insurance. Rural states historically have had more restrictive qualification criteria for public assistance. Likewise, welfare reform that limits the time one can receive benefits has had mixed results in rural areas. Particular rural concerns include fewer educational and employment opportunities and limited child care services for those trying to get off public assistance (Gamm & Hutchison, 2004; Gamm et al., 2003a, 2003b).

MAJOR HEALTH PROBLEMS

There are regional differences in the predominant health problems in rural communities, depending on environmental, genetic, industrial, and socioeconomic factors. Compared with urban areas, there are wider variations in rural areas in the rates of accidents, trauma, chronic illness, suicide, homicide, and use of alcohol and drugs, especially among some minority groups (Gamm & Hutchison, 2004; Gamm et al., 2003a, 2003b; USDHHS, 2000, 2007).

Accidents and Trauma

Trauma and violence pose serious threats of death and long-term disability in Americans, especially adolescent and young adult males. The leading cause of adolescent death is automobile accidents. Annually, thousands of others are severely injured because of alcohol-related accidents. In the United States, there are more than 125,000 individuals with trauma-induced paraplegia, a significant number of whom are between the ages of 15 and 24 years. Rural populations suffer more injuries from lightning, farm machinery, firearms, drowning, and accidents involving vehicles such as boats, snowmobiles, motorcycles, and all-terrain vehicles, although separate rural morbidity and mortality data are often unavailable for such accidents.

Occupational health is of particular concern in rural communities. Of the four most dangerous industries (agriculture, fishing, mining, construction), proportionally agriculture has the highest morbidity and mortality rates, although the number of persons actively engaged in farming has decreased. Not only is agricultural work inherently dangerous, but it must also be performed under adverse conditions, such as snow, mud, and extreme heat or cold, and workers must endure long hours. The agricultural labor force is extremely diverse with respect to age, work experience, education, and literacy levels. Because most farm enterprises are categorized as family farms, spouses, children, and other relatives often help with the work without much regard to competency, training,

or safety. Similarly, migrant workers (many of whom cannot read English) often consist of women and children of various ages who spend long hours working in fields without having been given Occupational Safety and Health Administration safety briefs. For these reasons, agriculture has by far the highest number of injuries and deaths among children of all industries (USDA, 2007a).

The number of agricultural accidents among women and children and the impact on the family when the male head of the household is involved in a serious injury or death are unknown. Family businesses are small, so they do not have workers' compensation insurance. Because health professionals are scarce, education regarding safety and injury prevention becomes an important responsibility of community health nurses who practice in rural communities (NRHA, 2004; Roberts & Dyer, 2004).

Chronic Illness

Rural residents in general are characterized by a relatively low mortality rate but a high rate of chronic illness. This increase in long-term health problems can be attributed to the greater percentage of poor elderly and other at-risk populations, poorer pregnancy outcomes, and the long-term consequences of non-fatal accidents. The most critically needed services in rural areas include preventive services such as health screening clinics, nutrition counseling, and wellness education to reduce the prevalence of chronic health problems. To provide care to those who have chronic health problems, there is an ever-increasing need for adult daycare, hospice and respite care, homemaker services, and meal deliveries to help chronically ill individuals who remain at home in geographically isolated areas (Gamm & Hutchison, 2004; Gamm et al., 2003a, 2003b; Morgan & Stewart-Fahs, 2007; Sawyer et al., 2006). Community health nurses in rural areas can be instrumental in advocating for the provision of such services.

There are special challenges in providing acute care services for the chronically impaired. Across the nation, there have been hospital closures; however, there has been a higher rate of closures among rural hospitals for some unusual reasons. For example, an out-of-community transfer of even one care provider, most often a physician, can mean that a small hospital must close its doors because of insufficient staff. The limited supply of and increasing demand for health professionals in general, and nurses in particular, will continue for some time. This shortage has a detrimental impact on providing a continuum of care to the chronically impaired who live in rural and underserved areas and creates an even greater demand for community health nurses.

Providing care to the chronically ill requires a move away from specialized acute curative medicine to a continuum of health care services. In rural areas, because of the current shortage of health care services, more facilities and personnel are needed to achieve an adequate level of service. Existing programs in urban as well as rural areas must become more effective by decentralizing services, providing more home services, and using mobile units. Nurses can have an important role in helping to address these concerns by providing available, accessible, and acceptable services. However, legislation must provide for direct third-party reimbursement for care provided by nurses prepared at the advanced level (Bushy, 2001, 2004).

Suicide and Homicide

Nationwide, among those 15 to 19 years of age, homicide and suicide are the two leading causes of death in males and the third and fourth leading causes of death in females. Each year, between 3000 and 5000 youths are murdered, and nearly an equal number commit suicide. Homicide is more likely to take place in the inner city, whereas suicide is more prevalent in suburban and rural settings. Often, however, it cannot be determined whether a vehicular or occupational accident was truly unintentional. Since the mid-1980s, a sharp upsurge has occurred in the rural suicide rate, especially among male adolescents and young men (Gamm & Hutchison, 2004; Gamm et al., 2003a, 2003b; Substance Abuse and Mental Health Services Administration [SAMHSA], 2003; USDHHS, 2000).

Because of the cluster or "copycat" phenomenon in self-inflicted death, in several towns the suicide rate has reached epidemic proportions, with three or more suicide incidents occurring in a very short time (after one suicide, there is an increased incidence of additional suicides in a community). In small towns or rural areas, where most people are fairly well acquainted with one another, a sudden death can be devastating to students and to the community as a whole. Many reasons are cited for the rise in rural suicides, including increasing economic hardships, changing community social structures, higher levels of drug and alcohol use, and lack of counseling and other social services. Community health nurses have an important role in educating the community to recognize self-destructive and risk-taking behaviors and advocating for crisis interventions to prevent those activities (Sawyer et al., 2006).

Alcohol and Drug Use

Recently, some rather unsettling information about alcohol use by Americans has come to light. Of particular interest are the following rural trends (Gamm, 2007; SAMHSA, 2003; Sawyer et al., 2006):

- Youths aged 12 to 17 years living in nonmetropolitan areas were more likely than youths in metropolitan areas to abuse or be dependent on alcohol or illicit drugs during the past year.
- In 2001, persons aged 12 years or older who lived in metropolitan areas were more likely than those in nonmetropolitan areas to abuse or be dependent on alcohol or illicit drugs during the past year.
- Arrests for drug abuse violations increased 54% in rural areas.
- Arrests for the use of cocaine and heroin increased 20% in rural areas.
- Most prison inmates in rural states abused alcohol, other drugs, or both.
- In rural areas children as young as 11 and 12 years of age are drinking as many as 14 to 18 beers on Friday and Saturday nights.

Nevertheless, compared with more populated areas, there are fewer health providers and services available per capita in rural areas to address chemical substance abuse. Consequently, community health nurses in rural settings should assume a proactive role with the community in planning, implementing, and evaluating primary prevention and follow-up intervention programs to educate the public about responsible alcohol consumption behaviors.

FACTORS INFLUENCING RURAL HEALTH

RURAL HEALTH CARE DELIVERY ISSUES

Discussion is underway by policy makers on ways to equitably allocate acute and primary preventive services among all Americans, especially those living in HPSAs, most of whom are in either rural counties or the inner city. Community health nurses who practice in rural areas, as well as those who provide outreach services to rural communities, should be aware of the concerns regarding the availability, accessibility, and acceptability of services. These interrelated delivery issues have serious implications for planning, implementing, managing, and evaluating community nursing services that target rural clients (BHPR, 2007; Brown & Swanson, 2003; Gamm, 2007; HRSA, 2003; Lee & Winters, 2006; Roberts & Dyer, 2004; Sawyer et al., 2006).

Availability of Services

Availability refers to the existence of services and sufficient personnel to provide those services. In rural areas, there are fewer physicians and nurses in general, as well as fewer family practice physicians, nurse practitioners, and specialists, especially obstetricians, pediatricians, psychiatrists, and social service professionals. Economically speaking, a sparse population limits the number and array of services in a given region. The per capita cost of providing special services to a few people often becomes prohibitive.

Accessibility of Services

Accessibility refers to the ability of a person to obtain and afford needed services. Accessibility of health care to rural families may be impaired by the following:

- Long travel distances
- Lack of public transportation
- Lack of telephone services
- A shortage of health care providers
- Inequitable reimbursement policies (e.g., diagnosis-related groups for Medicare)
- Unpredictable weather conditions
- Inability to obtain entitlements

Consider the case of a rancher with a high income who lives in a medically underserved frontier area of the United States and has a sudden heart attack. He may not have access to the most basic emergency care, although he has comprehensive medical insurance.

Access to funding sources to implement public health programs also can be hampered by the lack of grantsmanship on the part of those seeking aid. Successful grant writing requires practice and collaborative efforts between agencies to produce a fundable project. Political forces in small towns often oppose outside help because a grant writer is unable to quantify the immediate benefits to the local community of a proposed public health program for which funds are being sought. Resistance may be evidenced, for example, by the community's explicit preference for local government interventions and opposition to the perceived meddling of federal or state bureaucracies. As another example, a grant proposal to implement an innovative program to address the community health care needs of local subpopulations may not be supported by formal and informal community leaders. In rural areas power is often vested in an elite segment of the community. These individuals frequently remain unaware of the needs of the underprivileged. Sometimes, an affluent minority has more power than numerically greater ethnic groups in the community.

Insensitivity to others' needs on the part of leading community members can reinforce the stigma of seeking public assistance. Consequently, an individual who needs public services may avoid using them, even if they are available and accessible, out of concern that someone will tell others that he or she needs help. Community health nurses must recognize the stigma attached to the use of certain services, such as human immunodeficiency virus (HIV) testing, family planning, and chemical dependency services.

Acceptability of Services

Acceptability refers to the degree to which a particular service is offered in a manner congruent with the values of a target population. Given the wide diversity among rural families, acceptability of available community nursing services can be hampered by any of the following (Bushy, 2002, 2004; Sawyer et al., 2006):

- Traditions of handling personal problems without professional help (e.g., self-care practices such as using over-the-counter medications, exercising, ingesting alcohol, resting, praying)
- Beliefs about the cause of a disorder and the appropriate healer for it (e.g., medicine man, medicine woman, curandero, shaman)
- Lack of knowledge about a physical or emotional disorder and the value of formal services for prevention and treatment of the condition (e.g., being stoic and suffering in silence rather than seeking supportive care; only seeking care for emergencies rather than for health promotion or primary prevention)
- Difficulty in maintaining confidentiality and anonymity in a setting where most residents are acquainted with each other
- The urban orientation of most health professionals

With regard to urban orientation, many health professionals, including community health nurses, are educated in urban settings and have most, if not all, of their clinical experiences there. Therefore, they are not exposed to rural clients. When coupled with the stress experienced by many clients when seeking publicly funded care, cultural insensitivity can exacerbate a rural individual's mistrust of health professionals. Ultimately, a nurse's attitude affects the long-term health status of a client who may be embarrassed about his or her health problems. Embarrassment often is evidenced by a client's minimizing symptoms of illness and not seeking care when it is needed (i.e., health care is primarily sought for an acute illness or in an emergency). Therefore, it is prudent for schools of nursing to expose students to the rural environment and the people who live there. Rural clinical experiences for nurses will do much to create a climate of mutual sensitivity and trust between community health nurses and rural clients.

LEGISLATION AFFECTING RURAL HEALTH CARE DELIVERY SYSTEMS

Box 32-1 highlights some of the major legislation that has affected rural health care delivery. In rural communities, the issues of accessibility, availability, and acceptability of services and providers must always be considered when legislation is implemented. A program that is highly effective in a more populated area rarely can be lifted and transplanted as is to a rural environment. In some cases, legislated programs have resulted in highly innovative approaches that serve the population well. In other cases, mandated programs simply create other barriers that deter rural populations from using a much-needed service.

A successful program that serves as a good model is an immunization clinic held in conjunction with the county fair in an Appalachian community. This annual event is scheduled the week before school starts and attracts most county residents. Children's immunizations can be updated while adults undergo glaucoma and cholesterol testing. The program is promoted through word-of-mouth announcements to homemakers' clubs, notices in church bulletins, and public service announcements in the local media. Since the program's inception, the community has come to expect and accept the services that are offered at that particular time, as evidenced by the increasing numbers who seek care during the county event (Agency for Healthcare Research and Quality [AHRQ], 2003; BPHC, 2006).

Conversely, a poorly received program was one that involved American Indian children who were discharged from hospitals on apnea monitors. Using established protocols that were highly successful in the white community, health care providers made a dedicated effort to have young American Indian mothers comply with the prescribed regimen by placing their children on monitors while sleeping. In follow-up questioning the mothers reported adhering to all aspects of the program as instructed. However, after completing home visits, home health aides reported that the mothers were not following instructions. The program developers speculated that the mothers' verbal reports were motivated by fear of being reprimanded by caregivers or fear that their actions would be reported to IHS officials located on the reservation (Bushy, 2002).

Unfortunately, the program planners in this situation did not consider American Indians' beliefs related to the interference of biotechnology with a person's spirituality, nor did they consider the inherent role of extended family in caring for a child. In this particular tribe, grandmothers and aunts often provide the primary care to children in the extended family, but they were not included in the discharge planning. Other overlooked environmental considerations included the fact that it is not unusual for homes on the reservation to be without electricity or plumbing, and many American Indian families do not own a car. If the family does have access to a car, it may break down before they arrive at the hospital, or they may not be able to afford the gas. Program planners should have worked more closely with the community health nurses on the reservation to arrange transportation for families, or specialists might have taken their services to the IHS clinic on the reservation to make it easier for the women to get to the service location. Socioeconomic and cultural factors should always be considered when adapting a successful program to fit the needs and beliefs of a special population (IHS, 2007a, 2007b, 2007c).

A number of approaches have been legislated by the federal government to create innovative programs that are available, accessible, and acceptable to vulnerable rural populations (see Box 32-2 and references with website links at the end of this chapter). Of particular interest are the federally qualified health center (FQHC) program, which includes rural health clinics (RHCs) and migrant health centers (MHCs), and the

---

Box 32-1   Legislation Affecting Rural Health Care

1954 Transfer Act: Provided that all functions, responsibilities, authorities, and duties related to the maintenance and operation of hospitals and health facilities and the conservation of Indian health were to be administered by the Surgeon General of the U.S. Public Health Service

1957 Indian Health Assistance Act: Provided for construction of health facilities for American Indians

1958 Hill-Burton Act: Provided for construction of health care facilities where these were lacking; many rural communities built hospitals with these funds; a number of these hospitals currently are experiencing economic problems and are on the verge of closing

1962 Migrant Health Act: Authorized federal aid for clinics serving migratory agricultural workers and families

1964 Economic Opportunity Act: Provided a legal framework for the antipoverty program

1968 Neighborhood Health Centers: Extended grants to migrant health services

1970 Health Training Improvement Act: Provided expanded aid to allied health professionals

1971 Comprehensive Health Manpower Training Act: Increased federal programs for development of health manpower

1972 Act to Establish the Health Service Corps: Contained provisions to encourage health professionals to practice in areas designated as health professional shortage areas

1973 Health Maintenance Organization and National Health Planning and Resource Development Act: Increased health insurance coverage for the rural population

1975 Indian Self-Determination Act: Gave tribes the option of staffing and managing Indian Health Service programs in their communities and provided funding for improvement of tribal capability to contract for health care services

1976 National Consumer Health Information Act: Provided medical services in areas with an insufficient number of physicians

1976 Indian Health Care Improvement Act: Intended to elevate the health status of American Indians and Alaska Natives to a level equal to that of the general population by authorizing a higher budget for the Indian Health Service

1977 Rural Health Clinics Service Act: Provided medical services in areas with an insufficient number of physicians

1981 Planned Approach to Community Health (PATCH): Provided funding to states for delivery of preventive care and health promotion to rural communities

1981 Omnibus Budget Reconciliation Act: Consolidated various sets of categorical grant programs into block grants that served to increase state discretionary use of federal money (block grants for maternal and child health, services for disabled and other children with special health care needs, Supplemental Security Income services for disabled children, hemophilia treatment centers, and other programs aimed at specific groups or health problems)

1989 Omnibus Budget Reconciliation Act (OBRA): Initiated the federally qualified health center program to expand primary health care services in underserved areas by permitting recovery of reasonable costs for care provided to Medicare and Medicaid patients

1990 to present: Amendments added to existing health care legislation to revise policies

2002 to present: National Rural Initiative; Tommy Thompson, Secretary of Health and Human Services, instituted new efforts to improve and coordinate health services in conjunction with the states, local, and tribal governments

2002 Public Law No. 107-251: Provided funding and grant programs to improve health care outreach services, develop health networks, and improve the quality of small health care provider services in rural areas

2007 Public Law No. 110-23: Amended the Public Health Services Act to add requirements regarding trauma care and other health services for rural areas

---

IHS, because community health nurses play an active role in all of these federal initiatives (CMS, 2007a, 2007b).

Federally Qualified Health Centers

The FQHC program became a reality under the Omnibus Reconciliation Act (OBRA). It was designed to preserve and expand needed primary health care services in underserved areas by permitting legitimate recovery of reasonable costs from care provided to Medicare and Medicaid clients. The additional revenues are to be used to enhance and expand services in underserved communities, such as purchasing more time from a nurse practitioner, securing additional clinic sites, expanding specialty services like mental health, or enhancing the benefits and/or compensation of the clinic's personnel to help ensure retention. A detailed discussion of FQHC program requirements is beyond the scope of this chapter. However, a brief discussion of RHCs and MHCs is presented, because they serve underserved rural residents and migrant farmworkers.

Rural Health Clinics

RHC Public Law 95-210 was originally passed by Congress in 1977. Since then, Congress has passed several amendments to the act, but the intent of the legislation remains the same. Although the requirements change from time to time, essentially the act does the following:

- Encourages the use of mid-level practitioners (midwives, nurse practitioners, physician assistants) by providing reimbursement for their services to Medicare and Medicaid clients even in the absence of a full-time physician
- Creates a cost-based reimbursement mechanism for primary care services that can generate additional revenues for eligible rural practices
- Defines core RHC services that constitute comprehensive primary care to populations living in regions that are designated as rural and medically underserved or as HPSAs

An RHC can be located in several settings. For example, an RHC might be based in the outpatient department of a hospital, a freestanding clinic, or even a physician's office. The law allows an RHC's services to be tailored to best meet the needs of the local community. To become certified as an RHC under Medicare and Medicaid, an agency or clinic must meet the following criteria:

- Be located in a rural setting that is federally designated as an HPSA
- Be engaged primarily in the provision of outpatient primary medical care
- Employ at least one physician or nurse practitioner
- Meet applicable federal, state, and local requirements for Medicare and Medicaid health and safety requirements
- Be under the direction of a physician, who must be on site at least once every 2 weeks

Box 32-2   A Week in the Life of a Community Health Nurse in Rural Practice

Setting

The _____ District Health Unit is situated in the county seat of a county containing nine small towns in a rural Midwestern state. The county's population is approximately 10,000. The largest town has fewer than 1200 persons. There are seven schools in the county and a 15-bed hospital that provides obstetric, emergency, surgical, and medical-surgical services for clients of all ages. The community health nursing office is located in the medical clinic, which is adjacent to the hospital. The office hours are 8:00 AM to 5:00 PM. When there is no particular service scheduled, the community health nursing office is open to clients on a walk-in basis for services. Information on clinics is published in the county newspaper and announced on a radio station located in a nearby county.

Staff

RN (administrator): {½} time (0.5 FTE)

Job shared with:

RN (community health nurse): {½} time (0.5 FTE)
RN (community health nurse): as needed; responsible for monthly foot clinics; occasionally assists with in-town clinics
RN (community health nurse): as needed; teaches prenatal classes four times each year
Secretarial/reception services: shared with physician in the building

Community Health Nursing Services Provided

- Office visits—by appointment only
- Maternal health services—prenatal classes, in-hospital postpartum education classes, and follow-up home visits to new mothers and at-risk infants
- Healthy baby clinics
- Health promotion and education—by request and scheduled once each month (e.g., farm safety programs, baby-sitting classes, community health luncheons)
- Child/parent health nursing conferences
- Immunizations clinics
- Women's health clinics
- Senior health maintenance clinics
- Home visits—rural and city (health counseling and teaching; bedside and skilled nursing care; homemaker/home health aide referrals; maintenance nursing care)
- Screening for sexually transmitted diseases

Week's Schedule

Monday

8:00 AM	Home visits
9:00	Administrative office work:

- Plan community-wide senior wellness adventure scheduled in 8 weeks
- Order hepatitis vaccine for social services personnel who provide homemaker services
- Prepare presentation for county school administrators' meeting (next week)

- Plan and arrange for preschool screenings to be offered in all the schools

10:00	Immunization clinic
12:00 PM	Lunch
1:30	Child protection team meeting
3:15	Women's health clinic

Tuesday

8:00 AM	Prepare puberty talks for students in schools
9:00	Present puberty talk to fifth-graders in a school 15 miles from the community health nursing office
1:00 PM	Immunization clinic
2:30	Home visits
4:15	Infant hearing and ear clinic

Wednesday

8:00 AM	Home visits
1:00 PM	Preschool screening clinic for 4- to 5-year-olds (assisted by the part-time community health nurse and special education teacher)
1:30	Child parenting-nurturing meeting (in town)
2:00	School administrators' meeting (in town)
4:00	Home visit
7:30	Presentation on sexuality to Methodist church youth group (in town)

Thursday

8:00 AM	Home visits
10:00	Healthy baby clinic
11:00	Women's health clinic
12:00 PM	Give talk on farm safety at Farm Bureau luncheon meeting
1:00	Administrative office work:

- Prepare maternal child health grant
- Work on county health needs assessment
- Call Dr. _____ for standing orders

3:00	Immunization and hearing clinic
4:00	Blood pressure clinic
7:30	Give report at county commissioners' meeting

Friday

8:00 AM	Write article on farm safety for county newspaper
9:00	Home visits
11:00	Check _____ family for head lice
1:00 PM	Be at senior citizens' center (18 miles from community health nursing office) for monthly health maintenance clinic for 35 clients
3:00	Immunization clinic (out of town)
4:30	Get organized for next week

FTE, Full-time equivalent; *RN,* registered nurse.

- Have a mid-level practitioner (nurse practitioner, physician assistant, midwife) available to provide client care services in the clinic at least 50% of the time when the clinic is open
- Provide routine diagnostic services, including clinical laboratory services

- Maintain health records on all clients
- Have written policies governing the services that the clinic provides
- Have available drugs, blood products, and other necessary supplies to treat medical emergencies

- Have arrangements with other providers and suppliers to ensure that clinic clients have access to inpatient hospital care and to other physician and laboratory services not provided in the clinic

Migrant Health Centers

MHCs provide services only to migratory and seasonal agricultural workers and their families, generally on a fee-for-service basis. A sliding fee schedule is applied to those who are without insurance or who cannot pay the full charge for the services they receive. Depending on the health care needs of the community, an MHC provides services similar to those of an RHC. However, an MHC may also offer the following services if needed by a community:

- Environmental health services (e.g., rodent control, field sanitation, sewage treatment)
- Infectious and parasitic disease screening and control
- Accident prevention programs (including prevention of excessive pesticide exposure)

A few MHCs function only when migrant workers are in a given region to work in the agriculture industry. Services provided by these clinics tend to be limited in array and scope. Other MHCs operate year-round, particularly those in the South, where there is a year-round growing season. These clinics tend to provide a greater array of services designed to meet the particular needs of migrant families who may remain in the area as well as of those who migrate there for the season.

Indian Health Service

Another long-standing federal initiative in which community nurses have an important role is the IHS (2007a, 2007b, 2007c). Since 1955, the U.S. Department of Health and Human Services, primarily through the IHS branch of the Public Health Service, has been responsible for providing federal health services to American Indians and Alaska Natives under Public Law 83-568. The goal of the IHS is to raise the health status of American Indians and Alaska Natives to the highest possible level. The IHS works with *federally recognized tribes* to develop a unique health care delivery system to provide a range of health care services. Those services respect traditional healing beliefs and attempt to blend them with the latest advances in medical technology.

The IHS works with more than 560 federally recognized tribes located in 35 states. Their members live mainly on reservations and in rural communities, mostly in the western United States and Alaska (Figure 32-2). In keeping with the concept of tribal sovereignty, the Indian Self-Determination and Enhanced Education Act of 1975 (Public Law 93-638) gave tribes the option of staffing and managing IHS programs in their own communities. It also provides funding for the development of a tribe's capability to contract for services outside of IHS. Consequently, increasing numbers of American Indian and Alaska Native governments are exercising operational control of IHS hospitals, outpatient facilities, and other types of health care programs to better meet the needs of American Indian communities.

Although IHS recruitment materials state that practice in the service offers exposure to a diversity of health problems and transcultural enrichment, it has been difficult to recruit and retain qualified health providers who have the potential to deliver culturally consistent health care services. Health care providers who are culturally connected with a minority group are best equipped to provide meaningful care to them. Staffing with such providers has not been possible, for the most part, in the IHS. There is a critical shortage of American Indian nurses and physicians who are adequately prepared and available to work with the American Indian population in general, and with the various tribes in particular. Recruited professionals usually are of non-Indian origin, which has been a source of contention for caregivers as well as users of IHS services. On the one

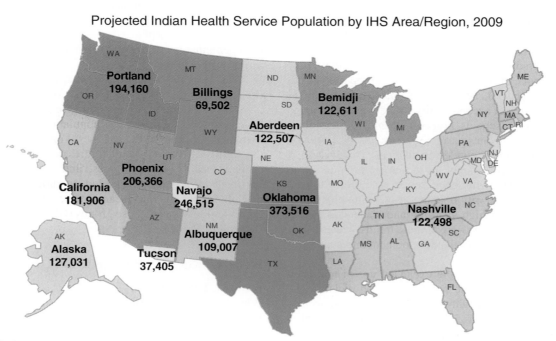

Projected Indian Health Service Population by IHS Area/Region, 2009

FIGURE 32-2 Projected Indian Health Service population by IHS area, fiscal year 2009. (From U.S. Department of Health and Human Services. [nd]. Budget in brief: Fiscal year 2009. Retrieved June 10, 2008 from *http://www.hhs.gov*.)

hand, IHS providers complain of treatment noncompliance, tardiness in seeking care, and broken clinic appointments on the part of American Indians (see Chapter 10). On the other hand, American Indians describe provider indifference and cultural intolerance toward them (e.g., verbal reprimands, impatience, inflexibility, and attitudes of superiority).

The problems become even more complex because nursing and medical personnel (who usually are white) tend to remain within the IHS only long enough to pay back National Health Service Corps (NHSC) education loans. Once loans are repaid, these individuals usually leave the IHS for more financially rewarding practice settings. Despite the legislated intent of the IHS, American Indian reservations are some of the least healthy areas in the United States, with a multitude of social and health-related problems, including high rates of unemployment, alcoholism, high-school dropout, poor perinatal outcomes, suicide, and homicide. Community health nurses have a major role in delivering care that is culturally and linguistically appropriate to American Indians across the country in urban as well as rural settings.

Federal Efforts to Augment Rural Health Resources

Legislation has been drafted to augment existing programs such as FQHCs (specifically RHCs and MHCs) and the IHS. Moreover, there is a trend in state and federal funding to make the needs of rural and frontier communities, particularly HPSAs, a priority. However, the actual dollars allocated for public health programs in rural areas have decreased in many cases. Currently, the focus is on accountability and innovation of programs, and this focus is enforced through allocation of federal and state funds (Coburn et al., 2007; Institute of Medicine, 2005; NRHA, 2004; ORHP, 2002).

One recent trend is the linking of federal training dollars to program outcomes. For example, when tax dollars are allocated to support an educational program, certain results should be expected relative to rural health care. Questions that are being asked include the following: Are the benefits of the program distributed to all of the state's residents, rural as well as urban? Do educational programs expose students to rural community practice? Are graduates remaining in the state? How many continue to practice in areas of need? Schools preparing health professionals in general, and nurses in particular, are mandated to assume greater accountability for outcomes of funded programs. Likewise, schools preparing health professionals who are applying for grants currently are required to provide student clinical rotations in underserved areas. The goal is not simply to educate professionals but to prepare providers who have the capability and willingness to increase access to care for underserved and minority populations. Community health nurses, because of their high visibility and leadership role in rural communities, must be aware of these trends, because they often are consulted regarding the development and support of public health programs.

Another emerging trend is the expanded use of mid-level primary care providers (nurse practitioners, physician assistants, midwives) in rural health care delivery systems as evidenced by legislation authorizing FQHCs. The trend is further supported by the NHSC (2007). This initiative provides scholarships and a loan repayment program for mid-level providers. The greatest challenge to implementing this initiative will be to develop and maintain health professional education programs in a time of federal and fiscal constraints. To effectively use declining resources, practicing health professionals and educational programs for health professionals will have to forge partnerships with rural communities to plan, implement, and evaluate programs that are available, accessible, and acceptable to populations who live there.

Program innovation in underserved areas is another trend, and this is essential for both providers and accrediting bodies (Institute of Medicine, 2005). In essence, a program must mesh with local lifestyles, values, and economic structures. In addition, program evaluations must reflect outcomes appropriate to a particular community or population. The Commonwealth Fund, Kellogg Foundation, and Robert Wood Johnson Foundation have led the movement by providing grants to universities to develop interdisciplinary education models and take them into rural communities. Federal programs such as the Rural Interdisciplinary Health Profession Training Program have fostered similar activities to expose students and professionals to the rural environment. These models have led to exciting new interactive telecommunication technologies that enable educational institutions to deliver classes directly to students living and working in even the most geographically remote settings. Telecommunications and computers hold great promise for linking rural professionals with their urban colleagues for the purpose of seeking consultation with health care specialists.

Congress and policy developers are looking to nurses to provide vital services to rural populations. For nursing to effectively respond to this opportunity, creativity is needed to ensure delivery of services to underserved regions of the United States. Nurses must be sensitive to the health beliefs of clients, however, and then plan and provide nursing care that fits with rural residents' value systems. For instance, how is health defined by a rural group? For a group of retired coal miners with black lung disease, it may mean being able to walk about at home using a portable oxygen tank. To an elderly woman with cancer in its late stages, it may mean being able to spend her last days in the local hospital to be near her family rather than having chemotherapy at a medical center located in a city some distance from home.

To address this challenge most effectively, information is needed about clients' perspectives. Although this may seem obvious to a community health nurse, most of the data that have been collected on rural populations are for reimbursement and policy-making purposes. Very little is known about the family systems of subcultures in rural areas in terms of their health beliefs, values, and perceptions of health. Pertinent information is needed on rural subpopulations to provide acceptable and meaningful community nursing programs and services to those groups (Glasgow et al., 2004; Lee & Winters, 2006).

RURAL LIFESTYLE AND BELIEF SYSTEMS

RURAL LIFESTYLE

What is it like to live in a small, rural town? What do nurses know about rural populations and their nursing needs? Although each community is unique, the experience of living in a small town is similar in all 50 states. The "typical" rural lifestyle is characterized by the following:

- Greater spatial distances between people and services
- An economic orientation toward the land and nature (agriculture, mining, lumbering, and/or fishing, all of which are classified as high-risk occupations)
- Work and recreational activities that are cyclic and seasonal
- Social interactions that facilitate informal, face-to-face negotiations, because most, if not all, residents are either related or acquainted

In brief, for rural residents, a small town is the center of trade for a region, and its churches and schools usually are the centers for socialization. This has implications for planning and implementing public health and community nursing programs for rural clients. In the following discussion, common themes and belief systems of rural groups are elaborated, particularly those related to self-reliance and self-care practices, a work ethic that is reinforced by rural economic structures, and patterns of utilization of social support services. These factors can either motivate or deter rural persons in seeking care (Long & Weinert, 1989; ORHP, 2002; Stein, 1989).

RURAL BELIEF SYSTEMS

Belief systems of rural people are complex and multifaceted, but common themes relate to their fatalism and subjugation by nature (e.g., rain and frost effects on crop outcome; effects of a hard winter on livestock) and an orientation to concrete places and things. Rural families tend to be more conservative politically, with a strong religious preference (church going), and this, too, affects their health beliefs.

In day-to-day activities, rural persons prefer to deal with someone they know rather than with a stranger. The preference for extended family ("kith and kin") can be advantageous in creating a support network (e.g., providing child care for a family during an illness). Familiarity, however, can also create some unusual problems. For instance, because most people in a rural area are acquainted, leaks in confidentiality can have serious consequences for someone who is seeking health care or social services (Gamm & Hutchison, 2004; Gamm et al., 2003a, 2003b; ORHP, 2002).

Informal community dynamics pose an even greater concern with regard to confidentiality. It is not unusual for rural people to report that, although they are well acquainted with most residents in the community, they feel there is no one they can trust and with whom they can discuss personal problems. This attitude stems from the fact that resident in small towns have a genuine interest in and question others about the well-being of neighbors and relatives. Public knowledge of personal problems can be devastating for all involved. In brief, social and economic structures can impose restrictions for those who desire to seek professional help for concerns with moral overtones, such as drug and alcohol dependence, an unplanned pregnancy, sexuality issues, conflicts in personal relationships, or behaviors associated with mental illness (Roberts & Dyer, 2004; SAMHSA, 2003; Sawyer et al., 2006).

Self-Reliance and Self-Care Practices

Self-reliance, which includes self-care practices, is a characteristic attributed to rural residents. Historically, self-care helped people to survive in austere, isolated, and rugged environments. Self-reliance is reflected in the statement, "We take care of our own," which implies a preference for receiving care from familiar people. "Neighborliness" and family support can be beneficial in promoting healthy behaviors, and a close-knit family can be highly supportive to a member who has a medical problem (e.g., chronic obstructive pulmonary disease or a pregnancy with complications).

Such support can be detrimental in some situations, however. For example, an individual with a drinking problem may be deterred from acknowledging the problem or seeking appropriate help because of family members' enabling behaviors. Emotional problems may be viewed by a family as a character flaw. Secrecy is reinforced by the rule of silence; that is, what happens in the family stays in the family. To preserve the standing of the family in the community, it becomes important not to let anyone in town know about a particular problem (e.g., substance abuse; domestic violence; incest; rape; an emotional disorder; a condition that may carry a stigma, including certain types of cancer and a positive result on an HIV blood test; and a decision about whether to terminate a pregnancy). Likewise, attempting to adhere to established family and community standards can be a source of tremendous stress for individuals who are struggling to develop their own sense of identity, especially adolescents and others with low self-esteem.

Work Ethic Reinforced by Economic Structures

Economic structures can also affect a person's health status and his or her health care-seeking behaviors. For example, family enterprises are characteristic of rural environments. Small businesses such as farms, ranches, and family-owned grocery stores and service stations generally do not provide employee benefits like health insurance. Concomitantly, some rural people define health as "the ability to work, to do what needs to be done." This attitude reinforces a work ethic and could be interpreted to mean that "illness is not being able to do one's usual work." Therefore, these people do not seek health care until they are too ill to work.

Economic structures and a work ethic ultimately influence a family's choice of leisure activities, its view of mental health, and its choice of health-promoting activities as well as primary prevention behaviors. For example, children may be taken to the physician for treatment of an illness at a time that coincides with the need to purchase repair parts for a piece of machinery in town. Similarly, services provided by the parish nurse may be openly welcomed by a congregation, but the services of an outreach worker at the county mental health clinic may not be welcomed by some of its members.

Patterns of Utilization of Social Support Services

Before implementing any kind of health care service, program planners must be sensitive to a target group's preferences regarding social support. Specifically, three levels of social support have been identified in the literature (Gamm, 2007; Sawyer et al., 2006; Stein, 1989). The first level includes services volunteered by family and friends. Although generally this help is not paid for, there is an expectation of reciprocity. The second level includes services that are provided by a group (e.g., civic organization, homemakers' club, faith community, chamber of commerce, 4-H club, or sports team). Members of the group may provide assistance to needy individuals and families in the community (e.g., volunteering time, providing food, and making financial contributions). Both of these social support levels offer a mutually understood "insurance policy" should a catastrophic event occur for an individual in the network. The third level of support includes formal government services, public health agencies, visiting or community nursing services, mental health centers, and school counseling services. Generally, remuneration by clients is expected for these services, albeit on a sliding scale.

When the patterns of utilization of the three levels of social support are compared, it is found that urban residents tend to prefer the third level, because they often do not have access to the informal systems that are more common in small towns. Historically, rural persons have learned to rely on the first two levels of social support as a way to cope with the hardships associated with geographical isolation. This pattern of help-seeking behavior has reinforced their ideas of self-reliance. Demographic changes have disrupted informal support networks and forced many rural residents to rely more on public support. Reluctance persists, however, because outreach services to a rural community are provided by professionals who often are strangers to the people who live there. At this time, one can only speculate on the long-term consequences of the recent influx of new residents into rural communities.

Rural Community/Public Health Nursing Practice

There is ongoing debate as to whether anything is unique about rural nursing practice, because nursing care is similar regardless of the setting (Bigbee & Crowder, 1985; Bushy, 2001; Case, 1991; Davis & Droes, 1993; Lee & Winters, 2006). Little information exists in periodicals or nursing texts on what makes community/public health nursing in rural settings different. Since 1990, however, most community/public nursing texts have included a chapter on rural nursing practice. The debate stems partly from some people's interpretation of "rural" as a geographic practice setting. Proponents of this view believe that nursing care is probably no different for rural clients than for other individuals, and that health problems and client care needs are similar regardless of the setting. Other nurses believe that rural practice should be designated as a specialty area, or at least a subspecialty, because of factors such as isolation, scarcity of resources, and the need for a wide range of practice skills that must be adapted to social and economic structures. The actual degree to which rural nursing has unique aspects probably lies somewhere between these two extremes. Often one or a few community health nurses provide a broad span of diverse services in rural communities (see Box 32-2).

Considering the wide variations of people and geographic settings in rural communities, how can nurses best be prepared to practice in health care settings in these environments? What entices nurses to elect to practice in these settings? Nurses being prepared for rural practice must be able to assess the community health needs in a region, including the particular causes of morbidity and mortality. Among current health care delivery issues, five factors emerge as salient themes for rural community health care: confidentiality, traditionally defined gender role behaviors, geographic and professional isolation, scarcity of resources, and legal considerations with regard to community health nurses' scope of practice.

Confidentiality

Confidentiality may be a concern for anyone who lives in a rural community, even those who say they enjoy being personally acquainted with others in the community. A nurse will probably know most clients as neighbors, friends, or friends of a friend or relative. As in all facets of professional life, familiarity has advantages and disadvantages. One nurse describes the experience in these terms:

Personally knowing a client and his or her family's lifestyle helps me to provide total care. After I provide care, I'm also able to keep track of the person's progress from direct reports by the person when I meet him or her in the store or on the street. Or, if the client is home bound, I get word-of-mouth reports from his or her family, friends, neighbors, or other members of his or her church. (D. R. B., personal communication, 1996)

The rural community usually holds nurses, like physicians, in high esteem, but this can make it difficult to have a life outside of work, as another nurse describes:

In an urban setting, when you leave work and drive your car out of the parking lot, you are just one more person in a city of a million people. In a rural area when you move your car out of the parking lot ... you are the same person as when you were in the parking lot. Everywhere you go you are seen as [a nurse]. ... This affects how you conduct yourself when you are downtown, too. (Davis & Droes, 1993, p. 167)

Personally knowing a client creates some concerns and frustrations, as illustrated by this community health nurse's remark:

Sometimes knowing your patients well allows you to make assumptions without a really valid evaluation. ... You can miss something that should actually have been caught. ... I just think other emotions can get in the way when you know someone well. (Davis & Droes, 1993, p. 166)

Maintaining confidentiality is often difficult, particularly when the clinic or agency is located in a public facility such as the county courthouse. Often the waiting room may be in a common hallway or area where clients are likely to be recognized. Moreover, announcements of specialty services such as sexually transmitted disease (STD) clinics, prenatal or family planning clinics, HIV testing, the Women, Infants, and Children (WIC) program, and immunization clinics are published in the local newspaper and church bulletins, announced over a local radio or television station, and posted in public places such as grocery stores, service stations, and grain elevators. Because most people in a small town are recognized by the cars that they drive, even parking lots can jeopardize confidentiality. Scheduling a clinic at a certain time also can impose problems. If an STD clinic is held on Friday mornings, for example, assumptions may be made about anyone seen in the building at that time, even if it is not to attend the clinic. Leaks in confidentiality result from such chance encounters, which can lead to a person's becoming stigmatized as the information quickly becomes public knowledge through the local rumor mill.

Maintaining confidentiality has implications for planning, providing, and evaluating community health services, such as determining an appropriate building and coordinating times to offer services (Coward et al., 2004; Roberts & Dyer, 2004; Sawyer et al., 2006). For example, prenatal or family planning clinics could be scheduled to coincide with an immunization clinic, and STD clinics and HIV testing could be offered on a walk-in basis. These suggestions may be difficult to implement, however, especially if there is only one nurse who is responsible for a large health district and visits the various communities in the area on a rotating schedule. Innovative approaches are required on the part of community health nurses in rural practice to address the community's concerns about anonymity and confidentiality.

TRADITIONALLY DEFINED GENDER ROLE BEHAVIORS

Persons in rural communities are more likely to adhere to traditional values, which often includes complying with expected gender role behaviors (Coward et al., 2004; Lee & Winters, 2006; Long & Weinert, 1989). In other words, they have defined ideas about what constitutes "men's work" versus "women's work." The activities comprising women's work, consistent with traditional values, are assumed to be "less important," because women generally are not monetarily compensated for their work. Activities such as managing a household and caring for and nurturing a spouse and children are defined as women's work—that is to say, these activities should be volunteered to maintain the family's well-being. A man, on the other hand, is expected to work for a salary and adequately support his family without any public assistance.

Nursing, too, because it is a predominantly female profession, tends to be viewed as women's work. In other words, nurses who live in rural communities may be expected to provide professional consultation at no cost to local people who drop by their homes or to respond to local traffic accidents. In one case in which there was no home health agency in the county, a physician referred clients being discharged from the county hospital (located in another town) to an unemployed nurse in the clients' home community. Instead of having a salaried position, this nurse was involved in the family business. The nurse received no compensation for her professional services.

In very small communities the identity of a woman is often based on her relationship to someone else—that is, a woman is considered the wife, sister, daughter, or mother of someone. This also holds true for nurses, who generally are women. Consequently, a new graduate who wants to work in a small town will have no identity of her own, even as a nurse. Directly and indirectly, assigned gender roles can contribute to the problems of retaining community health nurses in rural practice settings.

ISOLATION

Isolation, both geographic and professional, is another salient characteristic of rural community health nursing (Coward et al., 2004; Roberts & Dyer, 2004; Sawyer et al., 2006). Geographic isolation poses challenges to rural community health nurses because clients probably do not live nearby, as described in the following account by a nurse:

We had a situation in [our] county where we had a man coming home from the hospital after having a stroke. He was completely paralyzed on his left side. He came home one evening, and a nurse went out to the ranch the next morning to start services. We thought physical therapy and nursing and some aide services would be appropriate.

When she got there about 10 o'clock in the morning and was taking the history and assessment she found out that the man had driven into the nearest town the afternoon before. She asked him how he had driven with his left side completely paralyzed. He said when he got home, he realized that unless they drove that pickup, they were stranded. There was not anybody around for miles and miles.

So he thought it over, and he got a couple of his leather belts and put them together, climbed into his stick-shift-pickup, which was a feat in itself, and got it into first gear, got out on the road, slipped the belt around his left foot and when he was ready to change gears he just reached over with his right hand, pulled his foot up with the belt, dropped his left foot on the clutch, put it in second gear and went down the road.

Right away that precludes him from meeting the home-bound criteria for Medicare. All those services were not available to him. We provided services some other ways, but we were not able to get any Medicare benefits for him. (Davis & Droes, 1993, p. 163)

Although the nurse's account does not reveal the reason why the client went into town, the story does suggest a degree of self-sufficiency and autonomy as a way of coping with the isolation. This phenomenon is not always understood by those who are responsible for policy making or discharge planning of rural clients from urban-based hospitals.

Professional isolation is closely related to geographic isolation and can be perceived as positive, negative, or a combination of both. Many rural nurses enjoy the professional independence and creativity, which are not usually found in a larger practice setting. Others find that the responsibilities in a rural community health agency can be overwhelming. Often there is no immediately accessible network of professionals who can provide support and consultation on a particular matter of concern. Likewise, the lack of immediately available opportunities for establishing relationships with other professionals, or not having the "central office" nearby, can reinforce feelings of isolation.

For community health nurses, professional isolation requires an outstanding ability to evaluate and prioritize needs and the types of services that can be provided to the local population. The lack of physical access to other providers, education, and technology can potentially cause considerable role strain. Individuals who are uncomfortable when working alone or who lack the confidence to make independent nursing decisions probably would not fare well in a remote rural area. These individuals would likely be more comfortable in a less isolated setting (Bushy, 2001, 2004).

Telecommunications and electronic media are used to form networks that can provide support and consultation to professionals who are practicing in remote rural areas. Rapidly evolving technology has done much to reduce professional isolation among health care providers who practice in geographically isolated areas with a scarcity of resources. For instance, a cellular telephone or computer modem can be used to consult with a tertiary medical center, satellite or interactive telecommunications provide education to stay abreast of recent developments, and lifeline telemetry helps in monitoring clients so that problems can be recognized before an emergency occurs (Gamm, 2007; ORHP, 2002).

SCARCITY OF RESOURCES

Associated with the problems of geographic and professional isolation is the ever-present scarcity of human and financial resources in rural environments (Coward et al., 2004; Roberts & Dyer, 2004; Sawyer et al., 2006). This, too, has implications for community health nursing budgeted positions, salaries, support personnel, and services offered within an agency. Often community nursing positions are part time because in sparsely populated counties there is little funding that can be allocated for the salary and benefits required to hire a county nurse. Some involved in budget planning may rationalize that there are not enough people in the community to warrant a full-time equivalent nursing position. In some ways, this view is congruent with the national trend toward hiring "temporary workers," but in rural areas there may be no part-time nurses available for hire (Bushy, 2001; NRHA, 2004).

One reason that there are not more community nurses in rural agencies is that qualified personnel often are unavailable to fill vacant positions. Although salaries tend to be lower, the cost of living also may be less in a rural area. To address these problems, two or more counties sometimes organize a partnership, often referred to as a *health district*. In this arrangement one community health nurse provides services to both counties. This may be an ideal arrangement when distances between communities are not great. Problems can arise, however, when a health district spans great distances and there are natural barriers such as mountains, forests, or a lack of roads or telephone, plumbing, or electrical services.

LEGAL CONSIDERATIONS FOR COMMUNITY/ PUBLIC HEALTH NURSES' SCOPE OF PRACTICE

The expanded scope of practice has legal implications that a community health nurse considering rural practice must explore (Bushy, 2001, 2004; NRHA, 2004). Consideration and attention must be given to the state's requirements for advanced nursing practice and prescriptive privileges; the organizational relationship of the local health department to the state department of health; and specific mandates for specialty programs or services that are offered within the local health department, such as RHCs, MHCs, or contract services with the IHS.

The best way to approach the scope of nursing practice in a geographically and professionally isolated setting with associated scarce resources is to carefully review that state's nurse practice acts. These will provide a guide to the activities in which a nurse can legally engage. Likewise, all public agencies should have a health officer. This individual can provide additional guidelines for program goals as well as develop standing orders and protocols within an agency. In addition, it is prudent for community health nurses to establish a working rapport with other health care providers in the community. In professionally and geographically isolated communities, interdisciplinary rapport can provide a backup system and a referral network should unanticipated or emergency situations occur in the community nurse's practice.

Nurses in rural practice must be aware of local resources that can be used should an emergency arise. For instance, some nurses own a citizen's band radio or cellular telephone so they can contact a physician, hospital emergency department, or county sheriff if necessary. Others work closely with a faith community to organize home care for a client between nursing visits. Still other nurses encourage residents who live great distances from a health care facility to take an emergency medical training course. Finally, some rural community health nurses have assumed an active role in presenting community health needs to county commissioners or the district administrative board of a local or district health department. Several of these approaches have brought about significant improvement in the overall health status of communities.

As for community standards of practice, these are consistent with those established by the nursing profession. Providing safe quality care is mandated in all client-nurse relationships. In rural areas, however, achieving this outcome may require an innovative approach because of a lack of resources or great distances. For instance, informal support services may have to be coordinated by the nurse within a community to provide continuity of care for an individual who needs skilled home care and lives a great distance from the community nursing clinic. Community volunteers, however, must be knowledgeable about how to reach emergency services should these be needed. In brief, an effective community health nurse in a rural setting enhances residents' self-reliance by anticipating the types of services they might need and then teaching them how to access those services, which may be located great distances from their homes. The key to success in this endeavor is effective communication among nurses, clients, the community, and local health care providers.

A number of strategies have been used by community health nurses in rural settings to increase a population's self-reliance and self-care skills. Because schools and churches are viewed as socialization centers by rural residents, these facilities are an ideal setting in which to provide health promotion and health education programs. For example, programs on occupational safety, cardiopulmonary resuscitation, immunizations, and nutrition education are welcomed by most administrators and educators in local schools and by church leaders. Women's clubs also provide an opportunity to present health-related education, such as education on first aid interventions for emergencies, prenatal care, and breast and testicular self-examination.

Men tend not to be overtly receptive to health promotion education because women in rural environments usually make the final decisions regarding their families' health. Most women are eager for information that will help them in maintaining their families' health. However, some health-related topics are readily accepted by men attending service and civic club meetings. Interests vary depending on the predominant recreational and economic focus of the community (e.g., lumbering, mining, fishing, ranching, or farming). Generally, most men are interested in education related to safe pursuit of recreational activities (snowmobiling, firearm use, boating, fishing, motorcycling), safe operation of vehicles (trucks, automobiles, all-terrain vehicles), and prevention and treatment of occupational injuries (e.g., exposure to toxic products and first aid treatment of sports-related injuries, including cardiopulmonary resuscitation [CPR] and immediate care of trauma victims). They also may express an interest in mental health topics, especially depression and substance abuse.

Other approaches have been used to meet the health care needs of rural residents who live in HPSAs. For instance, screening clinics and specialized services such as immunizations and mammography can be brought to a community by van. This approach usually incorporates a team of specialists who can provide comprehensive diagnosis and care to residents in remote geographic areas. To be most effective, the visit by a mobile clinic should coincide with a community event such as a church bazaar, county fair, athletic tournament, or rodeo. To initiate such an endeavor requires active professional-community partnerships to effectively plan, implement, and evaluate services and programs based on the community's needs (BPHC, 2006).

BUILDING PROFESSIONAL-COMMUNITY PARTNERSHIPS

CONNECTING WITH THE COMMUNITY

There is increasing evidence that community members who are informed and active in planning their health care system are more likely to use and support that system. The community decision-making model offers tools to develop partnership arrangements and a consensus as to the most appropriate solution for a local problem (AHRQ, 2003; Gamm, 2007; Sawyer et al., 2006). It is important to stress that a partnership decision-making model in a rural area probably will be somewhat different from one in a larger community. In part, this relates to the dilemma associated with the fact that most residents are personally acquainted while at the same time wish to keep their health status confidential. The problem is even more complex because of the preference for informal (rather than formal) support services. In any setting, community health nurses with the skills to connect with a population can help empower the community to do the following:

- Establish a community health care priority list
- Involve large numbers of community members in considering and selecting their health care options
- Conduct health care needs assessments
- Incorporate business principles in social marketing
- Measure the local economic impact of the health system (particularly nursing care)
- Negotiate and evaluate ownership/sponsorship issues by getting local people involved in the planning

In many cases, longstanding problems can be resolved by the combined efforts of several organizations in a small community. Community health nurses would do well to establish partnerships to plan, implement, and evaluate a program or services. Partnership models take into account a population's lifestyle, health status, belief systems, and overriding health care delivery issues. Nurses must bear in mind that rural residents are known for their resourcefulness. Despite the lack of resources, historically most have fared rather well with self-care, neighborliness, and community support. Hence, partnership arrangements are not a new concept to rural communities.

BUILDING PROFESSIONAL-COMMUNITY PARTNERSHIPS

Because of the leadership roles community health nurses are expected to assume in rural communities, nurses must be familiar with the process of forming professional-community partnerships. This generally is a new experience for community health nurses and consumers alike. The next few paragraphs examine the process as it applies to rural community nursing practice (AHRQ, 2003; Coward et al., 2004; Roberts & Dyer, 2004; Sawyer et al., 2006).

Step 1: Identify the Problem Area

After a community problem is identified, the community health nurse can recruit a team of two to five individuals who share a common interest in addressing that concern. The issue of concern determines who will be involved in the preliminary discussions. For instance, because of the central importance of churches and schools in a rural community, leaders from those two institutions often can be counted on as key figures in organizing professional-community partnerships to address problems encountered by families with youths. Likewise, leaders in various civic and service clubs can be considered a community resource to help identify potential contact persons to begin discussions. Through dialogue, the informal group often becomes aware of others in the community who have similar interests, which hopefully leads to a more formal collaborative partnership (e.g., cooperative network, coalition, or alliance).

Step 2: Assess the Community's Perspective

Before developing a plan of action for a particular problem, it is wise for the group, with the guidance of the community health nurse, to undertake a community assessment pertaining to the problem. These data are useful in doing the following:

- Gaining the local perspective
- Assessing the degree of public awareness and support for the cause
- Identifying special-interest groups
- Identifying existing services to avoid duplication of programs
- Listing potential barriers and resources in the community

Data can be obtained by written or telephone surveys, personal interviews, the media, and national and state public health reports. The views of formal and informal community leaders, representatives from local organizations, and ordinary citizens should be included. Their ideas are critical elements in planning an effective and acceptable course of action for the problem of interest. Making these preliminary contacts is also an effective strategy to create community awareness of the problem, gain community support, and "test the water" regarding possible approaches to resolving the problem from the public's perspective. Essentially, seeking public input allows the community to feel ownership in the project, instead of viewing the situation as one in which "an outsider brings another bureaucratic program into town."

Step 3: Analyze the Data

Once the assessment is completed, the data must be analyzed, which includes identifying and prioritizing the issues of concern. The community health nurse, acting in a facilitator role, should make a dedicated effort to involve members of the community in this activity. When planning for an acceptable and effective public health program or community nursing service, the nurse should compare the listed concerns with available providers and existing community resources. All the information and suggestions provided by informants should be considered. The nurse should remember that local residents probably are more in tune with the needs and resources of their community than the nurse or other professional. Solutions that may seem farfetched to the nurse often are highly appropriate for the local population. In essence, creativity is required on the part of a community health nurse to implement a model program that meshes with local preferences.

Step 4: Develop a Long-Range Plan

After completing the data analysis, the professional and community partners can begin long-range planning. So that the program will be effective and accepted by the target group, the community health nurse should involve as many interested organizations and individuals as is feasible. For instance, a multicounty partnership focusing on a program for the prevention and treatment of hypertension might include the following activities:

- Preparing a list of possible target groups or clients
- Generating a list of potential community volunteers and professionals who can assist with the project
- Purchasing necessary materials to implement the program
- Creating an awareness of the program among target groups (e.g., individuals; families; attendees at senior centers; church and recreation groups; health care professionals; law enforcement personnel; and members of other religious, service, and civic clubs)
- Identifying potential sources of funding to implement the program

Step 5: Take Action

Once there is group consensus and a course of action is developed, the plan is implemented. The nurse must be willing to delegate responsibilities to interested community representatives. It is not unusual to find eager and willing volunteers among retired nurses, educators, social service personnel, and auxiliary members of local organizations. Remember that the best plans can go awry, especially when one is working with several individuals and groups. When a program is being planned and implemented, flexibility is critical so that changes can be made in the process as the situation requires. This strategy will go a long way toward providing community nursing services that are accessible, available, and acceptable to the target group.

Step 6: Evaluate the Program

As the program is developed and during its implementation, the nurse should plan for ongoing (formative) evaluation of the process as well as a final (summative) evaluation. Together, the two evaluation approaches are useful to measure the short- and long-term outcomes of the program and determine whether the problem has been adequately addressed. Partnership arrangements facilitate obtaining reliable and valid data, from the community's perspective, regarding the outcomes of the project (AHRQ, 2003; Coburn et al., 2007).

For instance, with a community nursing service, the short-term outcome might be a certain per capita utilization of services within a specified time frame. Long-term outcomes, however, may not be obvious for several years or more, as in the case of sex education provided to junior high students as an intervention to reduce the incidence of teenage pregnancies, a nutrition education program to prevent cardiovascular disease, and an integrated preconception program to improve pregnancy outcomes in the region. Community input is critical to assess both the short- and long-term outcomes of a project.

TRENDS AND ISSUES

There are many opportunities and challenges for community health nurses and other health care providers who choose to work in rural settings and for urban providers who provide care in their agencies or offer outreach services to rural populations in their catchment area. A few of the more critical issues that must be addressed by policymakers and health care providers alike are identified in Box 32-3. All of these issues and concerns have an impact on the provision of available,

---

| Box 32-3 | **Critical Issues to Address in Rural Health Care** |

Develop a consistent definition for rural. *Rural* has been defined as nonmetropolitan, nonurban, frontier, and farming areas. Different definitions lead to divergent approaches in program planning. Rural-Urban Continuum Codes may help resolve some of the confusion. Increased consistency in the definition of *rural* could lead to decreased fragmentation of services and increased sharing of ideas and resources.

Complete secondary compilations and analyses of existing databases into small regional units and according to subpopulations. For example, when examining rates of chronic obstructive pulmonary disease in a state, include a more detailed analysis that considers counties, towns, and ethnic subgroups as well. More comprehensive use of existing data will lead to a deeper understanding of the particular health concerns of diverse populations living in varied rural settings. In addition, outcome data are needed on managed care and the impact of managed care organizations on the health status of rural communities. This effort will do much to avoid duplication of assessment activities and will facilitate program planning and evaluation that is population oriented.

Resolve problems related to recruitment, retention, and training of health professionals for rural communities. Of particular concern are the inadequate numbers of primary health care providers and community health nurses who deliver basic preventive health care services to vulnerable rural populations, as specified by *Healthy People 2010*.

Eliminate the problematic professional liability crisis in rural America. More specifically, lack of obstetric care in rural communities

as a result of malpractice costs has almost eliminated even the most basic prenatal care in some areas of the country.

Identify mechanisms to accurately assess the quality of health care services and programs in rural America from the perspective of the people who use those services. Typically, existing programs for quality assurance, continuous quality improvement, and program evaluation incorporate complex technologic measures that are associated with large tertiary institutions. The comparatively low volume of clients who use services in a rural agency, combined with rural residents' beliefs and lifestyles, may render techniques used to measure program outcomes in larger agencies invalid and unreliable in rural settings.

Consider ethical issues that influence nursing care in rural communities. Potential issues center on poverty and the subsequent inability to pay for health care, inadequate access to services, and the lack of necessary and prepared health care providers and programs to meet even the most basic primary prevention needs in rural communities.

Disseminate pertinent information on rural nursing practice in general and community health nursing in particular. To date, most of the information that is available focuses on populations living in rural communities in the Appalachian Mountains, the Midwest, and intermountain regions. Information is critically needed about ethnic and racial minorities as well as other populations who live in other regions of the United States, especially groups living in the southeastern, northeastern, south central, and southwestern United States; Alaska; and Hawaii.

Compiled from Gamm, L., Hutchinson, L., Dabney, B., et al. (Eds.). (2003b). *Rural healthy people 2010: A companion document to Healthy People 2010* (Vol. 2). College Station, TX: Texas A & M University. Retrieved May 28, 2007 from http://www.srph.tamhsc.edu/centers/rhp2010.

accessible, and acceptable community health nursing services to rural populations.

To resolve the overriding health care delivery issues, health care providers in general and community/public health nurses in particular should form partnerships with rural communities. Health care professionals must talk with rural Americans to learn about what they believe to be their most pressing health care needs. Working together, as partners, they can develop effective solutions to meet rural America's public health and community health nursing needs and to achieve the goals specified in *Healthy People 2010* in a culturally and linguistically appropriate manner.

KEY IDEAS

1. Approximately 20% of Americans live in rural communities that have fewer than 20,000 residents. Access to health care is a problem for many of them. However, there has been a significant population and economic growth in many rural regions of the United States. The short- and long-term outcomes of this trend on rural communities continue to be monitored.

2. Compared with the total U.S. population, rural Americans tend to have higher rates of infant and maternal mortality, chronic disease, and occupational illnesses and injuries associated with agriculture, mining, and construction. Alcohol-related vehicle accidents are also a problem. Minority groups in rural areas have even more health problems, although major information gaps exist regarding their actual health status.

3. Many rural areas are designated as HPSAs because of inadequate numbers of health care providers and services.

4. Rural community/public health nurses are instrumental in providing a wide range of services to all age groups and addressing all levels of prevention. However, there are insufficient numbers of community/public health nurses in rural communities.

5. A higher percentage of persons are medically underinsured in rural areas than in nonrural areas; 40% of rural families live below the poverty level.

6. RHCs, MHCs, and the IHS are examples of federal initiatives to increase health care to vulnerable rural populations by using mid-level providers such as nurse practitioners, nurse midwives, and certified nurse anesthetists.

7. Community/public health nurses need to study the health beliefs and values of rural subpopulations and minority groups to provide more meaningful and appropriate nursing care.

8. Community/public health nurses provide culturally relevant care by honoring the values of rural residents, who tend to prefer informal support, are self-reliant, and often define health as the ability to work. It is a challenge to maintain confidentiality in areas where all residents know each other.

9. Successful rural community/public health nurses enjoy a high degree of professional independence and creativity that enables them to deal effectively with a scarcity of resources.

10. Partnerships between community/public health nurses and community members are essential to develop accessible, acceptable health care in rural areas.

CASE STUDY   Building a Professional Community Partnership

Johnson County, Tennessee, is located in the Appalachian Mountains in the northeastern-most corner of the state, with borders on North Carolina and Virginia. Two-lane, winding, twisting roads offer the only vehicular access to the county. Air travel is limited by foggy weather conditions common to this eastern mountain chain. Like many rural areas, Johnson County suffered in the rural recession during the 1980s. By 1988, unemployment in the county, influenced by the closing of several small industries, had reached 35%. The farm crisis affected the agricultural base of small crops, tobacco raising, and tree farming. Health care, once strong in the county, significantly diminished when the 60-bed Hill-Burton hospital facility in Mountain City, the county seat, closed. Only 3 physicians remained in the county by the end of 1988, down from a previous total of 12. The closest evening or emergency services were located at community hospitals in neighboring towns 36 miles away over dangerous mountain roads.

Step 1: Identify the Problem Area

Concerned with deteriorating economic, health, and social conditions in the county, a group of private citizens purchased at auction the equipment and supplies remaining in the defunct Johnson County Hospital and then donated the items back to the county.

The group, along with the Johnson County Commission, identified accessible health care as a vital component of protecting the county population and attracting new industry and residents to the area.

Step 2: Assess the Community's Perspective

A community assessment undertaken by an outside consulting firm identified the population's health care needs and available resources. The final report noted that the rates of preventable illnesses and conditions such as diabetes and cardiovascular and cerebrovascular problems; infant mortality; cancer; suicides; and accidents were 150% to 400% higher than national and state rates. The median per-capita income in the county was $8882, compared with $17,592 nationally and $14,736 statewide. Thirty-six percent of Johnson County high school students dropped out before graduation, which further limited economic potential in the community.

The following natural allies were identified from input to the consultants by a private-public community action group:

• The Health Science Division of East Tennessee State University, consisting of the School of Nursing, the School of Public and Allied Health, and the College of Medicine

• The Tennessee Department of Health through the First Tennessee Community Health Agency

Continued

CASE STUDY   Building a Professional Community Partnership—cont'd

Both of these agencies are headquartered in Johnson City, Tennessee, 47 miles and 1 hour travel time away from Johnson County.

Step 3: Analyze the Data

Analyses of formal and informal community assessment data were completed by an interdisciplinary team from the Health Science Division of East Tennessee State University. Their findings strengthened the decision by community leaders to invite the participation of nursing, medicine, and public health personnel in meeting the intense health care needs of the population. A partnership between the educational entities and the community held the potential for mutual benefit and the opening of new avenues of health care delivery appropriate to community needs. The East Tennessee State University School of Nursing, working through its Department of Family/Community Nursing, answered the expressed need of the community for primary health care during nontraditional hours.

Step 4: Develop a Long-Range Plan

The short- and long-range goals were identified and then formalized through a partnership relationship between the Johnson County Commission and the university's Health Science Division and School of Nursing. The long-term goals were to preserve the capability of the hospital to reopen and to attack the problems of joblessness and the lack of health care services.

Step 5: Take Action

With the support of key state and local leaders, the School of Nursing opened the Mountain City Extended Hours Health Center with the assistance of $176,500 in grant money from the First Tennessee Community Health Agency to help establish the community nursing practice and to offset the cost of indigent care provided by the center on a sliding scale. The Johnson County Hospital Board provided space in the vacant hospital that included two examination rooms, a waiting room, two offices, and bathroom facilities. Utilities, security, and some equipment were provided by the Johnson County Commission through the hospital board.

Site preparation for implementation of the clinic began in the summer. Trustees from the nearby Carter County Correctional Center worked with the School of Nursing project directors and the center's coordinator to prepare the long-unused site by moving equipment and furniture, cleaning, and painting. Many hours of intensive labor were required to empty, prepare, and refurbish the site.

During the preparatory months, protocols, policies, and procedures for carrying out the full range of functioning of a primary care clinic were developed. Services provided in the clinic included standard primary care options such as physical examinations, health counseling, and teaching; diagnosis and treatment of common recurring, acute, and chronic illnesses; and referral to more specialized health care providers when needed.

Application was made to and approved by the Tennessee Primary Care Board for site approval for nurse practitioner prescriptive privileges. Application was made for status as a rural community health clinic, which allowed nurse practitioner care to be reimbursed on a cost-for-service basis by Medicare and Medicaid.

Step 6: Evaluate the Program

The clinic opened as scheduled, and the number of clients who seek services has increased each month. A site visit after the clinic opened confirmed that the Mountain City Extended Hours Health Center met strict federal standards and qualified for certification as a rural community health clinic. The Office of Equal Opportunity ensured that the center was in compliance with civil rights regulations. Contracts with local industry to provide employee physical examinations, employee education, and drug screening have added to the center's revenue base. Major insurance carriers also provide reimbursement for some services. Community involvement through festivals and fairs, schools, and civic groups has led to a rapidly expanding client base. Newspaper articles and radio programs have increased the center's visibility and credibility. Faculties report that the nurse-managed clinic also has provided rich clinical experiences for students enrolled in the nursing program, as well as for students in other health care disciplines. Health status outcomes are being monitored.

Adapted from Edwards, J., Lenz, C., & East, J. (1993). Nurse-managed primary care: Serving a rural Appalachian population. *Family and Community Health, 16*(2), 52-57.

 See **Critical Thinking Questions** for this Case Study on the book's website.

LEARNING BY EXPERIENCE AND REFLECTION

Review the Case Study to answer questions 1 through 7.

1. From the discussion of the first two steps of partnership building, identify Johnson County's major public health concerns

2. Describe economic, cultural, and demographic factors that can influence the health status of Johnson County residents.

3. How do the goals of *Healthy People 2010* and *Rural Healthy People 2010* (three-volume companion document) apply to the approach used to address the problem in the Case Study?

4. What roles and responsibilities would a community/public health nurse in Johnson County have in building a professional-community partnership?

5. What specific concerns are related to impaired availability, accessibility, and acceptability of health care services and providers to residents of Johnson County?

6. What approaches or measures could be used to evaluate the short- and long-term outcomes of the Mountain City Extended Hours Health Center and the effectiveness of these outcomes?

7. What strategies could a community/public health nurse use to address concerns related to maintaining confidentiality in this small community?

8. How is *rural* defined or perceived in your community and practice setting?
9. How do the proposed concepts of rural nursing fit rural populations in your geographic region? (If possible, cite examples.)
10. Identify challenges, opportunities, and benefits of living and practicing as a community/public health nurse in a small and rural community.
11. Describe potential ethical concerns in community/public health nursing that might emerge from rural social and economic structures. Suggest some approaches that might be used to address those concerns.
12. Identify some of the health care problems of rural residents in your state.

STUDY AIDS   http://evolve.elsevier.com/Maurer/community/

Visit the Evolve website for this book to find the following study and assessment materials:

- Quiz
- Web Scenario
- Critical Thinking Questions and Answers for Case Studies
- Care Plans
- *Healthy People* Updates
- Glossary

REFERENCES

Agency for Healthcare Research and Quality. (2003). *Creating partnerships, improving health: The role of community based participatory research* (AHRQ Publication No. 03-0037). Retrieved May 28, 2007 from *http://www.ahrq.gov/research/cbprrole.htm*.

American Nurses Association. (1996). *Rural/Frontier Health Care Task Force: Rural/frontier nursing: The challenge to grow*. Washington, DC: Author.

Bigbee, J., & Crowder, E. (1985). The Red Cross Rural Nursing Service: An innovation of public health nursing delivery. *Public Health Nursing, 2*(2), 109-121.

Brown, D., Swanson, L. (2003). *Challenges for rural America in the twenty-first century*. University Park, PA: Pennsylvania State University Press.

Burbank-Schmitt, E. (2006). *America's nursing shortage*. Princeton, NJ: Robert Wood Johnson Foundation. Retrieved May 28, 2007 from *http://www.rwjf.org/pr/productlist.jsp?topicid=1318&catid=12*.

Bureau of Health Professions. (2007). *Health professional shortage areas*. Retrieved May 28, 2007 from *http://hpsafind.hrsa.gov*.

Bureau of Primary Health Care. (2006). *Migrant Health Program: National Advisory Council on Migrant Health recommendations*. Retrieved May 28, 2007 from *http://www.bphc.hrsa.gov/migrant/NACMHRecommendations.htm*.

Bushy, A. (2001). *Orientation to nursing in the rural community*. Thousand Oaks, CA: Sage.

Bushy, A. (2002). *Rural minority health resource book*. National Rural Health Association. Kansas City, MO: Project supported by the Office of Rural Health Policy, Health Resources Services Administration, and National Rural Health Association.

Bushy, A. (2004). *American Nurses Association continuing education program: Rural nursing: Practice and issues*. Retrieved May 28, 2007 from *http://nursingworld.org/mods/mod700/rural.pdf*.

Case, T. (1991). Work stresses of community health nurses in Oklahoma. In A. Bushy (Ed.), *Rural nursing* (Vol. II). Newbury Park, CA: Sage.

Centers for Medicare and Medicaid Services. (2007a). *Federally qualified health centers*. Retrieved May 28, 2007 from *http://www.cms.hhs.gov/center/fqhc.asp*.

Centers for Medicare and Medicaid Services. (2007b). *Rural health center*. Retrieved May 28, 2007 from *http://www.cms.hhs.gov/center/ru*.

Coburn, A., MacKinney, A., McBride, T., et al. (2007, March). *Choosing rural definitions: Implications for health policy* (Rural Policy Research Institute Health Panel, Issue Brief No. 2). Retrieved May 28, 2007 from *http://www.cdktest.com/rupri/Forms/RuralDefinitionsBrief.pdf*.

Coward, R., Davis, L., Gold, C., et al. (2004). *Rural women's health: Mental, behavioral, and physical issues*. New York: Springer.

Davis, D., & Droes, N. (1993). Community health nursing in rural and frontier counties. *Nursing Clinics of North America, 28*(1), 159-169.

Edwards, J., Lenz, C., & East, J. (1993). Nurse managed primary care: Serving a rural Appalachian population. *Family and Community Health, 16*(2), 52-57.

Gamm, L. (2007). Keynote address: *Rural Healthy People 2010* and sustaining rural populations. In L. Morgan & P. Stewart-Fahs (Eds.), *Conversations in the disciplines—Sustaining rural populations*. Binghamton, NY: Global Academic Publishing.

Gamm, L., & Hutchison, L. (Eds.). (2004). *Rural healthy people 2010: A companion document to Healthy People 2010* (Vol. 3). College Station, TX: Texas A & M University. Retrieved May 28, 2007 from *http://www.srph.tamhsc.edu/centers/rhp2010/Volume_3/Vol3rhp2010.pdf*.

Gamm, L., Hutchison, L., Dabney, B., et al. (Eds.). (2003a). *Rural healthy people 2010: A companion document to Healthy People 2010* (Vol. 1). College Station, TX: Texas A & M University.

Retrieved May 28, 2007 from *http://www.srph.tamhsc.edu/centers/rhp2010/Volume1.pdf*.

Gamm, L., Hutchison, L., Dabney, B., et al. (Eds.). (2003b). *Rural healthy people 2010: A companion document to Healthy People 2010* (Vol. 2). College Station, TX: Texas A & M University. Retrieved May 28, 3007 from *http://www.srph.tamhsc.edu/centers/rhp2010/Volume2.pdf*.

Gibbs, R. (2004). *Rural income, poverty and welfare: Rural poverty*. Washington, DC: United States Department of Agriculture. Retrieved May 28, 2007 from *http://www.ers.usda.gov/Briefing/IncomePovertyWelfare/ruralpoverty*.

Glasgow, N., Morton, L., Johnson, N. (2004). *Critical issues in rural health care*. Ames, IA: Blackwell.

Health Resources and Services Administration. (2003). *United States health personnel fact book*. Washington, DC: Author. Retrieved May 28, 2007 from *http://bhpr.hrsa.gov/healthworkforce/reports/factbook.htm#Registered%20Nurses%20&%20Licensed%20Practical%20Nurses*.

Indian Health Service. (2007a). *IHS fact sheets*. Retrieved May 28, 2007 from *http://info.ihs.gov/*.

Indian Health Service. (2007b). *Facts on Indian health disparities*. Rockville, MD: Author. Retrieved May 28, 2007 from http://info.ihs.gov/Files/DisparitiesFacts-Jan2007.doc.

Indian Health Service. (2007c). *IHS regional map*. Retrieved May 28, 2007 from *http://info.ihs.gov/Map.asp*.

Institute of Medicine, Committee on the Future of Rural Health Care, Board on Health Care Services. (2005). *Quality through collaboration: The future of rural health*. Washington, DC: National Academies Press. Retrieved May 28, 2007 from *http://www.iom.edu/?id=23359&redirect=0*.

Kaiser Foundation. (2003). *The uninsured in rural America*. Retrieved May 28, 2007 from *http://www.kff.org/uninsured/upload/The-Uninsured-in-Rural-America-Update-PDF.pdf*.

Lee, H., Winters, C. (Eds.). (2006). *Rural nursing: concepts, theory and practice* (2nd ed.). New York: Springer.

Long, K., Weinert, C. (1989). Rural nursing: Developing a theory base. *Scholarly Inquiry for Nursing Practice, 3*, 113-127.

Monk, D. (2007). Recruiting and retaining high-quality teachers in rural areas. *The Future of Children, 17*(1), 155-174. Retrieved May 28, 2007 from *http://www.futureofchildren.org/pubs-info2825/pubs-info_show.htm?doc_id=468970*.

Morgan, I., & Stewart-Fahs, P. (Eds.). (2007). *Conversations in the disciplines—Sustaining rural populations*. Binghamton, NY: Global Academic Publishing.

National Advisory Council on Migrant Health. (1993). *Under the weather: Farmworker health care*. Rockville, MD: Bureau of Primary Health Care.

National Health Service Corps. (2007). *About NHSC*. Retrieved August 30, 2003 from *http://nhsc.bhpr.hrsa.gov/about*.

National Rural Health Association. (2004). *Rural public health (NRHA Policy Brief)*. Retrieved May 28, 2007 from *http://www.nrharural.org/advocacy/sub/policybriefs/public_hlth.pdf*.

Office of Rural Health Policy. (2002). *One department serving rural America: HHS Rural Task Force: Report to the Secretary*. Washington, DC: Author. Retrieved May 28, 2007 from *http://ruralhealth.hrsa.gov/PublicReport.htm*.

Probst, J., Samuels, M., Jespersen, K., et al. (2002). *Minorities in rural America: An overview of population characteristics*. Columbia, SC:

University of South Carolina. Retrieved May 28, 2007 from *http://rhr.sph.sc.edu/report/MinoritiesInRuralAmerica.pdf*.

Randolph, R., Gual, K., & Slokfin, R. (2002). *Rural populations and health care providers: A map book*. Chapel Hill, NC: University of North Carolina. Retrieved May 28, 2007 from *http://www.shepscenter.unc.edu/research_programs/rural_program/mapbook2003/index.html*.

Roberts, L., Dyer, A. (2004). *Ethics in mental health care*. Washington, DC: American Psychiatric Publishing Company.

Sawyer, D., Gale, J., Lambert, D. (2006). *Rural and frontier mental and behavioral health care: Barriers, effective policy strategies, best practices*. National Association for Rural Mental Health. Retrieved May 28, 2007 from *http://www.narmh.org/publications/archives/rural_frontier.pdf*.

Stein, H. (1989). The annual cycle and the cultural nexus of health care behavior among Oklahoma wheat farming families. *Culture, Medicine, and Psychology, 6*, 81-89.

Substance Abuse and Mental Health Services Administration. (2003). Substance abuse or dependence in metropolitan and non-metropolitan areas. *The NHSDA Report*, 1-3. Retrieved May 28, 2007 from *http://www.oas.samhsa.gov/2k3/Urban/Urban.pdf*.

U.S. Bureau of the Census. (2000). *Census 2000 urban and rural classification*. Retrieved May 28, 2007 from *http://www.census.gov/geo/www/ua/ua_2k.html*.

U.S. Department of Agriculture. (2006). *Briefing rooms: Measuring rurality*. Retrieved

May 28, 2007 from *http://www.ers.usda.gov/Briefing/Rurality/*.

U.S. Department of Agriculture. (2007a, January). *Briefing rooms: Rural labor and education: Farm labor*. Retrieved May 28, 2007 from *http://www.ers.usda.gov/Briefing/LaborAndEducation/FarmLabor.htm*.

U.S. Department of Agriculture. (2007b, April). *Population dynamics are changing the profile of rural America*. Retrieved May 28, 2007 from *http://ers.usda.gov/AmberWaves/April07/PDF/Population.pdf*.

U.S. Department of Health and Human Services. (2000). *Healthy people 2010: Understanding and improving health* (2nd ed.). Washington, DC: U.S. Government Printing Office. Retrieved May 28, 2007 from *http://www.healthypeople.gov/*.

U.S. Department of Health and Human Services. (2006). *Healthy people 2010: Midcourse review*. Washington, DC: U.S. Government Printing Office.

U.S. Department of Health and Human Services. (2007, January). *2007 Annual report by the National Advisory Committee on Rural Health and Human Services to the Secretary of Health and Human Services*. Washington, DC. Retrieved May 28, 2007 from *ftp://ftp.hrsa.gov/ruralhealth/NACReport2007.pdf*.

U.S. Department of Health and Human Services U.S. Department of Health and Human Services. (nd). *Budget in brief: Fiscal year 2009*. Retrieved June 10, 2007 from *http://www.ihs.gov/09/budget/2009BudgetInBrief.pdf*.

SUGGESTED READINGS

Bushy, A. (2004). *American Nurses Association continuing education program: Rural nursing: Practice and issues*. Retrieved May 28, 2007 from *http://nursingworld.org/mods/mod700/rural.pdf*.

Davis, D., & Droes, N. (1993). Community health nursing in rural and frontier counties. *Nursing Clinics of North America, 28*(1), 159-169.

Long, K., & Weinert, C. (1989). Rural nursing: Developing a theory base. *Scholarly Inquiry for Nursing Practice, 3*, 113-127.

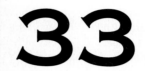

33 Community Mental Health

Verna Benner Carson

FOCUS QUESTIONS

What were the treatment breakthroughs and legislative changes that paved the way for the community mental health movement?

What is the philosophy of community mental health care?

Who are the severely mentally ill?

What are the needs of the severely mentally ill?

How are those needs met by community mental health?

What are the services available to meet the needs of the severely mentally ill?

What is nursing's role in community mental health?

CHAPTER OUTLINE

Advent of Community Mental Health Care
Legislative Changes in the 1960s
Moving Forward in the 1970s
Losing Ground in the 1980s
Doing More with Less in the 1990s
Surviving in the New Millennium
Philosophy of Community Mental Health Care
Care That Is Continuous and Comprehensive
Population Served by Community Mental Health Care

Prevalence of Mental Disorders
Who Are the Severely Mentally Ill?
What Are the Needs of the Severely Mentally Ill?
Services Provided in Community Mental Health Care
Types of Community Mental Health Services
Providers of Community Mental Health Services
Role of the Nurse in Community Mental Health Care
Focus on Prevention

The Nursing Process in Practice
Nursing Process: Community as Client
Nursing Process: Individual or Family as Client
Continuing Issues in Community Mental Health Care
Transformation of Mental Health Care
Inadequate Focus on Child Mental Health
Growing Elderly Population
Cultural Competence in Community Mental Health
Mandated Treatment for the Severely Mentally Ill

KEY TERMS

Catchment area
Community mental health centers
Congregate or sheltered housing
Day treatment
Deinstitutionalization

Institutionalization
Mobile treatment units
Primary prevention
Revolving-door cycle
Secondary prevention

Severely mentally ill
Single-room occupancy
Tertiary prevention

In this chapter the concept, history, and significance of community mental health care are explored. Persons who receive community-based psychiatric services are identified, services are discussed, and the role of nursing in community mental health care is examined. The chapter provides an evaluation of community mental health care today and a discussion of its future directions.

ADVENT OF COMMUNITY MENTAL HEALTH CARE

Before 1963, community mental health care was nonexistent in the United States. Severely impaired individuals were admitted

to psychiatric hospitals, where they frequently remained for the rest of their lives, forlorn, forgotten, and forsaken by family, professionals, and society. This all changed with the discovery of the phenothiazine drugs (e.g., chlorpromazine [Thorazine]). The effects of these drugs were nothing less than miraculous, because they eliminated or reduced the most challenging of psychiatric symptoms. Suddenly, discharge became not only a possibility but also a reality for many individuals. Although patients were dramatically improved, they were not ready to reenter the community, nor was the community prepared to receive them. Many patients lacked family support, and some still exhibited behaviors that interfered with social interactions.

Still other patients, accustomed to having needs met and decisions made by the institution, lacked the ability to function without institutional support. Therefore, these individuals were discharged from the state institution to a smaller institution, such as a nursing home or a group home. The condition of these individuals led to the recognition of the phenomenon of **institutionalization;** that is, long-term care in an institutional setting resulted in impaired social interaction, decision making, and independent living skills (Grob, 1994a).

As more and more individuals became ready for discharge, the need for supportive services in the community became increasingly apparent. As awareness of this need grew among mental health professionals and the lay public, so also grew the awareness that the community was lacking these supportive services.

LEGISLATIVE CHANGES IN THE 1960s

Concurrent with these changes, there were legislative mandates that focused psychiatry toward the community. In 1961, the Joint Commission on Mental Illness and Health published its report, which recommended that treatment of the mentally ill be moved from state hospitals to the community. The process of **deinstitutionalization** was underway with the goal of reducing the number of clients cared for in state hospitals by 50% over a two-decade period (Minkoff, 1978). In 1963, the U.S. government appropriated $150 million to fund **community mental health centers** through the Mental Retardation Facilities and Community Mental Health Centers Construction Act (Public Law 88-164, frequently referred to as the *Community Mental Health Act*). This money was to be matched by state funds over a 3-year period and used for the construction of comprehensive community mental health centers. For states to qualify for federal funding, they were required to provide five essential services: inpatient care, outpatient care, partial hospitalization, emergency care, and consultation and education. The expectation was that after 8 years, financial support of the centers would come from state and local funds and fees generated from services offered.

Before the system had a chance to get firmly established, while the available community resources were in the infancy stage of development, hospitals began to discharge large numbers of clients. Communities were unprepared to receive these clients. The system was fragile and incomplete. Financial support was lacking, housing and treatment facilities were scarce, and community attitudes were inhospitable to the individuals who were discharged. Psychiatric clients were feared, mocked, generally misunderstood, and stigmatized for conditions over which they had little or no control. Proposals for housing facilities in residential neighborhoods met with cries of indignation, alarm, and fear from residents. Communities felt that they had become "dumping grounds" for the large psychiatric hospitals. Former hospital residents, who were largely unwelcome and rebuffed, found that life outside the hospital was frightening and unappealing. They found themselves caught up in a **revolving-door cycle** of short inpatient stay, rapid discharge, and eventual repeat admissions.

Mary had been working as a registered nurse in a state mental hospital for several years when the first community mental health center was constructed in her area. She tells her story. "I was so excited—both for my clients and myself.

I believed that this was a new opportunity for them as well as me. Many of the folks that I worked with seemed capable of functioning in the outside world. And for me, working in the community seemed to offer a chance to practice nursing the way I thought it should be done. It didn't take me long to get on the community bandwagon, where I have been for many years. I was right about opportunity—but I never dreamed of all the roadblocks that had to be overcome. Community mental health care has more frustrations than I ever dreamed of. So many people are really ignorant about individuals with mental disorders and treat them horribly. And there have never been enough resources. Not just money—all resources are scarce. Yet, in spite of this I still believe we need to care for people in the midst of our communities. Now I see myself as a crusader for the rights of the mentally ill in the community. There are times when I think it's only my lone voice speaking out. But I'll keep doing it—probably as long as I'm able."

MOVING FORWARD IN THE 1970s

By the beginning of the 1970s, it was clear that there were real problems in the community mental health care movement. Among these problems was the fact that many state and local governments were not able to match federal funds. Some community mental health centers located in rural or poverty-stricken areas were unable to generate the necessary fees to be self-sufficient. Important services that generated little or no income, such as public education and consultation, began to suffer.

In 1977, President Jimmy Carter mandated a major reassessment of mental health needs. He established a 20-member President's Commission on Mental Health that included a nurse, Martha Mitchell, who was the Chairperson of the American Nurses Association Division on Psychiatric and Mental Health Nursing Practice. In 1978, the *Report to the President of the President's Commission on Mental Health* was published and focused on strengthening the community mental health care system as the foundation for the mental health system. This would involve improving community support systems, continuing the phase-out of large public hospitals, establishing a center with a focus on primary prevention within the National Institute of Mental Health, and improving the delivery of services to underserved and high-risk populations. The report also advocated other major changes in the delivery of mental health care. These suggestions included the following:

- Establishing national health insurance that includes coverage for mental health.
- Encouraging private insurance carriers to include mental health coverage (including outpatient care) in their packages.
- Providing funding to increase the number of mental health professionals, especially those who work with children, the elderly, and minorities.
- Developing advocacy programs for the chronically mentally ill.
- Protecting the rights of all persons in need of mental health services.
- Increasing support for research related to mental health and illness.
- Providing public health education to increase the public's understanding of mental health and illness.
- Centralizing the evaluation efforts of governmental agencies.

This commission's report was the first official high-level document to recognize the professional contributions of nurses to mental health care.

LOSING GROUND IN THE 1980s

In 1980, the Community Mental Health Systems Act was passed. It was designed to implement the recommendations of the President's commission and to coordinate the two-tiered mental health system that had evolved since the original 1963 legislation that mandated the establishment of community mental health centers. Those with severe mental disability still resided within state institutions, and those who were less disabled used the services of the community mental health centers.

The programs authorized by this legislation were to be implemented in 1982, but before this could occur, there was a significant retrenchment by the federal government in terms of its responsibilities in the area of mental health. The Ninety-seventh Congress essentially repealed the 1980 Community Mental Health Systems Act with the passage of the Reagan administration's Omnibus Budget Reconciliation Act (Public Law 97-35). This bill moved the authority for and administration of mental health programs from the National Institute of Mental Health to the individual states. Each state received a block grant to cover alcohol, drug abuse, and mental health services. As of 1984, federal funding for community mental health care and other mental health care delivery programs was terminated. Community mental health centers were mandated to provide only five essential services: outpatient care, partial hospitalization, 24-hour hospitalization and emergency care, consultation and education, and screening services. The continued existence of community mental health centers was dependent on state support, private funding, and the center's ability to earn revenue.

DOING MORE WITH LESS IN THE 1990s

As the 1990s unfolded it became clear that reliance on federal funding was inadequate. The political climate favored the support of "smaller" rather than "bigger" programs directed to meeting human needs. With so many programs competing for limited funds, community mental health care was challenged to do more with less. The trend moved increasingly toward managed care (Grob, 1994b), which ultimately meant less care for those with severe mental disabilities.

Another major innovation of the 1990s was the involvement of recipients of services in the planning efforts (Chamberlin & Rogers, 1990). The prime motivation for this change came from organizations of former hospital residents, which began in the early 1970s. Members have traditionally joined these groups as a way of reclaiming their voice and being heard by a system that has considered them incapable of defining their own needs. A primary goal of these groups is influencing public policy related to implementation of mental health programs. These groups (which include diverse local, regional, and national organizations) influenced the passage of legislation such as Public Law 99-660. This law requires the participation of various constituencies, including families, individuals with mental disorders, and professionals, in the planning of a community-based system of mental health care. It also provides a way for former residents of mental hospitals and their families to promote their vision regarding how care should and should not be given to people who suffer with mental disorders.

It became fashionable during the 1990s to refer to patients as *consumers,* a term that many formerly hospitalized patients find objectionable. The term *consumer* implies choice and power, a misnomer considering that clients in the mental health system are captive populations who have little choice regarding the services or the providers selected.

Additional changes in the 1990s included the closure of entire state psychiatric hospital systems with the wholesale transfer of large numbers of institutionalized severely mentally ill individuals into unprepared communities. At the same time, there was an increase in self-help programs, which are user-run programs that serve as drop-in centers and offer peer case management. Such services provide former patients with a feeling that they can make a difference to someone else, that they can give as well as receive, and that their lives have meaning.

SURVIVING IN THE NEW MILLENNIUM

Funding continues to be a major challenge to all community-based providers. According to Dr. C. Knight Aldrich, the federal government should provide for the full care of the severely mentally ill, "not as an experiment but as an ongoing responsibility as with the care of veterans" (Brickhouse, 2003, p. 2). Dr. Knight asserts that it is unrealistic to expect local communities to bear the cost of this care and state governments "have consistently made it evident that they cannot or will not adequately support care" (Brickhouse, 2003, p. 3). Today there are fewer than 50,000 people in state psychiatric hospitals. It is estimated that there are more than 900,000 with severe mental disorders—many of whom would be in state psychiatric hospitals if so many of these facilities had not been closed (Lowry, 2003, p. 3). Instead of receiving treatment, many live on the streets, where they comprise about one third of all the homeless, and many others reside in jails (Brickhouse, 2003). Refer to Chapter 21 for additional information about homelessness, poverty, and the mentally ill. Dr. Fuller Torrey, president of the Treatment Advocacy Center, states, "The Los Angeles County jail with 3400 mentally ill prisoners, is de facto the largest psychiatric inpatient facility in the United States. New York's Rikers Island jail, with 2800 mentally ill prisoners, is the second largest" (Lowry, 2003). The mental health objectives in *Healthy People 2010* are especially relevant to this large group of severely mentally ill individuals, who receive little to no treatment (see the *Healthy People 2010* box).

In 2002, the New Freedom Commission on Mental Health was created by President George W. Bush. The commission released its report to the President in July 2003. The report was entitled *Achieving the Promise: Transforming Mental Health in America.* Commissioners concluded that services for the mentally ill were fragmented and inefficient, particularly for the severely mentally ill. For example, services varied from state to state, with blurring of responsibility among agencies, programs, and levels of government. Many clients were noted to "fall through the cracks." Even those who received treatment had difficulty achieving financial independence because of limited job opportunities and the fear of losing health insurance in the workplace (President's New Freedom Commission on Mental Health, 2003). Despite the conclusions of this commission and its recommendations for change in the mental health system, the delivery of mental health services is largely under the domain of individual states without an overriding

■ HEALTHY PEOPLE 2010 ■
Mental Health Objectives

1. Reduce to 19% the proportion of homeless adults who have serious mental illness (SMI) (baseline: 25% of homeless adults aged 18 years and older had SMI in 1996).
2. Increase to 54% the proportion of persons with serious mental illnesses who are employed (baseline: 52% of persons aged 18 years and older with serious mental illnesses were employed in 2002).
3. Increase to 55% the proportion of juvenile residential facilities that screen admissions for mental health problems (baseline: 50% of facilities in 2000).
4. Increase the proportion of adults with mental health disorders who receive treatment.

Mental Disorder	2002 Baseline (%)	2010 Target (%)
Serious mental illness	62	68
Depression	58	64
Schizophrenia	60 (1984 baseline)	75
Generalized anxiety disorder	60	79

5. Increase to 57% the proportion of persons with co-occurring substance abuse and mental disorders who receive treatment for both disorders (baseline: 51% in 2002).
6. Increase to 51 the number of states and the District of Columbia with an operational mental health plan that addresses specialized mental health services for elderly persons (baseline: 18 states in 2000-2001).

From U.S. Department of Health and Human Services (USDHHS). (2000). *Healthy people 2010: Understanding and improving health* (2nd ed.). Washington, DC: U.S. Government Printing Office; and USDHHS. (2006). *Healthy people 2010: Midcourse review.* Washington, DC: U.S. Government Printing Office.

federal mandate for change (*New Freedom Commission on Mental Health State Implementation Activity,* 2004).

In 2007 and 2008, there was a push in the U.S. Congress for expansion of the mental health parity law passed in 1996 (Pear, 2007; U.S. Department of Labor, 2007). Currently health insurance provides less coverage and more restrictions for mental health care than for physical health care. Mental health parity means that insurance coverage for treatment of mental illness would be the same as for medical and surgical treatment (Krauss & O'Sullivan, 2007). Without mandated parity, those who suffer with severe mental illnesses will continue to be underserved in the United States. The issue of mental health parity remains unresolved.

Local communities faced with managing the needs of the severely mentally ill are taking matters into their own hands by passing state legislation. Unique partnerships among law enforcement agencies, providers of drug and alcohol services, mental health and retardation service providers, the National Alliance for the Mentally Ill (NAMI), consumer advocacy groups, and housing authorities have been formed to address the shortcomings of the community mental health system (Royer, 2003; Stratton, 2002). An example of a local community's taking action occurred in New York with the passage of Timothy's Law, signed by Governor George Pataki in December 2006. This state law went into effect in January 2007 as a result of local community efforts to address the inequities in mental health coverage.

The lightning rod for this community effort was the suicide in 2001 of a 12-year-old boy, Timothy O'Clair, who hanged himself in his bedroom closet. Timothy and his family had sought mental health care for almost 5 years. Because of the inequality between health care coverage for medical and mental health problems, Timothy's care was sporadic, expensive, and never adequate to help him achieve remission. To obtain better care for Timothy, Mr. and Mrs. O'Clair were forced to relinquish custody of the boy and place him in the foster care system so that Timothy would be eligible for Medicaid coverage and unrestricted access to mental health services. Once in the foster care system Timothy bounced around several placements and finally ended up in Northeast Parent Child Society, where he seemed to improve. He came home to celebrate his mother's birthday, and for 3 weeks he did well. Although the family continued to participate in therapy, Timothy became violent and threatened to kill himself—a threat he had made many times over the years. This last time he was serious, and while his dad was working and his mother was out with his brother, Timothy hanged himself (TimothysLaw.org, 2006).

Timothy's Law requires that all group health insurance and health maintenance organization–type plans provide at least 30 inpatient days and 20 outpatient visits per year for mental health treatment. The cost of this benefit to small businesses with 50 or fewer employees is subsidized by New York State's general fund. The law also requires large employers to provide unlimited treatment for adults and children who have biologically based mental disorders such as schizophrenia, bipolar and delusional disorders, major depression, panic disorders, obsessive-compulsive disorders, bulimia and anorexia, and psychotic disorders (New York State United Teachers, 2006).

Another community mental health issue facing the country in the new millennium is the mental health needs of veterans returning from the Iraq and Afghanistan conflicts who suffer from posttraumatic stress disorder (PTSD) (Hoge et al., 2004). Although many will be treated through the Veterans Administration system, problems related to the sequelae to PTSD will ripple throughout the community with an increase in divorce, joblessness, and homelessness (Vedantam, 2006).

PHILOSOPHY OF COMMUNITY MENTAL HEALTH CARE

The philosophy of community mental health care has a two-pronged focus. The first is to consider the community as client and attempt to improve situations in the community that detract from optimal mental health and could conceivably lead to mental illness. This focus is embodied in educational and consultation programs.

The second focus is to consider the individual within the community as client. To serve the individual, a full range of comprehensive services are provided. These include the following:

- Outpatient care
- Partial hospitalization
- Home care services
- 24-hour hospitalization and emergency care
- Screening services

Other services may also be available, including those designed to meet the needs of children, adolescents, and the elderly; alcohol and drug abuse services; and transitional services.

The community is defined in terms of a **catchment area,** which is a city or several rural communities whose total population ranges from 75,000 to 200,000 residents. The intent of this approach is to divide the larger population into manageable segments for the delivery of mental health services. Ideally, the system is small enough to allow collaboration among the components of the system.

CARE THAT IS CONTINUOUS AND COMPREHENSIVE

The stated goals of community mental health care are to provide care that is continuous and comprehensive. The goal of providing continuous care means ensuring that if individual clients are receiving care from different parts of the system, the providers are assuming responsibility for monitoring that care and assisting the clients in moving through the system. Ideally, there is a communication interface between programs so that individual clients do not feel that they are left to fend for themselves but rather that the road has been paved for them as they obtain a variety of needed services. Moving through the system should be smooth and appear seamless. Unfortunately, community mental health care has a long way to go before realizing the goal of providing continuity of care.

The goal of providing comprehensive care recognizes that the population of severely mentally ill have complex and multifaceted medical, nursing, and social needs, and each of these needs must be met using an integrated approach that is continually mindful of the holistic nature of the individual client.

POPULATION SERVED BY COMMUNITY MENTAL HEALTH CARE

Primarily, community mental health care serves the needs of those with severe mental illnesses. These illnesses are chronic with exacerbations and remissions as part of their course. Had it not been for the community mental health movement, many of those with severe mental illnesses might have been on the rolls of the mental institutions providing long-term care, especially the state psychiatric hospitals.

PREVALENCE OF MENTAL DISORDERS

The National Institute of Mental Health (2006) provides a summary of statistics describing the prevalence of mental disorders in the United States. According to this summary, an estimated 26.2% of Americans aged 18 years and older—about one in four adults—suffers from a diagnosable mental disorder annually. When this percentage is applied to the 2004 U.S. Census residential population estimate for those aged 18 years and older, this figure translates to 57.7 million people with mental disorders. Mental disorders are the leading cause of disability in the United States and Canada for individuals aged 15 to 44 years. Many individuals have more than one mental disorder at the same time. Table 33-1 shows the prevalence of selected psychiatric disorders in the United States.

WHO ARE THE SEVERELY MENTALLY ILL?

The **severely mentally ill** are a diverse group with a variety of diagnoses, including schizophrenia, major affective disorders,

and organic disorders secondary to trauma, disease, or substance abuse. They include the elderly with chronic and severe mental illnesses, who may reside independently with supportive family nearby or with a supportive network of caring people. This supportive network might include the landlord, the mailman, the local grocer, and others who look out for the welfare of the individual. Some of these elderly with severe mental illnesses live with family and friends; some live in supervised housing, such as foster care or nursing homes. Robert Bernstein, executive director of the Bazelon Center, believes that "many older people with mental illnesses or dementia are still isolated in nursing homes and other institutions, where they receive no more than custodial care" (Bernstein, 2003, p. 10).

Individuals with schizophrenia may hold jobs in the community during periods when symptoms are in remission; those with residual symptoms that interfere with their functional capacity rely on disability checks and sporadic employment. They also may reside in foster or group homes. Some seek shelter in decrepit urban hotels, whereas others take to the street and end up in shelters for the homeless. In rural areas, the chronically mentally ill may live in the woods, in abandoned buildings, or under bridges. Some of those with severe mental illnesses reside inappropriately in prisons.

Many are living with serious medical conditions, such as extreme obesity, diabetes, and cardiac and respiratory problems as well as hepatitis C, which occurs among those with severe mental illness at a rate of 10 times the national average (Goldbaum, 2003). Estimates are that 1.8% of Americans are infected with hepatitis C, and approximately 20% of those have severe mental illness (Patterson, 2003). The incidence of hepatitis C corresponds with the fact that many have complicating patterns of substance abuse—both issues are tied to the same risky behaviors that increase the likelihood of acquiring the bloodborne virus (see Chapters 8 and 25). For many of the severely mentally ill, substance abuse is a primary problem. For others, substance abuse may be an attempt to self-medicate to ease the pain of a difficult life (Bostelman et al., 1994; Conway et al., 1994; Drake & Mueser, 2000).

The population of severely mentally ill ranges in age from the very young who have never experienced long-term institutionalization to the very old who suffer from deinstitutionalization. All experience problems of being emotionally and mentally disabled and must live with the stigma of mental illness. Sheets and colleagues (1982) identified three subgroups among the young chronically mentally ill, those from 18 to 30 years of age. There is a high-functioning group, a passively accepting (low-energy, low-demand) group, and a group who actively deny that they have mental illness (high-energy, high-demand subgroup). Those who aggressively deny the reality of their illness have the most difficulty accepting any help, including supervised housing. They prefer the independence of hotels and the streets. Those who choose to live with limited interpersonal contact may withdraw, may neglect themselves, may stop taking their medications, and are especially vulnerable to exploitation by others. There are successes in working with these clients; some are persuaded to accept help within the community mental health care system, even to accept residential living arrangements (Wierdsma, et al., 2007). The following example illustrates the characteristics of a young adult who is severely mentally ill.

TABLE 33-1 Prevalence of Psychiatric Disorders in the United States

Disorder (Prevalence over 12 Months %)	Estimated Numbers of People Affected by Disorder
Schizophrenia (1.1%)	2.4 million Americans aged 18 years and older • Affects men and women equally. • May appear earlier in men than in women.
Any affective (mood) disorder—includes major depression, dysthymic disorder, and bipolar disorder (9.5%)	20.9 million Americans • Women affected 2 times more than men. • Depressive disorders may be appearing earlier in life in those born in recent decades than in the past. • Often co-occurs with anxiety and substance abuse.
Major depressive disorder (MDD) (6.7%)	14.8 million Americans aged 15-44 years • Leading cause of disability in U.S. and established economies world wide. • Nearly twice as many women as men suffer from major depressive disorder every year.
Bipolar affective disorder (2.6%)	5.7 million Americans aged 18 years and older • Affects men and women equally. • Median age of onset is 25 years.
Suicide	In 2004, 32,439 Americans died by suicide. More than 90% of people who complete suicide had a diagnosable mental disorder, most commonly a depressive disorder or a substance abuse disorder.
Anxiety disorders—includes panic disorder, obsessive-compulsive disorder, posttraumatic stress disorder, generalized anxiety disorder, and phobias (18.1%)	40 million Americans aged 18 years and older • Anxiety disorders frequently co-occur with depressive disorders, eating disorders, and/or substance abuse.
Panic disorder (2.7%)	6 million Americans aged 18 years and older • Typically develops in adolescence or early adulthood. • About 1 in 3 people with panic disorder develop agoraphobia.
Obsessive-compulsive disorder (OCD) (1%)	2.2 million Americans aged 18 years and older • First symptoms begin in childhood or adolescence.
Posttraumatic stress disorder (PTSD) (3.5%)	7.7 million Americans aged 18 years and older • Can develop at any time. • About 19% of Vietnam veterans experienced PTSD after the war. • Percentage high among first responders to 9/11 terrorist attacks on U.S. • Evidence suggests that 15.6% to 17% of veterans returning from duty in Iraq have PTSD (Hoge et al., 2004).
Generalized anxiety disorder (GAD) (3.1%)	6.8 million Americans aged 18 years and older • Can begin across life cycle; risk is highest between childhood and middle age.
Social phobia (6.8%)	15 million Americans aged 18 years and older • Typically begins in childhood or adolescence.
Agoraphobia (0.8%)	1.8 million Americans aged 18 years and older
Specific phobia (8.7%)	19.2 million Americans

Data from National Institutes of Mental Health. (2006, December 26). *The numbers count: Mental disorders in America*. Retrieved July 25, 2007 from *http://www.nimh.nih.gov/publicat/numbers.cfm*; and Hoge, C. W., Castro, C. A., Messer, S. C., et al. (2004). Combat duty in Iraq and Afghanistan, mental health problems, and barriers to care. *New England Journal of Medicine, 351*, 13-22.

My name is Sarah. I've been sick for a long time. I have been in every big mental hospital in my state. Once I ran away, and I was put in a hospital in another state. My family came and got me. They put me on medication that I don't like and gave me shock treatments. Sometimes I think I'm a human guinea pig. I'm living in a hotel now. My family doesn't see me too much—I think they feel fed up with me. But I do okay. Sometimes I go to the shelter for meals. Sometimes I don't eat. I go to the clinic for a shot of Prolixin [fluphenazine] every 2 weeks. I hate it, but I hate being in the big hospitals more. I have some friends. We hang out on the streets. Sometimes we drink together. Sometimes the police pick us up for being noisy. But I think they pick us up because they know we're crazy.

WHAT ARE THE NEEDS OF THE SEVERELY MENTALLY ILL?

The care needs of those with severe mental illnesses include the following:

• Basic life necessities
• A sense that life is meaningful
• Access to medications
• Support for family members
• Integrated nursing, medical, and social services

Basic Life Necessities

Included in basic life necessities are items such as food, clothing, both permanent and temporary housing, income maintenance, health care, and legal protection. Many of the chronically mentally ill are without these basic items.

A Sense That Life Is Meaningful

A sense that life is meaningful is an essential need for community adjustment, yet it is often denied to these individuals because they are discriminated against in their efforts to obtain employment as well as participate in recreational and other social activities. Multiple strategies, including skills training classes, job clubs, and sheltered employment, have been advanced for helping those with severe mental illness gain competitive employment. Unfortunately, these strategies have had limited success. Becker and Drake (2003) advocate supported employment in which clients are placed in jobs and then trained by on-site coaches using the Individual Placement and Support Method (IPS). This is a radically new approach to vocational rehabilitation for the severely mentally ill and is supported by empirical research demonstrating rates of competitive employment reaching 40% or more in programs using IPS compared with 15% in traditional mental health programs.

Resocialization and sheltered workshops also provide for time structuring and meaningful activities. Leisure and recreational activities are important to provide a healthy balance in life. Spiritual activities allow clients to connect not only with their God, but also with the meaning of their own lives in a broader context. Participation in peer support groups also provides individuals with the sense that their own suffering makes some sort of sense. As they are able to draw from their experiences to assist others similarly affected, they may be able to make sense out of life (Shoemaker, 2006).

Access to Medication

Access to medication is essential. This includes not only availability of reasonably priced medications, but also ongoing support for motivation to comply with the medication regimen, continual reassessment of dosage requirements and side effects, and active coordination with other aspects of treatment. The newer medications, when taken, do work. The treatment success rates for three serious mental illnesses are as follows (NAMI, 2000):

- Bipolar disorder: 80%
- Major depression: 65%
- Schizophrenia: 60%

Support for Family Members

Support for family members is critical to maintain an important element of the individual client's support network. The burden of caregiving on the family can be quite high; some family caregivers are at increased risk for physical illness. They benefit tremendously from encouragement, affirmation, education about their loved one's illness, and a collaborative attitude on the part of care providers that values and considers their opinions regarding what is in the best interests of the individual client (Shoemaker, 2006).

Integrated Nursing, Medical, and Social Services

Integrated nursing, medical, and social services are a tremendous need for those with severe mental illnesses. For this group to negotiate the maze of services necessary to facilitate community tenure, the system must do all that it can to facilitate this process (Shoemaker, 2006).

Additional Needs

In addition to the needs already described, those with severe mental illnesses have a great need for care, concern, and acceptance for who they are and at whatever their level of functioning (Shoemaker, 2006). This means that care providers must be aware of the nature of chronic mental illness, which is characterized by exacerbations and remissions, periods of apparent equanimity punctuated by major setbacks. This awareness must translate into patience, gentle encouragement, a willingness to help the client pick up the pieces and begin again, and an acceptance of the fact that the individual's level of functioning may be very impaired. Appropriate goals and interventions must begin where the client is at the moment and not where the care provider wishes the client to be.

Amanda had been in and out of mental hospitals for years. For a short time, she lived with her sister, a situation that caused Amanda great anxiety. When Amanda was anxious, she made a strange barking noise that made her sound like a seal. She also focused on strange somatic complaints, like having "pus running down my throat." While at her sister's house, Amanda became completely nonfunctional, staying in bed all the time and finding it impossible to communicate without making the "seal" sound. The sister's tolerance for this behavior wore down, and she placed Amanda in a boarding home. Amanda received psychiatric follow-up at a community mental health center. When Amanda was initially placed in the boarding home, Gina, her nurse therapist, worked with the care provider to establish appropriate goals for Amanda's care. It was clear that one of Amanda's needs was for increased diversional activities. Yet her level of functioning was so low that any aggressive effort to involve her in diversional activities precipitated her barking noises and somatic complaints. It was clear that Amanda was very anxious and that she coped with her anxiety by retreating. Gina helped the care provider arrive at a plan that seemed a bit unorthodox. Instead of focusing on keeping Amanda out of bed, the care provider gave her permission to go back to bed when she felt the need to do so. Amanda was required to tend to her personal needs and join the other residents for meals. After about a week, Amanda stopped making the barking noises. Receiving permission to retreat from others when she felt the need seemed to lessen her anxiety and allowed her to interact even more, but more at her own speed.

Certainly, it is not possible for one service to meet all of these needs. In fact, services to address many of these needs may have to be coordinated by the community mental health nurse, who assists the client in accessing a network of both professional and natural helpers. The professional helpers might include the following:

- Public welfare agencies
- Public health agencies
- General hospitals
- Home care agencies
- Mental health centers
- Courts
- Schools
- Faith communities
- Charitable organizations
- Child guidance centers
- Nursing homes
- Social service organizations
- Emergency/crisis services

The informal helpers might include the following:

- Family
- Friends
- Neighbors
- Neighborhood organizations
- Voluntary organizations
- Self-help groups
- Clergy
- Teachers
- Police
- Pharmacists
- Gas and electric person
- Landlord
- Anyone else who is interested in assisting and able to do so

SERVICES PROVIDED IN COMMUNITY MENTAL HEALTH CARE

A variety of services are made available to clients as part of community mental health care. Not all of these services are available in every community.

TYPES OF COMMUNITY MENTAL HEALTH SERVICES

Community Mental Health Centers

Community mental health centers are staffed by a variety of mental health professionals who provide individual, group, and family therapy to community residents. These services may be offered by a psychiatric nurse, a social worker, a psychologist, a mental health paraprofessional, or a psychiatrist.

Alternative Living Arrangements

Alternative living arrangements vary from the least restrictive to very restrictive. An example of an arrangement with few restrictions is a family placement. Some clients reside in **single-room occupancy** housing, in which they rent a room from a landlord. In this arrangement, they may share meals with other residents in the house, or they make seek food at restaurants, soup kitchens, and shelters. **Congregate or sheltered housing** also allows the client a good deal of freedom. In this arrangement, the client has a separate apartment and receives support in meal preparation, housekeeping chores, and errands. Other clients may need closer supervision and require placement in a group home or a foster care home. Still others who require 24-hour supervision and skilled nursing care may need a nursing home environment. Ideally the housing placement takes into consideration clients' strengths and abilities to live independently, to live safely, and to make decisions in their own best interest, as well as their requirements for supervision, and matches them with housing that allows them to be in a safe, healthy environment in which maximum independence is possible.

Support Groups

Support groups are self-help groups that focus on assisting individuals, families, or communities. The purpose of some may be to help individuals maintain their health, as with Alcoholics or Narcotics Anonymous. Others provide support to individuals and families who are dealing with a particular stress, such as the groups for families of persons with acquired immunodeficiency syndrome (AIDS). Some groups, such as the Seasons Support Group for the Survivors of Suicide, actually help restore mental health by bringing together people who have suffered similar tragedies.

Groups exist whose primary focus is to reform the mental health system. These groups are frequently composed of individual clients, their family members, and mental health professionals. Other groups define their goal as changing a particular aspect of community life. An example of this type of group is Mothers Against Drunk Drivers (MADD).

Day Treatment Centers

Day treatment centers are set up to provide meaningful social interaction, time structuring, and participation in recreational and learning activities to individuals who might otherwise be isolated or who lack the ability to structure their time independently. These **day treatment** centers also provide respite for family care providers, who benefit by having their loved ones spend a portion of their time at another facility.

Mobile Treatment Units

Mobile treatment units consist of professionals who go into the community to provide care. This type of service is appropriate for clients who are unable to keep clinic appointments and adhere to medication regimens as well as for crisis intervention. The treatment is basically delivered to the individual clients where they reside. This approach requires familiarity with the person's usual patterns of behavior, willingness to track down clients who may not be in their residence but instead be in a favorite neighborhood haunt, and a flexible approach on the part of the provider.

Psychiatric Home Care Services

Psychiatric home care services are services provided by a home care agency certified to care for clients with either Medicare or Medicaid coverage. A psychiatric nurse visits the individual's residence and provides assessment and observation, medication and behavioral management, psychoeducational interventions, and linkage to community-based services.

Community Services

Community services are services that contribute to the mental health of a community. Some may provide direct intervention with an individual, for example, a rape crisis center or Meals on Wheels. The focus may be on the family, as in family recreation centers; daycare centers for children, the disabled, or the elderly; or shelters for victims of domestic violence. The police and fire departments, public park services, social service departments, and educational groups are all examples of groups that serve the needs of the entire community (Shoemaker, 2006).

William, an elderly man diagnosed with chronic schizophrenia, regularly missed his clinic appointments. In fact, the only thing that the staff could depend on about William was that he was usually not compliant in keeping appointments or taking medication. After many hospitalizations, William was referred to the mobile treatment team. One of the nurses would track him down in his neighborhood. William's favorite hangout was a social club for men down the street from his boarding home. Usually when the nurse found William he would be laughing, happy, and generally enjoying life—always apologetic that the nurse had to come find him. However, once he was found, William was more than willing to step into a back room in the social club and get his injection of fluphenazine (Prolixin). By many people's standards, William was irresponsible and barely functional, but a successful plan of treatment had been developed that accommodated William's lifestyle and provided interventions that were useful to him.

PROVIDERS OF COMMUNITY MENTAL HEALTH SERVICES

A variety of health care professionals deliver care within the community. These include community mental health nurses, psychiatrists, psychologists, licensed professional counselors, case managers, social workers, recreational and physical therapists, and pharmacists. In addition, the client may receive care from mental health paraprofessionals who lack academic preparation but have life experiences, good interpersonal and communication skills, and common sense on which to draw. These workers may be supervised by a mental health professional such as the nurse. The client may also interact with government workers, religious leaders, educators, and a variety of others who in some way provide support. Family members, neighbors, and employers often play crucial roles in enabling the client to do well within the community (Wierdsma et al., 2007).

ROLE OF THE NURSE IN COMMUNITY MENTAL HEALTH CARE

Nurses with various levels of academic preparation, ranging from diploma or associate of arts degree to doctorate, practice within the community mental health setting. Education, experience, licensure, and certification directly influence professional responsibilities.

FOCUS ON PREVENTION

The principles of primary, secondary, and tertiary prevention are essential to community mental health work. These three principles provide direction for interventions carried out by nurses within the community setting.

Primary Prevention

Primary prevention occurs when the nurse focuses on preventing new occurrences of mental illness. To perform this role, the nurse develops interventions and programs that eliminate stresses which lead to or aggravate mental disorders. Examples include the following:

- Teaching parenting and sibling classes to assist new parents with a new or expanding family
- Offering support to self-help groups
- Providing mental health consultation to schools to strengthen resilience in children
- Providing mental health consultation to businesses and other community agencies
- Advocating within the political arena for the rights of the mentally ill

Box 33-1 describes a number of suicide prevention programs in which psychiatric nurses play an important role in primary prevention.

Secondary Prevention

Secondary prevention involves case finding and referrals, as well as treatment of a diagnosed disorder in a given individual.

BOX 33-1 Role of Psychiatric Nurses in Primary Suicide Prevention Programs

The Adolescent Suicide Awareness Program in New Jersey provides a continuous program focusing on intervention with school staff, parents, and students. The program is coordinated by the community mental health center and the school. The focus is on increasing awareness among teachers, parents, and students regarding depression, suicide warning signs, methods of helping the suicidal person, and community referral resources.

The Fairfax County (Virginia) Public Schools developed a program with the help of school staff, nurses, social workers, guidance counselors, and school psychologists. Parents, police, and other mental health professionals have also been involved. The program involves teacher training, parent education, and student support.

The Cherry Creek (Colorado) Schools provide crisis training for school psychologists, nurses, counselors, and social workers. Parents, teachers, and other school personnel are taught to recognize students at risk. The school curriculum includes a suicide prevention component.

The San Mateo (California) Schools make resources available to high-risk students. Teachers, nurses, and counselors are trained to identify and intervene in cases of adolescent depression and suicidal behavior. Student programs include an educational component, workshops, and peer counseling.

From Puskar, K., Lamb, J., & Norton, M. (1990). Adolescent mental health: Collaboration among psychiatric mental health nurses and school nurses. *Journal of School Health, 60*(2), 69–71.

Nursing interventions that exemplify secondary prevention include the following:

- Psychotherapy for individuals, families, and groups
- Crisis intervention, including hot line counseling
- Emergency mental health services
- Counseling for women who have been raped
- Support for victims of violence

Tertiary Prevention

Tertiary prevention involves rehabilitative services for clients diagnosed with psychiatric disorders. Discharge planning is an example of a nursing intervention directed at tertiary prevention. Assisting the client in making the transition between hospital and place of residence is another. Still others include making appropriate referrals to aftercare services or self-help groups, teaching clients and their families about medication management, and acting as an advocate.

THE NURSING PROCESS IN PRACTICE

Although there are many mental health professionals who work with persons with mental health conditions and mental disorders, the nurse occupies a unique position. Traditionally, nursing has concerned itself with the needs of the downtrodden, the underdogs, the forsaken of society. Certainly, the severely mentally ill fit this description. Nursing possesses a holistic view that recognizes the interaction among body, mind, and spirit and focuses on the nurse-client relationship as the vehicle through which change occurs. In addition to focus on the individual, nurses with bachelor's degrees or higher possess skills related to effective community work as well as family intervention. They are accustomed to interfacing with personnel in a variety of disciplines and have a great deal of ease and skill at crossing boundaries between lay and professional groups and marshaling resources. Nurses are oriented to assisting clients in moving from a dependent state to a relatively independent state of self-care. These skills are essential to helping the severely mentally ill to meet the multifaceted problems and needs that they confront.

In community mental health care, as in other areas of nursing, the nursing process is used to gain an understanding of the populations of individuals with mental disorders, to diagnose their needs, to determine appropriate outcomes, to plan effective and appropriate interventions, and to evaluate the results of the interventions. The one area that sets community mental health care apart is that sometimes the client is an individual or family, and sometimes the client is the community.

NURSING PROCESS: COMMUNITY AS CLIENT

The following discussion follows the application of the nursing process in the community setting.

Assessment

Community assessments can be focused in a number of different ways. For instance, the nurse might be interested in gauging community acceptance of a mental health initiative. The following questions are appropriate for this type of assessment:

- Do you believe that former residents of mental hospitals are able to function well in your community?
- Would you have any objections if an organization that you belonged to accepted someone with a severe mental disorder as a member?
- What would your feelings be if a person with a severe mental disorder moved next door to you?
- Do you think you could ever become friends with a person with a severe mental disorder?
- What would your feelings be about having a halfway house for mentally ill people located in your neighborhood? Next door to you?
- Would you offer an individual with mental illness assistance in obtaining a job at your place of employment?
- Do you think you would participate or support in some other way programs in your neighborhood designed to help the mentally ill person?

Diagnosis

The analysis of these answers leads to nursing diagnoses for the community. Some examples are the following:

- Knowledge deficit related to lack of understanding of the characteristics of the severely mentally ill.
- Anxiety related to misinformation about the severely mentally ill.
- Ineffective community coping related to the high stress level associated with perceptions of the severely mentally ill.

Outcome Identification

The expected outcomes for a community might be the following:

- After presentation of educational talks and materials, a random posttest of the community members will show significantly greater understanding of the characteristics of the severely mentally ill.
- The response to the posttest questions measuring affective and attitudinal issues will show a significant change toward greater acceptance of and more positive feelings about the severely mentally ill.
- Plans for the development and enhancement of existing resources and programs to meet the needs of the severely mentally ill will come from the community.

Development of a Plan for Intervention

The plan that is developed to achieve these community outcomes might rely heavily on education. The nurse, as program coordinator, might focus on public forums in schools, clinics, faith communities, neighborhood recreation centers, and health fairs as sites to begin education of the community. Possible short-term goals for such a plan might include those presented in Table 33-2.

Implementation

Interventions are limited only by the creativity and resources of those presenting such an educational program. The interventions to support this plan might include the following:

- Developing a brochure outlining the achievements of many that are severely mentally ill.

TABLE 33-2   Outcomes and Goals for Community Support of a Mental Health Institute

Expected Outcome	Short-Term Goals
1. After presentation of educational talks and materials, a random posttest of the community will show significantly greater understanding of the characteristics of the chronically mentally ill.	Community members will participate in a variety of educational programs offered throughout the community. Community members will take a pre-posttest to measure their level of knowledge about the chronically mentally ill.
2. The response to the posttest questions measuring affective and attitudinal issues will show a significant change toward greater acceptance and more positive feelings.	Community members will take a pre-posttest to measure their attitudes toward the chronically mentally ill.
3. Plans for the development and enhancement of existing resources and programs to meet the needs of the chronically mentally ill will come from the community.	Community members will participate in small focus groups to identify existing resources and programs within their community. Community members will participate in small focus groups to plan what resources are needed to support the chronically mentally ill. Community members will participate in small focus groups to plan how to develop the needed resources and programs to support the chronically mentally ill.

- Developing a slide and lecture presentation depicting the mentally ill in productive occupations contributing to the health of the community.
- Focusing on the spiritual benefits of caring for and being tolerant of those who are less fortunate.
- Explaining the economic benefits that a community receives when it cares for its own and does not send the severely mentally ill off to a state institution.

Evaluation of the Process and Outcomes

A project of this magnitude requires ongoing evaluation. Issues that must be evaluated include but are not limited to the following:

- Is the community assessment comprehensive enough? Are there areas that have not been explored?
- Is the planned teaching approach at an appropriate level for the community?
- Are the teaching materials effective?
- Are facilities available to offer the programs?
- Are community members adequately informed regarding the upcoming educational programs?

The final comprehensive evaluation of this particular approach is specified in the objectives. There are other ways, however, to gauge the effectiveness of a program (see Chapter 17). For instance, if a halfway house opened in a particular neighborhood, the nurse could collect statements from clients about how they were treated when they went for walks and frequented stores and other neighborhood establishments. These would be subjective data to support or refute the claim of success in a community-based intervention. (See the *Ethics in Practice* box in Chapter 27, which provides an example of restructuring the environment for those with severe mental illness.)

In addition to using the nursing process to help a community become more accepting of the severely mentally ill, the nurse might want to assess for the presence of a particular community need, such as dealing with substance abuse. Such data would form the basis of future community programs. The Case Study at the end of the chapter demonstrates how a psychiatric nurse used the nursing process in the development of a community substance abuse prevention program in Montana.

NURSING PROCESS: INDIVIDUAL OR FAMILY AS CLIENT

Assessment

To assess the individual or family within the community, it is essential to examine how well the client's basic needs are being met. As was noted earlier, the basic needs of the severely mentally ill include basic life necessities, a sense that life is meaningful, access to medication, support for family members, and integrated nursing, medical, and social services, among others. By observing and interviewing, the nurse can assess how well each of these needs is being met (Table 33-3).

Diagnosis: Determining Needs

Based on analysis of the assessment data, appropriate nursing diagnoses are identified for problems associated with each basic need. Possible nursing diagnoses for the person with problems in the area of *basic life necessities* are as follows:

- Bathing/hygiene self-care deficit related to low level of motivation.

TABLE 33-3   **Assessment of the Severely Mentally Ill Individual or Family**

Basic Need	Observation	Interview
Basic life necessities—areas such as nutrition, clothing, temporary and permanent housing, income, legal protection, and health care	The extent to which the patient is able to perform basic hygiene and activities of daily living Level of energy and motivation	What arrangements have you made to obtain daily meals? Describe a typical day's diet. Tell me about the place where you live. Who manages your living quarters? Cleaning? Laundry? What arrangements have you made to handle money? What is your source of income? How do you pay bills? Do you work? Tell me about your job. The people you work with. Your boss.
	General assessment of health status	Where do you go to see a doctor? What kind of doctor do you usually see? What symptoms make you go to see a doctor?
A sense that life is meaningful—areas such as structuring of time, diversional activities, a sense of purpose, support system, use of spiritual resources	The extent to which the patient can structure time, plan activities that she enjoys	How do you spend your time every day?
	The degree of social isolation (use the nurse-patient relationship as a barometer of the patient's social competence)	Do you think what you do makes a difference to anyone else? Do you think that you matter to anyone else?
	Verbalizations that indicate either hopelessness and a sense of despair or a feeling that life has some purpose	Tell me about something you do that gives you pleasure.
	Verbalizations that indicate that the patient is engaging in some enjoyable or purposeful activities	What kind of spiritual or religious activities do you participate in? Does anyone depend on you? If so, tell me about that relationship. Do you work? What do you do?

Continued

TABLE 33-3   Assessment of the Severely Mentally Ill Individual or Family—cont'd

Basic Need	Observation	Interview
Access to medication— whether the patient is on medication, what kind of medication, the presence of side effects, the patient's knowledge of the drug, the availability of the drug, compliance with the medication regimen	The extent to which the patient's behavior indicates effectiveness of the drug The extent to which the patient's behavior indicates the presence of side effects The number of doses left of the drug; does this correspond with the amount that should be remaining if the patient were compliant? Verbalizations that indicate an appropriate degree of understanding and compliance	Tell me about the medications you are taking. What are they? When are you supposed to take them? How much are you supposed to take? What effect does the medication have on you? Describe any problems you have run into while taking this medication. Tell me about the side effects of the medication. Are there any precautions you should be aware of when taking this medication? Are you attending the medication clinic? Where do you get your prescriptions filled? Do you have any difficulties with getting the prescriptions filled?
Support for family members—areas that are indicative of the patient's ego functioning, sense of self-esteem, and interpersonal relationships; the family's needs related to coping with the patient	The patient's general affect: does the patient appear depressed, angry, anxious? Verbalizations that indicate that the patient "feels bad" about himself Verbalizations that indicate fear of making decisions Verbalizations that indicate interpersonal problems Family member's affect and general response to the patient; does the family member appear angry or "fed up"? Does the family member act impatient or disdainful toward the patient?	Do you feel that you are "together"? If not, how do you feel? How would you describe your adjustment in the community? Boarding home? Family's home? Do you feel satisfied with the progress you are making? If not, tell me what you would like to change. Tell me about the people you spend your time with. What kind of relationships do you have? Are you satisfied with them? If not, what would you change? What problems are you (family member) experiencing on a day-to-day basis with. ... ? Are you (family member) able to arrange time away from the patient so that you get a break? How do you help the patient to feel that she is okay?
Integrated nursing, medical, and social services—needs for community services, availability of a support person to assist with transportation and other needs	The extent to which the patient is able to access community services independently Verbalizations indicative of a patient's sense of being overwhelmed in attempts to negotiate the health care and social service system Behaviors that indicate that other services are needed (e.g., Alcoholics Anonymous, adult daycare)	Who helps you to make appointments and get to them? What community service do you use in addition to this clinic? How would you go about getting information about [whatever community service is needed]? What would you think if I made a referral to. ... ? What do you know about [appropriate community resources]? Who assists you in dealing with [medical assistance, renewal of your pharmacy assistance card, access to other social programs]? Are you [family member] involved in any type of community support groups? Do you feel you are getting the help you need? Are there other service needs we can help you with? Are you experiencing other problems or concerns for which you would like care or assistance?

- Imbalanced nutrition: less than body requirements related to homelessness.
- Sleep pattern disturbance related to unstable living arrangements.
- Dressing/grooming self-care deficit related to low level of motivation.

Possible nursing diagnoses for the person with a deficient *sense that life is meaningful* are as follows:

- Spiritual distress related to conflict about God's role in permitting illness.
- Deficient diversional activity related to inability to structure time.
- Social isolation related to lack of social skills.

Nursing diagnoses for the person with problems of *access to medication* might be as follows:

- Deficient knowledge related to effects of medication, side effects of medication, and sources of financial aid to purchase medications.
- Nonadherence related to taking medication as prescribed.

Nursing diagnoses for the person with problems related to *support for family members* might be as follows:

- Disturbed thought processes related to noncompliance with antipsychotic medication regimen.
- Chronic low self-esteem related to repeated rejections by family, friends, and acquaintances.

- Ineffective individual coping related to changes in living arrangements, interpersonal difficulties, and the stress of daily living.

Nursing diagnoses for the person with needs for *integrated nursing, medical, and social services* might be as follows:

- Anxiety related to inability to negotiate the community mental health system.
- Decisional conflict related to which health-related services to access.
- Deficient knowledge related to how to access transportation to the clinic.

Outcome Identification

The expected outcomes for an individual or family receiving community mental health care for problems with *basic life necessities* may include successful demonstration of bathing and hygiene skills, acquisition of shelter, and getting adequate sleep and nutrition. Outcomes relevant for clients with a deficient *sense that life is meaningful* would include client recognition and resolution of spiritual conflicts, attendance at adult daycare, and successful initiation of conversations.

Clients with problems *accessing medications* might demonstrate outcomes that include the ability to identify each medication, understand its action and side effects, and follow the prescribed medication regimen. The expected outcomes for a client needing *support handling interpersonal relationships* might include identifying positive qualities of self, using new methods of coping with interpersonal conflict, and using strategies to deal with situational stress. For the client needing *integrated nursing, social, and medical services,* expected outcomes would include client use of support systems to access health care appointments and the ability to make and keep those appointments.

Expected outcomes are detailed in more measurable terms in the following discussion of planning interventions.

Planning of Interventions for Individuals

During the planning step, short-term objectives are identified that aim at achieving the expected outcomes previously identified. For the client with problems related to *basic life necessities,* short-term objectives might be as follows:

Expected Outcome	Short-Term Objectives
The client will demonstrate appropriate bathing and hygiene skills by the end of the fourth week.	The client will talk about reasons for not bathing and taking care of self. The client will state at least three benefits that accompany bathing and good hygiene. The client will wash his or her clothes. The client will brush his or her teeth. The client will bathe.
The client will access sheltered housing within 1 week.	The client will state the benefits of being in sheltered housing. The client will complete an application to enter sheltered housing.
The client will sleep at least 7 hours a night within 2 weeks.	The client will state three strategies to facilitate a good night's rest. The client will use at least one of the newly acquired skills before going to sleep.
The client will eat three meals a day by the end of 1 week.	The client will state the benefits of eating a balanced diet. The client will name two resources for obtaining healthy food.

For the client with a deficient *sense that life is meaningful,* short-term objectives might be the following:

Expected Outcome	Short-Term Objectives
The client will discuss spiritual conflicts with the nurse therapist and be able to come to resolution on this issue.	The client will talk about his or her spiritual beliefs. The client will discuss his or her views on God's role in this illness.
The client will attend an adult daycare center at least three times a week.	The client will visit an adult day treatment center. The client will agree to try out the center for a day to see if it works.
The client will demonstrate appropriate ways to initiate a conversation within 3 weeks.	The client will participate in social activities at the adult day treatment center. The client will practice initiating a conversation with a nurse.

For the client with a need for *access to medication,* short-term objectives might be as follows:

Expected Outcome	Short-Term Objectives
The client will be knowledgeable about his or her medications.	The client will state the reason for taking the medications. The client will state at least three side effects of the medications and how to deal with them.
The client will take all medications as prescribed within 2 weeks.	The client will state the schedule for taking medications. The client will state the benefits of taking medications. The client will set up a weekly adherence medication pack according to his or her schedule for taking medications.

For the client needing *support for family members,* short-term objectives might be the following:

Expected Outcome	Short-Term Objectives
The client will verbalize at least one positive quality about self by the end of the third week of therapy.	The client will do a sentence completion exercise: "My best qualities are _____." The client will discuss the feelings involved in performing this assignment.
The client will demonstrate that he or she has learned new responses for coping with interpersonal conflict.	The client will identify two areas of interpersonal conflict. The client will discuss his or her present responses to conflict. The client will evaluate present responses to conflict. The client will discuss how he or she would like conflicts to be resolved. The client will discuss three ways to resolve conflict differently.
The client will demonstrate deep breathing exercises as a means of dealing with situational stress.	The client will identify two sources of situational stress. The client will identify his or her current responses to this stress. The client will identify how he or she would like to respond to stress. The client will demonstrate the technique of deep breathing and relaxation as a strategy for dealing with situational stress.

For the client needing *integrated nursing, social, and medical services,* short-term objectives might be as follows:

Expected Outcome	Short-Term Objectives
The client will use the available support system to access health care appointments.	The client will identify resources in the community that might be beneficial to him or her. The client will initiate contact with one community agency.
The client will demonstrate the ability to make appropriate appointments and follow through with those appointments.	The client will state one reason for keeping follow-up mental health appointments. The client will call the community agency for a follow-up appointment.

Implementation of Nursing Plans for Individuals

The interventions used by the community mental health nurse are directed toward the individual as well as the community. The individual client-focused interventions fall into four categories:

- Teaching
- Case management
- Consulting
- Providing therapy
  The community-focused interventions include the following:
- Networking
- Crossing boundaries between the professional and lay communities
- Advocating

Teaching. Community mental health nurses are in an excellent position to teach the individual as well as the family and community as a whole about the following:

- Medication issues
- Stress management
- Illness
- The components of mental health
- Effective communication and interpersonal relationships
- Parenting
- Access to other health and social services
- Suicide awareness
- Drug and alcohol prevention
- Social skills and other issues that have an impact on the mental health of the individual as well as the larger group

Case Management. Case management is a modality of care that can be very effective in addressing the multifaceted and complex needs of the chronically mentally ill. Ideally the case manager does the following:

- Assesses client needs
- Compiles a plan for service
- Links clients with needed services
- Monitors the quality and appropriateness of services
- Advocates for the severely mentally ill

Unfortunately, funding has continued to be inadequate, and case managers find themselves overworked, poorly paid, and unable to change the system.

Consulting. The consultant role allows a psychiatric nurse to offer mental health services to agencies within the community such as schools, faith communities, or businesses. For instance, the nurse might consult on the development of a suicide prevention program for the local school system or the development of a stress management course for local business groups.

Providing Therapy. In the role of therapist, the advanced practice psychiatric nurse is concerned with both the individual and the family and may provide the appropriate therapy. For the most part, the therapy offered to the severely mentally ill and their families is supportive therapy in which the goals are symptom management, relationship building, and ego strengthening. An evaluation is made to determine whether individual or group therapy is the most appropriate modality for a particular person. For instance, Beth, a 19-year-old with chronic schizophrenia, had a great deal of difficulty tolerating the one-to-one relationship with her nurse. Beth was initially placed in a small group with the intention of developing such a relationship between her and the nurse therapist. Psychiatric nurse practitioners can prescribe medication therapy.

Part of the therapy role involves continual assessment to identify changes in the person's life that might be linked to symptomatic exacerbation. Many times, clients fail to report changes because they do not see the connection between stress and symptoms. A nurse therapist who seeks this type of information is in a position to intervene and to provide anticipatory guidance that may make the difference between the client's being able to cope or "falling apart." John's story provides a good example. Therapy skills are also directed at relieving the burden of caregiving felt by the family.

> John had been seeing his nurse Sheila every 2 weeks for about a year. On the last visit, Sheila observed that John seemed more scattered in his thinking. His appearance was disheveled, and he reported a return of the "voices" that had plagued him intermittently for years. Gentle questioning revealed that John was having difficulty with a fellow tenant who was stealing from him. Sheila asked whether John would like her to talk to the manager of the boarding home where he lived. John agreed that this might help. Sheila made a visit to John's home to discuss the problem with the manager. Together, Sheila, the manager, and John were able to work out an arrangement to secure John's personal belongings in an effort to cut down on the thievery. On the following visit to the community center, John was back to his "old self."

Coordinating and Networking. Networking helps community mental health nurses to coordinate services on behalf of populations of clients who need them. Nurses also attempt to create services where there are none.

Crossing Boundaries. Nurses seem to have the ability to cross the boundaries between the lay and professional communities to marshal resources and to communicate the needs of disadvantaged groups.

Advocating. The community mental health nurse needs to be an advocate for the needs of the severely mentally ill. Nurses serve as advocates not only for their own clients, but also in the policy making arena, where there is the potential to impact the whole system.

Evaluation

Evaluation criteria measure the extent to which the nurse's interventions are able to support the capacity of the severely mentally ill to remain functional and autonomous in the community.

CONTINUING ISSUES IN COMMUNITY MENTAL HEALTH CARE

There is consensus among mental health professionals that community mental health care has fallen short of the expectations to prevent mental disorders, to improve the quality of life for the severely mentally ill, and to counteract isolation and social disabilities resulting from institutionalization. Lack of funding along with poor coordination of available services leaves many clients without adequate treatment. The major criticisms of community mental health services are the following:

- Individuals are inappropriately discharged from more intense levels of service.
- The services are fragmented and sporadic.
- Families assume an inordinate burden of the care.
- There is minimal cost savings.
- Individuals are sometimes abandoned and enter the ranks of either the mentally ill homeless or the incarcerated.
- There is an increased likelihood of readmission to institutional care.

To address these problems there is a trend toward collaboration among a variety of community-based providers to deliver enhanced care. The ACCESS (Assertive Community Care and Effective Services and Supports) program and PACT (Program of Assertive Community Treatment) are examples of such collaborative attempts (NAMI, 2008; Randolph et al., 2002).

TRANSFORMATION OF MENTAL HEALTH CARE

During the first decade of the twenty-first century, several reports advocated for the transformation of the U.S. mental health system (Daniels & Adams, 2006; Institute of Medicine, 2006; USDHHS, 2005). Foremost among the recommendations is that the mental health system become more "person-centered, recovery-oriented [with] coordinated care for mental and substance use conditions" (Daniels & Adams, 2006, p. 29). Recommendations also call for health care purchasers to pay for "evidence-based illness self-management programs and peer support" (p. 30).

INADEQUATE FOCUS ON CHILD MENTAL HEALTH

Although one in five children and adolescents has symptoms of mental health disorders each year, an estimated two thirds of these young people are not receiving mental health services (Brauner & Stephens, 2006). Mental health disorders result in functional impairment in family, school, and community activities.

Existing services for children and youth are fragmented among primary care practices, school health services, the mental health system, child welfare agencies, and the juvenile justice system (Adelman & Taylor, 2006; Waxman, 2006). Also, services are focused on treatment of disorders rather than on prevention and promotion of child mental health (Hacker & Darcy, 2006).

Public health practitioners are responsible for assuring that (1) populations have access to care and (2) sound health policy and planning promote an effective mental health system. The public health community is only beginning to address issues related to child mental health. All community/public health nurses who work with families with children and populations of children and youth are in a position to promote child mental health. Advanced practice mental health nurses are needed to work with children with mental disorders.

GROWING ELDERLY POPULATION

Larger numbers of community-dwelling elderly with depression, organic brain impairment, and anxiety can be expected. Among the community-dwelling elderly, 8% to 15% have depressive symptoms; 38% of elders 85 years and older have moderately severe cognitive impairment; and 40% of those seeking treatment exhibit anxiety (Abrams & Young, 2006). In 2003, Medicare prescription changes increased access to psychotropic medications for many elderly. However, there are not enough providers of mental health services for the elderly. All nurses working with elderly populations need to screen for mental disorders, counsel, and refer appropriately. Advanced practice mental health nurses are especially needed to address mental health disorders in the elderly.

CULTURAL COMPETENCE IN COMMUNITY MENTAL HEALTH

Mental health and *mental illness* mean different things in various cultures. Stigma regarding mental illness and treatment exists in the U.S. mainstream and varies among cultures. In many cultures, treatment of mental and emotional conditions lies within the domain of folk healers or religious practices. These beliefs can act as barriers to seeking mental health treatment for those with mental illness. As the United States population continues to become more diverse, it will be even more important for community/public health nurses to explore cultural expectations.

Migration due to wars, environmental catastrophes, and persecution increases the numbers of refugees. Before 2001, 80,000 refugees were admitted to the United States annually. Refugee populations have a "high prevalence of severe mental disorders, including posttraumatic stress disorder, depression, substance abuse, somatization and traumatic brain injuries" (Savin et al., 2005, p. 225). Nurses with a public health team in a Colorado program screened over 1500 refugees for mental health disorders. Ten percent of those screened were referred for mental health services and over one third of those followed up (Savin et al., 2005).

MANDATED TREATMENT FOR THE SEVERELY MENTALLY ILL

Another continuing issue in community mental health is mandated treatment for the severely mentally ill. In 1999, New York passed Kendra's Law (New York Mental Hygiene Law 9.60), which allows courts to order certain individuals with brain disorders to comply with the prescribed treatment regimen while living in the community. This court-ordered treatment is called *assisted outpatient treatment* or *involuntary outpatient commitment* (Aebersold, 2001). The law was named in memory of Kendra Webdale. In January 1999, the 32-year-old Buffalo native was killed after being pushed into the path of a New York subway train by Andrew Goldstein, a man with severe mental illness who had a history of failing to adhere to his treatment regimen.

The advocates of this approach argue that those targeted for mandatory treatment lack awareness that they are ill and that once in treatment they are able to engage more fully in life. The critics of mandated treatment argue that the severely mentally ill have the "freedom" to choose their psychosis. Lowry (2003) argues that there is no liberty in psychosis and that it is medication which offers true freedom to those with severe mental illness.

Nurses are in a strategic position to influence community mental health care. They have proven to be cost-effective providers of care to the severely mentally ill, whose nursing needs are complex and multifaceted. Traditionally, nurses have held a view of clients that includes a holistic approach to assessing needs, recognition of the individual's and family's need for care, and a respect for the client's autonomy that encourages self-direction. These views provide nursing with a vantage point to advocate for change within the health care system and within the community. Such advocacy can influence reform within the system and decrease responses within the community that stigmatize and discriminate against people with psychiatric histories. It remains to be seen whether nursing will realize its potential as an agent of change in the community mental health care movement.

KEY IDEAS

1. Before 1963, community mental health care was nonexistent.
2. *Institutionalization* refers to the process in which an individual becomes dependent on an institution for care and decision making.
3. *Deinstitutionalization* refers to the process of preparing individual clients who have spent a great deal of time within the walls of an institution for life in the outside world.
4. Funding for community mental health care is dependent on the attitudes and actions of Congress, the President, and the states. It has never been sufficient for the needs of the mentally ill.
5. Community mental health care seeks to serve the needs of the severely mentally ill.
6. The severely mentally ill are a diverse group made up of people of all ages with many different psychiatric disorders.
7. The needs of the severely mentally ill include the need for basic life necessities; a sense that life is meaningful; access to medication; support for family members; and integrated nursing, medical, and social services.
8. Community mental health care focuses on the community, individual, and family.
9. The goal of community mental health care is to provide care that is continuous and comprehensive.
10. The nursing process can be applied to a community as a whole or to an individual or family within the community.

CASE STUDY   Developing a Community Substance Abuse Prevention Program: Use of the Nursing Process

Psychiatric nurse Britt Finley sought to develop a community substance abuse prevention program in Montana. She used the nursing process to develop a program that tackled alcohol abuse on several fronts simultaneously by involving the schools, law enforcement agencies, parents, and health professionals. To develop the program, Finley began by conducting a thorough *assessment*. She examined statistics related to the consumption of alcoholic substances in the community, then compared the data to national norms from several sources, including the Centers for Disease Control and Prevention. In the *diagnosis* step, Finley analyzed the data and came to the conclusion that the community was at substantial risk for health-related problems stemming from alcohol abuse. Finley therefore identified the following nursing diagnosis:

Ineffective community coping related to excessive consumption of alcoholic substances as evidenced by statistics demonstrating an incidence higher than the national norm for alcohol-related illnesses and alcohol-related accidents

The *outcome identification* step yielded the following expected outcome:

There will be evidence of a significant decrease in the purchase and consumption of alcoholic substances.

The *planning* step involved the participation of community leaders, who devised short-term goals. Those goals included the following:

1. Parents, teachers, and students will be educated about alcohol.
2. Chapters of Alcoholics Anonymous and Students Against Drunk Driving will be established.
3. Police will consistently enforce the minimum drinking age of 19 years.
4. The drinking age will be increased.
5. A statewide school policy will be instituted prohibiting drinking at extracurricular functions.
6. Employee assistance programs will be established at major employment sites.
7. In-service educational sessions will be provided for nursing and medical personnel to increase awareness of the problem.

In the *implementation* step, Finley used the following interventions: networking with concerned people, spreading the word about the dangers of alcohol, and widening the scope of people who were involved in making a commitment to the problem.

The *evaluation* step involved the use of a number of different approaches, including the following:

1. Surveying grade school and high school teachers to determine their perceptions of the extent of the problem
2. Examining statistics on alcohol-related traffic injuries
3. Examining student drinking patterns

Through each of these measures, the effectiveness of the program became clear.

From Finley, B. (1989). The role of the psychiatric nurse in a community substance abuse prevention program. *Nursing Clinics of North America, 24*(4), 121-136.

WEB   See **Critical Thinking Questions** for this Case Study on the book's website.

LEARNING BY EXPERIENCE AND REFLECTION

1. Conduct an informal survey in your community. Ask your family and neighbors how they would react to having a halfway house for the severely mentally ill established in their community.
2. Call a local community mental health center and ask what services are offered to clients.
3. Call the mental health association in your community. Ask if there are any self-help groups in your area. If there are, what services do they provide?
4. Visit a day treatment center. What types of clients use the center? What services are offered?
5. Reflect on your own experiences with the severely mentally ill. What aspect of nursing care are you comfortable with? What would improve your competence in addressing the needs of the severely mentally ill in your community?

COMMUNITY RESOURCES FOR PRACTICE

Information about each of the following organizations can be found on its website, which can be accessed through this book's website at *http://evolve.elsevier.com/Maurer/community/*.

National Alliance for the Mentally Ill (NAMI)
Depression, Awareness, Recognition, and Treatment Program (DART)
Depression and Related Affective Disorders Association
Medic Alert Foundation
Partnership for Health Care Change
Substance Abuse and Mental Health Services Administration

STUDY AIDS   http://evolve.elsevier.com/Maurer/community/

Visit the Evolve website for this book to find the following study and assessment materials:

- Quiz
- Web Scenario
- Critical Thinking Questions and Answers for Case Studies
- Care Plans
- *Healthy People* Updates
- Glossary

REFERENCES

Abrams, R., & Young, R. (2006, November-December). Crisis in access to care: Geriatric psychiatric services unobtainable at any price. *Public Health Reports, 121,* 646-649.

Adelman, H., & Taylor, L. (2006). Mental health in schools and public health. *Public Health Reports, 121*(3), 294-298.

Aebersold, A. (2001). Press kit: Kendra's law. New York. Retrieved October 16, 2003 from *http://www.psychlaw.org/PressRoom/presskits/Kendraslaw.htm*.

Becker, D. R., & Drake, R. E. (2003). *A working life for people with severe mental illness.* New York: Oxford University Press.

Bernstein, R. (2003). *Older people with mental illnesses remain unnecessarily segregated in nursing homes, institutional settings.* Retrieved May 2, 2008 from *http://www.bazelon.org/newsroom/archive/2003/3–10–03lastinline.htm*.

Bostelman, S., Callan, M., Rolincik, L. C., et al. (1994). A community project to encourage compliance with mental health treatment aftercare. *Public Health Reports, 109*(2), 153-157.

Brauner, C., & Stephens, C. (2006). Estimating the prevalence of early childhood serious emotional/behavioral disorders: Challenges and recommendations. *Public Health Reports, 121*(3), 303-310.

Brickhouse, B. (2003, January 17). *A national disgrace.* Retrieved October 14, 2003 from *http://www.virginia.edu/topnews/releases/disgrace-jan-17–2003*.

Chamberlin, J., & Rogers, J. A. (1990). Planning a community-based mental health system. *American Psychologist, 45*(11), 1241-1244.

Conway, A. S., Melzer, D., & Hale, A. S. (1994). The outcome of targeting community services: Evidence from the West Lambeth schizophrenia cohort. *British Medical Journal, 308*(6929), 627-630.

Daniels, A., & Adams, N. (2006). *From study to action: A strategic plan for transformation of mental care.* Retrieved August 18, 2007 from *http://www.healthcarechange.org*.

Drake, R. E., & Mueser, K. T. (2000). Psychosocial approaches to dual diagnosis. *Schizophrenia Bulletin, 26*(1), 105-118.

Finley, B. (1989). The role of the psychiatric nurse in a community substance abuse prevention program. *Nursing Clinics of North America, 24*(4), 121-136.

Goldbaum, E. (2003). Mental illness linked to diabetes. *University of Buffalo Reporter, 34*(23). Retrieved October 16, 2003 from *http://www.buffalo.edu/reporter/vol34/vol34n23/articles/BellnierDiabetes.html*.

Grob, G. N. (1994a). Mad, homeless and unwanted: A history of the care of the chronic mentally ill in America. *Psychiatric Clinics of North America, 17*(3), 541-558.

Grob, G. N. (1994b). Government and mental health policy: A structural analysis. *Milbank Quarterly, 72*(3), 471-500.

Hacker, K., & Darcy, K. (2006). Putting "child mental health" into public health. *Public Health Reports, 121*(3), 292-293.

Hoge, C. W., Castro, C. A., Messer, S. C., et al. (2004). Combat duty in Iraq and Afghanistan, mental health problems, and barriers to care. *New England Journal of Medicine, 351*(1), 13-22.

Institute of Medicine. (2006). *Improving the quality of health care for mental and substance-use conditions.* Washington, DC: National Academies Press.

Krauss, J., & O'Sullivan, C. (2007). Mental health parity: Will it ever happen? In D. Mason, J. Leavitt, & M. Chaffee (Eds.), *Policy and politics in nursing and health care* (5th ed.; pp. 311-322). St. Louis: Saunders.

Lowry, R. (2003). *Mistreating the mentally ill.* Retrieved May 2, 2008 from *http://www.townhall.com/columnists/RichLowry/2003/07/31mistreating_the_mentally_ill*.

Minkoff, K. (1978). A map of chronic mental patients. In J. Talbot (Ed.), *The chronic mental patient* (p. 1173). Washington, DC: American Psychiatric Association.

National Alliance for the Mentally Ill. (2000). Access to effective medications: A critical link to mental illness recovery. Retrieved May 2, 2008 from *http://www.nami.org* (type in name of publication).

National Alliance for the Mentally Ill. (2008). *Assertive Community Treatment (ACT).*

Retrieved May 2, 2008 from *http://www.nami. org/about/PACTFACT.html*.

National Institutes of Mental Health. (2006, December 26). *The numbers count: Mental disorders in America*. Retrieved July 25, 2007 from *http://www.nimh.nih.gov/publicat/numbers.cfm*.

New Freedom Commission on Mental Health state implementation activities. (2004). Retrieved July 29, 2007 from *http://www.nasmhpd.org/general_files/State%20table5.pdf*.

New York State United Teachers. (2006, December 14). *Legislative action center: Timothy's Law passes legislature, signed into law by governor*. NYSUT News Wire. Retrieved July 27, 2007 from *http://www.nysut.org/cps/rde/xchg/nysut/hs.xsl/legislation_5979.htm*.

Patterson, K. (2003). *Hepatitis C plagues mentally ill at a rate 10 times national average*. Retrieved September 20, 2003 from *http://www.heart-intl. net/HEART/120606/HepCPlague.htm*.

Pear, R. (2007, March 19). Proposals for mental health parity pit father's pragmatism against son's passion. *New York Times*. Retrieved July 26, 2007 from *http://query.nytimes.com/gst/fullpage. html?res=9B06E7D71630F93AA25750C0A961 9C8B63&sec=hea*.

President's New Freedom Commission on Mental Health. (2003). *Achieving the promise: Transforming mental health in America. Final report*. Rockville, MD: U.S. Department of Health and Human Services. Retrieved July 27,

2007 from *http://www.mentalhealthcommission. gov./reports/reports.htm*.

Puskar, K., Lamb, J., & Norton, M. (1990). Adolescent mental health: Collaboration among psychiatric mental health nurses and school nurses. *Journal of School Health, 60*(2), 69-71.

Randolph, F., Blasinsky, M., Morrissey, J. P., et al. (2002). Overview of the ACCESS Program. *Psychiatric Services, 53*(8), 945-948.

Report to the President of the President's Commission on Mental Health (Vol. 1). (1978). Washington, DC: U.S. Government Printing Office.

Royer, D. (2003). *Mental health care providers form alliance to avert crisis*. Retrieved October 1, 2003 from *http://www.bizjournals.com/memphis/stories/2003/07/28/focus4.html*.

Savin, D., Seymour, D., Littleford, L., et al. (2005). Findings from mental health screening of newly arrived refugees in Colorado. *Public Health Reports, 120*(3), 224-229.

Sheets, J. L., Prevost, J. A., & Reihman, J. (1982). Young adult chronically mentally ill patients: Three hypothesized subgroups. *Hospital and Community Psychiatry, 33*(3), 197-203.

Shoemaker, N. C. (2006). Mental health nursing in community settings. In E. Varcarolis, V. B. Carson, & N. C. Shoemaker (Eds.), *Foundations of psychiatric mental health nursing: A clinical approach* (5th ed.; pp. 85-96). St. Louis: Saunders.

Stratton, E. L. (2002, January 30). *Solutions for the mentally ill in the criminal justice system*.

Retrieved October 1, 2003 from *http://www. sconet.state.oh:us/Communications_Office/speeches/2002/0130cmc.asp*.

TimothysLaw.org. (2006). *Timothy's story*. Retrieved July 27, 2007 from *http://www. timothyslaw.org/timothys_story.htm*.

U.S. Department of Labor. (2007, February). *Mental Health Parity Act*. Retrieved July 26, 2007 from *http://www.dol.gov/ebsa/newsroom/fsmhparity.html*.

U.S. Department of Health and Human Services, Substance Abuse and Mental Health Services Administration. (2005). *Transforming mental health care in American: The federal action agenda: First steps*. Retrieved August 18, 2007 from *http://www.samhsa.gov/federalaction agenda/nfc_TOC.aspx*.

Vedantam, S. (2006, March 1). Veterans report mental distress. *Washington Post*, p. A01. Retrieved July 26, 2007 from *http://www.washingtonpost.com*.

Waxman, H. (2006). Improving the care of children with mental illness: A challenge for public health and the federal government. *Public Health Reports, 121*(3), 299-302.

Wierdsma, A. I., Poodt, H. D., & Mulder, C. L. (2007). Effects of community-care networks on psychiatric emergency contacts, hospitalization and involuntary admission. *Journal of Epidemiology and Community Health, 61*, 613-618.

SUGGESTED READINGS

Aquila, R., Malamud, T. J., Sweet. T., et al. (2006). *The store front, Fountain House, and the rehabilitation alliance*. Medscape General Medicine. Retrieved July 29, 2007 from *http://www.medscape. com/viewarticle/541401*.

Coombes, L. (2007). The lived experience of community mental health nurses working with people who have dual diagnoses: A phenomenological study. *Journal of Psychiatric and Mental Health Nursing, 14*(4), 382-392.

Herrman, J. (2007). News from NACCHO: When does mental health become public health? *Journal of Public Health Management Practice*,

13(5), 527-529. (Discusses public mental health preparedness related to disasters.)

Hunter, E. F. (2000). Telephone support for persons with chronic mental illness. *Home Healthcare Nurse, 18*(3), 172-179.

Institute of Medicine. (2006). *Improving the quality of health care for mental and substance-use conditions*. Washington, DC: The National Academies Press. (Executive summary available at *http://www.iom.edu/?id=30858*; full book available at *http://www.nap.edu/catalog. php?record_id=11470#toc*.)

Savin, D., Seymour, D., Littleford, L., et al. (2006). Findings from mental health screening of newly arrived refugees in Colorado. *Public Health Reports, 120*(3), 224-229.

U.S. Department of Health and Human Services, Substance Abuse and Mental Health Services Administration. (2005). *Transforming mental health care in American. The federal action agenda: First steps*. Retrieved August 18, 2007 from *http://www.samhsa.gov/federalactionagenda/nfc_TOC.aspx*.

Ergonomist
  issues, 242
  role, description, 255
Eskimos, 188
Ethical issues, 157–158
Ethical principles, consideration, 204
Ethical properties, 12
Ethics
  code. *See* Nurses
  law, relationship, 157–159
Ethnic groups
  differences, 284–285
  drug metabolism, variation, 285
  poverty rates, 537
Ethnic health
  disparities, factors, 537
  health care disparities, 275–277
Ethnic heritage, self-appraisal, 296
Ethnic influences, 537–538
Ethnicity, 275
  federal data, classification standards, 271
  race, interchange, 275
  reference, 275
  reflection, 407
  relationship. *See* Cancer
Ethnic minorities, infant mortality rates,
    276–277
Ethnocentric nursing care, 290
Europe
  nursing efforts, 33*t*
  visiting nursing, usage, 32
European Union Parliament, tobacco advertisement
    ban, 130
Evacuation, definitive medical care (relationship),
    567–568
Evaluation, 18. *See also* Adequacy; Appropriateness;
    Efficiency; Formative evaluation; Process;
    Summative evaluation
  data
    analysis, 456, 464
    collection, 456
    sources, 463
  measures. *See* Criterion-referenced evaluation
    measures
  methods/tools, 464–466
  planning, 456
  process, 454
  purpose, 454–455
  questions, 463
  questions/answers, 456–462
    list, 457*t*
  recording, 463–464
  report, 456
    data. *See* Written evaluation report
  research, 464
  responsibilities. *See* Communities
  results, implementation, 456
  standards, 456
  steps, 456
    list, 456
  strategies, selection, 519–521
Evidence-based home-visiting programs, future,
    321–322
Evidence-based practice, 25. *See also* Community/public
    health nursing
  incorporation, 383–384
  research findings, integration, 25
Evil eye. *See* Mal ojo
Examples, usage, 519*t*
Existing power structures, change, 20–21
Expectations, dissatisfaction, 463
Expected outcomes, delineation. *See* Health program
    planning
Experiential readiness, 514–515
  assessment, 515
  inclusion, 514
Experimental trials, 168
  definition, 168
Expert witnesses
  qualification, 156
  role, 156
  testifying, 20, 145
Exposure assessment, 243
Exposure history, taking, 244
Extended families, 690
External cues, impact, 477
External feedback, 411
External health risks, impact, 115

External influences, 7–8
  summarization, 407–408
External standards. *See* Care
  inclusion, 156
Extremely poor, consideration, 534
Eye contact
  importance, 282
  nonverbal communication, 282

F
Face-to-face interactions, 9
Facilities
  factor, 408–409
  influence, 408
Fair Housing Amendments (1988), 672
Faith communities
  health-promotion programs, 482
  locations, ideality, 482
Falls, unintentional injuries, 247
False-negative test results, 493
False-positive finding, 493
Familiarization approach. *See* Community assessment
Families. *See* Blended families; Extended families;
    Nuclear families; Reconstituted families
  abuse, prevention, 577
  adaptation, Double ABCX Model, 339
  age-appropriate subsystems, demonstration, 348
  appreciation, evolution, 327–328
  appreciation/cooperation, problems, 314
  approaches, integration, 340
  assessment, 347–350 Environment
    guide, 369
    guide, case study, 388
  autonomy, 305–306
  blame, 647
  boundary, 328
    variations, 334–335
  caregiver status, 283
  care unit, 329
  caring presence, fostering, 308–310
  case management, 346–347
    public health nursing perspective, 346–347
  change
    capacity, 366
    resistance, 365
  characteristics, 337
  children, inclusion, 690–693
  chronic problems, 377–381
  Circumplex Model, 337
  co-dependence, 647
  communication, change, 337
  communication themes, identification, 313
    efficiency, 313
  community/public health nurse, responsibilities,
      381–386
  comparison/contrast, 330–332
  competencies, identification, 356
  conflict reduction, 313–315
  conflictual relationships, example, 335–336
  confrontation. *See* Life cycle
  contact, nature, 342
  contract, formulation, 366
  contracting process, 311
  control, retention, 307
  coping
    ABCX Model, 337–338
    illustration, 338*f*
    behaviors, selection (nurse assistance), 361
    ineffectiveness, 353
    processes, adaptivity (increase), 386
    readiness, 353
    strategies, 362*t*
  crises, 318
    coping, 377
    definition, 377
    experience, 381
  cultural assessment, 289, 349–350
    guide, 291*t*
    list, 350
    requirement, 349–350
  data
    analysis, 350–359
    confidentiality, clarification, 315
  definition, 329–330
    variations, 330
  development, 332–333
    approach, 332
  developmental changes, teaching, 363–364

Families (*Continued*)
  developmental demands, nurse role, 363
  developmental tasks, 690–692
    achievement, 332
    list, 333*t*
  diagnoses, characteristics, 353
  differentiation, level, 335
    importance, 380
  direct care, 23
  disaster plan, 573
  dynamics, pregnancy (impact), 620
  dysfunction, 332, 647
  environment, identification, 314
  evaluation, 366–368
  family health nurses, intervention, 341
  focus, 305. *See also* Nurses
  forms, 330–331
    variation, 331
  framework, requirement, 342
  functioning
    continuum, 332
    definition, 357
    determination, 357
    levels, 337
    optimum, 332
    selection criteria, 357*t*
  functions, 332
    definition, 332
  goals
    accomplishment, fostering
      (practices), 308
    identification, problems, 383
  health
    community/public health nurse interest, 366
    programs, 480
  health maintenance
    assistance. *See* Environment
    role, 329
  health-promotion programs, evaluation
    criteria, 486
  health-related problems/goals, 304*t*
  health/social service agencies/providers, involvement
    (identification), 314
  hidden costs, 702
    accountability, 703
  historical frameworks, 332–340
  home care involvement, marital/family distress
    (development), 703
  identification, 313
  identified needs, priorities (determination), 359
  ill/disabled children, coping, 303
  illness
    coping, 361
    phases, 361–363
    reactions, 361
    requirements, 361
  illness/loss, coping (assistance), 360–363
  information
    recording, 348
    usefulness, 349
  information, hearing (ability differences), 363
  interaction processes/patterns, tracking, 366
  interactions/communication, 336–337
  internal dynamics
    change, coaching, 365–366
    disturbances, 352, 379–381
    disturbances, characteristics, 380
    outcome, sequencing/timing, 365–366
  internal relationships, problems, 365
  intervention strategies, usage, 23
  intimate relationships, importance, 329
  law, 153–154
  life, hierarchy, 336
  life cycle. *See* Poor
  lives, students (impact), 309
  map, 348
    diagramming usage, 348
    example, 348*f*
    usage, 336
  matters, 584
  models, 337
  needs, 342
    determination, 352
    determination, list, 354
    examination, 352
    identification, 359
    interventions, principles, 361*t*
  negative choices, 378

03/

Nelson Report October 2013

Pastor Jamal Bryant (Empowerment Temple)
Proverb
ACT 1:8
R   1 Samual 8:13
          Genesis 8

1 trillion Dollars in spending power

43 Million African American living in America

Our greatest weakness is we don't Know our own strength

Drug Store, Convenivant Stores   Dollar Stores

Smart Beauty Study (By Essence)
7$^{.5}$ billion Dollars a year on beauty products

The AA Woman has an average of 5-7 bottles of perfume, none
which has been manufactor by people that Cook like them.
10 Know Allergens that trigger hormonal disruption

03/ /14   Pastor Harold A. Jr.   New Shiloh Baptist Church
                                   Carter

Isaiha 55   Behold I have given him as a witness to the people. A
             leader and commander for the people.